Surgical Critical Care and Emergency Surgery

Surgical Critical Care and Emergency Surgery

Clinical Questions and Answers

Third Edition

Edited by

Forrest "Dell" Moore, MD, FACS
Associate Professor of Surgery
TCU & UNTHSC School of Medicine
Vice Chief of Surgery
Associate Trauma Medical Director
John Peter Smith Health
Forth Worth, TX, USA

Peter M. Rhee, MD, MPH, FACS, FCCM, DMCC
Professor of Surgery at New York Medical College
USUHS, and Morehouse College of Medicine
Chief of Acute Care Surgery and Trauma
Vice Chair of Surgery

Carlos J. Rodriguez, DO
Associate Professor of Surgery
TCU & UNTHSC School of Medicine
Director, Emergency General Surgery
Director, Surgical Research
John Peter Smith Health
Fort Worth, TX, USA

WILEY Blackwell

Registered Offices
John Wiley & Sons, Inc., 111 River Street, Hoboken, NJ 07030, USA
John Wiley & Sons Ltd, The Atrium, Southern Gate, Chichester, West Sussex, PO19 8SQ, UK

Editorial Office
9600 Garsington Road, Oxford, OX4 2DQ, UK

For details of our global editorial offices, customer services, and more information about Wiley products visit us at www.wiley.com.

Wiley also publishes its books in a variety of electronic formats and by print-on-demand. Some content that appears in standard print versions of this book may not be available in other formats.

Library of Congress Cataloging-in-Publication Data

Names: Moore, Forrest "Dell", editor. | Rhee, Peter M., 1961- editor. | Rodriguez,
  Carlos J., editor.
Title: Surgical critical care and emergency surgery : clinical questions
  and answers / edited by Forrest "Dell". Moore, Peter M. Rhee, Carlos J.
  Rodriguez.
Description: Third edition. | Hoboken, NJ : Wiley-Blackwell, 2022. |
  Includes bliographical references and index.
Identifiers: LCCN 2021029654 (print) | LCCN 2021029655 (ebook) | ISBN
  9781119756750 (paperback) | ISBN 9781119756767 (adobe pdf) | ISBN
  9781119756774 (epub)
Subjects: MESH: Critical Care–methods
  https://id.nlm.nih.gov/mesh/D003422Q000379 | Surgical Procedures,
  Operative–methods | Critical Illness–therapy | Emergencies | Emergency
  Treatment–methods | Wounds and Injuries–surgery | Examination
  Questions
Classification: LCC RD93 (print) | LCC RD93 (ebook) | NLM WO 18.2 | DDC
  617/.026–dc23
LC record available at https://lccn.loc.gov/2021029654
LC ebook record available at https://lccn.loc.gov/2021029655

Cover Design: Wiley
Cover Image: Courtesy of Peter Rhee

Set in 10/12pt Warnock Pro by Straive, Pondicherry, India

SKY10077845_061824

Contents

List of Contributors

Yousef Abuhakmeh, DO
MAJ, MC US Army
Banner University Medical Center
University of Arizona College of Medicine
Tucson, AZ, USA

Vishal Bansal, MD
Scripps Mercy Hospital
San Diego, CA, USA

Stephen L. Barnes, MD
Division of Acute Care Surgery, Department of Surgery
University of Missouri
Columbia, MO, USA

Elise Becker, MD
Naval Medical Center
San Diego, CA, USA

Christopher Bell, MD
William Beaumont Army Medical Center
El Paso, TX, USA

Patrick Benoit, DO
Walter Reed National Military Medical Center
Bethesda, MD, USA

Mauer Biscotti III, MD
Division of General Surgery, Department of Surgery
San Antonio Military Medical Center
San Antonio, TX, USA

Matthew J. Bradley, MD
Uniformed Services University of the Health Sciences
Program Director General Surgery Residency
Walter Reed National Military Medical Center
Bethesda, MD, USA

Matthew Bronstein, MD
Division of Trauma and Acute Care Surgery
New York Medical College
Westchester Medical Center
Valhalla, NY, USA

Kevin W. Cahill, MD
Christiana Care Health Care System
Newark, DE, USA

Catherine Cameron, MD
Landstuhl Regional Medical Center
Landstuhl, Germany

Jeremy W. Cannon, MD, SM
Division of Traumatology, Surgical Critical Care &
Emergency Surgery, Perelman School of Medicine at the
University of Pennsylvania
Philadelphia, PA, USA

Department of Surgery, F. Edward Hébert School
of Medicine, Uniformed Services University of the
Health Sciences
Bethesda, MD, USA

Luis Cardenas, DO, PhD
Department of Surgery
Christiana Care Health Care System
Newark, DE, USA

Brett M. Chapman, MD
LSUHSC-New Orleans
New Orleans, LA, USA

Elaine Cleveland, MD
William Beaumont Army Medical Center
El Paso, TX, USA

Jorge Con, MD
Division of Trauma and Acute Care Surgery
New York Medical College
Westchester Medical Center
Valhalla, NY, USA

Alan Cook, MD, MS
University of Texas at Tyler
Tyler, TX, USA

J. Craig Egan, MD
Phoenix Children's Hospital
Phoenix, AZ, USA

Brett D. Crist, MD
Department of Orthopaedic Surgery
University of Missouri
Columbia, MO, USA

Jeffrey P. Coughenour, MD
Division of Acute Care Surgery
Department of Surgery
University of Missouri
Columbia, MO, USA

Gregory J. Della Rocca, MD, PhD
Department of Orthopaedic Surgery
University of Missouri
Columbia, MO, USA

Harsh K. Desai, MD
Department of Surgery
Christiana Care Health Care System
Newark, DE, USA

Joshua Dilday, DO
Division of Acute Care Surgery
University of Southern California
LAC + USC Medical Center
Los Angeles, CA, USA

Jay J. Doucet, MD, MSc
Department of Surgery
University of California San Diego
San Diego, CA, USA

Therese M. Duane, MD
TCU & UNTHSC School of Medicine
Department of Surgery
Texas Health Resources
Fort Worth, TX, USA

Joseph DuBose, MD
Department of Surgery
Dell School of Medicine
University of Texas Austin
Austin, TX, USA

Drew Farmer, MD
Trauma Surgery, Surgical Critical Care
& Emergency Surgery
Perelman School of Medicine
University of Pennsylvania
Philadelphia, PA, USA

Adam D. Fox, DO
Division of Trauma and Critical Care Surgery
Rutgers New Jersey Medical School
University Hospital
Newark, NJ, USA

Charles J. Fox, MD
R Adams Cowley Shock Trauma Center
Division of Vascular Surgery
University of Maryland School of Medicine
Baltimore, MD, USA

Rondi Gelbard, MD
Division of Trauma and Acute Care Surgery
Department of Surgery
University of Alabama at Birmingham
Birmingham, AL, USA

Frederick Giberson, MD
Department of Surgery
Christiana Care Health Care System
Newark
DE, USA

Matthew A. Goldshore, MD, PhD, MPH
Department of Surgery
Perelman School of Medicine at the University
of Pennsylvania
Philadelphia, PA, USA

Rathnayaka M. K. Gunasingha, MD
Walter Reed National Military Medical Center
Bethesda, MD, USA

Juan P. Gurria, MD
Phoenix Children's Hospital
Phoenix, AZ, USA

Melike Harfouche MD
Division of Trauma and Acute Care Surgery
University of Maryland – Shock Trauma Center
Baltimore, MD, USA

Hang Ho, MD
Augusta University Medical Center
Augusta, GA, USA

Luke Hofmann, DO
Brooke Army Medical Center
San Antonio, TX, USA
F. Edward Hebert School of Medicine Uniformed
Services University
Bethesda, MD, USA

Romeo Ignacio, MD
Division of Pediatric Surgery
Rady Children's Hospital
San Diego, CA, USA

MAJ Jacob Swann, MD
Regions Hospital
Saint Paul, MN, USA

Douglas James, MD
Section of Trauma and Acute Care Surgery
Westchester Medical Center
Valhalla, NY, USA

Kirstie Jarrett, MD
Banner University Medical Center
Tucson, AZ, USA

Bellal Joseph, MD
Division of Trauma, Surgical Critical Care, Burns and
Acute Care Surgery
University of Arizona College of Medicine
Banner University Medical Center
Tucson, AZ, USA

Lewis J. Kaplan, MD, FCCM, FCCP
Division of Trauma, Surgical Critical Care and
Emergency Surgery, Department of Surgery, Perelman
School of Medicine, University of Pennsylvania
Philadelphia, PA, USA

Corporal Michael J. Crescenz VA Medical Center
Philadelphia, PA, USA

Lindsey Karavites, MD
Division of Acute Care Surgery
University of Southern California
LAC+USC Medical Center
Los Angeles, CA, USA

Joshua Klein, DO
Department of Surgery, Trauma & Acute Care Surgeon
Westchester Medical Center, Division of Trauma
& Acute Care Surgery
New York Medical College, Valhalla, NY, USA

Leslie Kobayashi, MD
Division of Trauma, Acute Care Surgery
Surgical Critical Care and Burns
University of California San Diego
San Diego, CA, USA

Narong Kulvatunyou, MD
Department of Surgery
University of Arizona School of Medicine
Banner University Medical Center
Tucson, AZ, USA

Raul Reina Limon, MD
Division of Trauma, Critical Care, Burns, and
Emergency Surgery
Department of Surgery
University of Arizona
Tucson, AZ, USA

Gary Lombardo, MD
Division of Trauma and Acute Care Surgery
New York Medical College
Westchester Medical Center
Valhalla, NY, USA

Ryan Malcom, MD
Division of Trauma and Acute Care Surgery
New York Medical College
Westchester Medical Center
Valhalla, NY, USA

Toni Manougian MD, MBA
Department of Critical Care Anesthesiology
New York Medical College
Westchester Medical Center
Valhalla, NY, USA

Matthew J. Martin, MD
Trauma and Acute Care Surgery Service
Scripps Mercy Hospital
San Diego, CA, USA

Kazuhide Matsushima, MD
Division of Acute Care Surgery
University of Southern California
LAC+USC Medical Center
Los Angeles, CA, USA

Adrian A. Maung, MD , FCCM
Yale School of Medicine
New Haven, CT, USA

Richard S. Miller, MD
Department of Surgery
TCU & UNTHSC School of Medicine
John Peter Smith Health
Fort Worth, TX, USA

William Mohr III, MD
Regions Hospital
Saint Paul, MN, USA

Ida Molavi, MD
Department of Trauma and Acute Care Surgery
Louisiana State University Health
Shreveport, LA, USA

Thomas Muse, MD
Department of Trauma and Acute Care Surgery
Department of Surgery
University of Alabama at Birmingham
Birmingham, AL, USA

Christopher S. Nelson, MD
Division of Acute Care Surgery
Department of Surgery
University of Missouri
Columbia, MO, USA

Omar Obaid, MD
Division of Trauma, Critical Care
Burns, and Emergency Surgery
Department of Surgery
University of Arizona
Tucson, AZ, USA

Thomas A. O'Hara, DO
Dwight D. Eisenhower Army Medical Center
Fort Gordon, GA, USA

Terence O'Keeffe, MB ChB
Augusta University Medical Center
Augusta, GA, USA

Kristine Tolentino Parra, MD
Naval Medical Center
San Diego, CA, USA

Gregory S. Peirce, MD
Womack Army Medical Center
Fort Bragg, NC, USA

Annalise Penikis, MD
University of Maryland Medical Center
Baltimore, MD, USA

Herb A. Phelan, MD, MSCS
Department of Surgery, LSU School of Medicine
New Orleans, LA, USA

Kartik Prabhakaran, MD
New York Medical College
Westchester Medical Center
Valhalla, NY, USA

Theodore Pratt, MD
Naval Medical Center
San Diego, CA, USA

Eric Raschke, DO
Madigan Army Medical Center
Tacoma, WA, USA

Shariq Raza, MD
Trauma Surgery, Surgical Critical Care
& Emergency Surgery
Perelman School of Medicine
University of Pennsylvania
Philadelphia, PA, USA

Peter M. Rhee, MD
Division of Trauma and Acute Care Surgery
New York Medical College
Westchester Medical Center
Valhalla, NY, USA

Daniel Roubik, MD
Brooke Army Medical Center
San Antonio, TX, USA

Navdeep Samra, MD
LSU Health
Shreveport, LA, USA

Jaideep Sandhu, MBBS, MPH
City of Hope National Medical Center
Duarte, CA, USA

Jarrett Santorelli, MD
Division of Trauma, Acute Care Surgery, Surgical
Critical Care and Burns
University of California San Diego
San Diego, CA, USA

Fariha Sheikh, MD
Division of Trauma and Critical Care Surgery
Rutgers New Jersey Medical School
University Hospital
Newark, NJ, USA

Jared Sheppard, MD
Division of Acute Care Surgery, Department of Surgery
University of Missouri
Columbia, MO, USA

Ilya Shnaydman, MD
Division of Trauma and Acute Care Surgery
New York Medical College
Westchester Medical Center
Valhalla, NY, USA

Elise Sienicki, MD
Naval Medical Center, San Diego, CA, USA

Brandt Sisson, MD
Naval Medical Center
San Diego, CA, USA

Michael C. Smith, MD
Division of Trauma and Surgical Critical Care
Vanderbilt University Medical Center
Nashville, TN, USA

Collin Stewart, MD
Banner University Medical Center
University of Arizona College of Medicine
Tucson, AZ, USA

Michelle Strong, MD, PhD
Trauma and Acute Care Surgeon
Austin, TX, USA

Jonathan Swisher, MD
LTC, MC US Army
William Beaumont Army Medical Center
El Paso, TX, USA

Andrew Tang, MD
University of Arizona College of Medicine
Banner University Medical Center
Tucson, AZ, USA

Anne Warner, MD
Department of Surgery
Christiana Care Health Care System
Newark, DE, USA

Cassandra Q. White, MD
Department of Surgery
Augusta University
Augusta, GA, USA

Andrew J. Young, MD
Division of Trauma, Critical Care and Burn
The Ohio State University
Columbus, OH, USA

Bardiya Zangbar, MD
Division of Trauma and Acute Care Surgery
New York Medical College
Westchester Medical Center
Valhalla, NY, USA

About the Companion Website

This book is accompanied by a companion website

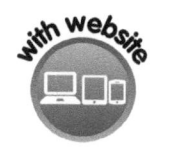

www.wiley.com/go/surgicalcriticalcare3e

The website features:

- Interactive multiple choice questions

Part One

Surgical Critical Care

1

Respiratory and Cardiovascular Physiology

Anne Warner, MD, Harsh Desai, MD, and Frederick Giberson, MD

Department of Surgery, Christiana Care Health Care System, Newark, DE, USA

1 In a patient who develops ARDS, the addition of PEEP in optimizing ventilatory support has which of the following effects?
   A Maximal alveolar recruitment with inspiration.
   B Decreasing mean airway pressure.
   C Decreased right ventricular afterload.
   D Improvement of functional residual capacity (FRC).
   E Increasing left ventricular afterload.

The use of positive end-expiratory pressure (PEEP) as part of the ARDS ventilatory strategy has been shown to improve the functional residual capacity (FRC) above the closing pressure of alveoli, thereby preventing alveolar collapse. PEEP maximizes alveolar recruitment at end expiration, not inspiration. The addition of PEEP increases inflation pressure, thereby increasing peak alveolar pressure and ultimately mean airway pressure. Increased PEEP increases pulmonary vascular resistance impeding right vascular stroke volume and thereby left ventricular filling. It also decreases the transmural pressure – the pressure needed to be overcome in order to eject stroke volume – thereby decreasing left ventricular afterload.

Answer: D

Briel M, Meade M, Mercat A, et al. Higher vs lower positive end-expiratory pressure in patients with acute lung injury and acute respiratory distress syndrome. *JAMA*. 2010; 303 (9): 865–873.

Schmitt JM, Viellard-Baron A, Augarde R, et al. Positive end-expiratory pressure titration in acute respiratory distress syndrome patients: impact on right ventricular outflow impedance evaluated by pulmonary artery Doppler flow velocity measurements. *Crit Care Med*. 2001; 29: 1154–1158.

2 Which of the following is NOT a component of the inflammatory cascade leading to lung injury in ARDS?
   A Injury to type I and type II epithelial cells within the alveoli.
   B Capillary endothelial dysregulation resulting in recruitment of neutrophils.
   C Sequestration of predominantly lymphocytes within the pulmonary microcirculation.
   D Release of cytoplasmic granules from neutrophil degranulation.
   E Exudation of protein-rich fluid into the distal airspaces.

The inflammatory cascade in ARDS is thought to be initiated by activation of circulating neutrophils by the release of IL-1 and TNF by macrophages and monocytes. Endothelial dysregulation attracts and retains neutrophils with subsequent sequestration within the pulmonary microcirculation. This occurs through adhesion of neutrophils to endothelial cells and neutrophil stiffening. Neutrophils then move into lung parenchyma and degranulate propagating injury to the type I and II epithelial cells within the alveoli allowing for exudation of protein-rich fluid, erythrocytes, and platelets into the distal airspaces.

Answer: C

Abraham E. Neutrophils and acute lung injury. *Crit Care Med*. 2003; 31(supp): S195–S199.

3 A 27-year-old man is undergoing exploratory laparotomy after presenting with a gunshot wound to the left flank. He is currently hemodynamically stable. The operative team has concern for possible ureteral

injury and asks that methylene blue be administered for identification of possible urine leak. Shortly after administration, the patient desaturates to SpO_2 of 82% with remaining hemodynamics remaining appropriate. What is the management for the etiology of this patient's desaturation event?

A *Perform a left tube thoracostomy.*

B *Immediate bronchoscopy.*

C *Abort the procedure.*

D *Manual bag mask ventilation.*

E *Watch and wait without immediate intervention.*

The multiple uses of methylene blue have been established including use in methemoglobinemia treatment as well as potential use in vasoplegic syndrome. In the operating room, methylene blue is often used to evaluate renal function and for potential leak in urologic procedures. However, one of the adverse effects of methylene blue is to decrease pulse oximetry readings.

Pulse oximeters are made up of a side containing two light emitting diodes that emit at 660nm and 940nm detecting deoxygenated and oxygenated hemoglobin, respectively. The light is captured after passing through the arteries in the finger by a probe on the other side of the oximeter. This is then passed through and alternating current amplifier to block nonpulsatile wave forms from veins. The ratio of oxygenated to total hemoglobin is used to calculate SpO_2. When administered, methylene blue transiently decreases the detected oxygenated hemoglobin as the methemoglobin fraction, usually a small percentage of total circulating hemoglobin, increases until processed out through the renal system. Therefore, for this patient, aborting the procedure is not necessary. The desaturation is transient and not caused by mucus plugging, which may require bronchoscopy, pneumothorax, which would require tube thoracostomy, or significant atelectasis, which may require bag mask ventilation.

Answer: E

Clifton J and Leikin JB. Methylene blue. *Am J Ther.* 2003; 10(4): 289–291.

Rong LQ, Mauer E, Mustapich TL, et al. Characterization of the rapid drop in pulse oximetry reading after intraoperative administration of methylene blue in open thoracoabdominal aortic repairs. *Anesth Analg.* 2019; 129(5): 142–145.

4 *A 65-year-old woman is in the post-anesthesia care unit following elective inguinal hernia surgery. Shortly after arriving, she is noted to have increasing shortness of breath and wheezing requiring administration of a nebulized beta agonist. The patient has a known history of COPD. Which of the following pulmonary function test patterns would be expected in a patient with COPD?*

A *FEV1 decreased; FVC decreased/normal; FEV1/FVC ratio decreased.*

B *FEV1 increased; FVC decreased; FEV1/FVC ratio increased.*

C *FEV1 decreased/normal; FVC decreased; FEV1/FVC ratio normal.*

D *FEV1 increased; FVC increased; FEV1/FVC ratio increased.*

E *FEV1 decreased; FVC decreased; FEV1/FVC ratio decreased.*

Pulmonary function testing is often used in preoperative evaluation, particularly prior to thoracic procedures. These can be used, in addition to history and exam, to identify obstructive versus restrictive lung processes. Three of the important measures are the forced vital capacity (FVC) – the total volume forcefully expired after maximal inspiratory effort; forced expiratory volume in 1 second (FEV1) – the volume of air forcefully expired after maximal inspiratory effort in 1 second; the FEV1/FVC ratio. In evaluating spirometry results, first step is to interpret the FEV1/FVC ratio. If less than the lower limit of normal, an obstructive pattern is suspected. If greater than lower limit of normal, the FVC is evaluated and if less than lower limit of normal, a restrictive process is considered. Obstructive diseases include COPD, asthma, and emphysema while restrictive lung diseases include neuromuscular disorders and interstitial lung diseases.

Answer: A

Barreiro TJ and Perillo I. An approach to interpreting spirometry. *Am Fam Physician.* 2004; 69(5): 1107–1115.

Pellegrino R, Viegi G, Brurasco V, et al. Interpretative strategies for lung function tests. *Eur Respir J.* 2005; 26:948–968.

5 *You are caring for a patient in your SICU who is post total abdominal colectomy and end ileostomy. Ileostomy output has been in excess of 1.5L daily with concomitant acute kidney injury noted on basic metabolic panel with continued required resuscitation. Which of the following represents the primary relationships between alveolar pressure (P_A), pulmonary arterial pressure (P_a), and pulmonary venous pressure (P_v) within the lung in a state of hypovolemia?*

A *$Pa > Pv > PA$ and $PA > Pv > Pa$*

B *$PA > Pv > Pa$ and $Pa > PA > Pv$*

C *$Pa > PA > Pv$ and $PA > Pa > Pv$*

D $PA > Pa > Pv$ and $Pv > Pa > PA$

E $Pa > PA > Pv$ and $Pa > Pv > PA$

The relationship between alveolar pressure, pulmonary arterial pressure, and pulmonary venous pressure represents the West zones of the lung. Zone 1, not seen in normal physiology, signifies alveolar dead space secondary to increased alveolar pressure causing arterial collapse ($P_A > P_a > P_v$). Zone 2 represents pulsatile perfusion ($P_a > P_A > P_v$) typically the upper portions of lung in a typical, upright person. Zone 3 represents the bulk of healthy lung tissue with continuous blood flow without

extrinsic compression ($P_a > P_v > P_A$). In a hypovolemic individual, as in this patient, decreased circulating volume converts Zone 3 tissue to Zone 1 and 2, increasing dead space.

Answer: C

West JB and Dollery CT. Distribution of blood flow and the pressure-flow relations of the whole lung. *J Appl Physiol*. 1965; 20(2): 175–183.

For questions 7–10, use the following figure to match the clinical scenario to the appropriate flow volume loop:

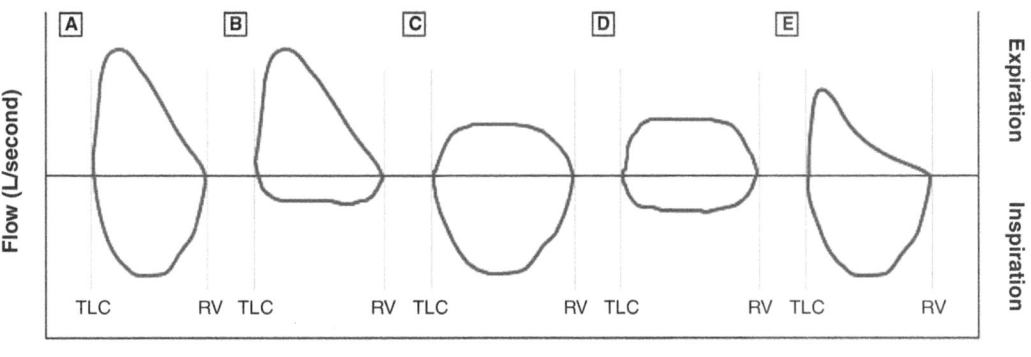
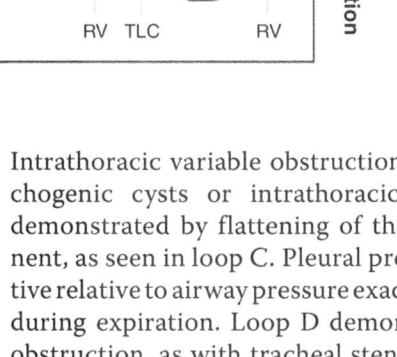

6   A 42-year-old man presents to the ICU following intubation for COPD exacerbation.

7   An 18-year-old woman diagnosed on bronchoscopy with intratracheal lipoma.

8   A recovered COVID-19 patient who develops tracheal stenosis following a 2 week intubation.

9   A 75-year-old male who undergoes emergent intubation following development of angioedema found to have R vocal cord paralysis.

Flow volume loops involve plotting inspiratory and expiratory flow on the Y-axis with volume on the X-axis, ideally during maximally forced inspiratory and expiratory effort. Flow volume loops are component of the information presented on mechanical ventilators as well and can aid in the diagnosis of airway obstruction. The normal loop is seen in loop A above representing a complete inspiratory and expiratory breath. Loop B demonstrates variable extrathoracic obstruction with a flattening of the inspiratory component. This is due to a combination of atmospheric extraluminal pressure and negative intraluminal pressure exacerbating extrathoracic obstruction as in vocal cord dysfunction and mobile tumors such as lipoma.

Intrathoracic variable obstruction, such as with bronchogenic cysts or intrathoracic tracheomalacia, is demonstrated by flattening of the expiratory component, as seen in loop C. Pleural pressure becomes positive relative to airway pressure exacerbating obstruction during expiration. Loop D demonstrates fixed airway obstruction, as with tracheal stenosis, causing flattening of both components of the loop. Finally, loop E demonstrates lower airway obstruction as seen in COPD and asthma. A scooped-out appearance to the loop comes from premature airway closure as heterogeneity of flow in expiration, i.e., areas with higher elastic recoil and lower airway resistance empty faster than diseased areas.

Answers: 6-E, 7-B, 8-C, 9-B

Loutfi SA and Stoller JK. Flow-volume loops. *UpToDate*. Retrieved November 16, 2020 from https://www.uptodate.com/contents/flow-volume-loops?search=flow%20volume%20loops&source=search_result&selectedTitle=1~59&usage_type=default&display_rank=1

Pellegrino R, Viegi G, Brusasco V, et al. Interpretative strategies for lung function tests. *Eur Respir J*. 2005; 26(5): 948–968.

10 A 72-year-old woman is admitted to the trauma ICU after presentation following high-speed MVC.

A pulmonary artery catheter is placed given the patient's refractory hypotension. Which of the following is consistent with cardiogenic shock?

	PCWP (mmHg)	CO (L/min)	SVR (dyne-sec/cm^5)	MVO$_2$ (%)
A	8	5	1200	70
B	4	3	1800	50
C	14	3	1800	50
D	8	8	1200	70
E	8	6	1800	70

Though used infrequently within the surgical ICU setting, the Swan-Ganz catheter is a useful adjunct in the diagnosis of undifferentiated shock. Normal values obtained, as in option A, show a pulmonary capillary wedge pressure (PCWP) 8–12 mmHg, cardiac output (CO) 5–7 L/min, systemic vascular resistance (SVR) 900–1300 dyne-sec/cm^5, and mixed venous oxygen (MVO$_2$) approximately 65%. Option B indicates severe hypovolemic shock with decreased PCWP, decreased CO, increased SVR, and decreased MVO$_2$. Option C indicates cardiogenic shock with increased PCWP, decreased CO, increased SVR, and decreased MVO$_2$. Option D indicates distributive shock with normal PCWP, increased CO, decreased SVR, and increased MVO$_2$. Option E indicates obstructive shock with normal PCWP, normal CO, increased SVR, and increased MVO$_2$.

Answer: C

Cecconi M, De Backer D, Antonelli M, et al. Consensus on circulatory shock and hemodynamic monitoring. Task force of the European Society of Intensive Care Medicine. *Intensive Care Med.* 2014; 40: 1795–1815.

11 *A 73-year-old female with past medical history of significant peripheral vascular disease, hypertension, and diabetes is admitted to the ICU with significant hypotension following a myocardial infarction in PACU after undergoing EVAR of a 6 cm AAA. STAT echocardiogram shows right-sided heart failure. Swan-Ganz catheter is placed with PCWP of 10 mmHg. What is the next appropriate intervention?*
A *Inotrope initiation.*
B *Vasopressor initiation.*
C *Placement of intra-aortic balloon pump.*
D *Volume resuscitation.*
E *Diuretic therapy.*

The initial treatment of choice following acute right heart failure following MI is fluid resuscitation until PCWP > 15 mmHg is reached. Following this, initiation of inotropes, such as dobutamine, is done. Diuretic therapy may play a role in normotensive individuals. Vasopressors may be used in hypotensive patients with the goal of increasing systemic vascular resistance without increasing pulmonary vascular resistance. Fluid resuscitation should be adequate before continuing to increase vasopressor use. The intra-aortic balloon pump is used in left heart failure, not right heart failure.

Answer: D

Ventetuolo CE and Klinger JR. Management of acute right ventricular failure in the intensive care unit. *Ann Am Thorac Soc.* 2014; 11(5): 811–822.

12 *An 83-year-old woman with past medical history of significant peripheral vascular disease, ESRD on peritoneal dialysis admitted following below knee amputation for acute limb ischemia. You are called to bedside for patient's mean arterial pressure of 55 mmHg. You note the systolic pressure is appropriate, but diastolic pressure remains low. Which of the following is part of the pathophysiology of diastolic heart failure?*
A *Adaptive myocyte remodeling.*
B *Volume overload of the ventricle.*
C *Cell loss secondary to increased oxygen demand.*
D *Impaired ventricular wall relaxation.*
E *Change of ventricle from elliptical to globular.*

Diastolic heart failure stems from incomplete relaxation of the ventricle. Three pathophysiologic pathways include impaired ventricular wall relaxation, as left atrial pressure exceeds left ventricular pressure causing pulmonary edema; increased stiffness of the ventricle secondary to increased wall thickness and decreased internal diameter often seen with poorly controlled hypertension; excess collagen deposition as myofibrils are laid in parallel secondary to ischemia, as seen with MI, impairing contractility. The pathophysiology of systolic failure involves adaptive myocyte remodeling, as occurs with CAD, changing ventricular shape resulting in an increasingly overloaded ventricle with decreasing contractility resulting in cell loss due to increased oxygen demand and eventual change of the ventricle from elliptical to globular.

Answer: D

Zile MR, Baicu CF and Gaasch WH. Diastolic heart failure – abnormalities in active relaxation and passive stiffness of the left ventricle. *NEJM.* 2004; 350: 1953–1959.

13 *You are utilizing central venous pressure monitoring to guide resuscitation of a patient with a 60% TBSA*

burn injury in your ICU. Which of the following components of the CVP waveform represents isovolumic contraction?
A c wave
B x descent
C a wave
D y descent
E v wave

CVP Waveform component	Mechanical event
a wave	Atrial contraction
c wave	Isovolumic contraction
v wave	Systolic filling of the atrium
x descent	Atrial relaxation, systolic collapse
y descent	Early diastolic filling, diastolic collapse

Answer: A

Magder S. Central venous pressure: a useful but not so simple measurement. *Crit Care Med.* 2006; 34: 2224–2227.

14 Which component of the cardiac cycle is represented by the answer given above?
A Early diastole
B Early systole
C End diastole
D Mid-systole
E End systole

The a wave occurs from right atrial contraction increasing venous pressure. Right ventricular contraction displaces the tricuspid valve into the right atrium, represented by the c wave. With the emptying of right ventricle, the right atrium relaxes and begins to fill, represented by the x descent. The v wave demonstrates the filled right atrium with increased atrial pressure. Finally, the y descent shows right ventricular filling as the tricuspid valve opens.

CVP Waveform component	Cardiac cycle event
a wave	End diastole
c wave	Early systole
v wave	Late systole
x descent	Mid-systole
y descent	Early diastole

Answer: B

Magder S. Central venous pressure: a useful but not so simple measurement. *Crit Care Med.* 2006; 34: 2224–2227.

15 Which of the following is NOT a physiologic effect of minimally invasive left ventricular assist device?
A Decreased left ventricular end diastolic pressure.
B Decreased left ventricular wall tension.
C Increased diastolic pressure.
D Increased mean arterial pressure.
E Increased pulmonary capillary pressure.

A minimally invasive left ventricular assist device is a miniature axial pump that allows blood to be aspirated from the left ventricle into the cannula component of the pump and expelled above the aortic valve into the ascending aorta. The device has been used for support in high-risk percutaneous coronary intervention as well as cardiogenic shock. The device works to unload the left ventricle reducing left ventricular end diastolic pressure and wall tension. This allows for decreased oxygen demand. Furthermore, it increased mean arterial pressure, diastolic pressure, and cardiac output, thereby improving both systemic and coronary blood flow. Finally, it decreases pulmonary capillary pressure and thereby right ventricular afterload.

Answer: E

Burzotta F, Trani C, Doshi S, et al. Impella ventricular support in clinical practice: collaborative viewpoint from a European expert user group. *Int J Cardiol.* 2015; 201: 684–691.

16 Which of the following is a physiologic impact of intra-aortic balloon pumps during systole?
A Increased systolic blood pressure.
B Decreased pre-systolic aortic pressure.
C Increase in the isometric phase of left ventricular contraction.
D Increased left ventricular wall tension.
E Decreased left ventricular ejection fraction.

The intra-aortic balloon pump follows the principle of counterpulsation i.e. inflation during diastole with deflation during systole. The physiologic impacts during the systolic phase include a decrease in aortic systolic pressure as well pre-systolic (end-diastolic) aortic pressure both of which contribute to decreased afterload by 10% and 30%, respectively; decrease in the isometric phase of left ventricular contraction, thereby reducing myocardial oxygen consumption; decreased left ventricular wall tension by 20%; increased left ventricular ejection fraction by up to 30%.

Answer: B

Parissis H, Graham V, Lampridis S, et al. IABP: history-evolution-pathophysiology-indications: what we need to know. *J Cardiothorac Surg.* 2016; 11(1): 122.

17 *Which of the following is an expected cardiovascular change during pregnancy?*
   A *Decreased heart rate.*
   B *Decreased cardiac output.*
   C *Increased peripheral vascular resistance.*
   D *Decreased ventricular distension.*
   E *Decreased systemic vascular resistance.*

Pregnancy results in increased heart rate, increased cardiac output, decreased peripheral vascular resistance, increased ventricular distension, and decreased systemic vascular resistance.

Answer: E

Hill CC and Pickinpaugh J. Physiologic changes in pregnancy. *Surg Clin N Am.* 2008; 88: 391–401.

18 *Which of the following is a mechanism by which vasodilators improve cardiac function in acute decompensated heart failure?*
   A *Increased ventricular preload.*
   B *Decreased stroke volume.*
   C *Increased ventricular afterload.*
   D *Increased cardiac output.*
   E *Increased ventricular filling pressure.*

The pathophysiology of acute heart failure involves increased myocardial oxygen demand with increased ventricular filling pressures, low cardiac output, and increased systemic vascular resistance. Nitroprusside and nitroglycerin remain two of the most potent vasodilators used in therapy. Nitrogylcerin is a venodilator working to decrease preload, decrease afterload, and myocardial oxygen demand. Nitroprusside is an arterial and venous dilator decreasing preload, afterload, myocardial oxygen demand as well as increasing stroke volume and cardiac output.

Answer: D

Carlson MD and Eckman PM. Review of vasodilators in acute decompensated heart failure: the old and new. *J Card Fail* 2013; 19(7): 478–493.

19 *Which of the following is an expected effect of increased intrapleural pressure from positive pressure ventilation?*
   A *Increased venous return.*
   B *Increased aortic pressure.*
   C *Baroreceptor dampening.*
   D *Increased systemic vascular resistance.*
   E *Increased preload.*

With positive pressure ventilation, increased intrapleural pressure results in initially increased aortic pressure causing compensatory reduction in systemic vascular resistance and left ventricular afterload by activated baroreceptors, thereby increasing cardiac output. Positive pressure additionally decreases venous return and, therefore, preload.

Answer: B

Alviar CL, Miller PE, McAreavey D, et al. Positive pressure ventilation in the cardiac intensive care unit. *J Am Coll Cardiol.* 2018; 72: 1532–1553.

20 *A 70-year-old woman in a motor vehicle collision undergoes a splenectomy for Grade IV laceration and receives four units of whole blood in the OR but arrives in the ICU tachycardiac and hypotensive. Point of care hemoglobin is 14.3 mg/dL 2 hours post-transfusion. Her abdomen was left open and minimal output is coming from her negative pressure abdominal dressing. She has multiple rib fractures and a radius fracture. Which of the following therapies would promote end-organ perfusion?*
   A *Decrease vasoactive drug doses (decrease peripheral vascular resistance).*
   B *Increase sedation and pain medications to decrease her heart rate.*
   C *Increase end-diastolic volume with volume resuscitation.*
   D *Increase contractility with positive inotrope.*
   E *Increase end-systolic volume.*

This patient has evidence of blunt chest trauma with multiple rib fractures and tachycardia. While she could have hypovolemic shock from her splenic injury and intraoperative blood loss, she remains hypotensive despite transfusions with a hemoglobin of 14.3 mg/dL making this less likely and no evidence of ongoing bleeding from her abdomen. This makes it less likely that further volume resuscitation with blood or crystalloid would be helpful. Blunt cardiac injury can occur with blunt chest trauma and is initially screened for with EKG and troponin assessment, followed by an echocardiogram. Blunt cardiac injury may be improved with positive inotropic medications.

Decreasing vasoactive drug doses would worsen hypotension and worsen end-organ perfusion. Vasopressors are often used in supportive treatment for blunt cardiac injury and may need to be increased to promote end-organ perfusion. Increasing sedation and pain medications may improve her tachycardia but would worsen her hypotension and end-organ perfusion. Increasing end-systolic volume would decrease her stroke volume and cardiac output further, worsening her end-organ perfusion.

Remember: $CO = HR \times SV$

$$SV = EDV - ESV$$

Answer: D

Levick JR. *An Introduction to Cardiovascular Physiology.* Butterworth and Co., London, 2013.

Clancy K, Velopulos C, Bilaniuk JW, et al. Screening for blunt cardiac injury: An Eastern Association for the Surgery of Trauma practice management guideline. *J Trauma Acute Care Surg.* 2012; 735: S301–S306.

21 *A 39-year-old man presents with a cold right leg and complains of nine days of symptoms. Following a thromboembolectomy and fasciotomy, he develops hypoxia with saturation of 87% and respiratory distress. An arterial blood gas shows: pH 7.47, $paO_2 = 50\,mm\ Hg$, $HCO_3 = 22\,mmol/L$, $pCO_2 = 30\,mm\ Hg$. Chest x-ray shows patchy consolidations bilaterally and he reports fever prior to admission and that he works in a skilled nursing facility during the pandemic.*

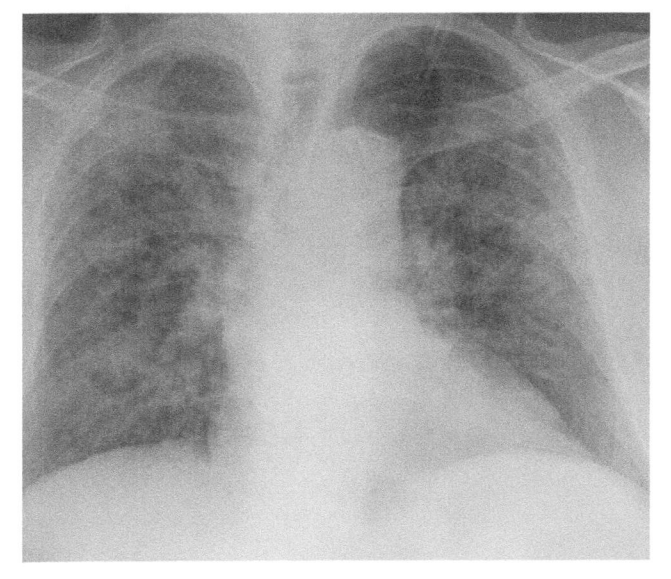

Based on the above results, his A-a gradient is (at sea level, water vapor pressure = 47 mm Hg):

A *150 mm Hg*
B *10 mm Hg*
C *38 mm Hg*
D *50 mm Hg*
E *62 mm Hg*

A-a gradient equals $PAO_2 - PaO_2$. His PaO_2 from the ABG is 50. The PAO_2 can be calculated from this equation:

$$PaO_2 = FiO_2 \left(P_B - P_{H_2O} \right) - \left(PaCO_2 / RQ \right)$$
$$= 0.21 \left(760 - 47 \right) - \left(30 / 0.8 \right)$$
$$PaO_2 = 112.5\,mm\,Hg$$

Therefore, A-a gradient $(PaO_2 - PAO_2)$ = 62.5 mm Hg.

Answer: E

Marino P. *The ICU Book*, 3rd ed., Lippincott Williams & Wilkins, Philadelphia, PA, chapter 19 2007.

22 *The patient above is placed on a nonrebreather mask with minimal improvement. What is the most likely etiology of the above patient's respiratory failure and appropriate intervention?*

A *Pulmonary embolism, anticoagulation.*
B *Hyperventilation from anxiety, benzothiazines.*
C *COVID-19 pneumonia, dexamethasone, and high-flow nasal canula.*
D *Neuromuscular weakness, reversal of paralytic.*
E *Pulmonary edema, acute kidney injury from rhabdomyolysis.*

Hypoxemia occurs in four conditions: low inspired oxygen, shunt, V/Q mismatch, and hypoventilation.

Hypoventilation would present with high CO_2 and normal A-a gradient. This could occur with oversedation, neuromuscular weakness, and residual anesthesia. Hyperventilation would cause tachypnea, low CO_2, but not hypoxia, so A-a gradient should be normal. Low inspired oxygen should have a low PO_2 and normal gradient. An acute PE or asthma exacerbation presents with V/Q mismatch with elevated A-a gradient and normal PCO_2. It should correct with administration of oxygen. Shunting (pulmonary edema or pneumonia) has an elevated A-a gradient that does not improve with oxygen administration. The patient is young for postoperative MI and has risk factors and a chest x-ray consistent with COVID-19 pneumonia, which could also increase his risk of thrombotic events since as an arterial thrombus.

Answer: C

Weinberger SE, Cockrill BA and Mande J. *Principles of Pulmonary Medicine*, 5th ed., W.B. Saunders, Philadelphia, PA, (2008).

NIH COVID-19 Treatment Guidelines. Therapeutic management of patients with COVID-19. www.covid19treatmentguidelines.nih.gov/therapeutic-management/ (accessed 15 December 20).

23 *A 63-year-old patient with history of hypertension and type 2 diabetes presents with acute respiratory distress syndrome from pneumococcal pneumonia and is being managed by the ICU team for severe ARDS. After appropriate sedation and analgesia, which of the following is NOT an appropriate strategy for management?*

A *Low tidal volume ventilation (4–8ml/kg IBW).*

B *Prone positioning <6 hours/day.*

C *Use of recruitment maneuvers.*

D *Higher PEEP levels with plateau pressures <30cm H2O.*

E *Very select use of high-frequency oscillatory ventilation.*

Acute respiratory distress syndrome management guidelines target management with low tidal volume ventilation, low inspiratory pressures with plateau pressures <30 cm H_2O, high PEEP levels are better than low PEEP levels, and prone positioning for at least 12-hour periods per day with improved mortality. Less than 6 hours of prone position per day would not be recommended as it is too short a time period.

Answer: B

Fan E., Del Sorbo L, Goligher EC, et al. An Official American Thoracic Society/European Society of Intensive Care Medicine/Society of critical care medicine clinical practice guideline: mechanical ventilation in adult patients with acute respiratory distress syndrome. *Am J Respir Crit Care Med.* 2017; 195 9: 1253–1263. https://www.thoracic.org/statements/resources/cc/ards-guidelines.pdf.

2

Cardiopulmonary Resuscitation, Oxygen Delivery and Shock

Kevin W. Cahill, MD, Harsh Desai, MD, and Luis Cardenas, DO, PhD

Department of Surgery, Christiana Care Health Care System, Newark, DE, USA

1   *A 72-year-old woman with a history of Child's B cirrhosis and supraventricular tachycardia is in the ICU following laparotomy for strangulated ventral hernia. She begins to complain of rapid heartbeat and is noted to be in an irregular, wide-complex ventricular tachycardia on EKG. She maintains pulse and adequate blood pressure. Which of the following is the best initial therapy to administer?*
   A   *Synchronized cardioversion.*
   B   *Adenosine 6 mg IV.*
   C   *Amiodarone 150 mg IV.*
   D   *Defibrillation.*
   E   *Vagal maneuvers.*

The 2020 ACLS guidelines differentiate between regular and irregular wide-complex tachycardia with and without pulse. In this instance, the patient is in an irregular wide-complex tachycardia, symptomatic, but stable as evidence by pulse and pressure. Given this hemodynamic stability, synchronized cardioversion and defibrillation are not the initial therapies (choices A, D). Adenosine and vagal maneuvers may be effective in regular ventricular tachycardia (choices B, E). Therefore, amiodarone is the best initial medication to administration often followed by infusion (choice C). Individuals with hemodynamically unstable ventricular tachycardia should not initially receive amiodarone. These individuals should be cardioverted. Amiodarone can be used regardless of the individual's underlying heart function and the type of ventricular tachycardia. It can be used in individuals with monomorphic ventricular tachycardia, but is contraindicated in individuals with polymorphic ventricular tachycardia as it is associated with prolonged QT intervals, which will be made worse with anti-arrhythmic drugs. Amiodarone is categorized as a class III anti-arrhythmic

agent, and prolongs phase 3 of the cardiac action potential. Amiodarone slows conduction rate and prolongs the refractory period of the SA and AV nodes. It also prolongs the refractory periods of the ventricles, bundles of His, and the Purkinje fibers without exhibiting any effects on the conduction rate. Serious side effects include interstitial lung disease and liver dysfunction with elevated liver enzymes.

Answer: C

Littmann L, Olson EG, Gibbs MA. Initial evaluation and management of wide-complex tachycardia: a simplified and practical approach. *Am J Emerg Med*. 2019; 37: 1340–1345.

Panchal AR, Bartos JA, Cabanas JG et al. Part 3: Adult basic and advanced cardiac life support: 2020 American Heart Association guidelines for cardiopulmonary resuscitation and emergency cardiovascular care. *Circulation*. 2020; 142 (suppl 2): S366–S468.

2   *Which of the following techniques has not been shown to be effective in airway management during cardiac arrest?*
   A   *Head tilt – chin lift*
   B   *Jaw thrust*
   C   *Cricoid pressure*
   D   *Nasopharyngeal airway*
   E   *Oropharyngeal airway*

Of the above maneuvers, cricoid pressure has not been shown to be effective during airway management in cardiopulmonary resuscitation. It may impede ventilation or placement of airway adjuncts such as a supraglottic airway as well as contribute to increased airway trauma.

Jaw thrust is preferred in patients with suspected spinal injury. Nasopharyngeal and oropharyngeal airways are particularly useful in cases of facial trauma though care must be taken with possible basilar skull fractures.

Answer: C

Carauna E, Chevret S, Pirracchio R. Effect of cricoid pressure on laryngeal view during prehospital tracheal intubation: a propensity-based analysis. *Emerg Med J.* 2017; 34 (3): 132–137.

Panchal AR, Bartos JA, Cabanas JG et al. Part 3: Adult basic and advanced cardiac life support: 2020 American Heart Association guidelines for cardiopulmonary resuscitation and emergency cardiovascular care. *Circulation*. 2020; 142 (suppl 2): S366–S468.

3   *In a patient experiencing PEA arrest, which of the following would not be a likely etiology?*
   A *Hypoglycemia*
   B *Hypoxia*
   C *Hypovolemia*
   D *Hypokalemia*
   E *Hypocalcemia*

Pulseless electrical activity is so named due to evidence of cardiac mechanical activity on echocardiogram or rhythm on EKG. The algorithm is similar to the asystole algorithm utilizing compressions and epinephrine. The traditional etiologies are described as "Hs" and "Ts." The "Hs" include hypoglycemia, hypoxia, hyper/hypokalemia, hypovolemia, acidosis, and hypothermia. Hypocalcemia can present with muscular and neurologic symptoms such as perioral numbness, cramping, fatigue, seizures, and irritability. Hypocalcemia may also be associated with increased risk of arrhythmias, but is not typically considered high on the initial differential of PEA arrest. The "Ts" taught as etiologies include tension pneumothorax, cardiac tamponade, toxins, pulmonary thrombosis, or coronary thrombosis. Evaluation for pneumothorax or tamponade includes rapid bedside physical exam as well as point of care ultrasound for rule out. Ultrasound may also reveal signs of thrombosis with right ventricular enlargement or free-floating thrombus.

Answer: E

Andersen LW, Holmberg MJ, Berg KM et al. In hospital cardiac arrest: a review. *JAMA*. 2019; 321 (12): 1200–1210.

Panchal AR, Bartos JA, Cabanas JG et al. Part 3: Adult basic and advanced cardiac life support: 2020 American Heart Association guidelines for cardiopulmonary resuscitation and emergency cardiovascular care. *Circulation*. 2020; 142 (suppl 2): S366–S468.

4   *Which of the following is the minimum chest compression fraction (defined as amount of time spent delivering chest compressions during CPR) shown to be associated with improved survival?*
   A *0–20%*
   B *21–40%*
   C *41–60%*
   D *61–80%*
   E *81–100%*

Optimal outcomes have been demonstrated with minimal pauses between compressions for pulse checks and breaths given during high-quality CPR. A compression fraction of at least 60% has been shown to be necessary for best outcomes. Animal studies previously conducted have demonstrated decreased coronary and cerebral perfusion when chest compressions are not being conducted resulting in worsened outcomes. Multiple retrospective analyses and cohort studies have resulted in many emergency agencies targeting a compression fraction of between 60 and 80% as a quality metric. This involves delivery of high-quality compressions of appropriate depth, 2 inches, and rate, at least 100/min.

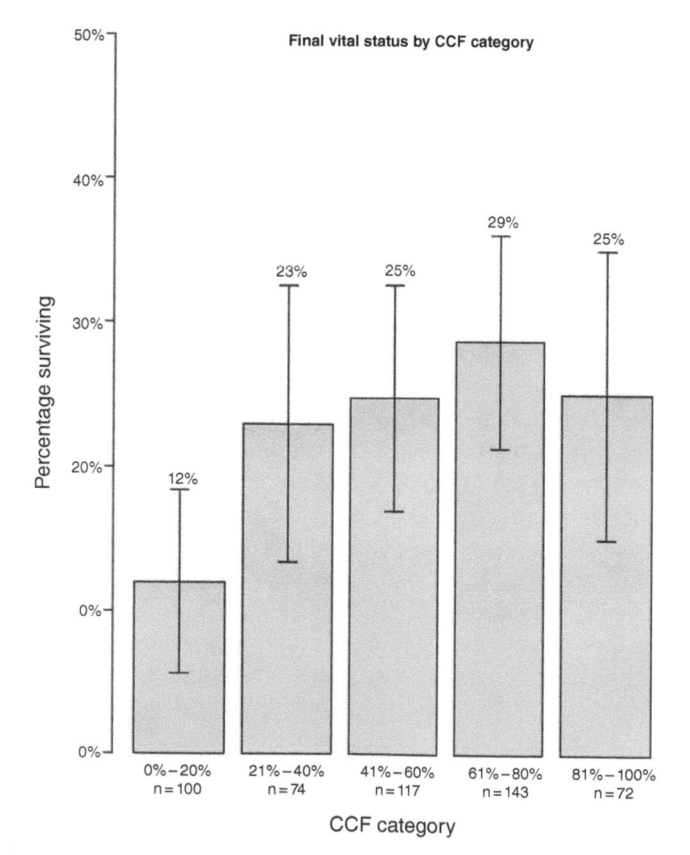

Answer: D

Christenson J, Andrusiek D, Everson-Stewart S et al. Chest compression fraction determines survival in patients with out of hospital ventricular fibrillation. *Circulation.* 2009; 120: 1241–1247.

Panchal AR, Bartos JA, Cabanas JG et al. Part 3: Adult basic and advanced cardiac life support: 2020 American Heart Association guidelines for cardiopulmonary resuscitation and emergency cardiovascular care. *Circulation.* 2020; 142 (suppl 2): S366–S468.

5 *Which of the following is considered the highest predictor of survival for in- and out-of-hospital CPR?*
   A *Age.*
   B *Shockable rhythm.*
   C *Arrest at home.*
   D *Arrest at night vs during the day.*
   E *Delayed EMS response time.*

On the whole, survivability is dependent on patient, system, event, and therapeutic factors. With increasing comorbidity and age, survivability decreases. System factors include time to arrival of EMS, time to initiation of CPR, and time to defibrillation. Event factors include preceding symptoms. Finally, therapeutic factors include availability of medications to treat suspected cause, time to ER, time to cath lab should it be required, etc. The greatest mortality risk with out of hospital cardiac arrest stems from unwitnessed arrests without bystander CPR often occurring at night in the elderly. Highest survivability stems from witnessed arrests with rapid initiation of bystander CPR and initial shockable rhythm, such as ventricular fibrillation.

Answer: B

Myat A, Song K-J, Rea T. Out of hospital cardiac arrest: current concepts. *Lancet.* 2018; 391: 970–79.

Navab E, Esmaelli M, Poorkhorshidi N et al. Predictors of out of hospital cardiac arrest outcomes in pre-hospital settings; a retrospective cross-sectional study. *Arch Am Emerg Med.* 2019; 7 (1): e36.

6 *A 70-year-old man is 2 weeks status-post laparoscopic sleeve gastrectomy and he undergoes witnessed cardiac arrest at home after complaint of new onset chest pain. Bystander CPR achieves ROSC after 10 minutes. He is now in the ICU, intubated, and on vasopressors for associated hypotension. Which of the following interventions has the strongest associated survival benefit in post-arrest care according to current resuscitation guidelines?*
   A *Maintain 100% FiO_2.*
   B *Pursuit of cardiac intervention when STEMI identified.*
   C *Use of corticosteroids.*
   D *Targeted temperature management to prevent fever.*
   E *Seizure prophylaxis.*

If a cardiac cause is suspected, pursuit of cardiac intervention such as with percutaneous coronary intervention (PCI) is strongly recommended. Hyperoxygenation therapy, the use of corticosteroids, and seizure prophylaxis have thus far shown no survival benefit (choices A, C, and E). Finally, targeted temperature management is currently recommended for post-arrest care with target of $32–36^{\circ}$ C. This is based on several studies showing potential neurologic benefit. Preventing fever has not yet been proven to improve outcome though the 2020 AHA guideline (choice D). Ischemic heart disease is a major cause of out of hospital cardiac arrest. Among patients who had been successfully resuscitated after out of hospital cardiac arrest and had no signs of STEMI, immediate angiography was not found to be better than a strategy of delayed angiography with respect to overall survival at 90 days.

Answer: B

Panchal AR, Bartos JA, Cabanas JG et al. Part 3: Adult basic and advanced cardiac life support: 2020 American Heart Association guidelines for cardiopulmonary resuscitation and emergency cardiovascular care. *Circulation.* 2020; 142 (suppl 2): S366–S468.

Yannapoulos D, Bartos JA, Aufderheide TP et al. The evolving role of the cardiac catherization laboratory in the management of patients with out of hospital cardiac arrest: a scientific statement from the American Heart Association. *Circulation.* 2019; 139 (12): e530–e552.

Lemkes JS, Janssens GN, van der Hoeven NW et al. Coronary angiography after cardiac arrest without ST-Segment elevation. April 11, 2019. *N Engl J Med.* 2019; 380: 1397–1407. DOI: https://doi.org/10.1056/NEJMoa1816897

7 *A 35-year-old, 26 week pregnant woman has cardiac arrest with CPR ongoing in the ED. CPR has been ongoing for 5 minutes. Which of the following has been shown to provide greatest benefit for achieving ROSC?*
   A *Corticosteroids.*
   B *Targeted temperature management.*
   C *Left lateral uterine displacement.*
   D *Fetal monitoring.*
   E *C-section.*

In conditions of cardiac arrest after pregnancy, rapid delivery of the fetus, typically by C-section, termed perimortem cesarean delivery (PMCD), has been shown to be associated with improved outcomes when CPR does not achieve ROSC. However, the decision must be made quickly as a review article states that if done within 10 minutes of arrest, it was associated with better maternal outcomes. It was also thought that it was beneficial to the mother in 31% of cases and was not harmful in any case. The review of the cases resulted in only 94 cases supporting that PMCD is rare. Corticosteroids have shown no benefit and targeted temperature management may be used after achievement of ROSC (choices A and B).The left lateral uterine displacement alleviates aortocaval compression in patients with hypotension, but delivery achieves this much more effectively (choice C). Fetal monitoring during maternal CPR is a distraction and may hinder care (choice D).

Answer: E

Einav S, Kaufman N, Sela HY. Maternal cardiac arrest and perimortem caesarean delivery: evidence or expert based? *Resuscitation.* 2012; 83 (10): 1191–1200.

Panchal AR, Bartos JA, Cabanas JG et al. Part 3: Adult basic and advanced cardiac life support: 2020 American Heart Association guidelines for cardiopulmonary resuscitation and emergency cardiovascular care. *Circulation.* 2020; 142 (suppl 2): S366–S468.

8   Which of the following scenarios causes a shift of the oxygen dissociation curve to the left?
  A A patient found unconscious in a basement apartment with malfunctioning heater.
  B Patient with pneumonia and fever of 102°C.
  C Patient with lactic acidosis from mesenteric ischemia.
  D Patient with depressed mental status taking slow, shallow breaths.
  E Patient returning from climbing Mt Everest where he had to stop and be treated for hypoxia after leaving base camp.

Everest where he had to stop and be treated for hypoxia after leaving base camp. The oxygen–hemoglobin dissociation curve is sigmoidal in shape based on allosteric interactions of each globin monomer binding oxygen. A shift to the right indicates decreased affinity favoring unloading of oxygen while a shift to the left achieves the opposite effect. The strength by which oxygen binds to hemoglobin is affected by several factors and can be represented as a shift to the left or right in the oxygen dissociation curve. A rightward shift of the curve indicates that hemoglobin has a decreased affinity for oxygen, thus, oxygen actively unloads. A shift to the left indicates increased hemoglobin affinity for oxygen and an increased reluctance to release oxygen. Several physiologic factors are responsible for shifting the curve left or right, such as pH, carbon dioxide (CO_2), temperature, and 2,3-Disphosphoglycerate. Carbon monoxide exposure, as can be seen in enclosed spaces with a malfunctioning heater, can result in a leftward shift. If the patient

was hypothermic or alkalotic, these conditions would also shift it toward the left.

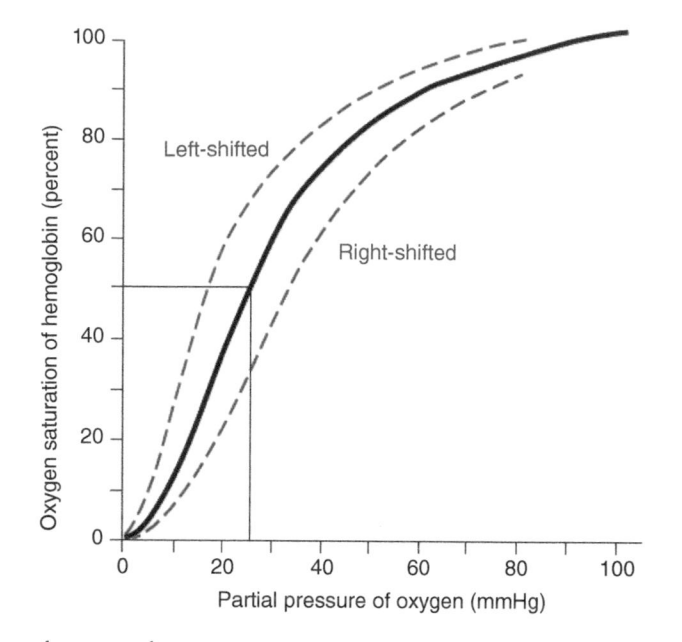

Answer: A

Woodson, RD. Physiologic significance of oxygen dissociation curve shifts. *Crit Care Med.* 1979; 7 (9): 368–373.

9   You are caring for a patient in the SICU, currently intubated after undergoing left upper lobectomy for tumor. Patient's current hemoglobin is 10g/dL, oxygen saturation 95%, and PaO_2 of 92 mmHg. What is the expected oxygen content (CaO_2)?
  A 0.9 mL/dL
  B 9 mL/dL
  C 13 mL/dL
  D 21 mL/dL
  E 140 mL/dL

Blood oxygen content is based on the following formula influenced by oxygen saturation, partial pressure of arterial oxygen, and patient's hemoglobin:

$$\begin{aligned} CaO_2 &= (1.34 \times Hb \times SaO_2) + (0.003 \times PaO_2) \\ &= (1.34 \times 10 \times 0.95) + (0.003 \times 92) \\ &= (12.73) + (0.28) \\ &= 13.01 \text{ or } 13 \text{ mL} / dL \end{aligned}$$

The single biggest factor for oxygen content is hemoglobin. Doubling of hemoglobin would double the oxygen content. Increasing the partial pressure of oxygen from 60 mmHg to 100 would increase saturation from 90 to 100% and would not be a large change in content. The doubling of partial pressure of oxygen from 60 mmHg to 120 mmHg would still only increase the content by 10% as the dissolved amount of oxygen in plasma is negated by the factor of 0.003. The constant of 1.34 is the amount of oxygen that one gram of hemoglobin carries at 1 atmosphere of pressure.

Answer: C

Crocetti J, Diaz-Abad M, Krachman SL. Oxygen content, delivery, and uptake. In GJ Criner, RE Barnette, GE D'Alonzo (Eds), *Critical Care Study Guide*. New York: Springer, 2010.

10 *Changes in which of the following components is the most influential in increasing oxygen delivery?*
   A *Cardiac output.*
   B *Hemoglobin level.*
   C *Oxygen saturation.*
   D *Oxygen dissolved in blood.*
   E *Systemic vascular resistance.*

As described in the question above, oxygen content is influenced by hemoglobin, oxygen saturation, and partial pressure of arterial oxygen. Of these, hemoglobin level, which has the greatest impact on oxygen content through binding, has the greatest impact on oxygen available to deliver to tissues. Arterial oxygen saturation and cardiac output are additional important factors in ensuring adequate oxygen delivery. Increased cardiac output as a compensatory mechanism can carry more oxygenated blood for delivery. Improved oxygen saturations ensure appropriate oxygen availability for hemoglobin binding. Changes in vascular resistance can influence oxygen diffusion. The least influential of the above choices given, the minimal contribution it makes to available oxygen, is partial pressure of arterial oxygen i.e. dissolved oxygen.

Answer: B

Marino P. *The ICU Book*, 4th edn. Philadelphia: Lippincott Williams & Wilkins, 2007.

11 *You are called to the PACU to evaluate a 64-year-old man with a history of metastatic lung cancer now s/p video-assisted thoracoscopic resection of the left upper lobe. His heart rate is 110 beats/min, blood pressure 70/42 mmHg. He appears tachypneic. On examination, he is cool and clammy, with evidence of peripheral cyanosis and prominent jugular venous distension. Anesthesia has successfully placed an arterial line and initiated several fluid boluses while awaiting your arrival; however, there has been no significant improvement in his hemodynamics. You note that his systolic blood pressure on the arterial line appears to decrease by at least 10 mmHg during respiration. While you prepare the appropriate*

intervention, what would be the best next step to help confirm the likely diagnosis?
   A *Chest X-ray*
   B *CT angiogram*
   C *CBC*
   D *EKG*
   E *Transthoracic echocardiogram*

This patient is exhibiting signs of cardiac tamponade, with evidence of pulsus paradoxus, jugular venous distension, and hypotension. The primary tool for diagnosis of cardiac tamponade is Doppler echocardiography, which in the presence of tamponade typically shows a circumferential pericardial fluid layer and compressed chambers with high ventricular ejection fractions. On inspiration, both the ventricular and atrial septa move leftward and reverse on expiration, due to the fixed pericardial volume. Right ventricular collapse is typically less sensitive but more specific for tamponade. The inferior vena cava is typically dilated with minimal respiratory variation. CT angiogram may demonstrate pericardial effusion, distension of the superior and inferior vena cavae, and reflux of contrast material into the azygos vein and inferior vena cava. However, these represent static images rather than the dynamic information presented by echocardiography. Chest x-ray may demonstrate an enlarged cardiac silhouette but is particularly unreliable in early/acute tamponade (choice A). Additionally, obtaining a CT scan is typically not portable, requiring transporting a hemodynamically unstable patient to obtain the study (choice B). A CBC would be of little use to obtaining this diagnosis (choice C). EKG may show evidence of pericarditis or electrical alternans but is unreliable in the diagnosis of tamponade (choice D).

Answer: E

Spodick DH. Acute cardiac tamponade. *N Engl J Med.* 2003; 349 (7): 684–90. doi: https://doi.org/10.1056/NEJMra022643. PMID: 12917306.

12 *A 27-year-old man presents after jumping from a diving board and striking the bottom of a pool with his upper body. On presentation, he has no sensation or motor strength of his lower extremities. On examination, he appears flaccid and you cannot elicit spinal reflexes. His heart rate is 54 beats/min, blood pressure 90/54, and respiratory rate 18. Despite appropriate fluid resuscitation, he remains hypotensive, though you identify no evidence of ongoing hemorrhage. What type of shock does this likely represent?*
   A *Obstructive*
   B *Distributive*
   C *Cardiogenic*
   D *Hypovolemic*
   E *Anaphylactic*

This patient demonstrates bradycardia, hypotension, and neurologic deficits in the setting of possible cervical or high thoracic spine trauma, suggesting he may have a component of neurogenic shock. This shock is a result of spinal cord injury with sudden loss of sympathetic tone with preserved parasympathetic activity and autonomic instability, leading to bradycardia and hypotension. These changes are typically seen with an injury to the spinal cord above T6. Disruption of the sympathetic division of the autonomic nervous system affects three areas of the cardiovascular system: coronary blood flow, cardiac contractility, and heart rate. There is systemic hypotension due to a decrease in sympathetic fiber-mediated arterial and venous vascular resistance, along with venous pooling and loss of preload, with or without bradycardia. The bradycardia is often exacerbated by suctioning, defecation, turning, and hypoxia. The hypotension places patients at increased risk of secondary spinal cord ischemia due to impairment of autoregulation. With preserved parasympathetic activity, this translates clinically into bradycardia (and possibly other cardiac arrhythmias) in the setting of profound hypotension. Trauma patients are hypotensive as a result of blood loss or intravascular hypovolemia but will mount an appropriate tachycardic response. Blood loss must be ruled out and treated appropriately before assuming that hypotension is due solely to spinal cord injury. It is common to have both blood loss and spinal cord injury. Initial management is composed of volume resuscitation to account for the increased intravascular space secondary to increased vasodilation, as well as vasopressors for blood pressure control. In addition to pressor support, chronotropic and inotropic support may be necessary. Norepinephrine is started initially but in refractory cases, epinephrine and vasopressin infusions may be required. Bradycardia usually responds to atropine and glycopyrrolate but in severe cases, dopamine infusion is required. When blood loss is a part of the presentation, volume resuscitation should be with blood products and not crystalloids. Spinal shock is often confused with neurogenic shock. Spinal shock, on the other hand, refers to loss of all sensation below the level of injury and is not circulatory in nature. Both may, however, coexist in a patient.

Answer: B

Stein DM, Knight WA. Emergency neurological life support: traumatic spine injury. *Neurocrit Care.* 2017; 27 (Suppl 1): 170–180.

Phillips AA, Krassioukov AV. Contemporary cardiovascular concerns after spinal cord injury: mechanisms, maladaptations, and management. *J Neurotrauma.* 2015; 32 (24): 1927–42. doi: https://doi.org/10.1089/neu.2015.3903. Epub 2015 Sep 1. PMID: 25962761.

13 *Shock is defined as:*
   A *Blood pressure less than 90 mm Hg.*
   B *Heart rate greater than 140 beats/min.*
   C *Urine output less than 0.5 ml/kg/hr.*
   D *Inadequate perfusion to meet end organ metabolic needs.*
   E *All of the above.*

Shock is defined by some as inadequate perfusion to meet end organ metabolic needs. Tissue and cellular hypoxia can be due to inadequate delivery, increased consumption, inadequate utilization, or a combination of these states. Although this is often reflected in hemodynamic changes such as hypotension, tachycardia, or oliguria, these are not sufficient criteria alone to diagnosis a patient as being in shock. A patient may present hypertensive, normotensive, or hypotensive. Conditions such as neurogenic shock may result in a patient with bradycardia despite inadequate perfusion. Shock can be further differentiated into hypovolemic, cardiogenic, obstructive, or restrictive (vasodilatory/distributive). Causes of obstructive shock include pulmonary embolism, tension pneumothorax, and pericardial tamponade. Causes of obstructive shock typically lead to decreased cardiac output and are sometimes included into the cardiogenic shock category. Identification of these sub categories of shock is crucial to guiding therapeutic intervention.

Cardiogenic shock
Extrinsic (tamponade)

Intrinsic (failure, ischemia)

Hemorrhagic

Distributive
Neurogenic

Answer: D

Kislitsina ON, Rich JD, Wilcox JE et al. Shock - classification and pathophysiological principles of therapeutics. *Curr Cardiol Rev.* 2019; 15 (2): 102–113. doi: https://doi.org/10.2174/1573403X15666181212125024. PMID: 30543176; PMCID: PMC6520577.

Vincent JL, De Backer D. Circulatory shock. *N Engl J Med.* 2013; 369: 1726.

14 *A 53-year-old woman with a history of ulcerative colitis controlled with 50 mg of oral prednisone daily undergoes a laparoscopic converted to open colectomy. Intra-operatively there are no complications noted and she receives appropriate fluid resuscitation. However, post-operatively she is noted to be febrile and hypotensive. This hypotension is refractory to additional fluid boluses or multiple vasopressors. On physical examination, her abdomen does not appear distended and she is appropriately tender. What would be the best next step in management of this patient?*
   A *Additional fluid boluses.*
   B *Adding on an additional vasopressor.*
   C *Return to the operating room for exploration.*
   D *Administer stress dose hydrocortisone.*
   E *Begin broad-spectrum antibiotics.*

This patient with a history of chronic adrenal suppression due to daily prednisone use presents with signs and symptoms consistent with an adrenal crisis. These events are typically brought on by an inability for the body to mount an appropriate response to an insult by generating endogenous cortisol secondary to chronic adrenal suppression. Unless administered appropriate exogenous glucocorticoids, they may exhibit evidence of hypotension refractory to typical interventions, abdominal pain, nausea/vomiting, and confusion. Additional fluid boluses or adding an additional vasopressor would not address the underlying pathology and has already been described as unsuccessful in this vignette (choices A, B). Initiating broad-spectrum antibiotics similarly does not address the underlying issue and would have no impact on this patient's hemodynamics (choice E). Septic shock would most likely develop later and not immediately. While a hypotensive patient post-operatively may be due to blood loss and ultimately require return to the operating room for exploration, in this case, failure to recognize the underlying adrenal crisis would result in unnecessary re-exploration (choice C).

Answer: D

Rushworth RL, Torpy DJ, Falhammar H. Adrenal Crisis. *N Engl J Med.* 2019; 381 (9): 852–861. doi: https://doi.org/10.1056/NEJMra1807486. PMID: 31461595.

15 *A 71-year-old patient has acute, non-perforated appendicitis. His BMI is 27 and otherwise healthy. Intra-operatively you begin with Veress needle insertion into the abdomen and begin to establish pneumoperitoneum with high flow rates. Your*

anesthesiologist immediately notes a marked decrease in the patient's end-tidal carbon dioxide and oxygen saturations as well as new onset tachycardia. You halt insufflation but the patient quickly becomes hemodynamically unstable. What is your best step to address the underlying pathology?
   A *Convert to open.*
   B *Place the patient in steep Trendelenburg and place a central line for therapeutic intervention.*
   C *Administer fluid bolus.*
   D *Start vasopressors.*
   E *Abort the procedure and transfer the patient to the ICU.*

This patient is demonstrating evidence of possible air embolism secondary to intravascular insufflation. The primary goal in this case is to prevent further gas entry into the venous system and reduce the amount of gas trapped in the heart. Placing the patient in Trendelenburg position maximizes blood flow to the brain and theoretically relieves right-sided heart airlock as well as prevent gas entry into the pulmonary artery. In a patient who is hemodynamically unstable secondary to an air embolism, a central line should be placed into the right atrium and attempts made to withdraw air from the right side of the heart. Converting to open would not address the underlying issue (choice A). Initiating fluids or vasopressors would briefly temporize the patient but would not address the underlying pathology (choices C, D). Aborting the procedure and taking a hemodynamically unstable patient to the ICU would not be correct as the underlying pathology should be addressed prior to leaving the operating room (choice E).

Answer: B

Sandadi S, Johannigman JA, Wong VL et al. Recognition and management of major vessel injury during laparoscopy. *J Minim Invasive Gynecol.* 2010; 17 (6): 692–702. doi: https://doi.org/10.1016/j.jmig.2010.06.005. Epub 2010 Jul 24. PMID: 20656569.

16 *A 32-year-old healthy man was passed out in a workplace fire but had minimal burns to the right hand. Given suspected inhalation injury, you take care to establish a definitive airway and transfer the patient to the ICU for additional monitoring. The patient is initially tachycardic and hypertensive but shortly thereafter develops bradycardia, hypotension, and cardiac dysrhythmias. On physical examination, his skin appears flushed with a cherry-red color. Labwork reveals a marked metabolic acidosis on arterial blood gas and serum lactate is 9 mmol/L. His carboxyhemoglobin level is normal. Which of the* *following would be most effective in addressing his underlying pathology?*

A *Aggressive fluid resuscitation*

B *Administration of hydroxocobalamin*

C *Vasopressor support*

D *Diuresis*

E *Continue supportive care*

This patient is showing evidence of possible cyanide poisoning with evidence of cardiovascular instability, marked metabolic acidosis, and classic "cherry-red" skin color. Although present in only a minority of patients, this finding is a result of impaired tissue oxygen utilization, resulting in high venous oxyhemoglobin concentration, and bright red appearance of the blood. Hydroxocobalamin is a precursor of Vitamin B12 that directly binds to intra-cellular cyanide, forming cyanocobalamin. This molecule is then readily excreted in the urine. This treatment acts rapidly, does not affect tissue oxygenation, and is relatively safe, making it a first-line agent for cyanide poisoning. The other answer questions do not address what is driving the patient's underlying pathology.

Answer: B

Hendry-Hofer TB, Ng PC, Witeof AE et al. A review on ingested cyanide: risks, clinical presentation, diagnostics, and treatment challenges. *J Med Toxicol.* 2019; 15: 128.

17 *A 37-year-old patient is admitted to the floor after suffering a femur fracture during a MVC. While he is stable over the next 24 hours, he shortly thereafter develops a new petechial rash on the non-dependent portions of his body, becomes hypotensive, confused, tachypneic, and is hypoxic on pulse oximetry. A chest x-ray is obtained but appears normal. A CT angiogram of the chest does not demonstrate any evidence of pulmonary thromboembolism. What would be the next step in management?*

A *Supportive care with fluid resuscitation and oxygenation*

B *Intravascular tPA lytic therapy*

C *Broad-spectrum antibiotics*

D *Vasopressors*

E *ECMO*

This patient is showing evidence of possible fat-embolism syndrome. This is a rare entity that can be encountered in patients 24–72 hours after an initial insult (long bone fracture in this patient). The triad of hypoxemia, neurologic abnormalities, and petechial rash is classic for fat-embolism syndrome, though non-specific. Fat embolism can also present with thrombocytopenia and this may help make a diagnosis. However, it remains a diagnosis of exclusion, primarily made clinically. Initial assessment is performed to exclude alternative diagnoses such as pulmonary embolism. There is no definitive treatment and therapy is primarily supportive while awaiting resolution. There is no role for intravascular lytic therapy or broad-spectrum antibiotics (choices B, C). While vasopressors and invasive ventilator support such as ECMO may be necessary in patients with refractory shock, they are not the initial step in management (choices D, E).

Answer: A

Stein PD, Yaekoub AY, Matta F et al. Fat embolism syndrome. *Am J Med Sci.* 2008; 336: 472.

18 *A 54-year-old patient with a history of diabetes mellitus on home metformin presents to your emergency department with shortness of breath, productive cough, and fever. On imaging, he is found to have a right lower lobe opacity consistent with pneumonia. He is hemodynamically stable but blood work is noted to have a lactic acidemia of 4 and his glucose is elevated to 300. His CBC is within normal limits and an EKG is normal. He is mentating well, making appropriate urine without evidence of tissue hypoperfusion. What best describes the patient's lactic academia?*

A *Type A lactic acidosis*

B *Type B lactic acidosis*

C *Septic shock*

D *Hemorrhagic shock*

E *Cardiac failure*

This patient is showing evidence of lactic acidosis in the absence of systemic hypoperfusion. Type A lactic acidosis is typically related to hypoperfusion secondary to hypovolemia, cardiac failure, sepsis, or cardiopulmonary arrest. Type B lactic acidosis occurs when there is no evidence of systemic hypoperfusion and may be related to impaired cellular metabolism (choice B). Both metformin use and diabetes mellitus have been implicated as associated with Type B lactic acidosis. This patient is showing no signs of septic, hemorrhagic, or cardiogenic shock (choices C, D, E).

Answer: B

3

ECMO

Mauer Biscotti III, MD[1], Matthew A. Goldshore, MD, PhD, MPH[2], and Jeremy W. Cannon, MD, SM[3,4]

[1] Division of General Surgery, Department of Surgery, San Antonio Military Medical Center, San Antonio, TX, USA
[2] Department of Surgery, Perelman School of Medicine at the University of Pennsylvania, Philadelphia, PA, USA
[3] Division of Traumatology, Surgical Critical Care & Emergency Surgery, Perelman School of Medicine at the University of Pennsylvania, Philadelphia, PA, USA
[4] Department of Surgery, F. Edward Hébert School of Medicine, Uniformed Services University of the Health Sciences, Bethesda, MD, USA

1 *A 45-year-old previously healthy man was a pedestrian struck by a motor vehicle resulting in multiple injuries including traumatic brain injury with a subarachnoid hemorrhage (SAH), multiple rib fractures, pulmonary contusion, hemothorax, splenic laceration, and a pelvic fracture. On postinjury day 5, he developed severe hypoxemic respiratory failure ($PaO_2:FiO_2$ ratio of 70 on FiO_2 of 1) and was diagnosed with an MRSA pneumonia. Workup for other causes of respiratory failure or sepsis was negative, and there was no evidence of SAH progression or torso hemorrhage on his most recent imaging. Which of the following should be performed before considering this patient for extracorporeal membrane oxygenation (ECMO)?*

A *High-frequency oscillatory ventilation*
B *Airway pressure release ventilation*
C *Prone positioning*
D *Rib fracture stabilization*
E *Decompressive laparotomy*

This patient is potentially a good candidate for venovenous extracorporeal membrane oxygenation (ECMO) for hypoxemic respiratory failure. The basic principles for determining a patient's candidacy for ECMO include lack of response to conventional ventilator management and rescue interventions for severe hypoxemic or hypercarbic respiratory failure, an underlying process that is potentially reversible, and no contraindications to ECMO. The ventilator should be optimized for acute respiratory distress syndrome (ARDS) management, and proning can be employed as a rescue intervention to optimize gas exchange. Chemical paralysis can also be used along with deep sedation, particularly in the setting of ventilator dyssynchrony. If the patient's oxygenation does not improve, ECMO is reasonable so long as his traumatic brain injury is not severe, his intracranial bleeding has stabilized, and there is no ongoing torso hemorrhage. The RESP score calculator can be used to quantify the patient's projected outcome on ECMO (https://www.elso.org/Resources/ECMOOutcome PredictionScores.aspx).

High-frequency oscillatory ventilation requires special expertise and does not offer any clear survival benefit for this patient. Airway pressure release ventilation (APRV) is better suited to awake patients with moderate respiratory failure and ventilator synchrony problems. Rib fracture stabilization should be performed earlier in the hospital course. The patient would not likely benefit from this procedure and also would be unlikely to significantly improve with this intervention. In the absence of abdominal compartment syndrome or refractory intracranial pressure elevation, decompressive laparotomy has no role in the management of this patient.

Answer: C

Brodie D, Bacchetta M. Extracorporeal membrane oxygenation for ARDS in adults. *N Engl J Med.* 2011;365(20):1905–14. doi: https://doi.org/10.1056/NEJMct1103720. PMID: 22087681.

Brodie D, Slutsky AS, Combes A. Extracorporeal life support for adults with respiratory failure and related indications: a review. *JAMA.* 2019;322(6):557–568. doi: https://doi.org/10.1001/jama.2019.9302. PMID: 31408142.

Bullen EC, Teijeiro-Paradis R, Fan E. How i select which patients with ARDS should be treated with venovenous extracorporeal membrane oxygenation. *Chest.* 2020;158(3):1036–1045. doi: https://doi.org/10.1016/j. chest.2020.04.016. Epub 2020 Apr 21. PMID: 32330459.

Cannon JW, Gutsche JT, Brodie D. Optimal strategies for severe acute respiratory distress syndrome. *Crit Care Clin.* 2017;33(2):259–275. doi: https://doi.org/10.1016/j. ccc.2016.12.010. PMID: 28284294.

ELSO Guidelines for Adult Respiratory Failure (2017). Extracorporeal Life Support Organization, Version 1. https://www.elso.org/Portals/0/ELSO%20Guidelines%20 For%20Adult%20Respiratory%20Failure%201_4.pdf (accessed 4 August 2017).

Schmidt M, Bailey M, Sheldrake J, et al. Predicting survival after extracorporeal membrane oxygenation for severe acute respiratory failure. The Respiratory Extracorporeal Membrane Oxygenation Survival Prediction (RESP) score. *Am J Respir Crit Care Med.* 2014;189(11):1374–82. doi: https://doi.org/10.1164/rccm.201311-2023OC. PMID: 24693864.

2 *A 62-year-old man with a history of alcoholic cirrhosis (MELD 18), active alcohol abuse, mild aortic valve insufficiency, type II diabetes, and obesity (BMI = 35) presents to the emergency department with an ST-elevation MI. He is immediately taken to the cardiac catheterization lab for percutaneous coronary intervention; a left anterior descending artery culprit lesion is successfully stented. However, postprocedure, he remains in profound shock on very high doses of intravenous epinephrine, norepinephrine, and vasopressin. Arterial blood pressure is 85/40 mm Hg. A bedside echocardiogram indicates significant left ventricular dysfunction with an ejection fraction of 25%. The cardiologist is requesting veno-arterial (VA) ECMO given the patient's shock state. Which of the following patient characteristics is the strongest contraindication for providing ECMO support?*

A *Age of 62*
B *Morbid obesity (BMI 35)*
C *Mild aortic valve insufficiency*
D *Alcoholic cirrhosis*
E *Immediately post-MI with LV dysfunction*

This patient is a poor candidate for several reasons; however, cirrhosis is the strongest contraindication to this therapy as it portends a poor overall outcome. Chronic end-organ dysfunction with no exit strategy (such as transplant for which this patient is not a candidate given his active alcohol abuse) is an absolute contraindication to ECMO.

Advanced age is a relative contraindication to ECMO, with age of 65 often used as a cutoff in older literature. However, VA ECMO in patients up to 75 years of age has proven safe and effective. Obesity is no longer a contraindication to ECMO, and in select patients it may even be protective. Severe aortic valve insufficiency is a relative contraindication to VA ECMO. Mild aortic valve insufficiency may require venting of the left ventricle with a microaxial pump, atrial septostomy, or LV drainage cannula, but it is not in itself a contraindication to VA ECMO. Cardiogenic shock after myocardial infarction is a reasonable indication for VA ECMO. It may also be considered in other forms of cardiogenic shock, including myocarditis, pulmonary embolism, and postcardiotomy. It may also be used to manage heart failure with a plan to bridge to permanent ventricular assist device placement or transplant.

Answer: D

Yannopoulos D, Bartos J, Raveendran G, et al. Advanced reperfusion strategies for patients with out-of-hospital cardiac arrest and refractory ventricular fibrillation (ARREST): a phase 2, single centre, open-label, randomised controlled trial. *Lancet.* 2020 Nov 12:S0140–6736(20)32338-2. doi: https://doi.org/10.1016/ S0140-6736(20)32338-2. Epub ahead of print. PMID: 33197396.

Lee SN, Jo MS, Yoo KD. Impact of age on extracorporeal membrane oxygenation survival of patients with cardiac failure. *Clin Interv Aging.* 2017 Aug 24;12:1347–1353. doi: https://doi.org/10.2147/CIA.S142994. PMID: 28883715; PMCID: PMC5576703.

Salna M, Chicotka S, Biscotti M III, et al. Morbid obesity is not a contraindication to transport on extracorporeal support. *Eur J Cardiothorac Surg.* 2018;53(4):793–798. doi: https://doi.org/10.1093/ejcts/ezx452. PMID: 29253111.

Makdisi G, Wang IW. Extra Corporeal Membrane Oxygenation (ECMO) review of a lifesaving technology. *J Thorac Dis.* 2015;7(7):E166–76. doi: https://doi. org/10.3978/j.issn.2072-1439.2015.07.17. PMID: 26380745; PMCID: PMC4522501.

3 *A 45-year-old previously healthy man was a pedestrian struck by a motor vehicle resulting in multiple injuries including traumatic brain injury with a subarachnoid hemorrhage (SAH), multiple rib fractures, pulmonary contusion, hemothorax, splenic laceration, and a pelvic fracture. On postinjury day 5, he developed severe hypoxemic respiratory failure (PaO$_2$:FiO$_2$ ratio of 70 on FiO$_2$ of 100%) and was diagnosed with an MRSA pneumonia. Workup for other causes of respiratory failure or sepsis was negative, and there was no evidence of SAH progression or torso hemorrhage on his most recent imaging. His hypoxemic respiratory failure did not improve with proning and neuromuscular* *blockade. What is the optimal ECMO cannulation strategy for this patient?*

A *Femoral venous drainage, carotid arterial reinfusion*

B *Femoral venous drainage, femoral arterial reinfusion*

C *Femoral venous drainage, jugular venous reinfusion*

D *Femoral venous drainage, femoral venous reinfusion*

E *Jugular venous drainage, right atrial reinfusion (dual lumen cannula)*

This patient has no evidence of cardiac failure, so veno-arterial cannulation is unnecessary. This approach increases the potential for an arterial injury or thromboembolic event, will significantly increase the patient's cardiac afterload, and may not provide adequate oxygenation.

The most common cannulation strategy for venovenous ECMO is femoral drainage and jugular reinfusion. A multistage, large-bore venous drainage cannula will adequately support the gas exchange needs for most adult patients (4–6 L/min flow) without risking flow limitations or recirculation that can be a problem with the bilateral femoral-femoral venovenous approach. Single site cannulation with a dual lumen cannula facilitates early ambulation for ECMO patients; it is commonly used for those awaiting a lung transplant.

Answer: C

Cannon JW, Gutsche JT, Brodie D. Optimal strategies for severe acute respiratory distress syndrome. *Crit Care Clin.* 2017;33(2):259–275. doi: https://doi.org/10.1016/j.ccc.2016.12.010. PMID: 28284294.

ELSO Guidelines for Adult Respiratory Failure (2017). Extracorporeal Life Support Organization, Version 1. https://www.elso.org/Portals/0/ELSO%20Guidelines%20For%20Adult%20Respiratory%20Failure%201_4.pdf (accessed 4 August 2017).

ELSO Guidelines for Cardiopulmonary Extracorporeal Life Support (2017). Extracorporeal Life Support Organization, Version 1. https://www.elso.org/Portals/0/ELSO%20Guidelines%20General%20All%20ECLS%20Version%201_4.pdf (accessed 4 August 2017).

4 *A 58-year-old man is on day 2 of veno-arterial ECMO support after an aspiration event led to a cardiac arrest. He is cannulated via his left common femoral vein for drainage and right common femoral artery for reinfusion. He is on a low-dose epinephrine infusion with a blood pressure of 110/60 mm Hg and a normal lactate level. He has no signs of renal, hepatic, or neurologic injury. On transthoracic echocardiography, his left ventricular ejection fraction has improved from 10% on day 1 to 30% on day 2. His left ventricular size appears normal with no obvious valvular abnormalities. He has responded well to furosemide and his fluid*

balance is 3L negative since initiation of ECMO. His pulmonary capillary wedge pressure is 12 mm Hg. His chest x-ray shows bilateral lower lobe infiltrates. However, his upper body peripheral oxygen PaO_2 is 40 mm Hg despite maximal ARDSnet appropriate ventilator settings, while his lower body PaO_2 remains > 200 mm Hg. What is the next best step in his management?

A *Place a left ventricular microaxial percutaneous ventricular assist device for left ventricular venting.*

B *Increase total VA ECMO flows to improve upper body saturation.*

C *Add a second-line inopressor in addition to epinephrine.*

D *Place a venous reinfusion ECMO cannula and convert the patient's configuration to VA-V ECMO.*

E *Perform an atrial septostomy for left ventricular unloading.*

Left ventricular venting is commonly employed in patients supported on peripheral VA ECMO when the native cardiac function is not robust enough to overcome the increased afterload generated by the VA ECMO circuit, which leads to left ventricular distention. This patient shows no signs of left ventricular distention with a normal PCWP, no signs of aortic or mitral insufficiency, and an improving ejection fraction. Performing LV decompression with a septostomy or mechanical device is likely unnecessary in this patient.

There is no evidence of renal or hepatic impairment and cardiac function has improved, making an increase in cardiac output, especially to the lower body (whether increased arterial flow or increased inopressor support), unnecessary. Rather, this patient is likely suffering from severe respiratory failure from aspiration pneumonitis rather than left-sided heart failure and pulmonary edema. While his lower body oxygen delivery is adequate, the oxygen delivery to the coronary and cerebral circulation is likely not, with a PaO_2 of 40 mm Hg. Addition of a venous reinfusion limb to convert to a hybrid VA-V ECMO circuit will provide additional oxygenation support and is the most useful next step.

Answer: D

Russo JJ, Aleksova N, Pitcher I, et al. Left ventricular unloading during extracorporeal membrane oxygenation in patients with cardiogenic shock. *J Am Coll Cardiol.* 2019;73(6):654–662. doi: https://doi.org/10.1016/j.jacc.2018.10.085. PMID: 30765031.

5 *While on venovenous ECMO, which of the following ventilator strategies should be used to provide lung protection and recovery?*

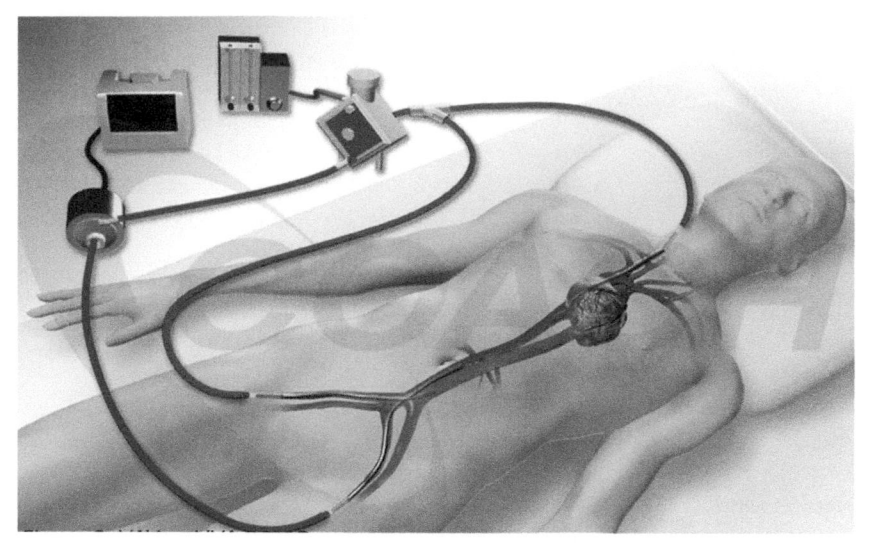

Figure 3.1 VA-V ECMO circuit. *Source:* From Biscotti M., Lee A,, Basner RC., et al. Hybrid configurations via percutaneous access for extracorporeal membrane oxygenation: a single-center experience. *ASAIO J.* 2014;60(6):635–42. with permission.

A *T-piece or tracheostomy collar*
B *High-frequency percussive ventilation*
C *High-frequency oscillatory ventilation*
D *Volume control 8 mL/kg ideal body weight*
E *Pressure control with PEEP of 10 cm H$_2$0*

Lung protective ventilation should continue after ECMO initiation. In fact, so-called ultra-lung protective ventilation is often feasible once the majority of the patient's gas exchange needs are provided by the ECMO circuit. The best current approach is likely reflected in the recently conducted EOLIA trial in which plateau airway pressure was limited to a maximum of 24 cm H$_2$O in conjunction with PEEP > = 10 cm H$_2$O (corresponding to a driving pressure < = 14 cm H$_2$O), respiratory rate of 10–30 breaths/min, and FiO$_2$ of 0.3–0.5. This can be achieved with either a volume control or a pressure control mode, but in our view, a pressure control mode is easier to apply in the setting of very low lung compliance. Often the tidal volumes will be much lower than 4 mL/kg, especially early after ECMO initiation. Furthermore, the respiratory rate should be minimized to further decrease ventilator-induced lung injury.

Early after ECMO initiation, patients may have significant air hunger and may also need moderate-to-deep sedation for a period of time. As a result, spontaneous modes of ventilation are not employed until the patient has shown some signs of stabilization or even recovery. High-frequency percussive ventilation can help with mobilizing secretions, particular in patients with inhalation injury, but this approach is not routinely used in ECMO patients. High-frequency oscillatory ventilation has no proven benefit in this population and may actually cause harm in some cases. Finally, volume control ventilation at this level typically results in extremely high driving pressures, especially early after ECMO initiation.

Answer: E

Abrams D, Schmidt M, Pham T, et al. Mechanical ventilation for acute respiratory distress syndrome during extracorporeal life support. Research and practice. *Am J Respir Crit Care Med.* 2020;201(5):514–525. doi: https://doi.org/10.1164/rccm.201907-1283CI. PMID: 31726013.

Brodie D, Bacchetta M. Extracorporeal membrane oxygenation for ARDS in adults. *N Engl J Med.* 2011;365(20):1905–14. doi: https://doi.org/10.1056/NEJMct1103720. PMID: 22087681.

ELSO Guidelines for Cardiopulmonary Extracorporeal Life Support (2017). Extracorporeal Life Support Organization, Version 1. https://www.elso.org/Portals/0/ELSO%20Guidelines%20For%20Adult%20Respiratory%20Failure%201_4.pdf (accessed 4 August 2017).

6 *A 30-year-old previously healthy man is placed on venovenous (VV) ECMO for severe COVID-19 pneumonia. On ECMO day 5, he is intubated but awake and interactive on minimal sedation. His morning chest x-ray demonstrates a new right-sided pneumothorax. After insertion of a tube thoracostomy, he continues to have a large, continuous air leak on ECMO day 7. His pulmonary compliance remains moderate-to-high, with a tidal volume of 7 mL/kg IBW on a positive end-expiratory pressure (PEEP) of 5, a driving pressure of 10 cm H$_2$O, a fraction of inspired oxygen (FiO$_2$) of 0.5, and a respiratory rate of 20 breaths/min. He remains on ECMO support with a sweep gas flow rate of 6 liters/min.*

His peripheral arterial blood gas shows a pH of 7.36, $PaCO_2$ of 47, and a PaO_2 of 78. What is the best management approach for this patient's mechanical ventilation?

A *Extubate to high flow nasal cannula.*

B *Increase PEEP.*

C *Convert to airway pressure release ventilation (APRV) with a P_{HI} of 30 and P_{LOW} of 0.*

D *Sedate, paralyze, and prone positioning.*

E *Increase tidal volumes.*

This patient has a persistent continuous air leak, which can be exacerbated by continuous positive pressure ventilation. Ventilator strategies to aid in healing of bronchopleural fistulae typically include lowering airway pressures and PEEP. Strategies that include increasing PEEP, tidal volumes, or APRV can lead to higher airway pressures, which may preclude lung healing. In select cases, extubation may be a reasonable strategy, provided the patient can be sufficiently supported without tracheal intubation.

Answer: A

Xia J, Gu S., Li M,s et al. Spontaneous breathing in patients with severe acute respiratory distress syndrome receiving prolonged extracorporeal membrane oxygenation. *BMC Pulm Med.* (2019);**19**:237. https://doi.org/10.1186/s12890-019-1016-2

7 *After initiating venovenous ECMO, which strategy is most likely to minimize bleeding while also preventing clot formation in the circuit or around the cannulas?*

A *Heparin bolus and infusion*

B *Low molecular weight heparin 1.5 mg/kg twice daily*

C *Argatroban infusion*

D *Dual antiplatelet therapy*

E *Withholding systemic anticoagulation for 24 hours*

Blood exposure to the surface of the gas exchange membrane and the circuit activates the intrinsic clotting cascade, the complement system, and platelets. This results in a state of both hyper- and hypo-coagulation. In some cases such as a recent intracranial bleed or solid organ injury, patients on venovenous ECMO may have anticoagulation withheld. However, in most cases, low-dose anticoagulation is used to preserve the gas exchange membrane's efficiency, increase the circuit longevity, and mitigate the risk of thromboembolic complications. Patients on veno-arterial ECMO are generally maintained on higher doses of anticoagulation given the more significant implications of an arterial thromboembolic event.

The most common anticoagulation approach is a heparin bolus upon cannula insertion (50–100 units/kg) followed by a continuous heparin infusion (7.5-20 units/kg/hr). Heparin titration has historically been performed based on activated clotting time (ACT) measured at the bedside (target 180–220 seconds); however, recent evidence suggests that either a PTT-based approach (1.5-2 times baseline) or an anti-Xa approach (0.25 units/mL) may be preferable.

Therapeutic low molecular weight injections are not typically performed on ECMO. Argatroban, a direct thrombin inhibitor, can be used but is generally reserved for patients with a history of, or concern for, HITT. Withholding anticoagulation can be done as described above, and some evidence suggests this may actually be safe for the entirety of a short ECMO run. However, this is not currently a standard approach. Likewise, dual antiplatelet therapy (DAPT) alone is not a standard approach although it may be used in patients with other indications for DAPT, which is more common in patients on veno-arterial ECMO.

Answer: A

ELSO Anticoagulation Guidelines (2017). Extracorporeal Life Support Organization, Version 2014. https://www.elso.org/portals/0/files/elsoanticoagulationguideline8-2014-table-contents.pdf (accessed 30 July 2021).

Kurihara C, Walter JM, Karim A, et al. Feasibility of venovenous extracorporeal membrane oxygenation without systemic anticoagulation. *Ann Thorac Surg.* 2020;110(4):1209–1215. doi: https://doi.org/10.1016/j.athoracsur.2020.02.011. Epub 2020 Mar 12. PMID: 32173339; PMCID: PMC7486253.

Parker RI. Anticoagulation monitoring during extracorporeal membrane oxygenation: continuing progress. *Crit Care Med.* 2020;48(12):1920–1921. doi: https://doi.org/10.1097/CCM.0000000000004635. PMID: 33255117.

Vandenbriele C, Vanassche T, Price S. Why we need safer anticoagulant strategies for patients on short-term percutaneous mechanical circulatory support. *Intensive Care Med.* 2020;46(4):771–774. doi: https://doi.org/10.1007/s00134-019-05897-3. Epub 2020 Jan 23. PMID: 31974917.

8 *Since the inception of ECMO technology in the 1970s, the rates of bleeding and thrombotic complications have decreased significantly, though they remain a significant cause of morbidity and mortality. Which factor is likely the most significant contributor to the observed decrease in bleeding and thrombotic complications over the past several decades?*

A *Novel anticoagulants including direct thrombin inhibitors*

B *Changes in ECMO device technologies*

C *The invention and use of thromboelastography*

D *More accurate assays for activated clotting time and activated partial thromboplastin time*

E *Discovery of modern-day antiplatelet therapy*

The use of novel anticoagulants and antiplatelet therapies in ECMO has been described but has not been studied sufficiently to make any recommendations for or against their use.

Use of TEG and ACT monitors, as well as protocols targeting low or high PTT goals, is often implemented; however, current evidence is insufficient to recommend one specific approach over the others. The improvements in ECMO circuit technology and heparin-coated cannulas have likely led to a decrease in total dose and duration of anticoagulation required and an improvement in circuit-related hemorrhagic or thrombotic complications.

Answer: B

Sklar MC, Sy E, Lequier L, et al. Anticoagulation practices during venovenous extracorporeal membrane oxygenation for respiratory failure. A systematic review. *Ann Am Thorac Soc.* 2016;13(12):2242–2250. doi: https://doi.org/10.1513/AnnalsATS.201605-364SR. PMID: 27690525.

9 *Acute kidney injury (AKI) is a common problem in patients requiring ECMO therapy. As such, the use of renal replacement therapy (RRT) is necessary in 40–60% of cases. Which of the following statements regarding use of RRT and ECMO is most accurate?*

A *RRT access should never be provided via an in-line approach with ECMO circuits. It should always be provided via separate vascular access.*

B *Fluid overload is an uncommon problem in the pediatric ECMO population and has no significant effect on morbidity and mortality.*

C *Uremia and electrolyte derangements are the most common indications for RRT initiation in both children and adults on ECMO.*

D *The polymethylpentene oxygenator used in ECMO circuits can also be used as a hemofilter to deliver RRT in patients with concomitant AKI.*

E *Negative fluid balance on RRT is independently associated with improved outcomes for both the adult and pediatric ECMO population.*

The most common indication for RRT in both adult and pediatric ECMO patients is fluid overload. Specifically, in the pediatric population, fluid overload is associated with increased mortality and longer duration of ECMO support. Further, several studies have associated a net negative fluid balance while on RRT with improved patient outcomes.

It is safe and feasible to provide RRT via either separate vascular access or direct integration into the ECMO circuit, depending on patient-specific circumstances. However, the polymethylpentene oxygenator will provide gas exchange but will not function as a hemofilter to provide RRT.

Answer: E

Ostermann M, Connor M Jr, Kashani K. Continuous renal replacement therapy during extracorporeal membrane oxygenation: why, when and how? *Curr Opin Crit Care.* 2018;24(6):493–503. doi: https://doi.org/10.1097/MCC.0000000000000559. PMID: 30325343.

Gorga SM, Sahay RD, Askenazi DJ, et al. Fluid overload and fluid removal in pediatric patients on extracorporeal membrane oxygenation requiring continuous renal replacement therapy: a multicenter retrospective cohort study. *Pediatr Nephrol.* 2020;35(5):871–882. doi: https://doi.org/10.1007/s00467-019-04468-4. Epub 2020 Jan 17. PMID: 31953749; PMCID: PMC7517652.

Dado DN, Ainsworth CR, Thomas SB, et al. Outcomes among patients treated with renal replacement therapy during extracorporeal membrane oxygenation: a single-center retrospective study. Blood Purif. 2020;49(3):341–347. doi: https://doi.org/10.1159/000504287. Epub 2019 Dec 19. PMID: 31865351; PMCID: PMC7212702.

10 *A 40-year-old man is placed on venovenous (VV) ECMO via a 25 Fr right femoral vein drainage cannula and a 17 Fr right internal jugular vein reinfusion cannula for refractory ARDS secondary to aspiration pneumonitis. He is 6' 2" tall and weighs 240 lbs (BMI 30.8 kg/m^2, BSA 2.35 m^2). His initial circuit flow is 5.0 L/min at an RPM of 4000 and drainage pressure of −120 cm H$_2$O; the ECMO specialist is unable to flow > 5.0 L/min because of excessively high drainage pressures (chatter) in the line. Over the next 48 hours, his SpO$_2$ remains at 70% on maximal ventilator settings with a hemoglobin of 14 g/dL; no signs of untreated sepsis, infection, or shock; normal biventricular function on echocardiogram, and a persistently elevated lactate. His circuit flows remain the same and the oxygenator health is excellent. What is the next most appropriate step?*

A *Consider adding an additional arterial reinfusion limb to provide increased ECMO support.*

B *Consider adding a 21 Fr venous reinfusion limb to provide increased ECMO support.*

C *Transfuse the patient to a supranormal hemoglobin to improve oxygen delivery.*

D *Begin aggressive intravenous fluid resuscitation to improve circuit venous drainage.*

E *Consider adding an additional drainage cannula to increase overall ECMO flows.*

Inadequate ECMO flows is a common problem, and because of fluid dynamics, venous drainage (access) insufficiency is typically the limiting factor rather than reinfusion cannula size. Venous drainage pressures more negative than −100 mm Hg are typically associated with "chatter" in the lines and, therefore, flow limitations. Conversely, flow is often not limited by reinfusion pressures until the reinfusion line pressure is > 300–400 mm Hg. In patients with drainage insufficiency, the addition of a venous or arterial reinfusion limb will not increase ECMO flows and will not provide any additional benefit.

Some ECMO physicians advocate for transfusions to normal hemoglobin levels, instead of using typical ICU transfusion practices with a transfusion threshold of 7 or 8 g/dL. However, supplementing the patient's already normal hemoglobin (14 g/dL) is unlikely to add additional benefit. Additionally, patients with severe ARDS typically benefit from volume removal rather than volume expansion. While fluid boluses may temporarily improve flows by improving venous drainage, this is not an effective long-term solution.

In patients with a large body size, they may require higher than typical ECMO flows, and addition of an extra drainage cannula via the contralateral femoral vein may improve total circuit flow capacity, which will mitigate the hypoxemia and resultant tissue hypoxia.

Answer: E

Dado DN, Ainsworth CR, Thomas SB, et al. Outcomes among patients treated with renal replacement therapy during extracorporeal membrane oxygenation: a single-center retrospective study. *Blood Purif.* 2020;49(3):341–347. doi: https://doi.org/10.1159/000504287. Epub 2019 Dec 19. PMID: 31865351; PMCID: PMC7212702.

11 *A 55-year-old man is emergently placed on femoral-femoral veno-arterial (VA) ECMO for a cardiac arrest caused by an acute MI. The culprit coronary lesion was stented in the cardiac catheterization lab, and he was taken to the ICU to recover. On hospital day 1, his post-oxygenator PaO$_2$ is 400 mm Hg and radial arterial PaO$_2$ is also 400 mm Hg. Transthoracic echocardiogram demonstrates a left ventricular ejection fraction of 10%. He remains intubated with a positive end-expiratory pressure (PEEP) of 5 cm H$_2$O and a fraction of inspired oxygen (FiO$_2$) of 40%. On hospital day 3, with the same ventilator settings, his right radial arterial line demonstrates a PaO$_2$ of 150 mm Hg and his post-oxygenator blood gas PaO$_2$ remains at 400 mm Hg. His lactate levels remain normal. The total ECMO flows have decreased by 0.5 L/min with the same device RPMs. What is the most likely explanation for this finding?*
    A *The oxygenator efficiency has decreased.*
    B *There is inadequate oxygen delivery to the tissue resulting in tissue hypoxia.*
    C *The patient now has severe ARDS.*
    D *The patient's heart and left ventricular ejection fraction are beginning to recover.*
    E *The right radial blood gas is likely venous.*

As the cardiac function improves in patients on peripheral VA ECMO, the native cardiac output will compete with retrograde aortic ECMO flow, thereby "pushing" left ventricular blood further across the aortic arch. This phenomenon of moving the mixing point more distally into the aortic arch demonstrates the "Harlequin syndrome" that is often seen with femoral-femoral veno-arterial ECMO. A sample of arterial blood from a right radial arterial line may demonstrate a more "normal" PaO$_2$ rather than the supranormal PaO$_2$ that is indicative of ECMO circuit blood, and this is often a sign that the cardiac function is beginning to recover. Because most modern ECMO circuits utilize an afterload-sensitive centrifugal pump, total VA ECMO flows will often decrease as cardiac function improves and the circuit afterload increases.

A high post-oxygenator PaO$_2$ suggests adequate and unchanged oxygenator function, and so long as end-organ perfusion remains normal, it is unlikely that tissue hypoxia is occurring.

A PaO$_2$:FiO$_2$ ratio > 300 does not meet clinical criteria for severe ARDS, and a PaO$_2$ > 100 mm Hg is unlikely to be from a venous blood sample.

Answer: D

Eckman PM, Katz JN, El Banayosy A, et al. Veno-Arterial extracorporeal membrane oxygenation for cardiogenic shock: an introduction for the busy clinician. *Circulation.* 2019;140(24):2019–2037. doi: https://doi.org/10.1161/CIRCULATIONAHA.119.034512. Epub 2019 Dec 9. PMID: 31815538.

12 *Which of the following sites of hemorrhage is most common during ECMO support?*
    A *Intracranial*
    B *Cannula site*
    C *Solid organ*
    D *Gastrointestinal*
    E *Pulmonary*

Bleeding complications occur in approximately 24% of ECMO patients. The ELSO registry records these complications. Participation in this registry is voluntary;

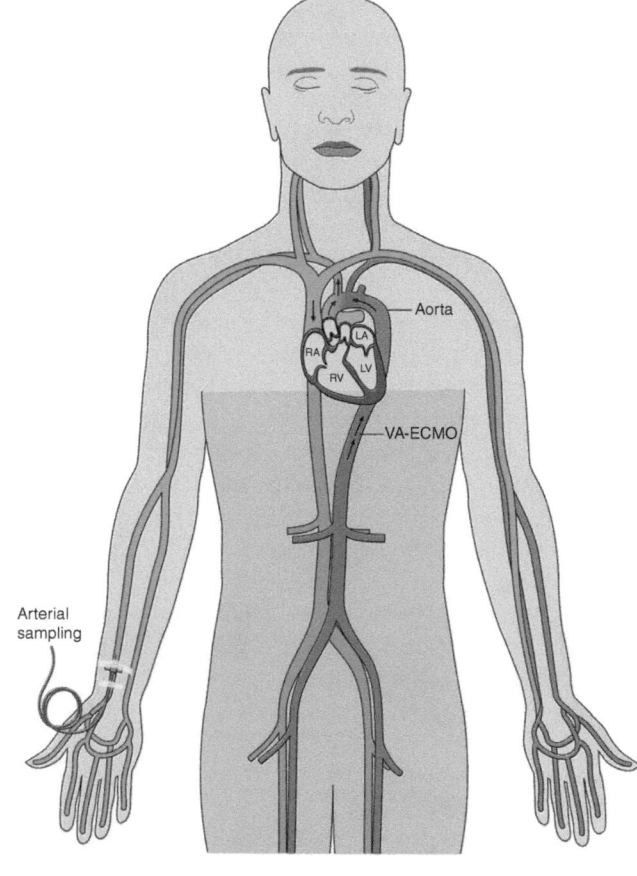

Figure 3.2 Harlequin syndrome. *Source:* From Eckman PM, Katz JN, El Banayosy A, et al. Veno-arterial extracorporeal membrane oxygenation for cardiogenic shock: an introduction for the busy clinician. *Circulation.* 2019;140(24):2019–2037, with permission.

however, in some instances, the exposure may not be 100% of patients resulting in an under-representation of certain types of bleeding complications (e.g. the percentage of surgical site bleeding may be artificially lowered by including nonsurgical patients in the denominator). However, it appears that cannula site hemorrhage is the most common bleeding complication (8%) followed by surgical site bleeding (7%), gastrointestinal bleeding (6%), pulmonary hemorrhage (4%), and central nervous system bleeding (3%).

Strategies for managing cannula site bleeding include prevention by under-sizing the insertion site incision for cannula insertion, application of topical hemostatics around the cannula site, placement of purse string sutures around the insertion site, or lowering the anticoagulation target.

Answer: B

Brodie D, Slutsky AS, Combes A. Extracorporeal life support for adults with respiratory failure and related indications: a review. *JAMA.* 2019;322(6):557–568. doi:

https://doi.org/10.1001/jama.2019.9302. PMID: 31408142.

13 *General and trauma surgeons are often called upon to consult on ECMO patients. Which statement about surgical procedures for ECMO patients is most accurate?*

   A *Intra-abdominal operations should not be performed on ECMO patients, as intraoperative mortality typically exceeds 50%.*

   B *Tracheostomy can be performed safely and effectively on ECMO patients.*

   C *The use of antifibrinolytic agents (such as aminocaproic acid or tranexamic acid) for mitigating bleeding in ECMO patients has not been described.*

   D *Interruption of anticoagulation for any period of time will result in immediate catastrophic circuit failure.*

   E *Caesarean section is absolutely contraindicated during ECMO support.*

Noncardiac surgical procedures on ECMO patients are common and are required in as many as 50% of patients. Most studies have not demonstrated increased mortality among patients who underwent surgical procedures. Use of ECMO in pregnancy is also well described with Caesarean sections successfully performed in patients on ECMO.

One of the most common procedures performed on ECMO patients is tracheostomy, and many reviews have demonstrated safety and efficacy of tracheostomy on ECMO patients. In fact, tracheostomy may decrease sedation requirements and decrease time on ECMO. Bleeding is still a risk; however, it is our approach to use electrocautery on the skin and soft tissue down to the trachea, turning the ventilator $FiO_2 < 60\%$ and then proceeding with a percutaneous tracheostomy technique.

Additionally, in many centers, antifibrinolytic medications are used prophylactically during surgical procedures or to treat bleeding complications in ECMO patients, and it is unlikely that short-term interruption of anticoagulation infusions will cause circuit failure.

Answer: B

Juthani BK, Macfarlan J, Wu J, et al. Incidence of general surgical procedures in adult patients on extracorporeal membrane oxygenation. *J Intensive Care Soc.* 2019 May;20(2):155–160. doi: https://doi.org/10.1177/1751143718801705. Epub 2018 Oct 2. PMID: 31037108; PMCID: PMC6475990.

Salna M, Tipograf Y, Liou P, et al. Tracheostomy is safe during extracorporeal membrane oxygenation support. *ASAIO J.* 2020;66(6):652–656. doi: https://doi.org/10.1097/MAT.0000000000001059. PMID: 31425269.

Buckley LF, Reardon DP, Camp PC, et al. Aminocaproic acid for the management of bleeding in patients on extracorporeal membrane oxygenation: four adult case reports and a review of the literature. *Heart Lung.* 2016;45(3):232–6. doi: https://doi.org/10.1016/j.hrtlng.2016.01.011. Epub 2016 Feb 20. PMID: 26907195.

Agerstrand C, Abrams D, Biscotti M, et al. Extracorporeal membrane oxygenation for cardiopulmonary failure during pregnancy and postpartum. *Ann Thorac Surg.* 2016;102(3):774–779. doi: https://doi.org/10.1016/j.athoracsur.2016.03.005. Epub 2016 May 4. PMID: 27154158.

14 *A 45-year-old woman is placed on femoral-femoral veno-arterial ECMO via a 25 Fr venous cannula in the left femoral vein and a 17 Fr arterial cannula in the right femoral artery. Six hours after cannulation, the patient remains on moderate-dose inopressors and is well supported with an ECMO flow of 3.5 L/min. The bedside nurse notices mottling of the right foot. What is the most likely etiology and reasonable next step?*

   A *The patient has a right femoral DVT and is developing phlegmasia cerulea dolens. She requires a venous thrombolysis procedure.*

   B *The patient has decreased cardiac output and requires an increase in inopressors.*

   C *The arterial reinfusion cannula has thrombosed and must be replaced immediately.*

   D *The arterial cannula is causing distal limb ischemia. A distal perfusion catheter should be placed emergently.*

   E *The patient has an ischemic foot and a below-the-knee amputation should be performed.*

The incidence of distal limb ischemia is 10–70% in peripheral VA ECMO patients. It is associated with an increased risk of morbidity and mortality. It must be recognized and treated urgently by placement of a distal perfusion catheter/cannula. If not recognized promptly, amputation may be required; however, reperfusion to the ischemic limb should be attempted prior to any consideration for amputation.

It is possible to have a DVT leading to phlegmasia in ECMO patients; however, it is more likely to occur in the leg with the venous cannula and unlikely immediately after cannulation.

It is unlikely that decreases in cardiac output or insufficient/absent ECMO flows would result in localized ischemia.

Answer: D

Bonicolini E, Martucci G, Simons J, et al. Limb ischemia in peripheral veno-arterial extracorporeal membrane oxygenation: a narrative review of incidence, prevention, monitoring, and treatment. *Crit Care.* 2019;23(1):266. doi: https://doi.org/10.1186/s13054-019-2541-3. PMID: 31362770; PMCID: PMC6668078.

15 *A 40-year-old man with severe influenza-induced ARDS is placed on venovenous ECMO via left and right common femoral veins. He requires ECMO for 12 days, and throughout his course is maintained on a continuous heparin infusion with an average activated partial thromboplastin time (aPTT) of 60 seconds. He is successfully decannulated after improvement in lung function, and then maintained on a continuous heparin infusion for 48 hours after decannulation. Two days after decannulation the patient has sudden-onset tachycardia, hypoxemia, and hypotension. There is no change in the physical exam, respiratory mechanics, or chest x-ray. What is the next most appropriate step?*

   A *Discontinue heparin as the patient may be bleeding from the cannulation sites.*

   B *Perform a transthoracic echocardiogram and consider CT chest to evaluate for a pulmonary embolism.*

   C *Place bilateral chest tubes.*

   D *Make the patient DNR after a family meeting.*

   E *Perform an emergent bronchoscopy.*

Venous thromboembolism is a very common complication after venovenous ECMO. It occurs in 30–50% of patients after decannulation, even despite appropriate anticoagulation. Pulmonary embolism should be high on every clinicians' differential diagnosis and should be ruled out and must be suspected and potentially treated.

Other causes of respiratory failure to include pneumothorax, worsening lung function, or mucous plugging are also common in patients recovering from severe lung disease and must be ruled out as well with physical exam, observation of respiratory mechanics, and chest x-ray.

Goals of care discussions are always valuable in the management of critically ill patients; however, in the young, recovering patient, a family meeting to address DNR status is probably premature.

Answer: B

Trudzinski FC, Minko P, Rapp D, et al. Runtime and aPTT predict venous thrombosis and thromboembolism in patients on extracorporeal membrane oxygenation: a retrospective analysis. *Ann Intensive Care.* 2016;6(1):66. doi: https://doi.org/10.1186/s13613-016-0172-2. Epub 2016 Jul 19. PMID: 27432243; PMCID: PMC4949188.

16 *Which of the following is the strongest clinical indication to discontinue ECMO support?*

   A *A patient is intubated for 16 days and requires a tracheostomy procedure.*

   B *Arterial blood gas demonstrates a pH of 7.36 and a $PaCO_2$ of 55 mm Hg on a sweep gas flow of 4 L/min.*

C *The patient has been on ECMO for 2 weeks.*

D *The patient is oozing blood from a left chest tube site and right femoral cannulation site.*

E *The patient has an SpO$_2$ of 96% and arterial PaCO$_2$ of 40 mm Hg on 0 L/min of VV ECMO sweep gas flow and low ventilator settings.*

As a rule of thumb, when extracorporeal support provides less than 30% of native cardiac or lung function, a trial off ECMO is indicated. If SpO$_2$ > 95%, and arterial PaCO$_2$ is < 50 mm Hg for > 60 min off of sweep flow, decannulation from VV ECMO is reasonable. Patients with an elevated PaCO$_2$ despite moderate sweep gas flow are likely not ready for a trial off ECMO.

The need for a surgical procedure alone is not an indication for decannulation. In some cases, ECMO is indicated to provide additional support to patients undergoing high-risk surgical procedures (such as complex airway or tracheal reconstructions or resections of anterior mediastinal masses). Additionally, prolonged duration of ECMO support should not be an isolated reason for decannulation.

A small amount of oozing from surgical sites is not uncommon in ECMO patients. Premature decannulation may be considered only in rare cases of uncontrollable bleeding.

Answer: E

ELSO Guidelines for Cardiopulmonary Extracorporeal Life Support (2017). Extracorporeal Life Support Organization, Version 1. Ann Arbor, MI, USA. www. elso.org (accessed 4 August 2017).

17 *A 35-year-old woman suffering from COVID-19 is decannulated from venovenous (VV) ECMO after 12 days. She remains on the ventilator and in the ECMO ICU. The family is asking what they can expect for her post-ECMO course. Which statement is most accurate?*

A *Approximately 40% of patients who are decannulated from ECMO will ultimately die in the hospital.*

B *She will require more sedation and higher ventilator settings in the coming days.*

C *Approximately 40% of patients will suffer from a DVT post-ECMO decannulation.*

D *Prior ECMO cannulation is a contraindication to future ECMO cannulation.*

E *Physical therapy is contraindicated in the week post-ECMO for fear of cannula site bleeding.*

The survival-to-discharge for all-comers in respiratory failure ECMO is approximately 60%, though this rate continues to improve year-to-year with improvements in ICU care and device technology; while the survival-to-discharge for cardiac failure ECMO is approximately 53%. Though data is limited and premature, the survival-to-discharge of ECMO patients with COVID-19 is 54%. While these survival rates are all encompassing and have been gathered over several decades, there are several prediction tools to attempt to elucidate anticipated survival for the individual patient; one of which is the RESP score. This model uses data points including age, duration of mechanical ventilation, immunocompromised status, among several other patient-specific data points.

Except in cases of severe device-related complications, patients decannulated from ECMO should be adequately and safely maintained on an amount of support that allows for expedient recovery, re-conditioning, and physical therapy. If it is anticipated that a patient requires neuromuscular blockade, increased sedation, and increased ventilator settings, then they should not be decannulated. The in-hospital mortality after ECMO decannulation is approximately 10%. In select cases, patients who were decannulated from ECMO may require a second ECMO run, and this is within reason.

Approximately 30–50% of patients decannulated from VV ECMO will suffer from a DVT, and screening for DVT is typically performed 48–72 hours post-ECMO decannulation.

Answer: C

ELSO Guidelines for Cardiopulmonary Extracorporeal Life Support (2017). Extracorporeal Life Support Organization, Version 1. Ann Arbor, MI, USA. www. elso.org (accessed 4 August 2017).

Trudzinski FC, Minko P, Rapp D, et al. Runtime and aPTT predict venous thrombosis and thromboembolism in patients on extracorporeal membrane oxygenation: a retrospective analysis. *Ann Intensive Care.* 2016;6(1):66. doi: https://doi.org/10.1186/s13613-016-0172-2. Epub 2016 Jul 19. PMID: 27432243; PMCID: PMC4949188.

Schmidt M, Bailey M, Sheldrake J, et al. Predicting survival after extracorporeal membrane oxygenation for severe acute respiratory failure. The Respiratory Extracorporeal Membrane Oxygenation Survival Prediction (RESP) score. *Am J Respir Crit Care Med.* 2014;189(11):1374–82.

18 *A 6-year-old previously healthy girl is admitted to the PICU after being involved in a house fire resulting in acute respiratory distress with severe hypoxemic respiratory failure. Which of the following would indicate a need for venovenous ECMO in this patient?*

A *PaO$_2$/FiO$_2$ > 100–150*

B *Oxygenation index (OI) > 40*

C *Mean airway pressure > 15 cmH$_2$O on high-frequency oscillatory ventilation*

D *Mean airway pressure > 15 cmH$_2$O on conventional ventilation*

E *Carboxyhemoglobin level of 10%*

When evaluating a patient's candidacy for extracorporeal support, the provider must consider the underlying pathology, the adequacy of gas exchange given the current mechanical ventilatory requirement, and the success/failure of adjunctive rescue therapies. Although significant variability in institutional protocols exists, salvage therapies for children on a conventional ventilator with mean airway pressure (MAP) > 20–25 cm H$_2$O includes use of high-frequency oscillatory ventilation (HFOV), nitric oxide, and prone positioning. MAP < 30 cm H$_2$O are tolerable while on HFOV. The PaO$_2$/FiO$_2$ is the ratio of arterial oxygen partial pressure to fractional inspired oxygen and is a clinical indicator of hypoxemia (normal PaO$_2$/FiO$_2$ > 300). An alternative measure of oxygenation is the oxygenation index (OI), which is calculated as the reciprocal of the PaO$_2$/FiO$_2$ times 100 times the mean airway pressure:

$$OI = \frac{1}{\left(\dfrac{PaO_2}{FiO_2}\right)} \times 100 \times MAP$$

$$OI = \frac{FiO_2}{PaO_2} \times 100 \times MAP$$

Severe respiratory failure as evidence by a sustained PaO$_2$/FiO$_2$ < 60–80 or OI > 40 predict high mortality and indicate a need for lung rescue with ECMO. For example, if the patient's PaO$_2$ were 60 mm Hg on an FiO$_2$ of 1 and MAP of 30 cm H$_2$O, the OI would be 50, which is a strong indication for ECMO initiation in the pediatric population.

Answer: B

Maratta C, Potera RM, van Leeuwen G, et al. Extracorporeal Life Support Organization (ELSO): 2020 pediatric respiratory ELSO guideline. *ASAIO J Am Soc Artif Intern Organs 1992*. 2020;66(9):975–979. doi: https://doi.org/10.1097/MAT.0000000000001223

Zabrocki LA, Brogan TV, Statler KD, et al. Extracorporeal membrane oxygenation for pediatric respiratory failure: survival and predictors of mortality. *Crit Care Med*. 2011;39(2):364–370. doi: https://doi.org/10.1097/CCM.0b013e3181fb7b35

19 *A newborn male infant with a fetal diagnosis of congenital diaphragmatic hernia (CDH) is admitted to the neonatal intensive care unit immediately after delivery where he is found to be acidotic (pH = 7.1)*

and hypoxemic (PaO$_2$ = 42 mm Hg). He is transitioned from a conventional ventilator to the high-frequency oscillatory ventilator. However, this results in minimal improvement in gas exchange with worsening metabolic acidosis and a rising lactate on escalating vasopressor support. What is the most appropriate ECMO cannulation strategy for this neonate?

A *Right femoral venous drainage, left femoral artery reinfusion*

B *Right femoral venous drainage, umbilical vein reinfusion*

C *Right femoral venous drainage, right carotid artery reinfusion*

D *Right internal jugular vein drainage, right carotid artery reinfusion*

E *Right internal jugular vein drainage and reinfusion with double-lumen bicaval catheter*

Extracorporeal support for VA ECMO requires veno-arterial access. In most situations, specific cannula selection occurs after surgical cut down with direct visual interrogation of the vessels of interest. Although some centers have started to implement percutaneous cannulation using Seldinger technique, this is best suited for femoral access that is inappropriate for children < 15 kg because of the size of the femoral vessels (answers A and C are therefore incorrect). Venous drainage via cannulation of the right internal jugular vein and reinfusion via the right common carotid artery is the standard approach for children < 15 kg (answer D). Right femoral venous drainage and umbilical vein reinfusion is not described as a mode of ECMO support. An umbilical vein catheter (UVC) can be used for infusions on a short-term basis but has not been described for ECMO support (answer B). Finally, right internal jugular venous drainage and reinfusion with a double-lumen bicaval catheter can be used for VV ECMO but is inappropriate to support the child necessitating both pulmonary and cardiac support (answer E).

Answer: D

Johnson K, Jarboe MD, Mychaliska GB, et al. Is there a best approach for extracorporeal life support cannulation: a review of the extracorporeal life support organization. *J Pediatr Surg*. 2018;53(7):1301–1304. doi:https://doi.org/10.1016/j.jpedsurg.2018.01.015

Wild KT, Rintoul N, Kattan J, et al. Extracorporeal Life Support Organization (ELSO): guidelines for neonatal respiratory failure. *ASAIO J Am Soc Artif Intern Organs 1992*. 2020;66(5):463–470. doi:https://doi.org/10.1097/MAT.0000000000001153

20 *Monitoring of which of the following anticoagulation assays is independently associated with prolonged circuit life in children on ECMO support?*

A *Fibrinogen*
B *Anti-factor Xa*
C *PTT*
D *ACT*
E *Platelets*

Anticoagulation is a critical component of ECMO management given the procoagulant properties of the ELCS circuit. Although clots in the circuit are the most common mechanical complications of ECMO, continuous anticoagulation with heparin or a direct thrombin inhibitor confers significant bleeding risk, the most catastrophic of which is intraventricular hemorrhage. In order to mitigate clotting and bleeding, anticoagulation monitoring is critical. Plasma anti-factor Xa (Anti-Xa) measures the anticoagulant impact of the heparin-AT3 complex. Higher anti-Xa levels have been independently associated with decreased circuit change due to clot formation in children on ECMO (answer B). In addition, monitoring protocols that include anti-Xa, thromboelastography, and antithrombin levels are associated with decreased blood product use, decreased hemorrhagic complications, and increased circuit duration when compared to standard monitoring protocols including only ACT, platelet count, protime/international normalized ratio (INR), and hemoglobin/hematocrit. Although fibrinogen, PTT, ACT, and platelets provide important information to inform anticoagulation management, all are poorly correlated with circuit thrombosis in children on ECMO.

Answer: B

Irby K, Swearingen C, Byrnes J, et al. Unfractionated heparin activity measured by anti-factor Xa levels is associated with the need for ECMO circuit/membrane oxygenator change: a retrospective pediatric study. *Pediatr Crit Care Med J Soc Crit Care Med World Fed Pediatr Intensive Crit Care Soc.* 2014;15(4):e175–e182. doi:https://doi.org/10.1097/PCC.0000000000000101

Northrop MS, Sidonio RF, Phillips SEM, et al. The use of an extracorporeal membrane oxygenation anticoagulation laboratory protocol is associated with decreased blood product use, decreased hemorrhagic complications, and increased circuit life. *Pediatr Crit Care Med.* 2015;16(1):66–74. doi:https://doi.org/10.1097/PCC.0000000000000278

21 *Which of the following parameters is evidence of myocardial recovery and thus a proxy of readiness for decannulation in a child supported on VA-ECMO for myocarditis?*
   A *Decreasing pulse pressure*
   B *Increasing systolic pressure*
   C *Left ventricular ejection fraction < 25% under low-flow conditions*
   D *Escalating requirement of ECMO sweep gas flow rate*
   E *Rising end-tidal CO_2 in children with systemic-to-pulmonary shunt*

Scant empirical data exists regarding the use of specific parameters to predict the readiness for decannulation of a child managed on ECMO. Moreover, although weaning protocols exist (i.e. wean ECMO flow to 100 mL/min and increasing ventilator support from rest to baseline settings), there is little data to support the appropriateness of one unit-based protocol over another. Data suggests that increased systolic pressure as well as increased pulse pressure and echocardiographic evidence of left ventricular ejection fraction > 25% are indicators of myocardial recovery. Escalating requirement of ECMO sweep gas flow rate implies increasing support requirements and would not be an evidence of myocardial recovery. Although a rising end-tidal CO_2 in children without systemic-to-pulmonary shunt can be a helpful parameter for prediction of successful wean, the presence of a systemic-to-pulmonary shunt would increase CO_2-rich blood passing through the lungs, thus confounding the measurement of $ETCO_2$.

Answer: B

Aissaoui N, Luyt C-E, Leprince P, et al. Predictors of successful extracorporeal membrane oxygenation (ECMO) weaning after assistance for refractory cardiogenic shock. *Intensive Care Med.* 2011;37(11):1738. doi: https://doi.org/10.1007/s00134-011-2358-2

Naruke T, Inomata T, Imai H, et al. End-Tidal carbon dioxide concentration can estimate the appropriate timing for weaning off from extracorporeal membrane oxygenation for refractory circulatory failure. *Int Heart J.* 2010;51(2):116–120. doi: https://doi.org/10.1536/ihj.51.116

Park B-W, Seo D-C, Moon I-K, et al. Pulse pressure as a prognostic marker in patients receiving extracorporeal life support. *Resuscitation.* 2013;84(10):1404–1408. doi: https://doi.org/10.1016/j.resuscitation.2013.04.009.

22 *Which of the following conditions is associated with the lowest ECMO-associated survival in neonates?*
   A *Bacterial pneumonia*
   B *Congenital heart disease*
   C *Meconium aspiration*
   D *Persistent pulmonary hypertension of the newborn*
   E *Persistent pulmonary hypertension of the newborn with hypoxic-ischemic encephalopathy*

Overall survival to hospital discharge is 73% for patients treated with ECMO for neonatal respiratory disease, approximately 35–45% for congenital heart disease, and 40–50% where ECMO is used for extracorporeal cardiopulmonary resuscitation. Persistent pulmonary hypertension of the newborn (PPHN) occurs secondary to infectious etiologies (pneumonia or sepsis), congenital disease (premature closure of the ductus or congenital diaphragmatic hernia), or genetic abnormalities (surfactant protein B deficiency) and results in pathologic vasoconstriction with resultant severe hypoxemia (with or without hypercapnia). ECMO survival for PPHN is approximately 80% even in the presence of hypoxemic-ischemic encephalopathy. Meconium increases the antibacterial milieu of amniotic fluid and predisposes to perinatal infection. Meconium aspiration syndrome (MAS) can also result in airway obstruction and/or a chemical pneumonitis with subsequent hypoxia. Although improvements in postnatal care and neonatal respiratory support have decreased the use of ECMO for management of MAS, survival for neonates cannulated for this indication remain high at 92%. Pneumonia is most commonly caused by group B beta-hemolytic Streptococcus or gram-negative organisms and is associated with a 60% ECMO survival. A number of prediction tools have been developed to assist with ECMO protocol development and clinical decision-making.

(https://www.elso.org/Resources/ECMOOutcome PredictionScores.aspx).

Answer: B

Agarwal P, Altinok D, Desai J, et al. In-hospital outcomes of neonates with hypoxic-ischemic encephalopathy receiving extracorporeal membrane oxygenation. *J Perinatol.* 2019;39(5):661–665. doi: https://doi.org/10.1038/s41372-019-0345-6

Allen KY, Allan CK, Su L, et al. Extracorporeal membrane oxygenation in congenital heart disease. *Semin Perinatol.* 2018;42(2):104–110. doi: https://doi.org/10.1053/j.semperi.2017.12.006

International Summary of the ELSO Registry Report (2017). Extracorporeal Life Support Organization (ELSO). Ann Arbor, Michigan: 2017. Published by ELSO online at www.ELSO.org

Lazar DA, Cass DL, Olutoye OO, et al. The use of ECMO for persistent pulmonary hypertension of the newborn: a decade of experience. *J Surg Res.* 2012;177(2):263–7. doi: https://doi.org/10.1016/j.jss.2012.07.058.

4

Arrhythmias, Acute Coronary Syndromes, and Hypertensive Emergencies

Ryan Malcom, MD

Division of Trauma and Acute Care Surgery, New York Medical College, Westchester Medical Center, Valhalla, NY, USA

1 *A 62-year-old woman with a smoking history was hospitalized with a bleeding duodenal ulcer. She has been managed nonoperatively thus far. On hospital day 2, she complains of chest pain and dyspnea. She is administered oxygen, nitroglycerin, and morphine. CBC, coagulation studies, and cardiac marker levels are drawn. The following is seen on a 12 lead EKG:*

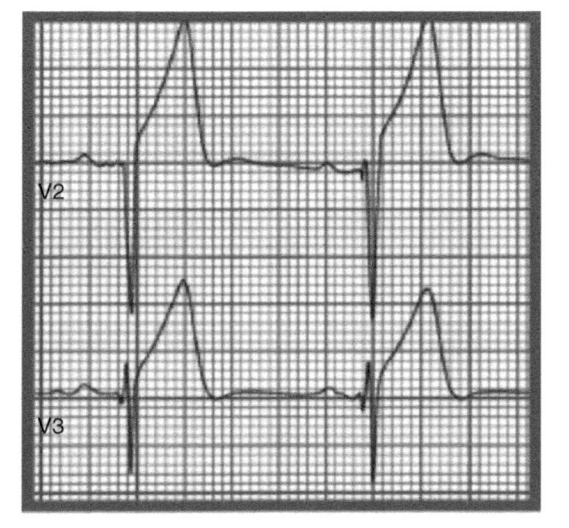

Figure 4.1 EKG.

The next best step in the treatment of this patient is:

    A *Immediate transfer to the catheterization laboratory*
    B *Administration of aspirin*
    C *Obtain chest x-ray*
    D *Fibrinolysis*
    E *Administration of ibuprofen*

The 12 lead EKG is central to the identification of ST-segment elevation myocardial infarction (STEMI). Elevated ST-segment elevation in two contiguous leads, or a new left bundle branch block (LBBB), characterizes STEMI. This patient has a STEMI. Usually, patients with STEMI have a complete occlusion of an epicardial coronary artery. To save heart muscle and reduce complications of myocardial infarction (MI), urgent treatment is required. The treatment of STEMI is early reperfusion therapy via either fibrinolysis or percutaneous coronary intervention (PCI). PCI is preferred if a catheterization laboratory is immediately available, otherwise fibrinolysis should be initiated. Transport to the catheterization laboratory should not be delayed for a CXR or cardiac marker lab results. This patient has a GI bleed, and therefore, fibrinolysis and aspirin are contraindicated. Nonsteroidal anti-inflammatory drugs (i.e. ibuprofen), excluding aspirin, are contraindicated because of increased risk of mortality with STEMI.

Answer: A

Antman EM, Anbe DT, Armstrong PW, et al. ACC/AHA guidelines for the management of patients with ST-elevation myocardial infarction. *J Am Coll Cardiol.* 2013;61:485–510.

Antman EM, Anbe DT, Armstrong PW, et al. ACC/AHA guidelines for the management of patients with ST-elevation myocardial infarction. *Circulation.* 2018

Pinto DS, Kirtane AJ, Nallamothu BK, et al. Hospital delays in reperfusion for ST-elevation myocardial infarction: implications when selecting a reperfusion strategy. *Circulation.* 2006;114(19):2019–2025.

Kimmel SE, Berlin JA, Reilly M, et al. The effects of nonselective non-aspirin non-steroidal anti-inflammatory medications on the risk of nonfatal myocardial infarction and their interaction with aspirin. *J Am Coll Cardiol.* 2004;43(6):985–990.

2 *A 57-year-old man with a history of coronary artery disease (CAD) has a bowel resection and ventral hernia repair for strangulated hernia. On postoperative day 3, he has new-onset chest pain. Which of the following most increases his risk for a major adverse cardiovascular event (MACE: death, nonfatal* *myocardial infarction, or urgent need for coronary revascularization)?*

A *New-onset chest pain lasting 10 minutes*
B *ST depression of 0.3 mm on his EKG*
C *Troponin I two times normal value*
D *Age greater than 50*
E *Male gender*

When chest pain is likely caused by CAD, there are assessments available for risk stratification. The Braunwald and thrombolysis in myocardial infarction (TIMI) risks scores are used for risk stratification. TIMI has become the primary tool for therapeutic recommendations. Neither recent surgery nor gender are included. Age does not become a predictor variable until age > 65 in the TIMI risk score. An ST depression is diagnostic when > 0.5 mm; less than 0.5 mm is nonspecific. In both scoring systems, elevated cardiac markers including troponin is a predictive variable and portend a high risk.

Answer: C

Antman EM, Cohen M, Bernink PJ, et al. The TIMI risk score for unstable angina/non-ST elevation MI: a method for prognostication and therapeutic decision making. *JAMA.* 2000;284(7):835–842.

Braunwald E, Antman EM, Beasley JW, et al. ACC/AHA guideline update for the management of patients with unstable angina and non–ST-segment elevation myocardial infarction--2002: summary article: a report of the American College of Cardiology/American Heart Association Task Force on Practice Guidelines (Committee on the Management of Patients With Unstable Angina). *Circulation.* 2002;106(14):1893–1900.

3 *The most important factor in improving survival during STEMI is:*
A *Early intubation*
B *Timely reperfusion*
C *Giving aspirin*
D *Smoking cessation*
E *IV metoprolol*

ST elevation begins after occlusion of a coronary artery. Myocardial cell death proceeds rapidly until re-establishment of blood flow. Reperfusion with fibrinolytic therapy and/or PCI can limit loss of heart muscle. The majority of infarct occurs by four hours after the onset of symptoms, and after 6 hours the infarct in nearly complete. Sudden cardiac death is most likely to develop during the first 4 hours after onset of symptoms. Reperfusion has

Predictor variable	Point value of variable	Definition
Age ≥65 years	1	
≥3 Risk factors for CAD	1	Risk factors • Family history of CAD • Hypertension • Hypercholesterolemia • Diabetes • Current smoker
Aspirin use in last 7 days	1	
Recent, severe symptoms of angina	1	≥ 2 anginal events in past 24 hours
Elevated cardiac markers	1	CK-MB or cardiac-specific troponin level
ST deviation ≥0.5 mm	1	ST depression ≥0.5 mm is significant; transient ST elevation ≥0.5 mm for <20 minutes is treated as ST-segment depression and is high risk; ST elevation ≥1 mm for >20 minutes places these patients in the STEMI treatment category
Prior coronary artery stenosis 50%	1	Risk predictor remains valid even if this information is unknown

Calculated TIMI risk score	Risk of ≥ 1 primary end point* in ≤ 14 days	Risk status
0 or 1	5%	Low
2	8%	
3	13%	Intermediate
4	20%	
5	26%	High

Abbreviations: CK-MB, MB fraction of creatine kinase; TIMI, Thrombosis in Myocardial Infarction; UA, unstable angina.
*Primary end points: death, new or recurrent myocardial infarction, or need for urgent revascularization.

Figure 4.2 TIMI risk assessment.

	High risk *Risk is high if patient has any of the following findings:*	Intermediate risk *Risk is intermediate if patient has any of the following findings:*	Low risk *Risk is low if patient has no high- or intermediate-risk features; may have any of the following:*
History	• Accelerating tempo of ischemic symptoms over prior 48 hours	• Prior MI *or* • Peripheral artery disease *or* • Cerebrovascular disease *or* • CABG, prior aspirin use	
Character of pain	• Prolonged, continuing (>20 min) rest pain	• Prolonged (>20 min) rest angina is now resolved (moderate to high likelihood of CAD) • Rest angina (<20 min) or relieved by rest or sublingual nitrates	• New-onset functional angina (Class III or IV) in past 2 weeks without prolonged rest pain (but with moderate or high likelihood of CAD)
Physical exam	• Pulmonary edema secondary to ischemia • New or worse mitral regurgitation murmur • Hypotension, bradycardia, tachycardia • S3 gallop or new or worsening rales • Age >75 years	• Age >70 years	
ECG	• Transient ST-segment deviation (≥0.5 mm) with rest angina • New or presumably new bundle branch block • Sustained VT	• T-wave inversion ≥2 mm • Pathologic Q waves or T waves that are not new	• Normal or unchanged ECG during an episode of chest discomfort
Cardiac markers	• Elevated cardiac troponin I or T • Elevated CK-MB	*Any of the above findings PLUS* • Normal	• Normal

Abbreviations: CABG, coronary artery bypass grafting; CK-MB, MB fraction of creatine kinase.

Figure 4.3 Braunwald risk assessment.

been shown to reduce mortality, preserve LV function, and limit the development of congestive heart failure. Intubation is not indicated in STEMI unless there is associated respiratory distress. Smoking cessation is a long-term preventive strategy and is not applicable acutely. Aspirin is indicated in the initial management and is complementary to fibrinolysis and reperfusion. Metoprolol may be helpful but is not the most important factor in improving survival.

Answer: B

O'Connor RE, Al Ali AS, Brady WJ, et al. Part 9: acute coronary syndromes: 2015 American Heart Association Guidelines Update for Cardiopulmonary Resuscitation and Emergency Cardiovascular Care. *Circulation.* 2015;132(18) (suppl 2):S483–S500.

Campbell RW, Murray A, Julian DG. Ventricular arrhythmias in first 12 hours of acute myocardial infarction: natural history study. *Br Heart J.* 1981;46(4):351.

4 *A 49-year-old mother of seven has a history of diabetes ellitus, hypertension, smoking, and 4 months ago underwent PCI with a paclitaxel-eluding stent placement for unstable angina. Her medications include aspirin, clopidogrel, metoprolol, HMG-CoA reductase inhibitor, metformin, and an angiotensin-converting enzyme (ACE) inhibitor. She now presents to your office with one episode of right upper quadrant pain and based on history, physical exam, labs, and ultrasound, you diagnose her with biliary colic and cholelithiasis. Of the following choices, which is the next best step in management?*

A *Delay the operation for 6 months.*
B *Stop aspirin and clopidogrel, and proceed with the operation in 5 days.*
C *Stop aspirin and clopidogrel, and proceed with the operation in 7 days with a preoperative heparin infusion as a bridge to surgery.*
D *Stop clopidogrel, continue aspirin, and proceed with surgery.*
E *Transfuse platelets, and proceed with surgery.*

In patients with coronary stents, dual antiplatelet therapy is recommended for at least one year to minimize the risk of stent thrombosis. Large observational studies suggest an increased risk of stent thrombosis for at least 6 months. A cholecystectomy is elective at this time. To stop, or adjust, dual antiplatelet therapy less than 6 months after placement of the stent risks thrombosis, and to operate on dual antiplatelet therapy increased bleeding complications. In the recommendations below, there are differences between bare-metal stents (BMS) and drug-eluding stents (DES). A biological explanation for these differences is the earlier endothelialization of bare-metal stents.

COR	LOE	Recommendations
I	B-NR	Elective noncardiac surgery should be delayed 30 days after BMS implantation and optimally 6 months after DES implantation.
I	C-EO	In patients treated with DAPT after coronary stent implantation who must undergo surgical procedures that mandate the discontinuation of P2Y$_{12}$ inhibitor therapy, it is recommended that aspirin be continued if possible and the P2Y$_{12}$ platelet receptor inhibitor be restarted as soon as possible after surgery.
IIa	C-EO	When noncardiac surgery is required in patients currently taking a P2Y$_{12}$ inhibitor, a consensus decision among treating clinicians as to the relative risks of surgery and discontinuation or continuation of antiplatelet therapy can be useful.
IIb	C-EO	Elective noncardiac surgery after DES implantation in patients for whom P2Y$_{12}$ inhibitor therapy will need to be discontinued may be considered after 3 months if the risk of further delay of surgery is greater than the expected risks of stent thrombosis.
III: Harm	B-NR	Elective noncardiac surgery should not be performed within 30 days after BMS implantation or within 3 months after DES implantation in patients in whom DAPT will need to be discontinued perioperatively.

Answer: A

Levine GN, Bates ER, Bittl JA, et al. 2016 ACC/AHA guideline focused update on duration of dual antiplatelet

therapy in patients with coronary artery disease. *Circulation.* 2016;134(10):e123–e155.

5 *This same patient turns 50-years-old 8 months after cardiac stent placement and needs a colonoscopy as recommended by her primary care physician. A sigmoid colon cancer is discovered. The most appropriate plan for her operation and antiplatelet medication is to:*
   A *Delay the operation for 4 months to perform at the same time as cholecystectomy.*
   B *Stop aspirin and clopidogrel, and operate after 7 days.*
   C *Stop aspirin and clopidogrel, operate after 7 days, and bridge with enoxaparin.*
   D *Stop clopidogrel, continue aspirin, and operate after 5 days.*
   E *Continue both clopidogrel and aspirin, and proceed with intraoperative platelet transfusion.*

At this time the surgery is for a malignancy and cannot wait months. The recommendation for urgent noncardiac surgery for a patient on dual antiplatelet therapy is to stop the clopidogrel and continue aspirin. This recommendation is based on expert opinion. For patients undergoing laparoscopic surgery, continuation of a single antiplatelet agent is not associated with an increased risk of preoperative bleeding. Since there is not an increased risk of bleeding, there is no indication for platelet transfusion. There is no role for enoxaparin bridge because it is not an antiplatelet agent. These are complex decisions and should be reached by consensus of the surgeon, cardiologist, anesthesiologist, and patient. When intraoperative platelet transfusion is given, it may cause thrombosing the stent.

Answer: D

Levine GN, Bates ER, Bittl JA, et al. 2016 ACC/AHA guideline focused update on duration of dual antiplatelet therapy in patients with coronary artery disease. *Circulation.* 2016;134(10):e123–e155.

Antolovic D, Rakow A, Contin P, et al. A randomised controlled pilot trial to evaluate and optimize the use of anti-platelet agents in the perioperative management in patients undergoing general and abdominal surgery—the APAP trial (ISRCTN45810007). *Langenbecks Arch Surg.* 2012;397(2):297–306.

Fujikawa T, Tanaka A, Abe T, et al. Does antiplatelet therapy affect outcomes of patients receiving abdominal laparoscopic surgery? Lessons from more than 1,000 laparoscopic operations in a single tertiary referral hospital. *J Am Coll Surg.* 2013;217(6):1044–1053.

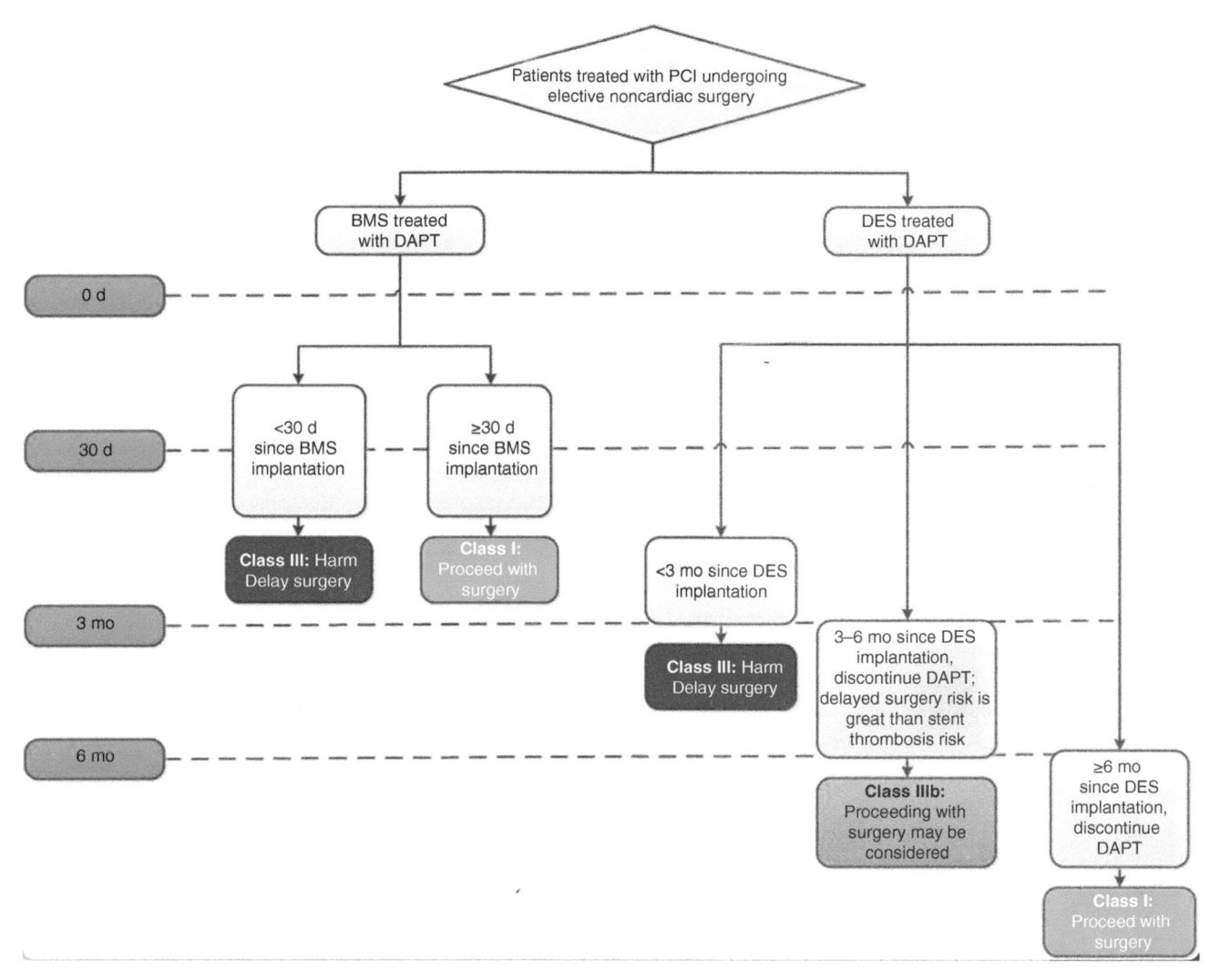

Figure 4.4 Elective noncardiac surgery in patients who undergo PCI and are on DAPT.

6 *You decide to perform a laparoscopic sigmoidectomy on the above patient in one week. In the perioperative period, she will continue to take her aspirin and beta-blocker medication. Which other medication should she continue to take perioperatively (before and after) to reduce mortality?*
   A *Clopidogrel*
   B *ACE inhibitor*
   C *Metformin*
   D *Furosemide*
   E *HMG-CoA reductase inhibitor*

Continuing clopidogrel may increase the risk of bleeding, and 6 months after stent placement, holding it for patients undergoing surgery has no increased mortality risk. Continuing metformin has not been shown to affect mortality, nor has continuing furosemide or ACE inhibitor, but continuing diuretics may make determining the patient's volume status more difficult. Perioperative (within 24 hours of elective surgery) continuation of HMG-CoA reductase inhibitors (statins) decreases mortality in patients undergoing noncardiac operations.

Answer: E

London MJ, Schwartz GG, Hur K, et al. Association of perioperative statin use with mortality and morbidity after major noncardiac surgery. *JAMA Intern Med.* 2017;177(2):231–242.

Mehran R, Baber U, Steg PG, et al. Cessation of dual antiplatelet treatment and cardiac events after percutaneous coronary intervention (PARIS): 2 year results from a prospective observational study. *Lancet.* 2013;382:1714–22.

7 *A 76-year-old man with a history of non-valvular atrial fibrillation on warfarin has a finding of right-sided colon cancer. He is scheduled for a right hemi-colectomy. His International Normalized Ratio is 2. His warfarin should be:*
  A *Continued through the preoperative period*
  B *Held for 5 days before surgery*
  C *Bridged with enoxaparin*
  D *Bridged with intravenous unfractionated heparin*
  E *Changed to daily aspirin*

This patient's CHA_2DS_2–VASc score is 2. While that makes him an anticoagulation candidate, it is not necessary to bridge for elective surgery if the CHA_2DS_2–VASc is 4 or less. Continuing warfarin would be an unacceptable bleeding risk. Temporary interruption of the anticoagulant should be the strategy to minimize post-operative bleeding risk. If this patient were a candidate for bridging therapy, then enoxaparin, IV unfractionated heparin, and fondaparinux are appropriate. After surgery he will need to go back on warfarin as his stroke risk is too high for treatment with aspirin alone.

If the patient has a CHA_2DS_2–VASc score of 5 to 6, and the procedure has no significant bleed risk, then bridging should be considered if the patient has had a prior stroke or TIA.

If the patient has a CHA_2DS_2–VASc score of 7–9, or a recent (within 3 months) ischemic stroke or TIA, bridging should be considered.

Bridging from warfarin with unfractionated heparin required holding the warfarin. Then start the parenteral anticoagulation therapy when the INR is no longer therapeutic. Discontinue the parenteral unfractionated heparin 4 hours prior to the procedure.

CHA2DS2–VASc acronym	Score
Congestive HF	1
Hypertension	1
Age ≥ 75 years	2
Diabetes mellitus	1
Stroke/TIA/TE	2
Vascular disease (prior MI, PAD, or aortic plaque)	1
Age 65 to 74 years	1
Sex category (i.e., female sex)	1
Maximum score	9

Answer: B

Doherty JU, Gluckman TJ, Hucker WJ, et al. 2017 ACC expert consensus decision pathway for periprocedural management of anticoagulation in patients with nonvalvular atrial fibrillation: A report of the American College of Cardiology clinical expert consensus document task force. *J Am Coll Cardiol.* 2017;69(7):871–898.

8 *The most common location of spontaneous ectopic foci as the underlying mechanism in paroxysmal atrial fibrillation is:*
  A *Left atrial appendage*
  B *Ligament of Marshall*
  C *Pulmonary veins*
  D *Right atrium*
  E *Superior vena cava*

Left atrial muscle extends into the pulmonary veins acting as a sphincter during atrial systole. Mapping of electrical activity preceding the onset of atrial fibrillation demonstrates in nearly 90 percent of patients that the point of origin is in the pulmonary veins. The other choices are all potential points of ectopic foci but less common. The left atrial appendage arises anteriolaterally, and its morphology may influence the risk of embolic stroke. The ligament of Marshall is on the epicardium between the left atrial appendage and left pulmonary veins and contains muscle fibers extending to the atrial myocardium, which can be a source of foci of atrial fibrillation. Rarely, ectopic foci of atrial fibrillation can originate in the right atrium or superior vena cava.

Answer: C

Haissaguerre M, Jais P, Shah DC, et al. Spontaneous initiation of atrial fibrillation by ectopic beats originating in the pulmonary veins. *N. Engl. J Med.* 1998;339: 659–666.

January CT, Wann LS, Calkins H. AHA/ACC/HRS focused update of the 2014 AHA/ACC/HRS guideline for the management of patients with atrial fibrillation: a report of the American College of Cardiology/American Heart Association Task Force on Clinical Practice Guidelines and the Heart Rhythm Society. *J. Am. Coll. Cardiol.* 2019;2019 doi: 10.1016

9 *Hypertensive emergency is defined as:*
  A *Malignant hypertension*
  B *Systolic blood pressure greater than 180 mm Hg*
  C *Diastolic blood pressure greater than 110 mm Hg*
  D *Hypertension-mediated organ damage*
  E *Mean arterial pressure greater than two times patient's baseline*

Patients with systolic blood pressure (SBP) > 180 or diastolic blood pressure (DBP) > 110 are usually defined as having hypertensive crisis. Pressures this high can result in acute injury including the heart, brain, lung, kidney, retina, aorta, and microvasculature. When there is organ damage, the condition is termed "hypertensive emergency." Malignant hypertension is an outdated term, which has been removed from blood pressure guidelines. Normal mean arterial pressure (MAP) is 70–100 mm Hg. MAP two times baseline is not a defined entity. A patient in hypertensive emergency should be placed in the ICU with intravenous blood pressure control. Hypertensive urgency is hypertension in the absence of organ failure. Those patients can be managed with oral agents with the goal of gradual normalization of blood pressure over days to weeks.

Answer: D

Peixoto AJ. Acute severe hypertension. *N Engl J Med.* 2019;381:1843.
Johnson W, Nguyen ML, Patel R. Hypertension crisis in the emergency department. *Cardiol Clin.* 2012;30:533.

10 *Hypertensive emergency is the consequence of:*
   A *Elevated systemic vascular resistance*
   B *High cardiac output*
   C *Renal failure*
   D *Tachycardia*
   E *Volume overload*

The most common precipitating factor in hypertensive crisis is noncompliance with medication in a patient with known hypertension. It is thought that humoral vasoconstrictors lead to an abrupt increase in systemic vascular resistance. This causes small vessel endothelial injury resulting in platelet and fibrin deposition and loss of vascular autoregulation. It is an afterload problem, not cardiac output problem. In most cases treatment should be directed at afterload reduction. Unless there is renal failure, continued hypertension results in natriuresis and volume contraction. Gentle volume expansion with saline may be indicated in some cases. Renal failure or tachycardia may or may not be present. Diuresis would result in worsening of the vasoconstriction.

Answer: A

Marik PE, Rivera R. Hypertensive emergencies: an update. *Curr Opin Crit Care.* 2011;17:569–580.
Peixoto AJ. Acute severe hypertension. *N Engl J Med.* 2019;381:1843.

11 *Treatment of hypertensive emergency should be more aggressive for which of the following conditions:*

   A *Ischemic stroke*
   B *Aortic dissection*
   C *Renal emergency*
   D *Lysergic acid diethylamide (LSD) overdose*
   E *Myocardial infarction*

Chronic hypertension leads to autoregulation of cerebral blood flow, necessitating higher pressures for adequate flow. Quick and excessive correction of blood pressure to a systolic below 100 to 120 mm Hg can potentiate injury and has an increased risk of death. In hypertensive emergency, blood pressure should be decreased by no more than 20–25% in the first hour, and then to 160/110 mm Hg during the next 2–6 hours. This applies to renal emergency, myocardial infarction, and sympathomimetic agents such as LSD. An exception is acute aortic dissection where the goal should be to lower the systolic blood pressure to 100 to 120 mm Hg within 20 minutes to reduce aortic shearing forces. Short-acting beta-blockers should be used, and a vasodilator like nitroprusside or nicardipine can be added if needed. Vascular or cardiothoracic surgery should be consulted as well. Patients with ischemic stroke should not have their blood pressure reduced unless it is greater than 220/120 mm Hg or if thrombolytic therapy is planned.

Answer: B

Mayer SA, Kurtz P, Wyman A, et al. Clinical practices, complications, and mortality in neurological patients with acute severe hypertension: the studying the treatment of acute hypertension registry. *Crit Care Med.* 2011;39:2330–2336.
Peixoto AJ. Acute severe hypertension. *N Engl J Med.* 2019;381:1843.

12 *The first line therapy for pheochromocytoma hypertensive crisis is:*
   A *Phentolamine*
   B *Metoprolol*
   C *Labetalol*
   D *Hydralazine*
   E *No treatment*

Hypertensive emergency from pheochromocytoma is catecholamine induced. It is treated with alpha-blockers such as phentolamine or direct vasodilators such as sodium nitroprusside or nicardipine. Paradoxically, beta-blockers including labetalol are contraindicated as sole therapy because they can lead to unopposed alpha-adrenergic action. Hydralazine may be a second-tiered therapy, but it is unpredictable and should be avoided as a first option in hypertensive emergency. Separately, arrhythmias in pheochromocytoma emergency can be treated with esmolol, but alpha-blockage should be in place first. Esmolol is preferred beta-blocker as it is titratable.

Answer: A

Young WF Jr. Adrenal causes of hypertension: pheochromocytoma and primary aldosteronism. *Rev Endocr Metab Disord.* 2007;8(4):309.

Peixoto AJ. Acute severe hypertension. *N Engl J Med.* 2019;381:1843.

13 *Which drug should be avoided in hypertensive emergencies in a pregnant patient:*
   A *Labetalol*
   B *Nifedipine*
   C *Metoprolol*
   D *Hydralazine*
   E *Nitroprusside*

Calcium channel blockers and hydralazine are safe in pregnancy. Though beta-blockers can cross the placenta, labetalol and metoprolol are safe in pregnancy; atenolol is not. The possibility of fetal cyanide poisoning has restricted the use of nitroprusside in pregnancy. When using nitroprusside, cyanide levels are typically monitored. While not an answer, angiotensin-converting enzyme (ACE) inhibitors also should not be used in pregnancy because of increased risk of fetal renal damage.

Answer: E

ACOG Committee Opinion No. 767: Emergent therapy for acute-onset, severe hypertension during pregnancy and the postpartum period. *Obstet Gynecol.* 2019;133:e174

Sass N, Itamoto CH, Silva MP, et al. Does sodium nitroprusside kill babies? A systematic review. *Sao Paulo Med J.* 2007;125:108.

14 *A 19-year-old man who is a long-distance runner has an irregular pulse on physical exam. An EKG demonstrates a PR interval that gets progressively longer until the final P wave elicits no response. The series then repeats every 4 beats. What is the appropriate treatment?*
   A *Atropine*
   B *Immediate transcutaneous pacing*
   C *Lidocaine*
   D *Elective transvenous pacing*
   E *No treatment*

In first-degree atrioventricular (AV) block, there is a prolonged PR interval. This is physiologically unimportant and does not require therapy; however, it may signal drug toxicity or conduction system disease. In second-degree AV block, some atrial impulses are conducted to the ventricles, and others are blocked. There are two types of second-degree AV block. The patient described has Mobitz type I (Wenckebach) block. It is the result of a conduction blockage in the AV node. The cause can be drug (digoxin) related or from intrinsic heart disease. It can also occur in endurance athletes. The AV node is supplied by the right coronary artery, so a Mobitz type I block can accompany an inferior myocardial infarction. The Mobitz type I block itself requires no treatment in a stable patient. Atropine and pacing might be effective but not indicated. Lidocaine has no role in the treatment of second-degree AV block.

Answer: E

Wenckebach KF. On the analysis of irregular pulses [article in German]. *Z Klin Med.* 1899;37:475–488.

Epstein AE, DiMarco JP, Ellenbogen KA, et al. American College of Cardiology Foundation, American Heart Association Task Force on Practice Guidelines, Heart Rhythm Society. 2012 ACCF/AHA/HRS focused update incorporated into the ACCF/AHA/HRS 2008 guidelines for device-based therapy of cardiac rhythm abnormalities: a report of the American College of Cardiology Foundation/American Heart Association Task Force on Practice Guidelines and the Heart Rhythm Society. *J Am Coll Cardiol.* 2013;61:e6–e75.

15 *A 52-year-old woman with a history of angina is admitted for a partial small bowel obstruction that resolves in 36 hours. She then develops new-onset bradycardia, and an EKG demonstrates a 2:1 atrioventricular (AV) block in addition to a bundle branch block. Carotid sinus stimulation improves the bradycardia; however, atropine worsens the bradycardia. Which type of AV block does this patient have?*
   A *There is no AV block*
   B *First-degree AV block*
   C *Type I second-degree AV block (Mobitz type I or Wenckebach)*
   D *Type II second-degree AV block (Mobitz type II or Infranodal)*
   E *Third-degree AV block*

There is an AV block. This patient has a second-degree AV block. A Mobitz type I block has increasing PR intervals until a QRS is dropped. A Mobitz type II has fixed PR intervals until a QRS is dropped. Often there is a widened QRS in Mobitz type II also, but in this patient with a 2:1 AV ratio, every other P wave is not conducted, which makes it difficult to diagnose the level of block. Vagal maneuvers such as carotid massage can be helpful in diagnosing the level. If the block is in the AV node

(Mobitz type I), carotid sinus massage may worsen the block. If the block is more distal at the bundle of His, or Purkinje fibers, (Mobitz type II) slowing the sinus rate may paradoxically improve the ratio of AV conduction and increase the ventricular rate. Conversely, atropine may increase the conduction rate across the AV node, which may paradoxically worsen the ratio of AV conduction if the block is at the His-Purkinje system (Mobitz type II). Third-degree AV block is complete dissociation between P waves and QRS, which is not the case in this patient, yet.

Answer: D

Epstein AE, DiMarco JP, Ellenbogen KA, et al. American College of Cardiology Foundation, American Heart Association Task Force on Practice Guidelines, Heart Rhythm Society. 2012 ACCF/AHA/HRS focused update incorporated into the ACCF/AHA/HRS 2008 guidelines for device-based therapy of cardiac rhythm abnormalities: a report of the American College of Cardiology Foundation/American Heart Association Task Force on Practice Guidelines and the Heart Rhythm Society. *J Am Coll Cardiol*. 2013;61:e6–e75.

16 *The above patient is hemodynamically stable and electrolytes are normal. What should be the next step in treatment?*
   A *Beta-blockade*
   B *Atropine*
   C *Transvenous pacing*
   D *Epinephrine*
   E *Transcutaneous pacing*

New-onset type II second-degree AV block (Mobitz type II) is usually associated with a pathologic lesion, often an occlusion of a septal branch off the left anterior descending coronary artery. It has a poorer prognosis than Mobitz type I (Wenckebach) and often progresses to third-degree or complete heart block. If the patient is unstable, the algorithm for bradycardia begins with atropine. Though in Mobitz type II, atropine should not be relied upon as discussed in the previous question. The next step should be transcutaneous pacing or beta-adrenergic support such as epinephrine or dopamine. The patient in question is stable and does not require these therapies at this time. Beta-blockade is not indicated in this patient. Because of the risk of progression to a third-degree AV block, transvenous pacing is the correct next step. Transvenous pacing is also indicated in third-degree block.

Answer: C

Epstein AE, DiMarco JP, Ellenbogen KA, et al. American College of Cardiology Foundation, American Heart Association Task Force on Practice Guidelines, Heart Rhythm Society. 2012 ACCF/AHA/HRS focused update incorporated into the ACCF/AHA/HRS 2008 guidelines for device-based therapy of cardiac rhythm abnormalities: a report of the American College of Cardiology Foundation/American Heart Association Task Force on Practice Guidelines and the Heart Rhythm Society. *J Am Coll Cardiol*. 2013;61:e6–e75.

17 *A 17-year-old basketball player presents with occasional palpitations, usually after exertion. He has the following EKG.*

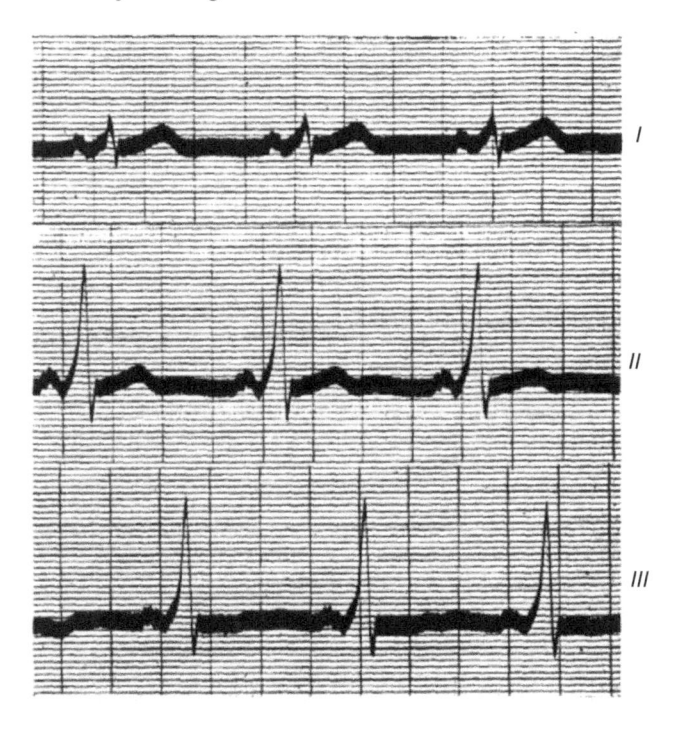

If this patient develops atrial fibrillation with rapid ventricular response, then he should be treated with:
   A *Adenosine*
   B *Amiodarone*
   C *Digoxin*
   D *Procainamide*
   E *Verapamil*

This patient has Wolff–Parkinson–White (WPW) syndrome. With WPW, there is a shortened P-R interval, less than 0.12 second, and a QRS complex widened by characteristic delta wave. The delta wave pre-excitation is caused by an accessory pathway (AP), the bundle of Kent. The AP may allow antegrade and retrograde conduction. These patients have a risk of developing atrial fibrillation with potential to degenerate to ventricular fibrillation related to a rapidly conducting AP. Agents commonly used to slow AV nodal conduction in atrial fibrillation can be harmful in patients with WPW. A paradoxic increase in ventricular rate is due to more atrial activity passing through the AP and less through the AV node. Adenosine, IV amiodarone, digoxin, and verapamil can lead to ventricular fibrillation. Procainamide is a class 1a anti-arrhythmic that will increase the refractory period and decrease conduction through the AP. If the patient is unstable, direct current cardioversion is recommended. Definitive treatment of WPW is catheter ablation of the AP.

Answer: D

Wolff L, Parkinson J, White PD. Bundle-branch block with short P-R interval in healthy young people prone to paroxysmal tachycardia. *Am Heart J*. 1930;5(6): 685–704

Simonian SM, Lotfipour S, Wall C, et al. Challenging the superiority of amiodarone for rate control in Wolff-Parkinson-White and atrial fibrillation. *Intern Emerg Med*. 2010; 5:421–6.

January CT, Wann LS, Alpert JS, et al. 2014 AHA/ACC/HRS guideline for the management of patients with atrial fibrillation: executive summary: a report of the American College of Cardiology/American Heart Association Task Force on practice guidelines and the Heart Rhythm Society. *Circulation*. 2014;130:2071.

18 An 88-year-old woman is in the ICU with pneumonia, ileus, and delirium. Her medications include furosemide, lisinopril, erythromycin, pantoprazole, enoxaparin, and haloperidol. After several hours with a prolonged QT interval (> 500 milliseconds) and then several runs of ventricular couplets, she develops a polymorphic ventricular tachycardia in the form of cyclic sinusoidal variation. She is appropriately resuscitated including treatment with 2 grams IV magnesium over 2 minutes and is back in sinus rhythm with prolonged QT interval. Which two drugs should be discontinued?
   A Erythromycin and haloperidol
   B Lisinopril and enoxaparin
   C Pantoprazole and erythromycin
   D Enoxaparin and haloperidol
   E Furosemide and lisinopril

This patient has torsades de pointes, the treatment of which is appropriate resuscitation and 1–2 grams IV magnesium over 2 minutes. It can be seen in several settings, including heart block or congenital syndromes, but can also be associated with drug treatments. Of the medications this patient is taking, erythromycin and haloperidol can cause torsades de pointes. The other medications do not. While furosemide does not cause torsades de pointes, it can lower potassium that increases the risk for torsades de pointes.

Answer: A

Roden DM. Drug-induced prolongation of the QT interval. *N Engl J Med*. 2004;350:1013.

Roden DM, Predicting drug-induced QT prolongation and tornadoes de pointes. *J Physiol actions*. 2016;594(9):2459–68.

19 A 35-year-old Asian man falls from heavy alcohol use, has a syncopal event, and lacerates his scalp. In the emergency room, bupivacaine is administered locally to suture repair his scalp laceration; however, during the repair he is combative. He is intubated and sedated with propofol. He subsequently develops spontaneous sustained ventricular tachycardia. He is resuscitated and his EKG is given below:

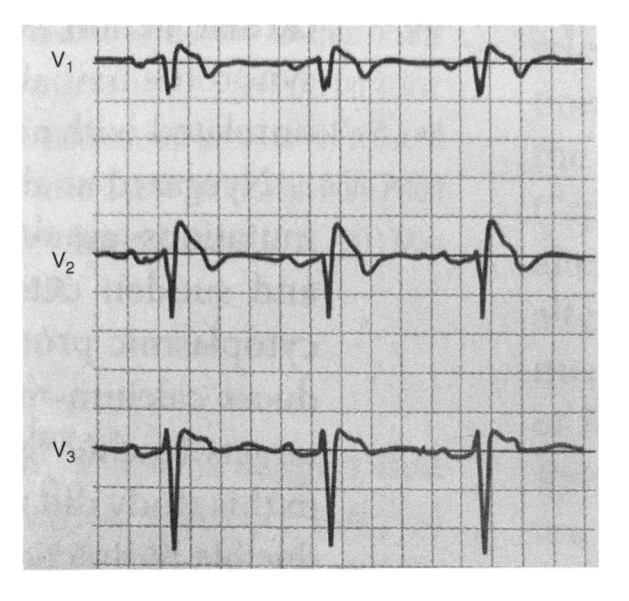

Definitive treatment for this patient's diagnosis is:
   A Observation
   B Avoidance of alcohol
   C Metoprolol
   D Cardiac catheterization with stent placement
   E Implantable cardiac defibrillator

There is a peculiar ST elevation in leads V1, V2, and V2 with a right bundle branch block, which characterizes Brugada syndrome. If it is suspected but not seen on EKG, an EKG on a sodium channel blocker test may help elucidate it. The symptoms of Brugada syndrome are syncope, and ventricular tachycardia or ventricular fibrillation, often while sleeping. Arrhythmias can be triggered by a large consumption of food or alcohol. Drugs that can trigger arrhythmias include bupivacaine, cocaine, alpha agonists (methoxamine), tricyclic antidepressants, lithium, and propofol. Definitive treatment requires an implantable cardiac defibrillator (ICD). The patient is at risk for sudden cardiac arrest, so observation is inadequate. Avoiding alcohol may be helpful in decreasing the risk of symptoms but is not definitive. Metoprolol is not indicated. There is no role for stent place because this is an electrical conduction disease, not ischemia.

Answer: E

Brugada J, Campuzano O, Arbelo E, et al. Present status of Brugada syndrome: JACC State-of-the-art review. *J Am Coll Cardiol.* 2018;72:1046.

Brugada P, Brugada J. Right bundle branch block, persistent ST segment elevation and sudden cardiac death: a distinct clinical and electrocardiographic syndrome. A multicenter report. *J Am Coll Cardiol.* 1992; 20: 1391–1396.

20 *An 81-year-old woman non-smoker has an episode of chest pain that lasts several hours. She rests at home and is able to sleep it off. 5 days later she has chest pain again and weakness. This time she goes to the hospital. She is found to be tachycardic and hypotensive with distended neck veins and has a pan-systolic murmur with ST elevations on EKG. She is taken for cardiac catheterization that demonstrates complete occlusion of her left anterior descending artery. An echocardiogram shows a left-to-right shunt. With medical treatment alone, what is the 30-day mortality for this condition?*

A *2%*
B *15%*
C *33%*
D *50%*
E *90%*

Ventricular septal defects occur in 0.2% of patients, typically the first week after a myocardial infarction. Advanced age and female sex are risk factors for its development. Diagnosis is determined clinically by a harsh systolic murmur and echocardiographic findings of a left-to-right shsunt, right ventricular dysfunction, or frank septal rupture. While the overall 30-day mortality is 75%, operative repair improves mortality to around 45%, down from about 90% for medical treatment alone. Surgical repair consists of a pericardial patch over the defect.

Answer: E

Crenshaw BS, Granger CB, Birnbaum Y, et al. Risk factors, angiographic patterns, and outcomes in patients with ventricular septal defect complicating acute myocardial infarction. GUSTO-I (Global Utilization of Streptokinase and TPA for Occluded Coronary Arteries) Trial Investigators. *Circulation.* 2000;101(1):27–32.

Omar S, Morgan GL, Panchal HB, et al. Management of post-myocardial infarction ventricular septal defects: a critical assessment. *J Interv Cardiol.* 2018;31(6): 939–948

5

Sepsis and the Inflammatory Response to Injury

Ilya Shnaydman, MD and Matthew Bronstein, MD

Division of Trauma and Acute Care Surgery, New York Medical College, Westchester Medical Center, Valhalla, NY, USA

1 *A 78-year-old woman recently discharged from the hospital after ventral hernia repair presents to the emergency department with a 5-day history of fever, chills, and productive cough. The patient's family reports poor oral intake and altered mental status. The patient's vital signs are temperature 38.5 °C; heart rate 125 beats/min; respiratory rate 30 breaths/min; blood pressure 80/60 mm Hg; and oxygen saturation 85% on room air. A chest radiograph demonstrates multifocal pneumonia and the urinalysis shows leukocyte esterase and nitrites. She is appropriately volume resuscitated and requires norepinephrine to maintain a mean arterial blood pressure of 65 mm Hg. Her serum lactate is 4 mmol/L.*
The patient's clinical condition can best be defined as:
A *Sepsis.*
B *Septic Shock.*
C *Severe Sepsis.*
D *Multiorgan dysfunction syndrome.*
E *Systemic inflammatory response syndrome (SIRS).*

The Society of Critical Care Medicine task force produced the new definition for sepsis and septic shock (Sepsis-3) in 2016. Sepsis is defined as life-threatening organ dysfunction caused by a dysregulated host response to infection. This is identified by a score of 2 points or more on the Sequential Organ Failure Assessment (SOFA) score and is associated with 10% mortality or greater. Patients with septic shock are defined as requiring a vasopressor to maintain a MAP > 65 mmHg and having a serum lactate level >2 mmol/L in the absence of hypovolemia and is associated with 40% mortality or greater (choice B). Severe sepsis (choice C) and Multiorgan dysfunction syndrome

(choice D) are not definitions recommended by the new guidelines. SIRS (choice E) is defined as two of the following: tachycardia (HR > 90 bpm), tachypnea (RR > 20 breaths/min), fever (>39 °C or <36 °C), and leukocytosis (WBC > 12 or <4 or >10% bands). SIRS would be correct if there was no identified or suspected source. A quick bedside score, qSOFA, can also be used (respiratory rate > 22/min, altered mental status or systolic blood pressure 100 mmHg or less). Using these new definitions, the patient has Septic Shock (choice B).

Answer: B

Gyawali B, Ramakrishna K, Dhamoon, A. Sepsis: the evolution in definition, pathophysiology, and management. *SAGE Open Med.* 2019;7:205031211983504. doi: https://doi.org/10.1177/2050312119835043.

Singer M, Deutschman CS, Seymour CW, et al. The third international consensus definitions for sepsis and septic shock (sepsis-3). *JAMA.* 2016;315(8):801.

2 *What is the first step in the initial management of the patient in the above question?*
A *Antibiotic Therapy.*
B *Transfer to Intensive Care Unit.*
C *Intravenous fluid bolus.*
D *Checking serum lactate level.*
E *Supplemental oxygen administration.*

Just as in trauma, the initial management of any critically ill patient should involve establishing an adequate airway, evaluating breathing (which may require supplemental oxygen and/or mechanical ventilation), and restoring adequate perfusion with volume resuscitation and/or vasopressors (choice E). The patient will also require antibiotics

Surgical Critical Care and Emergency Surgery: Clinical Questions and Answers, Third Edition.
Edited by Forrest "Dell" Moore, Peter M. Rhee, and Carlos J. Rodriguez.
© 2022 John Wiley & Sons Ltd. Published 2022 by John Wiley & Sons Ltd.
Companion website: www.wiley.com/go/surgicalcriticalcare3e

(choice A), ICU care (choice B), intravenous fluids (choice B) as well as measurement of serum lactate (choice D).

Answer: E

Rhodes A, Evans LE, Alhazzani W, et al. Surviving sepsis campaign: international guidelines for management of sepsis and septic shock: 2016. *Intensive Care Med.* 2017;43(3):304–377.

Holmes CL, Walley KR. The evaluation and management of shock. *Clin Chest Med.* 2003;24(4):775–789.

3 *An 80-year-old man is admitted to the surgical intensive care unit with perforated diverticulitis after a Hartmann procedure. He has received appropriate fluid resuscitation but is requiring high doses of norepinephrine and vasopressin. His labs are significant for white blood cell count 18 000/μL and hemoglobin 10 g/dL. Bedside critical care ultrasound demonstrates a non-collapsible inferior vena cava and an appropriate ejection fraction.*

   The next best intervention should be:
   A *Transfusion of 2 units packed red blood cells.*
   B *Continued fluid resuscitation.*
   C *Addition of Epinephrine.*
   D *Initiation of stress dose steroids.*
   E *Placement of intra-aortic balloon pump.*

Intravenous "low dose" corticosteroids (200 mg hydrocortisone daily) are recommended in patients with sepsis in which adequate fluid resuscitation and vasopressor therapy are unable to restore hemodynamic stability. Steroid use should also be considered in patients at risk of adrenal dysfunction due to exogenous steroid use. Packed red blood cell transfusion is recommended only when hemoglobin decreases to <7.0 g/dL in the absence of extenuating circumstances, such as myocardial infarction, severe hypoxemia, or acute hemorrhage (choice A). Additional intravenous fluids would not be helpful if the patient is already adequately fluid resuscitated as evidenced by his non-collapsible inferior vena cava (choice B). Intra-aortic balloon pump and epinephrine can be useful in cardiogenic shock, but the patient has an appropriate ejection fraction, indicating the absence of cardiogenic shock (choice C/E).

Answer: D

Annane D, Renault A, Brun-Buisson C, et al. Hydrocortisone plus fludrocortisone for adults with septic shock. *N Engl J Med.* 2018;378(9):809–818.

Rhodes A, Evans LE, Alhazzani W, et al. Surviving sepsis campaign: international guidelines for management of sepsis and septic shock: 2016. *Intensive Care Med.* 2017;43(3):304–377.

Cecconi M, De Backer D, Antonelli M, et al. Consensus on circulatory shock and hemodynamic monitoring. Task force of the European Society of Intensive Care Medicine. *Intensive Care Med.* 2014;40(12):1795–1815.

Hébert PC, Wells G, Blajchman, MA, et al. A multicenter, randomized, controlled clinical trial of transfusion requirements in critical care. Transfusion Requirements in Critical Care Investigators, Canadian Critical Care Trials Group. *N Engl J Med.* 1999;340(6):409–417. doi: https://doi.org/10.1056/NEJM199902113400601. Erratum in: N Engl J Med 1999 Apr 1;340(13):1056. PMID: 9971864.

4 *A 64-year-old man presents with left lower quadrant abdominal pain and fever. His exam does not show peritonitis. He has a white blood cell count of 16 000/μL. He undergoes CT abdomen & pelvis and is found to have diverticulitis with a 3 cm pelvic abscess. He is immediately started on antibiotics and undergoes percutaneous drainage by interventional radiology. How long should antibiotic therapy be continued?*
   A *7 days*
   B *4 days*
   C *10 days*
   D *Until his symptoms and fever resolve*
   E *Until his leukocytosis resolves*

Duration of therapy for complicated intra-abdominal infections is a frequent problem to manage for the acute care and critical care surgeon. Antimicrobial therapy guidelines continue to evolve from high-quality evidence. Traditionally, surgeons have treated patients until all evidence of SIRS have resolved, typically for 1–2 weeks (choice A/C/D/E). The Study To Optimize Peritoneal Infection Therapy (STOP-IT) trial was a multicenter randomized trial that examined 4 day therapy vs. 2 days after the resolution of physiologic abnormalities related to SIRS. The primary endpoint was surgical site infection, recurrent intra-abdominal infection, or death. There was no significant difference between the groups, so they concluded that a 4 day duration of antibiotic therapy was sufficient after obtaining source control.

Answer: B

Sawyer RG, Claridge JA, Nathens AB, et al. Trial of short-course antimicrobial therapy for intraabdominal infection. *N Engl J Med.* 2015;372(21):1996–2005.

5 *A 55-year-old male trauma patient who remained intubated 4 days after laparotomy undergoes bronchoscopy for suspected mucous plugging seen on a chest radiograph. Purulent secretions are encountered*

and a bronchoalveolar lavage (BAL) and quantitative culture is performed.

Which of the following supports a diagnosis of ventilator associated pneumonia (VAP)?

A *Negative gram stain but high clinical suspicion.*

B *Protected brush specimen culture growing 10^2 CFU.*

C *Bronchoscopic BAL culture growing 10^3 CFU.*

D *Endotracheal aspirate growing 10^4 CFU.*

E *Bronchoscopic BAL culture growing 10^5 CFU.*

Pulmonary cultures can be obtained via bronchoscopy BAL, protected brush specimen (PSB) or blind tracheal suctioning. The following criteria confirm a diagnosis of VAP: blind tracheal suctioning (endobronchial aspirate) $\geq 10^5$ CFU, PSB $\geq 10^3$ CFU, bronchoscopic BAL $\geq 10^4$ CFU (choice E). The trauma literature supports a diagnosis of VAP with BAL $\geq 10^5$ CFU/mL, while CDC uses $\geq 10^4$ CFU/mL.

Answer: E

Kalil AC, Metersky ML, Klompas M, et al. Management of adults with hospital-acquired and ventilator-associated pneumonia: 2016 clinical practice guidelines by the infectious diseases society of America and the American thoracic society. *Clin Infect Dis.* 2016;63(5):e61–e111.

Martin-Loeches I, Rodriguez AH, Torres A. New guidelines for hospital-acquired pneumonia/ventilator-associated pneumonia: USA vs. Europe. *Curr Opin Crit Care.* 2018;24(5):347–352.

Croce MA, Fabian TC, Mueller EW, et al. The appropriate diagnostic threshold for ventilator-associated pneumonia using quantitative cultures. *J Trauma: Inj, Infect, Crit Care.* 2004;56(5):931–936.

National Healthcare Safety Network, Center for Disease Control. Pneumonia (Ventilator-Associated [VAP] and Non Ventilator-Associated Pneumonia [PNEU]) Event. *Table 5: Threshold Values for Cultured Specimens Used in the Diagnosis of Pneumonia*, 2021.

Rea-Neto A, Youssef N, Tuche F, et al. Diagnosis of ventilator-associated pneumonia: a systematic review of the literature. *Crit Care.* 2008;12(2):R56.

6   *The BAL culture from the patient above grows an extended spectrum beta lactamase (ESBL) producing strain of Klebsiella. Which antibiotic would be most likely to be effective?*

A *Piperacillin/tazobactam*

B *Vancomycin*

C *Ampicillin/sulbactam*

D *Cefepime*

E *Meropenem*

Cefepime and piperacillin/tazobactam demonstrate antipseudomonal activity but have limited activity against ESBL organisms (choice A/D). Vancomycin has no activity against Klebsiella (choice B). Ampicillin/sulbactam is not effective for ESBL organisms or Pseudomonas (choice C). Carbapenems are first-line therapy for extended-spectrum beta-lactamase (ESBL) organisms (choice E).

Answer: E

Harris PNA, Tambyah PA, Lye DC, et al. Effect of piperacillin-tazobactam vs meropenem on 30-day mortality for patients with E coli or Klebsiella pneumoniae bloodstream infection and ceftriaxone resistance. *JAMA.* 2018;320(10):984.

7   *What is the next best step in management? A 52-year-old woman presents to the emergency department with right upper quadrant pain and weakness. On admission, her vital signs are temperature 39 °C; heart rate 130 beats/min; respiratory rate 22 breaths/min; blood pressure 80/50 mm Hg; oxygen saturation 97% on room air. On examination, she is disoriented and her skin is jaundiced. Laboratory studies demonstrate white blood cell count 20 000/μL and an elevated bilirubin. Ultrasound examination reveals cholelithiasis and intrahepatic biliary ductal dilatation.*

A *Emergent laparoscopic cholecystectomy.*

B *GI consultation.*

C *Parenteral antibiotic.*

D *ICU admission.*

E *Emergent MRCP.*

The patient is in septic shock from cholangitis. The Surviving Sepsis Campaign Guidelines recommend administration of IV antimicrobials to be initiated as soon as possible after recognition of sepsis and within 1 hour for both sepsis and septic shock (choice C). They recommend obtaining microbiological cultures prior to starting antimicrobial therapy; if doing so, results in no substantial delay in the start of antimicrobials. For fluid resuscitation, the guidelines recommend 30 mL/kg of IV crystalloid be given within the first 3 hours. The patient will require emergent decompression of the biliary tract with either ERCP (choice B), PTC, or surgical common bile duct decompression. While these choices would address source control, it would take time and initiating antibiotics should be done first. The patient should undergo cholecystectomy (choice A) during that hospitalization (non-emergently) after bile duct decompression, the cholangitis has resolved and the patient has stabilized. This patient is appropriate for admission to the ICU (choice D), but this would not be the next best step.

Table 5.1 Threshold values for cultured specimens used in the PVAP definition.

Specimen collection/technique	Values
Lung tissue	$\geq 10^4$ CFU/g tissue*
Bronchoscopically (B) obtained specimens	
Bronchoalveolar lavage (B-BAL)	$\geq 10^4$ CFU/mL*
Protected BAL (B-PBAL)	$\geq 10^4$ CFU/mL*
Protected specimen brushing (B-PSB)	$\geq 10^3$ CFU/mL*
Nonbronchoscopically (NB) obtained (blind) specimens	
NB-BAL	$\geq 10^4$ CFU/mL*
NB-PSB	$\geq 10^3$ CFU/mL*
Endotracheal aspirate (ETA)	$\geq 10^5$ CFU/mL*

CFU = colony-forming units, g = gram, mL = milliliter.
* Or corresponding, semiquantitative result (see FAQ no. 24 at the end of this protocol).

Answer: C

Rhodes A, Evans LE, Alhazzani W, et al. Surviving sepsis campaign: international guidelines for management of sepsis and septic shock: 2016. *Intensive Care Med.* 2017;43(3):304–377.

Mayumi T, Okamoto K, Takada T, et al. Tokyo guidelines 2018: management bundles for acute cholangitis and cholecystitis. *J Hepatobiliary Pancreat Sci.* 2018;25(1): 96–100.

8   A 45-year-old man is recovering in the surgical ICU after an exploratory laparotomy and small bowel resection for small bowel obstruction. On postoperative day 7, he is still unable to tolerate enteral nutrition and is started on total parenteral nutrition through his existing central line. Due to leukocytosis and persistent fevers, blood cultures demonstrating *Candida glabrata* fungemia were obtained on postoperative day 12.
   What is the next best step?
   A Remove the central line and immediately start fluconazole.
   B Remove the central line, start fluconazole, and initiate peripheral parenteral nutrition.
   C Remove the central line, start micafungin, obtain ophthalmology consultation.
   D Repeat blood cultures.
   E Obtain a CT scan.

Candidemia is usually the result of a central line-associated bloodstream infection. The Infectious Diseases Society of America (IDSA) currently recommends that all patients with documented candidemia undergo at least one dilated eye examination to rule out intraocular involvement. Intraocular candidiasis may require intravitreal antifungal therapy and/or vitrectomy. *Candida glabrata* is intrinsically resistant to azoles such as fluconazole (choice A), thus the antifungals of choice for *Candida glabrata* are echinocandins such as micafungin. Removal of the central line is appropriate, but appropriate treatment for candidemia (micafungin) is also required (choice B). Repeat cultures are also appropriate, but not the next best step as it does not treat the candidemia (choice D). A CT scan may be warranted to exclude an intra-abdominal source, but would not be the next best step (choice E).

Answer: C

Rodrigues CF, Silva S, Henriques M. Candida glabrata: a review of its features and resistance. *Eur J Clin Microbiol Infect Dis.* 2014;33(5):673–688.

Pappas, PG, Kauffman, CA, Andes, D, et al. Clinical practice guidelines for the management of candidiasis: 2009 update by the Infectious Diseases Society of America. *Clin Infect Dis.* 2009;48:503–535.

9   A 65-year-old woman with infected necrotizing pancreatitis and hypotension requires 6 L of crystalloid in her resuscitation. On physical exam, she is edematous and remains hypotensive.
   The major cause of vasodilation in sepsis appears to be mediated by:
   A Up-regulating fibrinolysis.
   B ATP-sensitive potassium channels in smooth muscle.
   C ATP-sensitive calcium channels in smooth muscle.
   D Increase in vasopressin.
   E G-arginine.

The major cause of vasodilation in sepsis appears to be mediated by ATP-sensitive potassium channels in smooth muscle. The result of their activation is increased permeability of vascular smooth muscle cells to potassium, and hyperpolarization of the cell membranes, preventing muscle contraction, leading to vasodilation. There is a relative deficiency of vasopressin in early sepsis. The endothelium is an endocrine organ, capable of regulating the function of the microcirculation and producing nitric oxide (NO), an endogenous vasodilator. Its major effects are to cause local vasodilation and inhibition of platelet aggregation. NO is produced from l-arginine by nitric oxide synthetase (NOS), and its actions are mediated by cGMP. There are two forms of the enzyme NOS, a constitutive form, produced as part of the normal regulatory mechanisms, and an inducible form, whose production appears to be pathologic. Inducible NOS (iNOS) is an off-shoot of the inflammatory response, by TNF and other cytokines. It results in massive production of NO, causing widespread vasodilation (due to loss of vasomotor tone) and hypotension, which is hyporeactive to adrenergic agents. NO has a physiological antagonist, endothelin-1, a potent vasoconstrictor whose circulating level is increased in cardiogenic shock and following severe trauma.

Answer: B

Jackson WF Ion channels and vascular tone. *Hypertension.* 2000;35(1 Pt 2):173–178.

Quayle, JM, Nelson, MT, Standen, NB ATP sensitive and inwardly rectifying potassium channels in smooth muscle. *Physiol Rev.* 1997;77(4):1165–1232.

10 *The removal of a central venous catheter alone could be effective in the treatment of a central line-associated bloodstream infection in which of the following organisms?*
   A *Pseudomonas*
   B *E. coli*
   C *Staphylococcus aureus*
   D *Klebsiella pneumonia*
   E *Staphylococcus epidermidis*

When treating catheter-related bloodstream infections (CLABSI), several factors are important to consider in the treatment algorithm. Staphylococcus epidermidis is often a contaminate and tends to behave in a nonvirulent manner. However, it is known to cause biofilms, so catheters must be removed. The use of antibiotics in a short course may be beneficial depending on the clinical condition of the patient.

Answer: E

Pérez Parra A, Cruz Menárquez M, Pérez Granda MJ A simple educational intervention to decrease incidence of central line-associated bloodstream infection (CLABSI) in intensive care units with low baseline incidence of CLABSI. *Infect Control Hosp Epidemiol.* 2010;31(9):964–967.

Pronovost P, Needham D, Berenholtz S, et al. An intervention to decrease catheter-related bloodstream infections in the ICU. *N Engl J Med.* 2006;355(26):2725–2732. Erratum in: New England Journal of Medicine (2007) 356 (25), 2660.

11 *A 60-year-old woman is admitted to the ICU from the operating room after undergoing an emergent right colectomy and end ileostomy for a perforated gangrenous cecum. Over the next 12 hours, she has escalating vasopressor requirements despite being adequately fluid resuscitated and is started on stress dose steroids. Despite all these measures, she remains*

in refractory shock. The addition of which therapeutic can best improve this patient's arterial pressure?
   A *Nitric oxide synthase inhibitor 546C88*
   B *Angiotensin II*
   C *Fludrocortisone*
   D *Vitamin C*
   E *Hypertonic saline*

The ATHOS-3 trials found that in patients with severe vasodilatory shock on high-dose catecholamine-based vasopressors and vasopressin, the administration of angiotensin II is associated with a 45% absolute increase in MAP response when compared to placebo. It has subsequently been approved for the treatment of refractory vasodilatory shock. Angiotensin II is a naturally occurring hormone secreted as part of the renin-angiotensin system that results in powerful systemic vasoconstriction. Angiotensin II is contraindicated in patients on ACE inhibitors. Nitric oxide synthase inhibitor 546C88 increased blood pressure in patients with septic shock but was associated with more frequent cardiovascular side effects and increased 28-day mortality (choice A). Fludrocortisone when used in conjunction with hydrocortisone has been demonstrated in the APROCCHSS trial to reduce mortality; however, it did not show an increase in MAP and subsequent trials questioned fludrocortisone's efficacy (choice C). Vitamin C has been shown to decrease organ dysfunction and mortality when administered early in combination with hydrocortisone and thiamine for patients with septic shock; however, it has not been shown to directly increase MAP (choice D). Hypertonic saline would increase intravascular volume, but would have no benefit in a patient who has been adequately resuscitated (choice E).

Answer: B

Khanna A, English SW, Wang XS, et al. Angiotensin II for the treatment of vasodilatory shock. *N Engl J Med.* 2017;377(5):419–430. doi: https://doi.org/10.1056/NEJMoa1704154. Epub 2017 May 21. PMID: 28528561.

López A, Lorente JA, Steingrub J, et al. Multiple-center, randomized, placebo-controlled, double-blind study of the nitric oxide synthase inhibitor 546C88: effect on survival in patients with septic shock. *Crit Care Med.* 2004;32:21–30.

Annane D, Renault A, Brun-Buisson C, et al. Hydrocortisone plus fludrocortisone for adults with septic shock. *N Engl J Med.* 2018;378(9):809–818. doi: https://doi.org/10.1056/NEJMoa1705716. PMID: 29490185.

Marik PE, Khangoora V, Rivera R, et al. Hydrocortisone, vitamin C, and thiamine for the treatment of severe sepsis and septic shock: a retrospective before-after study. *Chest.* 2017;151(6):1229–1238. doi: https://doi.org/10.1016/j.chest.2016.11.036. Epub 2016 Dec 6. PMID: 27940189.

12 A 71-year-old man with a history of poorly controlled diabetes presents to the ED for a foul-smelling
left lower extremity. He is found to be hypotensive
and tachycardic with altered mental status. He is
admitted to the ICU in septic shock and is awaiting
the OR for amputation. CMS has core measures for
septic shock and requires that the patient's volume
status be reassessed within 6 hours of admission.
Which of the following assessments qualifies for full
reassessment?

A Straight leg raise
B Point of care ultrasound
C Wedge pressure
D Central venous pressure
E Comprehensive physical exam

The Centers for Medicare and Medicaid Services core
measures require either a comprehensive physical examination or **two** other measures of volume status. The *comprehensive physical examination must include either:
focused examination documented by provider that
includes vital signs (including blood pressure, pulse, respiratory rate, and temperature), cardiopulmonary examination (heart and lung), capillary refill evaluation,
peripheral pulse evaluation, and skin examination; or two
of the following: central venous pressure measurement,
central venous oxygen measurement, bedside cardiovascular ultrasound, passive leg raise, or fluid challenge.*

Answer: E

Ford, H. *Severe Sepsis and Septic Shock: Management Bundle.*
Centers for Medicare and Medicaid Services, 2020.
ProCESS Investigators, Yealy DM, Kellum JA, et al. A
randomized trial of protocol based care for early septic
shock. *N Engl J Med.* 2014;370(18):1683–1693.
ARISE Investigators, ANZICS Clinical Trials Group, Peake
SL, et al. Goal-directed resuscitation for patients with early
septic shock. *N Engl J Med.* 2014;371(16):1496–1506.

13 A 63-year-old man with a past medical history of
depression for which he takes citalopram is admitted to the ICU following a motor vehicle collision. He
also has a history of anaphylaxis to cephalosporins
and vancomycin. After 10 days in the ICU, he
remains intubated and develops a fever to 39.9 °C.
Laboratory analysis shows hemoglobin level of
7.3 g/dL, white blood cell count 1500/μL, and platelet count 40 000/μL. Blood cultures from peripheral
blood and central venous catheters rapidly grow
gram-positive cocci in clusters. Rapid molecular
assay identifies the organism in the blood as
methicillin-resistant Staphylococcus aureus.
Sensitives are pending.

After removal of the central venous catheter, the
best antibiotic for this patient is?

A Linezolid
B Piperacillin/tazobactam
C Meropenem
D Daptomycin
E Vancomycin

Daptomycin and vancomycin are good options for MRSA
bacteremia. However, with the patient's history of anaphylaxis to vancomycin (choice E), daptomycin is preferred. Linezolid is not FDA-approved for Staphylococcus
aureus bacteremia as no significant data exist. Adverse
effects of Linezolid include worsening pancytopenia/
thrombocytopenia (choice A). Linezolid can also interact
with selective serotonin reuptake inhibitors (SSRIs) and
other drugs that may increase serotonin levels. This
patient is taking SSRIs (citalopram) and linezolid can predispose the patient to a higher risk of serotonin syndrome.
If a strain of Staphylococcus is resistant to oxacillin or
methicillin, it is resistant to all ß-lactam antibiotics,
including penicillins, cephalosporins, and carbapenems
(choice B/C). Piperacillin/tazobactam, ampicillin/sulbac-
tam, and meropenem do not have activity against MRSA.
Also, with the patient's history of anaphylaxis secondary
to cephalosporins, caution must be taken when administering penicillins or carbapenems.

Answer: D

Thwaites GE, Edgeworth JD, Gkrania-Klotsas E, et al.
Clinical management of Staphylococcus aureus
bacteraemia. *Lancet Infect Dis.* 2011;11(3):208–222.
Woytowish MR, Maynor LM. Clinical relevance of
linezolid-associated serotonin toxicity. *Ann
Pharmacother.* 2013;47(3):388–397.
Kelkar PS, Li JT. Cephalosporin allergy. *N Engl J Med.*
2001;345(11):804–809.

14 A 73-year-old man is admitted to the surgical ICU
after ground level fall leading to a subdural hematoma.
The patient's Glasgow coma score is 15. On admission,
he required placement of a urinary catheter. Three days
into hospitalization, although asymptomatic, he developed a fever which prompted a urinalysis and urine
culture to be sent during his workup. The urinalysis
demonstrates budding yeast and the culture grows
10^3 CFU Candida albicans.
What is the next best step?

A Start fluconazole
B Start micafungin
C Obtain ophthalmology consultation
D Remove the urinary catheter
E Flush the foley

Funguria is commonly seen in patients in the ICU. The most common pathogen is Candida species. Risk factors include an indwelling urinary catheter, immunosuppression, diabetes, TPN, and recent urologic procedures. In an asymptomatic patient, most candiduria is colonization and observation without antifungals is appropriate. This is confirmed by the urine culture demonstrating $< 10^5$ CFU. If a risk factor such as indwelling urinary catheter is present, the catheter should be removed or exchanged if still needed (Choice D). Persistent candiduria should prompt renal ultrasound or CT evaluation. Patients with candidemia should have an ophthalmologic evaluation to evaluate for endophthalmitis (choice C). *Candida albicans* is usually responsive to fluconazole (choice A), while other candida organisms such as glabrata should be treated with micafungin (choice B). Flushing the foley would not help with candiduria (choice E).

Answer: D

Kauffman CA, Fisher JF, Sobel JD, Newman CA. Candida urinary tract infections--diagnosis. *Clin Infect Dis.* 2011;52 Suppl 6:S452–S456.

Pappas PG, Kauffman CA, Andes D, et al. Clinical practice guidelines for the management of candidiasis: 2009 update by the Infectious Diseases Society of America *Clin Infect Dis.* 2009;48:503–535.

15 *A 59-year-old woman is admitted to the ICU after a sigmoid colectomy for perforated diverticulitis with end colostomy. On postoperative day 4, she is now having fever and chills. Two blood cultures are positive for vancomycin-resistant Enterococcus faecium. She is started on IV daptomycin.*

Which of the following laboratory parameters should be monitored for daptomycin toxicity?
A *Creatinine kinase*
B *Uric acid*
C *Activated partial thromboplastin time*
D *Platelets*
E *Amylase*

Clinical trials for daptomycin showed decreased skeletal muscle activity and increases in creatinine kinase levels. Daptomycin is approved in dose range 4–6 mg/kg every 24 hours, in patients with a creatinine clearance greater than 30 mL/min. The Infectious Diseases Society of America (IDSA) has endorsed higher doses for bacteremia and endocarditis. It is recommended to monitor creatinine kinase levels once weekly while on therapy (choice A). Uric acid (choice B), Ptt (choice C), Platelets (choice D), and Amylase (choice E) are not affected by daptomycin.

Answer: A

Bhavnani SM, Rubino CM, Ambrose PG, Drusano GL. Daptomycin exposure and the probability of elevations in the creatine phosphokinase level: data from a randomized trial of patients with bacteremia and endocarditis. *Clin Infect Dis.* 2010;50(12):1568–1574.

Arbeit RD, Maki D, Tally FP, et al. The safety and efficacy of daptomycin for the treatment of complicated skin and skin-structure infections. *Clin Infect Dis.* 2004;38(12):1673–1681.

Liu C, Bayer A, Cosgrove SE, et al. Clinical practice guidelines by the infectious diseases society of america for the treatment of methicillin-resistant Staphylococcus aureus infections in adults and children. *Clin Infect Dis.* 2011;52(3):e18–e55.

16 *Which of the following therapeutics has been found to help prevent Clostridium difficile-associated diarrhea?*
A *Prophylactic metronidazole*
B *Vancomycin enema*
C *Enteral nutrition*
D *Probiotics*
E *Proton pump inhibitors*

A recent Cochrane meta-analysis and systematic review and meta-analysis of 31 randomized controlled trials including 8672 patients, moderate certainty evidence suggests that probiotics are effective for preventing C. diff associated diarrhea. There is no evidence to suggest use of prophylactic oral, systemic or rectal antibiotic administration helps to prevent C. diff associated diarrhea. PPIs have been shown to be a risk factor for the development of C. diff.

Answer: D

Goldenberg JZ, Yap C, Lytvyn L, et al. Probiotics for the prevention of Clostridium difficile-associated diarrhea in adults and children. *Cochrane Database Syst Rev.* 2017;12:CD006095.

17 *A 24-year-old woman was involved in an ATV accident in which she collided with a tractor on her farm. She was found to have an extensive right lower extremity open fracture with large soft tissue defect and degloving injury. She was taken to the OR with orthopedics for washout and placement of external fixation. On hospital day 7, her wound was found to be black and necrotic appearing. Culture was found to be growing Mucormycosis. In addition to emergent surgical debridements, which of the following therapeutics should be initiated?*
A *Fluconazole*
B *Amphotericin B*
C *Caspofungin*
D *Voriconazole*
E *Liposomal amphotericin B*

Invasive fungal infections such as mucormycosis are a rare but serious complication of traumatic injury characterized by fungal angioinvasion and resultant vessel thrombosis and tissue necrosis. Risk factors for development in invasive fungal infections include large contaminated wounds from soil, gravel, and plant matter. Prompt recognition of the invasive infection is key although may be difficult to diagnose at first. Early treatment with aggressive surgical debridement and antifungals are key. The treatment of choice is Amphotericin B. Liposomal Amphotericin B has been shown to be equally efficacious with less adverse effects such as nephrotoxicity and less catheter-associated side effects (choice E). Fluconazole (choice A), Caspofungin (choice C), and Voriconazole (choice D) have no activity against Mucormycosis.

Type	Description
Type I	Clean wound <1 cm in diameter with simple fracture pattern and no skin crushing
Type II	A laceration >1 cm and <10 cm without significant soft tissue crushing. The wound bed may appear moderately contaminated
Type III	An open segmental fracture or a single fracture with extensive soft tissue injury >10 cm. Type III injuries are subdivided into three types
Type IIIA	Adequate soft tissue coverage of the fracture despite high-energy trauma or extensive laceration or skin flaps
Type IIIB	Inadequate soft tissue coverage with periosteal stripping
Type IIIC	Any open fracture that is associated with vascular injury that requires repair

Answer: E

Baldwin K, Babatunde O, Huffman G, Hosalkar H. Open fractures of the tibia in the pediatric population: a systematic review. *J. Child. Orthop.* 2009;3:199–208. doi: https://doi.org/10.1007/s11832-009-0169-6.

Lelievre L, Garcia-Hermoso D, Abdoul H, et al. Posttraumatic Mucormycosis. *Medicine*. 2014;93(24):395–404.

Kronen R, Liang SY, Bochicchio G, et al. Invasive fungal infections secondary to traumatic injury. *Int J Infect Dis.* 2017;62:102–111.

18 *A 25-year-old man was brought to the emergency room intoxicated after he was found at the bottom of a staircase. His GCS was 7 and he was intubated for airway protection. Upon intubation, he was found to have particulate matter and bile staining in his airway. A nasogastric tube was placed and chest x-ray confirms the position of the nasogastric and endotracheal tubes, but shows infiltrates in the right lower lobe. What is the most appropriate therapy for his aspiration?*

A *Fluconazole*
B *Piperacillin/tazobactam*
C *Vancomycin*
D *Piperacillin/tazobactam + vancomycin*
E *No antimicrobial therapy*

Aspiration is defined as the inhalation of oropharyngeal or gastric contents into the larynx and lower respiratory tract. Aspiration pneumonitis (Mendelson's syndrome) is a chemical injury caused by the inhalation of sterile gastric contents, whereas aspiration pneumonia is an infectious process caused by the inhalation of oropharyngeal secretions that are colonized by pathogenic bacteria. Aspiration of gastric contents results in a chemical injury of the tracheobronchial tree and pulmonary parenchyma, causing an intense parenchymal inflammatory reaction. The prophylactic use of antibiotics in patients in whom aspiration is suspected or witnessed is not recommended. Similarly, the use of antibiotics shortly after aspiration in patients in whom a fever, leukocytosis, or a pulmonary infiltrate develops is discouraged, since the antibiotic may select for more resistant organisms in patients with an uncomplicated chemical pneumonitis. With the presence of particulate matter in the airway, strong consideration for performing diagnostic/therapeutic bronchoscopy is warranted.

Answer: E

Marik PE. Aspiration pneumonitis and aspiration pneumonia. *N Engl J Med.* 2001;344(9):665–671. doi: https://doi.org/10.1056/NEJM200103013440908. PMID: 11228282.

19 *A 65-year-old man is recovering in the surgical ICU following subtotal colectomy and end ileostomy for severe clostridium difficile infection. He is receiving enteral nutrition via a nasogastric tube. He is having persistent gastric residuals of 250 mL.*
Which of the following is the best next step in management?
A *Discontinue enteral feeds for 2 hours and restart enteral nutrition at 50% of prior rate.*
B *Discontinue enteral feeds indefinitely and initiate TPN.*
C *Continue current rate of enteral feeding.*
D *Change to an elemental tube feed.*
E *Start promotility agents.*

Malnutrition is a major problem in the ICU. Critically ill patients are in a catabolic state requiring increased caloric demand. Trophic feeds in patients in septic shock have been demonstrated to lower mechanical ventilation days and length of stay. Enteral nutrition is frequently held for procedures, operations, and imaging studies. Multiple studies have shown that gastric residual volumes are unnecessary and only further contribute to malnutrition (choice A). TPN is not indicated with a functioning enteric tract (choice B). Elemental feeds are more costly and may help with absorption in patients with malabsorptive disease. They would have no effect on gastric motility (choice D). Promotility agents may decrease gastric residuals but do not affect mortality (choice E).

Answer: C

Reignier J, Mercier E, Le Gouge A, et al. Effect of not monitoring residual gastric volume on risk of ventilator-associated pneumonia in adults receiving mechanical ventilation and early enteral feeding: a randomized controlled trial. *JAMA.* 2013;309(3):249–256.

Patel JJ, Kozeniecki M, Biesboer A, et al. Early trophic enteral nutrition is associated with improved outcomes in mechanically ventilated patients with septic shock: a retrospective review. *J Intensive Care Med.* 2016;31(7):471–477.

McClave SA, Martindale RG, Vanek VW, et al. Guidelines for the provision and assessment of nutrition support therapy in the adult critically Ill patient: Society of Critical Care Medicine (SCCM) and American Society for Parenteral and Enteral Nutrition (A.S.P.E.N.). *JPEN J Parenter Enteral Nutr.* 2009;33(3):277–316.

20   *A 31-year-old woman is 32 weeks pregnant and works at a local grocery store at the deli counter. She presents to the hospital with high fevers, nuchal rigidity, and altered mental status. She is admitted to the ICU with the diagnosis of meningitis. CSF analysis is pending.*

What is the empiric antibiotic regimen of choice for this patient?
  A *Vancomycin and piperacillin/tazobactam*
  B *Vancomycin, ceftriaxone, and penicillin G*
  C *Vancomycin, ciprofloxacin, and ampicillin*
  D *Gentamicin, metronidazole, and amoxicillin*
  E *Vancomycin and cefotaxime*

Streptococcus pneumoniae followed by *Neisseria meningitidis* are the most common causative organisms for bacterial meningitis for the age group 16–50. Vancomycin and a third-generation cephalosporin should be used as empiric antibiotics (choice E). In pregnancy, there is also a risk of *Listeria monocytogenes* meningitis. Listeria is a facultative anaerobic gram-positive bacillus that is often transmitted via soft cheeses and smoked meats. The patient is at risk for this due to her occupation. Listeria is not susceptible to cephalosporins or vancomycin. A penicillin is necessary for adequate empiric coverage (choice B). Gentamicin and ciprofloxacin are pregnancy class D drugs and should be avoided during pregnancy (choice D).

Answer: B

Allerberger F, Wagner M. Listeriosis: a resurgent foodborne infection. *Clin Microbiol Infect* 2010;16(1):16–23.

Van de Beek D, de Gans J, Tunkel AR, Wijdicks EF. Community-acquired bacterial meningitis in adults. *N Engl J Med.* 2006;354(1):44–53.

6

Hemodynamic and Respiratory Monitoring

Jared Sheppard, MD, Christopher S. Nelson, MD, and Stephen L. Barnes, MD

Division of Acute Care Surgery, Department of Surgery, University of Missouri, Columbia, MO, USA

1 *A 19-year-old man suffering a gunshot wound (GSW) to the right chest is diaphoretic, hypotensive, tachycardic, and has decreased lung sounds in the right chest. He groans and localizes to painful stimuli. After placement of a thoracostomy tube, 1 L of dark blood is evacuated. Initial ABG shows:*

pH - 7.29

pCO_2 - 36

Bicarbonate: 17

Base excess: -8.6

Lactic acid: 5.3

Which of the above values is most concerning for shock in this patient?

A *pH*

B *PCO_2*

C *Bicarbonate*

D *Base excess*

E *Lactic acid*

The patient above clearly has significant blood loss from his GSW, such that he is in physiologic shock as a result of inadequate tissue perfusion. This can cause decreased GCS, and is consistent with his hypotension and tachycardia. Lactic acid is normally produced in excess by about 20 mmol/kg/day, which enters the bloodstream. It is then metabolized mostly by the liver and the kidney. Some tissues can use lactate as a substrate and oxidize it to carbon dioxide (CO_2) and water, but only the liver and kidney have the necessary enzymes to utilize lactate for the process of gluconeogenesis. In general, elevated lactate can be the result of increased production, decreased clearance, or both. The tissues which normally produce excess lactic acid include the skin, red cells, brain tissue, muscle, and the gastrointestinal (GI) tract. During heavy exercise, it is the skeletal muscles which produce the most excess circulating lactate, which normalizes in the absence of impaired hepatic metabolism. Inadequate perfusion causes inadequate oxygen delivery to the tissue beds, which prevents normal aerobic respiration on the cellular level. As a result, anaerobic respiration begins, which results in net 2ATP per molecule of glucose (compared with 32 net ATP with aerobic respiration), and produces lactate as a byproduct. This elevation in lactate is responsible for the changes in pH and subsequent base deficit exhibited by this patient. Shock and severe lactic acidosis (pH less than 7.2) are often comorbid, and this carries a mortality rate of about 50%. Survival is rare for severe lactic acidosis with shock when the pH had fallen under 7.0. The base deficit is also an indicator of severe shock; however, this choice is base excess.

Answer: E

Mayer K, Trzeciak S, Puri NK. Assessment of the adequacy of oxygen delivery. *Curr Opin Crit Care*. 2016;22(5):437–43. doi: 10.1097/MCC.0000000000000336. PMID: 27467272.

Bonanno FG. Hemorrhagic shock: The "physiology approach". *J Emerg Trauma Shock*. 2012;5(4):285–95. doi: 10.4103/0974-2700.102357. PMID: 23248495; PMCID: PMC3519039.

2 *A patient in the ICU is suffering from septic shock. Using the data available from a pulmonary artery catheter or an arterial line tracing, which of the following parameters are needed in order to calculate oxygen delivery (DO_2)?*

A *Pulmonary artery saturation, arterial saturation, cardiac output, oxygen consumption.*

B *Arterial pO_2, pulmonary artery pO_2, arterial saturation, cardiac output.*

C *Cardiac output, hemoglobin, arterial O_2 saturation, arterial pO_2.*

D *Stroke volume, hemoglobin, pulmonary artery pO_2, arterial saturation.*

E *None of the above.*

Tissues attempt to extract from blood the amount of oxygen required to maintain aerobic metabolism, thus mixed-venous O_2 tension falls when O_2 delivery (the product of cardiac output and arterial O_2 content) becomes insufficient for tissue needs. As a primary determinant of O_2 delivery, cardiac output measurements often prove helpful during selection of the appropriate ventilator settings (especially PEEP) for the patient with life-threatening hypoxemia. Depression of venous return may nullify any beneficial effect of improved pulmonary gas exchange in tissue oxygen delivery. A rational goal of resuscitative therapy in severe sepsis and shock is to restore balance between O_2 delivery and demand, and boosting cardiac output is fundamental to such an approach. Aggressive goal-oriented resuscitation in the earliest phase of management appears to improve mortality in septic patients. The oxygen delivery equation (below) expresses oxygen delivery in terms of cardiac output multiplied by the oxygen-carrying capacity of the blood. In order to calculate the oxygen delivery (DO_2) of a patient, cardiac output, hemoglobin, SaO_2, and PaO_2 must be known.

$$DO_2 = CO \times \{(1.34 \times Hgb \times SaO_2) + (0.003 \times PaO_2)\}$$

Answer: C

Mayer K, Trzeciak S, Puri NK. Assessment of the adequacy of oxygen delivery. *Curr Opin Crit Care*. 2016;22(5):437–43. doi: 10.1097/MCC.0000000000000336. PMID: 27467272.

3 *For a patient in hemorrhagic shock, when trying to increase oxygen delivery, which method is the most effective?*

A *Increasing hemoglobin*

B *Increasing preload*

C *Increase heart rate*

D *Increase oxygen content in the blood*

E *Increase the saturation of hemoglobin*

The oxygen delivery equation (below) is a function of cardiac output ($HR \times SV$), Hgb concentration, percent hemoglobin saturation with oxygen measured by blood gas (SaO_2), and percent of oxygen dissolved in the plasma itself, such that:

$$DO_2 = CO \times CaO_2$$

$$CaO_2 = \{(1.34 \times Hgb \times SaO_2) + (0.003 \times PaO_2)\}$$

$$DO_2 = CO \times \{(1.34 \times Hgb \times SaO_2) + (0.003 \times PaO_2)\}$$

However, this dissolved fraction of oxygen (PaO_2) factors only minimally into the overall oxygen delivery formula, as denoted by the 0.003 coefficient (Choice D). As such, while the PaO_2 is useful for determining various aspects of care (such as a P:F ratio in ARDS), it is essentially inconsequential in determining oxygen delivery. Typically, SaO_2 (oxygen saturation from blood gas) is used to calculate CaO_2. SPO_2 is oxygen saturation by pulse oximeter. Regarding goals of oxygen delivery, an indexed DO_2 (DO_2 divided by body surface area, denoted as DO_2i) of 400–600 mL/min/m^2 has been shown to be associated with increased survival. The most effective way to increase oxygen delivery is by increasing hemoglobin. When going from a hemoglobin of 6–8 would result in an increase of oxygen delivery by 33%. Increasing preload may increase cardiac output by increasing stroke-volume. It would be difficult to increase cardiac output easily by 33%. Increasing preload can often decrease PaO_2 (Choice B). Increasing heart rate is typically not a strategy used to increase cardiac output (Choice C). Increasing PaO_2 from 60 to 100 would only increase the saturation by 10% at the most as the saturation would only go from 90 to 100% (Choice E).

Answer: A

Lenkin AI, Kirov MY, Kuzkov VV, Paromov KV, Smetkin AA, Lie M, Bjertnæs LJ Comparison of goal-directed hemodynamic optimization using pulmonary artery catheter and transpulmonary thermodilution in combined valve repair: a randomized clinical trial. *Crit Care Res Pract*. 2012;2012:821218. doi: 10.1155/2012/821218.

Mayer K, Trzeciak S, Puri NK. Assessment of the adequacy of oxygen delivery. *Curr Opin Crit Care*. 2016;22(5):437–43. doi: 10.1097/MCC.0000000000000336. PMID: 27467272.

4 *A 36-year-old man following an MVC has open fractures of the bilateral lower extremities, as well as bruising across his lower abdomen and significant pain on abdominal exam. His vitals are as follows: HR 109, BP 125/95, SpO_2 98% on face mask, respiratory rate 18, and he is fully oriented and cooperative on exam. What percentage of total blood volume loss do you estimate the patient has experienced?*

A *<15%*

B *15–30%*

C *30–40%*

D *>40%*

E *Blood volume loss cannot be predicted in this patient*

The patient above has a narrowed pulse pressure (but is not yet hypotensive) and is tachycardic. He does not have any signs of overt shock (he is oriented and cooperative indicating adequate cerebral perfusion). Because of his tachycardia and narrowed pulse pressure with increased diastolic pressure, this would place him in class II shock, which is defined at 15–30% loss of total blood volume. By comparison, class I hemorrhagic shock is defined by less than 15% total blood volume loss, and typically does not have any significant vital sign abnormalities except for mild tachycardia. Class III hemorrhagic shock is achieved with 30–40% total blood volume loss, and will present with tachycardia, narrowed pulse pressure, hypotension, anxiety, and confusion. Therefore, a hypotensive patient from hemorrhagic shock has lost approximately 1.5–2 L of blood. Class IV hemorrhagic shock will have greater than 40% blood volume loss and will appear similar to class III but patients are typically lethargic instead of anxious. The astute clinician should recognize hemorrhagic shock long before the onset of hypotension, as by this point significant blood loss has already occurred. Instead, narrowed pulse pressure and tachycardia should be the first vital sign changes to point toward hemorrhage.

Answer: B

Bonanno FG. Hemorrhagic shock: The "physiology approach". *J Emerg Trauma Shock*. 2012;5(4):285–95. doi: 10.4103/0974-2700.102357. PMID: 23248495; PMCID: PMC3519039.

Lawton LD, Roncal S, Leonard E, Stack A, Dinh MM, Byrne CM, Petchell J. The utility of Advanced Trauma Life Support (ATLS) clinical shock grading in assessment of trauma. *Emerg Med J*. 2014;31(5):384–9. doi: 10.1136/emermed-2012-201813. Epub 2013 Mar 19. PMID: 23513233.

5 *A 16-year-old man trapped inside a house fire was found unconscious. He suffered a large laceration to his left lower extremity from some falling debris, and was intubated in the ED due to GCS of 6. His SpO_2 (from his pulse oximeter) shows 99%; however, his ABG drawn at the same time demonstrates a SaO_2 (from his blood gas) of 84%. You also note that he has pink nail polish on all of his fingernails. Which of the following could be a cause for this discrepancy?*

A *Acute blood loss anemia*

B *Carboxyhemoglobinemia*

C *Cyanide toxicity*

D *Positioning of the pulse oximeter on the patient's ear instead of his finger*

E *Nail polish*

Bedside pulse oximetry is a cornerstone of hemodynamic monitoring in the intensive care unit due to its noninvasive nature and accuracy. However, there are multiple situations in which readings can be erroneous. Once such example is sickle cell disease, which causes deformation of hemoglobin and decreases flow through the micro circulation, and thus causes an overestimation of readings. The clinical significance of these readings is often downplayed in studies. Acute blood loss anemia, by itself, seems to have no effect on oximetry readings

Table 6.1 Classes of hemorrhagic shock

Parameter	Class I	Class II (mild)	Class III (moderate)	Class IV (severe)
Approximate blood loss	<15%	15–30%	31–40%	>40%
Heart rate	↔	↔/↑	↑	↑/↑↑
Blood pressure	↔	↔	↔/↓	↓
Pulse pressure	↔	↓	↓	↓
Respiratory rate	↔	↔	↔/↑	↑
Urine output	↔	↔	↓	↓↓
Glasgow Coma Scale score	↔	↔	↓	↓
Base deficit*	0 to –2 mEq/L	–2 to –6 mEq/L	–6 to –10 mEq/L	–10 mEq/L or less
Need for blood products	Monitor	Possible	Yes	Massive transfusion protocol

*Base excess is the quantity of base (HCO_3^-, in mEq/L) that is above or below the normal range in the body. A negative number is called a base deficit and indicates metabolic acidosis.

Source: Data from: Mutschler A, Nienaber U, Brockamp T, et al. A critical reappraisal of the ATLS classification of hypovolaemic shock: does it really reflect clinical reality? *Resuscitation* 2013,84:309–313.

(Choice A). Most peripheral sensors use two wavelengths of light: those associated with oxygenated and deoxygenated hemoglobin. These light waves are in the near-infrared spectrum as these light waves can easily pass through bone and tissue. Thus, the light looks red as red light can passed through bone and tissue as well. The presence of carboxyhemoglobin and methemoglobin, which have differing specific wavelengths, causes an overestimation of oxygen saturation (Choice B). Cyanide toxicity would cause an inability to use oxygen as an electron acceptor in aerobic metabolism but would not change the SpO_2 (Choice C). Motion artifact has long been a reason for inaccuracy with peripheral sensors, and despite several attempts at correction, this remains a common cause of alarm that is not associated with actual patient decline (Choice D). Other causes of pulse oximetry inaccuracy include methylene blue, indocyanine green, indigo carmine, and black, blue, or green nail polish (Choice E).

Answer: B

Chan ED, Chan MM, Chan MM. Pulse oximetry: understanding its basic principles facilitates appreciation of its limitations. *Respir Med*. 2013;107(6):789–99. doi: 10.1016/j.rmed.2013.02.004. Epub 2013 Mar 13. PMID: 23490227.

6   *Following an MVC, A 47-year-old woman sustains a grade 4 splenic laceration and pelvic and femur fracture, for which she went immediately to the operating room. Following her operation, she remains intubated and is transferred to the surgical ICU for continued resuscitation and monitoring. She has a right internal jugular central line placed for CVP monitoring, as well as a right radial arterial line for monitoring of stroke volume variability. Which of the following measurements of stroke volume variability is consistent with insufficient intravascular volume?*

   A *2%*

   B *5%*

   C *10%*

   D *15%*

   E *Stroke volume variability is an unreliable predictor of intravascular volume status.*

Stroke volume variability is a naturally occurring phenomenon in which the arterial pulse pressure falls during inspiration and rises during expiration due to changes in the intrathoracic pressure secondary to negative pressure ventilation (i.e., spontaneous breathing). Variations over 10 mmHg have been referred to as pulses paradoxus. Reverse pulsus paradoxus is a same phenomenon with controlled mechanical ventilation. Stroke volume variability (SVV) is calculated from the percent variability in stroke volume between inspiratory and expiratory portions of the ventilator cycle. The differences in intrathoracic pressure from the ventilator directly affect the amount of venous return to the right ventricle, which determines the subsequent stroke volume (increased intrathoracic pressure decreases the amount of venous return, subsequently decreasing the stroke volume). This effect is magnified in states of volume deficiency, as the lower circulating volume is more subjected to the changes in intrathoracic pressure. A SVV of >13% has been shown to correlate well to a deficit in overall intravascular volume, and thus predicts an increase in stroke volume in response to fluid administration. Stroke volume variability can be measured from the arterial line using a variety of monitoring devices.

Answer: D

Pinsky MR. Functional hemodynamic monitoring. *Crit Care Clin*. 2015;31(1):89–111. doi: 10.1016/j.ccc.2014.08.005. PMID: 25435480; PMCID: PMC4250574.

Shi R, Monnet X, Teboul JL. Parameters of fluid responsiveness. *Curr Opin Crit Care*. 2020;26(3):319–26. doi: 10.1097/MCC.0000000000000723. PMID: 32332283.

7   *Pulse pressure variation (PPV), which quantifies the changes in arterial pulse pressure during mechanical ventilation, is one of the dynamic variables that can predict fluid responsiveness. In which of the following ventilated patients would PPV most reliably predict fluid responsiveness?*

   A *A 58-year-old woman with ARDS following an MVC.*

   B *A 93-year-old man with atrial fibrillation following total colectomy for stercoral ulcer.*

   C *A 27-year-old woman with abdominal compartment syndrome following a 63% total body surface area (TBSA) burn resuscitation.*

   D *A 68-year-old man with impending uncal herniation with a set respiratory rate of 35 breaths/min.*

   E *A 17-year-old man with complete transection at C4 following an MVC.*

Aortic pulse pressure is directly proportional to left heart stroke volume and aortic compliance. The variation in the pulse pressure (pulse pressure variation or PPV) should thus reflect stoke volume changes as a result of the respiratory cycle. With more intravascular volume, the respiratory influence on preload should diminish, and the variation in pulse pressure should similarly decrease. Several studies showed that PPV accurately predicts fluid responsiveness when patients are under controlled mechanical ventilation. Nevertheless, in many conditions encountered in the ICU, the interpretation of

PPV is unreliable (spontaneous breathing, cardiac arrhythmias) or doubtful (low V_T). However, there are certain instances in which the respiratory cycle does not significantly alter preload. If the patient has ARDS, he should be on low tidal volume lung-protective ventilation. Per ARDSNET protocol, a goal tidal volume of 6 mL/kg ideal body weight should be utilized in patients with ARDS. However, low tidal volumes have a less pronounced influence on preload, and several studies have shown that tidal volumes of at least 8 mL/kg are necessary for a reliable variation due to hypovolemia (Choice A). Atrial fibrillation (Choice B) likewise will alter pulse pressure due to changes in length between beats, thus changing the amount of time available for atrial/ventricular filling. This will result in intrinsic pulse pressure variation independent of volume status. In true abdominal compartment syndrome (Choice C), the increased abdominal pressure will prevent an adequate respiratory cycle, and similar to a patient with a set low tidal volume, this will result in significantly decreased effect on preload variation from hypovolemia. Increased respiratory rates (Choice D) can result in low PPV even in cases of sufficient intravascular volume, and thus PPV is not reliable when the heart rate/respiratory rate ratio is less than 3.6. The final patient (Choice E) may have altered hemodynamics secondary to neurogenic shock; however, this will not change the effect of respiratory cycle on ventricular filling. In medical critically ill patients, although no randomized controlled trial has compared PPV-based fluid management with standard care, the Surviving Sepsis Campaign guidelines recommend using fluid responsiveness indices, including PPV, whenever applicable. In conclusion, PPV is useful for managing fluid therapy under specific conditions where it is reliable. The kinetics of PPV during diagnostic or therapeutic tests is also helpful for fluid management.

Answer: E

Yang X, Du B. Does pulse pressure variation predict fluid responsiveness in critically ill patients? A systematic review and meta-analysis. Crit Care. 2014;18(6):650. doi: 10.1186/s13054-014-0650-6. PMID: 25427970; PMCID: PMC4258282.

Teboul JL, Monet X, Chemla D, Michard F. Arterial pulse pressure variation with mechanical ventilation. *Am J Res Crit Care Med.* 2019; 199(1):22–32. doi: 10.1164/rccm.201801-0088CI.

8 *A 32-year-old man is in your ICU following splenectomy and left hemicolectomy after he was kicked by a horse. On postop day 6, the patient is febrile, tachycardic, and hypotensive. Blood cultures are sent, and while awaiting results from gram stain and culture, you place invasive support and monitoring lines with a right internal jugular triple lumen central line and a left radial arterial line. In trying to evaluate whether his stroke volume will increase following fluid administration, you use ultrasound and observe his inferior vena cava during several inspiratory cycles. In regard to IVC diameter and respiratory variation, which of the following is true regarding IVC collapsibility?*

A *An IVC diameter variation of < 5% predicts an increase in SV in response to fluid administration.*

B *An IVC diameter variation of 5–8% predicts an increase in SV in response to fluid administration.*

C *An IVC diameter variation of 8–10% predicts an increase in SV in response to fluid administration.*

D *An IVC diameter variation of > 36% predicts an increase in SV in response to fluid administration.*

E *While used historically, the data do not clearly indicate that there is a consistent correlation between IVC variation and SV response to fluid administration.*

While IVC collapsibility or distensibility throughout the respiratory cycle (caval index) has been used for years as an adjunct to determine volume responsiveness in critically ill patients, the practice has demonstrated fairly poor reliability. In a systematic review and meta-analysis performed by Orso et al., 26 studies were evaluated that investigated the predictiveness of the caval index in both adult and pediatric intubated and non-intubated patients. While the caval index in intubated patients was more predictive than in non-intubated patients, there was not sufficient correlation among studies to show that IVC diameter throughout the respiratory cycle was a reliable method of predicting volume responsiveness.

Answer: E

Long E, Oakley E, Duke T, Babl FE; Paediatric Research in Emergency Departments International Collaborative (PREDICT). Does respiratory variation in inferior vena cava diameter predict fluid responsiveness: A systematic review and meta-analysis. *Shock.* 2017;47(5):550–9.

Orso D, Paoli I, Piani T, Cilenti FL, Cristiani L, Guglielmo N. Accuracy of ultrasonographic measurements of inferior vena cava to determine fluid responsiveness: A systematic review and meta-analysis. *J Intensive Care Med.* 2020;35(4):354–363. doi: 10.1177/0885066617752308. Epub 2018 Jan 17. PMID: 29343170.

9 *You are seeking an additional method to determine fluid responsiveness on the above patient, and one of your colleagues recommends attempting a noninvasive ventilator maneuver. Which of the following ventilator maneuvers can simulate a fluid challenge without actually administering volume?*

A *End-expiratory occlusion (EEO) test*
B *Deep inspiratory hold*
C *15-second elevated PEEP hold*
D *Increasing pressure support and decreasing PEEP*
E *Increasing tidal volume*

An end-expiratory occlusion test is done by increasing intrathoracic pressure during inspiration while on mechanical ventilation. The ventilation is stopped at end-expiration, at the level of positive end-expiratory pressure (PEEP). If done long enough, this increase in pressure results in decreased preload to the left ventricle and subsequently a reduced cardiac output. By performing end-expiratory occlusion (pausing mechanical ventilation at end-expiration for 15 seconds), the artificially reduced preload is eliminated, and so a preload increase is simulated. If there is significant change in stroke volume on bedside monitoring with inspiratory hold, this predicts that fluid administration would also increase stroke volume. A 2009 study by Monnet et al. evaluated EEO, passive leg raise, and a 500cc fluid bolus administration, and found that an increase in arterial pulse pressure > 5% during EEO was predictive of an increase in CO following volume administration. The other maneuvers listed would all decrease the left-sided preload and have the opposite effect.

Answer: A

Jalil BA, Cavallazzi R. Predicting fluid responsiveness: A review of literature and a guide for the clinician. *Am J Emerg Med*. 2018;36(11):2093–2102. doi: 10.1016/j.ajem.2018.08.037. Epub 2018 Aug 14. PMID: 30122506.

Monnet X, Osman D, Ridel C, Lamia B, Richard C, Teboul JL. Predicting volume responsiveness by using the end-expiratory occlusion in mechanically ventilated intensive care unit patients. *Crit Care Med*. 2009;37(3):951–6. doi: 10.1097/CCM.0b013e3181968fe1. PMID: 19237902.

10 *A 19-year-old man was injured in an MVC. He has a HR of 89 bpm, BP 134/78 mm Hg, SpO$_2$ 96%, RR 15 breaths/min, and the EMS crew relates that he was withdrawing to pain in all extremities, but was not opening his eyes or able to make any sounds, even with painful stimuli. A laryngeal mask airway was placed because endotracheal intubation was not successful. You exchange his laryngeal mask airway for an endotracheal tube in order to establish a definitive airway. Which of the following would be unreliable in confirming endotracheal intubation?*
A *Capnometry*
B *Bedside ultrasound*
C *Endotracheal tube fogging*

D *Flexible bronchoscopy*
E *Capnography*

Although routinely used, traditional methods for confirming the correct positioning of an endotracheal tube have limited reliability. These include stethoscopic audibility and symmetry of breath sounds and chest rise, direct visualization of the cords, ease of insufflation and recovery of tidal volume, tidal fogging and clearing of the endotracheal tube, palpation of the tube in the larynx, loss of voice, coughing and expulsion of airway secretions (Choice C), expansion of upper chest, and failure of the abdomen to progressively distend during gas delivery. To improve reliability and speed of placement, the physical detection of CO_2 during expiration by capnography and capnometry can be used (Choices A, E). CO_2 detection and measurement by these methods can occasionally and transiently be misleading. Minimal CO_2 is evolved or expelled during shock or circulatory arrest and some CO_2 may be liberated initially after esophageal intubation from gas trapped in the gastric pouch. However, this concentration falls rapidly as serial tidal volumes are delivered. When compressed, a large-capacity squeeze bulb affixed to the endotracheal tube will fail to fill easily if the tube is in the collapsible esophagus. Several studies have also established the efficacy of confirming endotracheal tube placement by direct trans-tracheal visualization with bedside ultrasound (Choice B). Although not always easily available, flexible bronchoscopy with visualization of the trachea would be confirmatory (Choice D).

Answer: C

Gottlieb M, Holladay D, Peksa GD. Ultrasonography for the confirmation of endotracheal tube intubation: A systematic review and meta-analysis. *Ann Emerg Med*. 2018;72(6):627–36. doi: 10.1016/j.annemergmed.2018.06.024. Epub 2018 Aug 14. PMID: 30119943.

Littlewood K, Durbin CG Jr. Evidenced-based airway management. *Respir Care*. 2001;46(12):1392–405; discussion 1406-7. PMID: 11728299.

11 *When inserting a pulmonary artery catheter, as the catheter is advanced from the right atrium into the right ventricle, which of the following pressures being recorded from the catheter changes the most?*
A *Diastolic*
B *Systolic*
C *Mean*
D *Central venous pressure*
E *All change equally*

When the catheter is inserted via the right internal jugular vein, the balloon is inflated 15 cm from the point of neck entry. From the RIJ approach, the RA is entered at approximately 25 cm, the RV at approximately 30 cm, and the PA at approximately 40 cm; the PCWP can be identified at approximately 45 cm. As a rule of thumb, the catheter tip should not require advancement of more than 20 cm beyond its current position before encountering the next vascular compartment. Coiling within the right ventricle and misdirection of the catheter should be suspected after reaching 45–50 cm and the appropriate PA waveform is not encountered. Fluoroscopy can be a helpful adjunct in difficult cases and is especially worthwhile to consider before attempting an insertion from the femoral site. When advancing the catheter from the RA to the RV, the systolic pressure will climb significantly owing to a functional tricuspid valve. During diastole, the valve is open, allowing for the diastolic pressure to remain the same between the RA and RV.

Answer: B

Whitener S, Konoske R, Mark JB. Pulmonary artery catheter. *Best Pract Res Clin Anaesthesiol* 2014;28(4):323–35. doi: 10.1016/j.bpa.2014.08.003. Epub 2014 Sep 8. PMID: 25480764.

Scheeren TWL, Ramsay MAE. New developments in hemodynamic monitoring. *J Cardiothorac Vasc Anesth.* 2019;33(Suppl 1):S67–72. doi: 10.1053/j.jvca.2019.03.043. PMID: 31279355.

12 *After correctly inserting the pulmonary artery catheter above, you attempt to determine the cardiac output, which is accomplished with the thermodilution principle. The patient with which of the following valvular abnormalities will have a falsely depressed reading?*
    A *Aortic stenosis*
    B *Aortic regurgitation*
    C *Mitral valve prolapse*
    D *Tricuspid stenosis*
    E *Tricuspid regurgitation*

Thermodilution is an indicator-dilution method of measuring blood flow. This method is based on the premise that, when an indicator substance is added to circulating blood, the rate of blood flow is inversely proportional to the change in concentration of the indicator over time. This can be accomplished by using a temperature change as an indicator. Using a pulmonary artery catheter, cold fluid is mixed in the right heart chambers and the cooled blood is ejected into the pulmonary artery and flows past the thermistor on the distal end of the catheter. The thermistor records the change in blood temperature over time. This information is sent to an electronic device that records and displays a temperature time curve. The area under the curve is inversely proportional to the rate of blood flow in the pulmonary artery, and this flow is equivalent to the cardiac output. Tricuspid regurgitation causes the cold indicator fluid to be recycled back and forth across the tricuspid valve (Choice E). This produced a prolonged, low-amplitude thermodilution curve, thus tricuspid regurgitation produces a falsely low thermodilution cardiac output. Aortic regurgitation, aortic stenosis, and mitral prolapse are left-sided heart abnormalities that can affect cardiac output but will not affect the thermodilutional method (Choices A, B, C). Similarly, tricuspid stenosis will still allow a steady rate of flow across the valve and will not affect thermodilution (Choice D).

Answer: E

Scheeren TWL, Ramsay MAE. New developments in hemodynamic monitoring. *J Cardiothorac Vasc Anesth.* 2019;33(Suppl 1):S67–72. doi: 10.1053/j.jvca.2019.03.043. PMID: 31279355.

Kobe J, Mishra N, Arya VK, Al-Moustadi W, Nates W, Kumar B. Cardiac output monitoring: Technology and choice. *Ann Card Anaesth.* 2019;22(1):6–17. doi: 10.4103/aca.ACA_41_18. PMID: 30648673; PMCID: PMC6350438.

13 *A 73-year-old woman undergoes a Roux-en-Y reconstruction for a perforated duodenal ulcer. She has an extended ICU stay complicated by ARDS and acute renal failure. A right internal jugular triple-lumen dialysis catheter is placed for CRRT. On hospital day 14, you notice erythema surrounding her right internal jugular triple-lumen central line. She also has had a rising leukocytosis and is febrile to 38.9 °C. Which of the following measures would have potentially helped to prevent this complication?*
    A *Placement of the central line in her right femoral vein.*
    B *Use of ultrasound during placement (assuming you placed the line without ultrasonographic guidance, and achieved access on the first stick).*
    C *Placement of a single lumen catheter vs a triple lumen catheter.*
    D *Use of a chlorhexidine-impregnated dressing.*
    E *Securement of the catheter with a suture rather than adhesive to prevent mobility of the line.*

Central line-associated blood stream infections (CLABSI) are a major risk of an indwelling central venous access, and major progress has been made with systemic guidelines implemented in most hospital systems to reduce their incidence. Placement of central lines in the subclavian vein has shown decreased rates of infection; however, other locations may be necessary for placement based on the patient's anatomy or injury pattern (Choice A). An increased number of passes before successful cannulation of the vein has been associated with increased risk of infection, and for this reason, ultrasound is recommended to achieve first-attempt vascular access (Choice B). In addition, ultrasound in real time use during the procedure has become the standard of care to decrease complications. While theoretical risk of infection increases with the number of lumens in a central line, this has not been borne out in literature (Choice C). Chlorhexidine-impregnated dressings significantly decrease the rate of infection, as do daily chlorhexidine baths of the line. While using a suture to secure a central line provides a more stable anchor, administering another wound (albeit small) to the skin from the needle also increases the risk of surrounding infection (Choice E).

Answer: D

Bell T, O'Grady NP. Prevention of central line-associated bloodstream infections. *Infect Dis Clin North Am.* 2017;31(3):551–9. doi: 10.1016/j.idc.2017.05.007. Epub 2017 Jul 5. PMID: 28687213; PMCID: PMC5666696.

Parienti JJ, Mongardon N, Mégarbane B, Mira JP, Kalfon P, Gros A, Marqué S, Thuong M, Pottier V, Ramakers M, Savary B, Seguin A, Valette X, Terzi N, Sauneuf B, Cattoir V, Mermel LA, du Cheyron D; 3SITES Study Group. Intravascular complications of central venous catheterization by insertion site. *N Engl J Med.* 2015;373(13):1220–9. doi: 10.1056/NEJMoa1500964. PMID: 26398070.

14 *In the above patient, which organism is most likely to be identified on a culture of the central line?*
   A *E. coli*
   B *Coagulase-negative staphylococci (CoNS)*
   C *E. faecalis*
   D *Pseudomonas*
   E *Clostridium*

Pathogen distribution and antimicrobial resistance, as reported to the National Healthcare Safety Network from 2011-2014 showed that among central line-associated blood stream infection (CLABSI), the most common causative pathogens were (in order): coagulase-negative staphylococci (20.9%), staphylococcus aureus (18.1%), Klebsiella spp (9.4%), Enterococcus faecalis (9.1%), Escherichia coli (7.4%), Enterobacter spp (5.5%), and Pseudomonas (3.4%). Multiple strategies have been studied and implemented to reduce the incidence of CLABSI, including antiseptic and antibiotic coating of the central lines; antiseptic/antibiotic impregnated catheters have been shown to result in a 2% absolute risk reduction of CLABSI. Another pillar of CLABSI prevention is catheter removal as soon as the catheter is no longer needed, as

well as catheter exchange when there is clinical concern of bloodstream infection. Prophylactic or scheduled catheter exchange versus removal when clinically indicated showed no difference in CLABSI rates, although procedure-related complications of catheter placement were more frequent in patients undergoing scheduled exchange.

Answer: B

Weiner-Lastinger LM, Abner S, Edwards JR, Kallen AJ, Karlsson M, Magill SS, Pollock D, See I, Soe MM, Walters MS, Dudeck MA. Antimicrobial-resistant pathogens associated with adult healthcare-associated infections: Summary of data reported to the National Healthcare Safety Network, 2015-2017. *Infect Control Hosp Epidemiol.* 2020;41(1):1–18. doi: 10.1017/ice.2019.296. Epub 2019 Nov 26. PMID: 31767041.

Bell T, O'Grady NP. Prevention of central line-associated bloodstream infections. *Infect Dis Clin North Am.* 2017;31(3):551–9. doi: 10.1016/j.idc.2017.05.007. Epub 2017 Jul 5. PMID: 28687213; PMCID: PMC5666696.

15 and 16:
A 78-year-old stunt pilot is involved in a training accident while attempting to land his plane. He sustains a large right subdural hematoma, right 1–9th rib fractures, left 2–7th rib fractures, bilateral pulmonary contusions, and a grade III liver laceration. Once in the ICU, a pulmonary artery catheter is placed, revealing the following values: MAP 60 mm Hg, PAP 40/20 mm Hg, PCWP 18 mm Hg, CVP 10 mm Hg, CO 4 L/min.

15 *In regards to determining his pulmonary vascular resistance (PVR):*
   A *It is a measurement obtained directly from the pulmonary artery catheter.*
   B *It can be calculated by (MAP – PCWP/CO) × 80.*
   C *It can be calculated by (mean PAP – LAP/CO) × 80.*
   D *It can be calculated by (LAP – PCWP/CO) × 80.*
   E *It can be calculated by (RAP – PCWP/CO) × 80.*

16 *The systemic vascular resistance (in dyne/sec/cm^{-5}) of the patient in the above question is:*
   A *840 dynes/seconds/cm^{-5}*
   B *1000 dynes/seconds/cm^{-5}*
   C *1300 dynes/seconds/cm^{-5}*
   D *1900 dynes/seconds/cm^{-5}*
   E *2200 dynes/seconds/cm^{-5}*

A major component of afterload is the resistance to ventricular outflow in the aorta and large, proximal arteries. The total hydraulic force that opposes pulsation flow is known as impedance. This force is a combination of 2 forces: a force that opposes the rate of change in flow (compliance), and a force that opposes mean or volumetric flow (resistance). Vascular resistance is derived by assuming that hydraulic resistance is analogous to electrical resistance. Ohm's law predicts that resistance to flow of an electric current (R) is directly proportional to the voltage drop across a circuit (V), and inversely proportional to the flow of current (I): R = V/I. This relationship is applied to the systemic and pulmonary circulations, creating the following derivations:

$$SVR = (MAP - CVP / CO) \times 80$$

$$PVR = (mean\ PAP - LAP / CO) \times 80$$

Systemic vascular resistance (SVR) reflects changes in the arterioles, which can affect emptying of the left ventricle. For example, if the blood vessels tighten or constrict, SVR increases, resulting in diminished ventricular compliance, reduced stroke volume, and ultimately a drop in cardiac output. The heart must work harder against an elevated SVR to push the blood forward, increasing myocardial oxygen demand. If blood vessels dilate or relax, SVR decreases, reducing the amount of left ventricular force needed to open the aortic valve. This may result in more efficient pumping action of the left ventricle and an increased cardiac output. If the SVR is elevated, a vasodilator such as nitroglycerine or nitroprusside may be used to treat hypertension. Diuretics may be added if preload is high. If the SVR is diminished, a vasoconstrictor such as norepinephrine, dopamine, vasopressin, or neosynephrine may be used to treat hypotension. Fluids may be administered if preload is low. Pulmonary vascular resistance (PVR) is similar to SVR except it refers to the arteries that supply blood to the lungs. If the pressure in the pulmonary vasculature is high, the right ventricle must work harder to move the blood forward past the pulmonic valve. Over time, this may cause dilation of the right ventricle, and require additional volume to meet the preload needs of the left ventricle. PVR can be calculated by subtracting the left atrial pressure (LAP) from the mean pulmonary artery pressure (PAP), divided by the cardiac output (CO) and multiplied by 80. To obtain the LAP pressure, a pulmonary artery catheter (PAC) is needed to perform a pulmonary artery occlusion pressure (PAOP), also known as pulmonary artery wedge pressure (PAWP). Normal PVR is 100–200 dynes/sec/cm^{-5}.

So, for question 15, PVR is equal to the difference between the PAP and the LAP divided by the cardiac output.

In question 16, the SVR is calculated by dividing the difference between the MAP and the CVP by the cardiac output and multiplying by the constant 80, such that: $[(60 - 10)/4] \times 80 = 1000$ dynes/seconds/cm^{-5}.

Answer: 15 – C, 16 – B

Kwan WC, Shavelle DM, Laughrun DR. Pulmonary vascular resistance index: Getting the units right and why it matters. *Clin Cardiol.* 2019;42(3):334–8. doi: 10.1002/clc.23151. Epub 2019 Feb 27. PMID: 30614019; PMCID: PMC6712411.

Wright SP, Granton JT, Esfandiari S, Goodman JM, Mak S. The relationship of pulmonary vascular resistance and compliance to pulmonary artery wedge pressure during submaximal exercise in healthy older adults. *J Physiol.* 2016;594(12):3307–15. doi: 10.1113/JP271788. Epub 2016 Mar 24. PMID: 26880530; PMCID: PMC4824842.

17 *A 43-year-old woman was assaulted with a baseball bat. She proceeds to the OR for laparotomy and splenectomy. She remains intubated, and postoperatively in the ICU, the chief resident places a right internal jugular vein central line to transduce CVP to assist in guiding resuscitation. Which of the following is true regarding the usefulness of CVP in predicting a response to fluid administration?*

A *CVP < 9 is predictive of an increase in stroke volume following IV fluid administration.*

B *CVP may be useful in predicting fluid responsiveness at extremes (e.g., <6 mm Hg or >15 mm Hg) but is not reliable for prediction of fluid responsiveness in middle ranges.*

C *An increase in CVP is indicative of an increase in cardiac output.*

D *CVP should be maintained as high as possible.*

E *CVP cannot adequately estimate the risk of extrathoracic organ congestion with fluid administration.*

Due to wide patient variability in Frank-Starling curves, using a single CVP number as a target for achieving increased SV is unrealistic, and has been shown to have limited clinical value in multiple studies (Choice A). However, using extremes of CVP may be useful to guide IVF administration. Eskesen et al. showed that significantly more patients with a CVP < 6 mm Hg responded to IVF than patients with a CVP > 15 mm Hg (Choice B). RA filling is dependent on a pressure gradient between mean systemic pressure and CVP, suggesting that as CVP rises, the cardiac output may actually decline (Choice C). Keeping CVP as low as possible while still allowing for adequate perfusion is associated with improved outcomes. In patients with ARDS, it has been shown that fewer days of mechanical ventilation were achieved when CVP was maintained as low as possible while still allowing adequate tissue perfusion following initial hemodynamic stabilization (Choice D). AKI has been shown to correlate with increased CVP in patients with CHF or sepsis. In patients undergoing hepatic operations, limiting CVP was associated with less risk of bleeding and improved outcomes. Of note, pulmonary edema does not appear to be linked to CVP (Choice E).

Answer: B

De Backer D, Vincent JL. Should we measure the central venous pressure to guide fluid management? Ten answers to 10 questions. *Crit Care*. 2018;22(1):43. Published 2018 Feb 23. doi:10.1186/s13054-018-1959-3.

Monnet X, Marik PE, Teboul JL. Prediction of fluid responsiveness: an update. *Ann Intensive Care*. 2016;6(1):111. doi:10.1186/s13613-016-0216-7.

18 *In the above patient, at what point during the respiratory cycle should CVP be measured in order to be most accurate?*
   A *End-inspiration*
   B *End-expiration*
   C *During an inspiratory hold*
   D *Only when PEEP is set at zero*
   E *CVP can reliably be measured at any point during the respiratory cycle.*

Intravascular pressure is the pressure of the blood inside the SVC measured at bedside, and is the pressure within the vessel lumen relative to the atmospheric pressure. Transmural pressure is the difference between the intravascular and intrathoracic pressures. As the intrathoracic pressure changes during the respiratory cycle, it will exert an effect on the measured intravascular pressure, and therefore the only time a truly accurate intravascular pressure can be measured is when the intrathoracic pressure is equal to atmospheric pressure. This only occurs at end-expiration.

Answer: B

Malbrain ML, De Waele JJ, De Keulenaer BL. What every ICU clinician needs to know about the cardiovascular effects caused by abdominal hypertension. *Anaesthesiol Intensive Ther*. 2015;47(4):388–99. doi: 10.5603/AIT.a2015.0028. Epub 2015 May 14. PMID: 25973663.

19 *An 86-year-old man with a history of CHF (last echocardiogram was performed 8 years ago, EF of 35%), atrial fibrillation, and pulmonary fibrosis is in your ICU following a left nephrectomy for renal cell carcinoma. On postoperative day 3, he has increased difficulty breathing and requires intubation. Post-intubation chest x-ray shows diffuse infiltrates and moderate pulmonary edema bilaterally. In order to ascertain whether his pulmonary edema is due to his heart disease, you utilize the portable ultrasound machine. Which of the following findings on bedside ultrasonography can reliably rule out pulmonary edema?*
   A *Lung pulse*
   B *Lung sliding*
   C *A-line pattern and absence of B-lines*
   D *A single B-line in one rib space*
   E *>3 B-lines on the same rib space*

Bedside ultrasonography is a noninvasive, readily available, and cost-effective method for real-time diagnosis in the ICU patient, and all critical care physicians should be comfortable and competent with routine use. Lung ultrasonography has greater diagnostic capability than physical exam, and can outperform plain film radiography in many instances. When evaluating for pneumothorax, the interface between the parietal and visceral pleura is seen between adjacent ribs; during a respiratory cycle, motion is seen if the two pleuras are in contact with each other (known as lung sliding), ruling out a pneumothorax at that location. Similarly, the pleural interface will show motion with cardiac motion, known as lung pulse. When evaluating the lung parenchyma itself, A-lines are seen in normal tissue, which are transversely oriented repeating reverberation artifacts with equal distances between them and the pleural line. B-lines, in contrast, are longitudinally oriented comet-tail-like lines that typically indicate pathology. In normal tissue, it is common to have occasional B-lines over the lower lateral chest and occasionally, single B-lines can be seen elsewhere; however, more than 3 B-lines in a single view is abnormal, reflecting an interstitial or alveolar irregularity. This can be due to both cardiogenic and non-cardiogenic causes (such as ARDS or interstitial lung disease). When a cardiogenic cause is present, the B-lines are typically diffuse due to a regular, smooth pleural surface. When a non-cardiogenic cause is present, the B-lines are nonhomogeneous with small subpleural areas of consolidation, owing to an irregular pleural surface. The presence of an A-line indicates that the pulmonary artery occlusion pressure is < 18 mm Hg, and can thus rule out cardiogenic pulmonary edema.

Answer: C

Koenig SJ, Narasimhan M, Mayo PH. Thoracic ultrasonography for the pulmonary specialist. *Chest*. 2011;140(5):1332–41. doi: https://doi.org/10.1378/chest.11-0348. PMID: 22045878.

(a)

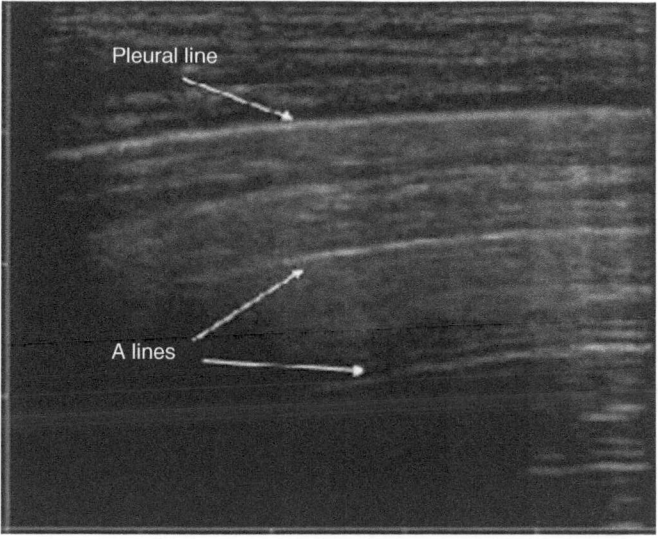

(b)

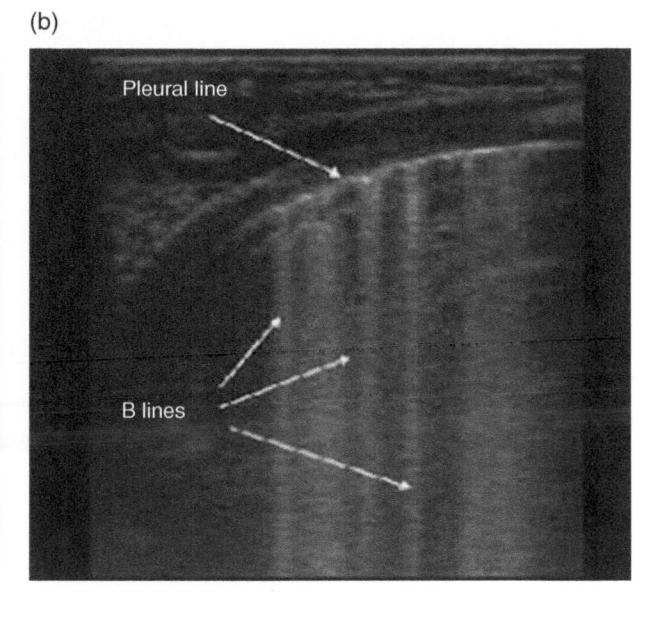

7

Airway and Perioperative Management

Jared Sheppard, MD, Jeffrey P. Coughenour, MD, and Stephen L. Barnes, MD

Division of Acute Care Surgery, Department of Surgery, University of Missouri, Columbia, MO, USA

1 *A 57-year-old man with a history of hypertension, hyperlipidemia, obstructive sleep apnea, and obesity (BMI 45 kg/m^2) is in your step down unit following a motor vehicle crash (MVC) 3 days ago, in which he sustained multiple bilateral rib fractures with associated pulmonary contusions. Initially, he required only nasal cannula to maintain a SpO$_2$ of 92%, but now requires heated high-flow nasal cannula at 70 L/min and 100% FiO$_2$, with a saturation of 86%. The decision is made to intubate. After giving RSI, you perform bag/mask ventilation to preoxygenate; however, you note significant difficulty with increasing his SpO$_2$. Which one of the following predicts difficulty of bag/mask ventilation?*

A *Age > 40 years*
B *BMI > 35 kg/m^2*
C *Neck circumference > 30 cm*
D *Facial hair*
E *Dentures*

Effective oxygenation and ventilation, while important, may be impossible in certain patient populations. While there is some dispute as to which factors are most predictive of bag-mask ventilation failure, Cattano et al. found the following to predict difficulty in BVM in the general surgical population: Age greater than 50 years old, BMI greater than 35, neck circumference greater than 40 cm, history of obstructive sleep apnea, history of difficult intubation, facial hair, and perceived short neck.

Answer: B

Saghaei M, Shetabi H, Golparvar M. Predicting efficiency of post-induction mask ventilation based on demographic and anatomical factors. *Adv Biomed Res.*

2012;1:10. doi: 10.4103/2277-9175.96056. Epub 2012 May 11. PMID: 23210069; PMCID: PMC3507007.
Cattano D, Killoran PV, Cai C, Katsiampoura AD, Corso RM, Hagberg CA. Difficult mask ventilation in general surgical population: observation of risk factors and predictors. *F1000Res.* 2014;3:204. Published 2014 Aug 27. doi: 10.12688/f1000research.5131.1.

2 *A 78-year-old woman with a history of COPD (80 pack-year history of cigarette smoking), peripheral vascular disease, hyperlipidemia, and malnutrition is admitted to your surgical ICU following a Whipple procedure for pancreatic adenocarcinoma, and remains intubated due to a mixed respiratory and metabolic acidosis. A medical student on service in the ICU asks if perioperative smoking cessation would have been of any value in this patient. You respond:*

A *Any amount of smoking cessation prior to a major operation has been shown to improve surgical site infection.*
B *Smoking cessation for at least 8 weeks duration has been shown to decrease cardiovascular complications.*
C *Smoking cessation for at least 4 weeks preoperatively reduces respiratory complications and wound-healing complications.*
D *Smoking cessation for 4 weeks only decreases wound-healing complications, but does not have a significant effect on respiratory complications.*
E *Smoking cessation for 2 weeks shows some reduction in wound-healing and respiratory complications.*

Smoking history drastically increases the chance of perioperative complication, especially in regard to wound-healing and respiratory complications. Wong et al. showed that 4 weeks of abstinence improved respiratory outcomes, while 2–3 weeks abstinence improved wound-healing complications without a significant effect on respiratory status. Mills et al. conducted a systematic review of randomized trials on smoking cessation and found that while 4 weeks smoking cessation had a significant improvement over less than 4 weeks, there was a nearly 20% increase in magnitude of effect for each week of cessation.

Answer: C

Mills E, Eyawo O, Lockhart I, Kelly S, Wu P, Ebbert JO. Smoking cessation reduces postoperative complications: a systematic review and meta-analysis. *Am J Med.* 2011;124(2):144–154.e8. doi: 10.1016/j.amjmed.2010.09.013. PMID: 21295194.

Wong J, Lam DP, Abrishami A, Chan MT, Chung F. Short-term preoperative smoking cessation and postoperative complications: a systematic review and meta-analysis. *Can J Anaesth.* 2012;59(3):268–279. doi: 10.1007/s12630-011-9652-x. Epub 2011 Dec 21. PMID: 22187226.

3 *A 59-year-old man with no significant past medical history is referred to your clinic for evaluation of an umbilical hernia. On exam, he has a reducible but tender umbilical hernia with an approximately 2 cm fascial defect. The decision is made to perform open repair. In preparation for his upcoming operation, what testing (if any) is indicated?*
   A *No testing is needed*
   B *Chest x-ray*
   C *Chest x-ray, EKG*
   D *Chest x-ray, EKG, CBC*
   E *Chest x-ray, EKG, CBC, BMP*

Appropriate perioperative cardiovascular evaluation is imperative for quality patient care. While traditionally certain tests were indicated solely based on patient's age, this practice has begun to fall by the wayside. According to current guidelines, a chest x-ray should be obtained for patients with signs or symptoms of cardiopulmonary disease, patients with COPD without a CXR in the past 6 months, and patients who smoke or who have had recent upper respiratory tract infections. EKG should be obtained for patients with signs and symptoms of cardiovascular disease. A CBC is indicated for patients at risk of anemia based on their history and physical exam, and those in whom significant blood loss is anticipated. BMP should be reserved for patients at risk of electrolyte abnormalities or renal impairment. A UA should be performed in patients undergoing urologic procedures or implantation of foreign material. A pregnancy test should be ordered for all women of reproductive age.

Answer: A

Feely MA, Collins CS, Daniels PR, Kebede EB, Jatoi A, Mauck KF. Preoperative testing before non-cardiac surgery: guidelines and recommendations. *Am Fam Physician.* 2013;87(6):414–418. PMID: 23547574.

Duceppe E, Parlow J, MacDonald P, Lyons K, McMullen M, Srinathan S, Graham M, Tandon V, Styles K, Bessissow A, Sessler DI, Bryson G, Devereaux PJ. Canadian cardiovascular society guidelines on perioperative cardiac risk assessment and management for patients who undergo noncardiac surgery. *Can J Cardiol.* 2017;33(1):17–32. doi: 10.1016/j.cjca.2016.09.008. Epub 2016 Oct 4. Erratum in: Can J Cardiol. 2017 Dec;33(12):1735. PMID: 27865641.

Siddaiah H, Patil S, Shelvan A, Ehrhardt KP, Stark CW, Ulicny K, Ridgell S, Howe A, Cornett EM, Urman RD, Kaye AD. Preoperative laboratory testing: implications of "Choosing Wisely" guidelines. *Best Pract Res Clin Anaesthesiol.* 2020;34(2):303–314. doi: 10.1016/j.bpa.2020.04.006. Epub 2020 Apr 22. PMID: 32711836.

4 *A 67-year-old woman with a history of atrial fibrillation, that is rate-controlled with metoprolol, presents with an acute episode of Hinchey III diverticulitis with associated peritonitis on exam. She is taken emergently to the operating room. Regarding perioperative beta blockade, which of the following is true?*
   A *While there is considerable controversy regarding initiating beta blockade in patients not currently on beta blockade, patients receiving a beta blocker should be continued on their home dose perioperatively.*
   B *Initiation of beta blockade during the perioperative period has been shown to reduce cardiovascular complications, while not changing overall mortality.*
   C *Initiation of a beta blockade during the perioperative period has been shown to reduce cardiovascular complications and improve mortality.*
   D *Patients with known CAD not currently on beta blockade and undergoing a high-risk operation should be initiated on a high-dose beta blocker.*
   E *Perioperative beta blockade should only be given to patients undergoing high-risk cardiac surgery, regardless of home prescription.*

Following Mangano's publication, beta blockade was considered one of the most effective means of protecting patients from adverse cardiac events during non-cardiac surgery. However, results were mixed in various trials that followed. The POISE trial was conducted as an attempt to demonstrate conclusive evidence for or against perioperative beta blockade. The trial, published in 2008, demonstrated cardiac protection, but also showed an increase in mortality, CVA, and hypotension in patients initiated on beta blockade in the immediate preoperative period. However, this study implemented high doses of beta blockade, and was thus criticized. Studies that followed have had mixed and similarly criticized results. What has been consistently shown is that there is benefit in continuing home beta blockade, and new beta blockade should likely be initiated in patients with high cardiac risk undergoing high-risk procedures, but high-dose beta blockade should be avoided.

Answer: A

POISE Study Group, Devereaux PJ, Yang H, Yusuf S, Guyatt G, Leslie K, Villar JC, Xavier D, Chrolavicius S, Greenspan L, Pogue J, Pais P, Liu L, Xu S, Málaga G, Avezum A, Chan M, Montori VM, Jacka M, Choi P. Effects of extended-release metoprolol succinate in patients undergoing non-cardiac surgery (POISE trial): a randomised controlled trial. *Lancet*. 2008;371(9627):1839–1847. doi: 10.1016/S0140-6736(08)60601-7. Epub 2008 May 12. PMID: 18479744.

Foex P, Sear JW. II. β-Blockers and cardiac protection: 5 yr on from POISE. *Br J Anaesth*. 2014;112(2):206–210. doi: 10.1093/bja/aet437. Epub 2013 Dec 15. PMID: 24343158.

Mangano DT, Layug EL, Wallace A, Tateo I. Effect of atenolol on mortality and cardiovascular morbidity after noncardiac surgery. Multicenter Study of Perioperative Ischemia Research Group. *N Engl J Med*. 1996;335(23):1713–1720.

5 *A 63-year-old man with a history of CAD status post CABG, HLD, HTN, and COPD is seen in your clinic for evaluation of a symptomatic right inguinal hernia, and the decision is made to perform an open repair. He states that he has had no shortness of breath or noted any cardiopulmonary symptoms. The patient asks if he should continue his daily aspirin and statin before his operation (scheduled for 14 days from now). You advise him:*

A *There are significant cardioprotective effects in continuing his statin through the perioperative period; however, he should hold his aspirin due to potential bleeding risk.*

B *Due to his history of CAD, he should continue his aspirin and statin, and should be started on a beta blocker in anticipation of his operation.*

C *The patient should continue his aspirin until 5 days before his operation, and should continue his statin through the perioperative period.*

D *While there is incomplete agreement, most expert panels recommend continuing aspirin for vascular procedures only, and continuing a statin throughout the perioperative period.*

E *The patient should continue his aspirin and statin and does not need to start a beta blocker.*

Perioperative aspirin should be continued for cardiac risk reduction unless there is a prohibitive bleeding risk. Statins have repeatedly demonstrated cardioprotective benefits in the perioperative period through an incompletely defined mechanism. Most evidence had shown benefit to statin use, but primarily in the vascular and cardiac surgery cohort. In 2017, London et al. demonstrated a significant risk reduction in 30-day all-cause mortality in patients exposed to statin on the day of surgery or the day following surgery, who underwent vascular, general, neurosurgical, orthopedic, thoracic, urologic, or otolaryngologic procedures.

Answer: E

Holt NF. Perioperative cardiac risk reduction. *Am Fam Physician*. 2012;85(3):239–246. PMID: 22335263.

London MJ, Schwartz GG, Hur K, Henderson WG. Association of perioperative statin use with mortality and morbidity after major noncardiac surgery. *JAMA Intern Med*. 2017;177(2):231–242. doi: 10.1001/jamainternmed.2016.8005. PMID: 27992624.

6 *A 34-year-old woman arrives in your trauma bay following an MVC in which she was the ejected driver. She was unresponsive at the scene, with hypotension and tachycardia noted by EMS. Upon arrival to the trauma bay, she has a GCS of 6 with a HR of 130, BP 106/89, SpO_2 of 91% on facemask, and has a respiratory rate of 28. She has scattered abrasions on her trunk, and FAST exam demonstrates fluid in the RUQ, as well as a gravid uterus. Which of the following is true in regard to this patient's pregnancy?*

A *Her pulmonary status and likelihood of first attempt success at intubation are unchanged compared to a nonpregnant counterpart.*

B *A chest tube should be placed approximately 3–4 rib spaces higher than in the nonpregnant patient.*

C *She is more susceptible to metabolic acidosis than a nonpregnant counterpart.*

D *This patient likely has a higher end-tidal CO_2 than a nonpregnant patient.*

E *Her risk of intra or retroperitoneal hemorrhage is lower than in a nonpregnant patient.*

The physiologic changes of pregnancy are important to know, especially in the trauma patient, and are summarized below:

Pulmonary: Pregnancy is associated with increased airway edema, O_2 consumption, and decreased RV and FRC. Therefore, intubation is technically more difficult and a patient may require a smaller endotracheal tube and additional airway adjuncts for successful airway management. It is important to properly preoxygenate prior to intubation. Increased tidal volume and minute ventilation lead to a compensated respiratory alkalosis, and elevation of the diaphragm in a gravid uterus requires chest tubes to be placed 1–2 rib spaces higher than in the nonpregnant patient.

GI: Decreased gastric emptying and LES tone lead to increased risk of aspiration.

CV: Increased plasma volume can delay recognition of hemorrhagic shock. Increased HR and decreased BP can alter the clinical picture in evaluating hypovolemic shock. Increased uterine and bladder blood flow, as well as increased vascular congestion, increased the risk of maternal hemorrhage with direct abdominal injury or retroperitoneal bleeding.

Renal: To compensate for pregnancy-associated respiratory alkalosis, the kidneys increase bicarbonate excretion. This leads to a decreased HCO_3, effectively reducing the capacity to buffer against a metabolic acidosis.

Answer: C

Sakamoto J, Michels C, Eisfelder B, Joshi N. Trauma in pregnancy. *Emerg Med Clin North Am*. 2019;37(2):317–338. doi: 10.1016/j.emc.2019.01.009. Epub 2019 Mar 8. PMID: 30940375.

Mendez-Figueroa H, Dahlke JD, Vrees RA, Rouse DJ. Trauma in pregnancy: an updated systematic review. *Am J Obstet Gynecol*. 2013;209(1):1–10. doi: 10.1016/j.ajog.2013.01.021. Epub 2013 Jan 17. PMID: 23333541.

Carroll MA, Yeomans ER. Diabetic ketoacidosis in pregnancy. *Crit Care Med*. 2005;33(10 Suppl):S347–S353. doi: 10.1097/01.ccm.0000183164. 69315.13. PMID: 16215358.

7   *A 28-year-old man presents to the trauma bay following a motorcycle crash in which he sustained significant head trauma. A CT brain from the referring facility demonstrates a large left-sided subdural hemorrhage with midline shift, and the patient has a GCS of 7, with a laryngeal-mask airway in place due to EMS being unable to perform endotracheal intubation. You prepare to establish a definitive airway in the trauma bay. Regarding induction medication selection in patients with traumatic brain injury (TBI), the optimal agents are:*

A   *Midazolam*
B   *Propofol*
C   *Etomidate*
D   *Ketamine*
E   *Both C and D*

While there are no absolute contraindications to any of the above medications for RSI in patients with TBI, the practitioner should be very aware of the consequences of each agent. Midazolam and propofol are both associated with a significant incidence of post-induction hypotension, subsequently worsening CPP and possibly increasing secondary brain injury. In fact, episodes of hypotension as short as 10 minutes have been shown to increase mortality in patients with TBI. However, administration of adequate oxygenation is also key – SpO2 of less than 90% is also associated with increased mortality. Etomidate and ketamine, on the other hand, have a significantly decreased incidence of post-administration hypotension and would be preferred for induction.

Answer: E

Shriki J, Galvagno SM Jr. Sedation for rapid sequence induction and intubation of neurologically injured patients. *Emerg Med Clin North Am*. 2021;39(1):203–216. doi: 10.1016/j.emc.2020.09.012. Epub 2020 Oct 31. PMID: 33218658.

8   *A 32-year-old man with a 4year smoking history (without COPD), hypertension controlled with losartan, and well-controlled type I diabetes mellitus is about to undergo emergent exploratory laparotomy for perforated appendicitis. Prior to making incision, the circulating nurse asks you to declare an American Society of Anesthesiologists (ASA) classification for this operation. The correct answer is:*

A   *2*
B   *2E*
C   *3*
D   *3E*
E   *4*

The American Society of Anesthesiologists developed this simple scale to describe the degree of a patient's medical illness. The numeric system was designed to ease communication between providers, provide a common language for documentation, and ease data abstraction for research. Because of variation among providers, it should not be used as the sole determinant of patient status and is not meant to act as an evaluation of perioperative risk.

ASA 1: Healthy patient; good exercise tolerance, excludes extremes of age.

ASA 2: Mild systemic disease, Mild diseases only without substantive functional limitations. Current smoker, social alcohol drinker, pregnancy, obesity (30 < BMI < 40), well-controlled DM/HTN, mild lung disease.

ASA 3: Severe systemic disease, Substantive functional limitations; one or more moderate to severe diseases. Poorly controlled DM or HTN, COPD, morbid obesity (BMI ≥40), active hepatitis, alcohol dependence or abuse, implanted pacemaker, moderate reduction of ejection fraction, ESRD undergoing regularly scheduled dialysis, history (>3 months) of MI, CVA, TIA, or CAD/stents.

ASA 4: Severe systemic disease, at least one severe disease that is poorly controlled or at end stage; possible risk of death; Recent (<3 months) MI, CVA, TIA or CAD/stents, ongoing cardiac ischemia or severe valve dysfunction, severe reduction of ejection fraction, shock, sepsis, DIC, ARD or ESRD not undergoing regularly scheduled dialysis.

ASA 5: Moribund patients not expected to survive more than 24 hours without surgery; ruptured abdominal/thoracic aneurysm, massive trauma, intracranial bleed with mass effect, ischemic bowel in the face of significant cardiac pathology or multiple organ/system dysfunction.

ASA 6: Brain-dead patients undergoing organ or tissue procurement procedures for transplantation.

An "E" is added to any case designated emergent.

The patient above has well-controlled disease of more than one body system, and requires emergent surgery, earning the designation ASA 2E.

Answer: B

Hurwitz EE, Simon M, Vinta SR, Zehm CF, Shabot SM, Minhajuddin A, Abouleish AE. Adding examples to the ASA-physical status classification improves correct assignments to patients. *Anesthesiology.* 2017;126:614–622.

Mayhew D, Mendonca V, Murthy BVS. A review of ASA physical status – historical perspectives and modern developments. *Anaesthesia* 2019;74:373–379.

9   You are waiting for your patient to arrive in the OR for a planned right inguinal hernia repair when anesthesia alerts you that they think you should reschedule your elective procedure due to uncontrolled hypertension. The patient currently has a BP of 178/100, and his only significant medical history is obesity, HTN, and HLD. He states that he has known about his hypertension for several months, but has not yet started his losartan that his PCP prescribed for him. He initially presented to the ED 3 days ago due to significant pain with his hernia and not being able to reduce it himself. Eventually, the surgical intern on call was able to reduce the hernia and the patient was discharged home. What is the appropriate course of action in this situation?

A   Cancel the case and reschedule for after he achieves better control with his prescribed regimen.

B   Admit the patient overnight for control of his blood pressure, with plans to operate the following day if he has responded to IV therapy.

C   Have a thorough discussion with the patient regarding risks and benefits, and proceed with the operation.

D   Administer high-dose beta blockade and, if successful, proceed with the operation.

E   This acute hypertension is likely due to pain and will likely resolve with sedation. Therefore, no intervention is needed.

While broadly encountered in the surgical population, there are no universal guidelines for case cancelation with hypertension in noncardiac cases. Based on risk stratification for adverse cardiac outcomes, several studies have shown that there is no benefit to delaying operations with stage 2 hypertension and accompanying target organ damage, or stage 3 hypertension (BP >180/110) without organ damage. In this scenario, the risk of delaying an operation (bowel incarceration, strangulation, or perforation, etc.) likely outweighs the risks of suffering a perioperative adverse outcome due to chronic hypertension. Sudden reduction in BP (as in choice B and D) can decrease perfusion pressure and are not recommended.

Answer: C

Sear JW. Perioperative control of hypertension: when will it adversely affect perioperative outcome? *Curr Hypertens Rep.* 2008;10(6):480–487. doi: 10.1007/s11906-008-0090-2. PMID: 18959836.

Vázquez-Narváez KG, Ulibarri-Vidales M. The patient with hypertension and new guidelines for therapy. *Curr Opin Anaesthesiol.* 2019;32(3):421–426. doi: 10.1097/ACO.0000000000000736. PMID: 31048597.

10   A 51-year-old man with alcoholic cirrhosis (MELD 19, weight = 50 kg) and a history of failed ventral hernia repair 7 years ago presents to the ED with severe abdominal pain, tachycardia, and acidosis. CT scan demonstrates incarcerated ventral hernia with surrounding air and fluid, consistent with perforated viscus. Laboratory studies are significant for a WBC of 17 000/mm³, Hgb of 12 g/dL, INR 3.1, and CO_2 of 15 mEq/L. Your chief resident asks what you would like to do prior to proceeding to the operating room to lower his bleeding risk. You respond:

A   Administer 2u fresh frozen plasma (FFP).

B   While the data are preliminary, prothrombin complex concentrate (KCentra) has shown encouraging results and may be of benefit.

C   Administer 10 mg IV Vitamin K.

D *Administer 15 mcg DDAVP.*

E *Proceed directly to the operating room as the emergent nature of his operation prohibits the time required to reverse his mildly elevated INR.*

Clearly, this patient requires an emergent operation, but requires reduction in his bleeding risk by treatment of his coagulopathy; accomplishing this is far from simple, however. Historically, reversal of coagulopathy of chronic liver disease (CCLD) was accomplished with FFP, with a dose of 10–15 mL/kg (which in this patient equates to 750 mL, and since there are 250 mL/unit of FFP, this would be 3 units). However, the data have fairly consistently shown that reversal of coagulopathy with FFP in this patient population is unreliable at best, with only transient changes in bleeding risk. Supratherapeutic doses of FFP can be given with slightly improved reversal; however, this exposes the patient to significant risk of volume overload, and should be avoided. IV vitamin K can be used to augment this reversal, but would be less effective in an emergent situation than FFP. DDAVP would be given at a rate of 3 mg/kg for treatment of uremic platelet dysfunction, but would be ineffective in correcting the INR in the above patient. A small study did demonstrate equivalence between DDAVP and FFP in bleeding reduction in patients with CCLD undergoing dental extraction, but there is currently no evidence to support DDAVP for acute reversal in this situation; furthermore, as previously mentioned, FFP is an unreliable reversal agent and so should not be the gold standard to which DDAVP is compared. PCC (KCentra) has more recently come to the market, and while there are no large-scale trials evaluating its role in coagulopathy of CCLD, several case reports and small studies have shown promising results. However, more research into its efficacy is needed.

Answer: B

Harrison MF. The misunderstood coagulopathy of liver disease: a review for the acute setting. *West J Emerg Med*. 2018;19(5):863–871. doi: 10.5811/westjem. 2018.7.37893. Epub 2018 Aug 8. PMID: 30202500; PMCID: PMC6123093.

Kujovich JL. Coagulopathy in liver disease: a balancing act. *Hematology Am Soc Hematol Educ Program*. 2015;2015:243–249. doi: 10.1182/asheducation-2015. 1.243. PMID: 26637729.

Pereira D, Liotta E, Mahmoud AA. The use of Kcentra® in the reversal of coagulopathy of chronic liver disease. *J Pharm Pract*. 2018;31(1):120–125. doi: 10.1177/0897190017696952. Epub 2017 Mar 15. PMID: 29278982.

Lesmana CR, Cahyadinata L, Pakasi LS, Lesmana LA. Efficacy of prothrombin complex concentrate treatment in patients with liver coagulopathy who underwent various invasive hepatobiliary and gastrointestinal procedures. *Case Rep Gastroenterol*. 2016;10(2):315–322. doi: 10.1159/000447290. PMID: 27482190; PMCID: PMC4945807.

11 *A 43-year-old woman presents to your trauma bay following an MVC. She is evaluated by standard ATLS protocol and is found to be hypotensive, tachycardic, and diaphoretic with a GCS of 14. FAST exam reveals fluid in Morrison's pouch. While preparing to bring the patient to the OR for exploration, the patient's husband alerts you that the patient takes rivaroxaban (Xarelto) for a provoked deep vein thrombosis 2 months ago. How should you proceed with her care?*

A *Administer prothrombin complex concentrate (PCC) and proceed to the operating room for exploration.*

B *Administer 15 mL/kg of FFP and proceed to the operating room for exploration.*

C *Proceed to the operating room immediately as hemodialysis is the only effective method of rivaroxaban (Xarelto) reversal.*

D *Administer platelets and proceed to the operating room for exploration.*

E *Administer protamine and proceed to the operating room for exploration.*

This patient requires an immediate operation to address her hemorrhagic shock. While proceeding to the operating room should not be delayed, her medication-induced coagulopathy should obviously be addressed. First-line reversal of direct factor Xa inhibitors (such rivarobaxan) is accomplished with prothrombin complex concentrate (PCC). Vitamin K antagonists (warfarin) is reversed with PCC first-line, and FFP as second-line therapy. Oral direct-thrombin inhibitors such as dabigatran are reversed with PCC first-line, with hemodialysis as second-line therapy. Heparin and LMWH can be temporarily and partially reversed with protamine. Aspirin and Plavix are treated with platelet transfusion, with desmopressin as a second-line option.

Answer: A

McCoy CC, Lawson JH, Shapiro ML. Management of anticoagulation agents in trauma patients. *Clin Lab Med*. 2014;34(3):563–574. doi: 10.1016/j.cll.2014.06.013. Epub 2014 Jul 19. PMID: 25168942.

12 *You evaluate a 74-year-old woman with a history of asthma and COPD who is brought to the trauma bay by EMS following a fall down a flight of stairs. Per EMS report, the patient had a GCS of 13 upon arrival for confused speech and localizing to pain only, and was initially hemodynamically normal. However, during transport, the patient became hypotensive and tachy-*

cardic. FAST exam in the trauma bay reveals fluid in the bilateral upper quadrants, as well as the pelvis, and she is taken immediately to the OR for exploration. During the operation, you are alerted that her thromboelastography (TEG) results are as follows:

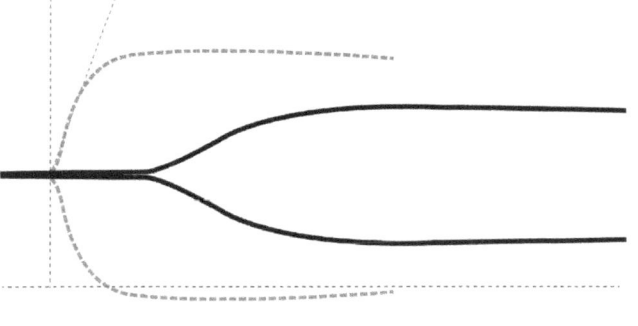

R (reaction time): Elevated
K (kinetics): Increased
α Angle: Decreased
MA (maximum amplitude): Decreased
LY30 (clot lysis): Normal

Based on these results, what intervention (if any) should be given?
A *Platelets only*
B *FFP and platelets*
C *TXA only*
D *Cryoprecipitate, platelets, and FFP*
E *Cryoprecipitate, FFP, and TXA*

This patient has an elevated reaction time (indicating that clot is taking longer than normal to form – which is a problem with coagulation factors, and as such should be treated with FFP), as well as an increased K (indicating the clot takes longer to reach a fixed strength – which indicates a fibrinogen deficiency and is thus treated with cryoprecipitate), and a decreased Alpha angle (indicating an elevated time of fibrin accumulation – which is a function of fibrinogen and platelet number, and is thus treated with cryoprecipitate and platelet transfusion). Additionally, the MA is decreased, indicating a decreased clot strength owing to platelet dysfunction, which can be addressed with platelet transfusion. An elevated LY30 indicates hyperfibrinolysis, which is reversed with TXA; however, the LY30 is normal in this patient.

Answer: D

Schmidt AE, Israel AK, Refaai MA. The utility of thromboelastography to guide blood product transfusion. *Am J Clin Pathol.* 2019;152(4):407–422. doi: 10.1093/ajcp/aqz074. PMID: 31263903.

13 *You are called to the intensive care unit to assist with a difficult airway in a patient with a sudden decline in mental status. The anesthesia resident has attempted intubation twice without success, and states he was unable to visualize the vocal cords on direct laryngoscopy. He is currently providing oxygenation and ventilation with bag-valve mask, and the SpO$_2$ is 91% and slowly rising. Which of the following should be performed?*
A *Consider placing a rescue device, such as laryngeal mask airway.*
B *Reattempt direct laryngoscopy with a different blade.*
C *Attempt to intubate over a blindly placed bougie.*
D *Continue with bag-mask ventilation until fully preoxygenated.*
E *All of the above.*

Establishment of an airway is critical in a patient who is unable to protect their airway. When difficulty is encountered, call for help, and follow your institution's difficult airway algorithm. Since more than 2 passes at intubation is associated with a significant increase in aspiration, hypothermia, and cardiac arrest, attempts should be made to optimize first-attempt success rate. This includes using an appropriate blade for direct laryngoscopy, providing adequate pre-oxygenation, optimizing hemodynamics, and choosing appropriate medication. A definitive airway is not always immediately needed – if appropriate oxygenation/ventilation is achieved with a laryngeal mask airway, then it should be used until a definitive airway is needed or ready to be placed.

Answer: E

Edelman DA, Perkins EJ, Brewster DJ. Difficult airway management algorithms: a directed review. *Anaesthesia.* 2019;74(9):1175–1185. doi: 10.1111/anae.14779. Epub 2019 Jul 21. PMID: 31328259.

Natt BS, Malo J, Hypes CD, Sakles JC, Mosier JM. Strategies to improve first attempt success at intubation in critically ill patients. *Br J Anaesth* 2016;117 Suppl 1:i60–i68. doi: 10.1093/bja/aew061. Epub 2016 May 24. PMID: 27221259.

14 *In the above patient, after placing an LMA, the patient begins to desaturate, and you notice that there is limited chest wall rise with inspiration. You then attempt another pass at direct laryngoscopy, and while you can see the vocal cords, you cannot pass the endotracheal tube. While attempting to provide adequate bag-mask ventilation, the patient has*

an SpO$_2$ of 78% which does not rise. The most appropriate next step is to:

A *Proceed with cricothyroidotomy*

B *Replace the LMA*

C *Proceed with percutaneous tracheostomy*

D *Proceed with open tracheostomy*

E *Re-dose your paralytic to improve ease of ventilation with bag-mask ventilation*

This difficult airway has now become a failed airway, and prompt action is needed to establish an airway before the patient arrests. A surgical airway is indicated. While tracheostomy could be performed, a cricothyroidotomy is still the procedure of choice given the more easily identifiable anatomy and closer proximity of skin to tracheal lumen.

Answer: A

Edelman DA, Perkins EJ, Brewster DJ. Difficult airway management algorithms: a directed review. *Anaesthesia* 2019;74(9):1175–1185. doi: 10.1111/anae.14779. Epub 2019 Jul 21. PMID: 31328259.

Natt BS, Malo J, Hypes CD, Sakles JC, Mosier JM. Strategies to improve first attempt success at intubation in critically ill patients. *Br J Anaesth*. 2016;117 Suppl 1:i60–i68. doi: 10.1093/bja/aew061. Epub 2016 May 24. PMID: 27221259.

15 *A 65-year-old man is in your intensive care unit following a motor vehicle crash in which he sustained pelvic fractures requiring percutaneous fixation, fractures of left ribs 1–7, and associated pulmonary contusions. His pain is well-controlled, and he is deemed fit to discharge to inpatient rehabilitation. Due to his pelvic fracture pattern, your orthopedic colleague requests that the patient be placed on DVT prophylaxis with warfarin for 6 weeks from the date of operation. Assuming anticoagulation is beneficial in this patient, your response should be:*

A *Place the patient on warfarin, and ensure an INR of 2–2.5.*

B *Place the patient on a NOAC.*

C *Place the patient on dual anti platelet therapy with aspirin and plavix.*

D *Place the patient on twice daily lovenox.*

E *Place the patient on aspirin alone.*

Many patients were historically were started on anticoagulation for the prevention of DVTs following orthopedic operations of the lower extremities. Over the past decade or so, there has been a trend to anticoagulate these patients with agents other than warfarin, due to fewer complications from bleeding, as well as decreased incidence of VTE in patients treated with alternate therapy. Aspirin has increasingly been studied as an alternate to low-molecular weight heparin and NOACs due to increased simplicity of administration, and multiple large-scale trials have shown aspirin to be non-inferior to other forms of anticoagulation.

Answer: E

Simes J, Becattini C, Agnelli G, Eikelboom JW, Kirby AC, Mister R, Prandoni P, Brighton TA; INSPIRE Study Investigators (International Collaboration of Aspirin Trials for Recurrent Venous Thromboembolism). Aspirin for the prevention of recurrent venous thromboembolism: the INSPIRE collaboration. *Circulation*. 2014;130(13):1062–1071. doi: 10.1161/CIRCULATIONAHA.114.008828. Epub 2014 Aug 25. PMID: 25156992.

Anderson DR, Dunbar MJ, Bohm ER, Belzile E, Kahn SR, Zukor D, Fisher W, Gofton W, Gross P, Pelet S, Crowther M, MacDonald S, Kim P, Pleasance S, Davis N, Andreou P, Wells P, Kovacs M, Rodger MA, Ramsay T, Carrier M, Vendittoli PA. Aspirin versus low-molecular-weight heparin for extended venous thromboembolism prophylaxis after total hip arthroplasty: a randomized trial. *Ann Intern Med*. 2013;158(11):800–806. doi: 10.7326/0003-4819-158-11-201306040-00004. PMID: 23732713.

Azboy I, Groff H, Goswami K, Vahedian M, Parvizi J. Low-dose aspirin is adequate for venous thromboembolism prevention following total joint arthroplasty: a systematic review. *J Arthroplasty*. 2020;35(3):886–892. doi: 10.1016/j.arth.2019.09.043. Epub 2019 Oct 5. PMID: 31733981.

15 *You are in the trauma bay during 5 simultaneous trauma activations. In order to most judiciously utilize your blood bank's resources, you are attempting to predict which patients will require a massive transfusion protocol (MTP). Which of the following patients is most likely to require MTP?*

A *A 19-year-old man with a GSW to the abdomen with negative FAST, SBP of 110 mm Hg, and HR of 100 beats/min.*

B *A 23-year-old woman involved in an MVC, with a positive FAST, SBP of 110 mm Hg, and HR of 100 beats/min.*

C *A 49-year-old man with a GSW to the abdomen with a negative FAST, SBP of 94 mm Hg, and HR of 115 beats/min.*

D *A 32-year-old man who was assaulted, with a positive FAST, SBP of 98 mm Hg, and HR of 130 beats/min.*

E *A 44-year-old woman with a stab wound to the LUQ with a negative FAST, SBP of 98 mm Hg, and HR of 110 beats/min.*

Identifying patients who will likely require MTP is essential in the trauma bay. The Assessment of Blood Consumption (ABC) scoring system relies on 4 non-weighted dichotomous parameters: penetrating mechanism, positive Focused Assessment with Sonography for Trauma (FAST), arrival systolic blood pressure (SBP) of 90 mm Hg or less, and arrival heart rate of 120 bpm or greater. Each positive parameter is given a score of 1, and the total score is evaluated out of 4. A score of 2 or greater predicts the need for MTP with a sensitivity of 75% and a specificity of 86%.

Answer: D

Maegele M, Brockamp T, Nienaber U, Probst C, Schoechl H, Goerlinger K, Spinella P. Predictive models and algorithms for the need of transfusion including massive transfusion in severely injured patients. *Transfus Med Hemother.* 2012;39(2):85–97. doi:10.1159/000337243.

Cotton BA, Dossett LA, Haut ER, Shafi S, Nunez TC, Au BK, Zaydfudim V, Johnston M, Arbogast P, Young PP. Multicenter validation of a simplified score to predict massive transfusion in trauma. *J Trauma.* 2010;69(Suppl 1):S33–S39. doi: 10.1097/TA.0b013e3181e42411. PMID: 20622617.

16 *A 37-year-old woman with a history of chronic cholecystitis undergoes a laparoscopic cholecystectomy which requires conversion to an open procedure due to significant inflammatory disease. The case is completed, and the patient is brought to PACU. While reviewing her postoperative labs, you note a blood glucose level of 190 mg/dL, as well as a mild acidosis and leukocytosis. In regard to her hyperglycemia, the following is true:*

   A *The patient is at increased risk of surgical site infection, as well as overall mortality, but her risk is less than that of a known diabetic.*

   B *The patient is at increased risk of surgical site infection, as well as overall mortality, but her risk is equal to that of a known diabetic.*

   C *The patient is at increased risk of surgical site infection, as well as overall mortality, and her risk is higher than that of a known diabetic.*

   D *The patient has an expected stress response to operation, and since she is not diabetic, no further intervention is required, and her risk of surgical site infection is not significantly increased.*

   E *There is no clear correlation between isolated episodes of hyperglycemia in non-diabetic patients, although there is a correlation for diabetic patients.*

There exists a dose-dependent relationship between blood glucose levels above 180 mg/dL and postoperative complications, including surgical site infection, length of stay, and overall mortality. Interestingly, this effect is more pronounced in patients who are non-diabetic than in patients who are diabetic. This is thought to possibly be due to several different causes, including a non-treatment bias in non-diabetics (patients with an established diagnosis of DM are more likely to receive insulin), and because hyperglycemia in non-diabetic patients is likely an indicator of a significant stress response, correlating with worse outcome. Glucose control should be maintained below 180, but overly restrictive control has been shown to have worse outcomes, especially in critically ill patients.

Answer: C

Kotagal M, Symons RG, Hirsch IB, Umpierrez GE, Dellinger EP, Farrokhi ET, Flum DR; SCOAP-CERTAIN Collaborative. Perioperative hyperglycemia and risk of adverse events among patients with and without diabetes. *Ann Surg.* 2015;261(1):97–103. doi: https://doi.org/10.1097/SLA.0000000000000688. PMID: 25133932; PMCID: PMC4208939.

Thompson BM, Stearns JD, Apsey HA, Schlinkert RT, Cook CB. Perioperative management of patients with diabetes and hyperglycemia undergoing elective surgery. *Curr Diab Rep.* 2016;16(1):2. doi: 10.1007/s11892-015-0700-8. PMID: 26699765.

17 *A 73-year-old woman with a history of rheumatoid arthritis (on 5 mg prednisone daily), carotid stenosis s/p carotid endarterectomy 4 years ago, and hypertension is in the ED with severe abdominal pain. Work up demonstrates diverticulitis with a significant amount of intra-abdominal free air. You post her for an emergent exploration. Regarding perioperative management of her steroids, which of the following is true?*

   A *She should receive 100 mg hydrocortisone/day for 2–3 days and resume normal oral therapy when she has return of bowel function.*

   B *She should receive 25 mg hydrocortisone at induction, and an IV equivalent of her home prednisone daily following her operation.*

   C *She should remain on the IV equivalent of her home prednisone.*

   D *She should receive 25 mg hydrocortisone at induction, and 100 mg hydrocortisone/day for 2–3 days and then resume her home equivalent.*

   E *She does not require any supplemental hydrocortisone and should hold her home dose.*

While "stress-dose steroids" are frequently given to patients on long-term glucocorticoid therapy due to fear of adrenal suppression, there is a fairly low yield of any data to support this. In patients who take less than 10 mg prednisone daily (or its equivalent), there is no indication for supplemental steroid in addition to whatever the patient's daily regimen is. For patients taking greater doses (>10 mg/day), there is no universally accepted regimen, but most recommendations are for 25–50 mg once on the day of surgery and continued at a similar rate for 2–3 days after surgery, with the goal to replace a physiologic dose of steroid. This can be assumed to be between 75–150 mg/day. If a patient has been off of daily steroids for greater than 3 months, they can be treated as if not on chronic steroids. Topical steroids are likewise not considered as necessitating perioperative steroid dosing.

Answer: C

MacKenzie CR, Goodman SM. Stress dose steroids: myths and perioperative medicine. *Curr Rheumatol Rep.* 2016;18(7):47. doi: 10.1007/s11926-016-0595-7. PMID: 27351679.

Chilkoti GT, Singh A, Mohta M, Saxena AK. Perioperative "stress dose" of corticosteroid: pharmacological and clinical perspective. *J Anaesthesiol Clin Pharmacol.* 2019;35(2):147–152. doi: 10.4103/joacp.JOACP_242_17. PMID: 31303699; PMCID: PMC6598572.

8

Acute Respiratory Failure and Mechanical Ventilation

Adrian A. Maung, MD[1] and Lewis J. Kaplan, MD[2,3]

[1] Yale School of Medicine, New Haven, CT, USA
[2] Division of Trauma, Surgical Critical Care and Emergency Surgery, Department of Surgery, Perelman School of Medicine, University of Pennsylvania, Philadelphia, PA, USA
[3] Corporal Michael J. Crescenz VA Medical Center, Philadelphia, PA, USA

1 *A 73-year-old woman is admitted to the intensive care unit after undergoing exploratory laparotomy and subtotal colectomy for C. diff colitis. Her past medical history is significant for smoking and clinically severe obesity with BMI 44.6 (height 160 cm, and weight 114 kg). She is hypotensive on a norepinephrine drip and mechanically ventilated on assist control volume mode of ventilation. The most appropriate initial tidal volume setting is:*

A *1100 mL*
B *684 mL*
C *312 mL*
D *520 mL*
E *912 mL*

The patient is at risk for developing acute respiratory distress syndrome based on her clinical condition as well as risk factors of smoking and morbid obesity. Low tidal volume ventilation, as described by ARDSnet, was the first intervention demonstrated to improve mortality in those with ARDS. Initial tidal volumes should be set at 6–8 mL/kg based on *predicted* (ideal) body weight. Based on the patient's height 160 cm, her predicted body weight is 52 kg thus answer C is the correct choice. Choice A is based on 10 mL/kg and actual weight. Choice B is 6 mL/kg but based on actual weight. Choice D is based on 10 mL/kg and ideal body weight and Choice E is 8 mL/kg and actual body weight.

Answer: C

Brower RG, Matthay MA, Morris A, et al. Ventilation with lower tidal volumes as compared with traditional tidal volumes for acute lung injury and the acute respiratory distress syndrome. *N Engl J Med.* 2000;342(18):1301–1308

Khan YA and Ferguson ND. *What is the Best Mechanical Ventilation Strategy in ARDS in Evidence-Based Practice of Critical Care*, 3rd Edition Elsevier 2020.

2 *48-year-old man has acute respiratory failure after a motorcycle crash. He is on low tidal volume, high PEEP ventilation with FiO_2 100% and his PaO_2 is 50 mm Hg. He is started on inhaled nitric oxide (NO). Based on the current evidence, the role of NO in acute respiratory failure is best characterized as:*

A *decreased mortality.*
B *improved oxygenation but not mortality*
C *decreased rate of acute kidney injury*
D *NO has no effect on oxygenation*
E *routine ARDS management*

Current clinical evidence does not support a role for inhaled NO in the routine management of ARDS. Although inhaled NO may improve oxygenation, it has not been shown to improve mortality (Answer B). NO has also been associated with increased rates of acute kidney injury.

Answer: B

Gebistorf F, Karam O, Wetterslev J, et al. Inhaled nitric oxide for acute respiratory distress syndrome (ARDS) in children and adults. *Cochrane Database Syst Rev.* 2016;(6):CD002787.

Ruan SY, Huang TM, Wu HY, et al. Inhaled nitric oxide therapy and risk for renal dysfunction: a systematic review and meta-analysis of randomized trials. *Crit Care.* 2015;19:137.

3 *27-year-old man with ARDS after debridement for necrotizing soft tissue infection of the perineum has worsening hypoxemia with PaO_2 90 mm Hg on 90% FiO_2 despite optimal low tidal volume ventilator settings and neuromuscular blockade. The next most appropriate step in his management would be:*

A *Inhaled nitric oxide*
B *High dose steroids*
C *ECMO rescue*
D *Prone positioning*
E *Continue current management and start prone positioning if there is no improvement after 72 hours.*

Clinical evidence supports the use of early prone positioning in patients with severe ARDS (answer D). The PROSEVA trial published in 2013 demonstrated an improved 28-day mortality with 16 hours of prone positioning per day (16% in the prone group vs 32.8% in control group). Most of the research has focused on early rather than a rescue role for severe ARDS and therefore waiting for 72 hours (choice E) would not be appropriate. Inhaled nitric oxide (choice A) has not been associated with improved outcomes. ECMO (choice C) has a role in the management of refractory hypoxemia but would not be the next step in the management of this patient. The role of early steroids remains controversial but there is no benefit to late (after 14 days) (choice B) steroid administration

Answer: D

Guérin C and Reignier J. PROSEVA study group. "Prone positioning in severe acute respiratory distress syndrome". *N Engl J Med.* 2013;368(23):2159–68. PMID: 23688302.

Guérin C, Albert RK, Beitler J, et al. Prone position in ARDS patients: why, when, how and for whom. *Intensive Care Med.* 2020;46(12):2385–2396. Epub 2020 Nov 10. PMID: 33169218; PMCID: PMC7652705.

4 *56-year-old woman who was initially admitted with necrotizing pancreatitis develops acute respiratory distress and hypotension. She is intubated and admitted to the intensive care unit. Over the next 24 hours, she is given 10 L of crystalloid for persistent hypotension and oliguria. She is on assist control volume-cycled ventilation (tidal volume 6 mL/kg, FIO2 30%, PEEP of 5) with an SpO2 of 98%. The ventilator is alarming for high pressure. Measurement of the pressures reveals a high peak airway pressure and a normal plateau pressure. The next step in management would be to:*
A *Decompressive laparotomy for abdominal compartment syndrome*
B *Neuromuscular blockade by continuous infusion*
C *Change to pressure support ventilation mode*
D *Adjust the ventilator alarm settings thresholds*
E *Inhaled bronchodilator therapy*

Elevated airway pressure can occur secondary to different pathologies that affect airway resistance and/or pulmonary compliance. The ventilator in many cases automatically reports the peak airway pressure but it is also important to measure the plateau pressure to distinguish between problems with pulmonary compliance (elevated plateau pressure) vs. problems with

airway resistance (difference between peak and plateau pressures). The patient in the clinical vignette is certainly at risk for development of abdominal compartment syndrome but a normal plateau pressure would point away from this diagnosis (choice A). A high peak pressure and normal plateau pressure is most suggestive of increased airway resistance that could be secondary to bronchospasm (Answer E), endotracheal tube occlusion, retained secretions and mucous plugging. Neuromuscular blockade (answer B) or a change to pressure support mode (answer C) would not address increased airway resistance. Ignoring the ventilator alarm (choice D) without further investigation is never a good idea.

Answer: E

Maung A and Kaplan L. Waveform analysis during mechanical ventilation. *Curr Probl Surg.* 2013; 50(10): 438–446. PMID: 24156841.

5 *Non-invasive ventilation in the critically ill patients is best supported by clinical evidence for this diagnosis:*
A *COPD exacerbation*
B *Acute Respiratory Distress Syndrome*
C *Post-extubation hypercarbic failure*
D *Hypercarbia due to severe traumatic brain injury*
E *Facilitating secretion clearance for pneumonia*

Multiple randomized trials have shown that non-invasive ventilation (NIV) decreases rates of intubation and improves mortality compared to standard therapy in patients with COPD exacerbation. (Answer A). NIV has also been shown to be helpful in acute cardiogenic pulmonary edema. There is currently conflicting (and even evidence that demonstrates deleterious effects) with using NIV in ARDS (choice b) and post-extubation failure (choice c). Contraindications to NIV include severe altered mental status (choice d) and copious secretions (choice e).

Answer: A

Plant PK, Owen JL and Elliott MW. Early use of non-invasive ventilation for acute exacerbations of chronic obstructive pulmonary disease on general respiratory wards: a multicentre randomised controlled trial. *Lancet* 2000;355(9219):1931–5. PMID: 10859037

Bourke SC, Piraino T, Pisani L, et al. Beyond the guidelines for non-invasive ventilation in acute respiratory failure: implications for practice. *Lancet Respir Med.* 2018;6(12):935–947. PMID: 30629932.

6 *The criterion that is most predictive of a successful attempt at liberation from mechanical ventilation is:*
A *Glasgow Coma Score of 8T*
B *Minute ventilation of 20 L/min*
C *Rapid Shallow Breathing Index of 40*
D *Maximal inspiratory pressure of −10 cm H_2O*
E *Calculated PaO_2/FiO_2 ratio of 125*

Although there is no single clinical predictor with the sensitivity and specificity to predict 100% successful liberation from mechanical ventilation, certain objective measures have been validated and used in combination as a screening tool. These include the rapid shallow breathing index < 105 breaths/min/L (answer C), minute ventilation < 10 L/min, an alert and appropriately interactive mental status, maximal inspiratory pressure less than –20 to –25 cm H_2O and a P/F ratio ≥ 150.

Answer: C

Baptistella AR, Sarmento FJ, da Silva KR, et al. Predictive factors of weaning from mechanical ventilation and extubation outcome: a systematic review. *J Crit Care.* 2018;48:56–62 PMID: 30172034.

7 *A 67-year-old woman with COPD is mechanically ventilated after undergoing cytoreductive surgery for ovarian cancer. She is on volume control ventilation with a decelerating waveform for gas delivery. Which of the following best describes the characteristics of the decelerating gas delivery waveform compared to a square waveform?*

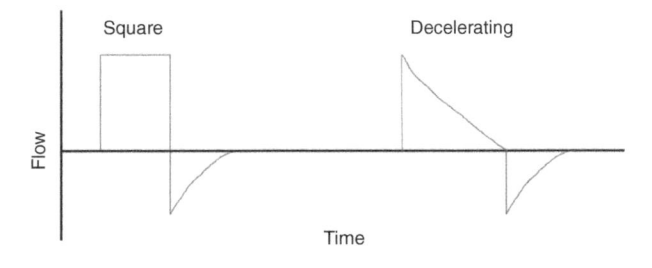

A *Higher peak airway pressure*
B *Higher likelihood of CO_2 retention*
C *Lower likelihood of CO_2 retention*
D *Shorter inspiratory time*
E *Lower mean airway pressure*

Two most commonly used gas flow waveforms in adults are square and decelerating. The square waveform is characterized by higher peak airway pressure, shorter inspiratory time (thus longer expiratory time) and lower mean airway pressure compared to the decelerating waveform (Choices: a, d and e). Since the expiratory time is shorter with the decelerating waveform, there is a higher likelihood of CO_2 retention (answer b) especially in patients who have preexisting limitation of expiratory flow such as COPD.

Answer: B

Maung A and Kaplan L Waveform analysis during mechanical ventilation. *Curr Probl Surg.* 2013;50(10): 438–446 PMID: 24156841.

8 *19-year-old woman has worsening respiratory failure over the past 48 hours. She is ten days after a motor vehicle collision resulting in multiple rib fractures, pulmonary contusions, and a grade 1 liver laceration. She is on low tidal volume ventilation, 100% FiO_2 with PaO_2/FiO_2 ratio of 71. She is being proned and was started on neuromuscular blockade. She is not on vasopressors and has a hemoglobin of 9 mg/dL The next most appropriate intervention would be:*
A *High frequency oscillation ventilation*
B *Veno-arterial ECMO*
C *Veno-venous ECMO*
D *Rib fracture fixation*
E *Helium-oxygen mixture*

Extracorporeal membrane oxygenation (ECMO) should be considered as salvage therapy in patients with refractory hypoxemia despite receiving standard care. In general, veno-venous ECMO (answer C) is utilized in patients who do not have severe cardiac dysfunction such as this patient and veno-arterial (choice b) is used in patients with hemodynamic compromise. Besides the inability to anticoagulated a patient, there are no specific absolute contraindications to ECMO. High frequency oscillatory ventilation (choice a) has been shown to have no benefit and possibly cause harm. Rib fracture fixation (choice d) remains an evolving therapy that is of optimal use in specific patient population but would not be appropriate in this patient due to severe ARDS. Helium-oxygenation mixture is sometimes utilized in cases with airflow resistance but would be contraindicated in this patient due to her high oxygen requirement.

Answer: C

Tillman BW, Klingel ML, Iansavichene AE, et al. Extracorporeal membrane oxygenation (ECMO) as a treatment strategy for severe acute respiratory distress syndrome (ARDS) in the low tidal volume era: a systematic review *J Crit Care.* 2017;41:64–71 PMID: 28499130.
Goligher EC, Munshi L, Adhikari NK, et al. High-frequency oscillation for adult patients with acute respiratory distress syndrome. a systematic review and meta-analysis. *Ann Am Thorac Soc.* 2017;14 (Suppl. 4):S289–S296 PMID: 29043832.

9 *Causes of postoperative respiratory failure in the immediate post-anesthesia period include which of the following:*
A *Inadequate reversal of neuromuscular blockade*
B *Opioid-induced respiratory depression*
C *Iatrogenic or negative pressure pulmonary edema*
D *Reduction in functional reserve capacity*
E *All of the above*

Early postoperative respiratory complications are common and may arise from multiple etiologies (answer e). General anesthesia and mechanical ventilation can lead to atelectasis and reduction in the functional reserve capacity of up to 50%, even in healthy individuals, especially if no PEEP is used during the procedure. Residual neuromuscular blockade can lead to impaired respiratory muscle strength and upper airway obstruction. Hypoxemia can be due to pulmonary edema, whether due to fluid resuscitation or negative pressure (identified more commonly in young, healthy, and muscular patients). Opioids, which are commonly administered both intraoperatively and postoperatively, can cause decreased respiratory drive, decreased level of consciousness, and upper airway obstruction due to a decrease in the supraglottic airway tone.

Answer: E

Karcz M and Papadakos PJ Respiratory complications in the postanesthesia care unit: a review of pathophysiological mechanisms *Can J Respir Ther Winter*. 2013;49(4): 21–9 PMID: 26078599.

Gupta K, Prasad A, Nagappa M, et al. Risk factors for opioid-induced respiratory depression and failure to rescue, a review. *Curr Opin Anaesthesiol.* 2018; 311:110–119 PMID: 29120929.

10 *A 46-year-old woman is invasively mechanically ventilated after developing pneumonia following a motorcycle crash. She is on assist control ventilation with oxygen saturations in the low 80s. Which of the following maneuvers would be most likely to improve her oxygenation.*
   A *Increase in tidal volume*
   B *Increase in respiratory rate*
   C *Change from square to decelerating waveform*
   D *Increase in expiratory time*
   E *Decrease in inspiratory time*

Oxygenation most closely correlates with mean airway pressure and reflects the area under the curve described by the gas-flow waveform. Change to a decelerating waveform (choice C) extends the inspiratory time and the area under the curve thus increasing the mean airway pressure. Increases in tidal volume (choice A) and respiratory rate (choice B) both increase the minute ventilation and likely CO_2 clearance but not oxygenation. Increase in expiratory time (choice D) increases the CO_2 clearance and maybe helpful in patients with significant airway resistance (e.g. asthma and COPD). This may however lead to poorer oxygenation due to decreased mean airway pressure. Decrease in inspiratory time (choice E) would lead to a lower mean airway pressure and possibly worse oxygenation.

Answer: C

Maung A and Kaplan L. Waveform analysis during mechanical ventilation. *Curr Probl Surg.* 2013; 50(10): 438–446 PMID: 24156841.

11 *A 52-year-old man is 6 days status-post ortho-topic liver transplantation and is evaluated by the rapid response team on the general floor for acute hypercarbic and hypoxemic respiratory failure as well as fever (T = 101.8° F) and hyponatremia (Na = 128 mEq/L). Which of the following modalities is the most appropriate for acute, pre-ICU management?*
   A *Diuretic administration*
   B *Oral endotracheal intubation*
   C *High-flow nasal cannula (HFNC)*
   D *Full face-mask BiPAP*
   E *Nasal mask CPAP*

This patient demonstrates acute respiratory failure in the setting of presumed volume overload. However, diuretic therapy will require some time to clear excess fluid in order to support oxygenation and CO_2 clearance. HFNC therapy and CPAP are much better at supporting oxygenation than CO_2 clearance - and the patient requires both. BiPAP may work but is less effective at immediate rescue in a patient who is anticipated to need higher PEEP, and a longer inspiratory time to support an increased mean airway pressure to correct hypoxemia. Also, BiPAP does not allow one to precisely control minute ventilation as does oral endotracheal intubation and mechanical ventilation regardless of patient location. This patient is expected to have an elevated CO_2 production based on fever and will therefore have a higher than usual minute ventilation requirement that is able to be met much better with invasive mechanical ventilation than with a non-invasive modality.

Answer: B

Moore S, Weiss B, Pascual JL, et al. Management of acute respiratory failure in the patient with sepsis or septic shock. *Surg Infect.* 2018; 19(2): 191–201; https://doi.org/10.1089/sur.2017.297.

12 *A 43-year-old woman is involved in a MVC. She sustains a grade 3 splenic laceration and flail chest with multiple rib fractures on the left side (3–9). She requires oral endotracheal intubation for acute respiratory distress. Which of the following management approaches is likely to result in the shortest duration of mechanical ventilation?*
   A *Paravertebral blocks*
   B *Multi-modal analgesics*

C *Liberation to helmet CPAP*
D *Epidural analgesic infusion*
E *Acute rib-fracture fixation*

While analgesics aid in managing pain, they do not restore thoracic cage stability. Furthermore, fracture stability also reduces pain. Only acute rib-fracture fixation accomplishes both goals. After fixation, liberation to helmet CPAP may be helpful in maintaining alveolar recruitment after general anesthesia and reducing work of breathing while in the PACU or SICU in the immediate peri-operative period.

Answer: E

Choi J, Gomez GI, Kaghazchi A, et al. Surgical stabilization of rib fracture to mitigate pulmonary complication and mortality: a systematic review and bayesian meta-analysis. *J Am Coll Surg.* 2020. DOI:https://doi.org/10.1016/j.jamcollsurg.2020.10.022

13 *During a disaster or pandemic when crisis standards have been activated, which of the following describes the best approach to allocating scarce resources such as ICU beds and invasive mechanical ventilators?*
   A *First-come-first-served*
   B *Youngest patients first*
   C *Maximum lives saved*
   D *Highest SOFA score first*
   E *Bedside clinician decision*

First-come-first-served is the approach when acute healthcare facilities operate using conventional standards and is in large part a libertarian approach. Age-based schemes use a life-cycle approach and may engender an element of ageism that does not incorporate the influence of underlying comorbid conditions such as malignancy. The highest SOFA score (higher score denotes greater organ failure) is an egalitarian approach and is characteristically inappropriate during crisis standards as those with the greatest illness will, in general, consume the greatest resources, including elements already in short supply and in a patient population with a reduced likelihood of survival. Maximum lives saved (greatest good for the greatest number) is the preferred approach as it is utilitarian and may be equitably supported by decision-making by a triage committee that is not directly involved in patient care.

Answer: C

Maves RC, Downar J, Dichter JR, et al. Triage of scarce critical care resources in COVID-19: an implementation guide for regional allocation an expert panel report of the Task Force for Mass Critical Care and the American College of Chest Physicians. *Chest.* 2020. https://doi.org/10.1016/j.chest.2020.03.063

14 *A 62-year-old clinically severely obese patient (BMI = 42) presents with presumed moderate COVID-19 pneumonia. CXR has ground glass opacities in mid - and lower lung fields. Room air ABG = pH 7.32, PaC0$_2$ 38, Pa0$_2$ 64; lactic acid = 3.2 mmol/L. Which of the following is the next most appropriate step in therapy after obtaining cultures, initiating fluid resuscitation, and administering empiric antibiotics as well as dexamethasone?*
   A *Initiate self-driven prone position therapy*
   B *Immediate oral endotracheal intubation*
   C *Begin helmet CPAP therapy*
   D *Non-contrast enhanced chest CT scan*
   E *Nebulized hypertonic saline and albuterol*

This patient has a body habitus that potentially precludes self-prone position therapy due to the risk of vomiting and aspiration. There is no acute need for airway control as CO_2 clearance is well-maintained and oxygenation may be addressed using other modalities. Non-invasive approaches also avoid iatrogenic ventilator-induced lung injury and ventilator-associated infection. A non-contrast enhanced CT scan of the chest may be useful from a diagnostic standpoint but will not help address the current clinical condition. Initial management of oxygenation using a continuous pressure but variable flow approach that also allows the patient to be seated upright is an ideal initial approach. There is heightened concern with nebulized medications in COVID-19 patients for possibly nosocomial transmission. This patient also does not have an indication for nebulized hypertonic saline at this time as hypertonic saline therapy in combination with albuterol is ideal for reducing the viscoelasticity of thick secretions but is not indicated to manage ground glass opacities.

Answer: C

Gaulton TG, Bellani G, Foti G, et al. Early clinical experience in using helmet continuous positive airway pressure and high-flow nasal cannula in overweight and obese patients with acute hypoxemic respiratory failure from coronavirus disease 2019. *Critical Care Explorations.* 2020;2(9). doi: 10.1097/CCE.0000000000000216

15 *In patients undergoing invasive mechanical ventilation, which of the following most strongly corelates with the risk of ventilator-induced lung injury?*
   A *Peak airway pressure = 35 cm H$_2$O pressure*
   B *Mean airway pressure = 14 cm H$_2$O pressure*

C *Positive End Expiratory Pressure = 12 cm H_2O pressure*

D *Plateau pressure = 28 cm H_2O pressure*

E *Driving pressure = 20 cm H_2O pressure*

Ventilator-induced lung injury (VILI) is often described as the impact of asymmetric distribution of a volume of gas into compliant alveoli that occurs over a short period of time and induces structural damage. That structural damage incites inflammation and leads to a process known as biotrauma that reflects activation of cytokines, the initiation of neutrophil trafficking, and the degradation of surfactant. As a result, alveolar interdependency is deranged, and regional time constants are lengthened. High tidal volumes are associated with these events as noted in the initial ARDSNet trials that led to the current common low tidal volume ventilation approach for ARDS. While high peak airway pressures may occur with inappropriate ventilator prescriptions, a peak pressure of 35 cm H_2O does not strongly correlate with VILI. Mean pressures of 14 cm H_2O may occur as the ventilator is adjusted to address hypoxemia, and a plateau pressure < 30 cm H_2O is an appropriate target.

PEEP of 12 is an acceptable pressure, is not associated with VILI and instead may define a patient population with a lung that is difficult to recruit. Driving pressures (plateau minus PEEP) > 15 appear strongly correlated with VILI and may be related to intra-tidal shear as well with rapid changes in pressure with breath cycling.

Answer: E

Williams EC, Motta-Ribeiro GC and Vidal Melo MF Driving pressure and transpulmonary pressure: how do we guide safe mechanical ventilation?. *Anesthesiol.* 2019; 131: 155–163 doi: https://doi.org/10.1097/ALN.0000000000002731.

16 *The square waveform for gas delivery during volume cycled ventilation is anticipated to be of benefit in which of the following patient populations?*
   A *Isolated traumatic brain injury*
   B *Blast injury pulmonary contusions*
   C *Abdominal compartment syndrome*
   D *Damage control open abdomen*
   E *Clinically severe obesity*

Blast injury-related pulmonary contusions lead to alveolar damage and collapse. Such patients benefit from alveolar recruitment to reduce hypoxic pulmonary vasoconstriction. A decelerating waveform – compared to a square waveform at the same peak flow rate for gas delivery – results in a longer inspiratory time and better matching of regional time constants as well as a lower peak airway pressure and a higher mean airway pressure. A higher mean airway pressure supports oxygenation. Since high peak airway pressures are a problem in those with the ACS, a square waveform is not ideal as it too is associated with higher peak pressures. With an open abdomen, using a decelerating waveform helps recruit the maximum number of alveolar units in preparation for abdominal wall closure and an increase in intra-abdominal pressure. A square waveform is associated with decreased recruitment by comparison. Since there are no valves between the brain and the right atrium, cerebral venous drainage is enhanced with more time at a lower intra-thoracic pressure – a direct consequence of a shorter inspiratory and a longer expiratory time, both of which are characteristic of the square waveform gas delivery profile. Those with clinically severe obesity demonstrate increased intra-abdominal pressure at baseline and therefore benefit from the use of a decelerating waveform to help reduce peak airway pressure and support postero-basal pulmonary recruitment as well.

Answer: A

Hamahata NT, Sato Rand Daoud EG Go with the flow-clinical importance of flow curves during mechanical ventilation: a narrative review. *Can J Respir Ther.* 2020;56: 11–20 doi: 10.29390/cjrt-2020-002. PMID: 32844110; PMCID: PMC7427988.

17 *A surgical ICU's data indicates that the mean length of time spent on mechanical ventilation is longer than desired. Which of the following is most likely to reduce the duration of mechanical ventilation for their patient population?*
   A *Emplacing a night-time intensivist*
   B *Using the ICU liberation bundle*
   C *Daily bedside physical therapy*
   D *Eliminating benzodiazepine use*
   E *Eliminating opioid analgesic use*

The goal of reducing the time spent on mechanical ventilation is a worthy goal for every ICU. This benefits from a multi-professional approach to care that empowers team members to work together across every shift to facilitate liberation from mechanical ventilation. Reduced time to liberation as well as increased ventilator free days are not associated with a night-time intensivist, physical therapy, nor eliminating a specific class of therapeutics. Both of those parameters are tightly tied to the A through F ICU liberation bundle that reduces ICU length of stay, duration of mechanical ventilation, delirium and coma, while engaging and empowering family members to participate in care and care planning. An important consequence of using the bundle is that patients often report more pain as sedating agents – including analgesics – are reduced to engage them in their own plan of care. This occurrence supports a multi-modal non-opioid approach to analgesia that helps address the opioid crisis as well. While it is unrealistic to eliminate opioid analgesic use, especially in the post-operative or post-injury patient, the use of opioids as the sole agent for sedation may be entirely abandoned in favor of other agents that target sedation as needed.

Answer: B

Pun BT, Balas MC, Barnes-Daly MA, et al. Caring for critically ill patients with the ABCDEF bundle: results of the ICU liberation collaborative in over 15,000 adults. *Critical Care Medicine*. 2019;47(1): 3. doi: 10.1097/ CCM.0000000000003482.

18 *The use of flexible bronchoscopy and bronchoalveolar lavage for the invasive diagnosis of pneumonia in the critically ill is associated with which of the following benefits?*
 A *Reduced FIO_2 requirement*
 B *Improved cardiac output*
 C *Increased anti-fungal agent use*
 D *Reduced antibiotic duration*
 E *Increased multi-drug resistance*

Flexible bronchoscopy and bronchoalveolar lavage (BAL) to invasively identify pneumonia confers the anticipated benefit of having confidence in the diagnosis of "no pneumonia". The lack of an infecting organism supports termination of empiric antibiotic therapy, reduced driving pressure for resistant organism genesis, and enhances an institutional approach to antibiotic stewardship. This in turn helps drive investigations into alternate explanations for the clinical findings and presentation. Flexible bronchoscopy for relief of lobar collapse from airway obstruction (but not BAL) is associated with reduced FIO_2 and improved cardiac output. Anti-fungal use is not increased by BAL, as those with risk factors for fungal pneumonia – and who have a compatible presentation – are generally empirically treated for fungal pathogens; guidelines to direct anti-fungal use have been articulated by a variety of organizations including the Infectious Disease Society of America.

Answer: D

Ranzani OT, Senussi T, Idone F, et al. Invasive and non-invasive diagnostic approaches for microbiological diagnosis of hospital-acquired pneumonia. *Critical Care*. 2019; 23(1): 51. https://doi.org/10.1186/ s13054-019-2348-2

19 *A 38-year-old patient with chest and abdominal blunt injury after a MVC has progressive ARDS and is managed using epinephrine and vasopressin infusions as well as glucocorticoid therapy for critical illness-related cortico-adrenal insufficiency. He has ongoing hypoxemic acute respiratory failure. Which of the following best supports pursuing cannulation for veno-venous extracorporeal membrane oxygenation (VV-ECMO)?*
 A *PaO_2/FIO_2 ratio of 135 on a FIO_2 of 0.7*
 B *Stabilized thoracic spine fractures*
 C *Inability to undergo prone position therapy*
 D *Increasing epinephrine dose for MAP support*
 E *Ejection fraction of 30%*

VV-ECMO provides oxygenation support and clears CO_2. It does not support cardiac performance. Therefore, an increasing need for vasopressor infusion or depressed ejection fraction does not drive one towards VV-ECMO but would instead favor veno-arterial ECMO. A PaO_2/ FIO_2 ratio of 135 on an FIO_2 of 0.7 indicates additional opportunity for oxygenation management such that ECMO is not required. Stabilized spine fractures should not generally influence the decision for VV ECMO. However, the inability to pursue standard care such as prone position therapy supports pursuing cannulation as rescue therapy, particularly in those with an escalating O_2 requirement or the progressive inability to clear CO_2.

Answer: C

Menk M, Estenssoro E, Sahetya SK, et al. Current and evolving standards of care for patients with ARDS. *Intensive Care Med*. 2020; 46:2157–2167. https://doi.org/10.1007/s00134-020-06299-6

20 *A patient with COPD has undergone an uneventful right hepatectomy for malignancy and arrives to the SICU intubated and mechanically ventilated. Settings are AC RR 12 breaths/minute, tidal volume 650 mL, FIO_2 50%, PEEP 5, decelerating waveform, peak flow rate = 60 LPM; P_{aw}peak = 32; P_{aw}mean = 8; SpO_2 = 96%; $ETCO_2$ = 42 torr and he is breathing with the ventilator. VS: T = 100.2°F, HR = 84 beats/minute, and BP = 132/74 mm Hg. One hour later, you are called for HR = 132 beats/minute, BP = 82/46, T = 98.9°F, SpO_2 = 84%, $ETCO_2$ = 58; RR = 20 breaths/minute. The most appropriate initial intervention is which of the following?*
 A *Return to the OR for hemorrhage control*
 B *Start a continuous epinephrine infusion*
 C *Therapeutic cardioversion for atrial fibrillation*
 D *Disconnect the patient from the ventilator*
 E *Emergency pleural decompression*

Patients with COPD often undergo surgery for unrelated conditions such as the patient in this question. Given that COPD eases gas entry but renders gas exit more difficult, such patients are at increased risk of gas trapping and increased intra-thoracic pressure. This is a particular risk on volume cycled ventilation when the patient's respiratory rate increases (anesthesia emergence, anxiety, pain, delirium, etc.) and their coupled expiratory time decreases. The physiology resembles tension pneumothorax in that venous return is compromised leading to decreased cardiac performance, but no pleural space occupying lesion is present. Instead, pulmonary overdistension is the issue in this unique patient population. Tachycardia and hypotension as well as hypoxemia and hypercarbia ensue, the former especially related to decreased pulmonary flow. Therefore, the *initial* therapy of choice is to disconnect from the ventilator and allow for exhalation.

Answer: D

Mosier JM and Hypes CD Mechanical ventilation strategies for the patient with severe obstructive lung disease. *Emerg Med Clin*. 2019; 37(3): 445–58. DOI: https://doi.org/10.1016/j.emc.2019.04.003

9

Infectious Disease

Rathnayaka M. K. Gunasingha, MD[1], Patrick Benoit, DO[1], and Matthew J. Bradley, MD[2]

[1] Walter Reed National Military Medical Center, Bethesda, MD, USA
[2] Uniformed Services University of the Health Sciences, Program Director General Surgery Residency, Walter Reed National Military Medical Center, Bethesda, MD, USA

1   *A 28-year-old man is found by police obtunded with a respiratory rate of four per minute in a local park. He was administered naloxone in the field and transported to the hospital. On arrival, he continues to be lethargic with a blood pressure of 90/54 mm Hg, heart rate of 103/min, respiratory rate of 16/min, and temperature of 101.1° F. Physical exam reveals a 3cm × 3cm area of erythema, fluctuance, and induration in his left antecubital fossa as well as tender nodules on his fingertips. Auscultation of his chest reveals a blowing diastolic murmur. A transthoracic echocardiogram is negative for any signs of endocarditis. The next steps in the management of this patient including blood cultures, fluid resuscitation, and I & D of abscess should include:*

A   *Transesophageal echocardiography, initiation of vancomycin*

B   *Transesophageal echocardiography, initiation of vancomycin and piperacillin-tazobactam*

C   *Transesophageal echocardiography*

D   *Metronidazole and piperacillin-tazobactam*

E   *Vancomycin and metronidazole*

This patient has 3 minor Modified Duke Criteria – (1) intravenous drug use, (2) fever > 100.4°F, and (3) Osler's nodes – that indicate possible endocarditis. Intravenous drug use is a risk factor for acquisition of infective endocarditis. The patient should receive a transesophageal echo (TEE) to evaluate his cardiac valves even though the transthoracic echocardiogram was negative as TEE is more sensitive for cardiac vegetations. *Staphylococcus aureus* is the most common organism that causes infective endocarditis, followed by *Viridans* group *Streptococci*, coagulase-negative *Staphylococci*, *Enterococcus* species, and *Streptococcus bovis*. Antibiotics should be started immediately after drawing blood cultures and should be broad to include MRSA coverage. Answer B is the correct choice as it provides broad-spectrum coverage as well as the TEE that is needed after a negative TTE in this patient whose presentation is suspicious for infective endocarditis. Answer A adequately covers for MRSA, but without a known causative organism, more broad-spectrum antibiotics should be initiated. Answer C is incorrect as it is critical that in cases of suspected endocarditis and sepsis that antibiotics be administered immediately after presentation. Answer D does not adequately cover against MRSA and is therefore incorrect. Answer E does not adequately cover gram-negative bacteria and is therefore inadequate as initial therapy for this patient. It is a strong recommendation to consult Infectious Disease to determine the optimal empirical antibiotic treatment. The fluctuance and induration at the patient's antecubital fossa indicate an abscess and must be drained as part of the treatment.

Surgical Critical Care and Emergency Surgery: Clinical Questions and Answers, Third Edition.
Edited by Forrest "Dell" Moore, Peter M. Rhee, and Carlos J. Rodriguez.
© 2022 John Wiley & Sons Ltd. Published 2022 by John Wiley & Sons Ltd.
Companion website: www.wiley.com/go/surgicalcriticalcare3e

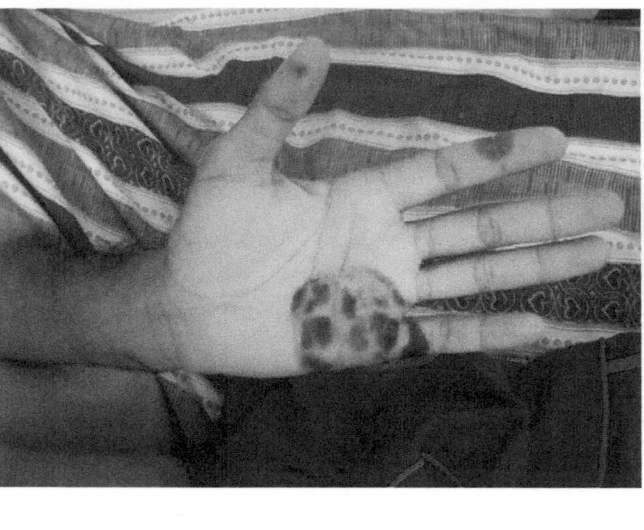 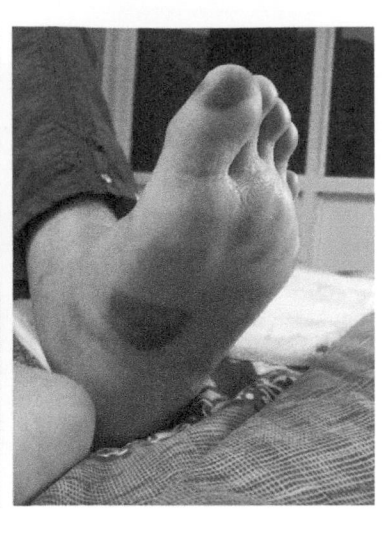

References for images:

Modified duke criteria

Pathological criteria
Positive histology or culture from pathological material obtained at autopsy or cardiac surgery
Major criteria
Two positive blood cultures with typical organism
Persistent bacteremia
Positive serology for Coxiella
Positive echocardiogram
1) Vegetation OR
2) Abscess OR
3) New regurgitation OR
4) Dehiscence of prosthetic valves
Minor criteria
Predisposing heart disease or IVDA
Fever > 38%
Immunological phenomena
Vascular phenomena
Microbiological evidence not fitting major criteria

Answer: B

Galindo R. Osler's nodes on hand. https://commons. wikimedia.org/wiki/File:Osler_Nodules_Hand.jpg. Published 2010. Accessed July 26, 2021.

Galindo R. Osler spots on foot. https://commons. wikimedia.org/wiki/File:Osler_Spots_foot.jpg. Published 2010. Accessed July 26, 2021

Baddour LM, Wilson WR, Bayer AS, et al. Infective endocarditis in adults: diagnosis, antimicrobial therapy, and management of complications: a scientific statement for healthcare professionals from the American Heart Association. *Circulation.* 2015;132(15):1435–1486. doi:10.1161/CIR.0000000000000296

Vogkou CT, Vlachogiannis NI, Palaiodimos L, et al. The causative agents in infective endocarditis: a systematic review comprising 33,214 cases. *Eur J Clin Microbiol Infect Dis.* 2016;35(8):1227–1245. doi:10.1007/s10096-016-2660-6

Wang A, Gaca JG, Chu VH. Management considerations in infective endocarditis: a review. *JAMA - J Am Med Assoc.* 2018;320(1):72–83. doi:10.1001/jama. 2018.75961.

Miller SE, Maragakis LL. Central line-associated bloodstream infection prevention. *Curr Opin Infect Dis.* 2012;25(4):412–422. doi:10.1097/QCO.0b013e3 28355e4da

Latif A, Halim MS, Pronovost PJ. Eliminating infections in the ICU: CLABSI. *Curr Infect Dis Rep.* 2015;17(7). doi:10.1007/s11908-015-0491-8

Noto MJ, Domenico HJ, Byrne DW, et al. Chlorhexidine bathing and health care-associated infections: a randomized clinical trial. *JAMA - J Am Med Assoc.* 2015;313(4):369–378. doi:10.1001/jama.2014.18400

2   *A 65-year-old man was admitted with acute pancreatitis and has been stable with intermittent tachycardia on the floor since his admission 2 days ago. Admission CT scan of the abdomen and pelvis showed edema and fat stranding around his pancreas. On the third day, he was noted to be more*

tachycardic, febrile with an increase of his leukocytosis. An interval CT scan demonstrates hypoattenuation of the pancreas, a large peri-pancreatic retroperitoneal fluid collection with air and surrounding fat stranding. The next best course of treatment is:

A *Start antibiotics with piperacillin-tazobactam.*

B *Start antibiotics and percutaneously drain the collection.*

C *Start antibiotics and surgery for emergent necrosectomy.*

D *Start antifungals and percutaneously drain the collection.*

E *Continue current treatment with IV fluid resuscitation.*

This patient has infected necrotizing pancreatitis based on the physiologic and laboratory changes and new findings on CT scan. Broad-spectrum antibiotics should be started since the fluid collection appears to be infected on clinical exam and on CT scan. In general, there is no indication to start antibiotics in necrotizing pancreatitis unless there is a culture-proven infection or a strong suspicion for infection (gas in collection, sepsis, and clinical deterioration). Prophylactic antibiotics should not be used for sterile necrosis. For infected pancreatic necrosis, a multicenter trial showed that a minimally invasive step-up approach (percutaneous drainage followed by minimal invasive retroperitoneal necrosectomy if needed) reduced major complications and death when compared to open necrosectomy. Answer A is incorrect because patient has indications for the need of drainage of the fluid collection. Answer C is not optimal as necrosectomy is now suggested to be reserved for failure of a step approach method. Answer D is incorrect because antifungals are not yet indicated. Answer E is incorrect because there is evidence of infection.

Answer: B

Da Costa DW, Boerma D, Van Santvoort HC, et al. Staged multidisciplinary step-up management for necrotizing pancreatitis. *Br J Surg.* 2014;101(1). doi:10.1002/bjs.9346

Baron TH, DiMaio CJ, Wang AY, et al. American Gastroenterological Association Clinical Practice Update: Management of Pancreatic Necrosis. *Gastroenterology.* 2020;158(1):67–75.e1. doi:10.1053/j.gastro.2019.07.064

van Santvoort HC, Besselink MG, Bakker OJ, et al. A step-up approach or open necrosectomy for necrotizing pancreatitis. *N Engl J Med.* 2010;362(16):1491–1502. doi:10.1056/nejmoa0908821

3 *A 68-year-old woman was injured in MVC and had exploratory laparotomy, small bowel resection, and splenectomy. She is now three weeks post-operative, and she has developed copious green fluid extruding from a newly opened wound on the superior aspect of her incision. Her abdomen is soft but exquisitely tender to palpation around the wound. A CT scan of the abdomen with oral contrast shows extravasation of the contrast through the abdominal wall. All of the following are important and necessary in the initial management of an enterocutaneous fistula except:*

A *Treatment and control of sepsis*

B *Fluid resuscitation*

C *Electrolyte repletion*

D *Effluent control and wound care*

E *Oral toleration of diet*

This patient has an enterocutaneous fistula, a very morbid complication after open surgery. Mortality is associated with sepsis, malnutrition, and fluid and electrolyte disturbances. It is important to control and treat sepsis as well as resuscitate the patient first. Effluent control and wound care are necessary to control output and prevent worsening and infection of any soft tissue wound. Nutrition is important for successful management of an EC fistula and can be a combination of enteral and parenteral, depending on nutritional needs and characteristics of the fistula. Oral toleration is not important initially and definitely not necessary. Characteristics of the fistula should be used to determine the appropriate nutrition source.

Answer: E

Evenson AR, Fischer JE. Current management of enterocutaneous fistula. *J Gastrointest Surg.* 2006;10(3):455–464. doi:10.1016/j.gassur.2005.08.001

Rosenthal MD, Brown CJ, Loftus TJ, et al. Nutritional management and strategies for the enterocutaneous fistula. *Curr Surg Reports.* 2020;8(6):1–10. doi:10.1007/s40137-020-00255-5

Gribovskaja-Rupp I, Melton GB. Enterocutaneous fistula: proven strategies and updates. *Clin Colon Rectal Surg.* 2016;29(2):130–137. doi:10.1055/s-0036-1580732

4 *A 32-year-old man with HIV is brought to the hospital post-ictal after a seizure while at home. He is now complaining of a stiff neck, nausea, and a constant headache. His temperature is 102.3°F, heart rate is 98,*

and blood pressure is 100/58. His ophthalmic exam reveals bilateral papilledema. What are the next steps for management after blood cultures, antibiotics, and fluids?

A *Lumbar puncture and place an ICP monitor*
B *Dexamethasone and lumbar puncture*
C *Dexamethasone and obtain a CT scan of head*
D *CT scan of head and place an ICP monitor*
E *DCT scan of head and mannitol*

This immunocompromised patient has signs and symptoms concerning bacterial meningitis. After blood cultures and broad-spectrum antibiotics are started, dexamethasone should be given to adult patients. A trial that evaluated outcomes in adult patients with bacterial meningitis found that negative outcomes, including death, were significantly lower in the group that received dexamethasone versus placebo; the group with streptococcus meningitis saw the most benefit. Hence, current recommendations state starting dexamethasone for any patients with possible streptococcal meningitis and continuing it only if culture results confirm the diagnosis. CT scan of the head should be obtained before a lumbar puncture since this patient has physical exam findings of elevated intracranial pressure (ICP), is immunocompromised, and had a new onset seizure within 1 week of presentation (choice A, B). There is a small (~1%) chance of herniation in adults with elevated ICP. A lumbar puncture is eventually necessary to identify the exact organism causing meningitis but is not done immediately (choice D). Mannitol may eventually be used to lower ICP prior to performing lumbar puncture. Initial empiric antimicrobial treatment for patients with suspected bacterial meningitis includes vancomycin in combination with either ceftriaxone or cefotaxime.

Answer: C

Predisposing factor	Common bacterial pathogens	Antimicrobial therapy
Age		
<1 month	*Streptococcus agalactiae, Escherichia coli, Listeria monocytogenes, Klebsiella* species	Ampicillin plus cefotaxime or ampicillin plus an aminoglycoside
1–23 months	*Streptococcus pneumoniae, Neisseria meningitidis, S. agalactiae, Haemophilus influenzae, E. coli*	Vancomycin plus a third-generation cephalosporin[a,b]
2–50 years	*N. meningitidis, S. pneumoniae*	Vancomycin plus a third-generation cephalosporin[a,b]
>50 years	*S. pneumoniae, N. meningitidis, L. monocytogenes, aerobic gram-negative bacilli*	Vancomycin plus ampicillin plus a third-generation cephalosporin[a,b]
Head trauma		
Basilar skull fracture	*S. pneumoniae, H. influenzae,* group A β-hemolytic streptococci	Vancomycin plus a third-generation cephalosporin[a]
Penetrating trauma	*Staphylococcus aureus,* coagulase-negative staphylococci (especially *Staphylococcus epidermidis*), aerobic gram-negative bacilli (including *Pseudomonas aeruginosa*)	Vancomycin plus cefepime, vancomycin plus ceftazidime, or vancomycin plus meropenem
Postneurosurgery	Aerobic gram-negative bacilli (including *P. aeruginosa*), *S. aureus,* coagulase-negative staphylococci (especially *S. epidermidis*)	Vancomycin plus cefepime, vancomycin plus ceftazidime, or vancomycin plus meropenem
CSF shunt	Coagulase-negative staphylococci (especially *S. epidermidis*), *S. aureus,* aerobic gram-negative bacilli (including *P. aeruginosa*), *Propionibacterium acnes*	Vancomycin plus cefepime,[c] vancomycin plus ceftazidime,[c] or vancomycin plus meropenem[c]

[a] Ceftriaxone or cefotaxime.
[b] Some experts would add rifampin if dexamethasone is also given.
[c] In infants and children, vancomycin alone is reasonable unless Gram stains reveal the presence of gram-negative bacilli.

van de Beek D, de Gans J, Spanjaard L, et al. Clinical
features and prognostic factors in adults with bacterial
meningitis. *N Engl J Med.* 2004;351(18):1849–1859.
doi:10.1056/nejmoa040845
Tunkel AR, Hartman BJ, Kaplan SL, et al. Practice
guidelines for the management of bacterial meningitis.
Clin Infect Dis. 2004;39(9):1267–1284. doi:10.1086/
425368
chart citation:
Tunkel AR, Hartman BJ, Kaplan SL, et al. Practice guidelines
for the management of bacterial meningitis. *Clin Infect
Dis.* 2004;39(9):1267–1284. doi:10.1086/425368

5 *A 77-year-old woman is transferred to the ICU with
increased work of breathing and desaturations. She
was admitted to the hospital after sustaining multiple
rib fractures from a ground-level fall and was being
treated for a hospital-acquired lobar pneumonia.
A new CT chest reveals a loculated pleural collection.
Which of the following is not an appropriate antibiotic
regimen?*

A *Gentamycin and metronidazole*
B *Vancomycin, cefepime, and metronidazole*
C *Vancomycin and piperacillin-tazobactam*
D *Vancomycin and meropenem*
E *Linezolid and piperacillin-tazobactam*

This patient has a hospital-acquired pneumonia complicated by an empyema. Antibiotic coverage for a pleural empyema in this setting should include coverage for gram-positive, gram-negative, and anaerobic organisms. In high-risk patients, coverage should also include MRSA and Pseudomonas. Aminoglycosides could possibly have poor pleural penetration and are inactivated in the setting of infection, so they are avoided as a class in treating empyema (choice A). In patients with hospital-acquired empyema, it is important to cover for anaerobes, MRSA, and Pseudomonas. Choice B is an appropriate antibiotic regimen as broad-spectrum coverage is present with vancomycin covering for MRSA, cefepime covering Pseudomonas, and metronidazole for anaerobic coverage. Choice C is appropriate as the piperacillin-tazobactam covers both Pseudomonas and anaerobes in addition to the MRSA coverage with vancomycin. Choice D is appropriate as the meropenem adequately covers Pseudomonas and anaerobes while the vancomycin covers MRSA. Choice E is an appropriate regimen with linezolid adequately providing MRSA coverage and piperacillin-tazobactam providing coverage against anaerobes and Pseudomonas. Further treatment with antibiotics can be tailored to the patient based on culture

and sensitivity data, and it is recommended that antibiotic treatment continue for at least two weeks following defervescence and source control of the empyema.

Answer: A

Shen KR, Bribriesco A, Crabtree T, et al. The American
Association for Thoracic Surgery consensus guidelines for
the management of empyema. *J Thorac Cardiovasc Surg.*
2017;153(6):e129–e146. doi:10.1016/j.jtcvs.2017.01.030
Rosenstengel A. Pleural infection-current diagnosis and
management. *J Thorac Dis.* 2012;4(2):186–193.
doi:10.3978/j.issn.2072-1439.2012.01.12
Thys JP, Vanderhoeft P, Herchuelz A, et al. Penetration of
aminoglycosides in uninfected pleural exudates and in
pleural empyemas. *Chest.* 1988;93(3):530–532.
doi:10.1378/chest.93.3.530

6 *A 56-year-old woman with asthma, who works in a
long-term healthcare facility, presents with fevers,
chills, generalized myalgias, and a severe cough for the
past four days. Over the last 24 hours, she has become
significantly more short of breath. Her rapid influenza
is positive, and her respiratory status continues to
deteriorate. Chest x-ray demonstrates a left lower lobe
consolidation. She is admitted to the ICU. What
should her treatment regimen include?*

A *Oseltamivir, vancomycin, piperacillin-tazobactam,
corticosteroids*
B *Oseltamivir, ampicillin-sulbactam, and corticosteroids*
C *Vancomycin and piperacillin-tazobactam*
D *Oseltamivir, vancomycin, and piperacillin-tazobactam*
E *Oseltamivir and daptomycin*

This patient may have **coinfection** with influenza and community-acquired pneumonia. In patients who test positive for influenza and are admitted to the hospital, anti-influenza treatment should be started, regardless of the duration of the illness before diagnosis. If this were a different patient who was being treated as an outpatient, administration of anti-viral therapy is only recommended within two days of symptom onset. Given the patient's employment in a long-term-care facility, she is at risk for MRSA, so initial coverage should be broad and cover MRSA as well as gram negatives. Daptomycin should not be used as it is inactivated by surfactant (choice E). Corticosteroids are not routinely prescribed for adults with severe CAP (choice A, B). Overall, the data for treatment with corticosteroids is conflicting with some showing a benefit and others showing no significant difference in outcomes. A meta-analysis of pneumonia due to influenza based on small studies, however, showed an increase in mortality in patients who receive corticosteroids. Corticosteroids are recommended to be used in patients with refractory septic shock. IDSA guidelines removed the term "healthcare-associated pneumonia (HCAP)" in 2016 and recommend that pneumonia be categorized as hospital acquired, community acquired, or ventilator associated. This patient has community-acquired pneumonia as she did not develop the pneumonia after being admitted to the hospital. She does, however, have risk factors for MRSA and Pseudomonas infection due to her job at a long-term healthcare facility. Because of this, she needs to be covered appropriately for MRSA and Pseudomonas infections.

Answer: D

Metlay JP, Waterer GW, Long AC, et al. Diagnosis and treatment of adults with community-acquired pneumonia. *Am J Respir Crit Care Med.* 2019;200(7):E45–E67. doi:10.1164/rccm.201908-1581ST

Uyeki TM, Bernstein HH, Bradley JS, et al. Clinical Practice Guidelines by the Infectious Diseases Society of America: 2018 Update on Diagnosis, Treatment, Chemoprophylaxis, and Institutional Outbreak Management of Seasonal Influenza. *Clin Infect Dis.* 2019;68(6):895–902. doi:10.1093/cid/ciy874

Davis BM, Aiello AE, Dawid S, et al. Influenza and community-acquired pneumonia interactions: the impact of order and time of infection on population patterns. *Am J Epidemiol.* 2012;175(5):363–367. doi:10.1093/aje/kwr402

Silverman JA, Mortin LI, VanPraagh ADG, et al. Inhibition of daptomycin by pulmonary surfactant: in vitro modeling and clinical impact. *J Infect Dis.* 2005;191(12):2149–2152. doi:10.1086/430352

7 *A 58-year-old man presents to the hospital with left lower quadrant pain for 3 days, subjective fevers at home, and anorexia. He reports that he has been having frequent liquid stools. His vital signs are normal except for his temperature of 100.4°F. He is tender to palpation in his left lower quadrant of his abdomen. He has a leukocytosis of 18×10^3 cells/mm^3 with 80% neutrophils. A CT of his abdomen shows a 6 cm rim-enhancing fluid collection and dots of free air in his pelvis. His most recent colonoscopy was 9 months ago and showed diverticulosis with no polyps or masses. The next best step in the management of this patient should be:*

A *Repeat colonoscopy*
B *Surgical drainage of the fluid collection*
C *Percutaneous drainage of the fluid collection*
D *PICC line placement for fluid resuscitation*
E *Sigmoidectomy and primary anastomosis*

This patient has Hinchey II diverticulitis with a pelvic abscess. Proper management is percutaneous drainage if amenable and initiation of a fluoroquinolone or cephalosporin and metronidazole. Initiation of broad-spectrum antibiotics, such as meropenem, should be reserved for patients with severe intra-abdominal infection or for healthcare-acquired intra-abdominal infection. A PICC line is not necessary in this patient as the duration of antibiotics following source control with percutaneous drainage should be four days and there is no need for parenteral nutrition at this point in time. A repeat colonoscopy would not be appropriate at this time and would likely further injure the diseased bowel. He will need a colonoscopy to rule out malignancy 6 to 8 weeks after resolution of his disease. Surgical drainage is an option for obtaining source control but is significantly more invasive than a percutaneous drain. Similarly, choice E is incorrect and sigmoidectomy in this patient should be reserved for disease refractory to treatment. Antibiotic choices for this patient should cover gram-negative aerobic and facultative bacilli as well as gram-positive streptococci. This is a community-acquired intra-abdominal infection, and there is no need to initiate anti-pseudomonal treatment in this patient. Ticarcillin-clavulanate, cefoxitin, ertapenem, or moxifloxacin are adequate single-agent choices. Treatment can also be dual agent with metronidazole in combination with cefazolin, cefuroxime, ceftriaxone, cefotaxime, levofloxacin, or ciprofloxacin. This patient's initial antibiotic regimen should be given intravenously; however, if he progresses to tolerating adequate nutrition by mouth, it is reasonable to convert the therapy to an oral antibiotic for the duration of the treatment.

Modified Hinchey classification

Stage	Definition
0	Mild diverticulitis
Ia	Pericolonic phlegmon/inflammation
Ib	Pericolic abscess
II	Pelvic/retroperitoneal/distant abscess
III	Purulent peritonitis
IV	Fecal peritonitis

Answer: C

Solomkin JS, Mazuski JE, Bradley JS, et al. Diagnosis and management of complicated intra-abdominal infection in adults and children: guidelines by the Surgical Infection Society and the Infectious Diseases Society of America. *Clin Infect Dis.* 2010;50(2):133–164. doi:10.1086/649554

Sawyer RG, Claridge JA, Nathens AB, et al. Trial of short-course antimicrobial therapy for intraabdominal infection. *N Engl J Med.* 2015;372(21):1996–2005. doi:10.1056/nejmoa1411162

8 *A 36-year-old man was in MVC, and his injuries include large areas of desquamation with dirt and vegetation over the wounds and multiple open fractures. He is taken to the operating room for a positive FAST in the setting of hypotension. He undergoes an exploratory laparotomy and splenectomy as well as external fixation of his open femur fractures with wound washout. On post-operative day 5, he becomes febrile and areas of his wound are noted to be black and necrotic. A biopsy is sent for histologic examination and returns mold with irregular non-septate broad hyphae. What is the best treatment course for this patient?*

A *Posaconazole*
B *Amphotericin B*
C *Lipid formulation of amphotericin B and perform serial wound debridements*
D *Posaconazole and perform serial wound debridements*
E *Micafungin and perform serial wound debridements*

This patient has an invasive fungal infection with Mucor, which has irregular non-septate broad hyphae. While rare, severely injured trauma patients can suffer from an invasive fungal infection. Mortality from this infection can be very high, so prompt debridement and antifungal therapy are important for success. Lipid formulation of amphotericin B (LAmB) is the antifungal of choice. LAmB has been shown to be more effective than other antifungals at treating Mucor, and the liposomal formulation has increased survivorship in patients with Mucor infections significantly (39%–67%). Other antifungals such as iatroconazole, voriconazole, and fluconazole do not have much effect against Mucor. Posaconazole has to be given in high and potentially toxic doses to treat Mucor and is not recommended as a first line option. It is, however, available to be used for refractory disease or for salvage therapy.

Choice A is incorrect as Posaconazole is not the first line treatment for Mucor, and it can be used if needed in refractory disease.

Choice B is incorrect as traditional formulations of amphotericin B have been shown to be significantly less effective against Mucor infections but it also lacks surgical debridement of the wound that plays a critical role in the treatment of the disease.

Choice D is incorrect as Posaconazole is not a first line treatment for this disease.

Choice E is incorrect as there is no data to suggest that micafungin is effective against Mucor.

Answer: C

Spellberg B, Ibrahim AS. Recent advances in the treatment of mucormycosis. *Curr Infect Dis Rep.* 2010;12(6):423–9. doi: 10.1007/s11908-010-0129-9. PMID: 21308550; PMCID: PMC2947016.

Kronen R, Liang SY, Bochicchio G, et al. Invasive fungal infections secondary to traumatic injury. *Int J Infect Dis.* 2017;62:102–111. doi:10.1016/j.ijid.2017.07.002

Ganesan A, Shaikh F, Bradley W, et al. Classification of trauma-associated invasive fungal infections to support wound treatment decisions. *Emerg Infect Dis.* 2019;25(9):1639–1647. doi:10.3201/eid2509.190168

Wilson W, Ali-Osman F, Sucher J, et al. Invasive fungal wound infection in an otherwise healthy trauma patient (Mucor Trauma). *Trauma Case Reports.* 2019;24:100251. doi:10.1016/j.tcr.2019.100251

9 *A 24-year-old man sustained multiple gunshot wounds to the abdomen. He was taken to the OR, given a dose of cefoxitin, and underwent an exploratory laparotomy. He was found to have multiple small bowel injuries and a colon injury, both of which had caused spillage of bowel content. The most appropriate duration of antibiotic therapy in this scenario should be:*

A *No more than 24 hours*
B *48 hours*
C *4 days*
D *7 days*
E *14 days*

The duration of antimicrobial therapy is controversial, but most studies have found that there is no difference in infection rates between a 24-hour course and a longer duration of therapy in patients that had penetrating abdominal trauma. Regardless, all patients with penetrating abdominal trauma should at least receive a single preoperative dose of broad-spectrum antibiotics. Traditionally, the most effective time to provide antibiotic dosing is prior to the time of bacterial contamination, but since this is not possible with abdominal trauma, it is recommended that the dose be given as soon as possible. Appropriate antibiotics for a patient with penetrating trauma will be broad spectrum with aerobic and anaerobic coverage. Second-generation cephalosporins are the recommended initial choice, and third-generation cephalosporins can be used as an alternative. It is important to also note that in patients with penetrating abdominal trauma who are also in hemorrhagic shock will need additional dosing of antibiotics with repeated dosing after 10 units of blood transfused.

Answer: A

Goldberg SR, Anand RJ, Como JJ, et al. Prophylactic antibiotic use in penetrating abdominal trauma. *J Trauma Acute Care Surg.* 2012;73(5 SUPPL.4): S321–S325. doi:10.1097/TA.0b013e3182701902

Jang JY, Kang WS, Keum MA, et al. Antibiotic use in patients with abdominal injuries: guideline by the Korean Society of Acute Care Surgery. *Ann Surg Treat Res.* 2019;96(1):1–7. doi:10.4174/astr.2019.96.1.1

Hospenthal DR, Murray CK, Andersen RC, et al. Guidelines for the prevention of infections associated with combat-related injuries: 2011 update: endorsed by the Infectious Diseases Society of America and the Surgical Infection Society. *J Trauma.* 2011;71(2 Suppl 2): S210–S234.

Rhodes A, Evans LE, Alhazzani W, et al. Surviving sepsis campaign. *Crit Care Med.* 2017;45(3):486–552. doi:10.1097/CCM.0000000000002255

Gordon AC, Mason AJ, Thirunavukkarasu N, et al. Effect of early vasopressin vs norepinephrine on kidney failure in patients with septic shock: the VANISH randomized clinical trial. JAMA - J Am Med Assoc. 2016;316(5): 509–518. doi:10.1001/jama.2016.10485

Russell JA, Walley KR, Singer J, et al. Vasopressin versus norepinephrine infusion in patients with septic shock. *N Engl J Med.* 2008;358(9):877–887. doi:10.1056/nejmoa067373

Demiselle J, Fage N, Radermacher P, Asfar P. Vasopressin and its analogues in shock states: a review. *Ann Intensive Care.* 2020;10(1):9. doi:10.1186/ s13613-020-0628-2

10 *A 68-year-old woman with diabetes, coronary artery disease, and peripheral vascular disease presents to the hospital 21 days after an emergent fem-femoral bypass. She is febrile and tachycardic with a white count of 16×10^3/microL. Her right groin incision is open with visible pus, and the area over the graft is erythematous and tender. A CTA shows increased soft tissue inflammation around the graft. What is the next best step?*

A *Obtain an ultrasound to assess blood flow velocities.*

B *Start intravenous ceftriaxone and flagyl.*

C *Start oral cephalexin.*

D *Explant the graft and replace with autologous vein.*

E *Start intravenous vancomycin and piperacillin-tazobactam.*

This patient has a graft infection. Gram-positive bacteria are the most causative organisms. Typically, the rate of vascular graft infection is 1.5–2.5%, but the infection rate of grafts in the groin can be as high as 6%. Not only does this patient have grafts in the bilateral groins, but her diabetes and the urgent nature of her initial procedure also increases her risk of graft infection.

While *Staphylococcus aureus* is the most common cause of vascular graft infection, there has been a documented rise of MRSA isolates from infected grafts as well as *Pseudomonas aeruginosa*, which is about 10% of graft infections. Because of this, a patient with a vascular graft infection should initially receive broad-spectrum antibiotic coverage extended to cover Pseudomonas and MRSA. Of the choices, only choice E (vancomycin and piperacillin-tazobactam) provides appropriate antibiotic coverage for this patient.

Ceftriaxone, metronidazole, and cephalexin do not cover MRSA. While obtaining an ultrasound can help assess blood flow, a CTA is 85–100% sensitive and 85–94% specific for graft infection and can be obtained quickly. There are some scenarios of surgical site infection after a vascular graft in which antibiotics, debridement, and wound care can be used to preserve an infected graft, and the graft will first need to be surgically explored before the decision for preservation or explant is made. If the decision is made to preserve the graft, a prolonged course of antibiotics will be required.

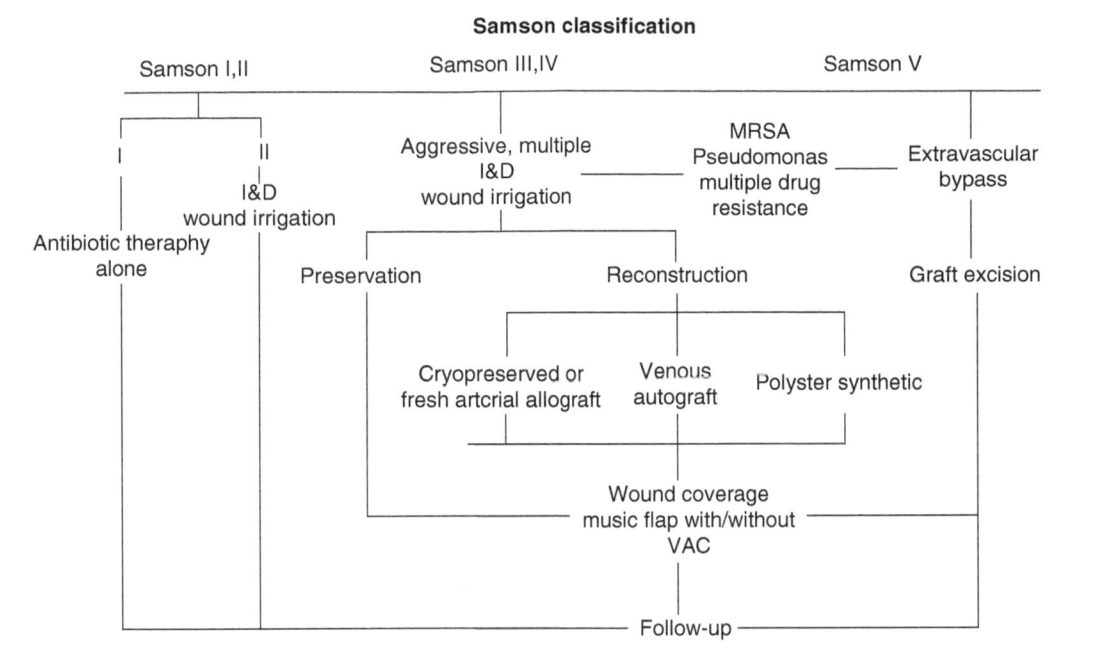

Samson classification

Antimicrobial therapy for extracavitary vascular graft infection

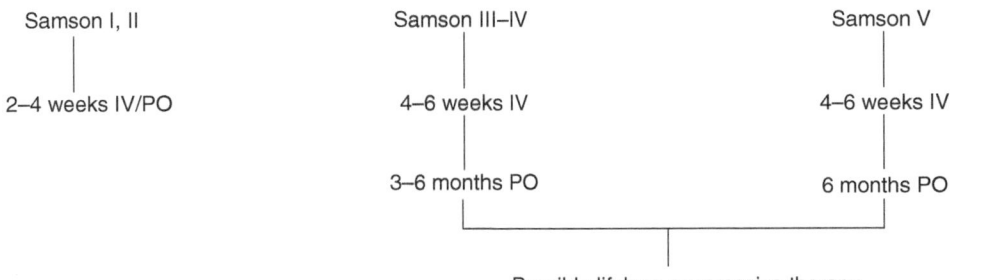

Possible lifelong suppressive therapy
- MRSA
- P. aeruginosa, multidrug resistant, Candida or other fungi
- Multiple surgical procedures for VGI
- Emergency surgery for VGI, reconstruction with rifampin-bonded graft
- Extensive perigraft infection
- Poor candidate for reoperation

Answer: E

Spelman D. Overview of infected (mycotic) arterial aneurysm - UpToDate. UpToDate. https://www. uptodate.com/contents/overview-of-infected-mycotic-arterial-aneurysm?search=infected vascular graft&source=search_result&selectedTitle= 1~20&usage_type=default&display_rank= 1#H1118621. Published July 2019. (accessed 3 December 2020).

Chakfé N, Diener H, Lejay A, et al. Editor's Choice – European Society for Vascular Surgery (ESVS) 2020 clinical practice guidelines on the management of vascular graft and endograft infections. *Eur J Vasc Endovasc Surg.* 2020;59(3):339–384. doi:10.1016/j. ejvs.2019.10.016

Kilic A, Arnaoutakis DJ, Reifsnyder T, et al. Management of infected vascular grafts. *Vasc Med (United Kingdom).* 2016;21(1):53–60. doi:10.1177/1358863X15612574

Wilson WR, Bower TC, Creager MA, et al. American Heart Association Committee on Rheumatic Fever, Endocarditis, and Kawasaki Disease of the Council on Cardiovascular Disease in the Young; Council on Cardiovascular and Stroke Nursing; Council on Cardiovascular Radiology and Intervention; Council on Cardiovascular Surgery and Anesthesia; Council on Peripheral Vascular Disease; and Stroke Council. Vascular Graft Infections, Mycotic Aneurysms, and Endovascular Infections: A Scientific Statement from the American Heart Association. *Circulation.* 2016;134(20):e412–e460. doi: 10.1161/CIR.0000000000000457. Epub 2016 Oct 13. PMID: 27737955.

11 *A 53-year-old man is in the ICU after a severe MVC. He has been on the ventilator for six days due to respiratory failure and lung contusion. He is noted to have increased inspiratory pressures, worsening hypoxemia, and purulent secretions. He has a white count of 16×10^3/microL and a progressive infiltrate on his chest x-ray. What is the appropriate duration of antibiotics to treat his ventilator-associated pneumonia?*

A *3 days*

B *5 days*

C *7 days*

D *10 days*

E *14 days*

Multiple studies have shown that short-course antibiotic regimens (7–8 days) increased the antibiotic-free days; when compared to longer duration of antibiotics (10–15 days), there was also no difference in mortality, duration of mechanical ventilation, or length of ICU stay. In turn, reducing antibiotic exposure reduces side effects, antibiotic resistance, and costs.

In patients with VAP, it is recommended that coverage includes *S. aureus*, *P. aeruginosa*, and gram-negative bacilli. Empiric treatment of MRSA and Pseudomonas should be employed if the patient has recent risk factors for drug-resistant infection including prior IV antibiotics use within 90 days, current septic shock, ARDS preceding the VAP, more than 5 hospital days preceding VAP diagnosis, and acute renal replacement therapy prior to the VAP onset. If the patient received IV antibiotics within the past 90 days, it is recommend that they be prescribed two agents that cover Pseudomonas in addition to an agent that covers MRSA.

Answer: C

Zilahi G, McMahon MA, Povoa P, et al. Duration of antibiotic therapy in the intensive care unit. *J Thorac Dis.* 2016;8(12):3774–3780. doi:10.21037/jtd.2016.12.89

Kalil AC, Metersky ML, Klompas M, et al. Management of adults with hospital-acquired and ventilator-associated pneumonia: 2016 clinical practice guidelines by the Infectious Diseases Society of America and the American Thoracic Society. *Clin Infect Dis.* 2016;63(5):e61–e111. doi:10.1093/cid/ciw353

Torres A, Niederman MS, Chastre J, et al. International ERS/ESICM/ESCMID/ALAT guidelines for the management of hospital-acquired pneumonia and ventilator-associated pneumonia. *Eur Respir J.* 2017;50(3). doi:10.1183/13993003.00582-2017

12 *An 83-year-old man with COPD, diabetes, and renal failure underwent resection of necrotic bowel from a closed-loop small bowel obstruction. He remains mechanically ventilated. On post-operative day six, he developed a fever to 102°F and a leukocytosis. A new right lobe infiltrate is seen on chest x-ray, and he is diagnosed with ventilator-associated pneumonia. Culture results are positive for Acinetobacter. What is the appropriate treatment?*

A *Piperacillin-tazobactam and gentamicin*

B *Vancomycin*

C *Colistin*

D *Meropenem*

E *Ciprofloxacin*

Acinetobacter is a gram-negative bacilli that is a common cause of late-onset VAP. Acinetobacter species are sensitive to carbapenems, ampicillin-sulbactam, and colistin. Carbapenems and ampicillin-sulbactam are preferred to colistin due to the risk of nephrotoxicity with colistin. Vancomycin is ineffective. Historically, ciprofloxacin has been effective in treating Acinetobacter, but the rate of ciprofloxacin-resistant Acinetobacter infections has been reported as high as 67% in recent years and is thus no longer considered an effective empiric treatment. Gentamicin is a viable treatment option for an Acinetobacter infection; however, the addition of piperacillin-tazobactam in choice A is unnecessary to treat this infection.

Answer: D

Kalil AC, Metersky ML, Klompas M, et al. Management of adults with hospital-acquired and ventilator-associated pneumonia: 2016 clinical practice guidelines by the Infectious Diseases Society of America and the American Thoracic Society. *Clin Infect Dis.* 2016;63(5):e61–e111. doi:10.1093/cid/ciw353

Wood GC, Hanes SO, Croce MA, et al. Comparison of ampicillin-sulbactam and imipenem-cilastatin for the treatment of Acinetobacter ventilator-associated pneumonia. *Clin Infect Dis.* 2002;34(11):1425–1430. doi:10.1086/340055

13 *A 35-year-old man suffers a 50% total body surface area third-degree burns after a house fire and has been in the burn ICU for the past 28 days. He has undergone multiple surgeries for his wounds and has been treated for a ventilator-associated pneumonia and a central line infection. Overnight, he develops a fever to 103°F and increased tachycardia and hypotension. On the changing of his dressings in the morning, the wound care nurse notes a sweet smell and areas of his torso wound appear to have a blue-green color. What is the appropriate treatment?*
   A *Cefepime and ciprofloxacin*
   B *Piperacillin-tazobactam*
   C *Colistin*
   D *Vancomycin*
   E *Tobramycin and amikacin*

This patient has an infected burn wound. *Pseudomonas aeruginosa*; the blue-green color and sweet, grape smell are characteristic. This patient with his prolonged hospital stay and previously treated infections is at risk for multidrug-resistant strains. Wound culture is important to obtain to determine susceptibility. For initial empiric therapy, while there is controversy in monotherapy versus combination therapy, combination therapy is used due to the high risk of drug resistance in Pseudomonas. In combination therapy, the goal is to use antibiotics with two different mechanisms of action (tobramycin and amikacin are both aminoglycosides and share the same mechanism of action, making this an inappropriate choice). Colistin, a polymyxin, should be preserved for serious infection with proven multidrug isolates. Vancomycin is not an appropriate choice since it does not cover Pseudomonas. While piperacillin-tazobactam covers Pseudomonas, it is a single agent.

Answer: A

Traugott KA, Echevarria K, Maxwell P, et al. Monotherapy or combination therapy? The Pseudomonas aeruginosa conundrum. *Pharmacotherapy.* 2011;31(6):598–608. doi:10.1592/phco.31.6.598

Micek ST, Lloyd AE, Ritchie DJ, et al. Pseudomonas aeruginosa bloodstream infection: importance of appropriate initial antimicrobial treatment. *Antimicrob Agents Chemother.* 2005;49(4):1306–1311. doi:10.1128/AAC.49.4.1306-1311.2005

Kang CI, Kim SH, Kim H Bin, et al. Pseudomonas aeruginosa bacteremia: risk factors for mortality and influence of delayed receipt of effective antimicrobial

therapy on clinical outcome. *Clin Infect Dis.* 2003;37(6):745–751. doi:10.1086/377200

14 *A 47-year-old man with obesity and diabetes suffers a deep laceration to his left thigh while working on his farm. He presents one day after the injury with severe pain in his left thigh, spreading erythema, and bullae. Necrotic muscle is visible in the wound, and he has crepitus on exam. The patient is started on broad-spectrum antibiotics and taken to the OR for debridement. Gram stains reveal a gram-positive rod. What is the most appropriate antibiotic regimen?*
   A *Vancomycin, piperacillin-tazobactam, and clindamycin*
   B *Vancomycin and clindamycin*
   C *Penicillin and clindamycin*
   D *Gentamycin and piperacillin-tazobactam*
   E *Penicillin and metronidazole*

Necrotizing soft tissue infections (NSTIs) have high morbidity and mortality. The goal is prompt recognition, antibiotics, and surgical debridement. Initially, it is important to start the patient on broad-spectrum antibiotics that include coverage for MRSA and anaerobes. Gram stains suggest infection with *Clostridium* species, which is a gram-positive rod. For Clostridium myonecrosis, the Infectious Disease Society of America (IDSA) currently recommends starting penicillin and clindamycin. Treatment should continue for 10–14 days after source control. Choices A, B, and D do not include penicillin – the appropriate antibiotic for Clostridium. Choice E does not contain clindamycin, which helps prevent exotoxin release.

Answer: C

Stevens DL, Bisno AL, Chambers HF, et al. Practice guidelines for the diagnosis and management of skin and soft tissue infections: 2014 update by the Infectious Diseases Society of America. *Clin Infect Dis.* 2014;59(2):e10–e52. doi:10.1093/cid/ciu296

Stevens DL, Bryant AE. Necrotizing soft-tissue infections. Longo DL, ed. *N Engl J Med.* 2017;377(23):2253–2265. doi:10.1056/NEJMra1600673

15 *A 47-year-old woman who is eight months status post a deceased-donor kidney transplant is admitted with nausea, vomiting, and watery diarrhea. She is tachycardic, afebrile, and normotensive with a leukopenia at 3×10^3/microL. Colon biopsies are positive for CMV. In addition to decreasing*

immunosuppression, which of the following should be started?

A *Oral valganciclovir*

B *IV ganciclovir*

C *IV foscarnet*

D *Oral ganciclovir*

E *Oral oseltamivir*

CMV is a major cause of infection in solid-organ transplant patients. The risk is highest in lung and small bowel transplant recipients. Biopsy is occasionally needed to confirm the presence of tissue-invasive disease if nucleic acid testing is negative. CMV is treated by decreasing immunosuppressive medications and starting appropriate antiviral therapy. IV ganciclovir is the first line therapy for gastrointestinal CMV. Oral valganciclovir, while effective for CMV, will not be effectively absorbed in a patient with GI disease (Choice A). IV foscarnet is a second-line therapy for treatment and is highly nephrotoxic (choice C). Oral ganciclovir and oseltamivir are not indicated in CMV infection. Oral ganciclovir should not be used for treating CMV disease as there is concern it may lead to emergence of ganciclovir resistance as its poor bioavailability leads to insufficient systemic levels. Oseltamivir is effective in treating influenza viruses, and there is no data to suggest that it would be an effective treatment for CMV infection.

Answer: B

Razonable RR, Humar A. Cytomegalovirus in solid organ transplantation. *Am J Transplant*. 2013;13(SUPPL.4): 93–106. doi:10.1111/ajt.12103

Eid AJ, Arthurs SK, Deziel PJ, et al. Clinical predictors of relapse after treatment of primary gastrointestinal cytomegalovirus disease in solid organ transplant recipients. *Am J Transplant*. 2010;10(1):157–161. doi:10.1111/j.1600-6143.2009.02861.x

16 *Which of the following practices is the least effective in reducing central line-associated bloodstream infection (CLABSI)?*

A *Appropriate hand hygiene and skin preparation*

B *Following a checklist during line insertion*

C *Daily bathing of ICU patients with chlorhexidine*

D *Removal of unnecessary lines*

E *Choosing the subclavian vein for a central line insertion*

Central line-associated bloodstream infection (CLABSI) is a frequent cause of hospital-associated infection. A multimodal approach has been shown to be effective in decreasing CLABSI. Hand hygiene is the most important practice in reducing healthcare-associated infections. Following a checklist during insertion ensures that steps, such as hand hygiene, skin preparation, and use of maximal sterile barrier precautions, should not be forgotten. The risk of developing a line infection increased with each day of use; reassessing their need daily helps remove a nidus for infection. The femoral site has the highest risk of infection followed by internal jugular and subclavian. Daily bathing of ICU patients with chlorhexidine did not demonstrate a reduction in CLABSIs, catheter-associated urinary tract infections (CAUTIs), ventilator-associated pneumonia, or *Clostridium difficile* in a randomized control trail.

Answer: C

Miller SE, Maragakis LL. Central line-associated bloodstream infection prevention. *Curr Opin Infect Dis*. 2012;25(4):412–422. doi:10.1097/ QCO.0b013e328355e4da

Latif A, Halim MS, Pronovost PJ. Eliminating infections in the ICU: CLABSI. *Curr Infect Dis Rep*. 2015;17(7). doi:10.1007/s11908-015-0491-8

Noto MJ, Domenico HJ, Byrne DW, et al. Chlorhexidine bathing and health care-associated infections: a randomized clinical trial. *JAMA - J Am Med Assoc*. 2015;313(4):369–378. doi:10.1001/ jama.2014.18400

17 *A 63-year-old female with type II diabetes and a recent HbA1c of 9.4 presents to the ED after she noted a foul odor emanating from the sole of her foot. Upon inspection of her foot, she noticed a large ulcer with surrounding erythema and purulence in the wound bed and presented to the ED. Upon evaluation in the ED, her WBC is 14.4 and she is afebrile. She denies being hospitalized or having a wound like this before.*

Next steps in care for this patient include:

A *Immediate culture of wound, initiation of meropenem, MRI of the foot*

B *Immediate culture of wound, initiation of vancomycin and piperacillin/tazobactam, MRI of the foot*

C *Cleansing and debridement of the wound followed by culture of the wound, initiation of ertapenem, MRI of the foot*

D *Cleansing and debridement of the wound followed by culture of the wound, initiation of ertapenem, x-ray of the foot*

E *Immediate initiation of vancomycin/piperacillin/ tazobactam, debridement and culture of the wound, x-ray of the foot.*

This patient has a diabetic foot infection and the wound should be evaluated and treated. Prior to antibiotic administration, the wound should be cleansed and debrided with the deep tissue from the wound sent for culture. Failure to do this can lead to the culturing of skin flora that may not be responsible for the infection. The wound should then be classified, and a probe-to-bone test can be used to help in making this decision. There are multiple ways to classify diabetic foot infections; two of the most frequently used classifications are mentioned below.

Following an adequate culture and classification of the wound, an antibiotic regimen can be started. This wound would be classified as a moderate diabetic foot infection and therefore should be treated with antibiotics. In a moderate diabetic foot infection, aerobic GPCs, MSSA, Streptococcus spp., Enterobacteriaceae, and other obligate anaerobes are the likely pathogens. These are all adequately covered by ertapenem. Initiation of vancomycin and piperacillin/tazobactam would be a correct answer if this patient had a severe diabetic foot infection. She does not require any further coverage for MRSA or pseudomonal infections as she does not have any current risk factors, nor is her illness severe enough to prompt broad-spectrum empiric antibiotic coverage.

Initial imaging of a diabetic foot infection should always be an x-ray of the foot, which is both sensitive and specific for osteomyelitis. If any diagnostic uncertainty remains following the x-ray, an MRI can be pursued.

Answer: D

Lipsky BA., Berendt AR, Cornia PB, et al. 2012 Infectious Diseases Society of America Clinical Practice Guideline for the Diagnosis and Treatment of Diabetic Foot Infections, *Clin Infect Dis.* 2012;5412: e132–e173, https://doi.org/10.1093/cid/cis346

18 *A 67-year-old male who has returned 6 weeks ago from a trip to New England where he had been trail-running in preparation from a marathon presents to the ED complaining of intractable fatigue, dark-reddish urine, and frequent high fevers at home. He reveals that he had pulled a small bug off his arm during his trip and that he did not notice any associated rash. He has splenomegaly on physical exam. His labs return showing a normocytic anemia with elevated transaminases. A Wright's/Giemsa stain of his peripheral blood demonstrates darkly stained rings with light blue cytoplasm within erythrocytes. The most likely disease responsible for his condition is:*
    A *Lyme disease*
    B *Babesiosis*

C *Rocky Mountain Spotted Fever*
D *Ehrlichiosis*
E *Anaplasmosis*

This patient has babesiosis, more specifically an infection with the parasite *Babesia microti. B. microti* is an intraerythrocytic parasite that is transmitted from ticks to vertebrates including humans. The disease contracted by the host can be broad with varying symptoms ranging from asymptomatic infection to a disease like malaria with severe hemolysis and death. Symptoms can take months after exposure to develop. Common signs and symptoms of babesiosis are fatigue, anemia, fevers, chills, night sweats, hemoglobinuria, transaminitis, weight loss, hepato/splenomegaly. Diagnosis is typically made with exposure to ticks, stained blood smears, and ELISA/PCR. The standard treatment for babesiosis is clindamycin and quinine. In a serious infection where clindamycin and quinine are not sufficient, there has been some benefit shown in erythrocyte exchange transfusion.

Lyme disease is the most common tick-borne illness in the United States and is also hosted by the *Ixodes* tick. It is known for its characteristic bull's-eye rash (erythema migrans), but this is not present in all cases. Lyme disease commonly presents with low-grade fevers and myalgias. The disease, however, can disseminate and affect the musculoskeletal, neurologic, and cardiovascular system. Most commonly, musculoskeletal symptoms are present in Lyme disease in the form of migratory joint and muscle pain. Anemia is not associated with Lyme disease, and this spirochete bacterium is not apparent on a peripheral blood smear. Treatment for Lyme disease is typically doxycycline for adults and amoxicillin for children.

Rocky Mountain Spotted Fever is a serious disease that is caused by *Rickettsia rickettsii* and transmitted after a tick bite. It is most common in the southeastern and south-central United States. This bacterium preferentially infects the vascular endothelial cells of small and medium vessels in the body. Patients typically present 4–10 days post exposure and have fever, headache, and a rash. Typically, patients are treated empirically based on their history and physical with doxycycline, but PCR can be performed to confirm diagnosis.

Ehrlichiosis is a tick-borne disease carried by the Lone Star Tick found in the south-central United States. Ehrlichiosis is associated with fever, headache, body aches, malaise, and chills but can include gastrointestinal symptoms, respiratory symptoms, and rash. Associated laboratory findings include leukopenia, thrombocytopenia, hyponatremia, and moderately elevated transaminases.

Diagnosis is made clinically or by PCR. Treatment is doxycycline.

Anaplasmosis is transmitted by the *Ixodes* tick and is found worldwide; it is caused by *Anaplasma phagocytophilum* – an obligate intracellular bacterium. Symptoms include fever, malaise, myalgias, and headache with some patients experiencing nausea, vomiting, diarrhea, cough, arthralgias, and confusion. Rash is uncommon in anaplasmosis. Anaplasmosis is visible on peripheral blood smear, and it can be seen within the neutrophils in aggregates called morulae. Doxycycline is the first line treatment for anaplasmosis.

Answer: B

Guzman N, Yarrarapu SNS, Beidas SO.. Anaplasma Phagocytophilum. [Updated 2021 Jan 5]. In: *StatPearls [Internet]*. Treasure Island (FL): StatPearls Publishing; 2021. Available from: https://www.ncbi.nlm.nih.gov/books/NBK513341/

Homer MJ, Aguilar-Delfin I, Telford SR III, et al. Babesiosis. *Clin Microbiol Rev*. 2000;13(3):451–69. doi: 10.1128/cmr.13.3.451-469.2000. PMID: 10885987; PMCID: PMC88943.

Snowden J, Simonsen KA, Rickettsiae Rickettsia. [Updated 2020 Nov 20]. In: *StatPearls [Internet]*. Treasure Island (FL): StatPearls Publishing; 2021. Available from: https://www.ncbi.nlm.nih.gov/books/NBK430881/

Snowden J, Bartman M, Kong EL, et al. Ehrlichiosis. [Updated 2020 Sep 17]. In: *StatPearls [Internet]*. Treasure Island (FL): StatPearls Publishing; 2021. Available from: https://www.ncbi.nlm.nih.gov/books/NBK441966/

Bratton RL, Whiteside JW, Hovan MJ, et al. Diagnosis and treatment of Lyme disease. *Mayo Clin Proc*. 2008;83(5):566–71. doi: 10.4065/83.5.566. PMID: 18452688

10

Pharmacology and Antibiotics

Michelle Strong, MD, PhD[1] and Elaine Cleveland, MD[2]

[1] *Trauma and Acute Care Surgeon, Austin, TX, USA*
[2] *William Beaumont Army Medical Center, El Paso, TX, USA*

1 *A 64-year-old man with a past medical history notable of hypertension, hyperlipidemia, peripheral vascular disease, and diabetes presents with copious purulent drainage coming from his right trans-metatarsal amputation site. He has been spiking fevers for the last two days; his white blood cell count is 24 000, and his blood pressure is 95/40 mm Hg. Previous cultures at the time of his amputation 3 months ago grew extended spectrum beta-lactamase (ESBL) Enterobacteriacea. What antibiotic should you start this patient on (assuming normal renal function)?*

   A *Ampicillin/sulbactam 3 gm every 6 hrs*
   B *Ceftriaxone 1gm every 24 hrs*
   C *Piperacillin/tazobactam 4.5 every 8 hrs (extended infusion)*
   D *Cefepime 2gm every 12 hrs*
   E *Meropenem 1 gm every 8 hrs*

ESBLs are plasmid-mediated enzymes that inactivate all β-lactam antibiotics including penicillins, third- and fourth-generation cephalosporins (ceftriaxone and cefepime, respectively), and monobactams. Carbapenems and cephamycin are effective against ESBLs. Detection of ESBLs is often difficult and some microbiology laboratories do not employ reliable methods, which may result in false susceptible reporting of ESBL strains to cefotaxime, ceftazidime, and ceftriaxone. Cefepime, a fourth-generation cephalosporin, does not appear to induce this type of chromosomal-mediated resistance to the same degree as ceftazidime, but is susceptible to the action of ESBLs. Most ESBLs also co-express resistance to other agents including aminoglycosides and fluoroquinolones. Carbapenems (specifically meropenem) are the most

effective agents against ESBLs. An ESBL E-test should be performed for this isolate, and the patient should be started on meropenem.

Answer: E

Ghafourian S, Sadeghifard N, Soheili S, et al. Extended spectrum Beta-lactamases: definition, classification and epidemiology. *Curr Issues Mol Biol.* 2015; **17**:11–21. Epub 2014 May 12.

Nathisuwan S, Burgess DS, Lewis JS. Extended-spectrum beta-lactamases: epidemiology, detection, and treatment. *Pharmacotherapy.* 2001; **21**(8):920–928. PMID: 11718498

McDaniel J, Schweizer M, Crabb V, et al. Incidence of Extended-Spectrum β-Lactamase (ESBL)- producing Escherichia coli and Klebsiella Infections in the United States: a systematic literature review. *Infect Control Hosp Epidemiol.* 2017; **38**(10):1209–1215. PMID: 28758612

2 *A 76-year-old woman with end-stage renal disease, uncontrolled diabetes, and pain control issues has been admitted to the ICU after undergoing an open right hemicolectomy. The procedure was uncomplicated, and the patient was extubated 3 hours after admission to the surgical intensive care unit. On examination, there is a nasogastric tube in place, and her vital signs are BP 110/60 mmHg, HR 85 beats/min, RR is 20 breaths/min, pulse oximetry 94% on 2L oxygen via nasal cannula, and she rates her pain on a 0–10 scale as 6.*

Which one of the following analgesics for postoperative pain management is the best choice for this patient?

A *Tramadol*
B *Ofirmev*
C *Oxycodone*
D *Morphine*
E *Celebrex*

Acetaminophen injection (Ofirmev®) is indicated for the management of mild-to-moderate pain and as an adjunct to opioid analgesics and other agents. Acetaminophen in metabolized by the liver and does not require adjustment in end-stage renal disease (ESRD). Patients report better pain control than with oral acetaminophen. Tramadol is metabolized to an active metabolite O-demethyl tramadol, which is excreted by the kidneys. Its elimination half-life is prolonged 2 times in patients with decreased glomerular filtration rate (GFR). Tramadol may be epileptogenic, especially with associated conditions that lower seizure threshold, such as with uremia. Respiratory depression is also described in patients with chronic kidney disease. Morphine should be used cautiously as morphine metabolites can accumulate, increasing therapeutic and adverse effects in patients with renal failure. Morphine and its metabolite can be removed with dialysis. Oxycodone should not be used in patients with renal failure. Oxycodone and its metabolites can accumulate causing toxic and CNS-depressant effects. There is no data on oxycodone and its metabolites removal with dialysis; however, oxycodone's half-life is significantly prolonged in ESRD. Celebrex is a nonsteroidal anti-inflammatory drug (NSAIDs), specifically a COX_2 inhibitor, used to treat pain and inflammation. NSAIDs may lead to reversible reduction in GFR. COX_2 is constitutively expressed in the kidney and has an important role in maintaining renal hemodynamics. Although potentially advantageous for patients at risk of bleeding, COX_2 inhibitors appear to exert similar effects on the kidney compared with traditional NSAIDs.

Answer: B

Davison SN. Pain in hemodialysis patients: prevalence, cause, severity, and management. *Am J Kid Dis.* 2003; **42**:1239–1247.

Foral PA, Ineck JR, Nystrom KK. Oxycodone accumulation in a hemodialysis patient. *South Med Journal.* 2007;**100**:212–214.

Kurella M. Analgesia in patients with ESRD: a review of available evidence. *Am J Kid Dis.* 2003; **42**:217–228.

Golembiewski J Intravenous acetaminophen. *J. Perianesth Nurs.* 2017; **32**(2):151–55.

3   *A 36-year-old man is involved in high-speed motor vehicle collision and was intubated in the field for a Glasgow Coma Scale (GCS) score of 4. His injuries include a severe traumatic brain injury with multiple*

intraparenchymal and intraventricular hemorrhages, multiple rib fractures bilaterally, bilateral pulmonary contusions, and a right femur fracture that is now in traction. Due to elevated intracranial pressures that have not been controlled, the patient is placed on a cisatracurium drip. Which statement is true regarding cisatracurium?
A *Primarily renally cleared.*
B *Cheaper cost compared to vecuronium.*
C *Is an aminosteroid-based neuromuscular blocking agent, similar to rocuronium.*
D *Associated with better outcomes in acute respiratory distress and traumatic brain injury.*
E *Fast onset of action and used for emergency airway management.*

Cisatracurium is a widely used nondepolarizing neuromuscular blocking agent (NMBA). Cisatracurium, an isomer of atracurium, undergoes spontaneous chemical degradation (not an enzymatic process) in a process known as Hofmann elimination. The cost of cisatracurium is substantially higher compared to other NMBA. Other NMBAs like pancuronium, rocuronium, and vecuronium are aminosteroid based and their elimination can be affected by hepatic or renal dysfunction. There are three randomized trials that have shown improvement with oxygenation in ARDS patients using cisatracurium. Two additional randomized trials found no decrease in intracranial pressure, mean arterial pressure, cerebral perfusion pressure, or cerebral blood flow velocity with cisatracurium. With atracurium, these parameters decreased and a subsequent rebound in elevated intracranial pressure was noted. Cisatracurium has a relatively slow onset, and should not be used for emergency airway management. Cisatracurium is often the paralytic of choice in patients with severe hepatic and renal dysfunction. Hofmann elimination is a temperature- and pH-dependent process, and therefore the rate of degradation is highly influenced by body pH and temperature; an increase in body pH favors the elimination process, whereas a decrease in temperature slows down the process.

Answer: D

Szakmany T, Minerva WT. Use of cisatracurium in critical care: a review of the literature. *Anestesiol.* 2015; **81**(4):450–60. Epub 2014 Apr 10.

Sparr HJ, Beaufort TM, Fuchs-Buder T. Newer neuromuscular blocking agents: how they compare with established agents? *Drugs.* 2001; **61**:919–942.

4   *A 37-year-old man is involved in an all-terrain vehicle (ATV) collision and has multiple left rib fractures, a left humerus fracture, and a grade II splenic*

laceration. Prior to his crash, he was taking alprazolam 2 mg three times a day. On post-trauma day 3, the patient is restless, shaking, tachycardic, diaphoretic, and having auditory hallucinations. Which is true regarding alprazolam withdrawal?

A *Alprazolam withdrawal is typically less severe compared to other benzodiazepines.*

B *Due to the long half-life, the abuse potential is lower compared to other benzodiazepines.*

C *Alprazolam has a slow absorption and high lipophilicity.*

D *Alprazolam uniquely affects dopaminergic function in the brain.*

E *Rebound anxiety is more commonly seen with diazepam withdrawal than with alprazolam withdrawal.*

Alprazolam has a high misuse potential and more severe withdrawal symptoms compared to other benzodiazepines. Alprazolam has unique pharmacokinetic properties since it is less protein-bound compared to other benzodiazepines resulting in rapid absorption, low lipophilicity, and short half-life. The half-life for alprazolam is 8–16 hours, while the half-life of diazepam is 22–72 hours (assuming healthy adult). In addition, alprazolam does not accumulate oxidative metabolites. Diazepam and its metabolites accumulate in the body and after discontinuation, there is a slow washout leading to less severe withdrawal symptoms. Alprazolam also crosses the blood-brain barrier and affects the dopaminergic function in the striatum leading to increased serotonin levels, thus, making it higher risk for abuse and misuse. Alprazolam withdrawal is more complicated and has a unique rebound anxiety associated with it.

Answer: D

Ait-Daoud N, Hamby AS, Sharma S, et al. A review of alprazolam use, misuse, and withdrawal. *J Addict Med.* 2018; **12**(1):4–10.

5 *A 38-year-old woman was involved in motorcycle crash and sustains a small subdural hematoma, an intraparenchymal hemorrhage, multiple right-sided rib fractures, right tibia and fibula fractures, and significant skin abrasions along right side of her body. She is intubated and sedated with dexmedetomidine drip in the ICU secondary to a Glasgow Coma Scale (GCS) score of 8. What is true regarding dexmedetomidine?*

A *It works on GABA receptors, like propofol.*

B *Side effects are mostly hemodynamic alterations such as hypotension, bradycardia, and hypertension.*

C *It is mainly eliminated via the kidneys and abnormal renal function can affect elimination.*

D *It has a long half-life, usually about 12 hours in healthy adults.*

E *In the ICU, it can be used for deep sedation and with paralytics.*

Dexmedetomidine is a selective α_2 adrenoceptor agonist that is used for its anxiolytic, sedative, and analgesic properties. Propofol and benzodiazepines both act on GABA receptors (Answer A). The side effects of dexmedetomidine are mainly hemodynamic changes, to include hypotension, sometimes hypertension, and bradycardia (Answer B). It is mainly hepatically eliminated and elimination can be impacted by hypoalbuminemia and liver failure. The half-life of dexmedetomidine is 2–3 hours in healthy adults and 2.2–3.7 hours in ICU patients (Answer D). It is approved for light to moderate sedation, not for deep sedation. It should not be used with paralytics in the ICU as it does not provide adequate sedation and cannot achieve the Richmond Agitation Sedation Score (RASS) of -4 or -5 that is recommended for paralytics (Answer E).

Answer: B

Weerink MAS, Struys MMRF, Hannivoort LN, et al. Clinical pharma-cokinetics and pharmacodynamics of dexmedetomidine. *Clin Pharmacokinet.* 2017; **56**(8):893–913.
Oddo M, Crippa IA, Mehta S, et al. Optimizing sedation in patients with acute brain injury. *Crit Care.* 2016; **20**(1):128.

6 *A 63-year-old man weighing 110 kg has a history of multiple pulmonary embolisms and is currently receiving warfarin therapy, presents with 3 hours of hematemesis. His vital signs are BP 86/45 mmHg, HR 121 beats/min, RR 22 breaths/min, and his temperature is 98.9°F. A nasogastric tube is placed with a large amount of bright red blood returned. His hemoglobin is 5.2 g/dL and his INR is 9.2. What is the most effective immediate reversal of his warfarin?*

A *Phytonadione 10 mg orally once.*

B *Four-factor prothrombin complex concentrate (PCC) 50 units/kg IV infused over 30 min.*

C *Tranexamic acid 1 gm IV over 10 minutes and followed by 1 gm IV over 8 hours.*

D *Fresh frozen plasma 15 mL/kg and repeat if INR > 3 on post-transfusion laboratory.*

E *Phytonadione 10 mg IV infusion daily for three days.*

This patient has an acute gastrointestinal hemorrhage complicated by supratherapeutic warfarin and hemodynamic instability. Reversal should be with four-factor PCC (Kcentra). Four-factor PCC contains factors IIa, VIIa, IXa, and Xa; proteins C, S, and Z; antithrombin III; and a small amount of heparin. Because of the heparin in the preparation, a patient with a history of heparin-induced thrombocytopenia, or an allergy to heparin, should not receive four-factor PCC (Kcentra). However, patients can receive *activated* four-factor PCC (FEIBA). Given his weight and elevated INR (INR > 6), the dose should be 50 units/kg, not to exceed 5000 units. For an INR 2–4, the dose should be 25 units/kg, not to exceed 2500 units; and for INR 4–6, the dose should be 35 units/kg, not to exceed 3500 units. While phytonadione (vitamin K) should be given intravenously (not orally - Answer A), the onset is 6–12 hours, and would not rapidly reverse this patient's severe supratherapeutic INR. Fresh frozen plasma requires large volumes, often has incomplete INR correction, has a risk of transfusion-related reactions, and requires extended time to achieve hemostasis, and therefore would not be ideal for a hemodynamically unstable patient. While tranexamic acid, an antifibrinolytic agent, has been shown to be beneficial in trauma and obstetric hemorrhage in studies such as CRASH 2 and WOMAN trial, respectively, it should not be used for warfarin reversal.

Answer: B

Daley, MJ, Bauer, SR. Shock Syndromes II: hypovolemic, critical bleeding, and obstructive. *2019 ACCP Critical Care Pharmacy Preparatory Review* and recertification Course. 2019

7   *Which of the following patients would be most appropriate for alvimopan?*
   A *A 46-year-old man with hypertension and hyperlipidemia who is scheduled to undergo a laparoscopic colostomy reversal with colorectal anastomosis.*
   B *A 63-year-old man with end-stage renal disease on dialysis and diabetes who is scheduled to undergo a sigmoid resection for cancer.*
   C *A 55-year-old woman with chronic back pain who is currently taking 15 mg morphine equivalents daily and is scheduled to have a laparoscopic gastric bypass.*
   D *A 36-year-old woman who is postoperative day 4 following a small bowel resection secondary to a small bowel obstruction and has a persistent ileus.*
   E *A 68-year-old man with COPD who is postoperative day 3 following a right hemicolectomy for cancer with end ileostomy and is now having 1500 mL/day output from his nasogastric tube.*

Alvimopan is a selective peripherally acting µ-opioid receptor antagonist that specifically targets peripheral µ receptors in the GI tract. It is used to accelerate time to upper and lower gastrointestinal (GI) recovery following large or small bowel resection surgery in patients who undergo a primary anastomosis. Alvimopan blocks the adverse effects of opioids on the GI tract without affecting overall analgesia. It has been shown to reduce time to GI transit and subsequently reduce hospital time. Alvimopan is indicated for planned inpatient surgery in patients undergoing partial bowel resection with primary anastomosis. Ideal dosing is a single 12 mg capsule 30 minutes to 5 hours prior to surgery, and then subsequent twice daily dosing beginning on postoperative day 1, for a maximum of 7 days (15 doses) or until discharge. Patients must remain inpatient while taking alvimopan. Alvimopan is contraindicated in patients who have received therapeutic dosing of opioids for more than 7 days prior to surgery, have severe hepatic impairment, or end-stage renal disease. It should not be used in patients with a small bowel obstruction or in those patients who will not undergo a primary anastomosis. Patient B is not a candidate due to end-stage renal disease. Patient C is not a candidate due to chronic high-dose opioid usage prior to surgery. Patient D is incorrect since she is postoperative from small bowel obstruction with a persistent ileus. Patient E is incorrect because he is postoperative, did not have a primary anastomosis, and is having high-volume nasogastric tube output.

Answer: A

Curran MP, Robins GW, Scott LJ, et al. Alvimopan. *Drugs.* 2008;**68**(14):2011–9.

Xu, LL, Zhou XQ, Yi PS, et al. Alvimopan combined with enhanced recovery strategy for managing postoperative ileus after open abdominal surgery: a systematic review and meta-analysis. *J Surg Res.* 2016; **203**:211–221.

Vaughan-Shaw PG, Fecher IC, Harris S, et al. A meta-analysis of the effectiveness of the opioid receptor antagonist alvimopan in reducing hospital length of stay and time of GI recovery in patients enrolled in a standardized accelerated recovery program after abdominal surgery. *Diseases Colon and Rectum.* 2012; **55**:611–620.

8   *Which one of the following definitions of pharmacokinetic and pharmacodynamic principles in the critically ill patient is correct?*
   A *Aggressive fluid resuscitation will not alter the volume of distribution in morbidly obese patients.*
   B *Metabolic clearance by the liver, mostly via the cytochrome P450 system, may be compromised in the critically ill patient by decreases in hepatic blood flow, intracellular oxygen tension, and cofactor availability.*
   C *Gut wall edema, changes in gastric or intestinal blood flow, concurrent administration of enteral nutrition, and incomplete oral medication dissolution has no effect on drug absorption.*

D *The response to antibiotics that have time-dependent killing pharmacodynamics would be improved by administering a higher dose of drug to increase the area under the inhibitory curve.*

E *Deceased in renal function decreases the half-life of medications cleared via the kidney and result in accumulation of drugs or their metabolites.*

Critically ill patients have alterations in medication pharmacokinetics and pharmacodynamics. Pharmacokinetics characterizes what the body does to a drug—the absorption, distribution, metabolism, and elimination of the drug. Pharmacodynamics is what the drug does to the body and describes the relationship between the concentration of drug at the site of action and the clinical response observed. Many factors affect drug absorption, distribution, and clearance in the critically ill patient. Failure to recognize these variations may result in unpredictable serum concentrations that may lead to therapeutic failure or drug toxicity. Drug absorption is altered by gut wall edema and stasis, changes in gastric and intestinal blood flow, concurrent medications and therapies such as enteral nutrition, and incomplete disintegration or dissolution of oral medications (Answer C). The volume of distribution describes the relationship between the amount of drug in the body and concentration in the plasma. Fluid shifts, particularly after fluid resuscitation, and protein binding changes that occur during critical illness, alter drug distribution (Answer A). Plasma protein concentrations may change significantly during critical illness and may affect the volume of distribution by altering the amount of the active unbound or free drug. Metabolic clearance by the liver is the predominant route of drug detoxification and elimination. With hepatic dysfunction that may occur in the critically ill patient, drug clearance may be decreased secondary to reduced hepatic blood flow, decreased hepatocellular enzyme activity, or decreased bile flow. A common pathway for drug metabolism is the cytochrome P_{450} system (Answer B). Critical illness may compromise this system by decreasing hepatic blood flow, intracellular oxygen, or cofactor availability. Antibiotics are usually categorized as having either concentration-dependent or time-dependent killing. The activity of concentration-dependent antibiotics increases as the peak serum concentrations of drug increase. Time-dependent antibiotics kill at the same rate regardless of the peak serum concentration that is attained above the MIC (minimum inhibitory concentration). Thus, an increase in dose is not associated with improved AUIC (area under the inhibitory concentration curve). Instead, increasing dosing frequency would improve antibiotic killing (Answer D). Decreases in renal function will prolong the half-life of drugs eliminated by the kidneys (Answer E).

Answer: B

Varghese JA, Robert JA, Lipman J. Pharmacokinetics and pharmacodynamics in critically ill patients. *Curr Opinion Anesth*. 2010; **23**(4):472–478.

Devlin JW, Barletta JF. *Principles of drug dosing in critically ill patients*. In *Critical Care Medicine* Parrillo JE and Dellinger RP (eds), 3rd edn, Mosby, Philadelphia, PA, 2008; pp. 343–76.

9 *Which statement is true regarding andexanet alfa, the factor Xa inhibitor reversal agent?*
  A *Reverses only direct-acting oral anticoagulants (DOACs) and not low-molecular-weight heparin.*
  B *There is concern for prothrombotic effects post-administration.*
  C *It is a monoclonal antibody that binds to factor Xa.*
  D *It has a long half-life and rarely requires redosing.*
  E *Dosing is based on the anticoagulant and the time from last dose.*

Andexanet alfa is a modified factor Xa protein (not a monoclonal antibody - Answer C) that directly binds to the factor Xa inhibitors in a 1:1 ratio to inactivate their anticoagulant response. Due to structural modifications, it does not have a direct prothrombotic effect (Answer B). Andexanet alpha reverses both direct- (DOACs) and indirect- (low-molecular-weight heparin) acting anticoagulants (Answer A). It has a short half-life of 1 hour and the infusion runs over 2 hours. In theory, the 2-hour time interval allows for a hemostatic plug to form and bleeding to stop. A rebound anticoagulation effect has yet to be found. In early studies, nearly 80% of patients had good or excellent hemostasis at 12 hours and did not require re-administration of andexanet alpha (Answer D). Andexanet alpha administration is based on the half-life of the anti-Xa inhibitor as well as when it was last taken. See chart below for dosing:

Anticoagulant	Last dose
Rivaroxaban	<10 mg: low dose >10 mg within 8 hours: high dose >10 mg after 8 hours: low dose
Apixaban	<5 mg: low dose >5 mg within 8 hours: high dose >5 mg after 8 hours: low dose
Enoxaparin (off-label)	High dose at any time
	Andexanet dosing
Low dose	400 mg bolus, 4 mg/min for 120 min
High dose	800 mg bolus and 8 mg/min for 120 min

If unsure time of last dose, assume high dose

Answer: E

Connolly SJ, Milling TJ Jr, Eikelboom JW, et al. Andexanet Alfa for acute major bleeding associated with factor Xa inhibitors. ANNEXA-4 investigators. *N Engl J Med.* 2016; **375**(12):1131–41.

10 *Which of these antipsychotics is matched with its proper description?*
   A *Haloperidol: atypical antipsychotic, fast onset, risk of QT interval prolongation, especially with IV formulation.*
   B *Olanzapine: atypical antipsychotic, renally cleared, risk of severe anticholinergic effects.*
   C *Quetiapine: atypical antipsychotic, hepatically cleared, risk of severe orthostatic hypotension.*
   D *Risperidone: typical antipsychotic, fast onset, risk of Parkinsonism.*
   E *Aripiprazole: atypical antipsychotic, slow onset, risk of QT interval prolongation.*

Olanzapine (Answer B), quetiapine (Answer C), and risperidone (Answer D) are atypical antipsychotics that are antagonists against D2, serotonin, histamine, and alpha-2 receptors. Due to action on multiple receptors, the risk of extrapyramidal symptoms is less compared to haloperidol, but each have an increased risk of orthostatic hypotension. Haloperidol (Answer A) is a typical antipsychotic, which is a potent antagonist of the dopamine D_2 receptor. Haloperidol has the strongest evidence for use in delirium and is available in oral (po), intramuscular (IM), and intravenous (IV) formulations. The IV form may cause QT interval prolongation. It also has minimal effects on vital signs and minimal interactions with other drugs. It has a moderate onset of action. All the antipsychotics are hepatically cleared. Olanzapine is the only atypical antipsychotic available in both IM and PO forms. Quetiapine has a high risk of orthostatic hypotension and is not recommended in emergency room settings for agitation. However, quetiapine is recommended for patients with Parkinson's disease because it has little or no risk compared to the other atypical antipsychotics. Aripiprazole (Answer E) is a partial dopamine agonist. It is available in oral, dissolvable, and IM forms. While it may be less effective compared to other antipsychotics, it is also less sedating and does not have any effect on QT interval prolongation.

Antipsychotic agents

Agent	Form	Half-life (hrs)	Clearance	Adverse effects	Effect on QT	Orthostatic hypotension	Antichol. effects	Sedation	Considerations
Haloperidol	PO, IM, IV	12–38	Hepatic	Akathisia, dystonia, Parkinsonism	IV: moderate	Mild	Mild	Mild	Minimal vital sign change, may worsen Parkinson's
Olanzapine	PO, SL, IM	21–54	Hepatic	Akathisia, Parkinsonism	Mild	Moderate	Severe	Moderate	Cancer-related nausea, do not combine with IV benzos, may worsen diabetes
Quetiapine	PO	6	Hepatic	Agitation	Mild	Severe	Moderate	Severe	Consider in Parkinson's disease
Risperidone	PO, SL	20	Hepatic	Parkinsonism	Mild	Severe	Mild	Moderate	Comes in dissolvable form
Aripiprazole	PO, SL, IM	75	Hepatic	Akathisia, agitation	None	Moderate	Mild	Moderate	Hypoactive delirium, no known QTC effect

Answer: C

Thom RP, Mock CK, Teslyar P. Delirium in hospitalized patients: risks and benefits of antipsychotics. *Cleve Clin J Med.* 2017; **84**(8):616–622.

11 *A 27-year-old man weighing 80 kg and otherwise healthy, presents with multiple gunshot wounds to the right thigh. There is no pulse distal to the injury and an expanding hematoma is present. He is taken urgently to operating room and is found to have 3 cm disruption of the superficial femoral artery at the mid-thigh. Proximal and distal control are achieved, saphenous vein graft is harvested from the contralateral groin, four-compartment fasciotomies are completed in the calf, and an end-to-end anastomosis is performed. Prior to performing the anastomosis, the patient is given 8000 units of heparin IV. Ninety minutes later,*

the patient has a palpable dorsalis pedis (DP) pulse; however, the fasciotomy sites and right groin are oozing considerably. How much protamine should be given to completely reverse the heparin?

A *Protamine 12.5 mg IV*

B *Protamine 25 mg IM*

C *Protamine 40 mg IV*

D *Protamine 50 mg IM*

E *Protamine 80 mg IV*

Protamine sulfate completely reverses the action of unfractionated heparin. Protamine is a highly cationic peptide that binds heparin or low-molecular-weight heparin to form a stable ionic pair. The ionic complex is then removed and broken down by the reticuloendothelial system (RES). Approximately 1 mg of protamine sulfate neutralizes 100 units of heparin. The half-life of heparin is about 60–90 minutes. Assuming normal renal function, there would be about 4000 units of heparin remaining in this patient (1 half-life), which would require 40 mg of IV protamine for complete reversal. Protamine can only be dosed IV and the maximum dose is 50 mg.

Answer: C

Dhakal P, Rayamajhi S, Verma V, et al. Reversal of anticoagulation and management of bleeding in patients on anticoagulants. *Clin Appl Thromb Hemost.* 2017; **23**(5):410–415.

12 *Which of these patients is most likely to develop propofol infusion syndrome?*

   A *A 23-year-old man receiving propofol 50 mcg/kg/min for 6 hours due to a subdural hematoma and intraparenchymal hemorrhage.*

   B *A 65-year-old woman receiving propofol 20 mcg/kg/min and norepinephrine 5 mcg/min for 24 hours following debridement for necrotizing fasciitis.*

   C *A 45-year-old man receiving propofol 60 mcg/kg/min and norepinephrine 10 mcg/min for 60 hours for alcohol induced necrotizing pancreatitis.*

   D *A 30-year-old woman receiving propofol 50 mcg/kg/min for 12 hours due to sustaining a subdural hematoma and following an exploratory laparotomy for splenectomy.*

   E *A 75-year-old man receiving propofol 30 mcg/kg/min for 8 hours following a Whipple procedure and inability to extubate due to COPD.*

Propofol infusion syndrome is a rare syndrome characterized by cardiac arrhythmias and rhabdomyolysis, which can manifest with elevated creatine phosphokinase (CPK) and potassium, lactic acidosis, and renal failure. The most significant risk factor for development of propofol infusion syndrome is high-dose propofol use for > 48 hours. Other risk factors include sepsis, head trauma, and status epilepticus. In addition, the use of vasopressors, glucocorticoids, mitochondrial disease, and carbohydrate depletion as seen with liver disease, starvation, or malnutrition can cause propofol infusion syndrome. Patient C is the only patient that received high-dose propofol for > 48 hours. He is also septic, receiving vasopressors, and likely has some element of liver disease given his alcohol use.

Answer: C

Mirrakhimov AE, Voore P, Halytskyy O, et al. Propofol infusion syndrome in adults: a clinical update. *Crit Care Res Pract.* 2015; **2015**:260385.

13 *Which of the following antiemetic medications is matched with its correct description?*

   A *Ondansetron: serotonin antagonist; adverse effects: headache, constipation.*

   B *Dexamethasone: corticosteroid; adverse effects: dry eyes, hypotension.*

   C *Promethazine: serotonin antagonist; adverse effects: sedation, dizziness.*

   D *Scopolamine: dopamine antagonist; adverse effects: dizziness, dry mouth.*

   E *Metoclopramide: dopamine antagonist; adverse effects: hyperglycemia, hypertension.*

Postoperative nausea and vomiting (PONV) is a common complication following surgery. As more procedures transition to outpatient surgery and enhanced recovery protocols try to minimize hospital stays, the management of postoperative nausea and vomiting becomes more important. Besides antiemetics, other strategies to reduce PONV include local nerve blocks, propofol induction and maintenance, minimizing perioperative narcotics, minimizing volatile anesthetics, avoiding nitrous oxide and reversal agents, and providing adequate perioperative hydration. Ondansetron is a serotonin antagonist and is usually well tolerated, though can cause headaches and constipation. Dexamethasone is a corticosteroid and can cause hyperglycemia and hypertension or hypotension. Promethazine is a histamine (H_1) antagonist and causes sedation and dizziness. Scopolamine is an anticholinergic which causes dry mouth, visual disturbances, and dizziness. Metoclopramide is dopamine antagonist which can cause sedation and hypotension.

Antiemetics

Drug group	Drugs	Dose	Timing for PONV	Adverse effects
Serotonin (5-HT$_3$ receptors) antagonists	Ondansetron	4–8 mg IV		
	Granisetron	1 mg IV	End of surgery	Headaches, constipation, raised LFTs
	Tropisetron	2 mg IV		
Corticosteroids	Dexamethasone	4–10 mg IV	After anesthesia induction	Increased glucose, hypo/hypertension
Butyrophenone	Droperidol	0.625 to 1.25 mg IV	After anesthesia induction	Extrapyramidal disturbances, Parkinson's, increased QT
Neurokinin antagonists (NK-1 receptors)	Aprepitant	40 mg PO	1–2 hour pre-op	Headaches, constipation, fatigue
Anticholinergics	Scopolamine	Patch	Pre-op	Dizziness, dry mouth, visual
Dopamine antagonists	Metoclopramide	10–25 mg IV	15 min prior to end of surgery	Sedation, hypotension
1st generation Antihistamine	Promethazine	12.5 to 25 mg PO/IM/IV	Post-op	Sedation, dizziness, extrapyramidal disturbances

Answer: A

Cao X, White PF, Ma H. An update on the management of postoperative nausea and vomiting. *J Anesth.* 2017; **31**(4):617–626.

14 *A 76-year-old man with hypertension, peripheral vascular disease, and diabetes is taking warfarin for atrial fibrillation. He also had a stroke 2 years ago. He will be undergoing a robotic low anterior resection for rectal cancer. What should be the management of his warfarin?*

   A *Stop warfarin 5 days prior to surgery, resume post-operative (POD) 2.*

   B *Stop warfarin 5 days prior to surgery, start weight-based enoxaparin 3 days prior to surgery, stop enoxaparin day of surgery, resume warfarin POD 1.*

   C *Stop warfarin 5 days prior to surgery, start weight-based enoxaparin 3 days prior to surgery, stop enoxaparin day before surgery, resume warfarin POD 1.*

   D *Stop warfarin 3 days prior to surgery, start weight-based enoxaparin 3 days prior to surgery, stop enoxaparin day before surgery, resume warfarin POD 2.*

   E *Stop warfarin 3 days prior to surgery, start weight-based enoxaparin 3 days prior to surgery, stop enoxaparin day before surgery, resume warfarin POD 5.*

Stopping anticoagulation medication prior to surgery must be weighed against the risk of thromboembolic events and the surgical bleeding risk. This patient has a high CHA$_2$DS$_2$-VASc score of 7 (hypertension -1, age > 75 - 2, diabetes -1, stroke -2, and vascular disease -1)

and is high risk for thromboembolic events, and therefore, should not have anticoagulation stopped completely (Answer A). This patient should be placed on enoxaparin therapy, which should be stopped the day before surgery (Answer C) and warfarin should be started POD 1, provided no/minimal bleeding risk. Weight-based enoxaparin should also be restarted 12–24 hours after surgery depending on bleeding risk, as it will take multiple days for warfarin to reach therapeutic levels.

BRIDGE trial anticoagulation protocol

Day (around procedure)	Protocol
–5	Stop warfarin
–3	Start bridging agent (LMWH)
–1	Stop bridging agent 24 hours prior to procedure
0	Procedure
1	Resume warfarin within 24 hours, resume bridging agent within 12 to 24 hours for low risk bleed
2 to 3	Resume bridging agent within 48–72 hours for high-risk procedure
5 to 10	Stop bridging agent when INR > 2

Answer: C

Barnes GD, Mouland E. Peri-procedural management of oral anticoagulants in the DOAC Era. *Prog Cardiovasc Dis.* 2018; **60**(6):600–606.

15 *A 45-year-old woman pedestrian was struck by a motor vehicle. She has a history of COPD and a penicillin allergy. She sustained bilateral rib fractures with a flail segment on the left, left pulmonary contusion, left diaphragmatic injury (status-post repair), and left open tibia and fibula fractures (also status-post repair). She was admitted to the surgical ICU 8 days ago. She has been difficult to wean from the ventilator and has had a central line and left chest tube in place since admission. She began spiking fevers 2 days ago and is now requiring vasopressors. Empiric cefepime, metronidazole, and vancomycin were started, but clinically she has not improved. Her bronchoalveolar lavage (BAL) and blood cultures have come back positive for Candida with species pending. What is the best treatment choice for this patient currently?*

A *Continue current antibiotics and give more time to improve*

B *Fluconazole 200 mg IV daily*

C *Voriconazole 4 mg/kg IV daily*

D *Caspofungin 70 mg IV x1 followed by 50 mg IV daily*

E *Flucytosine 50 mg/kg IV q6 hours*

Empiric antifungal therapy should be considered in critically ill patients with risk factors for invasive candidiasis and no other known cause of fever. This patient is not improving and cultures indicate fungal bacteremia and ventilator-associated pneumonia (VAP), thus, continuing the current antibiotic regimen would not treat this patient. Empiric antifungal therapy should be started as soon as possible in patients who have risk factors and who have clinical signs of septic shock. The preferred empiric therapy for suspected candidiasis in nonneutropenic patients in the ICU is an echinocandin (micafungin 100 mg IV daily, caspofungin 70 mg IV × 1 followed by 50 mg IV daily, anidulafungin 200 mg IV × 1 followed by 100 mg IV daily). Thus, Answer D is correct. Fluconazole at higher doses 800 mg IV ×1 followed by 400 mg IV daily is an acceptable alternative for patients who have not had recent azole exposure. B is incorrect because the dose is subtherapeutic. Voriconazole is used in much higher doses (6 mg/kg) BID × 2 then 3 mg/kg BID, but offers little advantage over fluconazole as initial therapy. Voriconazole is recommended as step-down therapy for selected cases of candidemia due to *Candida krusei*, for additional mold coverage and for neutropenic patients. Flucytosine is usually used in combination with other antifungals and reserved for very severe infections. It is used more commonly in combination with amphotericin B for central nervous system candidiasis. In addition, higher doses (100–200 mg/kg) in 4 doses over 24 hours are recommended.

Answer: D

Pappas PG, Kauffman CA, Andes AR, et. al. Clinical practice guidelines for the management of candidiasis: 2016 update by the Infectious Diseases Society of America. *Clinical Infectious Diseases*. 2016; **62**:e1–50.

16 *A 63-year-old woman is receiving rivaroxaban following a pulmonary embolism she had 5 months ago. She also has hypertension and hyperlipidemia. She has normal renal function. She will be undergoing a mastectomy with sentinel lymph node biopsy for stage 2 ductal carcinoma. How should her rivaroxaban be managed in the perioperative period?*

Last dose of the DOAC prior to elective procedure

Agent	Renal clearance	Low bleed risk	High or unknown bleed risk
Rivaroxaban, apixaban, edoxaban	CrCl > 30 mL/min	>24 hours	>48 hours
	CrCl 15–29 mL/min	>36 hours	>72 hours
	CrCl < 15 mL/min	>48 hours	Data lacking
Dabigatran	CrCl > 80 mL/min	>24 hours	>48 hours
	CrCl 50–80 mL/min	>36 hours	>72 hours
	CrCl 30–49 mL/min	>48 hours	>96 hours
	CrCl 15–29 mL/min	>72 hours	>120 hours
	CrCl < 15 mL/min	Unknown	Unknown

A *Stop rivaroxaban 5 days before surgery and restart POD 1.*

B *Stop rivaroxaban 2 days before surgery and restart POD 1.*

C *Stop rivaroxaban 5 days before surgery, start weight-based enoxaparin, and restart POD 1.*

D *Stop rivaroxaban 2 days before surgery, start weight-based enoxaparin, and restart POD 2.*

E *Stop rivaroxaban day of surgery and restart POD 2.*

This patient is at intermediate risk for thromboembolic events and should stop anticoagulation in the perioperative period without significant consequence. The direct-acting oral anticoagulants (DOACs) rarely need bridging therapy (Answers C & D). Provided normal renal function, rivaroxaban should be eliminated entirely by 35–55 hours, since its half-life is 7–11 hours (4–5 half-lives for 95% elimination). A mastectomy has a higher risk of bleeding compared to some other surgeries, thus, rivaroxaban should be stopped 2 days prior to surgery and resumed POD 1 provided no bleeding complications.

Answer: B

Barnes GD, Mouland E. Peri-procedural management of oral anticoagulants in the DOAC Era. *Prog Cardiovasc Dis.* 2018; **60**(6):600–606.

17 *A 45-year-old man was involved in a high-speed motor vehicle crash and has the following injuries: intra-parenchymal hemorrhage, diffuse axonal injury, T4 vertebral body fracture, T4 paraplegia, and multiple bilateral rib fractures. On hospital day 9, the patient remains intubated, spikes a fever, and has thick secretions from the endotracheal tube. Subsequent bronchial alveolar lavage is performed, and the culture grows vancomycin- resistant enterococcus (VRE). Blood cultures also grow 2/2 bottles with VRE. Which is the best choice of antibiotic to use?*

A *Cefepime*

B *Linezolid*

C *Daptomycin*

D *Piperacillin-tazobactam*

E *Meropenem*

Vancomycin-resistant enterococci (VRE) was first reported in 1986 and cases have been increasing in the ICU. In 2006 in the US, the rate of VRE was 0.6 per 1000 admissions. There is an increased risk of mortality with VRE bacteremia and treatment should be started promptly. Effective treatments for VRE include quinupristin-dalfopristin, linezolid, daptomycin, tigecycline, teicoplanin, and telavancin. Linezolid and daptomycin are the two most commonly used antibiotics

in the US for VRE. Linezolid (Answer B) is an oxazolidone that binds to the 50S ribosomal subunit, has been approved by the FDA for VRE treatment, has better tissue penetration than other antibiotics, especially lung penetration, and is bacteriostatic. Linezolid can suppress bone marrow, is expensive, and can interact with psychiatric medications, particularly monoamine oxidase inhibitors (MAOIs). Daptomycin (Answer C) is a novel cyclic lipopeptide that inhibits DNA and RNA synthesis and is bactericidal. It is not approved by FDA for VRE infections, though it is recognized as an appropriate treatment for some VRE infections; however, it should not be used to treat pneumonia because it is inactivated by alveolar surfactant. Daptomycin may cause *Clostridium difficile*, rhabdomyolysis, and thrombocytopenia. A meta-analysis showed linezolid treatment for VRE bacteremia had a lower mortality compared to daptomycin. Cefepime, piperacillin-tazobactam, and meropenem are not indicated for VRE.

Answer: B

Prematunge C, MacDougall C, Johnstone J, et al. VRE and VSE bacteremia outcomes in the Era of effective VRE therapy: a systematic review and meta-analysis. *Infect Control Hosp Epidemiol.* 2016; **37**(1):26–35.

Chuang Y-C, Wang J-T, Lin H-Y,et al. Daptomycin versus linezolid for treatment of vancomycin-resistant enterococcal bacteremia: systematic review and meta-analysis. *BMC Infectious Diseases.* 2014; **14**:687–695.

Kalil AC, et al Management of adults with hospital-acquired and ventilator-associated pneumonia: 2016 clinical practice guidelines by the Infectious Diseases Society of America and the American Thoracic Society. *Clin Infect Dis.* 2016; **63**(5):e61–e111. PMID: 27418577.

18 *Which of the following is the best practice to prevent antibiotic resistance in the ICU?*

A *Initially treating a septic shock patient of unknown etiology with monotherapy quinolones.*

B *Continuing antibiotics for at least 7 days for intra-abdominal sepsis after source control.*

C *Continuing vancomycin in a patient with ventilator-associated pneumonia due to E. coli.*

D *De-escalation of antibiotics based on culture results.*

E *Decrease the infusion time of intravenous antibiotics.*

Effective antimicrobial therapy is critical for the treatment of patients in the ICU and appropriate therapy decreases mortality as well as antibiotic resistance. The Surviving Sepsis campaign highlights starting antibiotics within an hour of emergency room admission or suspicion of sepsis and appropriate antimicrobial coverage of the suspected source. Sepsis of unknown origin requires active therapy against gram-positive and gram-negative pathogens. Common regimens are cefepime and vancomycin or piperacillin-tazobactam and vancomycin. Quinolones only (Answer A) provide narrow coverage for gram-negative bacteria and would not be appropriate for a septic patient of unknown origin. The Short Course Antimicrobial Therapy for Intraabdominal Infection (STOP-IT) trial showed there was no difference in outcomes between 4 days and 8 days of antibiotics after source control had been achieved. Another study showed longer antibiotic courses led to increased risk of secondary infections and higher mortality. Answer B is incorrect because the patient only needs 4 days of antibiotics. It is important to de-escalate antibiotics as soon as possible (Answer D). As vancomycin is used to cover gram-positive bacteria, and specifically methicillin-resistant *Staph aureus* (MRSA), vancomycin should be stopped as soon as it is known that the organism is not MRSA (Answer C). Answer E is incorrect because it is important to maintain minimum inhibitory concentration (MIC) of antibiotics. To achieve this, many beta-lactamase antibiotics (cefepime, piperacillin) have been switched to extended infusions.

Answer: D

Campion M, Scully G. Antibiotic use in the intensive care unit: optimization and de-escalation. *J Intensive Care Med.* 2018; **33**(12):647–655.

19 *An 82-year-old man was started on clindamycin for left lower extremity cellulitis. Eight days after starting antibiotics, he presents to the emergency department with severe diarrhea, fever, abdominal pain, and emesis. His vitals are: HR 130 bpm, BP 90/50 mmHg, and his WBC is 35 000. C. difficile PCR is positive. What is the best management of his C. difficile infection?*

A *Discontinue antibiotics only*
B *Discontinue antibiotics and start IV vancomycin*
C *Discontinue antibiotics and start PO metronidazole*
D *Discontinue antibiotics and start PO vancomycin*
E *Discontinue antibiotics and start IV rifampin*

Clostridium difficile infection (CDI) has increased in frequency and severity over the last decade. Minimizing antibiotics, especially clindamycin and fluoroquinolones, is the cornerstone of prevention. This patient has severe *C. difficile* infection, as he presents in septic shock. Based on current treatment regimens, the previous antibiotics need to be stopped and vancomycin 125 mg orally four times a day should be started. Discontinuation of antibiotics only (Answer A) is incorrect as this patient needs additional treatment since he is in septic shock. Answer B is incorrect since vancomycin should be given via the oral (PO) route and not the IV route. Vancomycin administered IV does not reach therapeutic levels in the colonic lumen. Answer C is incorrect since oral metronidazole is only for mild disease or if oral vancomycin is unavailable or contraindicated. Metronidazole, administered either orally or IV, only reaches low therapeutic levels in the colon; therefore, even a slightly elevated MIC of *C. difficile* for metronidazole may lead to therapy failure. Multiple studies have shown that monotherapy of IV metronidazole is inferior to monotherapy PO vancomycin for treatment of *Clostridium difficile.* If the patient advances to fulminant colitis, the regimen would be vancomycin 500 mg orally or via nasogastric tube four times a day and metronidazole 500 mg intravenously every eight hours. Surgery would also be indicated with fulminant colitis. Rifampin (Answer E) is incorrect because while it has been used previously, data is lacking on its efficacy and is currently not recommended.

Findoxamin, a novel macrolide antibiotic, bezlotoxumab, a monoclonal antibody against toxin TCDB, and fecal microbiota transplant, are gaining popularity, especially in recurrent infections. Surgical treatment, typically a total colectomy, are reserved for those patients with fulminant colitis, though patient selection and timing of operation can be challenging.

Answer: D

Guh AY, Kutty PK. Clostridioides difficile infection. *Ann Intern Med.* 2018; **169**(7):ITC49–ITC64.
Goldenberg JZ, Yap C, Lytvyn L, et al. Probiotics for the prevention of clostridium difficile- associated diarrhea in adults and children. *The Cochrane Database of Systematic Reviews.* 2017 Dec; 19(12):CD006095
Bignardi GE. Risk factors for clostridium difficile infection. *J Hosp Infect.* 1998;40(1):1–15. PMID: 9777516.
Bowman JA, Uteer GH. Evolving strategies to manage clostridium difficile infections. *J Gastrointest Surg.* 2020; 24(2):484–91.

20 *A 55-year-old otherwise healthy man presents to the emergency department with a large incarcerated umbilical hernia. He is brought to the operating room for open surgical repair. The patient was paralyzed with rocuronium to assist the reduction of the hernia. The surgery goes well and you tell the anesthesiologist that you are finished closing the fascia; however, a dose of rocuronium was just administered. Which statement is true regarding neuromuscular blocking agents (NMBAs) reversal?*

A *Neostigmine is an anticholinergic drug that is often used in conjunction with agents such as atropine and glycopyrrolate.*

B *The reversal agent available for succinylcholine is edrophonium.*

C *The mechanism of action of sugammadex includes chelating the NMBAs, making them inactive and removing them from the neuromuscular junction.*

D *Sugammadex is slower at reversing NMBA-induced paralysis than both neostigmine and edrophonium.*

E *Acetylcholinesterase inhibitors are reversal agents available for depolarizing NMBAs.*

Neuromuscular blocking agents (NMBAs) can be broken down into two main classes: depolarizing and non-depolarizing agents. Succinylcholine is the only member of the depolarizing class of NMBAs and there is no reversal agent available (Answer B). The nondepolarizing NMBAs are rocuronium, pancuronium, vecuronium, atracurium, and its isomer, cisatracurium. Neostigmine and other acetylcholinesterase inhibitors (Answer A – incorrect choice because neostigmine is an acetylcholinesterase inhibitor) were the only reversal agents available for nondepolarizing NMBAs (Answer E). These agents increase the endogenous amount of acetylcholine available for binding at the neuromuscular junction, thus, competitively counteract the NMBAs effect. Sugammadex is a novel class of drugs called selective relaxant binding agents (SRBAs). The mechanism of action is twofold: (1) encapsulating (chelating) steroid backboned NMBAs (rocuronium, pancuronium, vecuronium) making them inactive and removing them from the neuromuscular junction, thus restoring muscle function; (2) the NMBAs that are already bound to nicotinic receptors will dissociate from the receptor (Answer C). Sugammadex exerts its effect by forming very tight complexes at a 1:1 ratio with aminosteroid muscle relaxants (rocuronium > vecuronium >> pancuronium). The intermolecular (van der Waals') forces, thermodynamic (hydrogen) bonds and hydrophobic interactions make the sugammadex–rocuronium complex very tight. The resulting reduction in free-rocuronium plasma concentration creates a gradient between the tissue compartment (including the neuromuscular junction) and plasma-free rocuronium moves from tissue to plasma, with a reduction in nicotinic receptor occupancy at the neuromuscular junction. Multiple trials have found sugammadex is faster at reversing rocuronium- and vecuronium-induced paralysis than both neostigmine and edrophonium (Answer D) while having similar adverse event profiles as the traditional cholinesterase inhibitors. Atropine and glycopyrrolate (Answer A) are both anticholinergic drugs that are often used in conjunction with cholinesterase inhibitors (neostigmine and edrophonium) to help offset their cholinergic

effects such as bradycardia and excessive salivation. They have no role in NMBA reversal when used by themselves.

Answer: C

Abrishami A, Ho J, Wong J, et al. Sugammadex, a selective reversal medication for preventing postoperative residual neuromuscular blockade. *The Cochrane Library.* 2009 Oct; 7(4):CD007362.

Welliver, M, McDonough J, Kalynych N, et al. Discovery, development, and clinical application of sugammadex sodium, a selective relaxant binding agent. *Drug Des Devel Ther.* 2008; **2**: 49–59.

Keating, GM Sugammadex: a review of neuromuscular blockade reversal. *Drugs.* 2016; **76** (10):1041–1052.

21 *A 42-year-old man with no past medical history was in a motor vehicle crash and sustained a large subdural hematoma. The patient is intubated and taken to the operating room for a decompressive craniotomy. On postoperative day 6 while still intubated, the patient develops thick purulent-looking secretions, has a WBC 13 000, and a fever to 38.4°C. Blood cultures, urine cultures, and bronchial alveolar lavage are obtained. What should be the empiric therapy for his suspected ventilator-associated pneumonia?*

A *Vancomycin and ciprofloxacin*

B *Vancomycin and gentamicin*

C *Vancomycin and cefepime*

D *Ceftriaxone and azithromycin*

E *Ampicillin-sulbactam and doxycycline*

Per 2016 guidelines, antibiotic coverage for ventilator-associated pneumonia (VAP) should include an active agent against MRSA when risk factors for antimicrobial resistance is present (prior IV antibiotics within 90 days, septic shock at time of VAP, ARDS preceding VAP, 5 or more days of hospitalization prior to VAP, acute renal replacement therapy). This patient most likely received antibiotics prior to his craniotomy and has been in the hospital > 5 days, and therefore needs both MRSA and gram-negative coverage. This patient does not require double *Pseudomonas* coverage assuming he is in an intensive care unit that has antimicrobial resistance defined as < 10% of gram-negative isolates resistant to an agent considered for monotherapy. Fluoroquinolones and aminoglycosides (Answers A & B) should not be used as monotherapy for gram-negative coverage for ventilator-associated pneumonia. Answers D and E are both reasonable treatments for community-acquired pneumonia but are not appropriate for ventilator-associated pneumonia. In this case, cefepime would be preferred to piperacillin-tazobactam for gram-negative coverage as cefepime has CNS penetration and this patient has had neurosurgical intervention.

Answer: C

Kalil AC, Metersky ML, Klompas M,et al. Management of adults with hospital-acquired and ventilator-associated pneumonia: 2016 clinical practice guidelines by the Infectious Diseases Society of America and the American Thoracic Society. *Clin Infect Dis.* 2016; **63**(5): e61–e111.

Torres A, Niederman MS, Chastre J, et al. International ERS/ESICM/ESCMID/ALAT guidelines for the management of hospital-acquired pneumonia and ventilator-associated pneumonia: guidelines for the management of hospital-acquired pneumonia (HAP)/ ventilator-associated pneumonia (VAP) of the European Respiratory Society (ERS), European Society of Intensive Care Medicine (ESICM), European Society of Clinical Microbiology and Infectious Diseases (ESCMID) and Asociación Latinoamericana del Tórax (ALAT). *Eur Respir J.* 2017; **50**(3):1–26. PMID: 28890434.

22 *A 33-year-old man, otherwise healthy, has acute appendicitis and will be undergoing a laparoscopic appendectomy. He mentions both his father and brother have been diagnosed with malignant hyperthermia. The patient has never had surgery before and has not been tested for the gene. Which is the best plan for anesthesia?*
   A *Succinylcholine followed by isoflurane*
   B *Succinylcholine followed by desflurane*
   C *Rocuronium followed by sevoflurane*
   D *Rocuronium followed by propofol*
   E *Rocuronium followed by nitrous oxide*

Malignant hyperthermia is a rare autosomal dominant disorder which is characterized by skeletal muscle hypermetabolism following exposure to halogenated anesthetics, succinylcholine, or rarely, physiologic stress. The mutation is often found on the RYR1 gene. Exposure to halogenated gasses or succinylcholine causes uncontrolled release of calcium from the sarcoplasmic reticulum leading to sustained muscle contraction. Signs and symptoms are tachycardia, tachypnea, hypoxemia, hypercarbia, metabolic acidosis, hyperkalemia, cardiac dysrhythmias, hypotension, skeletal muscle rigidity, and hyperthermia. Earliest signs are often hypercarbia and tachypnea followed by hyperthermia. Treatment is to stop the inciting agent, call for help, administer dantrolene 2.5 mg/kg until the reaction subsides, increase tidal volume, start aggressive cooling measures, treat arrythmias (avoid calcium channel blockers), check electrolytes, and continue dantrolene 1 mg/kg every 4 hours for 24 to 48 hours. The gold standard test is the caffeine halothane contracture test. As this requires a muscle biopsy, genetic testing is becoming more common.

Succinylcholine and the halogenated gasses (isoflurane, desflurane, and sevoflurane) are known triggers for malignant hyperthermia, and should be avoided in this patient (Answers A, B, C). While nitrous oxide (Answer E) is not a halogenated gas, it is not typically used with laparoscopic surgeries as there is concern for bowel distension.

Answer: D

Watt S, McAllister RK. *Malignant Hyperthermia. Stat Pearls Publishing.* 2020

Ruffert H, Bastian B, Bendixen D, et al. Consensus guidelines on perioperative management of malignant hyperthermia suspected or susceptible patients from the European Malignant Hyperthermia group. *Br J Anaesth.* 2021; 126(1):120–130. doi: https://doi.org/10.1016/j. bja.2020.09.029. Epub 2020 Oct 31. PMID: 33131754

11

Transfusion, Hemostasis, and Coagulation

Lindsey Karavites, MD and Kazuhide Matsushima, MD

Division of Acute Care Surgery, University of Southern California, LAC+USC Medical Center, Los Angeles, CA, USA

1 *57-year-old man was brought into the trauma bay after a witnessed fall from his third-floor apartment onto the sidewalk. He is lethargic but arousable with blood pressure 80/40 mmHg and heart rate 135 beats/ min. He is noted to have a scalp laceration and bilateral lower extremity deformities with significant blood loss noted at the scene. What is one advantage of selecting low titer whole blood for his resuscitation over component therapy?*

A *24-hour survival benefit in the severely injured.*

B *Decreased 24-hour total transfusion requirement.*

C *Cost effectiveness of prolonged time to product expiration.*

D *Decreased transfusion reactions due to standardized safe antibody titer levels.*

E *No risk of post-transfusion hemolysis.*

Increasing retrospective data from the military medical community for use of whole blood in resuscitation have led to similar efforts in civilian trauma patients. Low titer whole blood may have institution specific definitions; however, it is generally considered unseparated blood collected from a donor with low titers of Ig M and/or IgG anti-A and anti-B. Implementation of cold-stored low-titer anti-A and anti-B group O whole blood (LTOWB) transfusion strategies are in place in civilian trauma centers but further prospective data are necessary to examine discrete comparisons of whole blood without simultaneous use of components, verification of appropriate safety, and determination of cost–benefit analyses. To date, the only randomized controlled pilot trial comparing the use of whole blood to component therapy demonstrated that those receiving whole blood required fewer blood products at 24 hours with no difference in mortality. Another recent study comparing between LTOWB vs. component therapy showed that the use of

LTOWB was significantly associated with a reduction in post-emergency department blood transfusion and improved 30-day survival. Additional advantages include ease of use with single bag product storage, reduced human error with administration, decreased transfusion reactions, although no standard safe antibody titer levels have been established, as well as avoidance of excessive volume, additives and anticoagulants.

Answer: B

Cotton, B.A, Podbielski, J., Camp, E., *et al.* (2013) Early Whole Blood Investigators: A randomized controlled pilot trial of modified whole blood versus component therapy in severely injured patients requiring large volume transfusions. *Ann Surg,* **258** (4), 527–532.

Williams, J., Merutka, D., Bai, Y., *et al.* (2019) Safety profile and impact of low-titer group O whole blood for emergency use in trauma. *J Trauma Acute Care Surg,* **88** (1), 87–93.

2 *When massive transfusion is indicated, the American College of Surgeons Trauma Quality Improvement Program currently recommends one unit of apheresis platelets to be given following the administration of how many units of packed red blood cells (PRBCs) in the setting of balanced component 1:1–1:2 (Plasma/ PRBCs) resuscitation?*

A *1*

B *2*

C *4*

D *6*

E *8*

Evidence currently supports a balanced transfusion strategy that targets a plasma:PRBC ratio approaching 1:1. There is no apparent increase in respiratory complications in the 1:1 group, despite prior retrospective associations between increased plasma transfusion and acute respiratory distress syndrome (ARDS). The latest massive transfusion guidelines from American College of Surgeons Trauma Quality Improvement Program (ACS-TQIP) recommends a 1:1–1:2 (plasma/RBCs) transfusion ratio with one unit of apheresis platelets given for every 6 units of RBCs transfused.

Answer: D

Cryer, H.G., Nathens, A.B., Bulger, E.M. (2014), American College of Surgeons Trauma Quality Improvement Program Massive Transfusion in Trauma Guidelines. facs.org/-/media/files/quality-programs/trauma/tqip/transfusion_guildelines.ashx.

3 *A 75-year-old woman with cirrhosis arrives in the trauma bay after being hit by a car while crossing the street. Her initial work up revealed two left-sided rib fractures and a grade 3 splenic laceration without evidence active extravasation. She is hemodynamically stable and her initial laboratory tests reveal a hemoglobin of 9.5 g/dL, hematocrit of 29%, platelet count of 125 000/mm3, and international normalized ratio of 3.1. While being managed nonoperatively in the intensive care unit, she becomes hypotensive. 1 unit of packed red blood cells (PRBCs) and 1 unit of fresh frozen plasma (FFP) are transfused. Shortly after the transfusions are completed, she develops tachycardia and dyspnea requiring supplement oxygen. Which of the following is the most diagnostic of transfusion-associated acute lung injury (TRALI) as the source of her new oxygen requirement?*
A *Bilateral infiltrate on chest radiography*
B *Heart Rate: 135*
C *PaO2/FiO2: 300*
D *Systolic Blood Pressure: 90*
E *Temperature 37.9*

The differential diagnosis of respiratory distress is broad in the setting of polytrauma, especially in those with known rib fractures and those requiring transfusions. Transfusion-related acute lung injury (TRALI) is defined by the documentation of acute hypoxemia with PaO_2/FIO_2 ratio (P/F) of less than 300 mm Hg, bilateral infiltrates on chest radiograph (in the absence of left atrial hypertension), and the absence of acute injury before transfusion. In addition, onset of transfusion-related acute lung injury is required to have occurred within 6 hours of the last transfusion. Transfusion-associated circulatory overload (TACO) was defined as acute onset or worsening respiratory distress during or up to 12 hours after transfusion, plus evidence of acute or worsening pulmonary edema and volume overload. Signs/symptoms

include fever, dyspnea, and hypotension. The treatment of TRALI is respiratory support, including measures to avoid worsening of lung injury. Transfusion of all types of blood products can cause TRALI. Pathogenesis is related to donor antibodies in the transfused blood and may also be related to modifications of stored blood. Measures to prevent TRALI include a restrictive transfusion policy, as well as blood bank measures such as predominant use of plasma from male donors.

Answer: A

Semple, J.W., Rebetz, J., and Kapur, R. (2019) Transfusion-associated circulatory overload and transfusion-related acute lung injury. *Blood*, **133** (17), 1840–1853.

4 *A 45-year-old man requires helicopter evacuation following a farming accident in which he was pinned under a peanut trailer experiencing crush injuries to his lower extremities. Transport time to nearest facility is approximately 35 minutes. His heart rate is 145 per minute, systolic blood pressure is 80 mmHg, and he appears confused. Prehospital providers obtained IV access and administered 1 L of crystalloid in the field. Repeat vitals en route demonstrate a heart rate of 125 and systolic blood pressure of 90. What additional resuscitation, if any, would offer the greatest survival benefit while traveling to the nearest hospital?*
A *Additional 1 L of crystalloid*
B *1 unit packed red blood cell (PRBC)*
C *1 unit fresh frozen plasma (FFP)*
D *1 unit PRBC + 1 unit FFP*
E *No additional resuscitation required*

More than one-third of preventable deaths due to hemorrhage occur in the field. Evidence gathered from the Prehospital Air Medical Plasma Trial and its secondary analysis, patients with signs of shock should receive prehospital blood products whenever available. Crystalloid alone appears to be inferior to blood products and has a dose–response increase in mortality in this setting. If both PRBC and plasma are available, patients should receive both, as reduction in mortality has been demonstrated. If only 1 product can be added, plasma should be favored, as there is level 1 evidence to support it. The additive benefit of PRBC and plasma also suggests that there may be a benefit to the use of whole blood in the prehospital setting. Finding a balance between organ perfusion and hemostasis is critical when resuscitating a severely injured trauma patient. Answer E would allow for permissive hypotension which would not be advisable for this patient given that his mechanism may have also resulted in a traumatic brain and/or spinal cord injury which have yet to be ruled out. Permissive hypotension is not recommended in the setting of central nervous system injury.

Answer: D

Guette, F.X., Sperry, J.L., Peitzman, A.B., *et al.* (2019) Prehospital blood product and crystalloid resuscitation in the severely injured patient: A secondary analysis of the prehospital air medical plasma trial. *Ann Surg.* doi: 10.1097/SLA.0000000000003324.

5 *Which of the following patients would receive the most benefit from administration of tranexamic acid (TXA)?*
   A *25-year-old male with massive transfusion protocol activated approximately 9 hours post fall from height.*
   B *80-year-old female with a nondisplaced pelvic fracture and stable vital signs on Warfarin.*
   C *35-year-old male with massive transfusion protocol activated for hemodynamic instability 1-hour after sustaining gunshot wounds to the chest.*
   D *8-year-old male receiving 1:1 component resuscitation immediately following motor vehicle collision.*
   E *65-year-old female with a history of stroke receiving 1:1 component resuscitation after being struck by a car.*

TXA is a synthetic derivative of the amino acid lysine that inhibits fibrinolysis by blocking the lysine binding site on plasminogen. In patients undergoing elective procedures, TXA has been shown to reduce the need for blood transfusion. The CRASH-2 trial, a randomized, placebo-controlled trial of TXA in trauma patients with significant bleeding, demonstrated a significant reduction in all-cause mortality, as well as deaths due to hemorrhage, in the patients who received TXA within 3 hours. Trial results have been met with both enthusiasm and controversy regarding the application antifibrinolytics for patients with traumatic bleeding. As a consequence, several high-quality randomized controlled trials are currently underway to help further elucidate the utility of TXA and other antifibrinolytics in traumatic injury, as well as other conditions with severe bleeding. Based on current evidence, TXA is most beneficial in the setting of trauma when empirically used in massive transfusion situations in those patients presenting within 3 hours of injury. Further trials are needed to refine and optimize TXA dosing regimens due to concern for seizures with higher dosing. There was no increase in vascular occlusive events in patients receiving TXA in the CRASH-2 trial. However, history of or risk factors predisposing to thromboembolic events is considered a relative contraindication, as is the use of TXA in patients with subarachnoid hemorrhages owing to the association with increased

cerebral ischemia. Although TXA has been studied extensively in the adult trauma patient, less evidence exists for children, and its use in the pediatric trauma population is not as widespread.

Answer: C

Ramirez, R.J., Spinella, P.C., and Bochicchio, G.V. (2017) Tranexamic acid update in trauma. *Crit Care Clin*, **33** (1), 85–99.
The CRASH-2 Collaborators (2010) Effects of tranexamic acid on death, vascular occlusive events, and blood transfusion in trauma patients with significant hemorrhage (CRASH-2): a randomized, placebo-controlled trial. *Lancet*, **376** (9734), 23–32.

6 *A 28-year-old man is taken emergently to the operating room for abdominal exploration after sustaining a gunshot wound to the right upper quadrant. On arrival, he was found to be in hemorrhagic shock and massive transfusion protocol was initiated. Intraoperatively, the bleeding is difficult to control, and diffuse oozing is noted as the case progresses. Rapid thrombelastography (TEG) is performed and reveals a prolonged R value, K value is slightly prolonged, α-angle is reduced, a normal maximum amplitude. What component replacement would aid in resuscitative efforts?*
   A *Cryoprecipitate*
   B *Platelets*
   C *Tranexamic acid*
   D *Fresh frozen plasma (FFP)*
   E *Platelets and cryoprecipitate*

Thrombelastography (TEG) has been used as a guide to blood product replacement for acutely bleeding patients and has been studied as an alternative to ratio-based mass transfusion protocols. TEG offers the advantage of real-time point of care testing of coagulation function in whole blood. A rapid TEG differs from conventional TEG because tissue factor is added to the whole blood specimen, resulting in accelerated reaction and subsequent analysis. See graphic representation and interpretation below (Figure 11.1 and Table 11.1). The R value, which is recorded as activated clotting time (ACT) in the rapid TEG specimen, reflects clotting factor activation and the time to onset of clot formation. Normal R time ranges from 5–10 minutes. A deficiency of clotting factors will result in a prolonged ACT, which can be treated by FFP transfusion. The K value is the interval from the beginning of clot formation to a fixed level of clot firmness measured at a standard 20 mm amplitude. It reflects the activity of thrombin which cleaves fibrinogen. Normal K time is 1–3 minutes. Similarly, the α angle reflects the rate of clot formation and is another measure

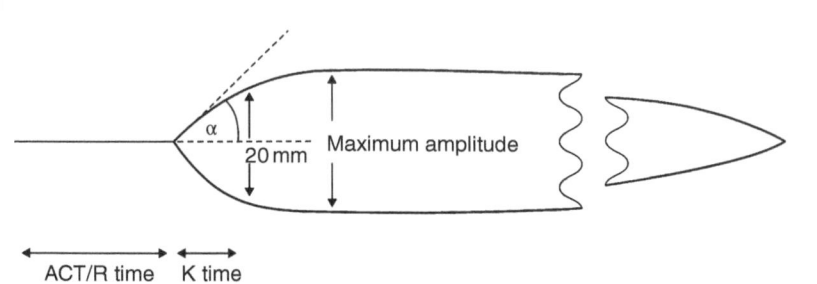

Figure 11.1 Normal thromboelastogram tracing

Table 11.1 Normal thromboelastogram tracing

Thromboelastogram (TEG) Interpretation

Components	Definition	Normal values	Problem	Treatment
R Time	Time to onset of clot formation	5–10 minutes	Coagulation factors	FFP
K Time	Time until fixed strength is reached	1–3 minutes	Fibrinogen	Cryoprecipitate
Alpha angle	Speed of fibrin accumulation	53–72°	Fibrinogen	Cryoprecipitate
Maximum amplitude	Highest vertical amplitude of the TEG	50–70 mm	Platelets	Platelets
Lysis at 30 minutes (LY30)	Percentage of amplitude reduction 30 minutes after maximum amplitude	0–8%	Excess fibrinolysis	Tranexamic acid

of fibrinogen activity. Normal α angle is 53–72°. A prolonged K value and a decreased α angle represent a fibrinogen deficit which can be treated by transfusion of FFP or cryoprecipitate. The maximum amplitude (MA) measures the final clot strength, reflecting the end result of platelet–fibrin interaction. Normal MA is 50–70 mm. If the MA is decreased after transfusion of FFP, then platelet transfusion should be considered. The patient described has a prolonged ACT as well as prolonged K time and decreased α angle. This is best treated by FFP transfusion to replace both the clotting factor deficiency and fibrinogen deficiency. If the K time remains prolonged after correction of the ACT, then cryoprecipitate can be given.

Answer: D

Inaba, K., Rizoli, S., Veigas, P.V., *et al.* (2015) 2014 consensus conference on viscoelastic test-based transfusion guidelines for early trauma resuscitation: report of the panel. *J Trauma Acute Care Surg*, **78** (6), 1220–1229.

Gonzalez, E., Pieracci, F.M., Moore, E.E., *et al.* (2010) Coagulation abnormalities in the trauma patient: The role of point-of-care thromboelastography. *Semin Thromb Hemost*, **36** (7), 723–737.

7 *Which of the following is not an advantage of rapid thrombelastography (TEG) in the setting of trauma?*

A *Viscoelastic assays better characterize trauma-induced coagulopathy when compared to conventional coagulation profiles.*

B *TEG can better direct massive transfusion than protocol-driven balanced ratio component therapy allowing for reduced product administration.*

C *TEG is the only clinically available means of detecting fibrinolysis accurately and in a point-of-care setting.*

D *TEG results are available within minutes.*

E *TEG has demonstrated survival benefit in guiding the management of thromboembolic events in the setting of post-injury hypercoagulability.*

TEG characterizes the life-span of a clot; from initial fibrin formation, to incorporation of platelets, to fibrinolysis. With results available within 10 minutes, an initial hemostatic assessment with TEG identifies patients at risk for post-injury coagulopathy upon arrival. The point-of-care variables that result enable the clinician direct management of patients in the trauma bay in real time while allowing for a data-driven, goal-directed hemostatic resuscitation. A recent clinical trial demonstrated that the use of TEG to guide massive transfusion in trauma patients, compared with conventional coagulation assays, resulted in a decrease in mortality while using fewer blood products. TEG is also currently used for patient-personalized administration of antifibrinolytics (e.g., tranexamic acid) based on LY30 parameters rather than administering TXA empirically when massive transfusion is required. Additionally, because TEG characterizes dynamic hypercoagulability and simultaneously reflects the antithrombotic effect of chemoprophylaxis, it may serve as a template for designing tailored thromboprophylaxis regimens; however additional studies are needed, and survival benefit has yet to be demonstrated.

Answer: E

Gonzalez, E., Moore, E.E., Moore, H.B., *et al.* (2016) Goal-directed hemostatic resuscitation of trauma-induced coagulopathy: A pragmatic randomized clinical trial comparing a viscoelastic assay to conventional coagulation assays. *Ann Surg*, **263** (6), 1051–1059.

Gonzalez, E., Pieracci, F.M., Moore, E.E., *et al.* (2010) Coagulation abnormalities in the trauma patient: The role of point-of-care thromboelastography. *Semin Thromb Hemost*, **36** (7), 723–737.

8 A 29-year-old man dropped off by his friend after crashing his all-terrain vehicle. Upon evaluation, he has altered mental status and a distended abdomen that is diffusely tender. His blood pressure is 80/60 mmHg and heart rate 140 per minute. He does not respond to initial resuscitation and massive transfusion protocol is activated. The time of his injury is unclear at this time and his initial thromboelastography (TEG) results reveal normal R time, normal k time, normal MA and LY30 greater than normal. What is the next best step in management?
  A Give 2 units of fresh frozen plasma
  B Administer 1g of tranexamic acid (TXA)
  C Give 1 unit of platelets
  D Give 10 units of cryoprecipitate
  E Give cryoprecipitate and platelets

TEG is useful in evaluating trauma-induced coagulopathy for goal-directed therapy. In this instance, the patient has massive transfusion requirements and time of injury is unclear. Rather, than empirically administering TXA, the TEG is useful in quickly identifying that this patient would likely benefit from its administration. LY30 greater than 3–5% is representative of hyperfibrinolysis. It seems intuitive that an antifibrinolytic medication should only be administered to those who have demonstrable hyperfibrinolysis; however, advocates for its empiric administration to all trauma patients exist. As evident by the CRASH-II trial, mortality benefit was seen in all trauma patients receiving TXA; however, this study also found that administration of tranexamic acid greater than 3 hours after injury was associated with increased mortality. Therefore, it is prudent to utilize TEG to ascertain those patients most likely to benefit from TXA.

Answer: B

Gonzalez, E., Moore, E.E., and Moore, H.B. (2017) Management of trauma-induced coagulopathy with thrombelastography. *Crit Care Clin*, **33** (1), 119–134.

9 A 35-year-old man is recovering in the intensive care unit 1 day after undergoing a damage control laparotomy for hemodynamic instability following a motorcycle crash in which he suffered a severe left pulmonary contusion, pneumothorax, femur fracture, grade 5 splenic laceration requiring splenectomy and destructive colon injury. He required massive transfusion as part of his resuscitation. Currently, his blood pressure is 110/75 mm Hg and heart rate 100. He is awake and breathing spontaneously on the ventilator with minimal support. His laboratory results reveal a hemoglobin of 7.9g/dL, platelets 40 000/mm³, prothrombin time 16 seconds, partial thromboplastin time 38 seconds, and fibrinogen 255 g/dL. He has remained stable and off vasopressors since admission to the ICU.

  Which product(s) should be transfused at this time?
  A Red blood cells, platelets, and plasma
  B Red blood cells, platelets, and cryoprecipitate
  C Tranexamic Acid
  D No products at this time
  E Red blood cells

Based on guidelines for enrollment in the current Pragmatic, Randomized Optimal Platelets and Plasma Ratios (PROPPR) study, criteria for stopping the massive transfusion protocol should include both anatomic (control of bleeding) and physiologic criteria (normalizing hemodynamic status). In this stable trauma patient without evidence of active bleeding, no blood products are needed at this time. A restrictive transfusion strategy maintaining hemoglobin at 7.0–9.0 g/dL has been shown to be as effective as a liberal transfusion strategy maintaining hemoglobin concentration at 10.0–12.0 g/dL. For those with an APACHE II score ≤ 20, 30-day mortality is significantly less with a restrictive strategy. In the absence of clinical bleeding, fresh frozen plasma transfusion may be associated with an increased incidence of acute lung injury. Evidence to support prophylactic platelet transfusion in critically ill patients without active bleeding is conflicting. Several authors have recommended avoidance of prophylactic platelet transfusion altogether, while others have recommended thresholds ranging from 10 000/mm³ to 100 000/mm³ for patients at risk of bleeding.

Answer: D

Holcomb, J.B., Tilley, B.C., Baraniuk, S., *et al.* (2015) Transfusion of plasma, platelets, and red blood cells in a

1:1:1 vs a 1:1:2 ratio and mortality in patients with severe trauma: The PROPPR randomized clinical trial. *J Am Med Assoc*, **313** (5), 471–482.

Hébert, P., Wells, B., Blajchman, M., *et al.* (1999) A multicenter, randomized, controlled clinical trial of transfusion requirements in critical care. *N Engl J Med*, **340** (6), 409–417.

10 *A 75-year-old woman is admitted to the intensive care unit following coronary artery bypass grafting. There were no complications during her surgery, and she is hemodynamically stable. Her postoperative labs reveal a hemoglobin of 8.1 g/dL. Which of the following supports implementing a restrictive transfusion strategy in this patient?*

A *Restrictive strategies reduce the risk of transfusion related reactions.*

B *Restrictive strategies reduce overall morbidity.*

C *Restrictive strategies improve survival.*

D *Restrictive strategies reduce the incidence of postoperative myocardial infarction.*

E *Restrictive strategies have demonstrated improvement in end-organ oxygen consumption.*

In a recent trial involving patients undergoing cardiac surgery, restrictive red-cell transfusion strategy (hemoglobin threshold of < 7.5 g/dL) was noninferior to a liberal strategy (hemoglobin threshold of < 9.5 g/dL in the operating room or intensive care unit) in regard to death and major disability (including myocardial infarction, stroke, and new-onset renal failure with dialysis) among postoperative patients who had a moderate to high risk of death. These outcomes were achieved with fewer units of blood being transfused. Contemporary evidence-based guidelines for all surgical patients also discourage liberally transfusing packed red blood cells (PRBCs) in most cases when bleeding has been controlled. Although transfusion of PRBCs was traditionally used to improve oxygen delivery, multiple studies have failed to demonstrate an improvement in end-organ oxygen consumption with transfusion. This may be partially explained by the decreased deformability and adverse microcirculatory effects of stored red blood cells. Risks associated with RBC transfusion include fluid overload, fever, acute transfusion reaction, increased rate of multi-organ failure, increased infection rates, transfusion-associated immunomodulation, human error with incorrect blood administration, transfusion-related acute lung injury (TRALI), and viral transmission.

Answer: A

Mazer, C.D., Whitlock, R.P., Fergusson, D.A., *et al.* (2017) Restrictive or liberal red-cell transfusion for cardiac surgery. *N Engl J Med*, **377** (22), 2133–2144.

Mirski, M.A., Frank, S.M., Kor, D.J., *et al.* (2015) Restrictive and liberal red cell transfusion strategies in adult patients: reconciling clinical data with best practice. *Crit Care Med*, **19** (1), 1–11.

11 *Given that mortality is improved with the rapid activation of massive transfusion protocol (MTP), but complications from unnecessary exposure to blood products can be devastating, prediction tools can be used to aid clinicians in the careful decision to initiate massive transfusion. Which of the following is not a metric of the Assessment of Blood Consumption (ABC) score used to trigger MTP?*

A *Heart rate > 120 per minute*

B *Systolic blood pressure < 90 mmHg*

C *Glasgow Coma Scale < 9*

D *Positive FAST (focused assessment with sonography for trauma)*

E *Penetrating injury to the torso*

There are no uniformly accepted criteria for activating an MTP. Several clinical factors have been validated as individual predictors of massive transfusion. The ABC score consists of four such factors (pulse > 120, SBP < 90, positive FAST, and penetrating torso injury), each assigned one point. A score of two or more warrants MTP activation. The ABC score overestimates the need for transfusion, with a positive predictive value of 50–55%, meaning that 45–50% of patients in whom MTP is activated will not need a massive transfusion. However, the ABC score is excellent at identifying patients who will not need massive transfusion, with a negative predictive value of less than 5%. Massive transfusion has been variably defined (e.g., ≥10 units packed red blood cells [PRBCs] over 24 hours, ≥3 units PRBCs per hour). Survival is improved by the timely administration of blood products in proper ratios.

Answer: C

Nunez, T.C., Woskresensky, I.V., Dossett, L.A., *et al.* (2009) Early prediction of massive transfusion in trauma: Simple as ABC (assessment of blood consumption). *J Trauma*, **66** (2), 346–352.

Callcut, R.A., Cotton, B.A., Muskat, P., *et al.* (2013) Defining when to initiate massive transfusion: a validation study of individual massive transfusion triggers in PROMMTT patients. *J Trauma Acute Care Surg*, **74** (1), 59–65.

12 *A 68-year-old intubated woman is being resuscitated in the intensive care unit after presenting in hemorrhagic shock following multiple episodes of hematemesis. She has received 6 units of packed blood cells (PRBCs) over the past 12 hours and her provider*

decides to administer plasma and platelets to balance her resuscitation efforts. What is the rationale for administering apheresis platelets over pooled platelets in this scenario?

A *Apheresis platelets have reduced risk of bacterial and viral contamination.*

B *Mortality is improved with use of apheresis platelets.*

C *Apheresis platelets are readily available and cost effective.*

D *Apheresis platelets have reduced risk of transfusion-related acute lung injury.*

E *Apheresis platelets have reduced risk of hemolytic transfusion reaction.*

A high ratio of platelets to PRBCs is defined variably in previous studies as approximately one unit of apheresis platelets for every 6–10 units of PRBCs transfused. Additionally, the PROPPR trial showed faster hemostasis and fewer deaths from hemorrhage in the group treated with a higher ratio of plasma and platelets to PRBCs. When massive transfusion is required, platelets should be transfused in an appropriate ratio without waiting for clinical laboratory results to confirm low platelet counts. No prospective study has demonstrated survival difference between apheresis and pooled donor platelets. One unit of apheresis platelets is obtained from a single donor, while pooled platelets are combined from six to eight donors. As a result, pooled platelets have a higher risk of bacterial contamination as well as viral transmission; however, there is no difference in transfusion-related lung injury. There is no difference in hemolytic transfusion reactions between the two.

Answer: A

Holcomb, J.B., Tilley, B.C., Baraniuk, S., *et al.* (2015) Transfusion of plasma, platelets, and red blood cells in a 1:1:1 vs a 1:1:2 ratio and mortality in patients with severe trauma: The PROPPR randomized clinical trial. *J Am Med Assoc*, **313** (5), 471–482.

Inaba, K., Lustenberger, T., Rhee, P., *et al.* (2011) The impact of platelet transfusion in massively transfused trauma patients. *J Am Coll Surg*, **211**, 573–579.

13 *An 85-year-old man is admitted to the intensive care unit following endovascular repair of a ruptured abdominal aortic aneurysm. He required a total of 12 units packed red blood cells intraoperatively. His postoperative labs reveal a calcium level of 6.1 mg/dL. Which of the following is not a consequence of his hypocalcemia?*

A *Muscle tremors*

B *Prolonged QT*

C *Hypotension*

D *Arrythmia*

E *T wave inversion*

Hypocalcemia is the most common abnormality associated with massive transfusion, occurring in >90% of patients receiving a massive blood transfusion. Stored blood is anticoagulated with citrate, which binds calcium and causes hypocalcemia after large-volume blood transfusion. Complications of hypocalcemia include prolonged QT, decreased myocardial contractility, hypotension, muscle tremors, pulseless electrical activity, and ventricular fibrillation. T wave inversion is classically associated with hypokalemia.

Answer: E

Sihler, K. and Napolitano, L. (2010) Complications of massive transfusion. *Chest*, **137**, 209–220.

14 *A 56-year-old man with a history of chronic atrial fibrillation is brought to the emergency department after being found down. He is unresponsive and promptly intubated. His blood pressure is 75/25 and there are no obvious external signs of trauma. A chest x-ray is performed for endotracheal tube confirmation and massive free air is noted under the bilateral hemidiaphragms. Stat laboratory results are most notable for white blood cell count of 23, hemoglobin of 12, hematocrit of 30, platelet count of 250, and an international normalized ratio of 3.1. Plans are made for emergent abdominal exploration. What is the fastest way to correct his coagulopathy in preparation for his procedure?*

A *Activate the massive transfusion protocol.*

B *Administer 4-factor prothrombin complex concentrate.*

C *Transfuse fresh frozen plasma.*

D *Transfuse fresh frozen plasma and administer vitamin K.*

E *No preoperative reversal is indicated as the case is a surgical emergency.*

Coagulopathy can delay or complicate surgical diseases that require emergent surgical treatment. Historically, warfarin reversal was achieved with rapid administration of fresh frozen plasma (FFP). In 2013, the US FDA approved a 4-factor prothrombin complex concentrate (PCC) for urgent warfarin reversal. PCC alone reduces INR and time to surgery effectively and safely in coagulopathic patients without an apparent increased risk of thromboembolic events, when compared to FFP use alone.

Answer: B

Goldstein, J.N., Refaai, M.A., Milling, T.J., *et al.* (2015) Four factor prothrombin complex concentrate versus plasma for rapid vitamin K antagonist reversal in patients needing urgent surgical or invasive interventions: a phase 3b, open-label, non-inferiority, randomized trial. *Lancet*, **385** (9982), 2077–2087.

Younis, M., Ray-Zack, M., Haddad, N.N., *et al.* (2018) Prothrombin complex concentrate reversal of coagulopathy in emergency general surgery patients. *World J Surg*, **42** (8), 2383–2391.

15 *A 26-year-old man is admitted to the surgical intensive care unit after an automobile struck his motorcycle. He is hemodynamically stable and found to have a grade 3 splenic laceration with no active extravasation and a left, displaced, mid-shaft fracture of the humerus. The fracture was reduced and leg placed in traction while he is being observed for his splenic laceration. Suddenly he becomes confused with progressive shortness of breath and hypoxia requiring intubation. A chest X-ray demonstrates diffuse bilateral infiltrates. Labs reveal a platelet count is 75 000/mm3, prothrombin time of 19 second, partial thromboplastin time of 50 second, oozing is noted from intravenous access sites, and blood is suctioned from his endotracheal tube. Which of the following test results would be consistent with the diagnosis of disseminated intravascular coagulation?*

A *Increased antithrombin level*
B *Elevated fibrin degradation products*
C *Decreased bleeding time*
D *Elevated fibrinogen level*
E *Decreased D-dimer*

Disseminated intravascular coagulation (DIC) is characterized by widespread microvascular thrombosis with activation of the coagulation system and impaired protein synthesis, leading to exhaustion of clotting factors and platelets. The end result is organ failure and profuse bleeding from various sites. DIC is always associated with an underlying condition that triggers diffuse activation of coagulation, most commonly sepsis, trauma with soft tissue injury, head injury, fat embolism, cancer, amniotic fluid embolism, toxins, immunologic disorders, or transfusion reaction. In this case, the patient appears to meet criteria for fat embolism syndrome which likely triggered his DIC. There is no single laboratory test that can confirm or rule out a diagnosis of DIC. A combination of tests in a patient with an appropriate clinical condition can be used to make the diagnosis. Low platelet count, elevated fibrin degradation products or D-dimer, prolonged prothrombin time, and low fibrinogen level are all consistent with a diagnosis of DIC.

Answer: B

Levi, M. (2007) Disseminated intravascular coagulation. *Crit Care Med*, **35** (9), 2191–2195.

16 *A 61-year-old man is admitted to the surgical intensive care unit with a diagnosis of ischemic colitis. Subcutaneous injection of unfractionated heparin was started for venous thromboembolism prophylaxis, and he is monitored closely with serial abdominal examinations. On hospital day five, he noted acute onset of left lower extremity pain and is found to have absent pedal pulses in the affected limb. His platelet count is noted to have dropped from 250 000/ mm3 to 90 000/mm3, and his creatinine has increased from 1.2 mg/dL to 2.8 mg/dL. He is taken to the operating room where he underwent thrombectomy of a white appearing clot in the right superficial femoral artery. He is diagnosed with Heparin Induced Thrombocytopenia (HIT) and started on argatroban postoperatively. What is the mechanism of action of argatroban?*

A *Direct factor Xa inhibitor*
B *Direct factor IIa inhibitor*
C *Indirect factor IIa inhibitor*
D *Binds antithrombin III*
E *Indirect factor Xa inhibitor*

HIT is a life-threatening disorder that occurs after exposure to unfractionated, or less commonly, low-molecular-weight heparin. HIT usually occurs after 5–10 days of heparin therapy and is caused by antibodies against the heparin-platelet factor 4 complex. Thrombotic complications occur in 20–50% of patients. The thrombus associated with HIT has been described as "white clot" with predominantly fibrin platelet aggregates and few red blood cells. Thrombocytopenia is common in the critically ill, and diagnosis of HIT can be difficult. Delays in obtaining test results often mean that management decisions must be made on the basis of clinical suspicion. Clinical findings that imply a diagnosis HIT are:

- Platelet fall of more than 50% from baseline, with platelet nadir > 20 000. Profound thrombocytopenia suggests a cause other than HIT.
- Onset on day 5–10 of heparin exposure.
- Thrombosis, skin necrosis, or an anaphylactoid reaction after heparin bolus.
- No other cause for the thrombocytopenia is present.

Treatment of HIT includes discontinuation of all sources of heparin and if anticoagulation is clinically warranted, use of a direct thrombin (factor IIa) inhibitor such as argatroban is recommended.

Answer: B

Greinacher, A. (2015) Heparin-induced thrombocytopenia. *N Eng J Med*, **373** (3), 252–261.

17 *An 18-year-old man is undergoing an exploratory laparotomy and right groin exploration for a gunshot wound to the right hip. Injuries to the right common femoral vein, bladder, and sigmoid colon are noted. Massive blood loss was reported at the scene and the patient was found to be in hemorrhagic shock on arrival. He has received 12 units of packed red blood cells, 12 units of fresh frozen plasma, and 2 units of apheresis platelets while in the operating room. His vital signs are: blood pressure 100/60 mm Hg, heart rate 120 beats/min, temperature 34.8 °C. Laboratory studies: hemoglobin 8.5 g/dL, platelets 100 000/mm3, prothrombin time 14 second, partial thromboplastin time 40 second. pH 7.1. His femoral vein has been ligated, bladder injuries were repaired, and sigmoid colon was resected. What is the next most appropriate treatment for his ongoing bleeding?*

A *Transfuse platelets, create a stoma, and close the abdomen.*

B *Transfuse fresh frozen plasma, perform primary anastomosis, and close the abdomen.*

C *No transfusion required, create stoma, and close the abdomen.*

D *External warming, primary anastomosis, and close the abdomen.*

E *Leave in discontinuity, place temporary abdominal closure device, and admit to surgical intensive care unit for external rewarming.*

This patient is severely hypothermic and acidotic. Following surgical control of bleeding and massive resuscitation, ongoing aggressive resuscitation is required to reverse the "lethal triad" of coagulopathy, acidosis, and hypothermia. Damage control operation should be performed with prompt admission to surgical intensive care unit for resuscitation and rewarming. Clotting factor and platelet deficiencies have been addressed during this resuscitation by maintaining 1:1 component replacement. Hypothermia < 35 °C is a strong independent risk factor for mortality in trauma patients, with more severe hypothermia conveying greater risk of mortality. Hypothermia contributes to coagulopathy through platelet and clotting factor dysfunction. Recommended measures for rewarming a patient with low body temperature include forced air warming, infusion of warmed fluids, under-body heating pads, radiant warmers, and humidified ventilation. If bleeding continues after aggressive warming and correction of clotting abnormalities, the patient must return to the operating room without further delay.

Answer: E

Inaba, K., Teixeira, P., Rhee, P., *et al.* (2009) Mortality impact of hypothermia after cavitary explorations in trauma. *World J Surg*, **33** (4), 864–869.

Perlman, R., Callum, J., Laflamme, C., *et al.* (2016) A recommended early goal-directed management guideline for the prevention of hypothermia-related transfusion, morbidity, and mortality in severely injured trauma patients. *Crit Care*, **20** (1), 1–11.

18 *A 22-year-old man was involved in a drive by shooting. He is noted to have multiple gunshot wounds to his back, abdomen, and extremities. He has a distended abdomen that is diffusely tender. His blood pressure is 80/60 mm Hg. What fluid should be administered while preparing for emergent laparotomy?*

A *Lactated ringers*

B *Hypertonic saline*

C *positive blood*

D *Type-specific blood*

E *Crossmatched blood*

The described physical exam findings are consistent with hemoperitoneum resulting in hemorrhagic shock; therefore, the patient requires emergent resuscitation and operative hemorrhage control to avoid mortality. Crystalloid solution should be minimized and resuscitation with blood products should be initiated without delay. Type O positive blood is readily available in most centers and can be used for emergent transfusion of male patients and women beyond childbearing age. If uncrossmatched blood resources are limited, type O negative blood may be used but is typically reserved for women of childbearing age to avoid the risk of Rh isoimmunization. Type O positive blood has been shown to be safe for transfusion in hemorrhaging trauma patients, with a very low rate of transfusion reaction. Advantages of using uncrossmatched type O blood include immediate availability before type-specific blood becomes available and avoidance of errors in multi-casualty situations. The safety of type O blood has been improved by prescreening donor blood for anti-A and anti-B antibodies, which can lead to hemolysis of native red blood cells.

Answer: C

Ball, C.G., Salomone, J.P., Shaz, B., *et al.* (2010) Uncrossmatched blood transfusions for trauma patients in the emergency department: incidence, outcomes and recommendations. *Can J Surg*, **54** (2), 111–115.

Dutton, R., Shih, D., Edelman, B., *et al.* (2005) Safety of uncrossmatched type-O red cells for resuscitation from hemorrhagic shock. *J Trauma*, **59** (6), 1445–1449.

19 *A 90-year-old man presents after a ground-level fall. He is found to have bruising on all extremities and a scalp laceration that requires suture repair for hemostasis. His daughter accompanies him to the emergency department and reports that he took dabigatran*

for his chronic atrial fibrillation 4 hours prior to the admission. Imaging reveals a moderate subdural hematoma. What is the best option for reversing effects of dabigatran?

A *No reversal is required if the INR is < 2*
B *Administer idarucizumab*
C *Administer platelets*
D *Administer fresh frozen plasma*
E *Administer cryoprecipitate*

Oral anticoagulants alternative to warfarin for reducing the risk of thromboembolic events in patients with chronic atrial fibrillation include rivaroxaban, apixaban, and dabigatran. Rivaroxaban and apixaban are factor Xa inhibitors. Dabigatran is a direct thrombin inhibitor. A major advantage of these medications is that they do not require routine INR monitoring. In clinical trials, bleeding events on these medications were comparable to, or lower than warfarin for similar indications. The major drawbacks of these agents are (1) their anticoagulation effect is not reliably measured by common laboratory tests, and (2) effects can be difficult to reverse. In 2016, the FDA approved idarucizumab as a specific reversal agent for dabigatran. Fresh frozen plasma (FFP) can be used to resuscitate patients on these medications who suffer low- to moderate-risk bleeding events. However, FFP is not a specific reversal agent. It takes time to infuse and cannot rapidly reverse coagulopathy. Administration of FFP can also lead to volume overload and transfusion reactions. For all of these reasons, FFP is not an ideal therapy. This patient has a life-threatening intracranial hemorrhage that requires rapid reversal of dabigatran. Idarucizumab is a monoclonal antibody fragment developed to rapidly, durably, and safely reverse the anticoagulant effect of dabigatran in emergency situations. PCC can also be considered to reverse dabigatran if idarucizumab is unavailable.

Answer: B

Pollack, C.V., Reilly, P.A., Van Ryn, J., *et al.* (2017) Idarucizumab for Dabigatran reversal – full cohort analysis. *N Engl J Med*, **377** (5), 431–441.

Faraoni, D., Levy, J.H., Albaladejo, P., *et al.* (2015) Updates in the perioperative and emergency management of non-vitamin K antagonist oral anticoagulants. *Crit Care*, **19**, 1–6.

12

Analgesia and Anesthesia
Toni Manougian, MD, MBA[1] and Bardiya Zangbar, MD[2]

[1] Department of Critical Care Anesthesiology, New York Medical College, Westchester Medical Center, Valhalla, NY, USA
[2] Division of Trauma and Acute Care Surgery, New York Medical College, Westchester Medical Center, Valhalla, NY, USA

1 *Which of the following effects of epidural analgesia is correct:*
   A *For patients without serious lung pathology, mid thoracic epidural analgesia has no effect on lung function.*
   B *Decreased gastric secretions, peristalsis, and enhanced gastric motility results from sympathetic splanchnic blockade at the T5-L1 level.*
   C *Renal blood flow is increased and an indwelling urinary catheter is always necessary when using continuous epidural analgesia.*
   D *Neuraxial analgesia (NA) has no effect on the surgical stress response. NA does not affect oxygen consumption, vasopressin, catecholamine, cortisol, or glucose levels.*
   E *Thoracic epidural catheters above T4 level are safe and unlikely to cause cardiovascular effects.*

All of the choices are false regarding thoracic epidural catheters except choice A. Pulmonary function is unaffected by thoracic epidural analgesia in patients with normal function. However, severe pulmonary disease is a relative contraindication for brachial plexus blocks. Brachial plexus blocks such as an interscalene block affect ipsilateral hemi-diaphragmatic excursion and reduce functional residual capacity and pulmonary function as much as 40%. Interestingly, the recurrent laryngeal nerve may also be blocked and can cause complete airway obstruction in a patient with existing vocal cord palsy. A blockade at the T5-L1 level will increase gastric secretions, peristalsis, and enhanced gastric motility due to increased parasympathetic activity and sympathetic splanchnic blockade making choice B incorrect answer. Renal blood flow is auto-regulated and unaffected by epidural analgesia. When thoracic epidural catheters are used, indwelling urinary catheters are not always required. Lumbar epidural analgesia however, can cause urinary retention, especially when blocking S2 to S4 spinal segments. Therefore, lumbar epidural catheters are more likely to affect bladder function than thoracic epidurals (choice C). One of the major benefits when choosing neuraxial analgesia (NA) is to blunt the sympathetic stress response. NA reduces oxygen consumption and decreases levels of vasopressin, catecholamines, cortisol, and glucose (choice D). Choice E is incorrect, because blocks at the T1-4 level result in sympathetic blockade and profound cardiovascular effects. Blocks at T1-T4 result in hypotension from both bradycardia and decreased cardiac contractility.

Answer: A

Mian A, Chaudhry I, Huang R, Rizk E, Tubbs RS, Loukas M. Brachial plexus anesthesia: A review of the relevant anatomy, complications, and anatomical variations. *Clin Anat.* 2014;27(2):210–21.
Basse L, Werner M, Kehlet H. Is urinary drainage necessary during continuous epidural analgesia after colonic resection? *Reg Anesth Pain Med.* 2000;25(5):498–501.

2 *A 45-year-old man is admitted to the ICU with pneumonia, fever, agitation, and confusion. He acutely becomes increasingly agitated and is treated with haloperidol. His vital signs are respiratory rate of 18/min, oxygen saturation 94%, heart rate 92/min, blood pressure 154/78 mmHg, and temperature 38.9 °C. He is sweating, drooling with painful contractions of the neck, and is salivating. Which of the following medications is the treatment of choice?*

A Benztropine (Cogentin)
B Lorazepam (Ativan)
C Metoclopramide (Reglan)
D Dantrolene (Ryanodex)
E Quetiapine (Seroquel)

The patient is exhibiting signs of a dystonic reaction and his symptoms are best treated with benztropine. Dystonic reactions are an unwanted effect after administration of neuroleptic medications. Dystonic reactions can occur immediately, or be delayed hours to days. Classic features of dystonic reaction to medications such as haloperidol are cholinergic symptoms such as increased salivation and spasmodic or sustained involuntary contractions of muscles in the face, neck, trunk, pelvis, extremities, or larynx. Dystonic reactions, while not usually life threatening, are distressing for patients and families. Benztropine, an anticholinergic agent, is used for symptomatic improvement (choice A). While some symptoms can be improved with benzodiazepines, this class of medication may worsen his confusion, blunt his respiratory drive, and contribute to ICU delirium, so choice B is not the best answer. Metoclopramide (Reglan) exerts an antiemetic effect by antagonist activity at central D_2 receptors in the chemoreceptor trigger zone and may potentiate the dyskinesia symptoms, so choice C is incorrect. Dantrolene (Ryanodex) is used in reversal of malignant hyperthermia and has no primary role in treatment of dystonic reactions (choice D). While haloperidol (Haldol) is associated with neuroleptic malignant syndrome, the side effects manifested is mental status change in the form of agitated delirium with confusion or catatonic signs and mutism. Other symptoms include muscular rigidity which can be demonstrated by moving the extremities and is characterized by "lead pipe rigidity" or stable resistance through all ranges of movement. Hypothermia is common and extremely high temperatures greater than 40 °C is common. Autonomic dysfunction in the form of tachycardia with hypertension and tachypnea along with dysrhythmias may occur. In the scenarios of induced neuroleptic malignant syndrome, dantrolene can be an antidote. Quetiapine (Seroquel) is a second-generation antipsychotic and known to be rare in causing extrapyramidal side effects and has no role in treatment of dystonic side effects (choice E).

Answer: A

Digby G, Jalini S, Taylor S. Medication-induced acute dystonic reaction: the challenge of diagnosing movement disorders in the intensive care unit. *BMJ Case Resp.* 2015;2015:bcr2014207215

Goff DC, Arana GW, Greenblatt DJ, Dupont R, Ornsteen M, Harmatz JS, Shader RI. The effect of benztropine on haloperidol-induced dystonia, clinical efficacy and pharmacokinetics: a prospective, double-blind trial. *J Clin Psychopharmacol* 1991;11(2):106–12.

3 *A 75-year-old woman underwent a cholecystectomy for a gangrenous gallbladder. Postoperatively, the patient appears calm and you would like to extubate the patient in the next 24 hours. Which of the following represents the best stepwise approach to pain and sedation?*

A *Short-acting narcotic infusion with fentanyl and propofol.*
B *Standing IV acetaminophen (Ofirmev), low-dose ketamine (Ketalar) infusion, and PRN hydromorphone (Dilaudid) IV push.*
C *Short-acting narcotic infusion with fentanyl, plus dexmedetomidine (Precedex) drip plus gabapentin (Neurontin) PO.*
D *Short-acting remifentanil and propofol infusions.*
E *Propofol infusion and dexmedetomidine (Precedex).*

Narcotic first regimens are common but undesirable because their adverse effects include ileus, delayed extubation, tolerance, and opioid-induced hyperalgesia. Narcotics also place patients at risk for withdrawal. For most patients, especially those you plan to extubate soon or those at risk for complications, narcotic infusions are not the first choice. A stepwise approach including multimodal analgesia with acetaminophen, intermittently dosed narcotics and ketamine (0.5 mg/kg IVP × 1 followed by 1–2 mcg/kg/min infusion) is recommended. The goal is to minimize opioid therapy when managing postsurgical adult patients in the ICU (conditional recommendation, very low quality of evidence) and ketamine can be used as an IV adjunct. Gabapentin is also available as part of stepwise approach. Acetaminophen and pain-dose ketamine infusions are excellent analgesics and can be added to an intermittently dosed narcotic plan as needed, making choice B the best answer. Choices A, C, and D are also incorrect because they rely on opioid infusions and do not represent the best stepwise approach. It is especially important to avoid continuous narcotic infusions in patients at high risk for opioid toxicity, such as those with sleep apnea or at patients at risk for ileus. Although dexmedetomidine (Precedex) has some pain effects as an alpha 2 agonist, its primary effect is sedation and would not be the best choice for pain in combination with propofol. The patient is calm and does not need two sedative agents, so choice (E) is also incorrect.

Answer: B

Devlin JW, Skrobik Y, Gélinas C, Needham DM, Slooter AJC, Pandharipande PP, Watson PL, Weinhouse GL, Nunnally ME, Rochwerg B, Balas MC, van den Boogaard M, Bosma KJ, Brummel NE, Chanques G, Denehy L, Drouot X, Fraser GL, Harris JE, Joffe AM, Kho ME, Kress JP, Lanphere JA, McKinley S, Neufeld KJ, Pisani MA, Payen JF, Pun BT, Puntillo KA, Riker RR, Robinson BRH, Shehabi Y, Szumita PM, Winkelman C, Centofanti

JE, Price C, Nikayin S, Misak CJ, Flood PD, Kiedrowski K, Alhazzani W. Clinical practice guidelines for the prevention and management of pain, agitation/sedation, delirium, immobility, and sleep disruption in adult patients in the ICU. *Crit Care Med.* 2018;46(9):e825–73.

4   *A 67-year-old woman is in the ICU on postoperative day 2 after laparotomy. Current medications include clonidine, quetiapine, hydromorphone, melatonin, and metoprolol. Her sleep pattern is altered and she shows signs of agitated delirium. Which of her medications increases her risk for aspiration?*

   A *Clonidine*

   B *Dexmedetomidine (Precedex)*

   C *Quetiapine (Seroquel)*

   D *Hydromorphone (Dilaudid)*

   E *Melatonin (N-acetyl-5-hydroxytryptamine)*

Antipsychotic medications such as haloperidol and quetiapine are used to manage delirium. These medications can increase the QTC interval but also antagonize dopamine signaling, which affects the swallow mechanism and increases the risk of aspiration. Therefore, choice C is correct.

Both clonidine (choice A) and dexmedetomidine (choice B) are useful adjuncts in pain management because of their effects at central α_2 receptors. Clonidine blocks sympathetic outflow, reduces arterial blood pressure, and ameliorates symptoms of alcohol and opiate withdrawal but does not increase aspiration risk. When used in epidural pain catheters, clonidine produces analgesia at the presynaptic and post junctional alpha 2 receptors. Dexmedetomidine (Precedex) produces centrally mediated sympatholytic sedation, anxiolysis, and analgesia. A transient increase in blood pressure during the loading dose of dexmedetomidine may occur, followed by hypotension which may be concerning for patients needing strict blood pressure control. A valuable characteristic of dexmedetomidine is the ability to produce sedation without respiratory depression. In some critically ill patients, night time sleep patterns are enhanced when patients are lightly sedated with dexmedetomidine. When compared to GABA agonists, dexmedetomidine resembles natural non-REM-type sleep.

Postsynaptic activation of α_2 receptors inhibits sympathetic activity, decreasing blood pressure and heart rate, having no effect on dopamine receptors or aspiration. According to the FDA, dexmedetomidine is indicated for initial sedation for the first 24 hours. Although not contraindicated, prolonged use of dexmedetomidine can lead to withdrawal effects like rebound hypertension, especially in higher doses. Hydromorphone (choice D) is an opioid receptor agonist used for severe pain. Hydromorphone is about 8–9 times more potent than morphine. Side effects of hydromorphone are pruritus,

sedation, constipation, nausea, and vomiting. Adverse effects are more pronounced with excessive dosages and include respiratory and cardiovascular depression, dependency, and ileus. An overdose of hydromorphone resulting in loss of consciousness could result in aspiration, but it does not contribute to aspiration in usual therapeutic doses.

Melatonin (N-acetyl-5-hydroxytryptamine) is a mild hypnotic and generally well tolerated and regarded as safe with few adverse effects. It is synthesized in the pineal gland and its release helps regulate sleep and circadian rhythms. The anterior hypothalamus regulates melatonin which has its effects at MT_2 and MT_1 receptors. Melatonin (M) receptors are ubiquitous, found in the brain, retina, throughout the cardiovascular system, in the liver, gallbladder, colon, and skin. The MT_1 receptor agonism is related to sleep onset. The most frequently reported adverse effects are daytime sleepiness, headache, dizziness, and hypothermia. Aspiration is not among reported adverse effects of melatonin, so choice E is incorrect.

Answer: C

Alexopoulou C, Kondili E, Diamantaki E, Psarologakis C, Kokkini S, Bolaki M, Georgopoulos D. Effects of dexmedetomidine on sleep quality in critically ill patients: a pilot study. *Anesthesiology.* 2014;121(4):801–7.

Besag FMC, Vasey MJ, Lao KSJ, Wong ICK. Adverse events associated with melatonin for the treatment of primary or secondary sleep disorders: a systematic review. *CNS Drugs* 2019;33(12):1167–86.

Herzig SJ, LaSalvia MT, Naidus E, Rothberg MB, Zhou W, Gurwitz JH, Marcantonio ER. Antipsychotics and the risk of aspiration pneumonia in individuals hospitalized for nonpsychiatric conditions: a cohort study. *J Am Geriatr Soc* 2017;65(12):2580–6.

DiBardino DM, Wunderink RG. Aspiration pneumonia: a review of modern trends. *J Crit Care.* 2015; 30(1): 40–8.

Longnecker D; Brown DL, Newman MF, Zapol W. *Anesthesiology*, Second Edition. New York: McGraw-Hill Professional; 2012. 1748 p. p.

5   *Which commonly prescribed medications in the intensive care unit is most likely to cause an unstable arrhythmia and sudden death?*

   A *Fentanyl, opioid analgesic*

   B *Meperidine (Demerol), opioid analgesic*

   C *Haloperidol (Haldol), typical antipsychotic*

   D *Dexmedetomidine (Precedex), alpha 2 agonist*

   E *Propofol, short-acting lipophilic intravenous general anesthetic*

Haldol (choice C) has a proven association with torsade de pointe and sudden death. Prolonged QT intervals can be congenital or acquired as in a patient receiving haldol, methadone, atypical antipsychotics, or antidepressants. Long QT associated with polymorphic ventricular tachycardia (PMVT) is called torsade de pointes. Factors that increase the QT and risk for torsades are rapid administration of QT prolonging drugs, coexisting myocardial ischemia, older age, recent dysrhythmia, hypomagnesemia, or hypokalemia. The first-line treatment of acquired QT prolongation with torsade de pointes is 2–4gm intravenous magnesium followed by infusion 1gm/h, replacement of potassium if needed, cardioversion or isoproterenol for bradycardia or pauses. PMVT without long QT can also be seen in acute coronary syndromes.

Fentanyl infusions typically in the range of 50–200mcg/h are used for sedation and pain control. Adverse effects of fentanyl include tolerance, constipation, hyperalgesia, and dependence. Fentanyl can cause hypotension; however, it is not associated with life-threatening arrhythmias (choice A). Similarly, meperidine (Demerol) is an opioid analgesic. Adverse effects of meperidine include respiratory and circulatory depression, lightheadedness, constipation, nausea, vomiting, and dependence. Meperidine does not have a known association with life-threatening arrhythmias (choice B).

Common side effects of the sedative-anxiolytic dexmedetomidine (Precedex) are sinus bradycardia and hypotension. Dexmedetomidine also provides some analgesic effects. It is a centrally acting sympatholytic alpha 2 agonist but it does not prolong the QT interval (choice D).

Propofol (choice E) is a hypnotic agent for induction of anesthesia or for sedation. It produces sedation through GABA potentiation. Some of the more serious adverse effects or propofol are hypotension from reduced systemic vascular resistance or direct myocardial depression and propofol infusion syndrome (PRIS). PRIS is a metabolic derangement manifested by metabolic acidosis, renal injury, and rhabdomyolysis. However, propofol is not usually associated with life-threatening arrhythmias or sudden death.

Answer: C

Ray WA, Chung CP, Murray KT, Hall K, Stein CM. Atypical antipsychotic drugs and the risk of sudden cardiac death. N Engl J Med. 2009;360(3):225–35.

Huffman JC, Stern TA. QTc prolongation and the use of antipsychotics: a case discussion. Prim Care Companion J Clin Psychiatry. 2003;5(6):278–81.

Milbrandt EB, Kersten A, Kong L, Weissfeld LA, Clermont G, Fink MP, Angus DC. Haloperidol use is associated with lower hospital mortality in mechanically ventilated patients. Crit Care Med. 2005;33(1):226–9; discussion 263-5.

Pandharipande PP, Pun BT, Herr DL, Maze M, Girard TD, Miller RR, Shintani AK, Thompson JL, Jackson JC, Deppen SA, Stiles RA, Dittus RS, Bernard GR, Ely EW. Effect of sedation with dexmedetomidine vs lorazepam on acute brain dysfunction in mechanically ventilated patients: the MENDS randomized controlled trial. JAMA. 2007;298(22):2644–53.

Riker RR, Shehabi Y, Bokesch PM, Ceraso D, Wisemandle W, Koura F, Whitten P, Margolis BD, Byrne DW, Ely EW, Rocha MG; SEDCOM (Safety and Efficacy of Dexmedetomidine Compared With Midazolam) Study Group. Dexmedetomidine vs midazolam for sedation of critically ill patients: a randomized trial. JAMA. 2009;301(5):489–99.

Biesenbach P, Mårtensson J, Lucchetta L, Bangia R, Fairley J, Jansen I, Matalanis G, Bellomo R. Pharmacokinetics of magnesium bolus therapy in cardiothoracic surgery. *J Cardiothorac Vasc Anesth.* 2018;32(3):1289–94.

Ling X, Zhou H, Ni Y, Wu C, Zhang C, Zhu Z. Does dexmedetomidine have an antiarrhythmic effect on cardiac patients? A meta-analysis of randomized controlled trials. PLoS One 2018;13(3):e0193303.

6 *A 120kg 82-year-old man with a past medical history of colon cancer, diabetes, and renal insufficiency is admitted to the ICU after a colectomy. Postoperatively, he had bilateral transversus abdominis (TAP) blocks placed. His creatinine clearance is estimated to be 52mL/min. Which of the following factors increase his risk for local anesthetic toxicity?*
   A *Renal insufficiency*
   B *Advanced age*
   C *Male sex*
   D *Obesity*
   E *Diabetes*

Local anesthetic toxicity (LAST) is a life-threatening event resulting from inadvertent intravascular administration or excessively dosed local anesthetic medications. The underlying mechanisms of LAST are multifactorial, but primarily manifest with cardiovascular and neurologic deterioration. The risk factors for LAST are extremes of age (choice B), pregnancy, low body weight, and pre-existing cardiovascular disease. The anesthetic medications should be based on ideal body weight. Renal insufficiency (choice A), gender (choice C), and diabetes (choice E) do not affect the likelihood of LAST. Obesity (choice D) could contribute if the dosage was based on actual rather than ideal body weight.

Answer: B

El-Boghdadly K, Pawa A, Chin KJ. Local anesthetic systemic toxicity: current perspectives. *Local Reg Anes.* 2018;11:35–44.

Neal JM, Barrington, MJ, Fettiplace MR, Gitman M, Memtsoudis SG, Mörwald EE, Rubin DS, Weinberg G The third American society of regional anesthesia and pain medicine practice advisory on local anesthetic toxicity: executive summary 2017. *Regional Anesth. Pain Med.* 2018;43(2):113–23.

7 *A 112 kg patient with a history of anxiety disorder has been admitted to the ICU. He is intubated and he is on multimodal sedation including a hydromorphone drip 3 mg/h for 7 days. To manage his ongoing sedation and acute pain needs, in addition to the current medications, including IV Tylenol, what is your next best action?*

A *Start a ketamine drip to provide dissociative analgesia, 5 mcg/kg/min.*

B *Start low-dose ketamine drip at 1–2 mcg/kg/min after a bolus and start to decrease hydromorphone (Dilaudid) by 20%.*

C *Increase the hydromorphone (Dilaudid) drip to 4 mg/h to provide both sedation and analgesia.*

D *Add lorazepam (Ativan) drip and increase the hydromorphone (Dilaudid) to 4 mg/h.*

E *Start a propofol infusion, switch hydromorphone (Dilaudid) to equianalgesic fentanyl.*

Higher doses of ketamine infusions contribute to the unwanted side effects including agitation, hallucinations, and somnolence. These psycho-mimetic effects are particularly worrisome in a patient who may be unable to communicate these effects. For this reason, choice A is incorrect. Sub-anesthetic doses of ketamine when added to a multimodal pain approach are opioid sparing and may attenuate unwanted side effects of ketamine (choice B). It is not appropriate to use narcotics as a single agent to control both pain and sedition (choice C) because tolerance develops, so increasing doses will be needed. Benzodiazepines are associated with ICU delirium and may contribute to delayed weaning from mechanical ventilation, so choice D is not the best choice. There is no indication to change from dilaudid to fentanyl (choice E).

Answer: B

Devlin JW, Skrobik Y, Gélinas C, Needham DM, Slooter AJC, Pandharipande PP, Watson PL, Weinhouse GL, Nunnally ME, Rochwerg B, Balas MC, van den Boogaard M, Bosma KJ, Brummel NE, Chanques G, Denehy L, Drouot X, Fraser GL, Harris JE, Joffe AM, Kho ME, Kress JP, Lanphere JA, McKinley S, Neufeld KJ, Pisani MA, Payen JF, Pun BT, Puntillo KA, Riker RR, Robinson BRH, Shehabi Y, Szumita PM, Winkelman C, Centofanti JE, Price C, Nikayin S, Misak CJ, Flood PD, Kiedrowski K, Alhazzani W. Clinical practice guidelines for the prevention and management of pain, agitation/sedation, delirium, immobility, and sleep disruption in adult patients in the ICU. *Crit Care Med.* 2018;46(9):e825–73.

Schwenk ES, Viscusi ER, Buvanendran A, Hurley RW, Wasan AD, Narouze S, Bhatia A, Davis FN, Hooten WM, Cohen SP. Consensus guidelines on the use of intravenous ketamine infusions for acute pain management from the American Society of Regional Anesthesia and Pain Medicine, the American Academy of Pain Medicine, and the American Society of Anesthesiologists. *Reg Anesth Pain Med.* 2018;43(5):456–66.

Radvansky BM, Shah K, Parikh A, Sifonios AN, Le V, Eloy JD. Role of ketamine in acute postoperative pain management: a narrative review. *Biomed Res Int.* 2015;2015:749837.

8 *A 30 year old patient with a history of substance abuse is admitted after a motor vehicle accident with left 3rd, 4th and 5th rib fractures and proximal tibia fracture. He takes buprenorphine 8 mg daily. What is the appropriate management of acute pain for a patient taking 8 mg buprenorphine daily?*

A *Always stop buprenorphine because it competes with opioid receptors.*

B *Continue buprenorphine in the same dose and order patient-controlled analgesia with dilaudid without basal rate.*

C *Request a femoral nerve block, avoid narcotics, and stop buprenorphine.*

D *Start dilaudid PCA with a basal rate and a demand dose of 0.5 mg every 10 minutes.*

E *Increase the dose of buprenorphine by 50% and start dilaudid 0.5 mg q4h prn.*

Buprenorphine is a lipophilic, semisynthetic opioid with partial agonist activity and high affinity for the mu receptor. Patients on buprenorphine maintenance therapy are frequently encountered in the ICU. In certain doses (more than 12 mg daily), buprenorphine can *block* the ability to use other opioids for breakthrough pain which does not occur at lower doses of buprenorphine (less than 8–12 mg daily sublingual dose). At low doses, there may be synergistic analgesia between buprenorphine and other opioids. Current opinion favors continuation of low-dose buprenorphine (either at full or reduced dose), so choice B is the correct answer. Patients on buprenorphine maintenance may have severe postoperative pain and experience buprenorphine-induced hyperalgesia. It may not be appropriate to stop buprenorphine at this dose (choices A and C). While regional anesthesia is ideal for this patient, given his type of injury, a femoral nerve block will mask symptoms of compartment syndrome that may result from tibial plateau fractures (choice C), so he may not be a candidate for regional anesthetic. Patient controlled analgesia (PCA) is another good choice but basal rates are not recommended due to risk of apnea, even in patients with tolerance (choice D). Basal rates increase both the overall amount of drug delivered and adverse effects without improving analgesia. There is no indication to increase the dose of buprenorphine (choice E).

Answer: B

Buresh M, Ratner J, Zgierska A, Gordin V, Alvanzo A. Treating perioperative and acute pain in patients on buprenorphine: narrative literature review and practice recommendations. *J Gen Intern Med.* 2020;35(12):3635–43. doi: 10.1007/s11606-020-06115-3. Epub 2020 Aug 21.

Goel A, Azargive S, Weissman JS, Shanthanna H, Hanlon JG, Samman B, Dominicis M, Ladha KS, Lamba W, Duggan S, Di Renna T, Peng P, Wong C, Sinha A, Eipe N, Martell D, Intrater H, MacDougall P, Kwofie K, St-Jean M, Rashiq S, Van Camp K, Flamer D, Satok-Wolman M, Clarke H. Perioperative Pain and Addiction Interdisciplinary Network (PAIN) clinical practice advisory for perioperative management of buprenorphine: results of a modified Delphi process. Br J Anaesth. 2019;123(2):e333–e342. doi: 10.1016/j.bja.2019.03.044. Epub 2019 May 29. PMID: 31153631; PMCID: PMC6676043.

Leighton BL, Crock LW. Case series of successful postoperative pain management in buprenorphine maintenance therapy patients. Anesth Analg. 2017;125(5):1779–83.

Chen KY, Chen L, Mao J. Buprenorphine-naloxone therapy in pain management. Anesthesiology. 2014;120(5):1262–74.

9   *A 62-year-old patient with chronic pain is admitted after Hartmann's procedure for diverticulitis. His chronic pain was controlled with 40 mg Oxycodone every 8 hours. He is intubated and you want to start a fentanyl drip post op in equianalgesic dose. What is the closest basal fentanyl dose?*

A *50 mcg/hr*
B *100 mcg/hr*
C *150 mcg/hr*
D *200 mcg/hr*
E *250 mcg/hr*

The first step in this calculation is to estimate the total daily narcotic dose and then convert this dose to an equivalent dose of oral morphine. Morphine is the reference point to convert between different narcotics to obtain the starting point for conversion. Each 20 mg of PO Oxycodone is equivalent to 30 mg PO Morphine. And IV to PO conversion rate of Morphine is 1 to 3. IV equianalgesic parenteral dose of Fentanyl to Morphine is 0.1–0.2 mg fentanyl per 10 mg morphine. This patient is taking 120 mg of oxycodone which converts to 180 mg of PO Morphine. 180 mg of PO morphine would be equal to 60 mg of IV morphine, and equianalgesic parenteral fentanyl dose would be 0.6–1.2 mg of Fentanyl daily (600–1200 mcg). Therefore, the hourly drip dose would be closest to 25–50 mcg/hr. Additionally, using higher than necessary continuous infusion rates (choices B through E) can cause opioid-induced hyperalgesia. Continuous opioid infusions at inappropriately high doses contribute to oversedation and delayed extubation. In context, a simple rule is that fentanyl is 100 x more potent than morphine. An infusion of 100 μg/h fentanyl is equivalent to 10 mg of morphine per hour.

Answer: A

Hurley RW, Hurley NM, Elkassabany and Wu CL. Acute Postoperative Pain. In: Miller RD, ed. *Miller's Anesthesia.* 9th ed. Philadelphia, PA: Elsevier Saunders.

Medication	Equianalgesic dose IV/IM	Equianalgesic dose PO	Typical adult starting dose IV	Typical adult starting dose PO
Morphine	10 mg	30 mg	5–10 mg q3-4h	15–30 mg q3-4h
Oxycodone		20 mg		5–10 mg q4-6h
Fentanyl	100 mcg (not patch)	25 mcg/h transdermal (patch) equivalent PO morphine dose 45–75 mg	50 mcg/h patch approx equal 1 mg/h morphine infusion	
Methadone	10 mg	20 mg	5–10 mg q12h	
Codeine		200 mg		30–60 mg q3-4h
Hydromorphone (Dilaudid)	1.5 mg	7.5 mg	1–2 mg q3-4h	4–8 mg q3-4h

10 *An 18-year-old boy is emergently intubated and exhibits masseter muscle spasm after induction with succinylcholine. He is in the OR for emergency surgery for a ruptured appendix. Which of the following additional symptoms would give you a heightened suspicion for malignant hyperthermia (MH)?*

A *Bradycardia*
B *End-tidal CO2 of 35 mmHG*
C *Rigidity of skeletal muscles of the limbs*
D *Erythema*
E *Diaphoresis*

The onset of malignant hyperthermia can be heralded by tachycardia, trismus or masseter muscle spasm, and arrhythmias. Although concerning, as few as 20% of patients with masseter spasm progress to malignant hyperthermia. Triggers for MH include succinylcholine and inhalation anesthetic gases such as desflurane. This susceptibility to these triggers is due to genetic mutations with the most common one being the RYR1 gene or dihydropyridine (DHP) receptors located within the t-tubule membrane. Monitoring for signs of MH such as increasing temperature, end-tidal CO2, and rigidity of skeletal muscles is key to prompt recognition. MH can be rapidly fatal and treatment with Dantrolene must be started immediately. Dantrolene is a direct skeletal muscle relaxant that blocks calcium release by antagonistic effect at the ryanodine receptor (RYR1). Metabolism is increased in malignant hyperthermia resulting in hypercarbia (choice B), hyperthermia, and tachycardia (choice A). In this scenario, masseter muscle spasm in combination with rigidity of other muscle groups makes the diagnosis of malignant hyperthermia likely (choice C). Erythema (choice D) or diaphoresis (choice E) is not specific for malignant hyperthermia.

Answer: C

Bandschapp O, Girard T. Malignant hyperthermia. *Swiss Med Wkly.* 2012;142:w13652.
Denborough M. Malignant hyperthermia. *Lancet.* 1998;352(9134):1131–6.
Sessler DI. Temperature Regulation and Monitoring. In: Miller RD, ed. *Miller's Anesthesia.* 8th ed. Philadelphia, PA: Elsevier Saunders.

11 *Which of the following medications is best reversed with Sugammadex (Bridon)?*

A *Succinylcholine (Anectine)*
B *Cisatracurium (Nimbex)*
C *Midazolam (Versed)*
D *Ropivacaine (Naropin)*
E *Rocuronium (Zemuron)*

Sugammadex (Bridon) is a dextran compound that surrounds and encapsulates the nondepolarizing aminos-teroid muscle relaxant rocuronium, allowing for reversal of its effects. It cannot reverse succinylcholine (Anectine), a depolarizing muscle relaxant which makes choice A incorrect. While sugammadex can reverse some other nondepolarizing medications, it has a lower affinity for the other aminosteroid paralytics such as vecuronium (Norcuron). Therefore, the quality of reversal depends on the class, amount of muscle recovery, and class of paralytic agent used. Choice B is incorrect because Sugammadex cannot reverse benzylisoquinolinium relaxants such as cisatracurium (Nimbex). Choice E is the correct answer here. Dosages to reverse rocuronium (Zemuron) are based on actual body weight and recovery at the motor end plate. For example, if two or more twitch responses to stimulation are present, 2 mg/kg of actual body weight is given. A higher dose, 4 mg/kg is needed if post tetanic stimulation is needed to produce a twitch response. For immediate reversal of rocuronium, 16 mg/kg is recommended. Train of four (TOF) monitoring is used to assess recovery from and depth of neuromuscular blockade. When using paralytic agents in the ICU, TOF monitoring should be used. Choice C, midazolam (Versed) is a benzodiazepine and can be reversed with flumazenil (Romazicon). Choice D, Ropivacaine (Naropin) is a local anesthetic and can be reversed with lipid emulsions in case of systemic toxicity.

Answer: E

Duvaldestin P, Kuizenga K, Saldien V, Claudius C, Servin F, Klein J, Debaene B, Heeringa M. A randomized, dose-response study of sugammadex given for the reversal of deep rocuronium- or vecuronium-induced neuromuscular blockade under sevoflurane anesthesia. *Anesth Analg.* 2010;110(1):74–82.
Hunter JM. Reversal of residual neuromuscular block: complications associated with perioperative management of muscle relaxation. Br J Anaesth. 2017;119(suppl_1):i53–i62.

12 *A 75-year-old woman is admitted to the ICU after axillary to bifemoral bypass. Patient complains of pain from anterior thigh to her toes and a quadratus lumborum block is performed. What is the most serious complication of this procedure?*

A *Hypertension*
B *Postdural puncture headache*
C *Hyperemia of the leg*
D *Numbness of the lumbar dermatomes*
E *Retroperitoneal hematoma*

Because the quadratus lumborum block (QL) is a deep block, complications to watch out for include direct injury to the kidney, lumbar arteries, leading to retroperitoneal hematoma and pleural penetration leading to

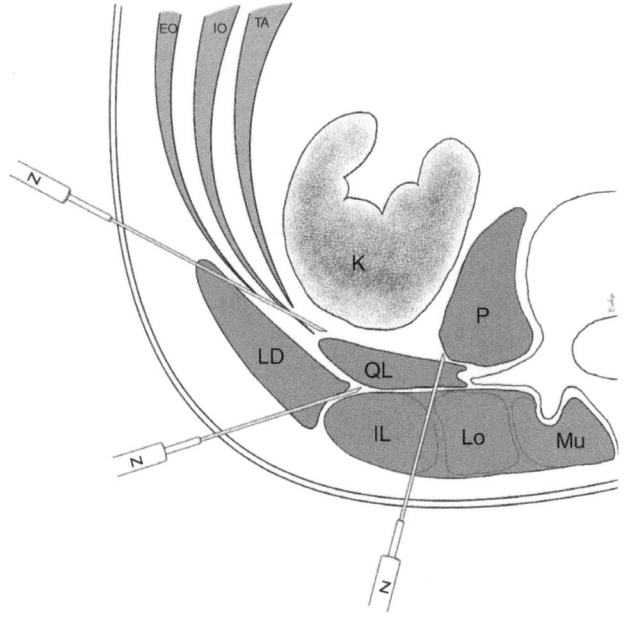

Figure 12.1 Quadratus lumborum block. QL: quadratus lumborum; EO: external oblique; IO: internal oblique; TA: transverse abdominis; K: kidney; P: psoas major; LD: latissimus dorsi; IL: iliocostalis lumborum; Lo: longissimus; Mu: multifidus.

pneumothorax (choice E). A prolonged motor block may result from anesthetic distribution to the lumbar plexus. Hypotension, which can result from the spread of local anesthetic to the paravertebral space, has also been described (choice A). Local anesthetic toxicity (LAST) is always a potential risk of any peripheral or neuraxial technique. Rupture of the dura mater causing postdural puncture headache is a complication of an epidural catheter placement (wet tap) and not a complication of QL block (choice B). Numbness of the lumbar dermatomes (choice D) is the desired effect and hyperemia of the leg is transient and not a complication (choice C) (Figure 12.1).

Answer: E

Elsharkawy H, El-Boghdadly K, Barrington M. Quadratus lumborum block: anatomical concepts, mechanisms, and techniques. *Anesthesiology*. 2019;130(2):322–335.

Krohg A, Ullensvang K, Rosseland LA, Langesæter E, Sauter AR. The analgesic effect of ultrasound-guided quadratus lumborum block after cesarean delivery: a randomized clinical trial. *Anesth Analg* 2018;126(2):559–565.

Blanco R, Ansari T, Girgis E. Quadratus lumborum block for postoperative pain after caesarean section: A randomised controlled trial. *Eur J Anaesthesiol*. 2015;32(11):812–8.

13 *A 60-year-old morbidly obese man with a difficult airway and obstructive sleep apnea was taken for* emergent laparotomy for peritonitis. After awake fiberoptic intubation with benzocaine and induction of anesthesia, the oxygen saturation reads and remains 85% with good signal quality. His lips appear cyanotic, and he has bilateral breath sounds. Which of the following is the most likely cause?

A *Carboxyhemoglobinemia*
B *Methemoglobinemia*
C *Cyanide toxicity*
D *Main stem intubation*
E *Hgb A1c level greater than 10%*

Acquired methemoglobinemia is potentially threatening and must be immediately recognized. The most common cause of methemoglobinemia is exposure to oxidizing agents such as benzocaine and nitroglycerine (choice B). When iron is ferrous oxidized to its ferric state, oxygen binding to hemoglobin is prevented which shifts the oxygen hemoglobin dissociation curve to the left. Excess methemoglobin leads to hypoxia, cyanosis, impaired aerobic respiration, and metabolic acidosis. Other etiologies are genetic deficiencies of cytochrome-b5 and cytochrome-b5 reductase. Unfortunately, pulse oximetry and arterial blood gases can be misleading in patients with methemoglobinemia. Co-oximetry is the gold standard. Treatment options for methemoglobinemia include supportive measures, methylene blue, and vitamin C which are potent reducing agents. Methylene blue is contraindicated in G6PD deficiency.

There are no triggering agents to cause Carboxyhemoglobinemia (i.e., Smoke inhalation with CO) and Cyanide toxicity (i.e., Smoke inhalation, Sodium Nitroprusside, Poisons) in this case which makes choices A and C unlikely. The patient is intubated fiber-optically and has bilateral breath sounds which makes choice D unlikely. Choice E indicates untreated diabetes mellitus and is therefore incorrect.

Answer: B

Guay J. Methemoglobinemia related to local anesthetics: a summary of 242 episodes. Anesth Analg. 2009;108(3):837.

Anderson CM, Woodside KJ, Spencer TA, Hunter GC. Methemoglobinemia: An unusual cause of postoperative cyanosis. *J Vasc Surg*. 2004;39(3):P686–690.

14 *Patient is a 70kg, 60-year-old man undergoing paravertebral nerve block due to multiple rib fractures in the ICU. Patient is hemodynamically stable before the block; however, becomes hypotensive and tachycardic 15 minute after the procedure is finished. You are suspecting local anesthetics toxicity. What would be the most appropriate treatment at this time?*

A *Vasopressin bolus followed by infusion*

B *Diltiazem (Cardizem) 5 mg bolus followed by infusion*

C *Lipid emulsion 20% 100 mL follow by infusion*

D *Propofol 100 mg*

E *Lorazepam (Ativan) 2 mg*

Local anesthetic systemic toxicity (LAST) can occur after inadvertent intravascular injection or increased vascular uptake of a local anesthetic (LA) agent. The mechanisms for the clinical responses seen are multifactorial, mostly affecting the central nervous and cardiovascular systems. Neurologic manifestations such as tinnitus, seizures, or confusion are most common but the cardiovascular effects can be devastating. LA medications accumulate in mitochondria and cardiac tissue with greater affinity relative to plasma and can manifest with profound shock and cardiac instability.

LA exerts its action at voltage-gated sodium channels, blocks calcium channels, and at higher concentrations inhibits other channels, enzymes, and receptors including the carnitine-acylcarnitine translocase receptor in mitochondria. This is the basis for treatment of LAST with lipid emulsion. Bupivacaine is more likely to cause cardiovascular collapse because it is more lipophilic and has a greater affinity for the voltage-gated sodium channels. Factors that increase the likelihood of toxicity are extremes of age, comorbidities, higher total dose of LA medication, and site of injection. The highest incidence of LAST is with paravertebral blocks.

Treatment of LAST includes 20% lipid emulsion which acts as a "lipid sink." Recommended dose is 100 mL over 2–3 minutes for patients at least 70 kg (1.5 mL/kg), followed by infusion of 250 mL over 20 minutes. The bolus can be repeated, and the infusion rate doubled if clinically not improved (choice C).

Further care includes supportive measures such benzodiazepines for treatment of seizures. Lorazepam (Ativan) can be administered if the patient is showing signs of seizure activity (choice E). Beta-blockers, calcium channel blockers (diltiazem), and vasopressin should be avoided (choices A and B). Epinephrine if needed should be administered at lower doses (less than 1 mg/kg). Propofol is not the best choice and can exacerbate hypotension (choice D).

Answer: C

Neal JM, Neal EJ, Weinberg GL. American Society of Regional Anesthesia and Pain Medicine Local Anesthetic Systemic Toxicity checklist: 2020 version. *Reg Anesth Pain Med.* 2020:rapm-2020-101986. doi: 10.1136/rapm-2020-101986. Epub ahead of print.

El-Boghdadly K, Pawa A, Chin KJ. Local anesthetic systemic toxicity: current perspectives. *Local Reg Anesth.* 2018;11:35–44.

15 *A 65-year-old polytrauma patient in the ICU with blunt cerebrovascular injury and rib fractures has severe pain which affects patient's respiratory efforts. Patient has a new lower extremity venous thromboembolic event. You place a pain consult for possible epidural anesthesia. Considering your plan for a neuraxial block, which of the following therapies should be avoided?*

A *Ketorolac (Toradol) and subcutaneous heparin*

B *ASA*

C *Enoxaparin (Lovenox)*

D *Heparin infusion*

E *Acetaminophen IV (Ofirmev)*

Because neuraxial techniques are increasingly used to manage pain in the ICU, intensivists need to understand the guidelines for management of anticoagulation as it affects the placement of epidural catheters. Serious complications associated with neuraxial anesthesia are epidural hematomas, epidural abscess, and nerve injuries. Absolute contraindications include patient refusal and severe coagulopathy. Relative contraindications are sepsis, thrombocytopenia, pre-existing nerve injury, placement in anesthetized adults, and anticoagulation. While none of the above medications alone are absolutely contraindicated (choices B, C, D, and E), a patient receiving more than one antithrombotic medication should not receive an epidural or spinal anesthetic technique (choice A). Non-steroidal anti-inflammatory medications are not contraindicated if used alone.

Answer: A

Horlocker TT, Vandermeuelen E, Kopp SL, Gogarten W, Leffert LR, Benzon HT. Regional anesthesia in the patient receiving antithrombotic or thrombolytic therapy: American Society of Regional Anesthesia and Pain Medicine Evidence-Based Guidelines (fourth edition). *Reg Anesth Pain Med.* 2018;43(3):263–309.

16 *Patient is a 65-year-old woman admitted to the ICU for TBI with past medical history of mitochondrial disease and lupus. Patient has been on long-term steroids. Patient is agitated and you suspect she has increased ICP. You are about to intubate the patient for airway protection. What would be the best choice for induction and intubation?*

A *Propofol*

B *Etomidate (Amidate)*

C *Lorazepam (Ativan)*

D *Fentanyl*

E *No induction, topicalize with benzocaine and plan for awake fiberoptic intubation*

Critically ill patients are often intubated emergently, and a rapid sequence technique is preferred if clinically deteriorating. Typically, clinicians combine sedative and paralytic agents although judgment is needed before deciding to use either class of drug. Fentanyl will provide a stable induction and can be used with succinylcholine for a rapid sequence intubation (choice D). Propofol lowers ICP and is also acceptable in traumatic brain injured patients. But in the setting of mitochondrial disease, it should be avoided as propofol infusion syndrome is thought to result from inhibition of mitochondrial enzymes in mitochondria and on mitochondrial membranes (choice A). A single low dose of propofol may be acceptable; however, it can cause vasodilation and hypotension and is not the best choice here. Etomidate, a sedative-hypnotic, is often used because it has relative cardiac stability when compared with propofol. Caution should be used with even a single dose of etomidate (Amidate) because it can cause adrenal insufficiency by inhibition of 11β-hydroxylase (choice B). Long-acting benzodiazepines such as lorazepam (Ativan) can delay a post intubation neurovascular exam and its use should be avoided (choice C). Awake fiberoptic intubation is unlikely to be tolerated in an agitated patient (choice E).

Answer: D

Niezgoda J, Morgan PG. Anesthetic considerations in patients with mitochondrial defects. Paediatr Anaesth. 2013;23(9):785–93.
Footitt EJ, Sinha MD, Raiman JA, Dhawan A, Moganasundram S, Champion MP. Mitochondrial disorders and general anaesthesia: a case series and review. *Br J Anaesth*. 2008;100(4):436–41.

17 *About 5 hours ago, a 35-year-old woman with a history of depression and anxiety, ingested an unknown amount of alcohol (ethanol), 20 tabs of alprazolam (Xanax), and methocarbamol (Robaxin). She is arousable to sternal rub. Blood pressure is 100/60 mmHg, heart rate is 68/min, respiratory rate is 8/min, and temperature is 36 °C. Which is the most appropriate intervention?*
   A *Intubation*
   B *Gastric lavage*
   C *Flumazenil (Anexate)*
   D *Fomepizole (Antizol)*
   E *Activated charcoal*

Since the patient ingested several medications, the best intervention is intubation and supportive care (choice A). Activated charcoal is not likely to be effective since the presentation is delayed, so activated charcoal and gastric lavage are not indicated (choices B, E). Flumazenil (Anexate) is an antidote for benzodiazepines but is contraindicated in a patient with chronic use of alprazolam. Flumazenil may precipitate withdrawal seizures in this case. It would be difficult to treat subsequent seizures after flumazenil since benzodiazepine receptors would be blocked (choice C). Benzodiazepine overdose may cause respiratory depression but risks of reversing benzodiazepines in chronic use outweigh potential benefits as it may precipitate seizure. Fomepizole (4-methylpyrazole, Antizol) competitively inhibits the first enzyme in the metabolism of ethylene glycol and methanol (alcohol dehydrogenase) which prevents their metabolism to toxic acids. The slower rate of metabolite production allows the liver to process and excrete the metabolites as they are produced; however, it is not indicated in acute ethanol toxicity. Do not give fomepizole in acute alcohol intoxication because fomepizole will compete for alcohol dehydrogenase (choice D) and impair metabolism. Methocarbamol (Robaxin) is a muscle relaxant.

Answer: A

Brent J, McMartin K, Phillips S, Aaron C, Kulig K; Methylpyrazole for Toxic Alcohols Study Group. Fomepizole for the treatment of methanol poisoning. *N Engl J Med*. 2001;344(6):424–9.
Seger DL. Flumazenil--treatment or toxin. *J Toxicol Clin Toxicol* 2004;42(2):209–16.
Chyka PA, Seger D, Krenzelok EP, Vale JA; American Academy of Clinical Toxicology; European Association of Poisons Centres and Clinical Toxicologists. Position paper: single-dose activated charcoal. *Clin Toxicol (Phila)*. 2005;43(2):61–87.

18 *Which of the following is a true statement regarding flumazenil (Anexate)?*
   A *It exerts a clinical effect by competitive antagonism at mu receptor.*
   B *It is a competitive inhibitor at GABA A receptors.*
   C *Flumazenil does not contribute to seizure activity in benzodiazepine tolerant patients.*
   D *It is a relatively long-acting medication.*
   E *Flumazenil consistently reverses respiratory depression caused by benzodiazepine overdose.*

Mu receptors are specific transmembrane neurotransmitter receptors that couple G proteins and are activated by opioids and are not affected in the presence of flumazenil (choice A). Naltrexone (Vivitrol) is a competitive antagonist to mu receptors. Flumazenil (Anexate) is structurally similar to midazolam and is a nonspecific competitive antagonist of the benzodiazepine receptor (GABA$_A$) in the central nervous system (CNS) (choice B). Flumazenil has a limited role in the management of benzodiazepine overdose, purportedly to avoid the need for procedure (i.e., intubation), and is contraindicated in the presence of a known seizure disorder or benzodiazepine dependence. It can reverse the effect of benzodiazepines in the CNS and precipitate seizures making choice C incorrect. Flumazenil rapidly undergoes hepatic metabolism to inactive metabolites and its half-life is not long, about 40–80 minutes, thus the duration of effect of a long-acting benzodiazepine or a large benzodiazepine dose can exceed that of flumazenil making choices D and E incorrect. However, in the right scenario, flumazenil as a reversal and rescue medication can be lifesaving. The recommended initial dose in adults is 0.2 mg IV given by slow push over 1–2 minutes. Doses can be repeated 0.2 mg, but one must watch for a maximum dose of 2 mg.

Answer: B

Kreshak AA, Cantrell FL, Clark RF, Tomaszewski CA. A poison center's ten-year experience with flumazenil administration to acutely poisoned adults. *J Emerg Med.* 2012;43(4):677–82.

Weinbroum AA, Flaishon R, Sorkine P, Szold O, Rudick V. A risk-benefit assessment of flumazenil in the management of benzodiazepine overdose. *Drug Saf* 1997;17(3):181–96.

Shalansky SJ, Naumann TL, Englander FA. Effect of flumazenil on benzodiazepine-induced respiratory depression. *Clin Pharm* 1993;12(7):483–7.

Seger DL. Flumazenil--treatment or toxin. *J Toxicol Clin Toxicol* 2004;42(2):209–16.

Murray L Little M Pascu O Hoggett KA. *Toxicology Handbook.* 3rd Edition. eBook ISBN: 9780729584951.

19 *A 40-year-old man with a history of depression is admitted to the ICU after laparotomy and lysis of adhesions. He was using a fentanyl PCA but developed autonomic dysfunction, confusion, and muscular rigidity. The PCA was stopped because it was suspected that he was exhibiting* **serotonin syndrome**. *When stable, you will need to rethink the pain management plan. What is the best course of action?*

A *Stop fentanyl PCA and order tramadol (Ultram)*

B *Continue fentanyl PCA and add methadone (Dolophine)*

C *Stop fentanyl PCA and order meperidine (Demerol)*

D *Stop the fentanyl PCA and order a morphine PCA*

E *Stop the fentanyl PCA and order oxycodone*

Some opioids including fentanyl, methadone, and demerol act as serotonergic agents that contribute to the development of **serotonin syndrome**. Medications in this class of opioids are the synthetic and semisynthetic opioids. Serotonin syndrome results from over-dosage or coadministration of narcotics with serotonin reuptake inhibitor antidepressants (SSRIs). Synthetic piperidine opioids are pro-serotonergic in their own right and can act as serotonin reuptake inhibitors. This class of narcotics includes fentanyl, methadone, oxycodone, meperidine

(Demerol), and tramadol (choices B, C, and E). Morphine is not in this class and does not inhibit serotonin reuptake (choice D) and is the correct answer. Clinical manifestations of serotonin syndrome results from increased postsynaptic stimulation of 5-hydroxytryptamine, 2A and 1A serotonin receptors in the central and peripheral nervous system. Since this patient has a history of depression and is receiving a synthetic opioid, serotonin syndrome is suspected.

Answer: D

van Ewijk CE, Jacobs GE, Girbes ARJ. Unsuspected serotonin toxicity in the ICU. *Ann Intensive Care.* 2016;6(1):85.

Pathan H, Williams J. Basic opioid pharmacology: an update. *Br J Pain.* 2012;6(1):11–16.

Pedavally S, Fugate JE, Rabinstein AA. Serotonin syndrome in the intensive care unit: clinical presentations and precipitating medications. *Neurocrit Care.* 2014;21(1):108–13.

20 *A 130 kg, 70-year-old man fell 2 weeks ago during a hiking trip and sustained a femur fracture and cervical spine injury. He has a history of heavy snoring and has a BMI of 38. His course was complicated by acute kidney injury but his GFR is now 35 and recovering. He is cooperative and comfortable on a PCA with hydromorphone (Dilaudid) 0.2 mg every 10 minutes. You prefer to do an awake bronchoscopy without intubation to evaluate his recent fever and infiltrate seen on the chest x-ray. Which of the following techniques is the best option for this procedure?*

A *Give a hydromorphone (Dilaudid) bolus and start a propofol infusion while maintaining spontaneous respirations.*

B *Topicalization is contraindicated; prepare to intubate for bronchoscopy using rocuronium and propofol.*

C *Topicalization of the recurrent and superior laryngeal nerves to anesthetize the tongue, epiglottis, vocal cords, and trachea.*

D *Topicalization of the hypoglossal nerve to anesthetize the base of the tongue and arytenoids and aryepiglottic folds.*

E *Bilateral superficial cervical plexus block.*

Different techniques are used to sedate and anesthetize the airway for an awake bronchoscopy using a variety of medications such as benzodiazepines, short-acting opioids (fentanyl, remifentanil), propofol, ketamine, or dexmedetomidine. In cooperative patients at risk for airway obstruction or difficult intubation, topicalization may be a good choice and should be considered. This can be achieved by anesthetizing the airway with regional techniques with or without sedation or in combination with inhaled anesthetic agents such as viscous lidocaine.

Sensation to the oropharynx, and larynx and trachea must be blocked to perform an awake fiberoptic bronchoscopy or intubation. There are several ways to achieve the necessary analgesia, but the sensory nerves should be anesthetized. The superior laryngeal nerve supplies sensory innervation to the base of the tongue, epiglottis and aryepiglottic folds, and arytenoids. It also supplies motor innervation to the external branch of the cricothyroid muscle. The recurrent laryngeal nerve supplies sensory innervation to the vocal cords and trachea (choice C).

The combination of narcotic bolus (Dilaudid) and propofol infusion is likely to result in apnea that would require intubation. Since this patient could have a difficult intubation (presence of cervical spine injury and a BMI of 38), this is not the best plan (choice A). Topicalization is not contraindicated in this patient and should be considered before intubation (choice A). The hypoglossal nerve is purely motor and does not need to be blocked (choice D). A superficial cervical plexus block provides anesthesia to the skin of the anterolateral neck and auricular areas and skin inferior to the clavicle. This block can be used in thyroid or clavicular surgery but would not anesthetize the airway or facilitate an awake bronchoscopy (choice E).

Answer: C

Elmaddawy AEA, Mazy AE. Ultrasound-guided bilateral superficial cervical plexus block for thyroid surgery: The effect of dexmedetomidine addition to bupivacaine-epinephrine. *Saudi J Anaesth*. 2018;12(3):412–8.

Simmons ST, Schleich AR. Airway regional anesthesia for awake fiberoptic intubation. *Reg Anesth Pain Med*. 2002;27(2):180–92.

21 *An 89-year-old man fell off a ladder and fractured ribs 3, 4, 5, and 6 on the left side. He is a smoker and has a history of chronic obstructive pulmonary disease (COPD). His pain score is 9/10 and he is taking shallow breaths. He takes antiplatelet medications for atrial fibrillation but cannot remember his last dose. His SpO2 reads 92% on a 30% face mask. His vital signs are stable. What intervention do you want to recommend to control his pain?*

A *Lidocaine patch*
B *Oxycodone*
C *Hydromorphone (Dilaudid) PCA*
D *Erector spinae block (ESP) plus hydromorphone (Dilaudid) PCA and gabapentin*
E *Intercostal nerve block (ICNB)*

Given his age and pre-existing COPD, this patient is at risk for pulmonary complications of thoracic trauma. He is in significant pain and appears to be splinting with hypoven-

tilation. The side effects of narcotics such as increased risk for ICU delirium, constipation, and nausea also make these agents a less attractive option when used alone (choices B and C). Erector spinae (ESP) blocks work through a combination of different mechanisms, particularly anesthetic spread to the thoracic paravertebral space. There is evidence to suggest that ESP block results in decreased postoperative pain and opioid requirement for a wide array of thoracic and abdominal procedures including in the management of rib fractures. Intercostal nerve blocks (ICNB) for multiple rib fractures require multiple injections of local anesthetics increasing the risk of toxicity. Choice E, ICNB alone is not the best choice as multimodal approach is recommended to control pain in patients with blunt thoracic trauma. Moreover, being on antiplatelet therapy increases the risk of bleeding for intercostal nerve block (choice E). Choice A, lidocaine patch would not provide sufficient pain relief and continued splinting with shallow breathing may contribute to atelectasis. The patch may cause some numbness to the skin but because of its superficial site of action, it does not decrease fracture pain. Erector spinae blocks in combination with narcotics and gabapentin would establish a multimodal pain control regimen and is conditionally recommended by latest EAST guidelines (choice D) (Figure 12.2).

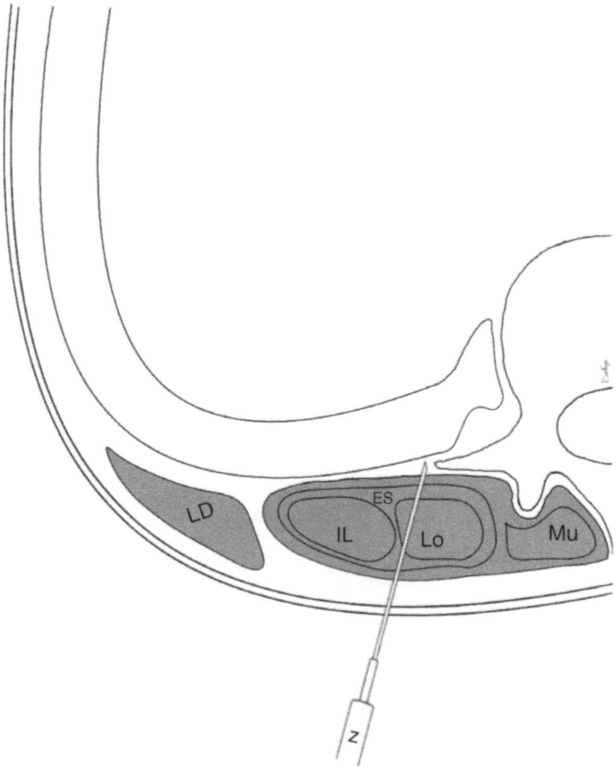

Figure 12.2 Erector spinae plane block. ES: erector spinae; LD: latissimus dorsi; IL: iliocostalis lumborum; Lo: longissimus; Mu: multifidus.

Answer: D

Galvagno SM Jr, Smith CE, Varon AJ, Hasenboehler EA, Sultan S, Shaefer G, To KB, Fox AD, Alley DE, Ditillo M, Joseph BA, Robinson BR, Haut ER. Pain management for blunt thoracic trauma: A joint practice management guideline from the Eastern Association for the Surgery of Trauma and Trauma Anesthesiology Society. *J Trauma Acute Care Surg.* 2016;81(5):936–51.

Saadawi M, Layera S, Aliste J, Bravo D, Leurcharusmee P, Tran Q. Erector spinae plane block: A narrative review with systematic analysis of the evidence pertaining to clinical indications and alternative truncal blocks. *J Clin Anesth.* 2020;68:110063.

22 *Considering the appropriateness of nerves blocked to the procedure performed, which patient's pain is more likely to be adequately controlled?*

    A *Abdominal wall reconstruction with bilateral TAP indwelling catheter.*

    B *Large bowel resection with bilateral TAP block injection.*

    C *Cervical fusion with erector spinae block single injection.*

    D *Esophageal reconstruction with a neurolytic celiac plexus block.*

    E *Shoulder surgery with axillary nerve block.*

Transverse Abdominis Plane (TAP) nerve blocks with indwelling catheters provide adequate somatic analgesia for abdominal wall surgery (choice A). In contrast, quadratus lumborum (QL) nerve blocks provide visceral in addition to somatic analgesia for the abdominal wall and the lower thoracic wall segments. This is because QL nerve blocks spread to the paravertebral space and sometimes achieve epidural spread. In large bowel resection, bilateral TAP block injections will not provide adequate analgesia for deep visceral pain (choice B). Erector spinae (ESP) block results in decreased postoperative pain and opioid requirement for a wide array of thoracic and abdominal procedures including in the management of rib

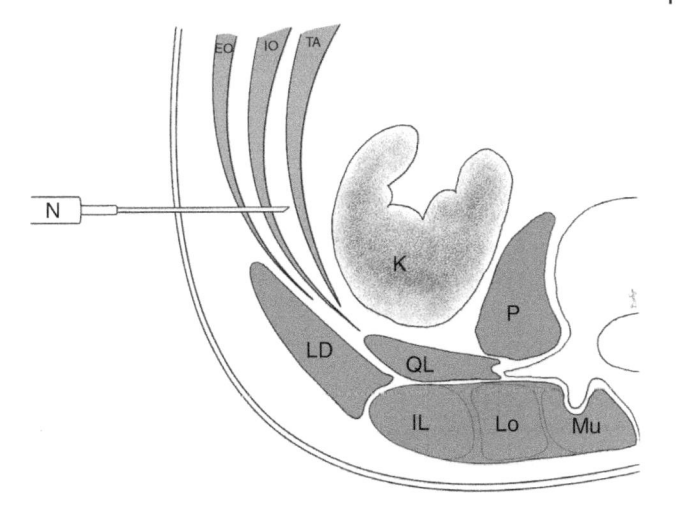

Figure 12.3 Transverse abdominis plane block. QL: quadratus lumborum; EO: external oblique; IO: internal oblique; TA: transverse abdominis; K: kidney; P: psoas major; LD: latissimus dorsi; IL: iliocostalis lumborum; Lo: longissimus; Mu: multifidus.

fractures. It does not relieve somatic pain for cervical fusion (choice C). Choice D, celiac plexus block places the either a local anesthetic or neurolytic solution directly on the celiac ganglion anterolateral to the aorta. When used, for example, to manage pain in terminal pancreatic cancer, a neurolytic agent is chosen. Choice E is incorrect since the axillary nerve block will not provide adequate coverage for the shoulder joint surgery. Axillary nerve block will provide adequate analgesia from the mid upper arm extending to the hand (Figure 12.3).

Answer: A

Tsai HC, Yoshida T, Chuang TY, Yang SF, Chang CC, Yao HY, Tai YT, Lin JA, Chen KY. Transversus abdominis plane block: an updated review of anatomy and techniques. *Biomed Res Int.* 2017;2017:8284363.

Saadawi M, Layera S, Aliste J, Bravo D, Leurcharusmee P, Tran Q. Erector spinae plane block: A narrative review with systematic analysis of the evidence pertaining to clinical indications and alternative truncal blocks. *J Clin Anesth.* 2020;68:110063.

13

Delirium, Alcohol Withdrawal and Psychiatric Disorders

Thomas Muse, MD and Rondi Gelbard, MD

Department of Trauma and Acute Care Surgery, Department of Surgery, University of Alabama at Birmingham, Birmingham, AL, USA

1   *A 77-year-old man with Parkinson's disease is admitted to the hospital after a fall at home, sustaining a femur fracture and multiple rib fractures. The day after admission, he undergoes femur fixation. The patient sleeps for most of the following day and that evening he frequently attempts to get out of bed despite redirection, pulls out an IV, and becomes combative with hospital staff. The ideal treatment of this patient's condition includes which of the following:*

   A *Diazepam*
   B *Haloperidol*
   C *Risperidone*
   D *Ziprasidone*
   E *Quetiapine*

This patient is most likely suffering from hyperactive delirium. Of the medications listed, quetiapine has the safest side effect profile for a patient with Parkinson's dementia and the treatment of delirium. Atypical antipsychotics are the preferred medical treatment of delirium in the elderly population, particularly those with Parkinson's. This is due to these medications having decreased likelihood of exacerbating extrapyramidal symptoms compared to typical antipsychotics. The likelihood of developing extrapyramidal symptoms is relative to the medications' potency for the D2 dopamine receptor. Of the atypical antipsychotics listed above (risperidone, ziprasidone, and quetiapine), the choice with the least potency for the D2 receptor is quetiapine. Benzodiazepines such as diazepam should be avoided in the elderly for treatment of delirium.

Answer: E

Devlin JW, Roberts RJ, Fong JJ, et al. Efficacy and safety of quetiapine in critically ill patients with delirium: a prospective, multicenter, randomized, double-blind, placebo-controlled pilot study. *Crit. Care Med.* 2010;38(2):419–427.

Alexopoulos GS, Streim J, Carpenter D, et al. Using antipsychotic agents in older patients. *J. Clin. Psych.* 2004;65(Suppl 2):5–99.

Fick DM, Agostini JV, and Inouye SK. Delirium superimposed on dementia: a systematic review. *J. Am. Geriatr. Soc.* 2002;50(10):1723–1732.

Inouye SK, Westendorp RG, and Saczynski JS. Delirium in elderly people. *Lancet* 2014;383(9920):911–922.

Lundstrom M, Edlund A, Bucht G, et al. Dementia after delirium in patients with femoral neck fractures. *J. Am. Geriatr. Soc.* 2003;51(7):1002–1006.

2   *A 72-year-old woman with no medical history presents to the emergency department as a passenger involved in a motor vehicle collision. Her injuries include five right-sided rib fractures, a sternal fracture, and a grade 2 liver laceration. A CT scan of her head at admission showed no evidence of intracranial hemorrhage. She is admitted to the ICU for pain control and pulmonary toilet. On hospital day three, she develops intermittent periods of confusion, disorientation to place and time, and believes her bedside nurse is her daughter. Her family members state that she has never behaved in this manner previously. Her vital signs are normal including a pulse oximetry reading of 99% on room air. Routine lab work including a metabolic panel and complete blood count are normal. Abdominal exam is unremarkable. The most appropriate initial evaluation of her condition includes which of the following:*

   A *MRI brain*
   B *Blood and urine cultures*
   C *Confusion Assessment Method for the ICU (CAM-ICU) score*

D *Ventilation/perfusion (V/Q) lung scan*
E *Repeat CT scan of the abdomen and pelvis with intravenous contrast*

This patient has developed acute delirium as indicated by the waxing and waning nature of her symptoms. She has many risk factors including advanced age, admission to the ICU, and acute pain due to trauma. The most appropriate initial evaluation is to perform a CAM-ICU assessment (Table 13.1). This tool has a high sensitivity and specificity for delirium and can even be used in ventilated patients. While confusion and hallucinations can be present in traumatic brain injury or degenerative brain disorders, the patient had a negative initial CT scan of the brain and no prior signs of dementia according to her family, thus a MRI of the brain is unlikely to be diagnostic. Geriatric patients may not mount a febrile response to commonly encountered infections such as urinary tract infections or pneumonia; however, this patient's vitals and lab work are normal and therefore infection is less likely. Ventilation/perfusion lung scans are used to determine the probability of pulmonary embolism. This patient has normal vital signs including oxygen saturation and therefore this test is unlikely to be helpful in this setting. This patient has a blunt solid organ injury and is at risk for intra-abdominal hemorrhage; however, with normal vital signs, lab work, and a benign abdominal exam, a repeat abdominal CT is unlikely to aid in diagnosis.

Table 13.1 Confusion assessment method to assess delirium (CAM).

Feature	Assessment
Acute onset and fluctuating course	Based on change from patient's baseline. Positive response to: "Is this mental status change acute?" "Is this mental status change fluctuating during the course of the day?"
Inattention	Positive response to: "Is there difficulty focusing attention, distractibility, or difficulty keeping track of what is being said?"
Disorganized Thinking	Positive response to: "Are there rambling, irrelevant conversation, unclear, illogical thoughts, frequent and unpredictable switching from subject to subject."
Altered level of Consciousness	Positive response if other than "alert" Normal = alert Hyper alert = vigilant Drowsy, easily aroused = lethargic Difficult to arouse = stupor Unarousable = coma
Delirium =	Features 1 AND 2 + either 3 OR 4

Answer: C

Devlin JW, Skrobik Y, Gelinas C, et al. Clinical practice guidelines for the prevention and management of pain, agitation/sedation, delirium, immobility, and sleep disruption in adult patients in the ICU. *Crit. Care Med.* 2018;46(9):e825-e873.

Adamis D, Rooney S, Meagher D, et al. A comparison of delirium diagnosis in elderly medical inpatients using the CAM, DRS-R98, DSM-IV and DSM-5 criteria. *Int. Psychogeriatr.* 2015;27(6):883–889.

3 *A 79-year-old man is hospitalized for three weeks following an antrectomy and Billroth II reconstruction for gastric outlet obstruction due to peptic ulcer disease. His hospital course was complicated by delayed gastric emptying requiring prolonged nasogastric tube decompression and parenteral nutrition. The patient spent over one week of his hospitalization in the ICU primarily due to hyperactive delirium which was difficult to manage. Of the following, which is true regarding the effects of delirium in this patient population:*
A *Delirium has no effect on inpatient mortality risk.*
B *The duration of delirium has no long-term effects on this patient's risk for mortality after discharge.*
C *His episodes of delirium could worsen the progression of any underlying degenerative brain disorders such as Alzheimer's dementia.*
D *Inpatient delirium episodes do not convey long-term risk on cognitive impairment.*
E *The patient is less likely to require transition to a skilled nursing facility upon discharge because of his prolonged hospital stay.*

This patient's prolonged hospital course and episodes of delirium convey a significant long-term survival and cognitive prognosis risk. Patients who suffer from delirium during their hospitalization have double the risk of death at 1 month and 6 months after discharge. The duration of delirium also conveys added risk of mortality, as increasing days adds increasing risk of death. Additionally, delirium encountered while inpatient has been shown to increase future cognitive decline and accelerate existing cognitive decline in dementia patients. Elderly patients with extended hospitalizations are at increased risk of discharge to a skilled nursing facility.

Answer: C

Girard TD, Jackson JC, Pandharipande PP, et al. Delirium as a predictor of long-term cognitive impairment in survivors of critical illness. *Crit. Care Med.* 2010;38(7):1513–1520.

Pandharipande PP, Girard TD, Jackson JC, et al; BRAIN-ICU Study Investigators. Long-term cognitive impairment after critical illness. *N. Engl. J. Med.* 2013;369(14): 1306–1316.

Goldberg TE, Chen C, Wang Y, et al. Association of delirium with long-term cognitive decline. A meta-analysis. *JAMA Neurology.* 2020;77:1373–1381.

Pisani MA, Kong SY, Kasl SV, et al. Days of delirium are associated with 1-year mortality in an older intensive care unit population. *Am. J. Respir. Crit. Care Med.* 2009;180(11):1092–1097.

4 *A 52-year-old woman with a history of hypertension and depression is being treated for acute uncomplicated diverticulitis with ciprofloxacin and metronidazole. By hospital day two, her abdominal pain has improved and her home medications (lisinopril and sertraline) are restarted. The following day, she develops recurrent nausea which is treated with ondansetron. That evening, she becomes delirious and is given 2 mg of IV haloperidol. An hour later, her telemetry shows intermittent polymorphic ventricular tachycardia with a characteristic twisting of the QRS complex. The patient feels dizzy but is otherwise awake, alert, and hemodynamically stable. What is the appropriate next step in management?*

A *Perform defibrillation.*

B *Begin an IV magnesium sulfate infusion and discontinue other possible offending medications.*

C *Administer a 1 liter crystalloid fluid bolus.*

D *Obtain a CT scan of the abdomen and pelvis with oral and IV contrast.*

E *Obtain an echocardiogram.*

This patient is experiencing intermittent torsades de pointes, a form of polymorphic ventricular tachycardia where the electrocardiogram tracing will show a characteristic twisting of the QRS complex above and below the isoelectric baseline. The most likely etiology for this patient's torsades de pointes is prolonged QT interval from administration of multiple medications which are known to cause QT prolongation. In this case, ciprofloxacin, sertraline, ondansetron, and haloperidol cause QT prolongation. Coadministration of multiple medications that prolong the QT interval increases the risk of developing QT prolongation. The correct management is to administer an IV magnesium sulfate infusion and to discontinue these medications. Defibrillation is inappropriate due to the patient being awake and hemodynamically stable. If the patient were to decline into ventricular fibrillation, then defibrillation would be appropriate. Worsening diverticulitis is unlikely to be the cause of her torsades de pointes and

obtaining a CT scan would only prolong treatment. An echocardiogram would not reveal the etiology of her arrhythmia and would also prolong treatment. A fluid bolus would not be helpful in this scenario.

Answer: B

Roden DM. Predicting drug-induced QT prolongation and torsades de pointes. *J. Physiol.* 2016;594(9): 2459–2468.

Thomas SH and Behr ER. Pharmacological treatment of acquired QT prolongation and torsades de pointes. *Br. J. Clin. Pharmacol.* 2016;81(3):420–427.

5 *A 27-year-old man was admitted to the ICU following a motorcycle collision with ejection. He was not wearing a helmet and sustained multi-compartment intracranial hemorrhages. His initial GCS was 7, and he was intubated and an intracranial pressure monitor was placed. On hospital day 10, he was unable to be liberated from the ventilator and a tracheostomy was performed. During the subsequent days, he was noted to have intermittent periods of agitation manifested by restlessness, thrashing in the bed, and pulling at lines and tubes. Between these episodes, he had periods of calmness where he was intermittently following commands. His agitation was treated with "as needed" doses of opioids and antipsychotics. In this scenario, which is the most reliable method of assessing this patient to avoid over- or under-sedation?*

A *Standard numerical rating pain scale (i.e., pain level 0 to 10).*

B *Wong-Baker FACES pain scale.*

C *Richmond Agitation-Sedation Scale (RASS) score.*

D *Monitoring vital signs alone and determining when the patient is in pain.*

E *Maintaining a continuous opioid infusion until the patient is no longer requiring mechanical ventilation.*

This patient sustained a severe traumatic brain injury. While recovering, these patients are often unable to convey their level of pain or anxiety with speech or purposeful movement. The Richmond Agitation-Sedation Scale (RASS) and other validated forms of assessing a patient's level of consciousness can aid in treatment of pain and anxiety in the critical care setting, especially in ventilated or non-verbal patients. Table 13.2 below outlines the scoring system of the RASS score. Standard numerical rating pain scales or visual analog pain scales such as the Wong-Baker FACES scale may not be feasible in ventilated or brain-injured patients. Even though monitoring objective data such as vital signs is important in evaluating a patient's level of pain and consciousness, it is not

Table 13.2 The Richmond Agitation-Sedation Scale (RASS).

Score	Term	Description
+4	Combative	Overtly combative, violent, immediate danger to staff
+3	Very agitated	Pulls or removes tubes or catheters, aggressive
+2	Agitated	Frequent non-purposeful movement, fights ventilator
+1	Restless	Anxious but movements not aggressive or vigorous
0	Alert and calm	Spontaneously pays attention to caregiver
−1	Drowsy	Not fully alert but has sustained (>10 s) awakening (eye contact) to voice
−2	Light sedation	Briefly (<10 s) awakens with eye contact to voice
−3	Moderate sedation	Any movement or eye opening to voice without eye contact
−4	Deep sedation	Any movement or eye opening to physical stimulation but not to voice
−5	Unarousable	No response to voice or physical stimulation

a reliable way of accurately assessing the brain injured patient. Monitoring vital signs alone may lead to under- or over-treating of pain and anxiety. Maintaining a continuous opioid infusion is not appropriate in this scenario and can potentially hinder weaning from mechanical ventilation.

Answer: C

Ely EW, Truman B, Shintani A, et al. Monitoring sedation status over time in ICU patients: reliability and validity of the Richmond Agitation-Sedation Scale (RASS). *JAMA* 2003;289(22):2983–2991.

Corrigan JD, Selassie AW, Orman JA. The epidemiology of traumatic brain injury. *J. Head Trauma Rehabil.* 2010;25(2):72–80.

Nakase-Thompson R, Sherer M, Yablon SA, et al. Acute confusion following traumatic brain injury. *Brain Inj.* 2004;18(2):131–142.

Trivedi V and Iyer VN. Utility of the Richmond Agitation-Sedation Scale in evaluation of acute neurologic dysfunction in the intensive care unit. *J Thoracic Disease.* 2016;8(5):E292–E294.

Robinson D, Thompson S, Bauerschmidt A, et al. Dispersion in Scores on the Richmond agitation and sedation scale as a measure of delirium in patients with subdural hematomas. *Neurocrit. Care.* 2019;30(3):626–634.

6   *A 55-year-old man with type 2 diabetes mellitus and chronic alcoholism presents to the emergency department in septic shock from a necrotizing soft tissue infection of the thigh and perineum. Treatment for his septic shock includes a 30 mL/kg intravenous fluid bolus, initiation of broad-spectrum antibiotics, and vasopressor administration. He is taken emergently to the operating room for debridement of the necrotic tissue. Over the next three days, he remains on the ventilator while returning to the operating room for multiple debridements. His septic shock resolves and an attempt is made to wean him from mechanical ventilation. Despite being awake, calm, and participatory, the patient fails multiple spontaneous breathing trials due to inadequate minute ventilation. Which of the following studies is most likely to reveal the etiology of his ventilator dependence?*

   A *Serum electrolytes*
   B *CT angiogram pulmonary embolism protocol*
   C *Diaphragm fluoroscopy ("Sniff Test")*
   D *Electrocardiogram and troponin level*
   E *MRI of the brain*

Hypophosphatemia is common in the ICU and is associated with failure to wean from mechanical ventilation. This effect is thought to be due to inadequate production of ATP and other phosphorylated intermediates which may decrease diaphragm contractility as well as inadequate 2,3-diphosphogycerate production causing a leftward shift of the oxygen–hemoglobin dissociation curve. One prospective cohort study showed an 18% greater risk of failure to wean from the ventilator if the serum phosphorus was < 1.05 mmol/L. Malnourished patients such as chronic alcoholics frequently present with low serum phosphorus levels. This patient has no evidence of a pulmonary embolism or myocardial infarction. While a fluoroscopic sniff test may show impaired diaphragm contractility, it is not going to give an explanation to the cause of failure to wean. An MRI of the brain is unlikely to aid in diagnosis of an awake patient who is unable to be liberated from the ventilator.

Answer: A

Amanzadeh J and Reilly RF Jr. Hypophosphatemia: an evidence-based approach to its clinical consequences and management. *Nat. Clin. Pract. Nephrol.* 2006;2:136–148

Alsumrain MH, Jawad SA, Imran NB, et al. Association of hypophosphatemia with failure-to-wean from mechanical ventilation. *Ann. Clin. Lab. Sci.* 2010;40(2):144–148

7 *A 23-year-old woman presents to the emergency department following a motor vehicle collision with unknown loss of consciousness. The patient's airway is intact; she has bilateral breath sounds and intact distal pulses. Physical exam reveals a forehead hematoma, cervical and abdominal seatbelt signs, a right wrist deformity, and left chest wall bruising. Pupils are dilated, speech is accelerated, and the patient repeatedly tries to sit up on the stretcher or roll over on her side. Her behavior is not aggressive toward hospital staff. Vital signs show heart rate 108 beats/minute, blood pressure 165/85 mm Hg, respiratory rate 18 breaths/minute, and oxygen saturation is 100% on room air. Chest and pelvis x-rays show no abnormalities. Urinary drug screen is positive for cocaine and methamphetamine. You suspect multiple potential sites of injury and would like to obtain CT scans, but the patient is uncooperative and refuses to lie still. What is the first-line treatment for this behavior?*

A *Naloxone*

B *Flumazenil*

C *Endotracheal intubation*

D *Midazolam*

E *Fentanyl*

This patient presents with a high-velocity blunt trauma mechanism in the setting of acute stimulant intoxication. Her primary survey is intact and secondary survey reveals multiple potential sites of hemorrhage (seatbelt sign, chest wall bruising, forehead hematoma). The patient's agitation and restlessness are preventing completion of the trauma workup to diagnose the extent of her injuries. Benzodiazepines such as midazolam or lorazepam are the first-line treatment of cocaine and methamphetamine intoxication and can be used to temporarily sedate the patient to complete the workup. Midazolam may be preferred due to its rapid onset, short time to peak effect, and short duration of effect. The addition of an antipsychotic, such as olanzapine or haloperidol, may be necessary in the setting of methamphetamine-induced psychosis. Naloxone and flumazenil are used to treat opioid and benzodiazepine overdose, respectively. Endotracheal intubation should not be used as the first-line treatment in this scenario. Although the patient may require analgesia with opioids such as fentanyl, the most appropriate treatment of her intoxication is with a benzodiazepine.

8 *The patient in the question above is diagnosed with a small subdural hematoma, multiple left rib fractures, a right radius and ulna fracture, and a grade 3 splenic laceration. She is admitted to the ICU for closer monitoring. Later that day, she develops a headache after*

her blood pressure increases to 205/112 mm Hg. All other vital signs remain within normal limits other than a heart rate of 110 beats/minute. An EKG shows sinus tachycardia and a stat CT of the head shows no change from the initial scan. Which of the following is the most appropriate next step in management?

A *Obtain a stat CT angiogram of the chest and abdomen*

B *Give 5 mg IV metoprolol*

C *Give 5 mg IV phentolamine*

D *Give 650 mg PO acetaminophen*

E *Consult cardiology for coronary angiography*

This patient has developed hypertensive urgency likely due to cocaine intoxication. The treatment of choice is IV phentolamine, an alpha-adrenergic antagonist. Beta-blockers such as metoprolol are contraindicated due to the lack of alpha-adrenergic blockade. This can result in unopposed alpha-adrenergic activity due to the cocaine which can acutely worsen hypertension and lead to stroke or myocardial infarction. This patient has no symptoms of an aortic or visceral dissection and thus a CT angiogram of the chest and abdomen is not beneficial. Similarly, although the patient is at risk of myocardial infarction, the EKG does not show a reason to proceed with coronary angiography at this time. The patient's headache is due to hypertensive urgency and therefore acetaminophen is unlikely to treat the symptoms.

Answer: D

Answer: C

Hadjizacharia P, Green DJ, Plurad D, et al. Methamphetamines in trauma: effect on injury patterns and outcome. *J. Trauma* 2009;66(3):895–898.

McCord J, et al. Management of cocaine-associated chest pain and myocardial infarction. *Circulation* 2008;117:1897–1907.

Stankowski RV, Kloner RA, and Rezkalla SH. Cardiovascular consequences of cocaine use. *Trends Cardiovasc. Med.* 2015;25(6):517–526.

Wodarz N, Krampe-Scheidler A, Christ M, et al. Evidence-based guidelines for the pharmacological management of acute methamphetamine-related disorders and toxicity. *Pharmacopsychiatry* 2017;50(3): 87–95.

9 *An 80-year-old woman is admitted to the hospital after sustaining a displaced femoral neck fracture after a ground level fall. She undergoes hip arthroplasty 12 hours after admission. Her pain is initially managed with intravenous morphine but she is subsequently transitioned to oral nonopioid analgesics. On* *postoperative day 3, she becomes acutely agitated and confused, with intermittent periods of somnolence. Her vital signs are normal and there are no focal deficits on neurologic examination. Which of the following is the most likely diagnosis?*

A *Acute ischemic stroke*

B *Delirium*

C *Opioid withdrawal*

D *Pulmonary thromboembolism*

E *Opioid overdose*

This patient is mostly likely experiencing delirium. Delirium is characterized by an acute change in cognition or fluctuating level of consciousness, and is often associated with an underlying medical condition or drug intoxication. It can have a variable presentation and is therefore often underdiagnosed. Studies have shown that postoperative delirium affects over 50% of patients over the age of 65, and the risk is even higher among geriatric patients admitted to the Intensive Care Unit. An acute stroke would most likely present as focal neurologic deficits rather than a fluctuating level of consciousness. There is no evidence of a pulmonary embolism in this patient with normal respiratory function and vital signs. This patient had not received morphine long enough to develop opioid dependence and therefore is at low risk of withdrawal. Given that she has already been transitioned to nonopioid analgesia, opioid overdose is unlikely.

Answer: B

Amador LF and Goodwin JS. Postoperative Delirium in the older patient. *J. Am. Coll. Surg.* 2005;200(5): 767–773.

Devlin JW, Skrobik Y, Gélinas C, et al. Clinical practice guidelines for the prevention and management of pain, agitation/sedation, delirium, immobility, and sleep disruption in adult patients in the ICU. Crit. Care Med. 2018;46(9):e825–e873.

Marcantonio ER. Delirium in Hospitalized older adults. N. Engl. J. Med.. 2017 12;(15):1456–1466.

10 *A 72-year-old man with dementia, atrial fibrillation, hypertension, neurogenic bladder, and depression is brought to the emergency department from his nursing facility for worsening agitation and confusion. Review of his medication list reveals that he takes lisinopril, apixaban, seroquel, and oxybutynin. His vital signs, laboratory tests, and chest radiograph are normal and an electrocardiogram is consistent with rate-controlled atrial fibrillation.*

Which of the following is the most appropriate initial step in management?

A *Increase the frequency of seroquel*

B *Start donepezil*

C *Obtain a CT scan of the head*

D *Discontinue anticholinergic medications*

E *Initiate an infectious workup*

Anticholinergic medications, including various antihistamines, antidepressants, and bladder antimuscarinics, can have significant adverse cognitive effects in the elderly. Studies have found that anticholinergic medications are associated with an increased risk of dementia, and alternative treatments should be considered. While occult infection or stroke can contribute to confusion and delirium in elderly patients (and should be ruled out), anticholinergic medications are the most likely cause of this patient's confusion in the absence of any signs or symptoms of infection. Seroquel is an atypical antipsychotic frequently used for delirium. It can have anticholinergic effects at high doses and should not be increased in this patient. Donepezil is an acetylcholinesterase inhibitor used for the treatment of Alzheimer's dementia and is not an appropriate treatment for delirium.

Answer: D

Coupland CA, Hill T, Dening T, et al. Anticholinergic drug exposure and the risk of Dementia. *JAMA Intern. Med.* 2019;179(8):1084–1093.

Egberts A, Moreno-Gonzalez R, Alan H, et al. Anticholinergic drug burden and delirium: a systematic review. J. Am. Med. Dir. Assoc. 2020: 22(1): 65–73

Pun BT, Balas MC, Barnes-Daly MA, et al. Caring for critically ill patients with the ABCDEF bundle: results of the ICU Liberation Collaborative in over 15,000 adults. Crit. Care Med. 2019;47(1):3–14

11 *A 46-year-old man is brought to the emergency department after being found wandering around his neighborhood, confused and intoxicated. On arrival, he appears thin and disheveled, and he has an ataxic gait and nystagmus on exam. Laboratory tests reveal a serum sodium level of 128 mEq/L and blood alcohol level of 240 mg/dL. Which of the following is the most appropriate next step in management?*

A *Administer intravenous thiamine*

B *Start hypertonic saline*

C *Give oral naltrexone*

D *Obtain a CT scan of the head*

E *Give ativan 2 mg IV*

This patient has clinical features of thiamine deficiency and should be given intravenous thiamine replacement. Thiamine deficiency is often seen among individuals with alcoholism and can manifest as Wernicke encephalopathy. The etiology is multifactorial and includes poor nutrition and reduced activity of thiamine-metabolizing enzymes in the brain. It can progress to irreversible neurologic and cognitive changes if not recognized early on. A CT of the head should be obtained at some point, but should not delay administration of thiamine. Hyponatremia is common among chronic alcoholic patients. Possible etiologies include beer potomania, cirrhosis, syndrome of inappropriate antidiuretic hormone (SIADH), hypovolemia or pseudo-hyponatremia from dyslipidemia. Symptoms typically occur at sodium levels below 120 mEq/L and it can often be corrected with free water restriction. Naltrexone is an opioid antagonist that blocks opioid receptors. It can reduce alcohol cravings and treat alcohol and opioid dependence, but would not be indicated for thiamine deficiency. Ativan would treat symptoms of alcohol withdrawal which this patient does not have.

Answer: A

Attaluri P, Castillo A, Edriss H, et al. Thiamine deficiency: an important consideration in critically ill patients. Am. J. Med. Sci. 2018;356(4):382–390.

12 *A 65-year-old woman with known alcohol use disorder and cirrhosis presents to the trauma bay after a motor vehicle collision. Her injury complex includes a thoracic wedge compression fracture, right intertrochanteric femur fracture, and small subarachnoid hemorrhage. Blood alcohol level on admission is 220 mEq/L. She is admitted to the ICU for closer monitoring and on hospital day 2 undergoes femur fixation. The following day, she becomes acutely agitated, diaphoretic, and tachycardic with a heart rate of 135 beats/minute. Her alcohol withdrawal score is 11. What is the next best step in management?*
   A *Initiate a beta-blocker for tachycardia*
   B *Start scheduled ativan 2 mg every 1 hour*
   C *Start chlordiazepoxide 50 mg PO*
   D *Start thiamine and ativan 2 mg IV every hour as needed for symptoms*
   E *Intubate and start heparin drip for suspected pulmonary embolus*

This patient is exhibiting signs and symptoms of alcohol withdrawal. Benzodiazepines are considered the first-line treatment for alcohol withdrawal. Data show that dosing based on objectively measured withdrawal symptoms, rather than fixed dose regimens, leads to lower total benzodiazepine dose and shorter duration of treatment. The most commonly used scale for measuring withdrawal and determining the need for therapy is the revised Clinical Institute Withdrawal Assessment for Alcohol (CIWA-Ar) scale. While chlordiazepoxide (Librium) has a longer half-life and low risk of dependence, a shorter acting benzodiazepine is preferred in the setting of known liver disease. A beta-blocker is not indicated as this patient's symptoms are most likely due to alcohol withdrawal. The patient is not hypoxic and the timing of onset and history is more consistent with alcohol withdrawal rather than a pulmonary embolism.

Answer: D

Daeppen JB, Gache P, Landry U, et al. Symptom-triggered vs fixed-schedule doses of benzodiazepine for alcohol withdrawal: a randomized treatment trial. *Arch. Intern. Med.* 2002;162(10):1117–1121.

Dixit D, Endicott J, Burry L, et al. Management of acute alcohol withdrawal syndrome in critically ill patients. Pharmacotherapy 2016;36(7):797–822.

Ibarra F. Single-dose phenobarbital in addition to symptom-triggered lorazepam in alcohol withdrawal. Am. J. Emerg. Med. 2020;38(2):178–181.

Sen S, Grgurich P, Tulolo A, et al. A symptom-triggered benzodiazepine protocol utilizing SAS and CIWA-Ar scoring for the treatment of alcohol withdrawal syndrome in the critically ill. *Ann. Pharmacother.* 2017;51(2):101–110.

13 *A 30-year-old man presents to the trauma bay after being struck by a car while attempting to cross a major intersection. He arrives confused and agitated. Laboratory results are notable for a blood alcohol level of 0.01% and a urine drug screen is positive for amphetamines and benzodiazepines. Imaging reveals multiple spine and pelvic fractures, a moderate pelvic hematoma without active extravasation, and a grade III splenic laceration. Shortly after admission to the ICU, he develops worsening agitation and claims that his nurse is trying to kill him. He begins speaking to people when no one is in his room and refuses to let anyone examine or approach him. Which of the following is the most likely explanation for his behavior?*
   A *An increase in brain dopamine activity*
   B *Blockage of the brain's dopamine receptor sites, thereby reducing dopamine activity*
   C *Decreased levels of norepinephrine*
   D *Increased cortisol levels*
   E *Benzodiazepine withdrawal*

This patient is exhibiting signs and symptoms of amphetamine psychosis, a syndrome in which high doses of amphetamines taken for prolonged periods of time result in symptoms of acute psychosis. Symptoms include severe agitation, paranoid and persecutory delusions, and hallucinations, and can be difficult to distinguish from a primary psychiatric disorder such as schizophrenia. More often, psychotic symptoms are subclinical and do not require intervention. The pathophysiology of amphetamine psychosis involves an increase in brain dopamine activity. Amphetamines act directly on the mesolimbic dopaminergic "reward system" by inducing release of dopamine, and to some extent norepinephrine, in the synaptic clefts. They also inhibit dopamine reuptake. Stress or trauma can induce an increase in circulating cortisol but this would not present with acute psychosis. Benzodiazepine withdrawal would more likely be characterized by irritability, anxiety, and tremors rather than acute psychosis.

14 *For the scenario above, which of the following is the next best step in management?*
  A *Initiate electroconvulsive therapy*
  B *Behavioral therapy*
  C *Start olanzapine*
  D *Initiate dexmedetomidine drip*
  E *Start disulfiram*

Treatment consists of supportive care during the acute intoxication phase, including hydration and managing blood pressure and heart rate until the drug is sufficiently metabolized. Antipsychotics help to reduce the symptoms of psychosis and control agitation. One study of 6 randomized controlled trials showed that aripiprazole, haloperidol, quetiapine, olanzapine, and risperidone were equally efficacious at treating the psychotic episodes. When psychosis persists after repeated use of stimulants, electroconvulsive therapy may be beneficial, but this would not be considered first-line treatment. While behavioral therapy would be helpful for preventing a relapse, this would not help to treat the acute psychosis. Dexmedetomidine is a sympatholytic drug that acts as an agonist of α_2-adrenergic receptors in certain parts of the brain and is often used as a sedative, but has not been studied for the treatment of amphetamine withdrawal. Disulfiram has been used for the treatment of cocaine dependence, not stimulant psychosis.

Answer: A

Answer: C

Fluyau D, Mitra P, Lorthe K. Antipsychotics for amphetamine psychosis. a systematic review. Front. Psych. 2019;10:740.

Bramness JG and Rognli EB. Psychosis induced by amphetamines. Curr. Opin. Psych. 2016;29(4): 236–241.

14

Acid-Base, Fluids, and Electrolytes

Joshua Dilday, DO[1], Catherine Cameron, MD[2], and Christopher Bell, MD[3]

[1] Department of Acute Care Surgery, University of Southern California, LAC + USC Medical Center, Los Angeles, CA, USA
[2] Landstuhl Regional Medical Center, Landstuhl, Germany
[3] William Beaumont Army Medical Center, El Paso, TX, USA

1 *A 73-year-old man with an extensive abdominal surgical history and multiple previous small bowel obstructions presents with several days of colicky abdominal pain. He cannot keep any food or water down and is vomiting multiple times over the past four days. Which is most likely this scenario?*

   A *Metabolic acidosis, hypokalemia, hyperchloremia, acidic urine*
   B *Respiratory alkalosis, hypokalemia, hyperchloremia, acidic urine*
   C *Metabolic alkalosis, hypokalemia, hypochloremia, acidic urine*
   D *Metabolic alkalosis, hypokalemia, hyperchloremia, alkaline urine*
   E *Metabolic acidosis, hypokalemia, hypochloremia, acidic urine*
   F *Respiratory acidosis, hypokalemia, hyperchloremia, alkaline urine*

The above patient is presenting with another small bowel obstruction. If the vomiting from a small bowel obstruction is significant, it can lead to acid/base and electrolyte abnormalities. The main problem is the severe dehydration. Proximal GI losses can cause a contraction metabolic alkalosis. Sodium is the key element as it tries to maintain intravascular volume through retention of water. During volume contraction, bicarbonate and sodium are reabsorbed to maintain volume and electrical balance as there is insufficient chloride. The body does all it can to hold on to the sodium and the distal convoluted tubules will compensate sodium reabsorption by excreting potassium, leading to hypokalemia. This continues until the potassium concentration is below tolerable levels at which point it starts to excrete hydrogen. The reabsorption of bicarbonate causes a loss of chloride and thus the hypochloremia. In this setting, the person is alkalotic but because they are urinating hydrogen ions despite being alkalotic, the kidneys are causing a "paradoxical aciduria". The chloride is also lost from GI losses. The first and foremost important treatment is the replenishment of water with any crystalloid solution. Answer A is incorrect as it is not metabolic acidosis nor hyperchloremia. B is incorrect because it is not hyperchloremic. Answer D is incorrect because it is not hyperchloremia as explained. Answers E and F are wrong due to previous explanations.

Answer: C

Khanna, A., & Kurtzman, N. A. (2001). Metabolic alkalosis. *Respiratory Care, 46*(4), 354–365.
Galla, J. H. (2000). Metabolic alkalosis. *Journal of the American Society of Nephrology, 11*(2), 369–375.
Luke, R. G., & Galla, J. H. (2012). It is chloride depletion alkalosis, not contraction alkalosis. *Journal of the American Society of Nephrology, 23*(2), 204–207.

2 *A 45-year-old woman is postoperative day 4 after a small bowel resection for adenocarcinoma. On examination, she has mild edema in her lower extremities. Her chest x-ray shows mild pulmonary congestive and an enlarged cardiac silhouette. She has been receiving D5 1/2 Normal Saline at 150 mL/hr. Her serum sodium level is 131 mEq/L and her urine output is 50–60 ml/hr. She has jugular venous distention and edema. The patient states that she takes diuretics at home on occasion when she develops edema in her legs. How would you treat her serum sodium?*

A *Increase IV fluids to 200 ml/hr*
B *Decrease IV fluids to 75 ml/hr*
C *Treat with thiazide diuretics*
D *Change her IV fluids to 3% hypertonic saline at 150 cc per hour*
E *Treat with loop diuretics, ACE inhibitors, and beta-blockers*

When addressing the disorder of hyponatremia, it is important to first classify the disorder based on volume status of hypovolemia, euvolemia, and hypervolemia. In general, hyponatremia is treated with fluid restriction in the setting of euvolemia, isotonic saline in the setting of hypovolemia, and diuresis in the setting of hypervolemia. Sometimes, a combination of these therapies may be needed based on the presentation. If the patient is hypovolemic from bowel obstruction, the therapy usually consists of isotonic or hypertonic saline. Euvolemic hyponatremia such as an SIADH is usually treated with fluid restriction and loop diuretics. Hypervolemic hyponatremia such as in patients with heart failure are treated with diuretics, angiotensin converting enzyme (ACE) inhibitors, and beta-blockers. With the addition of ACE inhibitors, congestive heart failure is treated and vasopressin secretion is reduced. One liter of normal saline will increase plasma sodium concentration by 1 mEq/L. Thus, treating hyponatremia in edematous patients with saline will only exacerbate the problem. The patient in this case is overloaded with fluids and thus choice A is incorrect. Decreasing IV fluids to 75 cc to restrict fluids may be helpful but restricting fluids is a better option and that is why choice B is incorrect. Choice C is incorrect because thiazide diuretics are contraindicated since it blocks reabsorption of sodium and chloride in the distal tubules and thus prevents the generation of maximally dilute urine. 3% hypertonic saline would in this case worsen the salt load and the hypervolemia. In a hypovolemic state, this may be a treatment option. If the patient is in a state of hypovolemia and hyponatremia and is symptomatic, a bolus of 100–150 mL of 3% hypertonic saline may be useful.

Answer: E

Adrogue, H. J., & Madias, N. E. (2000). Hyponatremia. *New England Journal of Medicine, 342*, 1581.

Braun, M. M., Barstow, C. H., & Pyzocha, N. J. (2015). Diagnosis and management of sodium disorders: hyponatremia and hypernatremia. *American Family Physician, 91*(5), 299–307.

Konstam, M. A., Kiernan, M. S., Bernstein, D., et al. (2018). Evaluation and management of right-sided heart failure: a scientific statement from the American Heart Association. *Circulation, 137*(20), e578–622.

3 *A 22-year-old man is admitted to the ICU after a motorcycle accident causing an ankle fracture, a mesenteric hematoma, and a splenic laceration. The patient received multiple saline boluses to maintain normal blood pressure. Despite multiple saline boluses, the patient remains hypotensive. On the way to the OR, massive transfusion protocol is initiated but the blood gas shows: pH 7.21, pCO2 32, pO2 70mm Hg, HCO3 16 mEq/L. Which of the following best describes his acid-base status?*
A *Primary metabolic alkalosis with respiratory compensation.*
B *Primary metabolic acidosis with combined respiratory alkalosis.*
C *Primary metabolic acidosis with respiratory compensation.*
D *Primary metabolic acidosis with combined respiratory acidosis.*
E *Primary respiratory alkalosis with metabolic compensation.*

The patient has a metabolic acidosis likely from lactic acidosis in addition to hyperchloremic acidosis due to multiple saline boluses in an attempt to control his hypotension. Excessive saline infusion can cause a hyperchloremic non-gap metabolic acidosis. The diagnosis of primary metabolic acidosis is made by the low pH and low plasma HCO_3. Once the determination of metabolic acidosis is made, it should be determined if a gap acidosis is present. However, since no electrolytes were given to determine a gap, the next determination should be appropriate respiratory compensation. This can be done utilizing Winters' formula [$pCO_2 = (1.5 \times HCO_3) + 8 \pm 2$]. The formula predicts the expected pCO_2 in a primary metabolic acidosis. If the measured pCO_2 is greater than expected, a superimposed respiratory acidosis is present. If the measured pCO_2 is less than expected, a combined respiratory alkalosis is present. In the case above, the expected $pCO_2 = (1.5 \times 18) + 8 \pm 2 = 35 \pm 2$. The measured pCO_2 in the above patient (34) is an expected respiratory compensation for primary metabolic acidosis. As a general rule of thumb, a change in the PCO2 by 10 results in a change in the pH by 0.08. For example, if the PCO2 was 30, the pH would be expected to be at 7.48. If the PCO2 was to be 50, then the pH would be 7.32. Thus, in the patient above, the respiratory compensation was not enough to normalized pH. Although many are biased against hyperchloremic metabolic acidosis caused by saline infusions, the numerous randomized clinical studies using hypertonic saline has not shown any clinically relevant complications from the iatrogenically caused hyperchloremic metabolic acidosis. Answers A and E are wrong because the patient is not alkalotic. Answer D is incorrect because the patient does not have respiratory acidosis. Answer B is incorrect as the patient is not alkalotic.

Answer: C

Bulger, E. M., May, S., Kerby, J. D., et al. (2011). Out-of-hospital hypertonic resuscitation after traumatic hypovolemic shock: a randomized, placebo controlled trial. *Annals of Surgery*, 253(3), 431–441.

Kellum, J. A. (2007). Disorders of acid-base balance. *Critical Care Medicine*, 35(11), 2630–2636

Winter, S. D., Pearson, J. R., Gabow, P. A., et al. (1990). The fall of the serum anion gap. *Archives of Internal Medicine*, 150(2), 311–313.

4   *A 75-year-old man with uncontrolled COPD from a 50 pack-year history of smoking is admitted to the ICU after a traumatic hip fracture. An admission ABG reveals pH 7.33; PaCO2 55 mmHg; PaO2 80 mmHg; HCO3 32 mEq/L.*

Which of the following is true regarding the acid-base status?

  A *Primary respiratory acidosis with metabolic acidosis.*

  B *Primary respiratory acidosis with metabolic compensation.*

  C *Primary metabolic acidosis with respiratory acidosis.*

  D *Primary respiratory acidosis without metabolic compensation.*

  E *Primary metabolic acidosis with respiratory compensation.*

The above patient has a respiratory acidosis as evidenced by his decrease in pH and increase in $PaCO_2$. Given the information that he has suboptimal COPD control, it can be assumed that he likely has a chronic respiratory acidosis. The adequate metabolic compensation in a chronic respiratory acidosis can be determined by the following equation:

$$HCO_3 = 24 + [0.4 \times (PaCO_2 - 40)]$$
$$HCO_3 = 24 + [0.4 \times (55 - 40)]$$
$$HCO_3 = 24 + [0.4 \times (15)]$$
$$HCO_3 = 24 + [6]$$
$$HCO_3 = 30$$

Thus, the expected bicarbonate level is within the correct range for compensation. If the patient were to have a combined metabolic acidosis, the bicarbonate would be lower than expected. As a general rule, a change in the PCO2 by 10 results a change in the pH by 0.08. For example, if the PCO2 was 30, the pH would be expected to be at 7.48. If the PCO2 was to be 50, then the pH would be

7.32. The patient above has a PCO2 of 55 and a pure respiratory acidosis would result in pH of lower than 7.27. Since the pH is higher than expected, there is some metabolic compensation. Answers A, C, and E are incorrect as the patient does not have metabolic acidosis. Answer D in incorrect as the patient does have metabolic compensation with a higher than normal bicarbonate level.

Answer: B

Kellum, J. A. (2007). Disorders of acid-base balance. *Critical Care Medicine*, 35(11), 2630–2636.

Plant, P. K., Owen, J. L., & Elliott, M. W. (2000). One year period prevalence study of respiratory acidosis in acute exacerbations of COPD: implications for the provision of non-invasive ventilation and oxygen administration. *Thorax*, 55(7), 550–554.

Winter, S. D., Pearson, J. R., Gabow, P. A., et al. (1990). The fall of the serum anion gap. *Archives of Internal Medicine*, 150(2), 311–313.

5   *A 16-year-old woman is admitted to the ICU after ingesting an unknown substance. An admission ABG shows pH 7.25; Na 143 mEq/L, K 4.6 mEq/L, Cl 99 mEq/L, HCO3 21, PaCO2 39 mm Hg.*

Which of the following is true regarding the acid-base status?

  A *Non-anion gap metabolic acidosis*

  B *Anion gap metabolic acidosis*

  C *Combined metabolic acidosis and respiratory acidosis*

  D *Respiratory acidosis*

  E *Normal gap metabolic acidosis*

The above patient has an anion gap metabolic acidosis. The first step in management of acidemia is determining whether it is respiratory or metabolic in nature. Since the bicarbonate level is low and in the same direction as the pH, a metabolic acidosis is present. The next step is to determine if an anion gap (AG) is present. The AG can provide information as to whether the acidosis is due to increased acid accumulation or bicarbonate loss. This can be determined by the equation AG = Na – (Cl + HCO_3). Normal AG ranges are 3–12 mEq/L. The above patient has an AG of 23 mEq/L (143-(99+21)), thus causing a high anion gap metabolic acidosis. Common causes of this can be remembered by the mnemonic – MUDPILES: (Methanol, Uremia, Diabetic ketoacidosis, Paraldehyde, Isoniazid. Iron, Lactic acidosis, Ethylene glycol, and Salicylates). This patient most likely ingested ethylene glycol which is antifreeze and found in the garage. Hyperchloremic metabolic acidosis is usually normal AG acidosis. Low AG is typically associated with hypoalbuminemia. Albumin constitutes 80% of the unmeasured anions. Answers A and E are incorrect because the patient has AG acidosis. Answers C and D are incorrect as the patient does not have respiratory acidosis as the PaCO$_2$ is 39 mm Hg.

The utilization of Winter's formula, [expected pCO$_2$ = $(1.5 \times HCO_3) + 8 \pm 2$], determined that there is an appropriate respiratory response. Expected pCO$_2$ = 31.5 +8 = 39.5. Thus, the respiratory response is appropriate.

Answer: B

Kellum, J. A. (2007). Disorders of acid-base balance. *Critical Care Medicine*, 35(11), 2630–2636

Kraut, J. A., & Xing, S. X. (2011) Approach to the evaluation of a patient with an increased serum osmolal gap and high-anion-gap metabolic acidosis. *American Journal of Kidney Diseases*, 58(3), 480–484.

6 A 27-year old man presents with a gunshot wound to the right anterior thigh with significant blood loss. His heart rate is 110 per minute and his systolic blood pressure is 90 mmHg. Which of the following is true regarding blood transfusion?

   A *Worsening base deficit is associated with need for blood product transfusion and outcome.*
   B *Transfusion should only be given if the hemoglobin falls below 7 g/dL.*
   C *Blood products such as fresh frozen plasma should only be given if the patient has demonstrable coagulopathy.*
   D *Lactate is not a useful marker of resuscitation.*
   E *Base deficit is not a useful in the initial phase of treatment.*

The above patient is in hemorrhagic shock as he is hypotensive and his shock index is greater than 1. Shock index is calculated by dividing the heart rate by systolic blood pressure and if the heart rate is greater than the systolic blood pressure, it is highly associated with need for blood products. The patient will undoubtedly need blood product resuscitation as crystalloids in hypotensive patients should be avoided. The principles of damage control resuscitation include permissive hypotension until hemorrhage is controlled. Control of hemorrhage is a priority over resuscitation. Early empiric use of blood products in a 1:1:1 (packed red blood cells, plasma, platelets) ratio. The early and empiric use of plasma is for volume resuscitation with blood-like products in order to minimize crystalloids and colloids and not necessarily to treat coagulopathy. The avoidance of coagulopathy by minimizing crystalloids is the main objective rather than treating coagulopathy. Withholding blood products until laboratory values show anemia will result in a delay in

treatment as these derangements may not be evident in acute hemorrhage. Lactate and base deficit have both been evaluated as beneficial biomarkers for both shock and resuscitation. Worsening base deficit and increasing lactate have been shown to be a useful biomarker associated with severity of shock and the need for blood products during resuscitation (answers A and D). Initially, they can both be a useful guide for resuscitation. They are also associated with numerous outcome variables including mortality.

Answer: A

Ibrahim, I., Chor, W. P., Chue, K. M., et al. (2018). Base deficit is superior to lactate in trauma. *The American Journal of Emergency Medicine*, 215(4), 682–685.

Hartman, M. (2016). Is arterial base deficit still a useful prognostic marker in trauma? A systematic review. *The American Journal of Emergency Medicine*, 34(3), 626–635.

Holcomb, J.B., Jenkins D., Rhee P., et al. (2007) Damage control resuscitation: directly addressing the early coagulopathy of trauma. *The Journal of Trauma*, 62(3), 307–310.

7 After recent chemotherapy of high-grade lymphoma, a 67-year-old man is admitted to the intensive care unit for signs and symptoms of tumor lysis syndrome. Which of the following would not likely be associated with this condition?

   A *Hypercalcemia*
   B *Hyperuricemia*
   C *Hyperphosphatemia*
   D *Elevated serum creatinine*
   E *Elevated LDH*

Tumor lysis syndrome (TLS) is a severe clinical condition that can affect both pediatric and adult patients with malignancy. TLS usually happens after initiation of chemotherapy and are more common in cases of lymphoma and leukemia. Burkitt's lymphoma, acute lymphocytic leukemia, and acute myeloid leukemia. The syndrome is characterized by massive release of intracellular ions such as potassium, phosphorus, and nucleic acids that have been metabolized into uric acid. The rapid accumulation of uric acid causes an obstructive uropathy. Answers B, C, D, and E are incorrect as these are all expected to be present in TLS. The hyperphosphatemia chelates the serum calcium, causing hypocalcemia (Answer A). In addition, calcium is found in the skeleton. Intracellular calcium is 100 000 times less than extracellular calcium. Lysis of cancer cells would not release calcium into the circulation.

Answer: A

Coiffier, B., Altman, A., Pui, C. H., et al. (2008). Guidelines for the management of pediatric and adult tumor lysis syndrome: an evidence-based review. *Journal of Clinical Oncology, 26*(16), 2767–2778.

Davidson, M. B., Thakkar, S., Hix, J. K., et al. (2004). Pathophysiology, clinical consequences, and treatment of tumor lysis syndrome. *The American Journal of Medicine, 116*(8), 546–554.

8 *A 43-year-old man is admitted to the ICU after exploratory laparotomy with splenectomy and repair of liver laceration. The patient also has multiple rib fractures with hemothorax, pelvic fracture, and multiple long bone fractures as well. He has on a pelvic binder and chest tubes. He received massive transfusions in the trauma bay and operating room. Which electrolyte abnormality and associated EKG finding would you expect this patient to have?*
   A *Hypokalemia – prolonged QT*
   B *Hypocalcemia – shortened QT*
   C *Hypocalcemia – prolonged QT*
   D *Hypokalemia – shortened QT*
   E *Hypomagnesemia – shortened QT*

Packed red cells contain citrate which is used as an anticoagulant and citrate binds with calcium in the bloodstream. As a result, a large transfusion of PRBCs will result in hypocalcemia. Hypocalcemia is typically transient after a transfusion because citrate undergoes rapid hepatic metabolism. The healthy adult liver metabolizes 3 g of citrate per 1 unit of blood administered every 5 minutes. Transfusions, however, may result in a large influx of citrate along with possible hypothermia and hypoperfusion of the liver which adds to the hypocalcemia. Massive transfusion usually results in hyperkalemia due to lysis of erythrocytes and not hypocalcemia (answers A and D). The added soft tissue trauma would most likely result in hyperkalemia rather than hypokalemia. Patient receiving massive transfusions will have citrate toxicity resulting in hypocalcemia which can shorten the myocardial action potential manifesting as prolonged QT on EKG along with tetany, decreased myocardial contraction, refractory hypotension, or arrhythmia. Hypercalcemia shortens the myocardial action potential resulting in a shortened QT interval. Hypokalemia will result in flattened T waves, prominent U waves, and prolonged QT. Answer B is incorrect because the patient will have prolonged QT interval and not shortened QT interval. Answer E is incorrect because while this may occur, it is not a consistent finding.

Answer: C

Byerly, S., Inaba, K., Biswas, S., et al. and Demetrios Demetriades (2020). Transfusion-related hypocalcemia after trauma. *World Journal of Surgery, 30*, 1–8.

Giancarelli, A., Birrer, K. L., Alban, R. F, et al. (2016). Hypocalcemia in trauma patients receiving massive transfusion. *The Journal of Surgical Research, 202*(1), 182–187.

RuDusky, B. (2001). ECG abnormalities associated with hypocalcemia. *Chest, 119*(2), 668–669.

9 *A 54-year-old woman with a history of alcohol abuse is admitted with severe acute pancreatitis. After 3 days in the hospital, the patient begins to complain of perioral numbness and muscle spasms. What is the next best step in treating this patient?*
   A *Replacing sodium by increasing IV fluids*
   B *Replacing calcium and IV infusion of Normal Saline*
   C *Replacing potassium and magnesium*
   D *Replacing calcium and magnesium*
   E *Replacing potassium and infusing Plama-Lyte A*

Acute severe pancreatitis can cause hypocalcemia as it precipitates calcium soaps in the abdominal cavity but glucagon-stimulated calcitonin release and decreased parathyroid hormone may play a role. It is used as one of the Ranson criteria for assessing severity of pancreatitis. Alcohol abuse can cause hypomagnesemia. Hypocalcemia can present as perioral numbness and tingling, carpopedal spasms, tetany, seizures, hypotension, and ventricular ectopy. Acute pancreatitis can also cause hypomagnesemia. The mechanism is thought to be due to the saponification of magnesium in necrotic fat, similar to that of hypocalcemia. Hypomagnesemia can also promote hypocalcemia by inhibiting parathyroid hormone secretion and reducing end-organ responsiveness. Hypocalcemia in the setting of hypomagnesemia is refractory to replacement of calcium alone, thus both calcium and magnesium need to be replaced.

Answer: D

Ahmed, A., Azim, A., Gurja, M., et al. (2016). Hypocalcemia in acute pancreatitis revisited. *Indian Journal of Critical Care Medicine, 20*(3), 173–177.

Cameron, J. L., & Cameron, A. (2017). *Current Surgical Therapy*. Mosby Elsevier.

10 *A 61-year-old man is admitted with nausea and vomiting. He has had a 25 lb weight loss over the last few months and is found to have an obstructing*

sigmoid colon mass and undergoes sigmoidectomy. Postoperatively he is started on TPN due to postoperative ileus. Four days later, he develops paresthesia, weakness, and thrombocytopenia. Which of the following electrolyte abnormalities would you expect in this patient?

A *Hypomagnesemia, hypokalemia, hypophosphatemia*
B *Hypocalcemia, hypomagnesemia, hyperkalemia*
C *Hypomagnesemia, hypokalemia, hypocalcemia*
D *Hypermagnesemia, hypophosphatemia, hypokalemia*
E *Hypomagnesemia, hypokalemia, hyperphosphatemia*

This patient has refeeding syndrome which results in hypomagnesemia, hypokalemia, and hypophosphatemia. Refeeding syndrome occurs in malnourished patients or patients undergoing high metabolic stress. Starvation results in catabolism of fat and muscle tissue. When refeeding is started, there is a shift from fat metabolism to carbohydrate metabolism causing an increased glucose load which in turn causes increased insulin release and decreased secretion of glucagon. Insulin stimulates glycogen, fat, and protein synthesis. This process requires minerals such as phosphate and magnesium and cofactors such as thiamine. Insulin stimulates the absorption of potassium into the cells through the sodium-potassium ATPase symporter, which also transports glucose into the cells. Magnesium and phosphate are also taken up into the cells. Water follows by osmosis. These processes result in a decrease in the serum levels of phosphate, potassium, and magnesium, all of which are already depleted. The clinical features of the refeeding syndrome occur as a result of the functional deficits of these electrolytes and the rapid change in basal metabolic rate. Answers D and E are wrong as it does not result in high levels of these elements. Answers B and C are incorrect because it does not cause hypocalcemia.

Answer: A

Mehana, H. M., Moledina, J., & Travis, J. (2008). Refeeding syndrome: what it is, and how to prevent and treat it. *BMJ*, 338(7659), 1495–1498

Silva, J. S., Seres, D. S., Sabino, K., et al. (2020). ASPEN consensus recommendations for refeeding syndrome. *Nutrition in Clinical Practice*, 35(2), 178–195

11   A 62-year-old veteran with a history of kidney stones presents to the emergency department with fatigue, confusion, and nausea. Work up reveals a calcium level of 13 mg/dL. What is the best initial management?

A *Administration of calcitonin*
B *Administration of zoledronate*
C *Administration of hydrocortisone*
D *Administration of plicamycin*
E *Hydration with normal saline*

This patient has acute hypercalcemia. Symptoms of hypercalcemia include nausea, constipation, ileus, nephrocalcinosis, polyuria, confusion, and depressed levels of consciousness. The signs and symptoms of hypercalcemia can be remembered by the phrase "moans, stones, groans, and bones." Initial treatment is hydration with normal saline and loop diuretics which is the fastest and most effective way to lower calcium levels. Hypercalcemia is usually accompanied by hypercalciuria which causes diuresis and eventually leads to hypovolemia. Correction of the hypovolemia promotes calcium excretion. Calcitonin, zoledronate, plicamycin, and hydrocortisone can all help decrease levels of calcium; however, they are not fast acting and do not help with acute correction; thus, hydration with normal saline and use of loop diuretics should be initiated first. The other answers are incorrect as the therapies take longer.

Answer: E

Ganesan, C., Weia, B., Thomas, I., et al. (2020). Analysis of primary hyperparathyroidism screening among veterans with kidney stones. *JAMA Surgery*, 155(9), 861–868.

Naples, R., Shin J. J., Berber, E., et al. (2019). Recognition of primary hyperparathyroidism: delayed time course from hypercalcemia to surgery. *Surgery*, 167(2), 358–364.

12   A 36-year-old factory worker is admitted after a piece of machinery fell on his lower extremity pinning him for several hours. He begins having dark urine output and you notice peaked T waves on his EKG. What electrolyte abnormality are you concerned about and what is the best initial step?

A *Hypercalcemia – hydration with normal saline*
B *Hyperkalemia – calcium gluconate*
C *Hyperkalemia – kayexalate*
D *Hypophosphatemia – hydration with normal saline*
E *Hypermagnesemia – hydration with normal saline*

This patient is suffering from hyperkalemia secondary to a crush injury. Hyperkalemia can result from the reperfusion of ischemia tissue. Answers A and D are incorrect because hypocalcemia, hyperphosphatemia, and hypovolemia can also be seen with crush injuries. He has EKG changes with peaked T waves. The best initial step is stabilizing the cardiac membrane with calcium gluconate.

Answer C is incorrect because while kayexalate does correct hyperkalemia, it takes hours to work. Answer E is incorrect because hypermagnesemia can also be seen with a crush injury, but the best initial step in treatment is similar to hyperkalemia with stabilization of the cardiac membrane by giving calcium gluconate.

Answer: B

Abid, M., Neff, L. P., Russo, R. M., et al. (2020). Reperfusion repercussions: a review of the metabolic derangements following resuscitative endovascular balloon occlusion of the aorta. *Journal of Trauma and Acute Care Surgery,* 89(2S Suppl 2), S39–S44.

Ayach, T., Nappo, R. W., Paugh-Miller, J. L., et al. (2015). Postoperative hyperkalemia. *European Journal of Internal Medicine, 26*(2), 106–111.

Brown, C. V. R, Rhee, P., Chan, L., et al. (2004). Preventing renal failure in patients with rhabdomyolysis: do bicarbonate and mannitol make a difference? *The Journal of Trauma, 56*(6), 1191–1196.

Malinoski, D. J., Slater, M. S., & Mullins, R. J. (2004). Crush injury and rhabdomyolysis. *Critical Care Clinics, 20*(1), 171.

13 *A 20-year-old woman with known history of gallstone presents to the ED with polyuria, abdominal pain, nausea, vomiting, fatigue, confusion, and fruity scented breath. She is found to have Na of 128 mEq/L and glucose of 615 mg/dL. What is the best initial treatment of her hyponatremia?*

A *Infusion of normal saline*
B *Infusion of hypertonic saline*
C *Fluid restriction*
D *Oral NaCl tabs*
E *Insulin infusion*

Diabetic ketoacidosis (DKA) is a serious problem that can happen in people with diabetes if the body runs out of insulin. When this happens, harmful substances such as ketones can build up in the body which can be life-threatening. DKA can cause complications such as hypokalemia, cerebral edema, pulmonary edema, and damage to the kidneys. Hyperglycemia causes osmotic shifts of water from the intracellular to the extracellular space, causing a relative dilutional hyponatremia. DKA will profoundly dehydrate the patient. During this time, both hyperglycemia and hyperosmolality drive a fluid shift that leads to intracellular dehydration and loss of electrolytes. The two most significant electrolytes depleted are sodium and potassium. This patient has sodium levels that are falsely low due to hyperglycemia. The measured sodium is lowered by 1.6 mEq/L for every 100 mg/dL of glucose above 100 mg/dL. Thus, once corrected, this patient's sodium is 136, which is within normal limits. Thus, the patients should just be initially treated for their elevated glucose levels.

Answer: E

Braun, M. M., Barstow, C. H., & Pyzocha, N. J. (2015). Diagnosis and management of sodium disorders: hyponatremia and hypernatremia. *American Family Physician, 91*(5), 299–307.

Sterns, R. H. (2018). Treatment of severe hyponatremia. *Clinical Journal of the American Society of Nephrology, 13*(4), 641–649.

14 *After admission for traumatic subdural hematoma and diffuse axonal injury, a 27-year-old man is found to have hyponatremia of 132 mEq/L with increased urine output of 200 mL/hr 4 days after admission. Upon further work up, he is found to have decreased serum osmality (250 mOsm/kg) and increased urine osmolality (175 mOsm/kg). Urine Na is 55 mEq. Despite aggressive fluid resuscitation, he continues to have hypotension and decreased skin turgor. Which of the following is his most likely diagnosis?*

A *SIADH*
B *Diabetes insipidus*
C *Cerebral salt wasting*
D *Diabetes mellitus*
E *Nephrotic syndrome*

The patient listed in this question is suffering from ongoing sodium and water loss after a head injury. He has evidence of hypovolemia and hyponatremia. Based upon his increased urine Na and increased urine osmolality with combined hypovolemic hyponatremia, he is most likely suffering from cerebral salt wasting (CSW). Although similar to CSW, SIADH presents with a euvolemic hyponatremia. This patient is clearly hypovolemic; thus, answer A is incorrect. Diabetes insipidus (DI) can also present after head trauma. However, DI presents with free water loss and causes hypernatremia with decreased urine osmolality, making answer B incorrect. Diabetes mellitus is not associated with a hypovolemic hyponatremia, making answer D incorrect. Nephrotic syndrome causes a hypervolemic hyponatremia with decreased urine Na, making answer E incorrect.

Answer: C

Braun, M. M., Barstow, C. H., & Pyzocha, N. J. (2015). Diagnosis and management of sodium disorders: hyponatremia and hypernatremia. *American Family Physician, 91*(5), 299–307.

Singh, S., Bohn, D., Carlotti, A. P., et al. (2002). Cerebral salt wasting: truths, fallacies, theories, and challenges. *Critical Care Medicine, 30*(11), 2575–2579.

Sterns, R. H., & Silver, S. M. (2008). Cerebral salt wasting versus SIADH: what difference? *Journal of the American Society of Nephrology, 19*(2), 194–196.

15 *A 50-year-old man is given a large amount of sodium phosphate for his bowel prep for a screening colonoscopy. He has no significant past medical history. He has labs drawn in the preoperative holding area and is found to have a phosphorous level of 7 mg/dL. He also has contraction of his facial muscles when his facial nerve is tapped (Chvostek sign). Which associated electrolyte abnormality would you expect in this patient?*

A *Hypocalcemia*
B *Hypercalcemia*
C *Hyperkalemia*
D *Hypermagnesemia*
E *Hyponatremia*

One of the common causes of hyperphosphatemia is from an exogenous source such as phosphate-based laxatives. Sodium phosphate is widely used as a bowel cleansing preparation. Its use is, however, not without risk. It can induce serious adverse effects like hypocalcemia, hyperphosphatemia, and renal failure. Hyperphosphatemia causes hypocalcemia by precipitating calcium, decreasing vitamin D production, and interfering with PTH-mediated bone resorption. Most symptoms associated with hyperphosphatemia are actually associated with a decrease in serum calcium levels. In this case, a 75-year-old man without known contraindications developed hypocalcemic tetany, hyperphosphatemia, and renal failure after oral sodium phosphate.

Answer: A

Tan, H. L., Lieu, Q. Y., Loo, S., et al. (2002). Severe hyperphosphatemia and associated electrolytes and metabolic derangement following the administration of sodium phosphate for bowel preparation. *Aneasthesia, 57*(5), 478–483.

Vincent, J. L., Abraham, E., Kochanek, P., et al. (2016). *Textbook of Critical Care E-Book*. Elsevier Health Sciences.

16 *A 68-year-old man is brought into the trauma bay following a motor vehicle collision where his car caught fire. He has extensive full thickness burns over both lower extremities and lower abdomen and back. During his resuscitation, he begins to experience respiratory distress. Rapid sequence intubation is performed with etomidate and succinylcholine. Shortly after intubation, the patient goes into cardiac arrest. Which of the following is the most likely electrolyte abnormality to lead to the above situation?*

A *Hypercalcemia*
B *Hypomagnesemia*
C *Hypocalcemia*
D *Hyperkalemia*
E *Hypokalemia*

Succinylcholine is a short-acting, depolarizing neuromuscular blocking agent that inhibits Na-K exchange pump. This can cause a small increase in serum potassium. Most of the time, the rise is minimal and is not associated with adverse reactions. However, patients with thermal injury, denervation of muscle (seen in patients with spinal cord injury or prolonged paralytic use), and severe infection can have life-threatening elevation of potassium with succinylcholine use. Rapid tissue necrosis, destruction of red cells, metabolic acidosis, rhabdomyolysis, and renal failure can all cause hyperkalemia. EKG changes seen in hyperkalemia include peaked T waves and can eventually lead to a widened QRS complex, heart block, ventricular fibrillation, and finally asystole. The use of succinylcholine in patients with hyperkalemia can result in cardiac arrest. Serum potassium levels greater than 5.5 mEq/L is a contraindication to the use of succinylcholine.

Answer: D

Huggins, R. M, Kennedy, W. K., Michael J. et al. (2003). Cardiac arrest From succinylcholine-induced hyperkalemia. *American Journal of Health-System Pharmacy, 60*(7).

Jeevendra Martyn, J. A., & Richtsfeldt, M. (2006). Succinylcholine-induced hyperkalemia in acquired pathologic states. *Anesthesiology, 104*, 158–169.

17 *A 32-year-old man is brought to the ED for confusion and lethargy following completion of an ultra-marathon. The patient is found to have a sodium of 120 mEq/L. He is admitted and started on hypertonic saline. The following day his symptoms have improved and he is found to have a sodium level of 145 mEq/L. On hospital day #2, he becomes encephalopathic and then subsequently develops seizures. What is the most likely cause of his symptoms?*

A *Too slow correction of sodium*
B *Too rapid correction of sodium*
C *Dehydration*
D *Cerebral edema*
E *Elevated lactic acid*

This patient is experiencing osmotic demyelination syndrome from too rapid correction of sodium. The risk of seizures from cerebral edema occurs at a sodium level of 120 mEq/L. A rapid correction of 5 mEq/L has been shown to significantly decrease the cerebral edema. New guidelines state that sodium levels should not be increased by greater than 8-10 mEq/L in a 24 hour period to decrease the risk of developing osmotic demyelination syndrome. (American guidelines recommend correcting sodium levels by less than 8 mEq/L per day and European guidelines suggest correcting sodium levels by less than 10 mEq/L per day in the first 24 hours and then less than 8 mEq/L per day in the subsequent days.) Answer A is incorrect because a slow correction would not result in osmotic demyelination syndrome. Answer C is incorrect as there is no indication that hypovolemia is ongoing. Answer D is incorrect because this is seen when hyponatremia is not corrected. Answer is incorrect because elevated lactic acid is not associated with osmotic demyelination syndrome.

Answer: B

Braun, M. M., Barstow, C. H., & Pyzocha, N. J. (2015). Diagnosis and management of sodium disorders: hyponatremia and hypernatremia. *American Family Physician*, 91(5), 299–307.

George, J. C., et al. (2018). Risk factors and outcomes of rapid correction of severe hyponatremia. *Clinical Journal of the American Society of Nephrology*, 6(7), 984–992.

Leise, M. D., & Findlay, J. Y. (2017). Hyponatremia in the perioperative period: when and how to correct. *Clinical Liver Disease*, 9(5), 111.

Sterns, R. H. (2018). Treatment of severe hyponatremia. *Clinical Journal of the American Society of Nephrology*, 13(4), 641–649.

18 *Regarding the use of colloid versus crystalloid resuscitation in the ICU for aggressive resuscitation, which of the following is the most correct?*
    A *Colloids can cause allergic reactions*
    B *Colloids are safer than crystalloids*
    C *Colloids and crystalloids are the preferred method for acute resuscitation*
    D *Crystalloids are safer*
    E *Colloids have not shown an improvement in overall survival compared to crystalloids*

There is no evidence from randomized controlled trials that resuscitation with colloids reduces the risk of death compared to resuscitation with crystalloids. Colloids are also more expensive. Crystalloids, while similar to colloids in terms of mortality, are not similar in terms of outcome when compared to blood products in other ways. Neither crystalloids nor artificial colloids are recommended for acute massive resuscitation as large volume resuscitation is best done with products that resemble blood.

Answer: E

Finfer, S., Bellomo, R., Boyce, N., et al. (2004). A comparison of albumin and saline for fluid resuscitation in the intensive care unit. *The New England Journal of Medicine*, 350(22), 2247–2256.

Joseph, B., Zangbar, B., Pandit, V., et al. (2014). The conjoint effect of reduced crystalloid administration and decreased damage-control laparotomy use in the development of abdominal compartment syndrome. *Journal of Trauma and Acute Care Surgery*, 76(2), 457–461.

Lewis, S. R, Pritchard, M. W, Evans, D. J., et al. (2018). Colloids versus crystalloids for fluid resuscitation in critically ill people. *Cochrane Database of Systematic Reviews*, 8(8).

19 *Which of the following is true regarding crystalloid resuscitation?*
    A *0.9% saline can be infused with blood while Plasma-Lyte cannot*
    B *Lactated ringers can be used when transfusing blood*
    C *Plasma-Lyte has lower risk of metabolic acidosis*
    D *Plama-Lyte should not be used in ongoing acidosis*
    E *Plasma-Lyte has the same concentration of potassium as 0.9% saline*

Compared to normal saline and lactated Ringer's, Plasma-Lyte is relatively a newer fluid choice for surgeons. It is closer to physiologic pH due to its included buffers (acetate and gluconate) and physiologic chloride content. It has been studied in patients with pre-existing acidosis and shown to be beneficial. Saline and Plasma-Lyte can be infused with blood as they both lack calcium. Ringer's lactate has calcium and should be run through a separate line. Although it has been shown that blood can be infused when mixed with Ringer's lactate, most blood banks and hospital policies still forbid it. Plasma-Lyte has a higher concentration of potassium compared to both normal saline and lactated Ringer's. Recent literature has shown that infusion-related metabolic hyperchloremic acidosis is decreased when using Plasma-Lyte compared to normal saline. Numerous prospective randomized multicenter trials have shown that hypertonic saline causes hyperchloremic metabolic acidosis but the outcome variables have not been adversely affected.

ELECTROLYTES	LACTATED RINGER	NORMAL SALINE	PLASMA-LYTE
POSITIVE mEq	*137*	*154*	*148*
Sodium	130	154	140
Potassium	4		5
Calcium	3		
Magnesium			3
NEGATIVE	*137*	*154*	*148*
Chloride	109	154	98
Lactate	28		
Acetate			27
Gluconate			23

Answer: C

Bulger, E. M., May, S., Kerby, J. D., et al. (2011). Out-of-hospital hypertonic resuscitation after traumatic hypovolemic shock: a randomized, placebo controlled trial. *Annals of Surgery*, 253(3), 431–441.

Chua, H. R., Venkatesh, B., Stachowski, E., et al. (2012). Plasma-Lyte 148 vs 0.9% saline for fluid resuscitation in diabetic ketoacidosis. *Journal of Critical Care*, 27(2), 138–145.

Young, J. B., Utter, G. H., Schermer, C. R., et al.(2014). Saline versus Plasma-Lyte A in initial resuscitation of trauma patients: a randomized trial. *Annals of Surgery*, 259(2), 255–262.

20 *A 50-year old, 70 kg man in the ICU with traumatic brain injury has: Na 160 mEq/L, K 4.3 mEq/L, Cl 105 mEq/L, HCO3 25 mEq/L, BUN 30 mg/dL, Cr 1.2 mg/dL, Uosm is 160 mOsm/L. On hospital day 3, he is arousable but disoriented and complaining of thirst. On examination, he has clear lung sounds bilaterally, heart rate of 95 beats/min, and a blood pressure of 140/80 mm Hg. His urine output is 300 mL/hr for the past 12 hours. What best explains his hypernatremia?*

A *Lack of renal response to antidiuretic hormone*

B *Lack of anterior pituitary gland release of antidiuretic hormone*

C *Overstimulation and release of antidiuretic hormone*

D *Lack of posterior pituitary gland release of antidiuretic hormone*

E *Excess resuscitation with saline*

Central diabetes insipidus (DI) is a lack of the hormone vasopressin or antidiuretic hormone (ADH) released from the posterior pituitary gland. Causes include head trauma, encephalopathy, and meningitis. Damage to the pituitary gland or hypothalamus from head injury can cause central diabetes insipidus. Central diabetes insipidus causes excessive production of very dilute urine (polyuria). Central DI differs from nephrogenic DI in that nephrogenic DI is a lack of end-organ responsiveness while central DI is a lack of ADH release. Central diabetes insipidus is also sometimes called neurogenic diabetes insipidus. It is confused with nephrogenic diabetes insipidus at times. Central DI manifests as polyuria with dilute urine in setting of hypertonic plasma. Urine osmolarity is often < 200 mosm/L. Failure of the urine osmolarity to increase after fluid restriction is diagnostic confirmation. Treatment is aimed at replacing free water deficits and vasopressin, an ADH analogue.

Answer: D

Capatina, C., Paluzzi, A., Mitchell, R., et al. (2015). Diabetes insipidus after traumatic brain injury. *Journal of Clinical Medicine*, 4(7), 1448–1462. doi: 10.3390/jcm4071448.

Makaryus, A. N. & McFarlane, S. I. (2006). Diabetes insipidus: diagnosis and treatment of a complex disease. *Cleveland Clinic Journal of Medicine*, 73(1), 65–71.

Robertson, G. L. (2016). Diabetes insipidus: differential diagnosis and management. *Best Practice & Research Clinical Endocrinology & Metabolism*, 30(2), 205–218.

21 *In the above patient, what is the free water deficit?*
  A *4.5 L*
  B *3.5 L*
  C *6 L*
  D *2 L*
  E *3 L*

The above patient has central diabetes insipidus, leading to a hypernatremic state. The patient is unable to concentrate urine due to decreased ADH. Hypernatremia due to free water loss is managed by free water replacement. The free water deficit must first be calculated to determine the amount of replacement. Free water deficit formula = $0.6 \ (kg) \times (Current \ Na/140 - 1) \rightarrow 0.6 \ (70) \times (160/140 - 1) = 6 \ L$.

Answer: C

Adrogué, H. J. & Madias, N. E. (2000). Hyponatremia. *New England Journal of Medicine*, 342(21), 1581–1589.

Marino, P. L. & Sutin, K. M. (2014). *The ICU Book*, 4th edn, Lippincot Williams & Wilkins, Philadelphia, PA.

Pokaharel, M., & Block, C. A. (2011). Dysnatremia in the ICU. *Current Opinion in Critical Care*, 17(6), 581–593.

15

Metabolic Illness and Endocrinopathies
Andrew J. Young, MD[1] and Therese M. Duane, MD[2]

[1] *Department of Trauma, Critical Care and Burn, The Ohio State University, Columbus, OH, USA*
[2] *TCU & UNTHSC School of Medicine, Department of Surgery, Texas Health Resources, Fort Worth, TX, USA*

1 *A 54-year-old obese woman with a history of end-stage renal disease on dialysis, atrial fibrillation on warfarin, and diabetes mellitus is admitted to the surgical intensive care unit after debridement of necrotic tissue from her right leg caused by calci phy-laxis. Anesthesia signs out that there was difficulty coming off vasopressor support at the conclusion of the case. She is intubated and sedated. The dressings are clean and dry. You note other lesions on her left leg that appear necrotic. You have begun to reconcile her medications. Which medication should **not** be continued?*

   A *Vancomycin*
   B *Phenylephrine*
   C *Oxycodone*
   D *Filgrastim*
   E *Warfarin*

Calciphylaxis is a difficult disease to treat. It typically occurs in patients with chronic kidney disease. Patients typically die from sepsis due to the wounds caused by calciphylaxis. The etiology of this disease has yet to be elucidated, but there are known risk factors. Medications that can cause this disease include warfarin, calcium, vitamin D, iron, and recombinant PTH. Thus, these should be stopped once the diagnosis of calciphylaxis is made. Answer E is correct. The other medications have not been associated with increased risk of calciphylaxis.

Answer: E

McCarthy JT, el-Azhary RA, Patzelt MT, et al. Survival, risk factors, and effect of treatment in 101 patients with calciphylaxis. *Mayo Clinic Proceedings* 2016;91(10):1384–1394. doi:10.1016/j.mayocp. 2016.06.025

Nigwekar SU, Thadhani R, and Brandenburg VM. Calciphylaxis. *The New England Journal of Medicine* 2018;378(18):1704–1714. doi:10.1056/NEJMra 1505292

2 *A 22-year-old man is admitted to the intensive care unit following a motorcycle collision. He was not wearing a helmet and suffered several small intracranial hemorrhages. It has been difficult maintaining adequate cerebral perfusion pressure although he has not required vasopressors. He has been receiving intravenous fluid, as well as enteral nutrition. On post-trauma day 4, his sodium is noted to be 156 mEq/L, and his urine output has increased to 120 mL/hr overnight. What is the best course of action at this time?*

   A *Change parenteral fluids to 0.9% normal saline.*
   B *Change parenteral fluids to 5% dextrose in water.*
   C *Add free water to his nasogastric tube.*
   D *Begin levothyroxine 100 mcg/daily.*
   E *Replace urine output milliliter per milliliter every 4 hours to maintain euvolemia.*

This patient has diabetes insipidus (DI), which is a deficiency of antidiuretic hormone (ADH). There are two types of DI – central and nephrogenic. This patient most likely has central DI from his brain injury. Administration of exogenous ADH helps differentiate between the two types of DI. If the patient responds to the ADH (urine out decreases and becomes more concentrated), then it is central DI. If the patient does not respond to the exogenous ADH, then it is nephrogenic. Initial treatment consists of increasing free water to try and correct the hyperosmolarity. There may also be elevated serum potassium and calcium. Free water administration may also correct these abnormalities. Initial administration of free water should occur enterally if access is available, thus answer C is correct, otherwise the next best choice is answer B. Answer A is incorrect because this may worsen the hypernatremia. This patient does not have thyroid insufficiency, so answer d is incorrect. While this patient may become hypovolemic due to the high urine output, there is no current recommendation for a specific fluid replacement protocol (answer E).

Answer: C

Capatina C, Paluzzi A, Mitchell R, et al. Diabetes insipidus after traumatic brain injury. *Journal of Clinical Medicine* 2015;4(7):1448–1462. doi:10.3390/jcm4071448

3   *A 63-year-old woman is admitted to the surgical intensive care unit following a sigmoid resection and Hartmann's procedure for diverticulitis complicated by feculent peritonitis. She is on two vasopressors and has received adequate fluid resuscitation. Her mean arterial blood pressure readings have been consistently above 65 mmHg and is making adequate urine. Should steroids be started and if so which one?*

   A *Hydrocortisone intermittent dosing*
   B *Hydrocortisone continuous infusion*
   C *Solumedrol*
   D *Dexamethasone*
   E *No steroids*

There is still much debate regarding steroids in septic shock; however, the current surviving sepsis guidelines recommend against start corticosteroids. In a patient who is responsive to fluid resuscitation and vasopressors, steroids should not be empirically started.

Answer: E

Rhodes A, Evans LE, Alhazzani W, et al. Surviving sepsis campaign: international guidelines for management of sepsis and septic shock: 2016. *Intensive Care Medicine* 2017;43(3):304–77. doi:10.1007/s00134-017-4683-6

Venkatesh B, Finfer S, Cohen J, et al. Adjunctive glucocorticoid therapy in patients with septic shock. *The New England Journal of Medicine* 2018;378(9):797–808. doi:10.1056/NEJMoa1705835

4   *A 58-year-old man has been admitted to the intensive care unit following a motor vehicle collision in which he sustained multiple long bone fractures, a colonic injury which was resected and a Hartmann's procedure was performed, and several small intraparenchymal hemorrhages. He had no known medical problems prior to this accident per his family. He is currently intubated with an orogastric tube. You wish to begin enteral feeds. At the same time, you order regular blood glucose checks with associated sliding scale insulin. The negative effects of hyperglycemia in critical illness include which of the following?*

   A *Worse outcomes in patients with traumatic brain injury*
   B *Hypercoagulable state*
   C *Poor gut motility*
   D *Risk factor for infection*
   E *All of the above*

While the exact target range for appropriate blood glucose level has had much debate, there is consensus that hyperglycemia can cause harm. Detrimental effects include worse outcomes in patients with traumatic brain injury, decreased gut motility potentially leading to bacterial overgrowth and translocation, and is a risk factor for infection (answer E).

Answer: E

Brealey D and Singer M. Hyperglycemia in critical illness: a review. *Journal of Diabetes Science and Technology* 2009;3(6):1250–1260. doi:10.1177/193229680900300604

Krinsley JS. Glycemic control in the critically ill: what have we learned since NICE-SUGAR? *Hospital Practice* 2015;43(3):191–197. doi:10.1080/21548331.2015.1066227

5   *A 54-year-old woman has been in the intensive care unit for the last week following a motor vehicle crash. She sustained multiple orthopedic injuries including bilateral femur fractures and a right humorous fracture. Neurologically, she has not had a Glasgow Coma Score (GCS) higher than 6 since her admission. She has been diagnosed with diffuse axonal injury (DAI). Her blood sugars have been slowly increasing over the last week with the most recent checks consistently over 200 mg/dL. A sliding scale insulin regiment is begun. What diagnosis in her past medical history might guide your insulin therapy?*

   A *Hypertension*
   B *Steroid use*
   C *Diabetes mellitus*
   D *Inflammatory bowel disease requiring immunomodulators*
   E *Hypothyroid*

Tight blood glucose control was first promulgated in 2001 with the publication of a trial that demonstrated that "tight" (80–110 mg/dL) blood glucose control improved mortality in the intensive care unit. Subsequent studies failed to reproduce this, and this was further debunked in 2009 with the publication of the NICE-SUGAR trial, which found that with moderate blood glucose control (a goal of <180mg/dL) have improved outcomes. However, later studies found that in patients with a history of diabetes, a higher blood glucose target was associated with better outcomes.

Answer: C

Finfer S, Bellomi R, Blair D, et al. Intensive versus conventional glucose control in critically ill patients. *The New England Journal of Medicine* 2009;360(13):1283–1297. doi:10.1056/NEJMoa0810625

Krinsley JS, Egi M, Kiss A, et al. Diabetic status and the relation of the three domains of glycemic control to mortality in critically ill patients: an international multicenter cohort study. *Critical Care* 2013;17(2):R37. doi:10.1186/cc12547

6   *A 32-year-old woman is admitted to the intensive care unit following a right robot-assisted adrenalectomy for an adrenal adenoma. A few hours postoperatively, she experiences hypotension, nausea, emesis, hypoglycemia, and confusion. The operative team tells you it was a glucocorticoid-secreting tumor that they removed. Which medication should she have been placed on prior to surgery?*
   A *Metoprolol and phenoxybenzamine*
   B *Hydrocortisone*
   C *Prazosin*
   D *Furosemide*
   E *Oxymetazoline*

The patient is experiencing an Addisonian crisis (primary adrenal insufficiency), which consists of hypotension, vomiting, diarrhea, hyperkalemia, hypercalcemia, fever, syncope, lethargy, and abdominal pain. Patients should be placed on replacement therapy prior to adrenalectomy and continue with therapy afterwards to prevent hypocortisolism. Therapy includes treatment for both mineralocorticoid and glucocorticoid deficiency (fludrocortisone and hydrocortisone, respectively). When a patient is in crisis, they require high-dose steroid therapy (hydrocortisone 100 mg every 8 hours), fluid resuscitation, electrolyte correction, and intensive care monitoring.

Answer: B

Charmandari E, Nicolaides NC, and Chrousos GP. Adrenal insufficiency. *The Lancet*. 2014;383(9935):2152–2167. doi:10.1016/S0140-6736(13)61684-0

7   *An 81-year-old woman arrives in the trauma bay in January following an unwitnessed ground level fall at her nursing home. Her Glasgow Coma Scale (GCS) is 8. On secondary exam, a heart rate of 42, blood pressure of 83/40, respiratory rate of 8, and temperature of 31 °C were found. A chest X-ray reveals a consolidation of the right lower lobe of her lung. She is intubated, resuscitated, and broad-spectrum antibiotics for a presumed pneumonia are begun, and she is admitted to the ICU. Additional imaging reveals only the right lung finding. Her TSH level is checked and found to be high. Myxedema coma is suspected. What is the best course of action?*
   A *Begin intravenous levothyroxine therapy alone.*
   B *Begin intravenous T4, T3, and hydrocortisone therapy.*
   C *Slowly correct electrolyte abnormalities prior to starting any hormone therapy.*
   D *Treatment of the infection with antibiotics alone is sufficient to correct any thyroid abnormalities.*
   E *Recheck TSH after normothermia is achieved before making the diagnosis of myxedema coma.*

Myxedema coma is a rare phenomenon, so one must have a high index of suspicion in order to make the diagnosis. The mortality rate is high given that there is usually a precipitating event (infection in this case), which can cloud the diagnosis. High TSH in the setting of profound hypothermia and unconsciousness should lead one to suspect the diagnosis. Admission to an intensive care unit is recommended along with concomitant treatment of respiratory failure, electrolyte abnormalities, vasoplegia, and cardiac depression. Treatment should focus on airway control due to patients having a mixed hypoxic and hypercapnic picture of respiratory failure. There is controversy surrounding whether or not to give T3 or T4, thus some recommend giving both. T3 will have a fast onset, while T4 will have a slow, steady onset depending on the patient's deiodinase activity.

Answer: B

Wartofsky L and Klubo-Gwiezdzinska J. Myxedema coma. In: Luster M, Duntas LH, Wartofsky L, eds. *The Thyroid and Its Diseases: A Comprehensive Guide for the Clinician*. Springer International Publishing; 2019:281–292. doi:10.1007/978-3-319-72102-6_20

8   *A 28-year-old woman underwent an uncomplicated laparoscopic appendectomy for acute appendicitis overnight. The next morning she is noted to be confused, hypertensive, tachycardic to 134, febrile to 102, complaining of chest pain, and difficulty breathing with new onset pedal edema and rales. A workup ensues. She is transferred to the intensive care unit and broad-spectrum antibiotics are started over the concern for sepsis. On review of her medical problems, it is noted that she had a history of Graves' disease for*

which she takes methimazole. It is unknown when she received her last dose. The most appropriate medication to give next is:

A Her home methimazole dose, 25 mg PO

B Potassium iodide, 5 drops PO

C Aspirin, 325 mg PO

D Hydrocortisone, 100 mg IV

E Oxygen, 2L nasal cannula per minute.

This patient is experiencing thyroid storm given her history of Graves' disease, tachycardia, signs of congestive heart failure, fever, and inciting event (surgery). While the patient should eventually have several of the medications listed in the answer choices, it is important to give these medications in the correct order: stop new thyroid gland synthesis with antithyroid medication (methimazole or propylthiouracil), treat with iodine therapy to stop thyroid hormone release (potassium iodide or Lugol's solution), and treat adrenergic symptoms (hydrocortisone and/or beta-blockers). Giving iodine therapy prior to antithyroid therapy may exacerbate a thyroid storm. Furthermore, there should be a delay of 30–60 minutes prior to giving iodine therapy. She had been taking methimazole for her Graves' disease, but she may have missed doses secondary to her disease process or perhaps her maintenance dose is not enough given this new stress. The safe course of action is to give the methimazole first, then wait 30–60 minutes to give the potassium iodide.

Patients with Graves' disease can be treated with either propylthiouracil or methimazole, although the FDA has issued a warning against propylthiouracil as it may cause hepatotoxicity. The cardiovascular effects of thyrotoxicosis can be severe and are treated with a beta-blocker. Propranolol is preferred as it also blocks T4 to T3 conversion at higher doses. Thyroid storm, while rare, can occur in patients with clinical or subclinical hyperthyroid disease following a precipitating event (e.g. infection, trauma). Mortality from thyroid storm ranges from 20 to 30%.

Answer: A

Burch HB. Life-threatening thyrotoxicosis: thyroid storm. *Endocrinology and Metabolism Clinics of North America* 1993;22(2):263–277. doi:10.1016/S0889-8529(18)30165-8

Nayak B and Burman K. Thyrotoxicosis and thyroid storm. *Endocrinology and Metabolism Clinics of North America* 2006;35(4):663–686. doi:10.1016/j.ecl.2006.09.008

9 A 20-year-old man with a history of cystic fibrosis is admitted to the surgical intensive care unit following a subcutaneous venous access port removal due to positive blood cultures. The port site was closed. He had been taking prednisone daily as a part of his cystic fibrosis treatment. Which of the following medications may help improve wound healing in this patient?

A Topical vitamin E

B Topical vitamin A

C Topical mitomycin C

D Oral doxycycline

E Topical hydrocortisone

Patients who are on steroids have impaired wound healing. Vitamin A is known to reverse many of the deleterious effects of steroids in wound healing, namely, the appearance of inflammatory cells, fibroblasts, deposition of ground substance, regeneration of capillaries, and epithelial migration. It should be noted that while steroids decrease wound contracture, vitamin A does not reverse this effect. While there are many animal models that demonstrate these effects of vitamin A, there is a lack of good randomized controlled trials to support the animal models. There are no studies to support topical vitamin E, mitomycin C, or hydrocortisone to improve wound healing. Topical steroids will most likely worsen this patient's wound healing.

Answer: B

Wicke C. Effects of steroids and retinoids on wound healing. *Archives of Surgery* 2000;135(11):1265–1270. doi:10.1001/archsurg.135.11.1265

Zinder R, Cooley R, Vlad LG, et al. Vitamin A and wound healing. *Nutrition in Clinical Practice* 2019;34(6):839–849. doi:10.1002/ncp.10420

10 A 24-year-old woman is in the intensive care unit following a motor cycle crash. She suffered several small intraparenchymal hemorrhages, as well as diffuse axonal injury. This morning her serum sodium is 124 mmol/L. Her plasma osmolarity 253 mOsm/kg and urine osmolarity is 467 mOsm/kg. Her thyroid-stimulating hormone level is 2.3 μIU/mL, and she has not received any loop diuretics. A cortisol level is checked and is noted to be 18 μg/dL. This patient most likely has:

A Sheehan's syndrome

B Hypothyroid

C SIADH

D Diabetes insipidus

E Addisonian crisis

This patient most likely has SIADH. SIADH is a diagnosis of exclusion: plasma osmolarity < 275 mOsm/kg, urine osmolarity > 100 mOsm/kg water, normal renal function, clinical euvolemia, elevated urinary sodium excretion, and absence of other potential causes – namely hypothyroidism, hypocortisolism, or recent diuretic use. Sheehan's syndrome is hypopituitarism caused by ischemic necrosis during hemorrhagic shock experienced by the mother in childbirth, so answer A is incorrect. The patient has a normal thyroid level, so answer B is incorrect. The clinical description is not consistent with diabetes insipidus in which the plasma osmolarity would be high and the urine osmolarity low, so answer D is incorrect. In an Addisonian crisis, the patient would present with hypotension, vomiting, diarrhea, hyperkalemia, hypercalcemia, fever, syncope, lethargy, and abdominal pain (answer E).

Answer: C

Moro N, Katayama Y, Igarashi T, et al. Hyponatremia in patients with traumatic brain injury: incidence, mechanism, and response to sodium supplementation or retention therapy with hydrocortisone. *Surgical Neurology* 2007;68(4):387–393. doi:10.1016/j.surneu.2006.11.052

Rajagopal R, Swaminathan G, Nair S, et al. Hyponatremia in traumatic brain injury: a practical management protocol. *World Neurosurgery* 2017;108:529–533. doi:10.1016/j.wneu.2017.09.013

11 *A 44-year-old man is admitted to the intensive care unit following a four-node parathyroidectomy with reimplantation for secondary hyperparathyroidism due to renal failure. He has a calcium level of 8.5 mg/dL six hours postoperatively. He is asymptomatic. Which of the following medications has been shown to decrease the need for parathyroidectomy in the patients with chronic kidney disease?*
A *Calcium carbonate*
B *Vitamin D*
C *Calcium Acetate*
D *Cinacalcet*
E *iPTH*

Patients with secondary hyperparathyroidism have abnormal regulation of several electrolytes including calcium and phosphate. This is due to the malfunction of calcium-sensing receptors in the parathyroid gland, which subsequently leads to abnormally high levels of parathyroid hormone (PTH). Calcimimetics (like cinacalcet) increase the sensitivity of the calcium-sensing receptors, thereby decreasing PTH when serum calcium increases. Calcium carbonate and vitamin D would in theory improve PTH levels; however, this treatment is limited by likely presence of hypercalcemia and hyperphosphatemia. Calcium acetate is a phosphorus-binding medication and plays an important part in electrolyte regulation in patient in chronic renal failure but does not address hypercalcemia or elevated PTH. Intact PTH (iPTH) is a peptide hormone, which is synthesized in the parathyroid gland.

Answer: D

Block GA, Bushinsky DA, Cheng S, et al. Effect of etelcalcetide vs cinacalcet on serum parathyroid hormone in patients receiving hemodialysis with secondary hyperparathyroidism: a randomized clinical trial. *Journal of the American Medical Association* 2017;317(2):156–164. doi:10.1001/jama.2016.19468

Rodríguez M, Goodman WG, Liakopoulos V, et al. The use of calcimimetics for the treatment of secondary hyperparathyroidism: a 10 year evidence review. *Seminars in Dialysis* 2015;28(5):497–507. doi:10.1111/sdi.12357

12 *A 24-year-old woman presents to the emergency department complaining of abdominal pain. She is found to have acute appendicitis; however, she is also noted to have significant derangement of her electrolytes, as well as a high blood glucose level (670 mg/dL). Additional laboratory values include a serum bicarbonate of 22 mEq/L, BUN 42, creatinine 1.2, negative urine acetoacetate, and pH of 7.32. In addition to acute appendicitis, what other diagnosis does she have?*
A *Diabetic ketoacidosis*
B *Diabetes Insipidus*
C *Addisonian crisis*
D *Thyroid storm*
E *Hyperglycemic hyperosmolar state*

The first clue that this is hyperglycemic hyperosmolar state (HHS) and not diabetic ketoacidosis (DKA) is lack of urine ketones (negative urine acetoacetate) and a lack of metabolic acidosis (pH 7.32). Key differences between HHS and DKA are described in the chart below. Thyroid storm, Addisonian crisis, and diabetes Insipidus are all incorrect as the patient exhibits none of the diagnostic criteria for these diseases.

Initial treatment should be focused on fluid resuscitation, correction of electrolyte abnormalities (specifically potassium), and improvement in hyperglycemia.

Variable	Diabetic ketoacidosis	Hyperglycemic hyperosmolar state
Plasma glucose	<600 mg/dL	>600 mg/dL
pH	≤7.3	>7.3
Bicarbonate level	≤18	>15
Urine or blood acetoacetate	Positive	Negative
β-hydroxybutyrate	>3 mmol/l	<3 mmol/l
Serum osmolality	Variable	>320 mmol/l
Anion gap	>12 mmol/l	<12 mmol/l
Mental status	Variable	Stupor/coma

Answer: E

Pasquel FJ and Umpierrez GE. Hyperosmolar hyperglycemic state: a historic review of the clinical presentation, diagnosis, and treatment. *Diabetes Care* 2014;37(11):3124–3131. doi: 10.2337/dc14-0984

Umpierrez G and Korytkowski M. Diabetic emergencies — ketoacidosis, hyperglycaemic hyperosmolar state and hypoglycaemia. *Nature Reviews. Endocrinology* 2016;12(4):222–232. doi: 10.1038/nrendo.2016.15

13 *A 56-year old man presents to the trauma bay after ground level fall. He is obtunded, but hemodynamically stable. Imaging reveals several right-sided rib fractures and a transverse process fracture of the third cervical vertebrae. Laboratory data shows a pH of 7.14, lactate of 1.5, sodium of 133, and bicarbonate level of 12. Finger stick shows a blood sugar of 538 mg/dL. A β-hydroxybutyrate level is 5.2 mmol/L. Treatment priorities include what?*

　A *Intravenous 0.9 % NaCl hydration, insulin, potassium repletion*

　B *Intravenous 0.45% NaCl hydration, insulin, phosphate repletion*

　C *Insulin, bicarbonate infusion, potassium repletion*

　D *Stress dose steroids, lactated ringers, levothyroxine*

　E *Insulin, bicarbonate infusion, phosphate repletion*

This patient is in diabetic ketoacidosis (DKA), which is diagnosed with a low pH, low bicarbonate level, and elevated serum β-hydroxybutyrate level. The patient is obtunded and likely fell due to his worsening diabetic ketoacidosis. β-hydroxybutyrate is specific for DKA and helps with distinguishing it from hyperglycemic hyperosmolar state (HHS). However, whether DKA or HHS is suspected, the treatment protocol is the same per the 2009 American Diabetes Association consensus statement. Priority should be given to adequate intravenous fluid administration starting with 0.9% NaCl at 500–1000 mL/h during the first 1–2 hours, insulin administration, and potassium repletion. Thus, the answer is A. Frequent serum potassium checks are required during the initial phases of resuscitation as exogenous insulin will cause potassium to shift to the intracellular space causing a prolonged Q-T interval leading to torsade de points, ventricular fibrillation, and sudden cardiac arrest. Answer B, C, and E are incorrect since phosphate and bicarbonate repletion are almost never required. Answer D is incorrect since the presentation is inconsistent with myxedema coma.

Answer: A

Kitabchi AE, Umpierrez GE, Miles JM, et al. Hyperglycemic crises in adult patients with diabetes. *Diabetes Care* 2009;32(7):1335–1343. doi:10.2337/dc09-9032

Umpierrez G and Korytkowski M. Diabetic emergencies — ketoacidosis, hyperglycaemic hyperosmolar state and hypoglycaemia. *Nature Reviews. Endocrinology* 2016;12(4):222–232. doi:10.1038/nrendo.2016.15

14 *A 23-year-old woman is in the surgical intensive care unit following a motor vehicle crash. She has multiple long-bone fractures, a pneumothorax with a chest tube in place, and an open abdomen after a damage control laparotomy with splenectomy and small bowel resection. She was intubated in the trauma bay for a low Glasgow Coma Score (GCS). Etomidate was used for induction. What is the mechanism of action of etomidate on the adrenal gland that causes reversible adrenal insufficiency?*

　A *Inhibition of cytochrome p450*

　B *Inhibition of adrenal mitochondrial activity*

　C *Suppression of the hypothalamic-pituitary-adrenal axis*

　D *Upregulation of triiodothyronine (T3)*

　E *Vasoconstriction on the suprarenal arteries*

While it is well established that there can be adrenal insufficiency following etomidate administration, the long-term effects are more difficult to show. As of late 2020, the most current studies have shown there is no change among multiple outcome indicators including ventilator days, days of hospitalization, and mortality. The mechanism of action is via inhibition of adrenal mitochondrial activity (answer B). Etomidate is metabolized via hepatic esterases. It has no effect on cytochrome p450, the hypothalamic-pituitary-adrenal axis, nor triiodothyronine. It does not affect blood flow to the adrenal glands.

Answer: B

Gu W-J, Wang F, Tang L, et al. Single-dose etomidate does not increase mortality in patients with sepsis: a systematic review and meta-analysis of randomized controlled trials and observational studies. *Chest* 2015;147(2):335–346. doi:10.1378/chest.14-1012

Wagner CE, Bick JS, Johnson D, et al. Etomidate use and postoperative outcomes among cardiac surgery patients. *Anesthesiology* 2014;120(3):579–589. doi:10.1097/ALN.0000000000000087

15 *A 38-year-old woman suffered a traumatic brain injury following a motorcycle crash the previous night. She is in the intensive care unit, intubated, with a ventriculostomy in place. She has bilateral femur fractures that have been reduced via external fixation. She remains hypotensive despite adequate*

resuscitation. A morning cortisol is drawn and shows a level of 10 µg/dL. This patient likely has:

A *Primary adrenal insufficiency*

B *Secondary adrenal insufficiency*

C *Normal adrenal function*

D *Central hypothyroidism*

E *Hypogonadism*

Secondary adrenal insufficiency is most likely to occur following traumatic brain injury (TBI) (answer b). A serum cortisol level is the first test to assess adrenal responsiveness following TBI; however, the cortisol level at which adrenal insufficiency is diagnosed is controversial. Lower than 15 µg/dL is diagnostic, but some literature suggests serum cortisol less than 36 ug/dL should be diagnostic. Adrenal function may vary widely in the first few days following traumatic brain injury, so not all patients require steroids for a low cortisol level. Instead, clinical findings, such as in this case in which the patient is hypotensive despite adequate resuscitation, should receive exogenous steroids. Due to the variation in adrenal function of TBI patients, cortisol should be rechecked if clinical deterioration occurs. There was no history of etomidate or direct injury to the adrenals, so answer a is incorrect. This patient likely does not have normal adrenal function given the cortisol level, thus answer c is incorrect. This patient is at risk for hypogonadism long term and should be considered if symptoms are present after the acute hospitalization for this disease (answer e).

Answer: B

Powner DJ, Boccalandro C, Alp MS, et al. Endocrine failure after traumatic brain injury in adults. *Neurocritical Care* 2006;5:10.

Wagner CE, Bick JS, Johnson D, et al. Etomidate use and postoperative outcomes among cardiac surgery patients. *Anesthesiology* 2014;120(3):579–589. doi:10.1097/ALN.0000000000000087

16 *A 67-year-old woman underwent a left adrenalectomy for a pheochromocytoma. In the intensive care unit, she has required low-dose vasopressor support to maintain an adequate blood pressure. In addition to hypotension in the postoperative period, what is an important biochemical marker that can be affected after removal of a pheochromocytoma?*

A *Blood glucose*

B *Calcium*

C *Potassium*

D *Thyroid stimulating hormone*

E *Sodium*

In addition to hypotension due to persistence of preoperatively prescribed antihypertensives and relative hypovolemia, patients may also experience hypoglyce-mia. This should be monitored closely and corrected should the patient experience hypoglycemia. Thus, answer A is correct. Patients may have additional electrolyte abnormalities, but do not necessarily need to be monitored at a higher frequency unless clinically indicated (answers B, C, and E). This question deals with a pheochromocytoma and the ensuing loss of catecholamines. Thyroid-stimulating hormone is not typically effected, so answer d is incorrect.

Answer: A

Adler JT, Meyer-Rochow GY, Chen H, et al. Pheochromocytoma: current approaches and future directions. *The Oncologist.* 2008;13(7):779–793. doi:10.1634/theoncologist.2008-0043

Williams DT, Dann S, and Wheeler MH. Phaeochromocytoma – views on current management. *European Journal of Surgical Oncology* 2003;29(6):483–490. doi:10.1016/S0748-7983(03)00071-4

17 *A 34-year-old man has been in the intensive care unit for 2 weeks following a helicopter crash. He has a severe traumatic brain injury (TBI), which was initially managed with an external ventricular drain (EVD). He also suffered multiple long bone fractures that were repaired via ex-fix shortly after the accident. He has had a tracheostomy placed, as well as a percutaneous endoscopic gastrostomy (PEG) feeding tube placed. During the first week, his sodium remained above 150 meq/L due to frequent boluses of hypertonic saline. Toward the end of this week, you have noticed that his serum sodium has continued to fall. This morning it is 128 meq/L. A urine sodium is added on to the morning labs and found to be > 40 meq/L. What should be the next step?*

A *Add salt and start fludrocortisone*

B *Add salt*

C *Fluid restriction*

D *Start hypertonic saline again*

E *Start desmopressin*

The two most common causes of hyponatremia in TBI patients are the syndrome of inappropriate antidiuretic hormone secretion (SIADH) and cerebral salt wasting (CSW). These can be difficult to distinguish in the TBI patient because fluid restriction often leads to an increase in serum sodium; however, restricting fluids for correction in hyponatremia can be dangerous and lead to cerebral infarction. Thus, salt-retaining therapy should be instituted with a mineralocorticoid like fludrocortisone. Given the patient has moderate hyponatremia (serum sodium of 125–129 meq/L), it is suggested to add enteric salt supplementation.

Answer: A

Mori T, Katayama Y, Kawamata T, et al. Improved efficiency of hypervolemic therapy with inhibition of natriuresis by fludrocortisone in patients with aneurysmal subarachnoid hemorrhage. *Journal of Neurosurgery* 1999;91(6):947–952. doi:10.3171/jns.1999.91.6.0947

Rajagopal R, Swaminathan G, Nair S, et al. Hyponatremia in traumatic brain injury: a practical management protocol. *World Neurosurgery* 2017;108:529–533. doi:10.1016/j.wneu.2017.09.013

18 *A 47-year-old woman with a history of diabetes mellitus, Graves' disease, and idiopathic pulmonary fibrosis has been admitted to the intensive care unit following a motor vehicle crash. She had computed tomography imaging of her head, cervical spine, chest, abdomen, and pelvis. She has a left humerus fracture, a left femur fracture, a grade II kidney laceration, and a grade III splenic laceration for which she underwent coil embolization of her splenic artery. She was intubated in the trauma bay due to desaturation. It is now hospital day 2, and she has become progressively more tachycardic and hypertensive despite multiple antihypertensive medications being given. She is now febrile to 104 degrees Fahrenheit. She has increased ventilator requirements with new bilateral haziness on chest X-ray. Overnight, she experienced atrial fibrillation and was given a bolus of amiodarone. You are concerned that she may be experiencing thyroid storm. What are the medications and in which order should they be given to a patient who is experiencing thyroid storm?*

A *Methimazole, potassium iodide, beta-blockade, hydrocortisone*

B *Potassium iodide, beta-blockade, propylthiouracil, hydrocortisone*

C *Hydrocortisone, beta-blockade, methimazole, potassium iodide*

D *Beta-blockade, propylthiouracil, potassium iodide, hydrocortisone*

E *Potassium iodide, methimazole, beta-blockade, hydrocortisone*

The order of therapy along with the appropriate medications is important for treatment of thyroid storm. Inhibition of thyroid gland synthesis of new thyroid hormone is a critical first step, so giving either methimazole or propylthiouracil should be done first. Second, potassium iodide (Lugol's solution) should be given next to block release of additional hormone release. The order of the next medications are not as critical, but the medications themselves are important to help medically support the patient. They include beta-blockade with propranolol

(which in addition to cardiac effects also decreases conversion of T4 to T3). Hydrocortisone should be used to treat hyperthermia, as well as decrease conversion of T4 to T3. Acetaminophen should be given for hyperthermia (not listed). Answers B, C, D, and E all contain the correct medications but in the incorrect order.

Answer: A

Burch HB. Life-threatening thyrotoxicosis: thyroid storm. *Endocrinology and Metabolism Clinics of North America* 1993;22(2):263–277. doi:10.1016/S0889-8529(18)30165-8

Nayak B and Burman K. Thyrotoxicosis and thyroid storm. *Endocrinology and Metabolism Clinics of North America* 2006;35(4):663–686. doi:10.1016/j.ecl.2006.09.008

19 *A 48-year-old woman is admitted to the intensive care unit following a motor vehicle crash. There was a prolonged extraction. She was intubated in the field for low Glasgow Coma Score (GCS). Workup revealed a splenic laceration for which she underwent a splenectomy, as well as a moderate-sized subdural hematoma for which she underwent craniotomy and evacuation. It is now 8 hours after her last operation and her urine output has increased to over 200 mL/h for the last three hours. What laboratory values would confirm a diagnosis of diabetes insipidus?*

A *Antidiuretic hormone (ADH) level*

B *Serum cortisol level*

C *Serum sodium, serum glucose, urine sodium, serum potassium*

D *Plasma osmolality, serum sodium, urine osmolality, serum glucose*

E *Antidiuretic hormone (ADH) level, serum and urine sodium, plasma osmolality*

There are no consensus guidelines for the diagnosis of diabetes insipidus. However, there are some basic criteria that need to be met in order to make the diagnosis. Greater than 200 mL/h for two consecutive hours or greater than 5 mL/kg/h for two consecutive hours should alert one to the possibility. Other causes such as hyperglycemia should be ruled out (thus, answers A, B, and E are incorrect). Other medications that may causes diuresis in traumatic brain injury patients (e.g. mannitol) should also be considered. If the patient has hypotonic urine (low osmolality: <300 mosm/kg; specific gravity < 1.005) along with hypernatremia (>145 mmol/L), and increased plasma osmolality (>300 mosm/kg), then the patient likely has diabetes insipidus. Potassium is not necessary for diagnosis (answer C), but should be followed closely during periods of excessive diuresis.

Answer: D

Boughey JC, Yost MJ, Bynoe RP. Diabetes insipidus in the head-injured patient. *The American Surgeon* 2004;70(6):500–503.

Capatina C, Paluzzi A, Mitchell R, et al. Diabetes insipidus after traumatic brain injury. *Journal of Clinical Medicine* 2015;4(7):1448–1462. doi:10.3390/jcm4071448

20 *A 23-year-old with Crohn's disease presents to the intensive care unit following a laparoscopic ileocecectomy. The case was uneventful; however, the patient remained hypotensive in the postanesthesia care unit requiring vasopressor support. Preoperatively, she was on adalimumab to treat her Crohn's disease, gabapentin for pain, oxycodone as needed for pain, and fluconazole for a fungal UTI. Prior to her treatment with adalimumab, she was on infliximab. During her assessment in the intensive care unit, the diagnosis of adrenal insufficiency is discussed. Why should this diagnosis be considered?*

A *Adalimumab can affect the pituitary function.*

B *There is high incidence of adrenal insufficiency in patients with inflammatory bowel disease undergoing operative intervention.*

C *Prolonged use of gabapentin has been shown to inhibit steroidogenesis via inhibition of 21-hydroxylase.*

D *The anti-TNF-α agent infliximab is a chimeric monoclonal antibody.*

E *Fluconazole has been associated with adrenal insufficiency.*

There are several medications, genetic disorders, and other pathologic mechanisms that may lead to adrenal insufficiency. Adrenal insufficiency has been described in with use of ketoconazole and fluconazole via inhibition of mitochondrial cytochrome P450-dependent enzymes (answer E). When adrenal insufficiency is being considered and the patient is hypotensive, glucocorticoid replacement should be initiated along with adequate fluid hydration. Adalimumab is not known to affect the pituitary gland (answer A). Surgery itself does not cause adrenal insufficiency in patients with inflammatory bowel disease; however, one should be cautious in treating this patient postoperatively if the patient has been on high dose or prolonged steroids to consider adrenal insufficiency if hypotension develops (answer B). Gabapentin has not been shown to effect steroidogenesis. While infliximab is a chimeric monoclonal antibody, it has no bearing on the status of the adrenal gland (answer D).

Answer: E

Albert SG, DeLeon MJ, and Silverberg AB. Possible association between high-dose fluconazole and adrenal insufficiency in critically ill patients. *Critical Care Medicine* 2001;29(3):668–670.

Charmandari E, Nicolaides NC, and Chrousos GP. Adrenal insufficiency. *The Lancet* 2014;383(9935):2152–2167. doi:10.1016/S0140-6736(13)61684-0

16

Hypothermia and Hyperthermia

Drew Farmer, MD and Shariq Raza, MD

Trauma Surgery, Surgical Critical Care & Emergency Surgery, Perelman School of Medicine, University of Pennsylvania, Philadelphia, PA, USA

1   *What is the fundamental difference between hyperthermia and fever?*
   A *Fever is secondary to infection whereas hyperthermia is not.*
   B *Fever is, by definition, 38.3 °C or greater, whereas hyperthermia is any temperature above a person's baseline temperature.*
   C *Fever occurs as a result of an altered set point of the body's normally functioning internal thermoregulatory system.*
   D *Fever is a pathologic condition, whereas hyperthermia may be an adaptive response to an environmental stress.*
   E *They are interchangeable terms.*

The fundamental difference between hyperthermia and fever is that fever is the result of a functioning thermoregulatory system working at an elevated set point. Hyperthermia is a condition in which the thermal set point is normal, but the thermoregulatory system is unable to adequately regulate heat exchange to achieve the desired temperature. (answer e.) Fever has many causes and is not limited to infection (answer a). While the Society of Critical Care Medicine does define fever as a body temperature above 38.3 °C (or 101 °F), the fundamental difference between fever and hyperthermia is related to the mechanism by which the temperature rises (answer b). Hyperthermia is the result of an inability to mount an adequate adaptive response to increased body temperature. Fever is often a physiologic response to a pathologic condition (answer d).

Answer: C

Marino PL and Sutin KM. *The ICU Book.* 3rd ed. Philadelphia: Lippincott Williams & Wilkins, 2007.

Society of Critical Care Medicine. *Fundamental Critical Care Support.* 5th ed., Society of Critical Care Medicine, 2012.

2   *A healthy 30-year-old woman prepares for a run on a hot, dry day. As she laces up her running shoes, her body temperature is 37 °C. What is her primary mode of heat loss?*
   A *Conduction*
   B *Convection*
   C *Evaporation*
   D *Radiation*
   E *Transduction*

In a healthy person in a physiologic state in a habitable environment, the majority (50–70%) of heat loss is via radiation of infrared rays from the skin. Conduction is the exchange of heat as kinetic energy by direct contact (i.e. the skin–air interface), and under normal conditions this accounts for only about 15% of heat loss. As the skin surface and the surrounding air temperatures equilibrate, heat transfer between the surfaces diminishes. Convection occurs by two processes – first, air movement over the skin replaces the warmed air with air that has not been warmed by conduction at the skin surface, and second, cutaneous vasodilation increases blood flow and surface area exposure to this interface. Each of these currents serves to maintain the energy gradient needed for heat exchange. At rest, evaporative heat loss occurs mainly through respiratory vapor and accounts for about 20% of total heat loss.

Answer: D

Rippe JM. *Irwin and Rippe's Intensive Care Medicine,* edited by Richard S. Irwin and James M. Rippe, Wolters Kluwer Health, 2011. *ProQuest Ebook Central,* https://

ebookcentral-proquest-com.proxy.library.upenn.edu/lib/
upenn-ebooks/detail.action?docID=2031844.

3 *The patient from the previous question goes on her run and after several miles in environmental temperatures >40 °C (104 °F), her skin is flush, she is dripping in sweat, and she begins to experience nausea, muscle cramps, and general dysphoria. She eventually is unable to continue due to a sensation of severe weakness and sits down by the side of the road to cool off in the wind. What is her primary mode of heat loss?*
   A *Conduction*
   B *Convection*
   C *Evaporation*
   D *Radiation*
   E *All of the above*

When the body experiences thermal stress, evaporation surpasses radiation (answer d) in its capacity for dissipating excess body heat. In particular, evaporation is not dependent upon ambient temperature to yield heat loss. Heat energy is used up during the conversion of liquid sweat into vapor. This is called the "latent heat of vaporization." Notably, for evaporative heat loss to occur, the sweat must evaporate. Therefore, significant evaporative heat exchange does not occur in conditions of high humidity (high vapor pressure) or when sweat is not allowed to evaporate from the skin surface (i.e. it is wiped away). Heat loss by conduction (answer a) and convection (answer b) rely upon ambient temperatures that are less than the body temperature. In the conditions described in the vignette, these would not be significant sources of heat loss.

Answer: C

Marino PL and Sutin KM. *The ICU Book*. 3rd ed. Philadelphia: Lippincott Williams & Wilkins, 2007.
Rippe JM. *Irwin and Rippe's Intensive Care Medicine*, edited by Richard S. Irwin and James M. Rippe, Wolters Kluwer Health, 2011. *ProQuest Ebook Central*, https://ebookcentral-proquest-com.proxy.library.upenn.edu/lib/upenn-ebooks/detail.action?docID=2031844.

4 *Given the patient's symptoms in the above vignette, what is her diagnosis and what is the recommended therapy?*
   A *Heat exhaustion: volume repletion*
   B *Heat exhaustion: volume repletion and cooling measures*
   C *Exertional heat stroke: volume repletion*
   D *Exertional heat stroke: volume repletion and cooling measures, supportive therapy for end-organ failure*

   E *Classic heat stroke: volume repletion, cooling measures, supportive therapy for end-organ failure*

The patient is suffering from heat exhaustion, a form of exertional heat illness. The recommended therapy for this illness is simply volume repletion and no cooling measures are usually needed as body temperature is typically ≤40 °C. The patient is not experiencing significant encephalopathy or other severe CNS dysfunction (which may include altered mental status, seizures, or persistent delirium) – hallmarks of exertional heat stroke (answers c and d). Classic heat stroke is characterized by hyperthermia with CNS derangements (not seen in this patient), whose pathology is non-exertional, but rather commonly stems from another medical comorbidity that prevents physiologic or behavioral response to hyperthermia. Examples include physical impairment or entrapment that prevents mobility to a cooler environment, psychiatric disorders, or drug (pharmaceutical or illicit) use, which may exacerbate dehydration and/or hyperthermia, or which may result in impaired mental status. A diagnosis of "heat injury" could be made if hyperthermia and end-organ damage are appreciated without severe neurologic dysfunction, but that was not seen in this patient.

Answer: A

Marino PL and Sutin KM. *The ICU Book*. 3rd ed. Philadelphia: Lippincott Williams & Wilkins, 2007.
Rippe JM. *Irwin and Rippe's Intensive Care Medicine*, edited by Richard S. Irwin and James M. Rippe, Wolters Kluwer Health, 2011. *ProQuest Ebook Central*, https://ebookcentral-proquest-com.proxy.library.upenn.edu/lib/upenn-ebooks/detail.action?docID=2031844.

5 *For exertional heat stroke, what is a safe and desirable cooling rate? At what body temperature should cooling be discontinued?*
   A *<0.1 °C/min: Stop at 39.5 °C*
   B *>0.1 °C/min: Stop at 39.5 °C*
   C *<0.1 °C/min: Stop at 38.5 °C*
   D *>0.1 °C/min: Stop at 38.5 °C*
   E *<0.1 °C/min: Stop at 36 °C*

For exertional heat stroke, the mainstay of therapy is rapid cooling (>0.1 °C/min) to a target temperature <39 °C prior to cessation of cooling measures. Conventional methods of external cooling include immersion in cold water (up to 0.35 °C/min cooling rate) or pouring large volumes of water over the body and fanning to maximize evaporative heat dissipation. Also available are commercially sold surface cooling systems that circulate cold fluid or cold air through blankets or pads that are wrapped around the patient. Invasive cooling systems use percutaneously placed central venous catheters in subclavian, internal jugular, or femoral veins, and temperature control is achieved by circulating cool saline in a closed loop through the catheter's balloon. Invasive cooling systems thus have a higher risk of catheter-related blood stream infections, however, can prove beneficial in difficult to cool patients such as those with high body mass index (BMI) (>30 kg/m^2).

Answer: D

Epstein Y and Yanovich R. Heatstroke. The New England Journal of Medicine 2019;380(25):2449–2459. doi: 10.1056/NEJMra1810762.

6 *A 74-year-old man presents with a temperature of 40 °C, labile blood pressure, "lead pipe" muscle rigidity, and altered mental status. The patient's wife says that she usually helps him with his medications, but she has been out of town for several days and came home to find him in this state. What is the best initial therapy for a patient?*
   A *Immediately restart a recently discontinued antipsychotic medication.*
   B *Immediately restart a recently discontinued dopaminergic medication.*
   C *IV fluid resuscitation.*
   D *Initiate Dantrolene therapy.*
   E *Initiate Bromocriptine therapy.*

This patient's presentation is consistent with neuroleptic malignant syndrome (NMS) – a condition that arises as a result of decreased dopaminergic activity at the D2 receptor in the central nervous system. This is most commonly a result of the use of dopamine antagonist medications such as antipsychotics, but can also be elicited by antiemetics, cocaine, amphetamines, or tricyclic antidepressants. Therefore, starting an antipsychotic would only exacerbate this condition, and the best initial therapy would be to remove the offending drug (answer a). Conversely, stopping dopaminergic medications such as bromocriptine, levodopa, or amantadine can result in NMS. Restarting these medications is the top priority in this patient. IV fluid resuscitation with the goal of slightly alkalinizing the urine may help mitigate the effects of rhabdomyolysis (answer c) but will not reverse the patient's condition. Dantrolene (answer d) and bromocriptine (answer e) may both be used in the treatment of NMS, but the most appropriate initial therapy in this patient is to immediately restart the dopaminergic medication.

Answer: B

Pileggi DJ and Cook AM. Neuroleptic malignant syndrome. *The Annals of Pharmacotherapy* 2016;50(11):973–981. doi: 10.1177/1060028016657553.

7 *A 25-year-old man presents to the emergency department with complaint of tremor, muscle rigidity, and subjective fever and sweats. On exam, the patient has mydriasis and horizontal ocular clonus. He is diaphoretic and has a notable hyperreflexia that is greater at the patellar tendon than in the upper extremities. His medical history is significant only for depression, which is actively treated by his primary care physician. He also reports that about 6 hours prior to his symptoms, he was using cocaine. Vital signs are as follows: Pulse, 133; BP, 165/94; SpO2, 99% on room air; Temp, 41.3 °C. Which of the following are true?*
   A *For this patient, intubation, sedation, and neuromuscular blockade with a nondepolarizing agent would be appropriate.*
   B *Dantrolene administration may be effective in improving the patient's fever and muscle rigidity, and may prevent rhabdomyolysis.*
   C *Benzodiazepines may exacerbate the patient's condition.*
   D *Physical restraints are recommended to prevent the hyper-reflexive patient from harming himself or others.*
   E *Removal of the offending agent and supportive care are adequate in the treatment of this patient.*

This patient has the classic signs of serotonin syndrome (SS), which may be distinguished from the other drug-induced hyperthermias with an accurate medication/drug history and the presence of hyperreflexia/clonus. Here the patient's synaptic serotonin levels were acutely elevated when he combined cocaine, which increases serotonin release, with his antidepressant medication, commonly a serotonin reuptake inhibitor (SSRI). Due to this patient's fever >41.1 °C, the patient meets criteria for neuromuscular blockade, which necessitates intubation and sedation. Depolarizing agents such as succinylcholine should be avoided as hyperkalemia with rhabdomyolysis is a concern (answer a). Dantrolene is not useful in the treatment of SS (answer b). Benzodiazepines are helpful in the treatment of SS by blunting the adrenergic response, improving agitation and muscle rigidity (answer c). Physical restraints result in isometric muscle contractions, which exacerbates lactic acidosis and hyperthermia, and should therefore be avoided (answer d). While removal of the offending agent and supportive therapy are paramount to the treatment of patients with drug-induced hyperthermia, this patient requires neuromuscular blockade and should also be treated with cyproheptadine, a 5-HT$_{2A}$ antagonist (answer e).

Answer: A

Boyer EW and Shannon M. The serotonin syndrome. N Engl J Med. 2005;352(11):1112–20. doi: 10.1056/ NEJMra041867. Erratum in: N Engl J Med. 2007 Jun 7;356(23):2437. Erratum in: N Engl J Med. 2009 Oct 22;361(17):1714.

8 Which of the following has been demonstrated concerning external cooling of intubated febrile patients in septic shock?
   A *External cooling yielded decreased vasopressor requirements in the first 12 hours of treatment.*
   B *External cooling was safe but not effective in changing 14-day mortality.*
   C *No significant difference in reversal of shock during the ICU stay.*
   D *Increased use of sedation and neuromuscular blockade.*
   E *Inhibition of viral replication.*

External cooling yielded decreased vasopressor requirements in the first 12 hours of treatment. The percentage of patients for whom vasopressor doses were decreased by 50% was higher in the cooling group. Furthermore, the cooling group had a significantly higher 14-day survival (answer b) and higher rates of shock reversal (answer c). Despite concerns for unwanted shivering or patient discomfort, the cooling group did not receive significantly more sedation or neuromuscular blockade (answer d). Finally, the study is not generalizable to viral infection, but fever is thought to inhibit viral replication and has been used as an argument against fever control (answer e).

Answer: A

Schortgen F, Clabault K, Katsahian S, et al. Fever control using external cooling in septic shock: a randomized controlled trial. American Journal of Respiratory and Critical Care Medicine 2012;185(10):1088–1095. doi: 10.1164/rccm.201110-1820OC

9 Which of the following patients should be considered for post-cardiac arrest therapeutic hypothermia/ targeted temperature management?
   A *A 32-year-old man who crashed his motorcycle into a tree and received approximately 4 minutes of BLS*

before ROSC. Noted to have a grade IV liver laceration and grade III spleen laceration.
   B *A 26-year-old G1P0 woman who had a cardiac arrest secondary to narcotic overdose and received 10 minutes of BLS prior to ROSC.*
   C *A 56-year-old man who presents after a near-drowning and an initial tympanic membrane temperature of 29 °C*
   D *A 74-year-old man who, despite being comatose prior to cardiac arrest, has an advance directive stating that he wishes to remain full code and pursue all life-saving measures.*
   E *A 68-year-old woman who presents after a witnessed cardiac arrest in which she received bystander CPR until EMS arrived. She was found to be in ventricular fibrillation and ACLS was performed on scene. Total downtime prior to ROSC was 16 minutes. She is comatose at the time of her presentation.*

TH/TTM should be considered for patients who experience a witnessed out-of-hospital cardiac arrest that is believed to be cardiac in origin, who are comatose (unable to follow commands) following ROSC. Hemorrhage/ risk of hemorrhage (answer a), pregnancy (answer b), hypothermia with initial TM temperature < 30°C (answer c), and prior comatose state (answer d) are all contraindications to TH/TTM. Additionally, TH/TTM may be contraindicated in cases of terminal illness and patients with blood coagulation disorders.

Answer: E

Society of Critical Care Medicine. *Fundamental Critical Care Support.* 5th ed., Society of Critical Care Medicine, 2012.

10 Which of the following is true concerning targeted temperature management (TTM)?
   A *The strongest evidence for benefit of TTM is in patients who have an in-hospital cardiac arrest.*
   B *TTM increases cerebral blood flow.*
   C *TTM may lead to hypovolemia and hypotension by inducing cold diuresis.*
   D *Colder temperatures and longer duration of cooling have been shown to increase pneumonia rates and impact patient survival.*
   E *Enteral feeding should be initiated when the patient is rewarmed.*

Hypovolemia and hypotension may occur as a result of diuresis induced by targeting temperatures 32–36 °C. The benefits of TTM are more controversial for in-hospital cardiac arrest than out-of-hospital cardiac arrest, which has much stronger supporting evidence (answer a). Cerebral blood flow and intracranial pressure decrease when patients undergo TTM (answer b). While "larger doses" of cooling seem to have a correlation with higher incidence of pneumonia, this has not been associated with differences in survival (answer d). Small volume enteral feeding (10 mL/h) is well tolerated during hypothermia. Rates may be increased as the patient enters the rewarming phase and further increased when normothermia is reached (answer e).

Answer: C

Kirkegaard H, Taccone FS, Skrifvars M, et al. Postresuscitation care after out-of-hospital cardiac arrest: clinical update and focus on targeted temperature management. Anesthesiology 2019;131(1):186–208. doi: 10.1097/ALN.0000000000002700.

11 *A patient presents after falling into an icy lake and being rescued by EMS. He has impaired mental status and is not shivering. What vital signs would you expect to find?*
   A *Temperature: 33 °C*
   B *BP: 80/45 mmHg*
   C *Pulse: 120 bpm*
   D *Temperature: 24 °C*
   E *Respiratory rate: 9 breaths/min*

The patient is in Stage II hypothermia characterized by impaired consciousness and little to no shivering. The expected body temperature range is 28–32 °C (answer a). Bradycardia (answer c) and bradypnea (answer e) are present, but hypotension is not expected (answer b).

Answer: E

Brown DJ, Brugger H, Boyd J, et al. Accidental hypothermia. The New England Journal of Medicine 2012;367(20):1930–1938. doi: 10.1056/NEJMra 1114208.

12 *Which of the following is the most effective rewarming technique in a hypothermic patient?*
   A *Hemodialysis*
   B *Cardiopulmonary bypass*
   C *Thoracic lavage*
   D *Veno-venous ECMO*
   E *Peritoneal dialysis*

Cardiopulmonary bypass has a potential rewarming rate of 9 °C/hr. In order from most effective to least effect: VA ECMO 6 °C/hr, VV ECMO 4 °C/hr, Thoracic lavage 3 °C/hr, Hemodialysis 2–4 °C/hr, and peritoneal dialysis 1–3 °C/hr.

Answer: B

Brown DJ, Brugger H, Boyd J, et al. Accidental hypothermia. The New England Journal of Medicine 2012;367(20):1930–1938. doi: 10.1056/NEJMra 1114208

13 *Which of the following is associated with perioperative hypothermia?*
   A *Acute kidney injury*
   B *Hypervolemia*
   C *Decreased risk of cardiac complications*
   D *Increased risk of surgical site infection*
   E *Rebound hyperthermia in the postoperative period*

Perioperative hypothermia is defined as a body temperature <36 °C. Increased rates of surgical wound infections and cardiac complications (answer c) have been associated with incidental perioperative hypothermia in patients undergoing noncardiac surgery. Perioperative hypothermia leads to vasoconstriction with relative tissue hypoxia, impaired migration of leukocytes to the wound bed, altered neutrophil phagocytosis, and changes in cytokine and antibody production. Systemic vasoconstriction also leads to elevated blood pressure and increased myocardial oxygen consumption. This increase in metabolic demand is thought to be responsible for the higher cardiac complication rate associated with PH. No increased rates of acute kidney injury (answer a), hypervolemia (answer b), or rebound hyperthermia (answer e) have been demonstrated. In a 2014 cohort study, for patients undergoing elective surgery, unintentional perioperative hypothermia was linked to increased incidence of mortality, sepsis, stroke, myocardial infarction, pneumonia, and length of hospital stay. For these reasons, it is recommended to actively warm patients in the perioperative setting to maintain a body temperature of >36 °C.

Answer: D

Billeter AT, Hohmann SF, Druen D, et al. Unintentional perioperative hypothermia is associated with severe complications and high mortality in elective operations. *Surgery* 2014;156(5):1245–1252. doi: 10.1016/j.surg.2014.04.024.
Forbes SS, Eskicioglu C, Nathens AB, et al. Best practice in general surgery committee, University of Toronto. evidence-based guidelines for prevention of perioperative hypothermia. *Journal of the American College of Surgeons*. 2009;209(4):492–503.e1. doi: 10.1016/j.jamcollsurg.2009.07.002.

14 *Which of the following is true of dantrolene sodium?*
   A *Its most common side effect is muscle weakness.*
   B *Its most serious side effect is renal injury.*

C *It binds to the MH1 receptor in the skeletal muscle sarcoplasmic reticulum.*

D *It can only be given in an IV form.*

E *The standard duration of therapy is 7 days.*

Muscle weakness (commonly seen as diminished hand grip strength) is the most common side effect of dantrolene sodium. Hepatocellular injury is the most concerning side effect (answer b), and to the extent that it can be avoided in patients with active hepatitis or cirrhosis, it should be. However, given to the threat of malignant hyperthermia, the contraindication is not absolute. It binds to the Ryanodine receptor RyR1 (answer c) in the sarcoplasmic reticulum of skeletal muscle, preventing the release of calcium stores into the cytoplasm of the myocyte, thus inhibiting muscle contraction. In cases of malignant hyperthermia, dantrolene is initially given as an IV bolus 1–2.5 mg/kg and every 5–10 minutes. Therapeutic effect may be appreciated 2–3 minutes after injection. The patient can be transitioned to an oral form (answer d), and the standard duration of therapy is between 24 and 72 hours (answer e) to prevent recurrence of MH.

Answer: A

Marino PL and KM Sutin. *The ICU Book*. 3rd ed. Philadelphia: Lippincott Williams & Wilkins, 2007.

Rippe JM. *Irwin and Rippe's Intensive Care Medicine*, edited by Richard S. Irwin and James M. Rippe, Wolters Kluwer Health, 2011. *ProQuest Ebook Central*, https://ebookcentral-proquest-com.proxy.library.upenn.edu/lib/upenn-ebooks/detail.action?docID=2031844.

15 *Which of the following is an independent risk factor for unintentional perioperative hypothermia in patients undergoing elective surgery?*

A *BMI < 25*

B *Age < 65 years*

C *Chronic renal impairment*

D *Female sex*

E *History of coronary artery disease*

Chronic renal impairment, anemia, and recent unintentional weight loss were found to be independent risk factors for unintentional perioperative hypothermia (PH). Other risk factors include severity of illness on admission, age > 65 years (answer b), male sex (answer d), and neurologic disorders. BMI < 25 (answer a) and coronary artery disease (answer e) have not been demonstrated to be independent risk factors. Unintentional PH has been associated with increased incidence of mortality, stroke, myocardial infarction, increased length of stay, pneumonia, and overall complication rate. Surgical site infection has been previously associated with unintentional PH. Early recognition of modifiable risk factors is necessary

to initiate preoperative patient optimization. Identification of non-modifiable risk factors enhances the clinician's diligence in taking proactive measures to prevent PH in the perioperative setting.

Answer: C

Billeter AT, Hohmann SF, Druen D, et al. Unintentional perioperative hypothermia is associated with severe complications and high mortality in elective operations. *Surgery* 2014;156(5):1245–1252. doi: 10.1016/j.surg.2014.04.024.

16 *Which of the following is true regarding reversing unintentional postoperative hypothermia?*

A *There is no difference between warm blanket and active rewarming in time to achieve normothermia.*

A *Use of warmed blanket is associated with decreased time to achieve normothermia compared to thermal insulation (reflective covering).*

B *Use of circulating hot water devices is associated with decreased time to achieve normothermia compared to forced air warming.*

C *Use of radiant heaters was associated with decreased time to achieve normothermia compared to forced air warming.*

D *Use of active rewarming resulted in about 40% decrease in the incidence of shivering when compared to use of an unwarmed blanket only.*

A 2014 Cochrane review examined different treatment modalities and their efficacy in the treatment of inadvertent postoperative hypothermia (PH). The review included 11 randomized trials and 699 adult patients. "Active rewarming" therapies included forced air warming, circulating hot water devices, radiant blankets, radiant warmers, and electric blankets. Overwhelmingly, active rewarming techniques are more effective at restoring normothermia and reducing shivering than other techniques such as warm or unwarmed cotton blankets (answer a). Among active rewarming techniques, forced air warming is associated with decreased time to achieving normothermia when compared to circulating hot water devices and radiant heaters (answers c and d). In one of the reviewed studies, shivering was seen in 100% of patients treated with unwarmed blanket vs. 58.3% of patients treated with active warming techniques.

Answer: E

Warttig S, Alderson P, Campbell G, et al. Interventions for treating inadvertent postoperative hypothermia.

Cochrane Database of Systematic Reviews 2014;20(11):CD009892. doi: 10.1002/14651858. CD009892.pub2

17 *Which of the following is true concerning thermal regulation in patients with significant burn injuries?*

  A *Because patients with significant burns are susceptible to hypothermia, elevated body temperatures are more likely to be secondary to infectious causes.*

  B *The hypothalamic temperature set point following a major burn is elevated.*

  C *Patients with large, healed skin grafts remain susceptible to hypothermia because grafted skin is a less-effective insulator than native skin.*

  D *Time to recover from hypothermia is not predictive of patient outcomes.*

  E *External cooling methods are particularly effective in the febrile burn patient and are a mainstay of therapy.*

The hypothalamic thermoregulatory set point is elevated in patients with significant burn injury. This is mediated by the release of pyrogenic cytokines IL-1 and IL-6, as well as surges in catecholamines. Because of this phenomenon, fever in the burn population is common and is not necessarily indicative of infection (answer a). However, burn patients are at increased risk for infection, and body temperature that is persistently >39°C warrants infectious workup. Once well-healed, skin grafts promote hyperthermia due to a diminished sweat response and impaired cutaneous vasodilation. These deficits in thermoregulation may persist for up to 8 years (answer c). Longer time needed to recover from hypothermia is associated with non-survival in adult burn patients (answer d). When treating fever in the burn patient, external cooling methods increase the metabolic rate through a process involving stress-response catecholamines, inflammatory cytokines, and increases in evaporative heat loss. The energy consumed by such a process can be profound at a time when the critically injured burn patient can ill-afford such losses.

Answer: B

Taveras LR, Jeschke MG, Wolf SE. Critical care in burns. In: Jeschke M., Kamolz LP., Sjöberg F., Wolf S. (eds) *Handbook of Burns*, Volume 1. Springer, Cham, 2020. https://doi-org.proxy.library.upenn.edu/10.1007/978-3-030-18940-2_20

17

Acute Kidney Injury
Cassandra Q. White[1], MD and Terence O'Keeffe, MB ChB[2]

[1] Department of Surgery, Augusta University, Augusta, GA, USA
[2] Augusta University Medical Center, Augusta, GA, USA

1 *Which of the following patients does not have a diagnosis of acute kidney injury?*
   A *77-year-old man with an increase in serum creatinine from 1.4 to 1.7 mg/dL in the past 48 hours.*
   B *24-year-old man with a serum creatinine that increased from 0.7 to 1.5 mg/dL in the past 48 hours.*
   C *32-year-old woman with anuria for 12 hours.*
   D *58-year-old man started on renal replacement therapy 24 hours prior.*
   E *45-year-old woman with urine output < 0.5 mL/kg/hr × 5 hours after exploratory laparotomy.*

Acute kidney injury is diagnosed in patients based on creatinine elevation (≥ 0.3 mg/dL) from baseline over a 48-hr period or by a period of oliguria (≤ 0.5 mL/kg/hr) over 6 hours.

Patients with stage 2 acute kidney injury have a serum creatinine that have doubled in 48 hours or have oliguria for over 12 hours.

Patients with stage 3 acute kidney injury have a serum creatinine that has tripled from baseline in 48 hours or have oliguria (≤ 0.3 mL/kg/hr) for over 24 hours or anuria for 12 hours. Patients initiated on renal replacement therapy are categorized as stage 3 also.

The only patient that does not meet the definition is option E as she has only been oliguric for under 6 hours.

Answer: E

Kellum JA. (2015) Diagnostic criteria for acute kidney injury. *Critical Care Clinics*, 31(4) pp. 621–632.

Ostermann M and Joanniidis M (2016) Acute kidney injury 2016: diagnosis and diagnostic work-up. *Critical Care*, 20, pp. 1–13.

2 *Which of the following patients with acute kidney injury (AKI) would most benefit from continuous renal replacement therapy?*
   A *94-year-old woman with a recent diagnosis of stage 3 AKI and potassium level of 5.5 mEq/L, but with a good prognosis.*
   B *58-year-old man with stage 3 AKI that is resistant to diuretic administration and a potassium level of 6.2 mEq/L.*
   C *48-year-old man with traumatic brain injury that is in septic shock secondary to pneumonia and anuric for 24 hours with a creatinine level of 3.5 mg/dL*
   D *28-year-old woman recovering from intra-abdominal sepsis with stage 1 AKI with improving creatinine levels.*
   E *54-year-old woman with chronic kidney disease who recently underwent angiography for claudication workup and stage 1 AKI.*

Approximately one third of critically ill patients will develop acute kidney injury. Of these patients, 30–70% may require renal replacement therapy. As the development of acute kidney injury is strongly associated with mortality in the critically ill, it is important to determine the etiology and tailor management promptly. While the timing of renal replacement therapy remains controversial, the initiation of therapy for diuretic-resistant volume overload, acidosis, severe hyperkalemia, and severe uremia is agreed upon. Patients without these signs/symptoms or evidence of improving renal function do not require any form of renal replacement therapy.

The patients in options A, D, E do not meet the thresholds for any form of renal replacement therapy.

The patients in options B and C meet criteria for renal replacement therapy; however, the patient in option B could most likely tolerate intermittent hemodialysis versus the patient in option C with a traumatic brain injury who is not hemodynamically stable. Continuous renal replacement would produce less disequilibrium compared to intermittent therapy and thus less risk of having episodes of cerebral hypoperfusion.

Answer: C

KDIGO Clinical Practice Guideline for Acute Kidney Injury (2012) Kidney International Supplements, 2(1), http://www.kdigo.org/clincal_practice_guidelines/pdf/ KDIGO%20AKI%20Guideline.pdf.

Tandukar S and Palevsky PM. (2019) Continuous renal replacement therapy: who, when, why, how. *Chest*, 155(3), pp. 626–638.

3 *In a patient with chronic kidney disease undergoing angiography, which of the following is superior to intravenous saline alone to prevent contrast-induced acute kidney injury?*
   A *N-acetylcysteine*
   B *IV sodium bicarbonate*
   C *Ascorbic acid plus saline*
   D *N-acetylcysteine plus IV sodium bicarbonate*
   E *No additional treatment (IV saline alone)*

Contrast-induced acute kidney injury is a problem that is commonly seen in both the outpatient and inpatient setting. Many methods have been studied to counteract this phenomenon including the use of pharmacologic agents to reduce oxidative stress of the kidney to prevent the injury from occurring. Many studies have been performed to assess using ascorbic acid (scavenger of reactive oxygen species), N-acetylcysteine (antioxidant), and sodium bicarbonate (alkalinization to prevent production of free oxygen radicals), none of which were superior to using IV saline. There are some studies that show some promise with using saline plus N-acetylcysteine; however, a randomized control trial performed in 2018 showed no benefit with N-acetylcysteine over placebo for preventing contrast-induced acute kidney injury.

Answer: E

Subramaniam RM, Suarez-Cuervo C, Wilson RF, et al. (2016) Effectiveness of prevention strategies for contrast-induced nephropathy: a systematic review and meta-analysis. *Annals of Internal Medicine*, 164(6), pp. 406–416.

Weisbord SD, Gallagher M, Jneid H, et al. (2018) Outcomes after angiography with sodium bicarbonate and acetylcysteine. *New England Journal of Medicine*, 378, pp. 603–614.

4 *Which of the following is NOT considered a perioperative risk factor for developing acute kidney injury in patients who undergo cardiac surgery?*
   A *Poor glycemic control*
   B *Need for emergent re-operation*
   C *Male sex*
   D *Cardiopulmonary bypass use and duration*
   E *Baseline renal function*

Based on many observational studies, susceptibility factors (i.e. risk) have been noted across various study populations. Patient characteristics that leave patients susceptible for developing acute kidney injury in the perioperative period include dehydration, advanced age, female gender, black race, chronic kidney disease, anemia, and diabetes mellitus. Trauma, burns, major noncardiac surgery, cardiac surgery requiring cardiopulmonary bypass, need for emergent re-operation are additional risk factors. Interestingly, male sex is a risk factor for AKI in NON-cardiac surgery patients, but females are more likely to develop AKI if they are undergoing a cardiac surgery procedure.

Answer: C

Hobson C, Singhania G, Bihorac A. (2015) Acute kidney injury in the surgical patient. *Critical Care Clinics*, 31(4), pp. 705–723.

KDIGO Clinical Practice Guideline for Acute Kidney Injury (2012) Kidney International Supplements, 2(1), http://www.kdigo.org/clincal_practice_guidelines/pdf/ KDIGO%20AKI%20Guideline.pdf.

5 *The use of furosemide to increase urine output in patients who are developing acute kidney injury has been demonstrated to:*
   A *Improve mortality*
   B *Should be started early in the development of AKI*
   C *Decrease the likelihood of requiring renal replacement therapy*
   D *Needs to be administered in high doses to be effective*
   E *Have minimal-to-no impact on the need for renal replacement therapy*

Although furosemide has been prescribed for decades now to patients who develop acute kidney injury to try and convert them from oliguric AKI to non-oliguric AKI, there is little-to-no convincing evidence that this has any impact on the need for CRRT or survival. There are conflicting reports in the literature that it may in fact reduce survival, although in meta-analyses this effect does not seem to be borne out. There is no data to support the use of higher doses or the use of earlier administration to increase success rates. There is minimal evidence to support the routine use of furosemide in the care of patients with AKI.

Answer: E

Bove T, Belletti A, Putzu A et al. (2018) Intermittent furosemide administration in patients with or at risk for acute kidney injury: meta-analysis of randomized trials. *PLoS One*, 13(4), p. e0196088

Kryzych LJ and Czempik PF. (2019) Impact of furosemide on mortality and the requirement for renal replacement therapy in acute kidney injury: a systematic review and meta-analysis of randomized trials. *Annals of Intensive Care*, 9, p. 85

6 *Use of **early** renal replacement therapy versus **delayed** renal replacement therapy for the management of severe acute kidney injury will:*
A *Decrease ICU mortality*
B *Increase in-hospital mortality*
C *Decrease cost of managing patients with acute kidney injury*
D *Potentially decrease hospital length of stay*
E *Lead to an increased risk of dialysis dependence at the time of hospital discharge*

For some time, there was growing evidence that early initiation of early renal replacement therapy led to improved survival. However, a recent systematic review demonstrated that there was no significant difference in mortality, ICU length of stay, hospital length of stay, or need for hemodialysis at the time of hospital discharge when early renal replacement therapy was compared to delayed initiation. In light of these facts among others, it was concluded that there was no advantage to starting early renal replacement therapy, especially as there were some patients with severe acute kidney injury that never were initiated on renal replacement therapy. Research has not been able to demonstrate a significant difference in hospital length of stay; however, early initiation of therapy may be associated with a shorter hospital stay due to the ability of some centers having the ability to discharge patients to another level of care (i.e. LTAC or rehab).

Answer: D

Gaudry S, Hajage D, Benichou N, et al. (2020) Delayed versus early initiation of renal replacement therapy for severe acute kidney injury. *Lancet*, 395(10235), pp. 1506–1515.

7 *A 68-year-old man with a PMHx of hypertension, hyperlipidemia, and BPH is POD #2 after an incisional hernia repair. He is given a PCA post-op for analgesic control. The nurse calls you to inform you that the patient has not voided since his foley was removed 6 hours prior. Bladder scan is unable to fully assess the bladder. Which of the following would NOT be included in the initial work-up of this patient?*
A *Abdominal CT scan*
B *MR urography*
C *Rectal exam*
D *Replacement of the foley catheter*
E *Ultrasonography of the GU tract*

Replacing the foley catheter will relieve the urinary retention in addition to quantifying the amount of urine produced in the postoperative period while you are continuing your workup. A rectal examination allows you to evaluate the patient's prostate for hypertrophy or the presence of a prostate cancer. Ultrasonography of the GU tract is a common screening modality and is highly sensitive for detecting hydronephrosis. While not the first choice in the workup of the patient, a CT scan can provide additional information regarding the anatomy of the urinary tract that is not elucidated by ultrasonography, as well as evaluating for renal calculi. MR urography is a useful modality for the investigation of obstructive uropathy in the pediatric population and would not be in the initial workup algorithm for this patient

Answer: B

Frøkiaer J and Zeidel ML. (2012) Urinary tract obstruction, in *Brenner and Rector's The Kidney*, 9th edition (editors, MW Taal, GM Chertow, PA Marsden, et al.), W.B. Saunders, Philadelphia, PA, pp. 1383–1410.

Morin CE, McBee MP, Trout AT, et al. (2018) Use of MR urography in pediatric patients. *Current Urology Reports*,19(11), p. 93.

8 *Fractional excretion of sodium (FENa) is traditionally used to discriminate the etiology of acute kidney injury. Results can be compromised by many factors including medication use, comorbidities, etc. Which of the following conditions listed does NOT affect the results of a FENa test?*
A *Cirrhosis*
B *Diuretic use*
C *Renal transplant*
D *Congestive heart failure*
E *Sepsis*

FENa is the most discriminating test to aid the clinician in determining the etiology (prerenal vs intrinsic) of acute kidney injury. However, as noted by several studies, there are some limitations to its utility. Conditions that affect sodium excretions (e.g. diuretics), non-oliguric ATN, liver failure, sepsis, and low-output heart failure can affect the calculation. Assuming that a healthy graft is utilized, a renal transplant patient should have normal function.

Answer: C

Makris K and Spanou L. (2016) Acute kidney injury: diagnostic approaches and controversies. *Clinical Biochemist Reviews*, 37(4), pp. 153–175.

Perazella MA and Coca SG. (2012) Traditional urinary biomarkers in the assessment of hospital-acquired AKI. *Clinical Journal of the American Society of Nephrology*, 7, pp. 167–174.

9 *A 45-year-old woman has sustained a liver laceration (grade III) after a motor vehicle collision and undergoes embolization. On HD #2, her urine output has diminished to 0.4 mL/kg/hr the last 12 hours. In trying to determine the etiology of her acute kidney injury, which of the following is NOT TRUE regarding the use of urinary biochemistry?*

A *FEUrea value is not affected by diuretic use.*
B *FEUrea < 35% is indicative of prerenal acute kidney injury.*
C *Sepsis can affect the FENa and FEUrea values.*
D *FEUrea is superior compared to FENa.*
E *A urine sodium concentration greater than 40 mEq/L occurs in ATN.*

Urea resorption occurs in the proximal segment of the nephron; thus, diuretics do not affect the FEUrea measurement due to their function distal to the proximal tubule. When FEUrea is utilized, a measurement that is <35% is indicative of prerenal azotemia. While it was initially believed that FEUrea was fairly reliable compared to FENa due to all of the conditions that can affect the FENa calculations, recent studies have shown that FEUrea is altered in the setting of advanced age and sepsis. Studies have also shown that FEUrea was shown to be discordant in critically ill patients. To date, there are no studies showing FEUrea superiority over FENa.

Urine sodium concentration > 40 mEq/L is consistent with ATN.

Answer: D

Makris K and Spanou L. (2016) Acute kidney injury: diagnostic approaches and controversies. *Clinical Biochemist Reviews*, 37(4), pp. 153–175.

Perazella MA and Coca SG. (2012) Traditional urinary biomarkers in the assessment of hospital-acquired AKI. *Clinical Journal of the American Society of Nephrology*, 7, pp. 167–174.

10 *A 48-year-old man comes into the trauma room after his thigh was crushed by a tree trunk falling onto it 4 hours prior. He complains of pain in his thigh and numbness in his leg extending from his knee distally to his foot. Laboratory studies are consistent with a diagnosis of rhabdomyolysis. Which of the following does not help prevent acute kidney injury progression?*

A *Aggressive hydration*
B *Administration of sodium bicarbonate*
C *Fasciotomy*
D *Prevention of renal hypoperfusion*
E *Elimination of drugs that lead to rhabdomyolysis*

Rhabdomyolysis is a complex medical condition secondary to the direct release of intracellular muscle components into the bloodstream and extracellular space from the damaged skeletal muscle. Acute kidney injury is a complication that can occur in about 33% of patients with rhabdomyolysis. As such, it is important that management includes maneuvers to prevent the progression to acute kidney injury such as aggressive fluid resuscitation, discontinuation of medications that cause rhabdomyolysis, discontinuation of nephrotoxic agents, and fasciotomy of involved extremity to limit progression of muscle damage. Urinary alkalinization with either sodium bicarbonate or sodium acetate has not been shown to prevent acute kidney injury progression, reduce the need for hemodialysis or decrease mortality.

Answer: B

Brown CV, Rhee P, Chan L, et al. (2004) Preventing renal failure in patients with rhabdomyolysis: do bicarbonate and mannitol make a difference? *Journal of Trauma*, 56(6), pp. 1191–1196.

Somagutta MR, Pagad S, Sridharan S, et al. (2020) Role of Bicarbonates and mannitol in rhabdomyolysis: a comprehensive review. *Cureus*, 12(8), p. e9742.

Torres PA, Helmstetter JA, Kaye AM, et al. (2015) Rhabdomyolysis: pathogenesis, diagnosis, and treatment. *The Oschsner Journal*, 15, pp. 58–69.

11 *Which of the following statements is correct regarding the use of diuretics in acute kidney injury?*

A *Utilizing furosemide as a continuous infusion (0.5 mg/kg/hr) is not associated with ototoxicity.*
B *Mannitol decreases the incidence of renal dysfunction by increasing urine output.*
C *Furosemide converts patients from an oliguric to non-oliguric state, which is associated with a decreased number of hemodialysis sessions if hemodialysis is needed.*
D *Administration of furosemide for acute kidney injury is associated with increased mortality.*
E *Administration of mannitol is comparable to saline in decreasing incidence of renal dysfunction.*

Volume overload is commonly seen in patients with acute kidney injury. In recent observational studies, it was noted that 59–70% patients received diuretics prior to being placed on renal replacement therapy in an attempt to remove this volume. Additionally, oliguric acute kidney injury has worse prognosis compared to non-oliguric patients, hence why diuretics are frequently prescribed. However, there was no difference in the number of hemodialysis sessions or mortality when diuretics were administered versus not administered. A downside of furosemide in particular is the development of ototoxicity at high doses. But when it was administered at a continuous infusion (0.5 mg/kg/hr), it was not associated with this side effect. Diuretic administration to prevent acute kidney is not supported in the literature and is noted to actually cause harm.

Mannitol, when administered, increases urine output; however, there is no data to support decreases in renal dysfunction. In fact, of the little data published, mannitol usage in diabetic patients leads to a higher incidence of renal dysfunction compared to saline alone.

Answer: A

KDIGO Clinical Practice Guideline for Acute Kidney Injury (2012) Kidney International Supplements, 2(1), http://www.kdigo.org/clincal_practice_guidelines/pdf/KDIGO%20AKI%20Guideline.pdf.

Van der Voort PH, Boerma EC, Koopman M, et al. (2009) Furosemide does not improve renal recovery after hemofiltration for acute renal failure in critically ill patients: a double blind randomized controlled trial. *Critical Care Medicine*, 37, pp. 533–538.

Wilczynski JA, Decaro MV, Marhefka GD, et al. (2020) Very high-dose furosemide continuous infusions: a case series. *Journal of Cardiac Failure*, 26(9), pp. 794–797.

12 *When vasodilators are used in the management of acute kidney injury, which of the following is true?*
   A *Dopamine has been shown to effectively reduce the need for renal replacement therapy.*
   B *Dopamine doesn't cause tachyarrhythmias at a rate of 3 mg/kg/min.*
   C *Patients given fenoldopam had a lower rate of developing acute kidney injury compared to dopamine.*
   D *Fenoldopam has minimal effect on blood pressure when targeted for acute kidney injury prevention.*
   E *Dopamine does not have an effect on intestinal blood flow.*

Both dopamine and fenoldopam were initially believed to be renal protective against acute kidney injury due to their effect on dopamine receptors leading to natriuresis. However, there have been multiple studies that have demonstrated that low-dose dopamine had no effect on renal function, need for dialysis, ICU length of stay, hospital length of stay, or mortality. Additionally, low-dose dopamine can trigger tachyarrhythmias and myocardial ischemia along with decreasing intestinal blood flow. Fenoldopam is a dopamine agonist that does not have systemic α- or β-adrenergic stimulation but has vasodilatory effects. There have been several studies that show that fenoldopam improves renal function when compared to dopamine; however, it is not recommended in the KDIGO guideline due to the trend of hypotension in the fenoldopam treatment group.

Answer: C

Gillies MA, Kakar V, and Parker RJ. (2015) Fenoldopam to prevent acute kidney injury after major surgery-a systematic review and meta-analysis. *Critical Care*, 19, p. 449.

KDIGO Clinical Practice Guideline for Acute Kidney Injury (2012) Kidney International Supplements, 2(1), http://www.kdigo.org/clincal_practice_guidelines/pdf/KDIGO%20AKI%20Guideline.pdf.

13 *In a patient with hyperkalemia, which treatments listed below will eliminate potassium from the body quickly?*
   A *IV insulin and glucose*
   B *Albuterol*
   C *Sodium zirconium cyclosilicate*
   D *Calcium chloride*
   E *IV furosemide*

Calcium chloride, while commonly given in the setting of hyperkalemia, is used for stabilization of the myocardium and thus decreasing the risk of developing ventricular arrhythmias. It is indicated when ECG changes are present.

IV insulin and albuterol have similar effect and onset of action. When administered, potassium shifts from the extracellular space to the intracellular space and thus decreases potassium levels. No potassium is eliminated from the body.

Sodium zirconium cyclosilicate and IV furosemide however eliminate potassium from the body through the GI tract and renally, respectively; however, potassium is eliminated from the body faster with IV furosemide compared to sodium zirconium cyclosilicate orally.

Answer: E

Garth D. (2011) Hyperkalemia in emergency medicine. eMedicine at Medscape.com: http://emedicine.medscape.com/article/766479-overview

Sterns RH, Grieff M, and Bernstein PL. (2016) Treatment of hyperkalemia: something old, something new. *Kidney International*, 89(3), pp. 546–554.

14 *A 62-year-old man is POD #1 after an open repair of a ruptured AAA. Patient is noted to be oliguric for the past 12 hours. Which of the following laboratory studies indicates a prerenal etiology?*
   A *BUN/Cr ratio of 18*
   B *The presence of granular casts in the urine*
   C *Urine osmolality of 100 mOsm/L*
   D *Urine sodium level of 12 mEq/L*
   E *FENa of 4%*

Determining the etiology of acute kidney injury can be difficult to distinguish in a critically ill patient. To aid with this diagnosis, urinary studies are often used. In patients with prerenal azotemia, the BUN/Cr ratio will typically be above 20 although this sharp cutoff has been called into question, as this variable more likely represents a continuum (see references). Nevertheless, higher BUN/Cr ratio is still considered indicative of a prerenal etiology for AKI. The presence of granular casts is seen in the setting of intrinsic causes of acute kidney injury. In prerenal AKI, the patient will also have an elevated urine osmolality (> 500 mOsm/kg), a low urine sodium (< 20 mEq/L), and a low FENa (< 1%) is usually seen.

Answer: D

Manoeuvrier G, Bach-Ngohou K, Batard E, et al. (2017) Diagnostic performance of serum blood urea nitrogen to creatinine ratio for distinguishing prerenal from intrinsic acute kidney injury in the emergency department. *BMC Nephrology*, 18(1), p. 173.

Ostermann M and Joannidis M. (2016) Acute kidney injury 2016: diagnosis and diagnostic workup. *Critical Care*, 20, p. 299.

Uchino S, Bellomo R, and Goldsmith D. (2012) The meaning of the blood urea nitrogen/creatinine ratio in acute kidney injury. *Clinical Kidney Journal*, 5(2), pp. 187–191.

15 *Which of the following is correct regarding nutritional support in patients with acute kidney injury?*
   A *Protein needs are the same regardless of need for renal replacement therapy.*
   B *The amount of nitrogen given daily should be decreased.*
   C *Total caloric intake should be no more than 25–30 kcal/kg/day.*
   D *Parenteral route is preferred over enteral route when continuous renal replacement therapy is used due to high protein loss.*
   E *High caloric intake should be administered in these patients due to increase in energy expenditure.*

Nutritional management is a multidisciplinary effort with acute kidney injury, especially in patient who are critically ill. Additionally, protein-calorie malnutrition is an independent predictor of in-hospital mortality in patients with acute kidney injury.

The amount of protein should not be restricted in these patients. Critically ill patients tend to have protein hypercatabolism due to inflammation, stress, and acidosis. As such, critically ill patients with acute kidney injury should have sufficient protein intake to maintain a metabolic balance. Additionally, the patient's protein needs vary depending on catabolic state or if the patient requires renal replacement therapy. Protein needs are generally higher in patients requiring dialysis or catabolic.

Energy consumption is not increased in this patient population. The goal of nutritional support is not to be in a negative nitrogen balance. Total caloric intake should be no more than 25–30 kcal/kg/day. It has been noted in some studies that achieving a caloric intake higher than this leads to a higher incidence of hyperglycemia, hypertriglyceridemia, and positive fluid balance.

Enteral feeding is the preferred route, even in the setting of continuous renal replacement. There is no data to support a parenteral route over enteral.

Answer: C

KDIGO Clinical Practice Guideline for Acute Kidney Injury (2012) Kidney International Supplements, 2(1), http://www.kdigo.org/clincal_practice_guidelines/pdf/KDIGO%20AKI%20Guideline.pdf.

McClave SA, Taylor BE, Martindale RG, et al. (2016) Guidelines for the provision and assessment of nutrition support therapy in the adult critically ill patient: Society of Critical Care Medicine (SCCM) and American Society for Parenteral and Enteral Nutrition (A.S.P.E.N.). *Journal of Parenteral Nutrition*, 40(2), pp. 159–211.

16 *A 39-year-old woman is being treated for sepsis from an intra-abdominal source. She has anuric for the last 12 hours and is about to be started on continuous renal replacement therapy. Which of the following strategies will NOT increase the survival of the filter?*
   A *Good vascular access*
   B *Regional sodium citrate use*
   C *Reduction of air-blood contact in the bubble trap*
   D *Routine use of saline flushes*
   E *High flow rates*

In patients requiring renal replacement therapy, patients are at risk for clotting the filter due to the activation of both the intrinsic and extrinsic pathways of the coagulation cascade by blood contacting the extracorporeal circuit. In order to prolong the filter in the circuit, systemic anticoagulants have been used in addition to regional sodium citrate use. Non-anticoagulant strategies used to prolong filter survival include high flow rates, having good functioning vascular access, reduction of blood–air contact in the bubble trap, and prompt reaction to alarms on the dialysis machine. Routine use of saline flushes does not increase filter survival.

Answer: D

Brain M, Winson E, Roodenburg O, et al. (2017) Non anti-coagulant factors associated with filter life in continuous renal replacement therapy (CRRT): a systematic review and meta-analysis. *BMC Nephrology*, 18(1), p. 69.

KDIGO Clinical Practice Guideline for Acute Kidney Injury (2012) Kidney International Supplements, 2(1), http://www.kdigo.org/clincal_practice_guidelines/pdf/KDIGO%20AKI%20Guideline.pdf.

17 Which of the following statements is CORRECT regarding patients on continuous renal replacement therapy utilizing sodium citrate as an anticoagulant?

A They have the same risk of hemorrhage as patients on systemic anticoagulation.

B Less monitoring requirements for titration compared to patients on systemic anticoagulation.

C A higher risk of metabolic derangements in the setting of impaired hepatic function.

D A higher incidence of filter failure compared to patients on systemic anticoagulation.

E A need for calcium replacement requiring monitoring.

Sodium citrate is the preferred anticoagulant utilized to increase the survival of the filter. In multiple studies, citrate was superior compared to systemic anticoagulation for filter survival.

Sodium citrate provides anticoagulation by forming a complex with ionized calcium, an essential component of the coagulation cascade, from circulation. If citrate reaches systemic circulation, it is metabolized in the liver releasing calcium and forming bicarbonate. Since it is administered regionally, there is a reduced risk of bleeding compared to systemic anticoagulation. However, due to extracorporeal calcium losses, exogenous calcium infusion should be part of the protocol for continuous renal replacement therapy. While there is monitoring of calcium levels, the citrate itself doesn't require monitoring compared to unfractionated or low-molecular-weight heparins. Due to the risk of citrate reaching systemic circulation, its use is contraindicated in patients with severely impaired liver function or shock with muscle

hypoperfusion. This is due to citrate accumulation leading to lower calcium levels from chelation.

Answer: C

KDIGO Clinical Practice Guideline for Acute Kidney Injury (2012) Kidney International Supplements, 2(1), http://www.kdigo.org/clincal_practice_guidelines/pdf/KDIGO%20AKI%20Guideline.pdf.

Kindgen-Milles D, Brandenburger T, Dimski T. (2018) Regional citrate anticoagulation for continuous renal replacement therapy. *Current Opinion in Critical Care*, 24(6), pp. 450–454.

Stucker F, Ponte B, Tataw J, et al. (2015) Efficacy and safety of citrate-based anticoagulation compared to heparin in patients with acute kidney injury requiring continuous renal replacement therapy: a randomized controlled trial. *Critical Care*, 19(1), p. 91.

18 A 22-year-old woman is admitted to the ICU for declining respiratory status due to a recently diagnosed pneumonia. It appears to be only susceptible to aminoglycosides. Which of the following is true regarding the use of aminoglycosides?

A Nephrotoxicity is only concerning in patients who are critically ill.

B Local (inhaled) administration has a lower rate of nephrotoxicity compared to systemic (intravenous) administration.

C Single-dose daily regimens are preferable compared to multiple daily-doses in the critically ill.

D Daily-dose regiments do not require monitoring.

E Peak levels are used to assess aminoglycoside accumulation to minimize risk of acute kidney injury.

Aminoglycosides are bactericidal antibiotics that remain effective against gram-negative bacteria and selected gram-positive bacteria. Despite their many favorable attributes, nephrotoxicity, ototoxicity, and neuromuscular blockade are the downsides of their use, in both critically ill patients and those with normal renal function. They can be administered as a single-dose daily regimen or as a multiple-dose daily regimen. In patients with steady state and normal renal function, a single-dose daily regimen is recommended to minimize toxicity. However, in critically ill patients, a multiple-dose daily regimen is recommended due to the changing pharmacokinetics and pharmacodynamics in this patient population. Regardless of dose regimen, monitoring of serum levels is required, and for maximal effectiveness, peak levels should be 10-fold greater than the MIC. Trough levels are used to monitor for medication accumulation, which is highly associated with nephrotoxicity. Local administration of aminoglycosides (such as to the lungs via the inhaled route) provides high levels of the antibiotic with minimal systemic concentration compared to systemic administration.

Answer: B

Avent ML, Rogers BA, Cheng AC, et al. (2011) Current use of aminoglycosides: indications, pharmacokinetics and monitoring for toxicity. *Internal Medicine Journal*, 41(6), pp. 441–449.

KDIGO Clinical Practice Guideline for Acute Kidney Injury (2012) Kidney International Supplements, 2(1), http://www.kdigo.org/clincal_practice_guidelines/pdf/KDIGO%20AKI%20Guideline.pdf.

Paquette F, Bernier-Jean A, Brunette V, et al. (2015) Acute kidney injury and renal recovery with the use of aminoglycosides: a large retrospective study. Nephron, 131(3), pp. 153–160.

19 *In a patient with severe hyperkalemia (potassium > 6.5mEq/dL) and widened QRS complexes, which of the following is the BEST treatment algorithm?*

  A *Inhaled albuterol, intravenous bicarbonate, and dialysis*

  B *Intravenous calcium gluconate, inhaled albuterol, intravenous insulin and glucose, with furosemide if the potassium remains above 6.0 mEq/dL*

  C *Intravenous sodium bicarbonate, inhaled albuterol, followed by kayexalate*

  D *Intravenous calcium gluconate, Intravenous insulin and glucose, and dialysis*

  E *Inhaled albuterol, kayexalate, and intravenous furosemide*

While all the medications listed above are effective in lowering the potassium levels, the fact that the patient has an EKG with widened QRS complexes is concerning and mandates rapid treatment. Calcium gluconate will have the most rapid effect by stabilizing the myocardium, decreasing the risk of arrhythmias. It is usually only indicated when EKG changes are present. Intravenous insulin will drive potassium back into the cells and the effects occur within 30 minutes of administration. Glucose is given simultaneously to prevent hypoglycemia. Albuterol has a similar effect and onset of action as that of intravenous insulin. Sodium bicarbonate raises pH, which results in potassium shifts into the intracellular space. Furosemide can be effective by inducing potassium loss through the kidney if the patient can still make urine, but the onset of action is slower, and large doses may be needed in AKI. Dialysis may indeed be necessary but will usually require placement of a dedicated intravenous catheter to be performed and usually is reserved for those patients in which the above measures are not effective.

Answer: B

Lindner G, Burdmann E, Clase C, et al. (2020) Acute hyperkalemia in the emergency department: a summary from a kidney disease: improving global outcomes conference. *European Journal of Emergency Medicine*, 27(5)–, pp. 329–337.

Palmer BF, Carrero JJ, Clegg DJ, et al. (2020) Clinical management of hyperkalemia. *Mayo Clinic Proceedings*, S0025-6196(20), p. 30618-2.

20 *Which of the following is CORRECT regarding the use of pharmacologic agents to treat acute kidney injury?*

  A *Dopamine has been shown to improve urine output and decrease the need for dialysis.*

  B *Fenoldopam is only effective in treating contrast-induced nephropathy.*

  C *Steroids can be useful in patients with AKI secondary to glomerulonephritis.*

  D *Activated protein C was highly effective in reversing AKI in sepsis.*

  E *Levosimendan is effective in reducing the risk of AKI after cardiac surgery.*

The search for effective pharmacologic agents that can ameliorate or reverse AKI has continued for a long time, with no clear effective agents. Both dopamine and fenoldopam, although initially felt to be promising, have been shown conclusively to have no effect on survival or the need for renal replacement therapy. Steroids have a specific indication in the treatment of rapidly deteriorating AKI due to glomerulonephritis and should be considered only in those circumstances. Although Xigris or activated protein C was seen anecdotally to improve renal function in patients with sepsis, overall this agent was ineffective in treating sepsis and came with a poor risk–benefit ratio and has been discontinued since 2011. While levosimendan has been investigated as an inotropic agent in patients at risk undergoing cardiac surgery, there is little conclusive evidence in its favor. There are multiple agents currently being developed, but no specific pharmacological agent that is approved for use in AKI at this time.

Answer: C

Hulse M and Rosner MH. (2019) Drugs in development for acute kidney injury. *Drugs*, 79, pp. 811–821.

Kyung Jo S, Rosner MH, and Okusa MD. (2007) Pharmacologic treatment of acute kidney injury: why drugs haven't worked and what is on the horizon. *CJASN*, 2(2), pp. 356–365.

18

Liver Failure

Bellal Joseph, MD[1] and Omar Obaid, MD[2]

[1] Division of Trauma, Surgical Critical Care, Burns and Acute Care Surgery, University of Arizona College of Medicine, Banner University Medical Center, Tucson, AZ, USA
[2] Division of Trauma, Critical Care, Burns, and Emergency Surgery, Department of Surgery, University of Arizona, Tucson, AZ, USA

The following vignette applies to questions 1–6

A 40-year-old man presents to the emergency department complaining of severe abdominal pain, nausea, and intractable vomiting for the last 8 hours. The most recent vomitus contained blood and bile-stained fluid. He is somnolent and markedly jaundiced. His wife says that they recently had a major disagreement and a few hours later she found him writhing in pain on the bathroom floor, with 3 unmarked pill bottles lying empty nearby. After much counseling, the patient finally agrees to have his blood taken for some tests.

Question 1:

His LFTs are in the 1000s IU/L and his INR is 3.2. He has no prior history of liver disease. What is the definition of acute liver failure?

A *Signs of severe liver injury, encephalopathy, and impaired liver synthetic function (INR greater than 1.5), with the onset of range of symptoms occurring in less than 26 weeks, in a patient without pre-existing liver disease or cirrhosis.*

B *Signs of severe liver injury, renal failure, and portal hypertension, with the onset of range of symptoms occurring in less than 12 weeks, in a patient without pre-existing liver disease or cirrhosis.*

C *Mixed hyperbilirubinemia, AST and ALT levels greater than 500 IU/L, and signs of cardiogenic shock, with the onset of range of symptoms occurring*

in less than 12 weeks, in a patient without pre-existing liver disease or cirrhosis.

D *The onset of acute encephalopathy in cirrhotic patients with impaired liver function tests, with the onset of worsening symptoms occurring over more than 26 weeks.*

E *None of the above.*

Question 2:

In the developed world, what is the most common cause of drug-induced acute liver failure?

A *Antituberculous drugs, such as isoniazid*
B *Antiretroviral drugs, such as didanosine*
C *Lipid-lowering medications, such as statins*
D *Acetaminophen*
E *Antiepileptic drugs, such as valproic acid*

Acute liver failure (ALF) is a rare but life-threatening disease. The most widely accepted definition of ALF is signs of acute severe liver injury (such as hyperbilirubinemia, and markedly raised LFTs), an abnormal liver synthetic function (such as an INR ≥ 1.5), and any degree of encephalopathy in a patient without cirrhosis or pre-existing liver disease. The timeframe for ALF is less than 26 weeks for the development of the full range of symptoms and signs. If it occurs over a longer period, it is characterized as chronic liver failure (CLF). ALF may then be further subdivided into hyperacute (< 7 days), acute (7–21 days), and subacute (> 21 days but < 26 weeks). Although there may additionally be signs and symptoms of renal failure (due to hepatorenal syndrome) or cardiogenic shock (as ALF frequently leads to multi-organ failure), the presence of encephalopathy is a cornerstone of diagnosis. Cirrhosis, pre-existing liver disease, and portal hypertension are all inconsistent with a diagnosis of ALF. The exceptions to this strict definition of ALF include patients with Wilson disease, vertically acquired hepatitis B virus, and Budd-Chiari syndrome where there is underlying cirrhosis or liver disease; illness duration has been less than 26 weeks overall. Hyperbilirubinemia and deranged LFTs are markers of severe liver injury, but are not prerequisites for a diagnosis.

This patient has taken a large number of unknown pills; however, in the *developed* world, the most common cause of drug-induced, and indeed of all causes of ALF, is acetaminophen toxicity. Although the other options are all possible causes of drug-induced ALF, they are not as common as acetaminophen. Conversely, in the *developing* world, virus-induced ALF has been implicated as the most common cause of ALF, particularly hepatitis B virus (HBV).

Q1 Answer: A

Q2 Answer: D

Bernal W, Auzinger G, Dhawan A, Wendon J. Acute liver failure. *The Lancet* 2010;376(9736):190–201.

Khan R, and Koppe S. Modern management of acute liver failure. *Gastroenterology Clinics* 2018;47(2):313–326.

Lee WM, Larson AM, and Stravitz RT. AASLD position paper: the management of acute liver failure: update 2011. *Hepatology* 2011;55(55):965–967.

Question 3:

Regarding N-acetylcysteine:
- A *Its use is not recommended for acute liver failure.*
- B *Its use is only recommended for acetaminophen-induced liver failure.*
- C *Its use is especially recommended in acetaminophen-induced liver failure but also provides a survival benefit in other causes of acute liver failure if administered before the onset of advanced encephalopathy.*
- D *Its use is recommended for all causes of acute liver failure and should be prescribed for up to 10 days.*
- E *Its main mechanism of action is to act as a pro-inflammatory agent that supports the immune system and prevents nosocomial infections in patients with acute liver failure.*

N-acetylcysteine acts by replenishing reduced glutathione stores in the liver and has general anti-inflammatory properties. The replenishment of reduced glutathione in the liver counteracts the depletion caused by toxic metabolites of acetaminophen, and the anti-inflammatory properties aid in reducing the cytokine surge and inflammation associated with ALF. Although especially beneficial in cases of acetaminophen-induced ALF, its use is also recommended in all other causes of ALF, as long as advanced (grade III or IV) encephalopathy has not yet developed. It may only be prescribed for up to 5 days, as there is a risk of significant immunosuppression due to its anti-inflammatory properties.

Answer: C

Albalawi MA, Albalawi SA, Albalawi THS, Almuhawwis KS, Alswilem AM, Aldakhil F, et al. Evaluation of recent updates regarding acetaminophen-induced acute liver failure. *Archives of Pharmacy Practice* 2019;1:56.

Lee WM, Hynan LS, Rossaro L, Fontana RJ, Stravitz RT, Larson AM, et al. Intravenous N-acetylcysteine improves transplant-free survival in early stage non-acetaminophen acute liver failure. *Gastroenterology* 2009;137(3):856–864.e1.

Smilkstein MJ, Knapp GL, Kulig KW, Rumack BH. Efficacy of oral N-acetylcysteine in the treatment of acetaminophen overdose. *New England Journal of Medicine* 1988;319(24):1557–1562.

Question 4:

The patient is diagnosed with acute liver failure. He becomes unconscious and unresponsive. His blood test reveals very high levels of acetaminophen. He is intubated, mechanically ventilated, and given IV fluids and N-acetylcysteine. His right pupil is dilated and nonreactive. The attending physician is concerned about raised ICP in this patient. Which of the following indicate a higher risk for intracranial hypertension in a patient with acute liver failure?
- A *Shorter symptom-to-encephalopathy interval, and higher grades of encephalopathy*
- B *Younger age and vasopressors*
- C *Renal impairment*
- D *Sustained arterial ammonia of greater than 150–200 μmol/L*
- E *All of the above*

Question 5:

Regarding possible intracranial hypertension in this patient:
- A *An ICP monitor should be placed to quantitatively measure the ICP.*
- B *He should be given barbiturates to induce a coma.*
- C *He should be given corticosteroids to reduce cerebral vasogenic edema.*
- D *He should be hyperventilated and given either mannitol or hypertonic saline.*
- E *All of the above are appropriate.*

Patients with ALF are at high risk for intracranial hypertension. There is a strong body of evidence that suggests raised ammonia levels in ALF cause encephalopathy, cerebral edema, and subsequent intracranial hypertension. Although invasive intracranial ICP monitoring is often recommended for other patients with raised ICP, it is not usually recommended in patients with ALF due to their poor coagulation status and the risk of an intracranial bleed. In addition, barbiturate coma induction would also be unwise as it would worsen encephalopathy. Although corticosteroids are routinely administered to reduce vasogenic edema in infectious and malignant causes of intracranial hypertension, they are not routinely recommended in ALF because of the immunosuppression associated with their use and a lack of survival benefit. The only exception to the use of corticosteroids to treat intracranial hypertension in ALF is when the cause of ALF is biopsy- or biomarker-proven autoimmune hepatitis. Hypertonic saline and mannitol are optimal for treating intracranial hypertension in ALF, especially hypertonic saline as ALF patients are often hyponatremic. Hyperventilation is a temporizing measure as its effects on ICP do not last longer than 3–6 hours. Therapeutic hypothermia and propofol sedation can also help improve ICP and stabilize the patient for liver transplantation.

A 2007 prospective study on 265 ALF patients admitted to a specialized Liver Intensive Therapy Unit (LITU) concluded that shorter symptom-to-encephalopathy interval, higher grades of encephalopathy, younger age, a requirement for vasopressors, renal impairment, sustained arterial ammonia greater than 150–200 μmol/L all were independently associated with a higher risk of developing intracranial hypertension in ALF patients.

Q4 Answer: E

Q5 Answer: D

Bernal W, Auzinger G, Dhawan A, Wendon J. Acute liver failure. *The Lancet* 2010;376(9736):190–201.

Bernal W, Hall C, Karvellas CJ, Auzinger G, Sizer E, Wendon J. Arterial ammonia and clinical risk factors for encephalopathy and intracranial hypertension in acute liver failure. *Hepatology* 2007;46(6):1844–1852.

Lee WM, Larson AM, Stravitz RT. AASLD position paper: the management of acute liver failure: update 2011. *Hepatology* 2011;55(55):965–967.

Maher SZ and Schreibman IR. The clinical spectrum and manifestations of acute liver failure. *Clinics in Liver Disease* 2018;22(2):361–374.

Mohsenin V. Assessment and management of cerebral edema and intracranial hypertension in acute liver failure. *Journal of Critical Care* 2013;28(5):783–791.

Question 6:

The patient is no longer having any ongoing bleeding. However, his INR is still 3.2. There are no invasive procedures planned for the patient currently. With regards to his coagulation status, what should the next step in management be?

A *Subcutaneous vitamin K infusion*
B *Fresh frozen plasma transfusion*
C *Prothrombin complex concentrate transfusion*
D *Recombinant factor VIIa infusion*
E *Platelet transfusion*

In a recent update, the American Association for the Study of Liver Diseases (AASLD) recommended 5–10 mg of subcutaneous vitamin K administration for all patients with ALF, as coagulopathy remains a cornerstone of diagnosis. Although platelet and coagulation factor levels (especially factor VIIa) are commonly deranged in ALF, the routine use of platelet, fresh frozen plasma, prothrombin complex concentrate, or recombinant factor VIIa transfusion is not recommended unless there is ongoing bleeding, platelet counts are less than 10,000/mm^3, or if there is an invasive procedure planned. The risk of transfusion-related acute lung injury and volume overload must be avoided in patients with ALF.

Answer: A

Flamm SL, Yang Y-X, Singh S, Falck-Ytter YT, Lim JK, Rubenstein JH, et al. American Gastroenterological Association Institute guidelines for the diagnosis and management of acute liver failure. *Gastroenterology* 2017;152(3):644–647.

Lee WM, Larson AM, Stravitz RT. AASLD position paper: the management of acute liver failure: update 2011. *Hepatology* 2011;55(55):965–967.

Munoz SJ, Stravitz RT, Gabriel DA. Coagulopathy of acute liver failure. *Clinics in Liver Disease* 2009;13(1):95–107.

Pereira SP, Rowbotham D, Fitt S, Shearer MJ, Wendon J, Williams R. Pharmacokinetics and efficacy of oral versus intravenous mixed-micellar phylloquinone (vitamin K1) in severe acute liver disease. *Journal of Hepatology* 2005;42(3):365–370.

Question 7:

A 25-year-old woman has been admitted to the ICU after becoming severely ill within 4 hours of picking and consuming some mushrooms from the woods near her house in San Francisco. She was diagnosed with Amanita phalloides mushroom poisoning. Which of the following is a promising new treatment option for this condition?

A *Ribavirin*
B *Glutathione*
C *IV vitamin C*
D *IV silibinin*
E *IV sodium gluconate*

Intravenous silibinin (also known as milk thistle or silymarin) is an experimental treatment option currently being investigated by the FDA for the treatment of mushroom-induced ALF. It has already been approved for use in Europe and treatment can be obtained free of charge in the US if the patient enrolls in the current trial. Moreover, the AASLD recommends the addition of penicillin G and N-acetylcysteine to the management plan of such patients.

Answer: D

Hruby K, Csomos G, Fuhrmann M, Thaler H. Chemotherapy of Amanita phalloides poisoning with intravenous silibinin. *Human Toxicology* 1983;2(2):183–195.

Khan R and Koppe S. Modern management of acute liver failure. *Gastroenterology Clinics* 2018;47(2):313–326.

Lee WM, Larson AM, Stravitz RT. AASLD position paper: the management of acute liver failure: update 2011. *Hepatology* 2011;55(55):965–967.

Question 8:

High serum ammonia levels in ALF have been implicated in the pathogenesis of hepatic encephalopathy, cerebral edema, and intracranial hypertension. Lactulose and rifaximin are commonly used to reduce levels of serum ammonia by decreasing bacterial ammonia load that is absorbed by the patient's gastrointestinal tract. Which of the following is a major concern when administering lactulose or rifaximin to patients with ALF?

A *Rifaximin may worsen hepatorenal syndrome in ALF.*

B *Lactulose may get absorbed systemically and cause cardiac arrhythmias.*

C *Lactulose may lead to diarrhea and ileus.*

D *Rifaximin may disrupt the gut microbiome.*

E *Lactulose and rifaximin can be used indiscriminately in patients with ALF.*

The American Association for the Study of Liver Diseases (AASLD) recommends that in patients with ALF, during "early stages of encephalopathy, lactulose may be used either orally or rectally to effect a bowel purge, but should not be administered to the point of diarrhea, and may interfere with the surgical field by increasing bowel distention during liver transplantation." Since patients with ALF frequently require liver transplantation, lactulose must be used with caution. Ileus and abdominal distension due to lactulose overuse can lead to significant difficulties during abdominal surgeries. Rifaximin has not been known to worsen hepatorenal syndrome. While the chronic use of rifaximin may lead to disruption of gut microbiome as with most antibiotics, it would not be a major concern in patients with ALF. Lactulose is not absorbed systemically.

Answer: C

Flamm SL, Yang Y-X, Singh S, Falck-Ytter YT, Lim JK, Rubenstein JH, et al. American Gastroenterological Association Institute guidelines for the diagnosis and management of acute liver failure. *Gastroenterology* 2017;152(3):644–647.

Lee WM, Larson AM, Stravitz RT. AASLD position paper: the management of acute liver failure: update 2011. *Hepatology* 2011;55(55):965–967.

Question 9:

A 25-year-old college student is admitted to the ICU after being diagnosed with acute hepatitis B virus infection-induced acute liver failure. He is somnolent and lethargic but momentarily becomes alert and aggressive. He is not oriented to person, place, or time. His speech is slurred, and he has noticeable nystagmus. He follows the resident's command and extends his arms and hands outward, which start flapping uncontrollably. According to the West Haven criteria, how severe is this patient's hepatic encephalopathy?

A *Grade I*

B *Grade II*

C *Grade III*

D *Grade IV*

E *Grade V*

The West Haven criteria were developed for grading hepatic encephalopathy in chronic liver failure and cirrhosis. However, they are frequently employed in assessing the central neurologic status of ALF patients as well. This patient fits into West Haven Grade III encephalopathy, as he is not yet comatose but is markedly somnolent, still occasionally responds to commands, is grossly disoriented and confused, and demonstrates asterixis (flapping of outstretched hands). There are only four grades of encephalopathy in this system.

Hepatic encephalopathy grade	Signs and symptoms
I	Sleep disturbance
	Mild confusion
	Impaired cognition
	Elevated or depressed mood
	Tremors
II	Moderate confusion
	Disorientation only to time
	Irritability and personality changes
	Slurred speech, impaired handwriting

Hepatic encephalopathy grade	Signs and symptoms
III	Marked confusion
	Disoriented to time, place, and person
	Lethargic, somnolent, but arousable and still able to follow commands
	Bizarre, inappropriate behavior
	Marked anxiety, paranoia, anger, or rage
	Nystagmus, ataxia, slurred speech
	Asterixis
	Abnormal deep tendon reflexes
IV	Comatose, cannot follow commands
	May have dilated pupils or loss of cranial reflexes
	Signs of herniation
	Flexor or extensor posturing
	Complete loss of deep tendon reflexes

Answer: C

Amodio P, Montagnese S, Gatta A, Morgan MY. Characteristics of minimal hepatic encephalopathy. *Metabolic Brain Disease* 2004;19(3–4):253–267.

Conn H, Leevy C, Vlahcevic Z, Rodgers J, Maddrey W, Seeff L, et al. Comparison of lactulose and neomycin in the treatment of chronic portal-systemic encephalopathy: a double blind controlled trial. *Gastroenterology* 1977;72(4):573–583.

Parsons-Smith B, Summerskill W, Dawson A, Sherlock S. The electroencephalograph in liver disease. *The Lancet* 1957;270(7001):867–871.

Weissenborn K. Hepatic encephalopathy: definition, clinical grading and diagnostic principles. *Drugs* 2019;79(1):5–9.

The following vignette applies to questions 10–12

A 54-year-old man is brought to the emergency department because he has been vomiting blood for the last 3 hours. Over the last 6 months, he has had multiple similar occurrences. He has a history of Child Class B alcoholic cirrhosis. He has a 35 pack-year smoking history and has been drinking 2 glasses of whiskey daily for the last 30 years. He is pale and diaphoretic. His pulse is 103 beats/min and blood pressure is 101/69 mm Hg. On abdominal examination, there is marked distension, hepatomegaly, and shifting dullness to percussion.

Question 10:

His hemoglobin concentration is 9.8 g/dL, leukocyte count is 5 000/mm³, and platelet count is 120 000/mm³. He is given IV fluids and octreotide. What is the next best step in management?

   A *Propranolol*
   B *Endoscopic band ligation*
   C *Packed red blood cell transfusion*
   D *Intravenous ceftriaxone*
   E *Balloon tamponade*

The initial management of a patient with hematemesis who is suspected of having esophageal variceal bleeding should focus on airway management, fluid resuscitation, coagulation status stabilization, prophylactic antibiotics, octreotide, or terlipressin therapy to reduce portal hypertension, and proton pump inhibitor therapy. Patients with chronic liver disease may present with hepatic encephalopathy, and this places them at high risk of aspiration and aspiration pneumonia, thus airway management and proton pump inhibitor therapy may be warranted. Fluid resuscitation and coagulation status are vital, and blood products (packed red blood cells, prothrombin complex concentrate, recombinant factor VIIa, etc) may need to be administered if there is massive bleeding, the patient is hemodynamically unstable, or if the hemoglobin concentration is less than 7 g/dL. If this is not the case, as in our stable patient, fluid resuscitation and subcutaneous vitamin K should be administered instead. Patients with chronic liver disease or cirrhosis are at high risk of superimposed infection and spontaneous or secondary bacterial peritonitis, and subsequent sepsis during hospitalization, and thus prophylactic antibiotics are also required. Octreotide and terlipressin are both vasoactive medications that can cause a reduction in portal venous pressure, thus reducing the pressure gradient for ongoing variceal bleeding. Once all these measures have been adopted, management may proceed with upper endoscopy for a definitive diagnosis of esophageal varices.

Answer: D

Corley DA, Cello JP, Adkisson W, Ko WF, Kerlikowske K. Octreotide for acute esophageal variceal bleeding: a meta-analysis. *Gastroenterology* 2001;120(4): 946–954.

Chen P-H, Chen W-C, Hou M-C, Liu T-T, Chang C-J, Liao W-C, et al. Delayed endoscopy increases re-bleeding and mortality in patients with hematemesis and active esophageal variceal bleeding: a cohort study. *Journal of Hepatology* 2012;57(6):1207–1213.

Ejlersen E, Melsen T, Ingerslev J, Andreasen RB, Vilstrup H. Recombinant activated factor VII (rFVIIa) acutely normalizes prothrombin time in patients with cirrhosis during bleeding from oesophageal varices. *Scandinavian Journal of Gastroenterology* 2001;36(10):1081–1085.

Hou MC, Lin HC, Liu TT, Kuo BIT, Lee FY, Chang FY, et al. Antibiotic prophylaxis after endoscopic therapy prevents rebleeding in acute variceal hemorrhage: a randomized trial. *Hepatology* 2004;39(3):746–753.

Lo EA, Wilby KJ, Ensom MH. Use of proton pump inhibitors in the management of gastroesophageal varices: a systematic review. *Annals of Pharmacotherapy* 2015;49(2):207–219.

Question 11:

The patient is given IV fluids, ceftriaxone, omeprazole, and subcutaneous vitamin K. After receiving these, the patient's blood pressure is now 110/75 mm Hg. However, the hematemesis continues. An upper endoscopy is performed and reveals 2 bleeding esophageal varices and multiple non-bleeding varices. What is the next best step in management?

A *Endoscopic band ligation*

B *Balloon tamponade*

C *Endoscopic injection sclerotherapy*

D *Trans-jugular intrahepatic portosystemic shunt procedure*

E *Emergency liver transplantation*

Further management often depends on the patient's hemodynamic status. Hemodynamically unstable patients require emergency treatment and balloon tamponade would be the treatment of choice. In the case of hemodynamically stable patients, as is the case in our example, the next best step after direct visual diagnosis of bleeding esophageal varices would be band ligation. Endoscopic injection sclerotherapy would be an alternative to band ligation, but banding is preferred as the first-line. If despite these measures, bleeding cannot be controlled, a transjugular intrahepatic portosystemic shunt procedure is warranted. Emergency liver transplantation may also be considered as a last resort if available.

Answer: A

Laine L, El-Newihi HM, Migikovsky B, Sloane R, Garcia F. Endoscopic ligation compared with sclerotherapy for the treatment of bleeding esophageal varices. *Annals of Internal Medicine* 1993;119(1):1–7.

Laine L and Cook D. Endoscopic ligation compared with sclerotherapy for treatment of esophageal variceal bleeding: a meta-analysis. *Annals of Internal Medicine* 1995;123(4):280–287.

Rodrigues SG, Cárdenas A, Escorsell À, Bosch J, editors. *Balloon tamponade and esophageal stenting for esophageal variceal bleeding in cirrhosis: a systematic review and meta-analysis. Seminars in liver disease*; 2019: Thieme Medical Publishers.

Question 12:

After endoscopically ligating the two bleeding esophageal varices, the patient's hematemesis stops. However, the patient is concerned about recurrence. In addition to alcohol cessation and propranolol therapy, what is the optimal secondary prophylaxis strategy for esophageal varices?

A *Endoscopic ligation of remaining varices every 1–2 weeks until all are removed.*

B *Terlipressin therapy.*

C *Trans-jugular intrahepatic portosystemic shunt procedure.*

D *Endoscopic injection sclerotherapy of remaining varices every 1–2 weeks until all are removed.*

E *Propranolol and alcohol cessation alone are adequate.*

After the patient survives the initial hospitalization, and there is no longer ongoing variceal bleeding, secondary prophylaxis for future variceal bleeds must be undertaken. Alcohol cessation would be very appropriate in our patient, as it would stop the progression of his liver disease and lead to reduced liver inflammation and portal hypertension. Non-selective beta-blockers like propranolol block beta-adrenergic receptors in the gastrointestinal tract, leading to splanchnic vasoconstriction and reduced portal venous blood, reducing portal venous pressure. Terlipressin is not approved for secondary prophylaxis of variceal bleeds in the US. Although nitrates such as isosorbide dinitrate can synergistically reduce portal venous pressure when given with beta-blockers, they have not been found to decrease the risk of mortality or rebleeding when compared to beta-blocker therapy alone. For complete secondary prophylaxis, in addition to beta-blocker therapy and alcohol cessation, endoscopic variceal ligation (EVL) should be performed every 1–2 weeks until all the varices have been removed, and regular upper endoscopic examinations should be performed every 3–6 months thereafter. The rebleeding rate is lowest with this combination (15%), as opposed to EVL alone (30–45%) or propranolol alone (40–45%). Although a TIPS procedure would markedly reduce portal hypertension and variceal bleeds, it would also lead to a worsening of hyperammonemia and lead to an increased risk of hepatic encephalopathy development. As such, TIPS procedures would be considered only if initial therapy proved inadequate.

Answer: A

Angelico M, Carli L, Piat C, Gentile S, Capocaccia L. Effects of isosorbide-5-mononitrate compared with propranolol on first bleeding and long-term survival in cirrhosis. *Gastroenterology* 1997;113(5):1632–1639.

Lo G-H. The role of endoscopy in secondary prophylaxis of esophageal varices. *Clinics in Liver Disease* 2010;14(2):307–323.

García-Pagán JC, Feu F, Bosch J, Rodés J. Propranolol compared with propranolol plus isosorbide-5-mononitrate for portal hypertension in cirrhosis: a randomized controlled study. *Annals of Internal Medicine* 1991;114(10):869–873.

Ravipati M, Katragadda S, Swaminathan PD, Molnar J, Zarling E. Pharmacotherapy plus endoscopic intervention is more effective than pharmacotherapy or endoscopy alone in the secondary prevention of esophageal variceal bleeding: a meta-analysis of randomized, controlled trials. *Gastrointestinal Endoscopy* 2009;70(4):658–664.e5.

The following vignette applies to questions 13–15:

A 48-year-old man is admitted to the intensive care unit (ICU) after presenting with severe dyspnea and cyanosis. He was diagnosed 10 months ago with Child-Pugh Class C cirrhosis due to chronic hepatitis C virus infection and is currently undergoing antiviral treatment with high viral loads. His oxygen saturation was 64%, respiratory rate was 25 breaths/min. His abdomen is grossly distended, with hepatomegaly and fluid thrill. His arterial blood gas analysis shows a PaO_2 of 49 mm Hg.

Question 13:

He says that over the last 12 weeks he has had many similar episodes that are becoming more frequent and severe. His condition usually improves when he lies down and worsens when he sits or stands. What is the test of choice to diagnose hepatopulmonary syndrome?

   A *Computed tomography pulmonary angiography (CTPA)*
   B *Pulmonary capillary wedge pressure (PCWP) measurement with Swan-Ganz catheter*
   C *Ventilation-perfusion scan*
   D *Contrast echocardiogram*
   E *Lung MRI*

Question 14:

The diagnostic study in question 13 is performed, which shows intrapulmonary vasodilation. A diagnosis of hepatopulmonary syndrome is made. Which of the following can be offered to the patient as a treatment strategy?

   A *Long-term oxygen with or without positive pressure ventilation as supportive measures until a liver transplant is possible*
   B *Inhaled bosentan (endothelin-1 antagonist) therapy*
   C *Inhaled prostacyclin therapy*
   D *Atenolol therapy*
   E *IV methylprednisolone*

This patient presents with dyspnea, platypnea (worsening of shortness of breath upon sitting or standing up and improves upon lying down), and orthodeoxia (worsening of oxygen saturation upon standing up), along with a history of HCV-induced cirrhosis. Hepatopulmonary syndrome is characterized by hypoxemia, dyspnea, othodeoxia, platypnea, and intrapulmonary vasodilation in the presence of cirrhosis and portal hypertension. The exact mechanism is not clearly understood; however, it is believed that translocation of bacterial endotoxins occurs in the setting of portal hypertension and liver damage. This is thought to lead to the release of inflammatory cytokines and pulmonary vasodilators (in particular, nitric oxide), which results in inappropriate intrapulmonary vasodilation. Alveolar-arterial gradient more than 15 mm Hg in adults or more than 20 mm Hg in geriatric patients while in a seated position, in the setting of advanced liver disease, suggests the diagnosis. The gold standard test for this condition is a contrast echocardiogram using agitated saline contrast. It will reveal intrapulmonary vasodilation. Another test that can be performed is a lung perfusion scintigraphy using Tc-99m MAA, which can help quantify the degree of intrapulmonary vasodilation. Treatment largely revolves around supportive measures using long-term oxygen support with or without positive pressure ventilation until definitive therapy can be achieved with liver transplantation. Bosentan and prostacyclin are both pulmonary vasodilators and would actually worsen this patient's condition. Methylprednisolone, which can exert anti-inflammatory effects, would not address this patient's pulmonary vasodilation. Atenolol, a cardioselective beta-blocker, would only cause a worsening of this patient's cardiac output without improving his respiratory function.

Q13 Answer: D

Q14 Answer: A

Grilo-Bensusan I and Pascasio-Acevedo JM. Hepatopulmonary syndrome: What we know and what we would like to know. *World Journal of Gastroenterology* 2016;22(25):5728.

Hoeper MM, Krowka MJ, Strassburg CP. Portopulmonary hypertension and hepatopulmonary syndrome. *The Lancet* 2004;363(9419):1461–1468.

Lange PA and Stoller JK. The hepatopulmonary syndrome. *Annals of Internal Medicine* 1995;122(7):521–529.

Rodriguez-Roisin R, Agusti A, Roca J. The hepatopulmonary syndrome: new name, old complexities. *Thorax* 1992;47(11):897–902.

Question 15:

Upon further investigations, the patient is found to have a lesion in the left lobe of the liver suspicious for a hepatocellular carcinoma, along with 3 nodules in the left lung. The patient also reveals that he has been depressed and drinking large amounts of alcohol every day for the last year. Which of the following would constitute an absolute contraindication to liver transplant in this patient?

A *PaO$_2$ < 50 mm Hg on arterial blood gas analysis (ABG)*

B *Extrahepatic malignancy*

C *Active alcohol/substance abuse*

D *Active, uncontrolled viremia*

E *All of the above*

All of the listed option choices are absolute contraindications to liver transplantation. Cardiopulmonary failure is a very important absolute contraindication in patients with liver failure, as it indicates low possibility of organ and patient survival. One of the manifestations of cardiopulmonary failure would be consistent hypoxemia on arterial blood gas analysis. Prolonged, consistent, and severe hypoxemia in the setting of hepatopulmonary syndrome must be treated before consideration for liver transplant can begin. Active alcohol or substance abuse, extrahepatic malignancy, and active viral replication are all absolute contraindications to liver transplantation. In addition, some relative contraindications to liver transplantation include advanced age, acquired immunodeficiency syndrome, cholangiocarcinoma, and diffuse portal vein thrombosis.

Answer: E

Mahmud N. Selection for liver transplantation: indications and evaluation. *Current Hepatology Reports* 2020:1–10.

Varma V, Mehta N, Kumaran V, Nundy S. Indications and contraindications for liver transplantation. *International Journal of Hepatology* 2011;2011.

19

Nutrition Support in Critically Ill Patients

Ida Molavi, MD[1] and Jorge Con, MD[2]

[1] *Department of Trauma and Acute Care Surgery, Louisiana State University Health, Shreveport, LA, USA*
[2] *Division of Trauma and Acute Care Surgery, New York Medical College, Westchester Medical Center, Valhalla, NY, USA*

1 Based on current guidelines and recommendations, what should the glycemic control target be in the critically ill patient?
   A ≤ 200 mg/dL
   B ≤ 160 mg/dL
   C ≤ 180 mg/dL
   D ≤ 80–120 mg/dL
   E ≤ 80–160 mg/dL

Hyperglycemia in the critically ill patient is multifactorial and can be attributed to the activation of the sympatho-adrenal system and the stress response triggering catecholamine and glucocorticoid production. These hormones in turn trigger glucagon release, which subsequently causes an increase in gluconeogenesis and glycogenolysis, leading to insulin resistance and decreased insulin production. Although a result of the body's compensatory mechanism, this can lead to an array of complications including a suppressed immune system and increased risk of infection. A large, single-center landmark trial revealed that tight glycemic control (80–110 mg/dL) with insulin infusion in the postoperative period was associated with reduced mortality, ICU length of stay, and sepsis. Tight glycemic control, however, does carry the risk of severe hypoglycemia, negating the benefits. Based off the results of the NICE-SUGAR study, the Society of Critical Care Medicine (SCCM) and the American Society for Parenteral and Enteral Nutrition (ASPEN) nutritional guidelines recommend a glycemic range of 150–180 mg/dL and 140–180 mg/dL, respectively.

Answer: C

McClave, S. A., Taylor, B. E., Martindale, R. G., et al. (2016). Guidelines for the provision and assessment of nutrition support therapy in the adult critically ill patient Society of Critical Care Medicine (SCCM) and American Society for Parenteral and Enteral Nutrition (ASPEN). *Journal of Parenteral and Enteral Nutrition*, 40(2), 159–211.

NICE-SUGAR Study Investigators, Finfer, S., Chittock, D. R., Su, S. Y., et al. (2009). Intensive versus conventional glucose control in critically ill patients. *The New England Journal of Medicine*, 360(13), 1283–1297.

Van den Berghe, G., Wouters, P., Weekers, F., et al. (2001). Intensive insulin therapy in critically ill patients. *The New England Journal of Medicine*, 345(19), 1359–1367.

2 Prealbumin, retinol-binding protein, and transferrin may be useful as nutritional markers. Which of the following is true regarding these proteins?
   A The half-life of prealbumin is longer than that of transferrin.
   B They are positive acute phase proteins.
   C Albumin has a half-life of 120 days.
   D Prealbumin and retinol-binding protein are positive acute phase proteins, while transferrin is a negative acute phase protein.
   E They do not accurately represent nutrition status in the critical care setting.

Acute phase reactants (APR) are proteins whose plasma concentrations either increase or decrease by at least 25% percent during inflammatory states. Such proteins are termed either positive or negative acute phase reactants, accordingly. This is guided by the hepatic reprioritization of protein synthesis away from negative APRs and toward positive APRs. The negative acute phase proteins are albumin, prealbumin, retinol-binding protein, and transferrin. Their serum concentrations fall immediately after injury, and in proportion to injury severity. Albumin has a half-life of 20 days, transferrin 8 days, and prealbumin <2 days. Continued and prolonged production of acute phase proteins in critically ill patients may be an indicator of ongoing sepsis and tissue damage, and is associated with higher mortality rates. Recent studies have revealed that these acute phase reactants characterize an underlying inflammatory response and do not accurately represent nutritional status in the critical care setting.

Answer: E

Evans, D. C., Corkins, M. R., Malone, A., et al. & ASPEN Malnutrition Committee (2020). The use of visceral proteins as nutrition markers: an ASPEN position paper. *Nutrition in Clinical Practice*, doi:10.1002/ncp.10588.

McClave, S. A., Taylor, B. E., Martindale, R. G., et al. (2016). Guidelines for the provision and assessment of nutrition support therapy in the adult critically ill patient Society of Critical Care Medicine (SCCM) and American Society for Parenteral and Enteral Nutrition (ASPEN). *Journal of Parenteral and Enteral Nutrition*, 40(2), 159–211.

Raguso, C. A., Dupertuis, Y. M., & Pichard, C. (2003). The role of visceral proteins in the nutritional assessment of intensive care unit patients. *Current Opinion in Clinical Nutrition and Metabolic Care*, 6(2), 211–216.

3   Which of the following statements is true regarding antioxidants?
   A Antioxidants are not recommended in critically ill patients.
   B Only vitamin C is an antioxidant.
   C Antioxidants should be used only in burn patients.
   D Selenium supplementation does not affect the mortality of critically ill patients.
   E Selenium is the most effective antioxidant.

Antioxidant vitamins (including vitamins A, E, and C) and trace minerals (including selenium, zinc, and copper) may improve patient outcome, especially in burns, trauma, and critically ill patients. It has been demonstrated that antioxidant and trace element supplementation is associated with a significant reduction in overall mortality. Infectious complications, length of stay, and duration of mechanical ventilation were not significantly different between patients placed on such antioxidant supplements and controls receiving placebo. Selenium is one of the micronutrients with antioxidant capabilities. Plasma concentration of selenium is decreased in septic patients, and it is believed to be one of the most potent antioxidant agents in clinical setting. The current recommendation is to provide a combination of antioxidant vitamins and trace minerals, especially including sele-

nium, to all critically ill patients receiving specialized nutrition therapy.

Answer: E

Crimi, E., Liguori, A., Condorelli, M., et al. (2004). The beneficial effects of antioxidant supplementation in enteral feeding in critically ill patients: a prospective, randomized, double-blind, placebo-controlled trial. *Anesthesia and Analgesia*, 99(3).

Huang, T. S., Shyu, Y. C., Chen, H. Y., Lin, L. M., Lo, C. Y., Yuan, S. S., Chen, P. J., et al. (2013). Effect of parenteral selenium supplementation in critically ill patients: a systematic review and meta-analysis. *PLoS One*, 8(1), e54431.

McClave, S. A., Taylor, B. E., Martindale, R. G., et al. (2016). Guidelines for the provision and assessment of nutrition support therapy in the adult critically ill patient Society of Critical Care Medicine (SCCM) and American Society for Parenteral and Enteral Nutrition (ASPEN). *Journal of Parenteral and Enteral Nutrition*, 40(2), 159–211.

4   A severely injured 70-year-old man is admitted to the ICU for severe necrotizing pancreatitis. The following nutritional strategies are correct:
   A Probiotics are of no benefit to pancreatitis patients receiving enteral nutrition.
   B Patients with moderate-to-severe acute pancreatitis benefit from parenteral nutrition over enteral nutrition.
   C Jejunal feeding is superior to gastric feeding regarding tolerance and clinical outcomes.
   D Strategies to improve tolerance to enteral nutrition include: early start of enteral nutrition, feeding distally, and near fat-free elemental diets.
   E Parenteral nutrition should be started when enteral nutrition has not been feasible after 72 hours from onset of pancreatitis.

In patients with mild acute pancreatitis, initiation and advancement of an oral diet is recommended over specialized enteral or parenteral nutrition. In patients with moderate-to-severe acute pancreatitis, enteral nutrition should be initiated within the first 24–48 hours of admission, at a trophic rate, and advanced to goal as fluid volume resuscitation is completed. Measures to improve tolerance to enteral nutrition should be initiated if necessary.

Use of enteral nutrition is preferred to parenteral nutrition because of decreased infectious morbidity, hospital LOS, need for surgical intervention, and mortality. Several randomized controlled trials comparing gastric with jejunal feeding in severe acute pancreatitis showed no significant differences between the two.

Measures to improve tolerance to enteral nutrition in patients with moderate-to-severe acute pancreatitis include starting enteral nutrition as soon as possible and within the first 48 hours of admission, feeding more distally in the gastrointestinal tract, changing from a standard polymeric formula to one that contains small peptides and medium chain triglycerides or to one that is a nearly a fat-free elemental formulation, and switching from bolus to continuous infusion.

Current guidelines suggest use of probiotics be considered in patients with severe acute pancreatitis who are receiving early enteral nutrition based on evidence that it may decrease sepsis and multi-organ dysfunction in this population.

If the patient is well nourished, supplemental parenteral nutrition (PN) should be considered after 7 days if unable to meet >50–60% of energy and protein requirements by the enteral route. If the patient is nutritionally at-risk and unlikely to achieve desired EN goal, PN should be considered within 3–5 days of admission. PN should be initiated as soon as feasible for patients with baseline moderate-to-severe malnutrition in whom oral intake or enteral nutrition is not possible or sufficient; therefore, answer E is wrong.

Answer: D

Cao, Y., Xu, Y., Lu, T., Gao, F., et al. (2008). Meta-analysis of enteral nutrition versus total parenteral nutrition in patients with severe acute pancreatitis. *Annals of Nutrition & Metabolism*, 53(3–4), 268–275.

Chang, Y. S., Fu, H. Q., Xiao, Y. M., et al. (2013). Nasogastric or nasojejunal feeding in predicted severe acute pancreatitis: a meta-analysis. Critical Care (London, England), 17(3), R118.

McClave, S. A., Taylor, B. E., Martindale, R. G., et al. (2016). guidelines for the provision and assessment of nutrition support therapy in the adult critically ill patient Society of Critical Care Medicine (SCCM) and American Society for Parenteral and Enteral Nutrition (ASPEN). *Journal of Parenteral and Enteral Nutrition*, 40(2), 159–211.

Wang, G., Wen, J., Xu, L., et al. (2013). Effect of enteral nutrition and ecoimmunonutrition on bacterial translocation and cytokine production in patients with severe acute pancreatitis. *The Journal of Surgical Research*, 183(2), 592–597.

Worthington, P., Balint, J., Bechtold, M., et al. (2017). When is parenteral nutrition appropriate? *Journal of Parenteral and Enteral Nutrition*, 41(3), 324–377.

5 A 68-year-old woman with a history of hypertension, diabetes, and body mass index of 45 is admitted to the intensive care unit after a traumatic brain injury. She is intubated and is expected to remain intubated for the next few days. Which of the following statements is true?

A The optimal protein requirement for this patient is 1 g/kg/day.

B The caloric intake should not exceed 60–70% of her target energy requirement.

C Feeds should be advanced to 100% of target energy requirement within 24–48 hours of admission.

D Enteral nutrition should be held until post-admission day 7.

E The caloric intake should be 45 kcal/kg actual body weight/day.

Initiating early enteral nutrition within 24–48 hours of admission is essential in the critically ill patients who cannot sustain volitional intake, regardless of BMI. Current guidelines recommend high-protein hypocaloric feeding in obese critically ill patients. Hypocaloric feeding in this patient population may decrease ventilator days and length of stay in the unit while improving insulin sensitivity. The goal of enteral nutrition should not exceed 60–70% of target energy requirement as measured by indirect calorimetry in the obese critically ill patient (answer C is therefore wrong). If indirect calorimetry is not available, 11–14 kcal/kg actual body weight per day should be the goal in order to minimize the metabolic complications of overfeeding. A critically ill patient with a BMI of 30–40 should receive 2 g of protein/kg/day, while patients with a BMI of greater than 40 should receive 2.5 g protein/kg/day as part of an overall hypocaloric feeding regime.

Answer: B

McClave, S. A., Taylor, B. E., Martindale, R. G., et al. (2016). Guidelines for the provision and assessment of nutrition support therapy in the adult critically ill patient Society of Critical Care Medicine (SCCM) and American Society for Parenteral and Enteral Nutrition (ASPEN). *Journal of Parenteral and Enteral Nutrition*, 40(2), 159–211.

Jiang, H., Sun, M. W., Hefright, B., et al. (2011). Efficacy of hypocaloric parenteral nutrition for surgical patients: a systematic review and meta-analysis. *Clinical Nutrition (Edinburgh, Scotland)*, 30(6), 730–737.

6 The response to stress and injury consist of three phases: the ebb phase, the catabolic flow phase, and the anabolic flow phase. Which of the following is true:

A The anabolic flow phase is driven by cytokine mediators released by lymphocytes and macrophages in the cellular immune reaction, dominated by interleukin-6 (IL-6).

B The ebb phase is dominated by catabolism, typically lasts 3–10 days, but may last longer.

C The catabolic flow phase is dominated by circulatory changes that require resuscitation (with fluid, blood, and blood products) over a period of 8–24 hours.

D The ebb phase should be treated with fluid, blood, and blood products.

E The catabolic phase emerges as the patient's metabolism shifts to synthetic activities and reparative processes.

The response to stress and injury consists of three phases, the ebb phase, the catabolic flow phase, and the anabolic flow phase. Each of these phases has distinct changes that require specific interventions in order to eliminate or minimize the consequences of illness and/or injury. The ebb phase is dominated by circulatory changes that require resuscitation (with fluid, blood, and blood products) over a period of 8–24 hours. The catabolic flow phase, dominated by catabolism, typically lasts 3–10 days, but may last longer. The anabolic flow phase emerges as the patient's metabolism shifts to synthetic activities and reparative processes. The catabolic flow phase is driven by cytokine mediators released from lymphocytes and macrophages in the cellular immune reaction, dominated by interleukin-6 (IL-6). The release of these mediators is proportional to the intensity of the injury, but the release of cytokines themselves is upregulated by hormonal and humoral events. The early nonspecific response to systemic tissue injury that is responsible for the reprioritization of protein synthesis in the liver is termed the acute phase response (APR). Depending on the magnitude and the severity of the injury, APR is characterized by an exponential increase in positive acute phase proteins and a decrease in negative acute phase proteins. The regulation of APR, a complex process, depends on many factors. Tissue injury or infection leads to a local inflammatory response, which in turn leads to the release of many cytokines at the site of inflammation; the cytokines are eventually carried to the liver, where they act on the hepatocytes. Crystalloids, blood, and blood products may be required for the initial resuscitation based on the severity and the magnitude of the injury.

Answer: D

Latifi, R. (2011). Nutritional therapy in critically ill and injured patients. *Surgical Clinics*, 91(3), 579–593.

Şimşek, T., Şimşek, H. U., & Cantürk, N. Z. (2014). Response to trauma and metabolic changes: posttraumatic metabolism. *Ulusal Cerrahi Dergisi*, 30(3), 153–159.

Varela, M. L., Mogildea, M., Moreno, I., & Lopes, A. (2018). Acute inflammation and metabolism. *Inflammation*, 41(4), 1115–1127.

7 A 68-year-old man presents with perforated cancer of the ascending colon and is in septic shock. He is taken to the operating room for a right hemicolectomy and end-ileostomy. His NUTRIC score is 3. He remains intubated in the intensive care unit, requiring minimal vasopressor for hemodynamic support. Which of the following statements is true?

A Withhold enteral nutrition, initiate parenteral nutrition within the first 7 days of ICU admission

B Withhold enteral nutrition, initiate parenteral nutrition after 7 days of ICU admission

C Initiate trophic enteral feeds and advance as tolerated

D Initiate trophic enteral feeds, supplemented with parenteral nutrition within the first 7 days of admission

E Withhold enteral feeds while the patient is on vasopressors

In the critically ill septic patient, splanchnic perfusion to the bowel is reduced. Patients are therefore at risk for subclinical bowel ischemia, reperfusion injuries, and bowel perforation. This may steer clinicians away from initiating enteral feeds in the septic patient. A recent single-center retrospective trial of mechanically ventilated patents with septic shock revealed that trophic enteral feeds, while on low-dose vasopressors, was associated with decreased mortality, duration of mechanical ventilation, and ICU stay. Guidelines recommend considering early enteral nutrition in those undergoing withdrawal of vasopressor support, while monitoring for signs of intolerance (e.g. increasing base deficit or lactate, abdominal distention, decreased passage of flatus, and stool). Enteral nutrition, however, should be avoided in the hemodynamically unstable patient requiring high doses of vasopressors.

Proper nutrition is essential in the management of trauma and surgical critical care patients. One way to assess the nutritional risk in this patient population is the Nutrition Risk in the Critically Ill (NUTRIC) score. This scoring system is capable of determining nutritional status and disease severity, while linking starvation, inflammation, nutritional status, and outcomes. The system utilizes 6 variables to formulate which patients will benefit more from aggressive protein-energy provisions, and include age, APACHE II score, SOFA score, number of comorbidities, IL-6 levels, and days from hospital to ICU admission. Patients with a score of greater than 5 out of a maximum of 10 are most likely to benefit from aggressive nutritional therapy.

The above patient has a low NUTRIC score and low nutrition risk while on minimal vasopressor support, therefore trophic enteral feeds should be initiated. Supplemental parenteral nutrition should be considered after 7–10 days if unable to achieve >60% of energy and protein requirements by the enteral route alone. If the scenario was different in that the patient was determined to be at high nutrition risk while on high vasopressor support where enteral nutrition was not feasible, then parenteral nutrition should be initiated within 7–10 days of admission.

Answer: C

Mancl, E. E., & Muzevich, K. M. (2013). Tolerability and safety of enteral nutrition in critically ill patients receiving intravenous vasopressor therapy. *Journal of Parenteral and Enteral Nutrition*, 37(5), 641–651.

McClave, S. A., Taylor, B. E., Martindale, R. G., et al. (2016). Guidelines for the provision and assessment of nutrition support therapy in the adult critically ill patient Society of Critical Care Medicine (SCCM) and American Society for Parenteral and Enteral Nutrition (ASPEN). *Journal of Parenteral and Enteral Nutrition*, 40(2), 159–211.

Patel, J. J., Kozeniecki, M., Biesboer, A., et al. (2016). Early trophic enteral nutrition is associated with improved outcomes in mechanically ventilated patients with septic shock: a retrospective review. *Journal of Intensive Care Medicine*, 31(7), 471–477.

8 A patient with a traumatic brain injury has been receiving enteral nutrition in the ICU for the past week. You are being called because of a gastric residual of 400 mL. Which of the following statements is correct?

A Bundled interventions including chlorhexidine mouthwash has been shown to decrease nosocomial respiratory infections.

B Head of bed elevated 30–45 degrees, although routine, has not been shown to decrease the incidence of pneumonia.

C A gastric residual volume of 350 mL should always prompt cessation of feeds and further evaluation.

D Gastric residual volumes correlate well with gastric emptying.

E Scheduled monitoring of gastric residual volumes (GRV) should be part of routine care.

Gastric residual volumes (GRVs) do not correlate well with the incidence of pneumonia, regurgitation, or aspiration. In a trial using a highly sensitive and specific marker for aspiration, GRVs (over a range of 150–400 mL) were shown to be a poor predictor of aspiration. Results from four randomized controlled trials indicate that raising the threshold to stop feeds for GRVs from 50–150 mL to 250–500 mL did not increase the incidence of regurgitation, aspiration, or pneumonia. Current recommendations do not support checking GRVs, and to use a threshold of > 500 mL GRVs to stop enteral nutrition if compelled to do so. Studies in which chlorhexidine oral care was included in bundled interventions showed significant reductions in nosocomial respiratory infections. Elevating the head of the bed 30°–45° was shown in to reduce the incidence of pneumonia from 23 to 5%.

Answer: A

Drakulovic, M. B., Torres, A., Bauer, T. T., et al. (1999). Supine body position as a risk factor for nosocomial pneumonia in mechanically ventilated patients: a randomised trial. *The Lancet*, 354(9193), 1851–1858.

McClave, S. A., Taylor, B. E., Martindale, R. G., et al. (2016). Guidelines for the provision and assessment of nutrition support therapy in the adult critically ill patient Society of Critical Care Medicine (SCCM) and American Society for Parenteral and Enteral Nutrition (ASPEN). *Journal of Parenteral and Enteral Nutrition*, 40(2), 159–211.

McClave, S. A., Lukan, J. K., Stefater, J. A., et al. (2005). Poor validity of residual volumes as a marker for risk of aspiration in critically ill patients. *Critical Care Medicine*, 33(2), 324–330.

9 A 78-year-old smoker with COPD sustains a ground level fall and multiple bilateral rib fractures and he remains intubated after one week. Which of the following regarding his nutrition is correct?

A High-fat low-carbohydrate formulations are designed to increase CO_2 production.

B Specialty high-fat/low-carbohydrate formulations should be used.

C Fluid-restricted energy-dense formulations should not be used in respiratory failure.

D Enteral formulations with an anti-inflammatory profile typically include omega-3 fatty acids, borage oils, and antioxidants.

E Serum phosphate concentrations do not affect respiratory failure.

The predominant fuel type affects the respiratory quotient (RQ), which is the ratio of carbon dioxide produced over oxygen consumed. The RQ for fat is 0.7 and for glucose is 1.0. In patients with acute respiratory failure, increased carbon dioxide production can complicate the ventilator weaning process. One school of thought behind using high-fat low-carbohydrate formulations is to decrease CO_2 production and hence assist with the weaning process. Although an early small trial showed that high-fat/low-carbohydrate formulations reduced duration of mechanical ventilation, these findings were not reproduced in subsequent randomized controlled trials and are therefore not recommended. Using a high fat-to-carbohydrate ratio becomes clinically significant in lowering CO_2 production only in the overfed ICU patient. Instead, efforts should be made to avoid total energy provision that exceeds energy requirements, as lipogenesis significantly increases CO_2 production, which poorly tolerated in patients prone to CO_2 retention (COPD).

Phosphate deficiency is associated with respiratory muscle weakness and failure to wean from mechanical ventilation. Fluid-restricted formulations may be considered for patients with fluid accumulation, pulmonary edema, and renal failure. Six randomized controlled trials have evaluated the use of additives or formulas with an anti-inflammatory lipid profile (omega-3 fatty acids, borage oilS, and antioxidants) in patients with ARDS, ALI, and sepsis. However, studies were heterogeneous and because of conflicting data, are not currently recommended to be routinely used in patients with ARDS/ALI in the ASPEN guidelines 2016.

Answer: D

Bech, A., Blans, M., Raaijmakers, M., et al. (2013). Hypophosphatemia on the intensive care unit: individualized phosphate replacement based on serum levels and distribution volume. *Journal of Critical Care*, 28(5), 838–843.

McClave, S. A., Taylor, B. E., Martindale, R. G., et al. (2016). Guidelines for the provision and assessment of nutrition support therapy in the adult critically ill patient Society of Critical Care Medicine (SCCM) and American Society for Parenteral and Enteral Nutrition (ASPEN). *Journal of Parenteral and Enteral Nutrition*, 40(2), 159–211.

Mesejo, A., Acosta, J. A., Ortega, C., et al. (2003). Comparison of a high-protein disease-specific enteral formula with a high-protein enteral formula in hyperglycemic critically ill patients. *Clinical Nutrition*, 22(3), 295–305.

10 A 64-year-old woman with a history of alcoholic cirrhosis and on the transplant list is admitted for hepatic failure. Regarding nutritional therapy in this patient, the following is correct:

A Actual weight is superior to dry weight or usual weight in calculating energy and protein needs in patients with cirrhosis and hepatic failure.

B Branched-chain amino acids are of no benefit for encephalopathic patients in the ICU already receiving luminal-acting antibiotics and lactulose.

C Protein restriction may reduce risk from hepatic encephalopathy.

D Parenteral nutrition is contraindicated in cirrhosis.

E Branched-chain amino acids include lysine, isoleucine, serine, and valine.

Patients with chronic liver disease are at a higher nutrition risk. In this patient population, dry weight should be used over actual weight to determine energy and protein needs given the complications of ascites, intravascular volume depletion, portal hypertension, hypoalbuminemia, and edema.

Although protein restriction was historically used to reduce risk from hepatic encephalopathy, such a strategy may worsen nutrition status, decrease lean muscle mass, and ironically lead to less ammonia removal. Branched-chain amino acids (leucine, isoleucine, and valine) are essential amino acids with a stimulatory effect on ammonia detoxification to glutamine, and their plasma levels are decreased in liver failure. There is no evidence to suggest that a formulation enriched in branched-chain amino acids improve patient outcomes compared with standard whole-protein formulations in critically ill patients with liver disease. In patients with hepatic encephalopathy already receiving first-line therapy (antibiotics and lactulose), there is no evidence to date that adding branched-chain amino acids will further improve mental status or coma grade.

Enteral nutrition is preferred over parenteral nutrition in liver failure as long-term parenteral nutrition can worsen existing cirrhosis and liver failure. In clinical trials, enteral nutrition has been associated with decreased infection rates and fewer metabolic complications in patients with liver disease and after liver transplantation, when compared with parenteral nutrition. However, current guidelines recommend initiating parenteral nutrition in moderately or severely malnourished patients with liver failure who cannot be nourished sufficiently by oral and/or enteral route (answer D is therefore wrong).

Answer: B

Bémeur, C., Desjardins, P., & Butterworth, R. F. (2010). Role of nutrition in the management of hepatic encephalopathy in end-stage liver failure. *Journal of Nutrition and Metabolism*, 2010.

Bischoff, S. C., Bernal, W., Dasarathy, S., et al. (2020). ESPEN practical guideline: clinical nutrition in liver disease. *Clinical Nutrition*, 39(12), 3533–3562.

McClave, S. A., Taylor, B. E., Martindale, R. G., et al. (2016). Guidelines for the provision and assessment of nutrition support therapy in the adult critically ill patient Society of Critical Care Medicine (SCCM) and American Society for Parenteral and Enteral Nutrition (ASPEN). *Journal of Parenteral and Enteral Nutrition*, 40(2), 159–211.

11 A 48-year-old man with morbid obesity is admitted to the intensive care unit with septic shock one week after undergoing a Hartmann's procedure. Fluid resuscitation, antibiotics, and vasopressors are immediately initiated. Abdominal CT reveals a pelvic abscess, which is drained percutaneously. Which of the following adequately predicts this patient's daily energy requirements?

A Nutrition Risk in Critically Ill (NUTRIC) score
B Harris-Benedict equation
C Indirect calorimetry
D Sequential Organ Failure Assessment (SOFA) score
E Toronto formula

The metabolic response in critically ill surgical patients and burn patients is characterized by an increase in resting energy expenditure. Underfeeding or overfeeding this patient population can adversely affect outcomes, hence proper nutritional support represents one of the most important cornerstones in their management. Indirect calorimetry is considered the gold standard in determining energy expenditure, but it requires specialized equipment and personnel. This method provides a measurement of both resting energy expenditure and respiratory quotient by measuring whole-body oxygen and carbon dioxide gas exchange. Predictive equations do not accurately assess the true caloric needs. The Harris-Benedict equation is a predictive tool designed to provide an estimate of basal metabolic rate, which is a minimum number of calories required for basic function at rest. The Toronto formula is used to predict energy expenditure in burn patients.

The NUTRIC score utilizes 6 variables to formulate which patients will benefit more from aggressive protein-energy provisions and include age, APACHE II score, SOFA score, number of comorbidities, IL-6 levels, and days from hospital to ICU admission. Patients with a score of greater than 5 out of a maximum of 10 are most likely to benefit from aggressive nutritional therapy. The SOFA score quantifies the severity of illness based on the degree of organ dysfunction serially over time and is not used to estimate a patient's nutritional needs when used by itself.

Answer: C

Boullata, J., Williams, J., Cottrell, F., et al. (2007). Accurate determination of energy needs in hospitalized patients. *Journal of the American Dietetic Association*, 107(3), 393–401.

McClave, S. A., & Snider, H. L. (1992). Invited review: use of indirect calorimetry in clinical nutrition. *Nutrition in Clinical Practice*, 7(5), 207–221.

McClave, S. A., Taylor, B. E., Martindale, R. G., et al. (2016). Guidelines for the provision and assessment of nutrition support therapy in the adult critically ill patient Society of Critical Care Medicine (SCCM) and American Society for Parenteral and Enteral Nutrition (ASPEN). *Journal of Parenteral and Enteral Nutrition*, 40(2), 159–211.

12 A 58-year-old man with a history of morbid obesity is admitted to the intensive care unit with Fournier's gangrene, requiring multiple trips to the operating room for debridement. His postoperative course is complicated with pneumonia and difficulties weaning from the ventilator. You decide to perform indirect calorimetry to assess his nutritional status. What does a respiratory quotient of 1.4 imply regarding this patient's overall nutrition?

A The patient is in starvation.
B The patient is receiving appropriate nutritional support.
C The patient is being overfed.
D The patient is being underfed.
E Hypermetabolism.

The respiratory quotient (RQ) is the ratio of carbon dioxide production to oxygen consumption and corresponds to the predominant fuel type being utilized. The RQ for fat is 0.7, for glucose 1.0, and for protein 0.8. In starvation, the caloric intake is inadequate to meet the metabolic demands of the body. Hence, alternate fuel sources are used as an adaptive mechanism to preserve lean body mass and minimize protein wasting. An RQ of 0.7 is when fat becomes the primary source of fuel after depletion of glycogen stores and exhaustion of gluconeogenesis in starvation. An RQ of greater than 1 indicates potential overfeeding and lipogenesis, which leads to increased production of carbon dioxide that in turn may contribute to difficulties with weaning mechanical ventilation. Hypermetabolism is characterized by an increase in oxygen consumption and energy expenditure as the body's response to major stressors such as in pancreatitis, severe burns, poly-trauma, or brain injury. Hypermetabolism clinically manifests itself with hyperglycemia, elevated serum lactate, and a net negative nitrogen balance. The body utilizes a mixed oxidative fuel source, resulting in an RQ ranging from 0.80 to 0.95.

Answer: C

Barton, R. G. (2014). Nutrition support. In: Parillo, J. E., & Dellinger, R. P., eds. *Critical Care Medicine: Principles of Diagnosis and Management in the Adult*. Philadelphia, PA: Elsevier Saunders, 1421–1435.

Druck, P. (2005). Nutritional support in critical illness. In: Abrams, J., Druck, P., & Cerra, F. B., eds. *Surgical*

Critical Care. 2nd ed. Boca Raton, FL: Taylor & Francis, 43–62.

McClave, S. A., Lowen, C. C., et al. (2003). Clinical use of the respiratory quotient obtained from indirect calorimetry. *Journal of Parenteral and Enteral Nutrition*, 27(1), 21–26.

13 A 23-year-old presents with multiple gunshot wounds to the abdomen. He is found to have three different sites of injury to the small bowel. The affected sites were resected and he was left in discontinuity during the initial damage control surgery. He is re-anastomosed during the subsequent exploration; however, he has a prolonged postoperative ileus requiring parenteral nutrition. Which of the following statements is true?

A Glutamine is an essential amino acid because it cannot be synthesized in sufficient quantities during periods of stress.

B Glutamine is involved in many immune functions, but not in the production of heat shock proteins.

C Glutamine is contraindicated in critically ill patients except traumatic brain injury and perioperative SICU patients.

D Glutamine is classified as a branch-chain amino acid and should be given to patients with liver failure.

E Glutamine serves as the primary fuel for colonocytes and other slowly proliferating cells.

Glutamine is an amino acid that serves as the primary fuel for small bowel enterocytes and other rapidly proliferating cells, such as cells in wounds. Butyrate is the primary fuel source for colonocytes and slowly proliferating cells. Glutamine is classified as a nonessential amino acid because the human body can synthesize it in sufficient quantities. Yet, during periods of stress, the body's requirements may exceed its capacity to synthesize glutamine. Branched chain amino acids include leucine, isoleucine, and valine. Answer D is therefore wrong. Glutamine is involved in many immune functions, including the production of heat shock proteins. Studies have shown that supplementation with glutamine may lead to a decrease in nosocomial infections in patients with systemic inflammatory response and a decrease in pneumonia, sepsis, and bacteremia in trauma patients. Parenterally administered glutamine has been associated with a decrease in gram-negative bacteremia. The addition of glutamine to enteral nutrition has been recommended for TBI and perioperative patients in the SICU in the 2016 Society of Critical Care Medicine (SCCM)/American Society for Parenteral and Enteral Nutrition (ASPEN) nutritional guidelines.

Answer: C

Garrel, D., Patenaude, J., Nedelec, B., et al. (2003) Decreased mortality and infectious morbidity in adult burn patients given enteral glutamine supplements: a prospective, controlled, randomized clinical trial. *Critical Care Medicine*, 31 (10), 2444–2449.

McClave, S. A., Taylor, B. E., Martindale, R. G., et al. (2016). Guidelines for the provision and assessment of nutrition support therapy in the adult critically ill patient Society of Critical Care Medicine (SCCM) and American Society for Parenteral and Enteral Nutrition (ASPEN). *Journal of Parenteral and Enteral Nutrition*, 40(2), 159–211.

Wischmeyer, P.E., Lynch, J., Liedel, J., et al. (2001) Glutamine administration reduces gram-negative bacteremia in severely burned patients: a prospective, randomized, double-blind trial versus isonitrogenous control. *Critical Care Medicine*, 29 (11), 2075–2080.

14 Which of the following patients would benefit from arginine-supplemented immunonutrition?

A 57-year-old man admitted to the intensive care unit with pancreatitis and septic shock

B 36-year-old woman admitted to the intensive care unit with polytrauma

C 18-year-old man with familial adenomatous polyposis presenting for abdominal perineal resection

D B and C

E None of the above

Immune-modulating formulas for enteral feeding, also known as immunonutrition, contain nutrients such as glutamine, arginine, omega-3 fatty acids, nucleotides, and antioxidants, added to standard enteral formulas. Immune-modulating formulas are hypothesized to reduce the inflammatory response while enhancing the immunologic response. Studies to date have revealed mixed outcomes with immunonutrition. Current guidelines from the Society of Critical Care Medicine and the American Society for Parenteral and Enteral Nutrition recommend that immune-modulating formulations be considered in select patient populations (trauma, major elective surgery, head and neck cancers, burn). Arginine is considered a conditionally essential amino acid with reduced availability during sepsis and tissue injury. Through its role in the urea cycle, arginine takes part in the synthesis of other amino acids, urea, and nitric oxide. Arginine is important for cell-mediated immunity. It is required for the growth and function of T lymphocytes in cultures. in vivo, arginine retards thymic involution by encouraging production of thymic hormones and thymocyte proliferation. Arginine also promotes leukocyte-mediated cytotoxicity. Growth hormone receptors are widely distributed in the immune system, and by releasing growth hormone, arginine may increase the cytotoxic activity of macrophages, neutrophils, NK cells, and cytotoxic T cells. Arginine supplementation can, in theory, contribute to excessive nitric oxide production, which may cause unwanted vasodilation and hypotension in the septic patient (answer A is wrong). Current guidelines from the Surviving Sepsis Campaign recommend against the use of arginine to treat sepsis and septic shock.

Answer: D

Heyland, D., Muscedere, J., Wischmeyer, P.E., et al. (2013) A randomized trial of glutamine and antioxidants in critically ill patients. *New England Journal of Medicine*, 368, 1489–1497.

McClave, S. A., Taylor, B. E., Martindale, R. G., et al. (2016). Guidelines for the provision and assessment of nutrition support therapy in the adult critically ill patient Society of Critical Care Medicine (SCCM) and American Society for Parenteral and Enteral Nutrition (ASPEN). *Journal of Parenteral and Enteral Nutrition*, 40(2), 159–211.

Rhodes, A., Evans, L. E., Alhazzani, W., et al. (2017). Surviving sepsis campaign: international guidelines for management of sepsis and septic shock: 2016. *Intensive Care Medicine*, 43(3), 304–377.

15 Which of the following statements is true regarding nutrition in critically ill patients?

A Parenteral nutrition should be delayed until day 7 in the malnourished patient to minimize risk of line sepsis.

B Immune-modulating formulas for enteral feeding are the standard of care for critically ill septic patient.

C Early parenteral nutrition decreases mortality in the critically ill patient.

D Initiation of enteral nutrition within 24–48 hours of admission is the optimal choice in the critically injured trauma patients.

E Enteral nutrition should not be initiated in a patient with an open abdomen.

Proper nutritional support is essential in the treatment of critically ill patient. Current guidelines recommend initiating enteral nutrition within 24–48 hours of admission to the intensive care unit for optimal management. In comparison to parenteral nutrition, enteral nutrition not only promotes functional and structural integrity of the gut, but it has also been shown to reduce the rate of infectious complications. An open abdomen is not a contraindication to enteral nutrition. In fact, initiating enteral nutrition in this patient population has been shown to decrease complications and mortality while increasing fascial closure. Immune-modulating formulas for enteral feeding have been hypothesized to decrease the inflammatory response while improving the immune response. Current guidelines from the Society of Critical Care Medicine and the American Society for Parenteral and Enteral Nutrition recommend immunonutrition in select patient populations such as patients with traumatic brain injury and perioperative patients in the surgical intensive care unit. The guidelines, on the other hand, recommend against immunonutrition in patients with septic shock given the increase in mortality.

The general indications for the use of parenteral nutrition are (1) provision of adequate nutrition for as long as necessary intravenously when use of the gastrointestinal tract is impractical, inadequate, ill-advised, or impossible; (2) reduction of mechanical and secretory activity of the alimentary tract to basal levels in order to achieve a state of "bowel rest"; (3) provision of specially tailored formulas to improve nutritional status in patients with kidney or liver failure; and (4) reduction of the urgency for surgical intervention in patients who might eventually require operation, but in whom prolonged, progressive malnutrition will greatly increase the risk of the operation and postoperative complications. With respect to timing of parenteral nutrition, in patients at low nutrition risk, parenteral nutrition should not be started until after hospital day 7. Early initiation of parenteral nutrition in this patient population has been associated with higher complications and delayed recovery. On the other hand, early parenteral nutrition is recommended in high nutrition risk patients, as it has been associated with decreased nosocomial infections and shorter duration of mechanical ventilation.

Answer: D

Burlew, C. C., Moore, E. E., Cuschieri, J., et al. (2012). Who should we feed? Western Trauma Association multi-institutional study of enteral nutrition in the open abdomen after injury. *The journal of trauma and acute care surgery*, 73(6), 1380–1388.

Casaer, M. P., Mesotten, D., Hermans, G., et al. (2011). Early versus late parenteral nutrition in critically ill adults. *The New England Journal of Medicine*, 365(6), 506–517.

McClave, S. A., Taylor, B. E., Martindale, R. G., et al. (2016). Guidelines for the provision and assessment of nutrition support therapy in the adult critically ill patient Society of Critical Care Medicine (SCCM) and American Society for Parenteral and Enteral Nutrition (ASPEN). *Journal of Parenteral and Enteral Nutrition*, 40(2), 159–211.

Patel, J. J., Kozeniecki, M., Biesboer, A., et al. (2016). Early Trophic enteral nutrition is associated with improved outcomes in mechanically ventilated patients with septic shock: a retrospective review. *Journal of Intensive Care Medicine*, 31(7), 471–477.

Rhodes, A., Evans, L. E., et al. (2017). Surviving sepsis campaign: international guidelines for management of sepsis and septic shock: 2016. *Intensive Care Medicine*, 43(3), 304–377.

16 A 52-year-old woman is admitted to the intensive care unit following a motor vehicle collision. Her injuries include pulmonary contusions and a ruptured right ventricle requiring sternotomy and repair. She was well nourished prior to hospital admission. She is weaning from mechanical ventilation and tolerating low-dose enteral nutrition via a nasogastric tube, achieving 50% of her estimated caloric requirements. Which of the following statements is true?

A Post-pyloric feeding access must be established prior to initiation of enteral nutrition.

B Supplemental parenteral nutrition should be initiated within 7–10 days of admission.

C Parenteral nutrition should not be initiated as the patient is receiving enteral nutrition.

D Supplemental parenteral nutrition should be initiated after 7–10 days of admission.

E Enteral nutrition should be discontinued and parenteral nutrition initiated.

The level of infusion of enteral feeds within the gastrointestinal tract can be gastric or post-pyloric. Although post-pyloric/small bowel enteral nutrition (EN) decreases the risk of pneumonia, there is no difference in mortality or length of stay. Therefore, early enteral feeds should not be delayed if timely obtainment of post-pyloric enteral access is not feasible. Therefore, answer A is wrong.

Early initiation of EN, preferably within 24–48 hours of admission, is recommended in the critically ill patient who is unable to maintain volitional intake. If the patient is well-nourished, supplemental parenteral nutrition (PN) should be considered after 7 days if unable to meet >50–60% of energy and protein requirements by the enteral route. If the patient is nutritionally at-risk and unlikely to achieve desired enteral intake, PN should be considered within 3–5 days of admission. Lastly, PN should be considered as soon as feasible in a patient with baseline moderate-to-severe malnutrition when enteral intake is not sufficient.

Initiating supplemental PN earlier than recommended in a patient who is able to tolerate some enteral nutrition does not improve outcomes and may even be detrimental. The randomized control trial by Casaer et al. revealed that when compared to early supplemental PN, delayed initiation of supplemental PN led to fewer infections, shorter duration of mechanical ventilation, and renal replacement therapy, as well as shorter length of stay in the ICU and lower health care costs.

Early enteral (EN) nutrition promotes gut integrity and systemic immunity while reducing oxidative stress. In addition to this, EN is preferred to parenteral nutrition given its beneficial effects, as well as reduction in infectious morbidity and ICU length of stay. Enteral nutrition is therefore preferred over parenteral nutrition whenever possible. Once the nutrition requirements delivered by EN advance toward goals, supplemental PN should be discontinued. Answer E is therefore wrong.

Answer: D

Casaer, M. P., Mesotten, D., Hermans, G., et al. (2011). Early versus late parenteral nutrition in critically ill adults. *The New England Journal of Medicine*, 365(6), 506–517.

Heyland, D. K. (2012). Early supplemental parenteral nutrition in critically ill adults increased infections, ICU length of stay and cost. *BMJ Evidence-Based Medicine*, 17(3), 86–87.

McClave, S. A., Taylor, B. E., Martindale, R. G., et al. (2016). Guidelines for the provision and assessment of nutrition support therapy in the adult critically ill patient Society of Critical Care Medicine (SCCM) and American Society for Parenteral and Enteral Nutrition (ASPEN). *Journal of Parenteral and Enteral Nutrition*, 40(2), 159–211.

Worthington, P., Balint, J., Bechtold, M.et al. (2017). When is parenteral nutrition appropriate? *Journal of Parenteral and Enteral Nutrition*, 41(3), 324–377.

17 Which of the following is true regarding lipid use in critically ill patients?

A Omega-3 and not omega-6 fatty acids are currently used in total parenteral nutrition formulas.

B There is no biochemical test to diagnose fatty acid deficiency.

C Lipid emulsions should be avoided in critically ill patients in the first week of the ICU stay.

D Essential fatty acid deficiency occurs if patients do not receive lipids within the first seven days.

E None of the above.

Intravenous lipid emulsions are a key component of parenteral nutrition, serving as both a source of essential fatty acids (omega-3 and omega-6), as well as nonprotein calories. Essential fatty acids play a key role in structural stability of membranes, as well as in generation of cellular signaling molecules. Humans lack the ability to synthesize these fatty acids and must therefore be obtained from other sources. Essential fatty acid deficiency can manifest through nonspecific biochemical changes that should raise suspicion, such as a rise in triene:tetraene ratio, liver function tests, and triglyceride levels.

The nature of the lipids that should be administered is currently the focus of much debate; so is the question of whether or not such innovations as structured lipids and triglycerides of varying chain lengths are of any benefit. A study by Dudrick et al. proved that the fear of essential fatty acid deficiency, if fatty emulsions are not given to critically ill and injured patients, is unfounded. In that study, designed to arrest and eliminate atherosclerotic plaque formation in patients with severe heart disease, total parenteral nutrition (TPN) was administered, with no lipids, for 3 months. None of the patients on TPN without lipids developed fatty acid deficiency, as measured by the triene:tetraene ratio and by clinical examinations. A subsequent study found that trauma patients on TPN with no lipids had better clinical outcomes than patients on TPN with lipids. The latest guidelines of the American Society for Parenteral and Enteral Nutrition call for no fat, or limited fat, in the first week in the ICU.

Answer: C

Mogensen, K. M. (2017). Essential fatty acid deficiency. *Practical Gastroenterology*, 41(6), 37–44.

McClave, S. A., Taylor, B. E., Martindale, R. G., et al. (2016). Guidelines for the provision and assessment of nutrition support therapy in the adult critically ill patient Society of Critical Care Medicine (SCCM) and American Society for Parenteral and Enteral Nutrition (ASPEN). *Journal of Parenteral and Enteral Nutrition*, 40(2), 159–211.

Schneider P. J. (2006). Nutrition support teams: an evidence-based practice. *Nutrition in Clinical Practice*, 21(1), 62–67.

18 A 54-year-old man is admitted to the surgical intensive care unit with septic shock after undergoing a partial colectomy for perforated colon cancer. Which of the following is an optimal method to assess his risk for adverse events that can be modified with aggressive nutritional therapy?
    A Measuring triceps skinfold thickness
    B Nutrition Risk in the Critically Ill (NUTRIC) score
    C Serum transferrin and prealbumin levels
    D Serum albumin level
    E None of the above

The American Society for Parenteral and Enteral Nutrition (ASPEN) guidelines recommend all trauma and critical patients undergo a full assessment of nutritional risk within the first 48 hours of admission.

Nutrition Risk in the Critically Ill (NUTRIC) score is particularly suited for the trauma and critically ill population as it can determine nutritional status and disease severity. This scoring system is designed to quantify the risk of critically ill patients' developing adverse events that may be modified by aggressive nutrition therapy. The scoring system incorporates the following six variables: age, APACHE II score, SOFA score, number of comorbidities, days from hospital to ICU admission, and interleukin-6 levels. A score of greater than 5 out of 10 is associated with worse clinical outcomes and is likely to benefit from aggressive nutrition therapy. Triceps skin fold thickness utilized as a proxy for total body fat, and hence a measure of nutritional status. However, it is not a reliable indicator of nutritional status as it is observer dependent and can vary with conditions such as edema, dehydration, and old age. Serum albumin, prealbumin, and transferrin are a reflection of the acute phase response and not an accurate indicator of the nutritional status in the critically ill.

Answer: B

Heyland, D. K., Stephens, K. E., Day, A. G., et al. (2011). The success of enteral nutrition and ICU-acquired infections: a multicenter observational study. *Clinical nutrition (Edinburgh, Scotland)*, 30(2), 148–155.

McClave, S. A., Taylor, B. E., Martindale, R. G., et al. (2016). Guidelines for the provision and assessment of nutrition support therapy in the adult critically ill patient Society of Critical Care Medicine (SCCM) and American Society for Parenteral and Enteral Nutrition (ASPEN). *Journal of Parenteral and Enteral Nutrition*, 40(2), 159–211.

19 Regarding nutritional therapy in burns, the following is correct:
    A Protein needs are increased and should be in the range of 1.5–2 g/kg/d.
    B Indirect calorimetry is almost never needed as other predictive formulas are just as accurate.
    C Supplementation of enteral nutrition with parenteral nutrition is of benefit.
    D Nutrition should be held until > 48 hours, at the onset of the catabolic phase.
    E None of the above.

Indirect calorimetry remains the gold standard for estimating energy expenditure in patients who are critically ill, including burn patients. If indirect calorimetry is not available, various published predictive equations have been used in the past, although their accuracy in burn patients is poor. In an evaluation of 46 predictive equations published between 1953 and 2000, Dickerson et al. found none of them to be precise in estimating energy expenditure measured by indirect calorimetry in 24 patients with >20% total body surface area burns. A trial evaluating the role of supplemental parenteral nutrition showed that patients receiving both parenteral and enteral nutrition had a higher incidence of infection and increased mortality compared with patients receiving enteral nutrition alone. The 2001 American Burn Association guidelines, the 2013 ESPEN guidelines, and ASPEN 2016 guidelines all recommend the provision of 1.5–2 g of protein/kg/d for patients with burn injury. Based on expert consensus, very early (within 4–6 hours of injury) initiation of enteral nutrition in burn patients is recommended.

Answer: A

Dickerson, R. N., Gervasio, J. M., et al. (2002). Accuracy of predictive methods to estimate resting energy expenditure of thermally-injured patients. *JPEN. Journal of Parenteral and Enteral Nutrition*, 26(1), 17–29.

McClave, S. A., Taylor, B. E., Martindale, R. G., et al. (2016). Guidelines for the provision and assessment of nutrition support therapy in the adult critically ill patient Society of Critical Care Medicine (SCCM) and American Society for Parenteral and Enteral Nutrition (ASPEN). *Journal of Parenteral and Enteral Nutrition*, 40(2), 159–211.

Rousseau, A. F., Losser, M. R., Ichai, C., & Berger, M. M. (2013). ESPEN endorsed recommendations: nutritional therapy in major burns. *Clinical Nutrition*, 32(4), 497–502.

20   Which of the following statement about TPN is true?

   A Dr. Stanley Dudrick described the growth of intravenously fed mice that experienced normal weight gain and normal growth, as compared with their orally fed counterparts.

   B The rate of TPN use in the critical care setting has increased in recent years.

   C TPN cannot give clinicians the ability to parenterally fulfill patients' ongoing requirement for calories, protein, electrolytes, vitamins, minerals, trace elements, and fluids.

   D TPN is imperative in all critically ill patients.

   E Early nutritional support via TPN has the potential to reduce disease severity, diminish complications, and decrease the intensive care unit (ICU) length of stay.

In 1967, Dudrick et al. described the growth of intravenously fed beagle puppies that experienced normal weight gain and normal growth, as compared with their orally fed counterparts. When enteral nutrition is not feasible or adequate, early nutritional support via

TPN has the potential to reduce disease severity, diminish complications, and decrease the intensive care unit (ICU) length of stay. When enteral nutrition is not possible, TPN gives clinicians the ability to parenterally fulfill patients' ongoing requirement for calories, protein, electrolytes, vitamins, minerals, trace elements, and fluids. TPN use has been studied in patients with a wide array of clinical conditions, such as trauma, cancer, inflammatory bowel disease, short gut syndrome, radiation enteritis, poor wound healing, and gastrointestinal (GI) fistula. Yet few well-designed, randomized, controlled trials of the efficacy of TPN in critically ill and injured patients have been conducted. It is well known that 20–40% of critically ill and injured patients exhibit some form of malnutrition. Of that subgroup, 85–90% can be treated with enteral nutrition. In the remaining 10–15%, enteral nutrition is contraindicated; TPN, delivered intravenously, provides the only support. Many interacting biologic and clinical factors are responsible for the development of malnutrition in critically ill and injured hospitalized patients, including a history of pre-injury or disease-specific causes, the hypercatabolic states associated with trauma, sepsis, cancer, and surgical interventions. Rhee et al. showed that the rate of TPN use in the critical care setting has declined; intensivists continue to encounter many cases where enteral feeding fails and TPN is imperative.

Answer: E

Dudrick, S. J., Wilmore, D. W., Vars, H. M., et al. (1968). Long-term total parenteral nutrition with growth, development, and positive nitrogen balance. Surgery, 64(1), 134–142.

Latifi, R., & Dudrick, S. J. (2003). *The Biology and Practice of Current Nutritional Support*, 2nd Edition. Georgetown, Texas: Landes Bioscience, 208–215.

Rhee, P., Hadjizacharia, P., Trankiem, C., et al. (2007). What happened to total parenteral nutrition? The disappearance of its use in a trauma intensive care unit. *The Journal of Trauma*, 63(6), 1215–1222.

Worthington, P., Balint, J., Bechtold, M., et al. (2017). When is parenteral nutrition appropriate? *Journal of Parenteral and Enteral Nutrition*, 41(3), 324–377.

Ziegler, T. R. (2009). Parenteral nutrition in the critically ill patient. *The New England Journal of Medicine*, 361(11), 1088–1097.

21   A 34-year-old man sustains a subdural hematoma, pulmonary contusion, and pelvic fracture following a motor vehicle crash. He is admitted to the intensive care unit for continuation of care and mechanical ventilation. Which of the following statements is true?

A Food coloring in enteral nutrition can be used as a marker for aspiration.

B There is no role in starting prokinetics in high-risk patients.

C Post-pyloric feeding has been shown to reduce the risk of aspiration pneumonia.

D Targeting 24-hour feeding volumes is equal to targeting hourly rates.

E High-risk patients and those intolerant to bolus feeds should not receive continuous feeds.

A Cochrane review by Alkhawaja et al. revealed that post-pyloric feeding, when compared to gastric feeding, had a 30% lower rate of pneumonia. There was, however, insufficient evidence to show that other clinically important outcomes such as duration of mechanical ventilation, mortality, and length of stay were affected by the level of tube feeds. Therefore, post-pyloric feeding is preferred in ICU patients when feasible. It is acceptable to start gastric feeds initially if post-pyloric access is not readily available; however, recommendations suggest beginning with jejunal feeding in patients with any of the following features: recurrent aspiration of gastric contents, esophageal dysmotility with a history of regurgitation, or delayed gastric emptying.

Volume-based feeding protocols in which 24-hour or daily volumes are targeted instead of hourly rates have been shown to increase volume of nutrition delivered. This is due to the fact that it empowers nurses to increase the feeding rate as needed to make up for the volume lost as a way to address the challenges of frequent interruptions. Therefore, volume-based protocols enable a greater volume of enteral nutrition to be delivered compared to a fixed hourly rate protocol.

Adding prokinetic agents such as erythromycin or metoclopramide have been shown to improve gastric emptying and tolerance of enteral nutrition but has resulted in little change in clinical outcome for ICU patients. Besides food coloring being found to be associated with mitochondrial toxicity, the US Food and Drug Administration (FDA), through a Health Advisory Bulletin (September 2003), issued a mandate against the use of blue food coloring as a monitor for aspiration in patients receiving enteral nutrition.

Answer: C

Alkhawaja, S., Martin, C., Butler, R. J., & Gwadry-Sridhar, F. (2015). Post-pyloric versus gastric tube feeding for preventing pneumonia and improving nutritional outcomes in critically ill adults. *Cochrane Database of Systematic Reviews*, (8).

Heyland, D. K., Murch, L., Cahill, N., et al. (2013) Enhanced protein-energy provision via the enteral route feeding protocol in critically ill patients: results of a cluster randomized trial. *Critical Care Medicine*, 41(12), 2743–2753.

Heyland, D. K., Drover, J. W., MacDonald, S., et al. (2001). Effect of postpyloric feeding on gastroesophageal regurgitation and pulmonary microaspiration: results of a randomized controlled trial. *Critical Care Medicine*, 29(8), 1495–1501.

McClave, S. A., Taylor, B. E., Martindale, R. G., et al. (2016). Guidelines for the provision and assessment of nutrition support therapy in the adult critically ill patient. *Journal of Parenteral and Enteral Nutrition*, 40(2), 159–211.

22 A 24-year-old critically ill man has a prolonged ileus postoperatively after multiple penetrating small-bowel injuries and resections. The decision is made to initiate total parenteral nutrition in the intensive care unit. His actual body weight is 80 kg, height 71 inches, and BMI 24.6. kg/m^2. Patient's estimated protein needs are 2–2.5 g/kg/day and total calories of 25–30 kcal/kg/day (Note: protein = 4 kcal/g; carbohydrate = 3.4 kcal/g; lipid = 10 kcal/g). Which of the following represents his calculated nutritional needs?

A Protein: 70 g/d; Dextrose: 300 g/d; Lipids 65 g/d; rate of 105 mL/hr

B Protein: 180 g/d; Dextrose: 225 g/d; Lipids 40 g/d; rate of 80 mL/hr

C Protein: 105 g/d; Dextrose: 500 g/d; Lipids 45 g/d; rate of 90 mL/hr

D Protein: 180 g/d; Dextrose: 300 g/d; Lipids 65 g/d; rate of 100 mL/hr

E Protein: 105 g/d; Dextrose: 300 g/d; Lipids 90 g/d; rate of 65 mL/hr

Total parenteral nutrition (TPN) can serve as an essential therapeutic modality for a variety of indications. TPN prescriptions can be challenging with possible adverse effects, hence steering clinicians away. Appropriate and safe prescription of TPN is a critical first step and an essential component in utilizing parenteral nutrition. TPN is an admixture of solutions containing dextrose, amino acids, electrolytes, vitamins, and minerals. Lipid emulsion can be infused separately or added to the main mixture.

One simple approach to calculating the requirements and components of TPN is as follows (calculations are based on actual body weight, unless BMI > 30 kg/m^2; if the patient is obese, then you would use ideal body weight):

Step 1: Calculating the protein needs depends on the patient's physiologic status. Per the Society of Critical Care Medicine/American Society of Parenteral and Enteral Nutrition (SCCM/ASPEN) Guidelines for the Provision and Assessment of Nutrition Support Therapy in the Adult Critically Ill Patient, this patient is critically ill. Protein requirements recommended for critically ill trauma patients are 2–2.5 g/kg/day. In our scenario:

80 kg actual body weight × 2–2.5 g/kg/d = 160–200 g/d
1 g protein = 4 kcal energy
180 g/d × 4 kcal = 720 kcal/d from protein

Step 2: Calculating the nonprotein calories also depends on the patient's physiologic status. Due to the patient's critical illness, the SCCM/ASPEN guidelines recommend 25–30 kcal/kg/day. In our scenario:

80 kg actual body weight × 30 kcal/kg/d = 2400 total kcal/d
2400 kcal/d − 720 kcal/d from protein = 1680 kcal/day of nonprotein calories

Step 3: Lipids typically make up 20–30% of the total daily caloric content in parenteral nutrition.

Lipids = 0.2 − 0.3 × 2400 kcal/d = 480 kcal/d to 720 kcal/d
1 g of lipids = 10 kcal which would give 48–72 grams of lipids per day
To simplify from the example, 65 g of lipids would be 650 kcal/d

Step 4: Calculating grams of dextrose. 2400 kcal/d − (720 kcal/d of protein + 650 kcal/d of lipids) = 1030 kcal/d of dextrose.

1 g dextrose = 3.4 kcal
1030 kcal/d ÷ 3.4 kcal = 302.9 g of dextrose, which can be rounded to 300 g of dextrose a day

Step 5: To calculate the total fluids needed per day, an average of 30 mL/kg/day may be used. In our scenario:

80 kg actual body weight × 30 mL/kg/d = 2400 mL total volume of fluids required daily, which would give you a rate of 100 mL/hr

Answer D

McClave, S. A., Taylor, B. E., Martindale, R. G., et al. (2016). Guidelines for the provision and assessment of nutrition support therapy in the adult critically ill patient. *Journal of Parenteral and Enteral Nutrition*, 40(2):159–211.

Mundi, M. S., Nystrom, E. M., Hurley, D. L., & McMahon, M. M. (2017). Management of parenteral nutrition in hospitalized adult patients. *Journal of Parenteral and Enteral Nutrition*, 41(4):535–549.

20

Neurocritical Care

Kevin W. Cahill, MD and Frederick Giberson, MD

Department of Surgery, Christiana Care Health Care System, Newark, DE, USA

1 *The early resumption of high-dose statin therapy in a hospitalized patient following ischemic stroke results in:*
   A *No difference in outcome when compared to holding statin therapy or delaying resumption.*
   B *An equivalent benefit when compared with resuming a lower dose statin.*
   C *A significant worsening of patient outcomes.*
   D *Strong association with increased post-stroke survival, even compared to low-dose therapy.*
   E *No significant effect on clinical outcomes.*

A large retrospective study of 17 hospitals (Flint et al.) found that those patients who underwent statin withdrawal in the hospital had a substantially greater risk of death. Although the use of low-dose statins appears to be beneficial, those taking high-dose statins (>60 mg/day) compared to low-dose (<60 mg/day) have been shown to have a greater survival benefit. Multiple trials have demonstrated statin therapy is associated with a marked improvement in patient outcomes in ischemic stroke.

Answer: D

Flint AC, Kamel H, Navi BB, Rao VA, Faigeles BS, Conell C, Klingman JG, Sidney S, Hills NK, Sorel M, Cullen SP, Johnston SC. Statin use during ischemic stroke hospitalization is strongly associated with improved poststroke survival. *Stroke* 2012;43(1):147–154. 10.1161/STROKEAHA.111.627729.

Flint AC, Kamel H, Navi BB, Rao VA, Faigeles BS, Conell C, Klingman JG, Hills NK, Nguyen-Huynh M, Cullen SP, Sidney S, Johnston SC. Inpatient statin use predicts improved ischemic stroke discharge disposition. *Neurology* 2012;78(21):1678–1683. 10.1212/WNL.0b013e3182575142

2 *When compared with placebo, the use of benzodiazepines in the treatment of out-of-hospital patients with status epilepticus has shown a trend toward:*
   A *Higher rates of respiratory compromise*
   B *Lower rates of respiratory compromise*
   C *Higher rate of resulting neurologic deficit at hospital discharge*
   D *Lower rate of resulting neurologic deficit at hospital discharge*
   E *Unchanged duration of status epilepticus*

Out-of-hospital use of benzodiazepines in the treatment of status epilepticus is associated with a trend toward lower out-of-hospital complications than placebo, as demonstrated in a randomized, double-blind by Alldredge BK et al. The rates of respiratory or circulatory complications after the study treatment were 10.6% for the lorazepam group, 10.3% for the diazepam group, and 22.5% for the placebo group. Though the use of out-of-hospital benzodiazepines resulted in a statistically significant decreased duration of out-of-hospital status epilepticus, it did not ultimately affect the rate of resulting neurologic deficit at hospital discharge. Additionally, a more recent study examined pre-enrollment data from the Established Status Epilepticus Treatment Trial (ESETT) and found that many of those patients with status epilepticus who were considered to "fail" benzodiazepine receive lower than guideline recommended dosages. This trial found that approximately 76% of patients received lower than recommended first doses of benzodiazepine treatment for status epilepticus, suggesting this delay may place patients at high risk for longer seizures and poor outcomes.

Surgical Critical Care and Emergency Surgery: Clinical Questions and Answers, Third Edition.
Edited by Forrest "Dell" Moore, Peter M. Rhee, and Carlos J. Rodriguez.
© 2022 John Wiley & Sons Ltd. Published 2022 by John Wiley & Sons Ltd.
Companion website: www.wiley.com/go/surgicalcriticalcare3e

Answer: B

Alldredge BK. A comparison of lorazepam, diazepam, and placebo for the treatment of out-of-hospital status epilepticus. *New England Journal of Medicine* 2001;345(9):631–637.

Sathe AG, Underwood E, Coles LD, Elm JJ, Silbergleit R, Chamberlain JM, Kapur J, Cock HR, Fountain NB, Shinnar S, Lowenstein DH, Rosenthal ES, Conwit RA, Bleck TP, Cloyd JC. Patterns of benzodiazepine underdosing in the Established Status Epilepticus Treatment Trial. *Epilepsia* 2021;62(3):795–806. 10.1111/epi.16825.

3   *The medication of choice for initial treatment of status epilepticus is:*
    A *IV lorazepam*
    B *IV midazolam*
    C *IV phenobarbital*
    D *IV phenytoin*
    E *IV magnesium*

A double-blind study at 16 VA medical centers and 6 affiliated university hospitals over 5 years randomly assigned patients with generalized convulsive status-epilepticus to receive intravenous lorazepam, phenobarbital, phenytoin, or diazepam followed by phenytoin. Treatment was considered successful if all clinical and electrical evidence of seizure activity halted within 20 minutes of infusion and did not recur within 60 minutes. Lorazepam was demonstrated to have the highest rate of treatment success. More recently, a systematic review by the Japan Resuscitation Council Task Force in 2020 performed a meta-analysis and found that IV lorazepam had a statistically significant superior effect for seizure cessation when compared with diazepam.

Answer: A

Kobata H, Hifumi T, Hoshiyama E, Yamakawa K, Nakamura K, Soh M, Kondo Y, Yokobori S; Japan Resuscitation Council (JRC) Neuroresuscitation Task Force and the Guidelines Editorial Committee. Comparison of diazepam and lorazepam for the emergency treatment of adult status epilepticus: a systemic review and meta-analysis. *Acute Medicine & Surgery*. 2020;7(1):e582. 10.1002/ams2.582.

Treiman DM, Meyers PD, Walton NY, Collins JF, Colling C, Rowan AJ, Handforth A, Faught E, Calabrese VP, Uthman BM, et al. A comparison of four treatments for generalized convulsive status epilepticus. Veterans affairs status epilepticus cooperative study group. *New England Journal of Medicine* 1998;339(12):792–798.

4   *For which of the following side effects of benzodiazepines is flumazenil a <u>reliable</u> reversal agent?*
    A *Respiratory depression*
    B *Hypoventilation*
    C *Sedative effects*
    D *Cardiac depression/hemodynamic instability*
    E *Benzodiazepine-induced amnesia*

Although flumazenil has been shown to reverse the effects of benzodiazepine-induced ventilatory depression, it appears to be inconsistent particularly in pediatric use, those with liver disease or those who have concurrently received an opioid. While flumazenil has been shown to reliably reverse the sedative effect of benzodiazepines, the duration of flumazenil tends to be shorter than that of the most commonly used benzodiazepines. Flumazenil has no significant effect on cardiovascular parameters when administered to patients with stable ischemic heart disease and does not completely and consistently reverse benzodiazepine-induced amnesia.

Answer: C

Marraffa J, Cohen V, Howland MA. Antidotes for toxicological emergencies: a practical review. *American Journal of Health-System Pharmacy* 2012; 69(3):199–212.

Roche Pharmaceuticals. Flumazenil (Romazicon) data sheet. Revised April 2010.

5   *Which of the following side effects are less commonly seen in atypical (second generation) antipsychotic drugs when compared to first-generation antipsychotics?*
    A *Anticholinergic effect*
    B *QTc prolongation*
    C *Hyperprolactinemia*
    D *Akathisia*
    E *Weight gain*

All the listed side effects are associated with atypical antipsychotic agent use. Anticholinergic symptoms include constipation, urinary retention, blurred vision, or dry mouth. All antipsychotics, including atypical, cause prolongation of ventricular repolarization, which can lead to torsades and sudden cardiac death. Antipsychotics block the normal inhibition of dopamine production on pituitary mammotropic cells in the hypothalamus, leading to higher levels of prolactin. This may be asymptomatic or may be associated with gynecomastia, galactorrhea, acne, infertility, or loss of bone density. Akathisia can subjectively be described as a feeling of inner restlessness and inability to remain still for long. Second-generation antipsychotics have often been distinguished from first-generation antipsychotics by the decreased risk of extrapyramidal side effects such as akathisia. Despite a relative decreased risk compared to first-generation antipsychotics, a review of the literature demonstrated that second-generation drugs still lead to akathisia with rates ranging from 2.9 to 13.0%. Weight gain is more common in the second-generation antipsychotics than in some first generation.

Answer: D

Chow CL, Kadouh NK, Bostwick JR, VandenBerg AM. Akathisia and newer second-generation antipsychotic drugs: a review of current evidence. *Pharmacotherapy* 2020;40(6):565–574. 10.1002/phar.2404.

Muench J, Hamer AM. Adverse effects of antipsychotic medications. *American Family Physician* 2010;81(5):617–622.

Solmi M, Murru A, Pacchiarotti I. Safety, tolerability, and risks associated with first- and second-generation antipsychotics: a state-of-the-art clinical review. *Therapeutics and Clinical Risk Management* 2017; 13:757–777.

6 *Which of the following is a known side effect of barbiturate overdose?*
 A *Hypertension*
 B *Tachycardia*
 C *Polycythemia vera*
 D *Hypokalemia*
 E *Increased vascular tone*

Hypotension is a common side effect of barbiturate due to medullary depression, peripheral vasodilation, and myocardial depression. Inadvertent intra-arterial administration of barbiturates has resulted in ischemia and gangrene of the extremity. Rather than leading to excessive RBC production, phenobarbital has been implicated in drug-induced megaloblastic anemia, thought to be induced by decreased absorption of folic acid. Multiple case reports have identified the development of persistent hypokalemia in certain patients undergoing barbiturate infusion, particularly those patients with severe traumatic brain injury. Multiple various mechanisms have been suggested for this effect, including inhibition of voltage-dependent potassium channels, inhibition of ATP-dependent potassium channels of the B-cells of the pancreas leading to excessive insulin secretion or excess mineralocorticoid secretion and catecholamine surge leading to hypokalemia. One recent study examined the incidence of dyskalemia in patients with traumatic brain injuries treated with barbiturate therapy. This study found that 62% of patients treated with barbiturate therapy developed mild-to-moderate hyperkalemia (2.6–3.5 mEq/L); 16.2% of patients developed severe hypokalemia (<2.5 mEq/L). It was noted that 66% of patients with severe hypokalemia who had received

aggressive potassium supplementation went on to develop severe hyperkalemia after cessation of barbiturate therapy. This suggests that the barbiturate-induced redistributive hypokalemia reverses quickly with cessation of therapy, placing those who undergo aggressive supplementation at higher risk for developing rebound hyperkalemia.

Answer: D

Aytuluk HG, Topcu H. Severe hypokalemia and rebound hyperkalemia during barbiturate coma in patients with severe traumatic brain injury. Neurocirugía (Asturias, Spain). 2020;31(5):216–222. 10.1016/j.neucir.2019.12.003.

Mintzer DM, Billet SN, Chmielewski L. Drug-induced hematologic syndromes. *Advances in Hematology*. 2009;2009:495863. 10.1155/2009/495863.

Neil MJ, Dale MC. Hypokalaemia with severe rebound hyperkalaemia after therapeutic barbiturate coma. *Anesthesia & Analgesia* 2009;108(6):1867–1868. 10.1213/ane.0b013e3181a16418

Vangerven M, Delrue G, Brugman E, Cosaert P. A new therapeutic approach to accidental intra-arterial injection of thiopentone. *British Journal of Anaesthesia* 1989;62(1):98–100.

7 *Targeted hypothermia after ventricular fibrillation-associated cardiac arrest has been shown to improve neurologic outcomes in patients who are unconscious after resuscitation. Hypothermia appears to improve outcomes through reduced cerebral metabolic demand, decreased free radical generation, and reduced inflammatory response following reperfusion. However, more significant hypothermia can have markedly adverse effects. What side effects are associated with significant hypothermia?*
 A *Hyperkalemia*
 B *Cardiac dysrhythmia*
 C *Decreased urine output*
 D *Hepatic failure*
 E *Hypoglycemia*

Targeted-temperature management has been associated with hypokalemia, not hyperkalemia. More severe hypothermia has been associated with the development of cardiac dysrhythmias; ventricular tachycardia or ventricular fibrillation being the most common. This is most common if the patient is severely hypothermic (<30 degrees Celsius). In patients who are both hypothermic and unstable due to an additional mechanism, rewarming is the treatment of choice given that defibrillation and medications appear to have decreased reliability until the patient is adequately rewarmed. Cold diuresis has been observed to be a side effect of therapeutic hypothermia. This is thought secondary to the redirection of blood from the extremities due to peripheral vasoconstriction. This relative increase in core fluid volume leads to higher blood pressure. The corresponding renal response to elevated renal perfusion leads to increased urine output. Hypothermia is not associated with increased risk of hepatic failure. Hypothermia decreases insulin secretin and increases insulin resistance, leading to hyperglycemia in patients receiving targeted-temperature management. As patients are rewarmed, they may develop significant hypoglycemia.

Answer: B

Haase, KK et al. Variability in glycemic control with temperature transitions during therapeutic hypothermia. *Critical Care Research and Practice* 2017;2017:4831480. 10.1155/2017/4831480

Hoek T. 2010 American Heart Association guidelines for cardiopulmonary resuscitation and emergency cardiovascular care. *Circulation* 2010;122:5829–586.

Piktel JS, Cheng A, McCauley M, Dale Z, Nassal M, Maleski D, Pawlowski G, Laurita KR, Wilson LD. Hypothermia modulates arrhythmia substrates during different phases of resuscitation from ischemic cardiac arrest. *Journal of the American Heart Association* 2017;6(11):e006472.

Raper, JD, Wang, HE. Urine output changes during postcardiac arrest therapeutic hypothermia. *Therapeutic Hypothermia and Temperature Management* 2013;3(4):173–177. 10.1089/ther.2013.0015

8 *A 27-year-old man presents with fever and complains of back pain and lower extremity weakness. He endorses a history of intravenous drug use for the past six months. What is the most likely causative organism?*
   A *Pseudomonas aeruginosa*
   B *Staphylococcus aureus*
   C *Escherichia coli*
   D *Actinomyces*
   E *Candida albicans*

Staphylococcus aureus is the most common causative agent found in epidural abscesses, typically accounting for greater than 40% of all organisms identified in multiple studies. One retrospective study from 2017 of 11 cases of epidural abscess found that of those 84% of cases in which a causative organism was identified, Staphylococcus remained the predominant pathogen. Although increasingly associated with epidural abscesses in those with a history of intravenous drug use, Pseudomonas remains a less likely organism. With a history of intravenous drug use or urinary tract infections, *Escherichia coli* may be seen, although with a comparatively low incidence. Actinomyces or Candida species are rarely associated with epidural abscesses.

Answer: B

Darouiche RO. Spinal epidural abscess. *New England Journal of Medicine* 2006;355(19):2012–2020. 10.1056/NEJMra055111.

Kaufman DM, Kaplan JG, Litman N. Infectious agents in spinal epidural abscesses. *Neurology* 1980;30:844–850.

Vakili M, Crum-Cianflone NF. Spinal epidural abscess: a series of 101 cases. *The American Journal of Medicine* 2017;130(12):1458–1463. 10.1016/j.amjmed.2017.07.017.

9 *What is the disadvantage when using midazolam for neurologically compromised patients?*
   A *Limited disturbance of cerebral and vascular tone*
   B *Anticonvulsant activity*
   C *Coupled decrease in cerebral metabolic demand with a decrease in cerebral blood flow*
   D *Prolonged sedative effects when used as an infusion*
   E *Rapid onset of action*

Benzodiazepines cause minimal alteration in cerebral and vascular tone, making them useful for treating neurologically ill patients. This class of drugs has potent anticonvulsant effects and are the initial pharmacologic treatment of choice for urgent control of seizure activity. The treatment of agitation with adequate sedation in neurologically ill patients at risk for intracranial hypertension is crucial. Benzodiazepine treatment results in decreased cerebral metabolic demand along with an associated decrease in cerebral blood flow. This decrease in the cerebral metabolic demand may improve the resulting cerebral oxygen supply to demand ratio despite potential decreased cerebral blood flow, making their use advantageous. Though single doses are typically well tolerated, continuous infusions may result in the accumulation of an active metabolite, alpha 1-hydroxy-midazolam. This may result in more prolonged sedation than desired. This has been noted to be exacerbated in patients with renal dysfunction, the obese, and those with hypoalbuminemia.

Answer: D

Barr J, Fraser GL, Puntillo K, et al.; American college of critical care medicine: Clinical practice guidelines for the management of pain, agitation, and delirium in adult patients in the intensive care unit. *Critical Care Medicine* 2013;41:263306.

Mirski MA, Lewin JJ 3rd. Sedation and analgesia in acute neurologic disease. *Current Opinion in Critical Care* 2010;16(2):81–91. 10.1097/MCC.0b013e328337495a.

10 *In patients who attain return of spontaneous circulation (ROSC) after cardiac arrest, which of the following physical examination, test, or imaging findings has the highest specificity for predicting poor neurologic outcomes?*

A *Status myoclonus < 48 hours after ROSC*

B *Unreactive burst suppression immediately following ROSC*

C *Diffuse anoxic brain injury on MRI*

D *Bilateral absent pupillary light reflex at > 72 hours from ROSC*

E *Early EEG reactivity*

Although the presence of an early post-anoxic status myoclonus is typically associated with poor neurologic outcome, in some cases it may be associated with neurologic recovery. Myoclonus is considered to be a less reliable predictor than pupillary light reflex and is recommended to be used only in conjunction with other markers such as EEG recording to rule out benign forms of post-anoxic myoclonus such as Lance-Adams syndrome. Malignant EEG patterns such as burst suppression have been shown to predict poor neurologic outcomes with high specificity, but most studies have looked for the presence of this pattern on EEG recorded a median 77 hours after ROSC. Given these confounders and that until recently, there was a lack of consistent classification of different EEG patterns associated with poor neurologic outcomes, the European Resuscitation Council and European Society of Intensive Care Medicine Guidelines for 2015 stated only to consider malignant EEG patterns in association with other predictors. MRI has been shown to be accurate for predicting poor neurologic outcome in small studies, but the methods used thus far are highly heterogeneous. Given the relative paucity of patients studied, as well as the lack of standardization, brain imaging studies for prognostication should only be used in combination with other predictors. Though the sensitivity of bilaterally absent pupillary light reflex at >72 hours from ROSC is low, it is highly specific for predicting poor neurologic outcomes (false positive rate < 5%). Early post-resuscitation EEG reactivity is a predictor of good neurologic outcome.

Answer: D

Sandroni, C., D'Arrigo, S. & Nolan, J.P. Prognostication after cardiac arrest. *Critical Care* 2018;22:150. https://doi.org/10.1186/s13054-018-2060-7.

Westhall E, Rossetti AO, van Rootselaar AF, Wesenberg Kjaer T, Horn J, Ullen S, Friberg H, Nielsen N, Rosen I, Aneman A, et al. Standardized EEG interpretation accurately predicts prognosis after cardiac arrest. *Neurology* 2016;86:1482–1490.

11 *A 28-year-old non-helmeted motorcyclist has a GCS of 6 (E2 V1T M3) due to severe traumatic brain injury (TBI). Non-contrast head CT demonstrates bifrontal contusions, scattered subarachnoid hemorrhage bilaterally, and global cerebral edema. An intracranial pressure (ICP) monitor is placed with an opening pressure of 34 mm Hg and sustained intracranial pressure of 28 mmHg. ABG shows a $PaCO_2$ of 38 mm Hg and sodium level is 143 mEq/L. The most appropriate next step in management to control ICP is:*

A *Hypoventilation to $PaCO_2$ less than or equal to 32 mm Hg*

B *Dexamethasone 4 mg IV every 6 hours*

C *Evacuation of intracranial hemorrhage*

D *Induction of pentobarbital coma*

E *250 mL bolus of 3% saline*

Brief elevations in ICP in TBI patients, especially when associated with stimulus, do not require specific intervention. But sustained elevation in ICP is associated with poor neurologic outcomes and death and should be treated. Hypertonic saline and mannitol are important early treatment options in TBI with intracranial hypertension caused by cerebral edema. Bolus hypertonic saline or mannitol is generally favored over continuous infusion, though the available evidence for bolus versus infusion are mixed in adult patients. Steroids are contraindicated in TBI with intracranial hypertension as the evidence indicates no survival nor good functional outcome benefit, and increased morbidity secondary to skin breakdown, gastritis or ulcer, and infection. In the scenario presented, there is no evacuable extra-axial hematoma. If a subdural or epidural hematoma is causing symptomatic mass effect, surgical evacuation would be first-line treatment. Pentobarbital coma remains a third-line option for refractory ICP elevation but has become largely displaced with craniectomy for decompression in some centers.

Answer: E

Carney N, Totten AM, O'Reilly C, et al. Guidelines for the management of severe traumatic brain injury, 4th edition. *Neurosurgery* 2017;1(80):6–15. 10.1227/NEU.0000000000001432.

12 *A 55-year-old woman is admitted to the ICU with depressed level of consciousness. Her GCS is 12. Workup reveals a tumor in the right middle cranial fossa with significant surrounding vasogenic edema. The most appropriate next step in management to prevent worsening mental status is:*

A *Dexmedetomidine infusion titrated to RASS less than or equal to one*

B *Phenobarbital 100 mg IV every 12 hours*

C *Dexamethasone 4 mg IV every 6 hours*
D *Levetiracetam 500 mg IV every 12 hours*
E *250 mL bolus of 3% saline*

Sedation, pain control, and prophylaxis or treatment of seizures are important adjuncts to the treatment of patients with symptomatic brain tumors, but do not directly affect cerebral edema. Cerebral edema associated with brain tumors is vasogenic edema, which is responsive to steroid therapy. This is in contradistinction to edema associated with traumatic brain injury, which is a combination of cytotoxic and vasogenic edema. Cytotoxic edema is not responsive to steroids, and the risks of steroid treatment therefore outweighs any potential benefit. Hypertonic saline has not been demonstrated to reduce cytotoxic edema nor outcomes with patients with brain tumors and edema, and therefore is not recommended.

Answer: C

Carney N, Totten AM, O'Reilly C, et al. Guidelines for the management of severe traumatic brain injury, 4th edition. *Neurosurgery* 2017;1(80):6–15. 10.1227/NEU.0000000000001432.
Koenig M. Cerebral edema and elevated intracranial pressure. *Continuum* 2018;24:1588–1602.

13 *Decompressive craniectomy in traumatic brain injured patients with medically refractory cerebral edema results in:*
   A *Improved odds of good functional recovery*
   B *Increased mortality*
   C *Greater incidence of vegetative state in survivors*
   D *No effect on survival*
   E *Greater need for other ICP-directed interventions*

Craniectomy should be considered as a third-line treatment for refractory ICP in traumatic TBI patients with global or multifocal brain injuries and cerebral edema with elevated ICP refractory to medical intervention. Decompressive Craniectomy in Diffuse Traumatic Brain Injury (DECRA) and Randomised Evaluation of Surgery with Craniectomy for Uncontrollable Elevation of Intracranial Pressure (RESCUEicp) are two recent clinical trials evaluating decompressive craniectomy in this patient population. In the DECRA trial, early decompressive craniectomy resulted in lowered ICP, but patients had worse neurologic outcomes in the early surgery arm. The RESCUEicp trial randomly selected patients with severe TBI with refractory ICP elevation to undergo decompressive craniectomy as a third-line treatment versus medical control of high ICPs. RESCUEicp demonstrated some benefits to decompressive craniectomy with higher odds of survival and lower odds of severe disability, but there was no effect on the odds of good recovery

and more patients survived in the vegetative state in the decompression group. Craniectomy remains a recommended option supported by weak evidence as third-line intervention for refractory ICP, with an understanding of a higher chance of survival but also of survival in a vegetative state.

Answer: C

Cooper DJ, Rosenfeld JV, Murray L, et al. Decompressive craniectomy in diffuse traumatic brain injury. *The New England Journal of Medicine* 2011;364(16):1493–1502. 10.1056/NEJMoa1102077.
Hutchinson PJ, Kolias AG, Timofeev IS, et al. Trial of decompressive craniectomy for traumatic intracranial hypertension. *The New England Journal of Medicine* 2016;375(12):1119–1130. 10.1056/NEJMoa1605215.

14 *A 62-year-old woman is admitted to the ICU with aneurysmal subarachnoid hemorrhage (aSAH). The care team is concerned about her risk for developing cerebral artery vasospasm. Interventions that reduce the likelihood of onset of vasospasm include:*
   A *Hypertension*
   B *Hemodilution*
   C *Hypervolemia*
   D *Dexamethasone*
   E *Nimodipine*

Aneurysmal SAH not infrequently causes cerebral artery vasospasm, which may result in cerebral ischemia. The traditional use of hypertension, hypervolemia, and hemodilution has been curtailed due to the lack of supporting evidence for the latter two interventions. Induced hypertension retains a role in the **treatment** of vasospasm associated with controlled aSAH but has no evidence-based role in prophylaxis. While maintenance of euvolemia may reduce the risk for vasospasm, hypervolemia, hemodilution, and hypervolemia do not. Steroids have no role in prevention or treatment of vasospasm in aSAH. While there is some conflicting evidence that the calcium channel blocker nimodipine affects the incidence of angiographic or symptomatic vasospasm, it has been demonstrated to improve patient outcomes in aSAH and has become a standard of care. Its action may be related to dilation of small arteries not seen on angiograms, inhibition of ischemia through other means, reductions of calcium-dependent toxicity or a combination thereof and remains to be fully elucidated.

Answer: E

Barker FG, Ogilvy CS. Efficacy of prophylactic nimodipine for delayed ischemic deficit after subarachnoid hemorrhage: a meta-analysis. *Journal of Neurosurgery* 1996;84:405.

Dankbaar JW, Slooter AJ, Rinkel GJ, Schaaf IC. Effect of different components of triple-H therapy on cerebral perfusion in patients with aneurysmal subarachnoid hemorrhage: a systematic review. *Critical Care*. 2010;14:R23. https://doi.org/10.1186/cc8886.

Gathier CS, Dankbaar JW, van der Jagt M, Verweij BH, Oldenbeuving AW, Rinkel GJ, et al.; HIMALAIA Study Group. Effects of induced hypertension on cerebral perfusion in delayed cerebral ischemia after aneurysmal subarachnoid hemorrhage: a randomized clinical trial. *Stroke*. 2015;46:3277–3281. 10.1161/STROKEAHA. 115.010537.

15 *A 22-year-old pedestrian was struck by an automobile resulting in a left femur fracture and moderate traumatic brain injury with low-volume left-sided subdural hematoma. Pneumatic compression boots were placed on the bilateral lower extremities. The consulting neurosurgeon requests withholding chemical venous thromboembolism (VTE) prophylaxis (prophylactic anticoagulation) for five days. Which of the following is most likely to reduce symptomatic pulmonary embolism within 90 days from injury?*

A *Hypervolemia*

B *Removal of the pneumatic compression device from the injured extremity*

C *Placement of IVC filter within 72 hours of admission*

D *Early mobilization and initiation of chemical VTE prophylaxis 24–48 hours after a stable head CT*

E *Avoidance of sitting position*

Early mobilization decreases the risk for deep venous thrombosis and pulmonary embolism (DVT/PE), as well as pneumonia. Removal of the compression device from the injured extremity would likely increase his risk for DVT/PE. A recent multicenter trial of early (within the first 72 hours of hospital admission) placement of an IVC filter in severely injured patients with contraindication to chemical prophylaxis for up to seven days showed no significant improvement in the incidence of PE or mortality in the filter placement arm. Anecdotal evidence may suggest a role for hypovolemia and seated position in development of DVT (and possibly therefore extension to PE), but there is no strong evidence to support this, and hypervolemia certainly plays no role in prevention.

Answer: D

Ho KW, Rao S, Honeybul S, et al. A multicenter trial of vena cava filters in severely injured patients. *The New England Journal of Medicine* 2019;381:328–337. 10.1056/ NEJMoa1806515.

16 *A 72-year-old woman on warfarin for atrial fibrillation has a hypertensive intracranial hemorrhage resulting in a large (> 15 mL in volume) intraparenchymal hematoma. Recommended interventions to improve functional outcome include:*

A *Administration of activated factor VII*

B *Evacuation of cerebellar hematomas in patients with hydrocephalus from ventricular obstruction*

C *Reduction of blood pressure to a normal range (systolic blood pressure 110–130 mmHg)*

D *Minimally invasive thrombolysis and evacuation of hematoma*

E *Prophylactic levetiracetam*

Hydrocephalus is an indication for evacuation of cerebellar hematomas. Early reversal of coagulopathy reduces ultimate hematoma volume and likely improves outcome. Activated Factor VII has been used for emergent reversal of coagulopathy but has limited effect for warfarin-induced coagulopathy. Prothrombin complex concentrate is the preferred reversal agent for warfarin, often with vitamin K supplementation. Though fresh frozen plasma reverses warfarin coagulopathy, dosing may be inaccurate, reversal takes longer, and the volume infused may be problematic with patients with heart disease. Guidelines recommend acute reduction of systolic blood pressure to 140 mm Hg in patients with baseline moderate hypertension and slower, incremental reduction, possibly to a higher target, for patients with baseline severe hypertension. More aggressive reduction may result in brain ischemia while inadequate reduction increases risk for recurrent hemorrhage. The recent MISTIE III trial of minimally invasive thrombolysis and evacuation showed safety of the procedure but no improvement in good functional outcome for patients with moderate-to-large intracerebral hematomas. Seizure prophylaxis is not recommended for patients with spontaneous intracerebral or intracerebellar hemorrhage.

Answer: B

Hanley D, Thompson R, Rosenblum M, et al. Efficacy and safety of minimally invasive surgery with thrombolysis in intracerebral haemorrhage evacuation (MISTIE III): a randomised, controlled, open-label, blinded endpoint phase 3 trial. Lancet. 2019;393: 1021–1032. 10.1016/ S0140 6736(19)301953.

Hemphill III JC, Greenberg S, Anderson C, et al.; on behalf of the American Heart Association Stroke Council, Council on Cardiovascular and Stroke Nursing, and Council on Clinical Cardiology Stroke. Guidelines for the management of spontaneous intracerebral hemorrhage. *Stroke* 2015;46. 10.1161/STR. 0000000000000069.

17 *A 45-year-old man with a history of hypertension and tobacco use presents to the ED with sudden onset of severe headache, which started six hours earlier. He has no recent history of trauma. His GCS is 15. Non-contrast head CT is normal. The most appropriate next step in management of this patient is:*

A *Diagnostic lumbar puncture*

B *Symptom treatment followed by discharge*

C *CTA of head*

D *Imitrex*

E *Magnesium sulfate*

This scenario presents a classic encounter with the patient with aneurysmal subarachnoid hemorrhage (aSAH). The challenge is distinguishing this etiology from other causes of headache such as migraine or cluster headache. A minimal amount of subarachnoid hemorrhage from aneurysm rupture may not be seen on head CT, which alone does not adequately rule out aSAH. This patient is at increased risk because of hypertension and tobacco use. An aSAH may be missed with only symptomatic treatment and discharge. A diagnostic lumbar puncture is warranted to look for blood in the cerebrospinal fluid. CTA of the head may demonstrate an aneurysm but will not indicate rupture, causing subarachnoid hemorrhage. Imitrex and magnesium sulfate are useful treatments for some types of headache but are not indicated in the treatment of aSAH.

Answer: A

Connolly ES Jr, Rabinstein AA, Carhuapoma JR, et al. Guidelines for the management of aneurysmal subarachnoid hemorrhage: a guideline for healthcare professionals from the American Heart Association/American Stroke Association. *Stroke* 2012;43(6):1711–1737. 10.1161/STR.0b013e3182587839.

Suarez JI, Tarr RW, Selman WR. Aneurysmal subarachnoid hemorrhage. *The New England Journal of Medicine* 2006; 354(4):387–396. 10.1056/NEJMra052732.

Thompson BG, Brown RD Jr, Amin-Hanjani S, et al. Guidelines for the management of patients with unruptured intracranial aneurysms: a guideline for healthcare professionals from the American Heart Association/American Stroke Association. *Stroke* 2015;46(8):2368–2400. 10.1161/STR.0000000000000070.

18 *An 18-year-old man with ASIA A, C4 quadriplegia after a dive into shallow water has a bradycardic arrest on ICU day 4. He is intubated and mechanically ventilated. He has been on tube feeds for three days without a bowel movement and had a Foley catheter removed on ICU day 3. After initial resuscitation to return of spontaneous circulation, the next best step in management is:*

A *Glycopyrrolate infusion*

B *Insertion of transvenous pacer*

C *Bladder and rectal decompression*

D *Epinephrine infusion*

E *Tube thoracostomy*

Neurogenic shock, characterized by bradycardia and hypotension, results from decreased sympathetic nervous tone as compared to parasympathetic tone. This can be exacerbated by gastric, urinary bladder, or rectal distention, resulting in severe bradycardia including bradycardic arrest. While transvenous pacing, glycopyrrolate, and even epinephrine infusion have a role in treating bradycardia secondary to high spinal cord injury, the next best step for this patient would be ensuring decompression of his stomach, bladder, and rectum. Care should be taken during placement of decompression tubes or with digital rectal exam and decompression as this may worsen bradycardia. A tube thoracostomy would be appropriate for this patient if signs or symptoms of tension pneumothorax are evident.

Answer: C

Fehlings M, Tetreault L, Wilson J et al. A clinical practice guideline for the management of acute spinal cord injury: introduction, rationale, and scope. *Global Spine Journal* 2017;7(3 Suppl): 84S–94S. 10.1177/2192568217703387.

Yue J, Winkler E, Rick J et al. Update on critical care for acute spinal cord injury in the setting of polytrauma. *Neurosurgical Focus* 2017;43(5):E19.

19 *A 43-year-old woman with myasthenia gravis is admitted to the ICU due to hypoventilation. The intervention least likely to improve her outcome is:*

A *Intubation and mechanical ventilation for vital capacity less than 20 mL/kg*

B *Administration of pyridostigmine if not intubated*

C *Plasma exchange up to five times over the next 7–10 days*

D *IVIG for five days*

E *Magnesium repletion*

Patients with myasthenic crisis are at high risk for respiratory failure requiring intubation and mechanical ventilation. Useful indicators for progression of respiratory compromise include a vital capacity less than 30 mL/kg and a negative inspiratory force less than 30 cm H_2O. IVIG and plasma exchange are recommended for treatment of myasthenic crisis. There is no clear superiority of one treatment over the other, with each having limitations. Plasma exchange is contraindicated in patients with sepsis, and IVIG is contraindicated in patients with renal failure. Plasma exchange may be more effective in a subset of myasthenic patients positive for antimuscle specific kinase antibody. Steroids or other immunosuppressive therapies (not choices provided above) are also indicated for myasthenic crisis. Various medications including beta-blockers and magnesium impair neuromuscular transmission and should be avoided when feasible.

Answer: E

Damian M, Srinivasan R. Neuromuscular problems in the ICU. *Current Opinion and Neurobiology* 2017;30(5).

Sanders DB, Wolfe GI, Benatar M at al. International consensus guidance for management of myasthenia gravis. *Neurology* 2016;87:419–425. 10.1212/WNL. 0000000000002790.

20 *Recommendations for evaluation and management of blunt cerebrovascular injury (BCVI) include all the following except:*
   A *Routine stenting as an adjunct to antithrombotic therapy in patients with Grade II or III BCVI*
   B *Screening imaging for patients with cervical spine injuries associated with low risk for BCVI*
   C *Systemic anticoagulation with heparin*
   D *Antithrombotic therapy with aspirin*
   E *Screening imaging for patients with GCS less than or equal to 8 and normal head CT*

Screening imaging with CT angiography of the neck is recommended for patients with both low- and high-risk cervical spine injuries (low and high risk for blunt cerebrovascular injury) because of its accuracy and low risk for complication, versus high risk for neurologically impairing stroke if BCVI is not found and treated. Screening is also recommended for blunt trauma patients with unexplained GCS less than or equal to 8. While antithrombotic therapy is used in most institutions for prevention of stroke in patients with BCVI, systemic anticoagulation with heparin is also effective, with protocols for each varying by institution. Routine stenting as an adjunct to antithrombotic therapy for patients with BCVI Grades III and IV is not recommended but may be useful for higher grades, including to facilitate embolization.

Answer: A

Kim D, Biffl W, Bokhari S, et al. Evaluation and management of blunt cerebrovascular injury. *The Journal of Trauma* 2020;88(6):875–887.

Shahan CP, Sharpe JP, Stickley SM, Manley NR, Filiberto DM, Fabian TC, Croce MA, Magnotti LJ. The changing role of endovascular stenting for blunt cerebrovascular injuries. *Journal of Trauma and Acute Care Surgery* 2018;84(2):308–311.

21

Venous Thromboembolism

Brett M. Chapman, MD[1] and Herb A. Phelan, MD, MSCS[2]

[1] LSUHSC-New Orleans, New Orleans, LA, USA
[2] Department of Surgery, LSU School of Medicine, New Orleans, LA, USA

1   *A 21-year-old man is admitted to the trauma ICU following a motorcycle crash in which he suffered multiple bilateral rib fractures and a grade V splenic injury. He required activation of the massive transfusion protocol (MTP) due to his profound hypotension in the trauma bay and was taken emergently to the operating room for an exploratory laparotomy and splenectomy. On postoperative day 3, he develops redness and pain of the left calf. A lower extremity venous duplex ultrasound shows a nonocclusive thrombus in the popliteal vein. Which of the following regarding venous thromboembolism (VTE) risk and blood product transfusion is CORRECT?*

   A   *RBC transfusion does not increase risk of hypercoagulability and VTE.*

   B   *RBC transfusion increases VTE risk in adults but not the pediatric patient population.*

   C   *Patients who receive massive transfusion protocol have a decreased risk of VTE.*

   D   *RBC transfusions have a dose-response effect with increased risk of VTE at higher transfusion requirements.*

   E   *RBC storage time prior to transfusion has no physiologic effects on VTE risk.*

The risk of VTE in critically ill patients is increased in those receiving blood product transfusions. A recent meta-analysis by Wang et al. that included more than 3.5 million patients found an odds ratio of 2.95 in development of VTE among patients who received preoperative blood transfusion compared to those who did not. An analysis by Goel et al. of the American College of Surgeons National Surgical Quality Improvement Program (ACS-NSQIP) registry from 2014, including greater than 750,000 patients who received at least one perioperative RBC transfusion, found an association with RBC transfusion and VTE (OR 2.1), DVT (2.2), and PE (1.9) independent of other risk factors and across all surgical subspecialties analyzed. Additionally, a significant dose-response effect was observed with increased odds of VTE as the number of RBC transfusion events increased – OR 2.1 for 1 event, OR 3.1 for 2 events, and OR 4.5 for 3 or more events compared to no intraoperative or postoperative RBC transfusions (p < 0.001 for trend). A similar increased VTE risk is seen in pediatric patients. A study of approximately 20 000 neonates, 80 000 infants, and 380 000 children found that VTE was significantly more common in all age groups – OR 4.1 in neonates, OR 2.4 in infants, and OR 2.2 in children. Weight-based volume of RBCs transfused was associated with VTE in a dose-dependent manner. Patients receiving massive fluid and blood product resuscitation after major hemorrhage due to trauma display a complex coagulation disorder that is multifactorial in nature. Coagulopathy is often perceived as hemorrhagic, but it is important to recognize that extensive hemodilution affects procoagulants, as well as anticoagulants, profibrinolytic, and antifibrinolytic elements. Studies on VTE risk in patients who survive MTP show an odds ratio of 2–3 compared to those who did not receive MTP. There are several effects of RBC storage that can increase the risk of VTE. Free hemoglobin from hemolyzed cells scavenge nitric oxide. Its decreased concentration leads to endothelial dysfunction and contributes to intravascular thrombosis.

Answer: D

Bradburn EH, Ho KM, Morgan ME, D'Andrea L, Vernon TM, Rogers FB. Massive transfusion protocol and subsequent development of venous thromboembolism: statewide analysis. *The American Surgeon* 2021; 87:15–20.

Surgical Critical Care and Emergency Surgery: Clinical Questions and Answers, Third Edition.
Edited by Forrest "Dell" Moore, Peter M. Rhee, and Carlos J. Rodriguez.
© 2022 John Wiley & Sons Ltd. Published 2022 by John Wiley & Sons Ltd.
Companion website: www.wiley.com/go/surgicalcriticalcare3e

Dhillon NK, Smith EJT, Ko A, Harada MY, Yang AR, Patel KA, Barmparas G, Ley EJ. The risk factors of venous thromboembolism in massively transfused patients. *The Journal of Surgical Research* 2018; 222:115–121.

Goel R, Patel EU, Cushing MM, et al. Association of perioperative red blood cell transfusions with venous thromboembolism in a North American registry. *JAMA Surgery* 2018; 15:826–833.

Lin SY, Chang YL, Yeh HC, Lin CL, Kao CH. Blood transfusion and risk of venous thromboembolism: a population-based cohort study. *Thrombosis and Haemostasis* 2020; 120:156–167.

Wang C, Kou H, Li X, Lan J. Association between preoperative blood transfusion and postoperative venous thromboembolism: review meta-analysis. *Annals of Vascular Surgery* 2020; 28:S0890-5096(20)31076-1.

Wirtz MR, Schalkers DV, Goslings JC, Juffermans NP. The impact of blood product ratio and procoagulant therapy on the development of thromboembolic events in severely injured hemorrhaging trauma patients. *Transfusion* 2020; 60(8):1873–1882.

2   *A 68-year-old man presents to the emergency department via EMS with worsening left lower extremity edema and bluish discoloration from the proximal thigh to the toes for the past 5 hours. He had a fall from standing 2 weeks ago and suffered an isolated hip fracture. He was discharged home on postoperative day 3 with home health physical therapy. His daughter reports that he has been refusing to work with PT and has been in bed since discharge. His motor exam is intact on your assessment, but he has loss of sensation in the toes. You start a heparin infusion immediately. What is the best next step in management?*

   A   *Guillotine above-knee amputation*
   B   *Common femoral vein thrombectomy*
   C   *Placement of an inferior vena cava filter*
   D   *Venography and catheter-directed and/or mechanical thrombolysis*
   E   *Systemic thrombolysis*

Phlegmasia cerulea dolens is an uncommon complication of acute iliofemoral DVT that can result in loss of limb or life. Extreme venous hypertension leads to obstructed arterial flow and critical limb ischemia. It is characterized by marked swelling of the lower extremity with pain and cyanosis. Sensorimotor deficits soon follow if not recognized and treated promptly. Development of gangrene and necessity of amputation are unfortunately common in this disease process. It is seen most commonly in the 5th and 6th decades of life and in the left lower extremity due to compression of the left common iliac vein by the right common iliac artery. The immediate goals are bed rest, elevation of the affected extremity, and heparin administration followed by intervention to aggressively reduce the thrombus load and prevent further thrombus propagation. This can be accomplished via various techniques including catheter-directed thrombolysis (CDT), pharmacomechanical thrombolysis (PMT), and open thrombectomy. There is no consensus on a management algorithm, but most authors suggest a graduated approach from endovascular to open surgical treatments based on the extent of acute ischemia. This patient has Rutherford class IIa acute ischemia with minimal sensory impairment and intact motor function. His limb is potentially salvageable with prompt therapy. Of note, he should be considered for fasciotomies given his ischemic time prior to presentation. Common femoral vein thrombectomy and immediate amputation should be reserved for more extensive sensorimotor deficits and unsalvageable limbs, respectively. CDT has not been shown to increase the rate of embolization, so empiric IVC filter placement is not routine practice.

Answer: D

Broderick C, Watson L, Armon MP. Thrombolytic strategies versus standard anticoagulation for acute deep vein thrombosis of the lower limb. *Cochrane Database of Systematic Reviews.* 2021; 19;1:CD002783.

Chinsakchai K, Ten Duis K, Moll FL, de Borst GJ. Trends in management of phlegmasia cerulea dolens. *Vascular and Endovascular Surgery* 2011; 45:5–14.

Fleck D, Albadawi H, Shamoun F, Knuttinen G, Naidu S, Oklu R. Catheter-directed thrombolysis of deep vein thrombosis: literature review and practice considerations. *Cardiovascular and Diagnosis Therapy* 2017; 7(Suppl 3):S228–S237.

Pouncey AL, Gwozdz AM, Johnson OW, Silickas J, Saha P, Thulasidasan N, Karunanithy N, Cohen AT, Black SA. AngioJet pharmacomechanical thrombectomy and catheter directed thrombolysis vs. catheter directed thrombolysis alone for the treatment of iliofemoral deep vein thrombosis: a single centre retrospective cohort study. *European Journal of Vascular and Endovascular Surgery* 2020; 60:578–585.

3   *A 32-year-old pregnant woman at 27 weeks estimated gestational age is admitted following a motor vehicle collision during which she sustained fractures of right ribs 3–6 and a right inferior pubic ramus fracture. Her nurse is preparing to administer chemical DVT prophylaxis on hospital day 1. Which of the following is INCORRECT about VTE in pregnancy?*

   A   *Women have a 4- to 5-fold increase in venous thromboembolism risk during pregnancy and the postpartum period.*

B *DVT occurs with equal frequency in each trimester and the postpartum period.*

C *PE is more common during pregnancy than the postpartum period.*

D *During pregnancy, 80–90% of DVTs occur in the left lower extremity.*

E *VTE accounts for approximately 10% of all maternal deaths.*

VTE complicates 0.5–3.0 per 1000 pregnancies and is the leading cause of maternal mortality in the United States. All of the factors in Virchow's Triad (hypercoagulability, vascular injury, and venous stasis) occur in pregnancy. Pregnant or postpartum women carry a relative risk of 4.3 for VTE compared to nonpregnant women. Cesarean delivery also significantly increases risk of VTE compared to vaginal delivery with an odds ratio of 13.3. DVT occurs with equal frequency in each trimester and the postpartum period. The vast majority of DVTs in pregnancy occur in the left lower extremity, which accounts for 80–90% of cases. Of those, approximately 70% occur in the iliofemoral distribution, which are more prone to embolization. In nonpregnant patients, left lower extremity DVTs account for 55% of cases with 10% in the iliofemoral vein. DVT and PE during pregnancy or the postpartum period require anticoagulation similar to the general population. Unfractionated heparin (UFH) and low-molecular-weight heparin (LMWH) are safe during pregnancy with LMWH replacing UFH as the therapy of choice due to minimal excretion in breast milk and lower rates of adverse events (heparin-induced thrombocytopenia, symptomatic osteoporosis, bleeding, and allergic reactions). Warfarin is contraindicated during pregnancy due to teratogenicity.

Answer: C

Blanco-Molina A, Trujillo-Santos J, Criado J, et al., for the RIETE Investigators. Venous thromboembolism during pregnancy or postpartum: findings from the RIETE Registry. *Thrombosis and Haemostasis* 2007; 97:186–190.

Creanga AA, Syverson C, Seed K, Callaghan WM. Pregnancy-related mortality in the United States, 2011–2013. *Obstetrics and Gynecology* 2017; 130:366–373.

Heit JA, Kobbervig CE, James AH, Petterson TM, Bailey KR, Melton LJIII. Trends in the incidence of venous thromboembolism during pregnancy or postpartum: a 30-year population-based study. *Annals of Internal Medicine* 2005; 143:697–706.

Pomp ER, Lenselink AM, Rosendaal FR, Doggen CJ. Pregnancy, the postpartum period and prothrombotic defects: risk of venous thrombosis in the MEGA study. *Journal of Thrombosis and Haemostasis* 2008; 6:632–637.

4 *A 16-year-old man presents to the emergency department as the restrained front seat passenger in a high-speed motor vehicle collision with airbag deployment. A thorough trauma workup reveals a left sacroiliac disruption, pubic symphysis widening to 3 cm, left midshaft tibial fracture, and right distal tibia and fibula fractures. Which of the following statements about this patient is true?*

A *Patients under age 18 should not receive chemical DVT prophylaxis.*

B *The patient should be started on chemical prophylaxis with low-molecular-weight heparin every 12 hours.*

C *Patients with an Injury Severity Score (ISS) ≥ 10 should receive chemical DVT prophylaxis.*

D *The patient should have intermittent pneumatic compression devices (IPCs) and graduated compression stockings (GCSs) placed for VTE risk management.*

E *The patient should receive active surveillance with DVT ultrasound in lieu of chemical DVT prophylaxis.*

Prepubertal patients are generally a low-risk population for VTE, a phenomenon thought to be due to a lack of sex hormones. Older children and adolescents have a VTE risk that approaches their adult counterparts. The Pediatric Trauma Society and the Eastern Association for the Surgery of Trauma joint practice management guideline recommend pharmacologic prophylaxis be considered for children older than 15 years of age and younger in postpubertal children with an Injury Severity Score greater than 25. Particular injury patterns that are high risk for VTE (i.e. pelvic fracture, long bone fracture, TBI) should be given consideration as well. Intermittent pneumatic compression devices and graduated compression stockings should be placed for mechanical VTE prophylaxis in the absence of an injury pattern contraindication. Several studies have investigated serial ultrasound surveillance in the absence of chemical VTE prophylaxis with no identified clinical benefit.

Answer: B

Landisch RM, Hanson SJ, Cassidy LD, Braun K, Punzalan RC, Gourlay DM. Evaluation of guidelines for injured children at high risk for venous thromboembolism: a prospective observational study. *Journal of Trauma and Acute Care Surgery* 2017; 82(5):836–844.

Liras IN, Rahbar E, Harting MT, Holcomb JB, Cotton BA. When children become adults and adults become most hypercoagulable after trauma: an assessment of admission hypercoagulability by rapid thrombelastography and venous thromboembolic risk. *Journal of Trauma and Acute Care Surgery* 2016; 80(5):778–782.

Mahajerin A, Petty JK, Hanson SJ, Thompson AJ, O'Brien SH, Streck CJ, Petrillo TM, Faustino EV. Prophylaxis against venous thromboembolism in pediatric trauma: a practice management guideline from the Eastern Association for the Surgery of Trauma and the Pediatric Trauma Society. *Journal of Trauma and Acute Care Surgery* 2017;82(3):627–636.

5 Which of the following is true regarding low-molecular-weight heparins (LMWH)?
   A The effects of LMWH are more unpredictable than natural or unfractionated heparin (UFH).
   B The incidence of heparin-induced thrombocytopenia is approximately 5% with LMWH compared to 1% with UFH.
   C The therapeutic effect of LMWH can be measured with the partial thromboplastin time (PTT), activating clotting time (ACT), or anti-factor Xa assay.
   D LMWH is contraindicated in patients with a GFR 30–50 mL/min due to its renal clearance.
   E The risk of heparin-induced thrombocytopenia is reduced with fondaparinux due to its lack of affinity for platelet factor 4.

Unfractionated heparin (UFH) consists of multiple molecular chains of various lengths and molecular weights. Low-molecular-weight heparin (LMWH) have only short chains with the class of drug being obtained by fractionation or depolymerization of UFH. Due to the lower degree of variation, the effects of LMWH are more predictable than UFH. LMWH also has a lower risk of heparin-induced thrombocytopenia (HIT) at 1% compared to 5% with UFH. The effects of LMWH cannot be measured using PTT or ACT, but rather with an anti-Xa level. Recent studies suggest that anti-Xa monitoring for therapeutic levels is beneficial, particularly in patients at the extremes of weight. Also, many patients are subtherapeutic at the standard dosing of LMWH common in many institutions. LMWHs are contraindicated in severe renal impairment – defined by a creatinine clearance (CrCl) < 30 mL/min – due to their renal metabolism. There are no dose adjustments required in normal renal function (CrCl ≥ 80 mL/min), mild renal impairment (CrCl 50–79 mL/min) or moderate renal impairment (CrCl 30–49 mL/min).

Answer: E

Lee AY, Levine MN, Baker RI, Bowden C, Kakkar AK, Prins M, Rickles FR, Julian JA, Haley S, Kovacs MJ, Gent M; Randomized Comparison of Low-Molecular-Weight Heparin versus Oral Anticoagulant Therapy for the Prevention of Recurrent Venous Thromboembolism in Patients with Cancer (CLOT) Investigators. Low-molecular-weight heparin versus a coumarin for the prevention of recurrent venous thromboembolism in patients with cancer. *The New England Journal of Medicine* 2003; 349(2):146–153.

Lim W, Dentali F, Eikelboom JW, Crowther MA. Meta-analysis: low-molecular-weight heparin and bleeding in patients with severe renal insufficiency. *Annals of Internal Medicine* 2006; 144(9):673–684.

PROTECT Investigators for the Canadian Critical Care Trials Group and the Australian and New Zealand Intensive Care Society Clinical Trials Group, Cook D, Meade M, Guyatt G, Walter S, Heels-Ansdell D, Warkentin TE, Zytaruk N, Crowther M, Geerts W, Cooper DJ, Vallance S, Qushmaq I, Rocha M, Berwanger O, Vlahakis NE. Dalteparin versus unfractionated heparin in critically ill patients. *The New England Journal of Medicine* 2011; 364(14): 1305–1314.

6 Which of the following statements regarding irreversible hypercoagulable states is INCORRECT?
   A Hyperhomocysteinemia provokes thrombus formation via endothelial injury, inflammation, and oxidative stress.
   B Antiphospholipid antibody syndrome provokes thrombosis in both arteries and veins, as well as pregnancy-related complications (i.e. spontaneous abortion, stillbirth, preterm delivery, or severe preeclampsia).
   C Antithrombin III deficiency is confirmed by levels less than 70%.
   D Factor V Leiden results in a factor V variant that is more easily degraded by activated protein C.
   E Protein C deficiency is associated with an 8- to 10-fold increase in VTE risk with no associated increase in arterial thrombosis risk.

Hyperhomocysteinemia has an estimated prevalence of 5–7% in the general population. It is associated with increased cardiovascular, cerebrovascular, and thromboembolic events. Elevated levels of homocysteine can increase the risk of atherosclerosis by causing endothelial injury, promoting an inflammatory response, and increasing oxidative stress. Antiphospholipid antibody syndrome is an autoimmune hypercoagulopathy caused by antiphospholipid antibodies. Diagnosis requires either DVT, arterial thrombus, or pregnancy-related complications (i.e. spontaneous abortion, stillbirth, preterm deliver, or severe preeclampsia), as well as presence of at least one of the antiphospholipid antibodies (i.e. lupus anticoagulant, anticardiolipin, β2-glycoprotein-1). Lifelong anticoagulation is required once diagnosis is confirmed. Antithrombin III deficiency can be a rare hereditary or acquired disorder with a prevalence of 0.02–0.2% in the general population and 1–5% of patients with VTE. These patients carry a 50% risk of VTE development by age 50. Antithrombin III deficiency is defined as less than 70% of normal on reference testing. Protein C deficiency is a rare thrombophilia seen in 0.1–0.5% of the population that is associated with an 8- to 10-fold increase in relative risk of VTE without an increase in arterial thrombosis risk. It is vitamin K-dependent and inhibits factors V and VIII, which are prothrombotic. Deficiency of protein C leads to relative increase in the activity of factors V and VIII and increased thrombus formation. Factor V Leiden is the most common hereditary hypercoagulable disorder in the Caucasian population with a prevalence of 1–5% overall and 10–20% in patients with VTE. It is a point mutation in factor V that impairs binding of protein C, which leads to a decreased ability to deactivate the prothrombotic factor V and subsequent hypercoagulable state. Most patients are heterozygous for the gene which carries a 7-fold increase in lifetime thrombosis risk.

Answer: D

Lee M, Hong KS, Chang SC, Saver JL. Efficacy of homocysteine-lowering therapy with folic Acid in stroke prevention: a meta-analysis. *Stroke* 2010; 41:1205–1212.

Pabinger I, Thaler J. How I treat patients with hereditary antithrombin deficiency. *Blood* 2019; 26:134.

Park WC, Chang JH. Clinical implications of methylenetetrahydrofolate reductase mutations and plasma homocysteine levels in patients with thromboembolic occlusion. *Vascular Specialist International* 2014; 30:113–119.

7 *You are on call overnight and receive a call on a 62-year-old woman who is admitted to the surgical intensive care unit following an open abdominal aortic aneurysm repair 5 days ago. She is doing well overall but remains deconditioned and working with physical therapy. She is on mechanical and chemical DVT prophylaxis with enoxaparin. She was resting comfortably on 2 liters of nasal cannula throughout the day before developing sudden onset tachycardia, shortness of breath, and chest pain. You obtain a CTA of the chest that reveals a segmental right upper lobe pulmonary embolism. Upon further investigation, you notice a 50% decrease in platelet count in the past 36 hours. Which of the following statements about HIT is CORRECT?*

A *IgG, IgA, and IgM antibodies contribute to the pathogenesis of HIT.*

B *A positive platelet factor 4 ELISA should be confirmed with a serotonin release assay.*

C *Type I HIT is an autoimmune, antibody-mediated reaction.*

D *Risk of HIT development is dependent on heparin product exposure in the preceding 7 days.*

E *Type II HIT is only present at least 5 days following heparin product exposure.*

Heparin-induced thrombocytopenia (HIT) is a potentially severe complication occurring in up to 5% of patients following exposure to any form of heparin product that is characterized by a fall in platelet count and a hypercoagulable state. The potential thromboembolic consequences are heightened by the wide use of heparin products for treatment and prophylaxis for VTE, line flushes, and heparin-coated catheters. HIT is categorized into two types. Type I HIT is a non-immune-mediated reaction that can occur as early as day 1 of therapy. This type is by far the most common and typically consists of a mild reaction that is not associated with any complications. Platelet counts will spontaneously correct to normal even in the setting of continued heparin therapy. Type II HIT is an immune, antibody-mediated reaction that usually occurs 5–14 days after receiving heparin. It can, however, manifest as soon as day 1 of therapy if heparin products have been used in the past 100 days, as there can be circulating antibodies from the prior exposure. This reaction is very severe and causes a significant hypercoagulable state that predisposes the patient to potentially life-threatening VTE events. HIT causes thromboembolic complications in up to 50% of patients with an associated mortality rate of up to 30%. HIT is more likely to occur with unfractionated heparin than low-molecular-weight heparin. HIT occurs when antibodies to the heparin-platelet factor 4 (PF4) complex bind the FC receptor on the platelet surface and lead to platelet activation. Fondaparinux does not cause HIT due to its lack of affinity for PF4. Activated platelets then release pro-thrombotic substances (i.e. thrombin) and PF4, which creates a cyclical effect that can only be broken when heparin is discontinued and heparin-PF4 complexes are no longer formed. No amount of heparin is too small to cause HIT. It is, however, more likely to occur in exposure to higher doses of heparin products and longer duration of therapy. A clinical diagnosis of HIT should be confirmed with the platelet factor 4 (PF4) ELISA and serotonin release assay (SRA). The ELISA immunoassay detects the presence of antibodies. The test is highly sensitive with a high negative predictive value, meaning a negative result can rule out a diagnosis of HIT. The PF4 ELISA has low specificity, however, and is prone to false positives because the test captures the presence of IgA and IgM antibodies that do not play a role in HIT in addition to IgG antibodies that are central to the pathophysiology. A confirmatory SRA should be obtained for any positive PF4 ELISA.

Answer: B

Cuker A, Arepally GM, Chong BH, Cines DB, Greinacher A, Gruel Y, Linkins LA, Rodner SB, Selleng S, Warkentin TE, Wex A, Mustafa RA, Morgan RL, Santesso N. American Society of Hematology 2018 guidelines for management of venous thromboembolism: heparin-induced thrombocytopenia. *Blood Advances* 2018; 2:3360–3392.

Fathi M. Heparin-induced thrombocytopenia (HIT): Identification and treatment pathways. *Global Cardiology Science and Practice* 2018; 2018:15.

Stoll F, Gödde M, Leo A, Katus HA, Müller OJ. Characterization of hospitalized cardiovascular patients with suspected heparin-induced thrombocytopenia. *Clinical Cardiology* 2018; 41:1521–1526.

8 *A 32-year-old woman who is admitted to the trauma service after an MVC in which she sustained a femur fracture. In the course of taking her history, she states that she has had five pregnancies, four of which have ended with a miscarriage. Her prenatal care was delivered by a midwife in the village in which she lived before recently immigrating to the U.S. and has never discussed this with a physician. In considering the possibility of antiphospholipid syndrome (APS) and what it would do to her VTE risk profile, which statement is INCORRECT?*

   A *Almost one half of APS patients present with a catastrophic thrombotic event.*

   B *In APS, arterial thrombosis tends to recur on the arterial side and venous thrombosis tends to recur on the venous side.*

   C *Livedo reticularis, cutaneous ulcers, thrombocytopenia, hemolytic anemia, cardiac valvular disease, and nephropathy, while common manifestations of the disease, are not included in the current classification criteria.*

   D *Presence of the antiphospholipid antibody on a single determination constitutes a diagnosis of the syndrome.*

   E *The syndrome is referred to as "primary APS" when it occurs by itself and as "secondary APS" when it occurs in conjunction with another autoimmune condition.*

Antiphospholipid antibodies can occur in 5–10% of healthy donors, but these titers normally disappear over time. The diagnostic criteria for APS involve a characteristic clinical picture of thrombosis and a persistent antiphospholipid antibody titer on two separate occasions at least 12 weeks apart. Patients diagnosed with APS have high rates of recurrent thrombosis after discontinuation of anticoagulation for a period of years. Therefore, the consensus treatment is to continue anticoagulation indefinitely. Beginning an anticoagulation regimen can be difficult as the syndrome is known for occasionally interfering with standard assays. This necessitates specific inquiries with your hematology lab as to whether INR reagents resistant to this effect are being used and potentially following functional factor II and X assays. For reasons that are unclear, recurrences of thrombosis in APS tend to occur on the same side of the circulation as the original event. Efforts are currently underway to develop a comprehensive set of classification criteria that will likely include other clinical manifestations and stratification using multi-criteria decision analysis.

Answer: D

Garcia D, Erkan D. Diagnosis and management of the antiphospholipid syndrome. *The New England Journal of Medicine* 2018; 378:2010–2021.

Sammaritano LR. Antiphospholipid Syndrome. *Best Practice & Research. Clinical Rheumatology* 2020;34: 101463.

9 *Which of the following is INCORRECT regarding the recommendations in the 2020 American Society of Hematology (ASH) guidelines on VTE?*

   A *As opposed to the 2016 American College of Chest Physician (ACCP) guidelines, direct oral anticoagulants (DOACs) are dealt with extensively in the ASH guidelines.*

   B *Conditional recommendations include the preference for home treatment over hospital-based treatment for uncomplicated DVT and PE at low risk for complications.*

   C *When making the decision to initiate a naïve VTE patient on DOAC therapy, the ASH guidelines rank the preferred DOAC to be used as follows: 1. dabigatran, 2. rivaroxaban, 3. apixaban, and 4. edoxaban.*

   D *For patients with PE with echocardiography showing right ventricular dysfunction and no hemodynamic compromise, the ASH guideline panel suggests anticoagulation alone over routine thrombolysis in addition to anticoagulation.*

   E *For VTE patients in whom thrombolysis is considered appropriate, the ASH guidelines recommend using catheter-directed thrombolysis over systemic thrombolysis*

The recommendation for home treatment of uncomplicated VTE is obviously conditional upon the requirement that they have no other conditions that would require hospitalization. Further, it does not apply to patients with VTE who have limited or no support at home and cannot afford medications or have a history of poor compliance. The ASH makes no recommendations of one DOAC over another. For patients with RV dysfunction and normal hemodynamics, while not to be done routinely, thrombolysis is reasonable to consider if the risk for bleeding is low in select younger patients or for patients at high risk for decompensation due to concomitant cardiopulmonary disease.

Answer: C

Kearon, C, Akl, EA, Ornelas, J, et al. Antithrombotic therapy for VTE disease: CHEST guideline and expert panel report. *Chest* 2016; 149:315–352.

Ortel TL, Neumann I, Ageno W, et al. American Society of Hematology 2020 guidelines for management of venous thromboembolism: treatment of deep vein thrombosis and pulmonary embolism. *Blood Advances* 2020; 4:4693–4738.

10 *A 37-year-old man is admitted after suffering a grade II spleen injury in a motor vehicle collision. He is hemodynamically stable, and you undertake a course of nonoperative management. On post-injury day 3, he develops acute shortness of breath and a workup reveals a pulmonary embolism. What should be the next step in your management?*

A *Placement of a permanent vena cava filter.*

B *Placement of a retrievable vena cava filter.*

C *Immediate initiation of systemic anticoagulation.*

D *Performance of splenectomy followed by systemic anticoagulation.*

E *An echocardiogram to assess for signs of right heart strain followed by initiation of systemic anticoagulation at 5 days post-injury if no heart strain is found.*

Prophylactic and therapeutic anticoagulation in patients with nonoperatively managed solid organ injuries is a controversial topic with a paucity of data to support any opinion. Santaniello and colleagues examined a series of 20 patients with blunt aortic injuries and concomitant grade I or II spleen or liver injuries, which were being managed nonoperatively. All these patients underwent systemic heparinization with bypass during the repair of their blunt aortic injuries at a mean of 1.5 days post-injury, and the authors reported no failures of splenic/liver nonoperative management. In a multicenter retrospective study of patients presenting with solid organ injury while on anticoagulation, Bhattacharya et al. found no significant difference in AAST injury grade, rates of initial nonoperative management, rates of failure of nonoperative management, length of stay, or

mortality. Further, others have shown that low-molecular-weight heparin can be used as prophylaxis at 48 hours post-injury without an increase in transfusion requirement or failure rates. While extrapolation of data should always be undertaken with caution, in the setting described above, systemic anticoagulation would seem to be suitable management by post-injury day 3. Because "C" is a safe option, which is the least invasive and does not involve a delay in care, it represents the best answer.

Answer: C

Bhattacharya B, Askari R, Davis KA, et al. The effect of anticoagulation on outcomes after liver and spleen injuries: a research consortium of New England centers for trauma (ReCONECT) study. *Injury* 2020; 51(9):1994–1998.

Joseph B, Pandit V, Harrison C, Lubin D, Kulvatunyou N, Zangbar B, Tang A, O'Keeffe T, Green DJ, Gries L, Friese RS, Rhee P. Early thromboembolic prophylaxis in patients with blunt solid abdominal organ injuries undergoing nonoperative management: is it safe? *American Journal of Surgery* 2015; 209(1):194–198.

Santaniello JM, Miller PR, Croce MA, et al. Blunt aortic injury with concomitant intra-abdominal solid organ injury: treatment priorities revisited. *The Journal of Trauma.* 2002; 53(3):442–445.

11 *After a helmeted motorcycle collision, a 37-year-old man suffers a left tib/fib fracture and two left-sided rib fractures. He undergoes ORIF of his tibia on the day of injury, and his convalescence is slow due to pain. One week post-op, he develops a swollen left leg, and an ultrasound confirms that he has a DVT extending from the popliteal vein into the distal superficial femoral vein. He is started on therapeutic anticoagulation with enoxaparin and discharged home two days later. He misses several clinic appointments with you and does not follow up until 4 months after injury. At that time, he is complaining of a painful, swollen, heavy leg. On exam, the leg has normal skin color with no breakdown and is swollen and mildly tender to palpation. As you begin to explain his condition to him, which of the following statements about post-thrombotic syndrome (PTS) would be INCORRECT?*

A *The Compression Elastique Evaluation du Syndrome post Thrombotique (CELEST) Trial demonstrated that high-strength (ankle pressure 35 mm Hg) were superior to low-strength (ankle pressure 25 mm Hg) external compression garments to prevent PTS after proximal DVT.*

B *PTS develops in 20–50% of patients following a leg DVT despite treatment with anticoagulation and is severe in 5–10% of cases.*

C *Symptoms of PTS usually occur within 3–6 months after DVT, but can occur up to 2 years later.*

D *Studies have shown that the quality of life of patients suffering from PTS is poorer than patients of similar age with arthritis, chronic lung disease, or diabetes.*

E *There are no diagnostic criteria for PTS, instead relying on the characteristic clinical picture.*

Controversy exists around the ability of external compression garments to prevent PTS development. Two RCTs have published contradictory findings, although both were riddled with methodologic errors and compliance issues. The French CELEST trial is ongoing at the time of this writing, and will hopefully shed light on this complex subject. Thrombosis damages the deep venous valves and frequently renders them incompetent. This results in venous reflux and venous hypertension. Venous hypertension in turn can affect segments of veins and valves not involved in the original area of thrombus. This is the fundamental pathophysiology of PTS, which is characterized by pain, heaviness, and edema of the involved extremity. When it occurs in the leg, these symptoms are exacerbated by standing and ambulating. As the disease becomes more severe, it can progress to subcutaneous atrophy, hyperpigmentation, and ulceration. This condition markedly diminishes quality of life, particularly given the fact that it often affects younger patients and affects their ability to earn a livelihood.

Answer: A

Galanaud JP, Genty-Vermorel C, Rolland C, et al. Compression stockings to prevent postthrombotic syndrome: Literature overview and presentation of the CELEST trial. *Research and Practice in Thrombosis Haemostasis* 2020; 4:1239–1250.

Rabinovich A, Kahn SR. The postthrombotic syndrome: current evidence and future challenges. *Journal of Thrombosis and Haemostasis* 2017; 15:230–241.

12 *Which of the following statements about D-dimer is INCORRECT?*

A *Elevated D-dimer levels are associated with increased severity of COVID-19 infection.*

B *In the setting of low-to-intermediate risk, a negative D-dimer value can rule out PE with a sensitivity of 95% and a negative predictive value of 99% and no further testing is necessary.*

C *Because D-dimer increases with age, diagnostic criteria for VTE should employ age stratification.*

D *When patients stop anticoagulation after DVT or PE, D-dimer loses its predictive strength.*

E *D-dimers accuracy in predicting risk is even higher in patients with congenital thrombophilias.*

The hyperinflammation and coagulopathy seen in COVID-19 infection is associated with a wide derangement in various hemostasis parameters, including D-dimer, prothrombin time, and thrombocytopenia. These tests serve as potential prognostic markers of severe disease and/or mortality. When anticoagulation after VTE is stopped, D-dimer is a useful predictor of recurrence. While the negative predictive value of a normal D-dimer is very good, its lack of specificity and elevation by general states of hypercoagulability has limited its use as a sole tool for the positive diagnosis of PE.

Answer: D

Favaloro EJ, Thachil J. Reporting of D-dimer data in COVID-19: some confusion and potential for misinformation. *Clinical Chemistry and Laboratory Medicine* 2020; 58:1191–1199.

Weitz J, Fredenburgh JC, Eikelboom JW. A Test in context: D-Dimer. *Journal of the American College of Cardiology* 2017; 70:2411–2420.

13 *While on call, you are asked to evaluate a homeless woman who appears to be approximately 50 years old. She presents with abdominal pain, abdominal wall ecchymosis, a productive cough, and hypoxia. She is confused and a poor historian. As you are making preparations to explore her, you are notified that she has tested positive for COVID-19 on the ER's screening. After intubation in a negative pressure room with universal precautions including the use of powered air-purifying respirators (PAPRs), you take her to the operating room where you find a mesenteric rent and a twelve-inch segment of ischemic small bowel. You perform an uneventful resection with a hand-sewn anastomosis and transport her to the SICU postoperatively on the ventilator. Regarding her risk for VTE in the setting of presumed active COVID-19 infection, which of the following statements is INCORRECT?*

A *Most studies suggest that approximately 20% of COVID-19 patients admitted to the ICU will develop VTE.*

B *A case series of postmortem COVID-19 autopsies found that PE was the direct cause of death in 33%.*

C *The risk of VTE appears to be similar between patients admitted to the ICU with COVID-19 or those admitted to the ICU with severe influenza.*

D *The role of antiphospholipid antibodies in the coagulopathy seen in COVID-19 infection is unknown.*

E *When routine ultrasound surveillance is conducted on patients in the ICU with COVID-19 infection, the rate of detected VTE raises goes up to almost 70% despite appropriate prophylactic regimens.*

Evidence is mounting that severe COVID-19 seems to be associated with a hypercoagulable state with a potential impact on thromboembolism risk, but the nature and extent of these abnormalities is not clear. The risk appears to be proportional to the severity of the disease, and therefore a common finding across studies is a higher rate of VTE in COVID-19 patients in the ICU versus those being cared for on a regular ward. It is distressing that the risk in ICU patients persists despite appropriate pharmacologic and mechanical prophylaxis. A French analysis of 107 subjects admitted to the ICU with COVID-19 showed a PE rate of 20.6%, while a similar cohort with influenza had a PE rate of 7.5%.

Answer: C

Al-Ani F, Chehade S, Lazo-Langner A. Thrombosis risk associated with COVID-19 infection. A scoping review. *Thrombosis Research* 2020; 192:152–160.

Llitjos JF, Leclerc M, Chochois C, et al. High incidence of venous thromboembolic events in anticoagulated severe COVID-19 patients. *Journal of Thrombosis and Haemostasis* 2020.

Wichmann D, Sperhake JP, Lutgehetmann M, et al. Autopsy findings and venous thromboembolism in patients with COVID-19: a prospective cohort study. *Annals of Internal Medicine* 2020.

14 *A frail 62-year-old woman is on a novel oral anticoagulant (NOAC) as an outpatient for treatment of a DVT. She is admitted to the SICU after falling down four cement stairs outside her front door and sustains fractures of ribs 4 through 9 on the left. You consult the pain service to place an epidural catheter for pain control. According to the 2018 guidelines from a consortium of six American and European anesthesia organizations, which of the following statements about her NOAC in this setting is INCORRECT?*

A *The NOAC should be stopped for 5 half-lives before placing the epidural.*

B *When the NOAC is stopped, bridge therapy with heparin or a low-molecular-weight heparin is contraindicated.*

C *After the epidural is placed, the NOAC may be restarted after 24 hours.*

D *If the risk of VTE is very high, half the usual NOAC dose may be given 12 hours after the epidural is placed.*

E *Depending on the NOAC, the time interval between cessation of the NOAC and performance of the procedure can be between 3 and 6 days.*

Novel oral anticoagulants (NOACs) include apixaban (Eliquis), dabigatran (Pradaxa), rivaroxaban (Xarelto), and edoxaban (Lixiana). The recommendations for NOAC management by the American Society of Regional Anesthesia and Pain Medicine, European Society of Regional Anaesthesia and Pain Therapy, American Academy of Pain Medicine, International Neuromodulation Society, North American Neuromodulation Society, and the World Institute of Pain state that a bridge with a heparin product is permissible upon NOAC cessation as long as the bridge therapy is held 24 hours before the epidural is placed. Dabigatran should be stopped for 4 days in patients with normal renal function and 6 days in those with impaired renal function. Rivaroxaban should be stopped for at least 65 hours, edoxaban for 70 hours, and apixaban for 75 hours.

Answer: B

Narouze S, Benzon HT, Provenzano D, et al. Interventional Spine and Pain Procedures in Patients on Antiplatelet and Anticoagulant Medications (2nd ed.): Guidelines From the American Society of Regional Anesthesia and Pain Medicine, the European Society of Regional Anaesthesia and Pain Therapy, the American Academy of Pain Medicine, the International Neuromodulation Society, the North American Neuromodulation Society, and the World Institute of Pain. *Regional Anesthesia and Pain Medicine* 2018; 43:225–262.

15 *You see a 43-year-old woman in clinic who is very anxious after seeing a commercial on late-night TV for a legal firm soliciting clients who have received an IVC filter. She reports that she was told she had an IVC filter placed during an ICU admission for an MVC in 1997 and hands you a copy of her medical records, which state that a Greenfield filter was placed prophylactically due to her injury burden and a perceived contraindication to pharmacologic prophylaxis. She reports no problems since her discharge from rehab that same year, and she had two term pregnancies in the five years after discharge. A plain film in your clinic demonstrates a strut fracture of one limb of the filter. What should be your recommendation?*

A *Elective operative removal*

B *Elective endovascular removal*

C *Referral to the emergency room for a stat CT scan of the abdomen*

D *Referral to the emergency room for a CT scan of the chest*

E *Expectant management*

A discussion of risk/benefit with this patient should emphasize the technical difficulties associated with attempting endovascular removal as the filter will endothelialize within a matter of months. Open removal for the sake of peace of mind should be absolutely ruled out as intraoperative exsanguination is a serious possibility. The strut fracture probably occurred during her term pregnancies as the enlarging uterus collapses the Greenfield filter, which subsequently re-expands postpartum. If a strut is broken but does not have any missing pieces, imaging of the chest is not warranted. Additionally, in the face of an asymptomatic patient, there are no indications for abdominal imaging beyond the film in clinic. She should also be made aware that the longest follow-up of her type of filter is a mean of only about 9 years. On the whole, though, the most prudent course of action would seem to be reassurance. Discussions about continued follow-up with imaging should be individualized to the patient since any risks associated with contemplated removal would only grow with time, prompting the question of what would be done if new information was gleaned while remaining asymptomatic.

Answer: E

Greenfield LJ, Proctor MC. Twenty-year clinical experience with the Greenfield filter. *Cardiovascular Surgery* 1995; 3:199–205.

Phelan HA, Gonzalez RP, Scott WC, et al. Long-term follow-up of trauma patients with permanent prophylactic vena cava filters. *The Journal of Trauma* 2009; 67:485–489.

16 Which of the following statements about the Factor V Leiden mutation is incorrect?

   A *Five percent of Caucasians are heterozygous for the mutation.*

   B *The mutation causes resistance to activated protein C.*

   C *Long-term anticoagulation with a vitamin K antagonist is recommended for patients who are heterozygous for the mutation.*

   D *Venous thromboses are more common than arterial thromboses in patients with Factor V Leiden mutation.*

   E *Venous thrombosis after general surgical or orthopedic procedures does not appear to be increased in patients heterozygous for the Factor V Leiden mutation when they are managed with well-reasoned protocols for VTE prophylaxis.*

Five percent of Caucasians are heterozygous for the mutation, making it the most common inherited hypercoagulable state, as approximately 1 person in 5000 is homozygous for the disorder among the general population. Platelets carry an endogenous protein

C inhibitor, which makes arterial thrombosis less common. The preponderance of the literature suggests that for patients undergoing major general surgical or orthopedic procedures, the incremental risk carried by possession of the mutation is overwhelmed by well-reasoned prophylaxis measures. Therefore, there is no basis for altering their perioperative management based on a history of Factor V Leiden. The same cannot be said for arterial thrombosis after a vascular procedure, however. Asymptomatic heterozygosity for Factor V Leiden does not constitute an indication for intervention.

Answer: C

Nicholson M, Chan N, Bhagirath V, Ginsberg J. Prevention of venous thromboembolism in 2020 and beyond. *Journal of Clinical Medicine* 2020; 9(8):2467.

Zhang S, Taylor AK, Huang X, Luo B, Spector EB, Fang P, Richards CS; ACMG Laboratory Quality Assurance Committee. Venous thromboembolism laboratory testing (factor V Leiden and factor II c.*97G>A), 2018 update: a technical standard of the American College of Medical Genetics and Genomics (ACMG). *Genetics in Medicine* 2018; 20(12):1489–1498.

18 *In considering VTE risk after urgent laparoscopic cholecystectomy (LC), ventral hernia repair (VHR), and partial colectomy (PC), which of the following statements is CORRECT?*

   A *The VTE risk is related to the procedure itself, not whether the procedure was performed on an emergent or elective basis.*

   B *Upon discharge, the risk of VTE continues to be high, with more than 30% of VTEs among patients with an urgent LC occurring after admission.*

   C *The higher rates of VTE seen after urgent LC are explained primarily by missed dosing of chemoprophylaxis.*

   D *The risk of urgent case status on postoperative VTE development is inconsistent as LC shows a higher VTE risk while VHR and PC show no increase above baseline.*

   E *The higher risk for VTE of urgent procedures is explained by the finding that patients requiring urgent LC, VHR, or OC are sicker at baseline, and the effect disappears when baseline health is controlled for.*

While missing doses of chemoprophylaxis are certainly a factor in higher VTE rates, the inflammation and tissue disruption seen after emergent surgery are also significant contributors to the higher rates of VTE seen compared to when the same procedure is performed electively. The effect of tissue disruption also explains why higher rates of VTE are seen after a given procedure is performed open rather than laparoscopically. LC, VHR, and PC all show increased rates of VTE as compared to their elective counterparts.

Answer: B

Ross SW, Kuhlenschmidt KM, Kubasiak JC, et al. Association of the risk of a venous thromboembolic event in emergency vs elective general surgery. *JAMA Surgery* 2020; 155:503–511.

22

Transplantation, Immunology, and Cell Biology
Jarrett Santorelli, MD and Leslie Kobayashi, MD

Division of Trauma, Acute Care Surgery, Surgical Critical Care and Burns, University of California San Diego, San Diego, CA, USA

1 *A 57-year-old woman is admitted to the intensive care unit (ICU) with hepatic encephalopathy requiring intubation and management of cerebral edema. Her body mass index (BMI) is 41 kg/m, her albumin is 1.9 g/dL, and prealbumin is 9 mg/dL. A feeding tube is placed for enteral nutrition. Regarding nutrition in cirrhotic and pretransplant patients, which of the following is true?*

   A *A preoperative BMI < 20 is associated with improved outcomes following transplant.*

   B *A preoperative BMI > 40 is associated with improved outcomes following transplant.*

   C *Preoperative energy intake should target a goal of 30–35 kcal/kg/day.*

   D *Immuno-enhanced nutrition has been associated with improved outcomes following transplant.*

   E *Percutaneous gastrostomy (PEG) tube is the preferred route for long-term enteral access in cirrhotic patients.*

It is well known that nutrition has a central prognostic and therapeutic role in the management of patients with liver disease. Based on available published data, patients should have an energy intake of 30–35 kcal/kg/d and a protein intake of 1.2–1.5 g/kg/d. In a well-conducted prospective trial measuring total body nitrogen, the nocturnal administration of oral nutritional supplements has been shown to be more effective in improving total body protein status than daytime oral nutritional supplements. Patients undergoing liver transplantation who are underweight or severely obese experience significantly higher rates of morbidity and mortality in comparison with patients in the middle BMI categories. Across different eras of liver transplantation, underweight and severe obesity are independent predictors of death in a multivariable analysis. Despite some promising small studies of immuno-enhanced nutritional supplementation particularly in the burn ICU population, there is no good evidence to support their use in patients with

end-stage liver disease (ESLD) either pre- or post-transplant. Anti-inflammatory oils have also not been demonstrated to have any substantial benefit when compared to standard enteral nutrition. While there is definite evidence that enteral nutrition is superior to parenteral nutrition, PEG tubes are not recommended in patients with ESLD. The presence of ascites, abdominal wall, gastric and esophageal varices, as well as the coagulopathy present in many ESLD patients, makes the risks of placement and infection/dislodgement after placement prohibitive.

Answer: C

Dick AAS, Spitzer AL, Seifert CF, *et al.* Liver transplantation at the extremes of the body mass index. *Liver Transplantation* 2009; 15(8): 968–977.

Plauth M, Bernal W, Dasarathy S, *et al.* ESPEN guidelines on clinical nutrition in liver disease. *Clinical Nutrition* 2019; 38(2): 485–521.

2 *A 37-year-old male is postoperative day (POD) 3 from orthotopic liver transplant (OLT) and his postoperative course has been unremarkable after successful extubation on POD 1. Today was his first day working with physical therapy and getting out of bed. He reports to you after the session that he noticed some weakness and moderate swelling and pain with movement in his right calf. Ultrasound of the bilateral lower extremities reveals a deep venous thrombosis (DVT) of the right popliteal vein. Regarding venous thromboembolic (VTE) complications in live transplant patients, which of the following is true?*

   A *Rates of VTE are higher after liver transplant than after other major abdominal procedures.*

   B *Chemoprophylaxis is associated with reduced rates of VTE after OLT.*

   C *Comorbid conditions such as end-stage renal disease and diabetes are associated with lower risk of VTE following OLT.*

D *Treatment factors such as veno-venous bypass and central venous catheters have not been shown to increase risk of VTE in OLT patients.*

E *Conventional laboratory measures of coagulation are good measures of VTE risk and can be relied upon to guide timing of VTE chemoprophylaxis.*

Venous thromboembolism (VTE), with deep vein thrombosis (DVT) and pulmonary embolism (PE) as the most common manifestations, is a serious and potentially fatal complication of major abdominal surgery and is estimated to occur in 5–10% of patients. The most common risk factors for VTE are hospitalization (52%), cancer (48%), and surgery (42%). Numerous risk factors for VTE exist in patients who undergo orthotopic liver transplantation (OLT) including critical illness, prolonged periods of bedrest, indwelling central venous catheters, and veno-venous bypass. Recent studies have also demonstrated an increased risk of VTE in transplant recipients with diabetes, previous history of VTE, end-stage renal disease (ESRD), patients discharged to rehabilitation centers, receiving factor VII during surgery, or having postoperative pneumonia. A marked reduction of both procoagulant factors (II, V, VII, IX, X, XI, XII), anticoagulant factors (anti-thrombin III, protein C, and protein S), an increase in von Willebrand factor (vWF), and a reduced level of ADAMTS13 are the specific features of cirrhosis and bring the patient to a new hemostatic balance. Elevated tissue plasminogen activator and a deficiency of thrombin-activatable fibrinolysis inhibitor have been associated with laboratory changes typical of hyperfibrinolysis and an increased risk of bleeding. However, cirrhosis has also been associated with reduced fibrinolysis, as shown by the decreased plasminogen and increased plasminogen activator inhibitor. The contrasting results explain the ongoing debate regarding the absence or presence of a hyperfibrinolytic state in patients with liver disease, even if the balance of fibrinolysis is probably restored by the parallel changes in profibrinolytic and antifibrinolytic drivers. In addition, patients may also suffer from microvascular consumption causing further decreases in AT-III levels. Despite this balanced hemostatic condition, cirrhosis results in the prolongation of standard coagulation tests, which usually do not analyze the complex interplay between pro- and anticoagulants and thus do not provide an accurate evaluation of the alteration in the in vivo hemostatic balance. Prothrombin time (PT), activated partial thromboplastin time (aPTT), and International Normalized Ratio (INR) provide only a measure of procoagulant factors and are insensitive to the plasma levels of anticoagulant factors, so they are unreliable to depict the hemostatic status of patients with end-stage liver disease.

Compared to patients undergoing other major abdominal surgeries, OLT patients have comparable to somewhat lower rates of VTE. Chemoprophylaxis, when utilized, has been associated with reduced risk of VTE after OLT. Chemoprophylaxis has also been associated with lower rates of portal vein thrombosis. Chemoprophylaxis has not been associated with higher mortality or complications.

Answer: B

Feltracco P, Barbieri S, Cillo U, *et al.* Perioperative thrombotic complications in liver transplantation. *World Journal of Gastroenterology* 2015; 21(26): 8004–8013.

Nachal R, Subramanian R, Karvellas CJ, *et al.* Guidelines for the management of adult acute and acute-on-chronic liver failure in the ICU: cardiovascular, endocrine, hematologic, pulmonary and renal considerations: executive summary. Critical Care Medicine 2020; 48(3): 415–419.

Salami A, Qureshi W, Kuriakose P, *et al.* Frequency and predictors of venous thromboembolism in orthotopic liver transplant recipients: a single-center retrospective review. *Transplantation Proceedings* 2013; 45(1): 315–319.

Yip J, Bruno DA, Burmeister C, *et al.* Deep vein thrombosis and pulmonary embolism in liver transplant patients: risks and prevention. *Transplantation Direct* 2016; 2(4):e68.

3 *A 73-year-old man with a medical history significant for hypertension, diabetes, and gastroparesis previously requiring total parenteral nutrition (TPN), and end-stage renal disease (ESRD) is now POD 10 from renal transplant. The patient has had increasing work of breathing and required intubation; his*

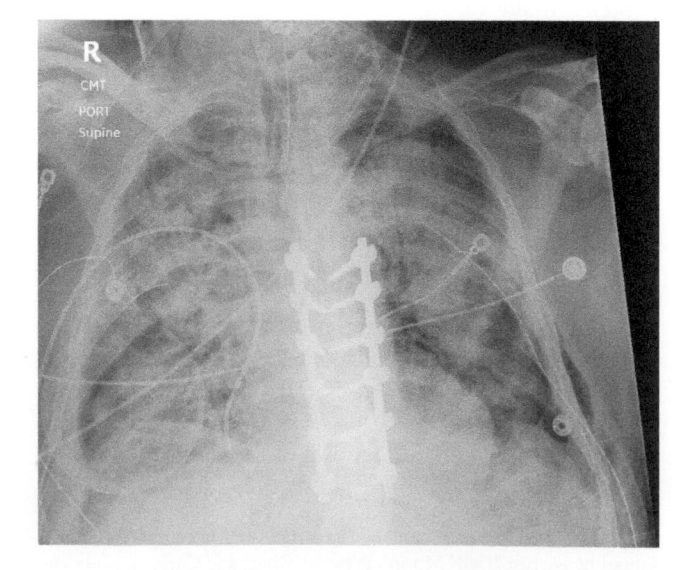

post-intubation x-ray is seen below. Further workup including bronchoscopy with bronchoalveolar lavage and CT scan of the chest demonstrated an invasive fungal disease (IFD). The patient was started on caspofungin. Regarding IFD following solid organ transplant, which of the following is true?

A *IFD are common complications following solid organ transplant.*

B *IFD do not impact mortality following transplant.*

C *Of all solid organ transplant recipients, IFD are most common following renal transplant.*

D *Candida and Aspergillus are the most common causes of IFD.*

E *IFD most often occur early following transplant, with the majority of infections occurring <90 days after surgery.*

Invasive fungal disease (IFD) is one of the critical opportunistic infections afflicting solid organ transplant (SOT) recipients. IFD contributes to relatively high morbidity and mortality compared to its low incidence, due to multiple causes, which include fungal virulence and delayed diagnosis in SOT patients. While still uncommon, incidence of IFD is increasing slightly over time. The incidence of IFD among kidney transplant recipients is commonly known to be the lowest among all SOT recipients, reported as 1–10%. The patients with highest risk for IFD are small bowel, lung, and liver recipients. The period of the highest risk for the development of IFD is known to be the period of intense immunosuppression, from one to six months after SOT. Recent studies reported that the majority of IFD cases developed later than six months after kidney transplantation (KT). Candida and Aspergillus species are the most common organisms, with non-albicans species increasing in frequency.

Answer: D

Lum L, Lee A, Vu M, Strasser S, Davis R. Epidemiology and risk factors for invasive fungal disease in liver transplant recipients in a tertiary transplant center. *Transplant Infectious Disease* 2020; e13361.

Pappas PG, Alexander BD, Andes DR, *et al*. Invasive fungal infections among organ transplant recipients: results of the Transplant-Associated Infection Surveillance Network (TRANSNET). *Clinical Infectious Diseases* 2010: 50(8): 1101–1111.

Seok H, Huh K, Cho SY, *et al*. Invasive fungal diseases in kidney transplant recipients: risk factors for mortality. *Journal of Clinical Medicine* 2020; 9(6):1824.

4 *A 45-year-old woman is POD 11 from combined OLT and kidney transplant and is doing well on the floor when she develops a fungal urinary tract infection and is started on fluconazole. Over the next several days, the patient's urine output drops and the patient's creatinine begins to rise. She also appears sleepy on rounds and when asked how she feels complains of a headache. The patient's vital signs have remained stable except for mild hypertension. Lab abnormalities also include worsening hyperglycemia and new hyperkalemia. Which of the following agents is the most likely cause of these signs and symptoms? (Table 22.1).*

A *Prednisone*

B *Mycophenalate mofetil*

C *Tacrolimus*

D *Gabapentin*

E *Oxycodone*

This patient is demonstrating the most worrisome toxicity of tacrolimus, which is nephrotoxicity. Other typical symptoms of calcineurin inhibitor (CNI) toxicity include altered mental status, hypertension, hyperglycemia, and hyperlipidemia. CNIs are both the savior and Achilles heel of kidney transplantation. Though CNI have significantly reduce rates of acute rejection, their numerous toxicities can plague kidney transplant recipients. CNIs function as immunosuppressants by blocking T-cell activation by binding to specific receptors and blocking calcineurin, a calcium-dependent phosphatase within T-cells. Though CNIs have been successful in preventing acute kidney transplant rejection, their use has been described as a significant contributing factor in acute and chronic allograft injury and ultimately allograft loss – with virtually universal presence of CNI nephrotoxicity on allograft biopsy by 10 years after kidney transplant. CNIs are metabolized by cytochrome P450 3A4 (CYP3A4) in both the liver and small intestine, and clearance is primarily from biliary excretion and fecal elimination. Any medications that inhibit CYP3A4 will increase drug concentrations, and in contrast, medications that induce CYP3A4 will decrease drug

Table 22.1 Common pharmacologic CYP3A4 inhibitors and inducers.

Inhibitors	Inducers
Cannabidiol	Carbamazepine
Diltiazem	Phenytoin
Verapamil	Phenobarbital
Erythromycin	Rifampin
Ketoconazole	Rifabutin
Fluconazole	Efavirenz
Clotrimazole	Dexamethasone
Ritonavir	

concentrations. Azole antifungals like fluconazole are commonly encountered inhibitors of CYP3A4 and will result in increased levels of tacrolimus and increased toxicity. While steroids, narcotics, and gabapentin may all contribute to altered mental status and increased somnolence, they are unlikely to affect renal function and both narcotics and gabapentin are more likely to result in decreased blood pressure than hypertension. Mycophenolate mofetil (MMF) is a first-line drug in the maintenance of immunosuppression after solid organ transplant and has the benefit of low toxicity and minimal side effect profile. Side effects of MMF include gastrointestinal distress and pancytopenia. In contrast to CNIs, nephrotoxicity and neurotoxicity are rare with MMF.

Answer: C

Farouk SS, Rein JL. The many faces of calcineurin inhibitor toxicity- What the FK? *Advances in Chronic Kidney Disease* 2020; 27(1): 56–66.
Vanhove T, Annaert P, Kuypers DR. Clinical determinants of calcineurin inhibitor disposition: a mechanistic review. *Drug Metabolism Reviews* 2016; 48(1):88–112.

5 *A 47-year-old woman with medical history significant for hypertension, diabetes, and ESLD secondary to alcoholic cirrhosis is now POD 0 from OLT. Regarding immunosuppression regimens in liver transplant recipients, which of the following is TRUE?*

 A *Tacrolimus results in improved graft survival and mortality compared to cyclosporine when used for maintenance immunosuppression.*

 B *Steroids have improved mortality and graft failure compared to basiliximab when used for induction immunosuppression.*

 C *Tacrolimus causes fewer adverse events compared to cyclosporine.*

 D *Tacrolimus has reduced risk of post-transplant diabetes compared to cyclosporine when used for maintenance immunosuppression.*

 E *Tacrolimus plus sirolimus reduces mortality and graft loss compared to tacrolimus alone when used for maintenance immunosuppression.*

Both tacrolimus and cyclosporine are classified as calcineurin inhibitors (CNIs) and are often used in maintenance immunosuppression following SOT. Tacrolimus binds to FK binding protein-12 and blocks proliferation of calcineurin, preventing interleukin-2 (IL-2) expression/production, thus preventing an immune response from lymphocytes. Tacrolimus is superior to cyclosporine in increasing patient and graft survival. Fewer episodes of acute cellular rejection and steroid-resistant rejection have also been seen with tacrolimus use in the

first-year post-transplant compared to cyclosporine. Tacrolimus is preferred at most transplant centers because of its greater potency and improved cardiovascular side-effect profile. While cyclosporine and tacrolimus have similar nephrotoxicity, tacrolimus has a greater diabetogenic effect than cyclosporine. Based on low-quality evidence, basiliximab induction may decrease mortality and graft failure compared to glucocorticosteroid induction in people undergoing liver transplantation. Based on low-quality evidence from a single small trial from direct comparison, tacrolimus plus sirolimus increase mortality and graft loss at maximal follow-up compared with tacrolimus.

Answer: A

Best LMJ, Leung J, Freeman SC, *et al.* Induction immunosuppression in adults undergoing liver transplation: a network meta-analysis. *Cochrane Database of Systematic Reviews* 2020; 1(1): CD013203.
Haddad EM, McAlister VC, Renouf E, *et al.* Cyclosporin versus tacrolimus for liver transplanted patients. *Cochrane Database of Systematic Reviews* 2006; 18(4):CD005161.
Rodrique-Peralvarez M, Guerrero-Misas M, thorburn D, *et al.* Maintenance immunosuppression for adults undergoing liver transplantation: a network meta-analysis. *Cochrane Database of Systematic Reviews* 2017; 3(3):CD011639.

6 *A 67-year-old female with Childs C cirrhosis secondary to hepatitis B has been in the ICU for several weeks with acute-on-chronic liver failure, requiring intubation for respiratory failure and hepatic encephalopathy, and hepatorenal syndrome requiring continuous renal replacement therapy. She is currently on the wait list to receive a liver transplant. Which of the following are risk factors for poor outcomes following transplantation?*

 A *Hypernatremia*

 B *Mechanical ventilation*

 C *High Sequential Organ Failure Assessment (SOFA) score*

 D *High Model of End-stage Liver Disease (MELD) score*

 E *Occurrence of acute-on-chronic liver failure*

Acute-on-chronic liver failure (ACLF) is a recently described entity in chronic liver disease defined by acute hepatic decompensation, organ failure, and a high risk of short-term mortality. Although there is not a universal agreement about the definition of ACLF, there is a wide agreement that ACLF is a distinct syndrome that is different from chronic, progressive hepatic decompensation. In most cases of ACLF, patients present initially with clinical manifestations of a decompensating event, usually renal impairment, worsening of abdominal ascites, jaundice, or hepatic encephalopathy, often precipitated by bacterial infection. Child-Pugh and Model for End-Stage Liver Disease (MELD) scores were initially the only available tools to predict outcomes in patients with ACLF. The use of these scores has limitations as they do not include measures of extrahepatic organ failure nor markers of systemic inflammation, both key features of ACLF. While increasing number of organ system failures is correlated with poor outcomes neither high MELD/Child-Pugh nor SOFA scores have been found to independently predict mortality following OLT. Older age, hyponatremia, and mechanical ventilation have been associated with higher mortality after OLT. The role of liver transplantation in ACLF remains a topic of debate. While liver transplantation is potentially the only curative intervention in such advanced patients, ACLF is also associated with higher post-operative complications and longer ICU and hospital stays compared with non-ACLF recipients. However, one-year survival was not significantly different when comparing transplanted patients with ACLF grade 3 to grades 1–2, or no ACLF.

Answer: B

Artu F, Lovet A, Ruiz I, *et al*. Liver transplantation in the most severely ill cirrhotic patients: a multicenter study in acute-on-chronic liver failure grade 3. *Journal of Hepatology* 2017; 67(4): 708–715.

Karvellas CJ, Bagshaw SM. Advances in management and prognostication in critically ill cirrhotic patients. *Current Opinion in Critical Care* 2014; 20(2): 210–217.

Sundaram V, Jalan R, Wu T, *et al*. Factors associated with survival of patients with severe acute-on-chronic liver failure before and after liver transplantation. *Gastroenterology* 2019; 156(6): 1381–1391.

7   *A 35-year-old African-American woman has just undergone living-related renal transplant for ESRD. She was on dialysis for 2 years prior to transplant and her medical history includes type 2 diabetes, hypertension, and hyperlipidemia. She is a past smoker. She is currently in the ICU still requiring intermittent dialysis for delayed graft function (DGF). Which of the following is a risk factor for reduced long-term survival?*

   A   *Black race*
   B   *Obesity (body mass index ≥ 30)*
   C   *Younger age*
   D   *Living-related donor graft*
   E   *Type 2 diabetes*

The burden of chronic kidney disease (CKD), end-stage renal disease (ESRD), and kidney transplant in the US non-Hispanic Black (NHB) population cannot be overstated. Based on the 2010 Census and 2014 USRDS data, NHBs represent 12.6% of the US population, yet 32.2% of those with ESRD, 33.9% of those on the kidney transplant waiting list, and 22.2% of those that received a kidney transplant are NHB. Following transplant, NHBs are at significantly higher risk of graft loss. The most recent US-based data from the United Network of Organ Sharing (UNOS) registry data demonstrates NHB kidney transplants have a 5-year graft/patient survival rate of 61%, which compares to 74% in non-Hispanic White (NHW); a 13% absolute lower graft survival rate. However, NHBs do not have worsened survival following kidney transplant, in fact mortality was found to be significantly lower compared to NHWs prior to adjustment and comparable after adjustment. Type 2 diabetes is one of the commonest causes of ESRD worldwide. While transplantation is the treatment of choice, restricted access to transplantation for ESRD patients with diabetes seems to be a worldwide problem. Despite an improvement in the relative survival of patients with type 2 diabetes in the general population, a recent study found no evidence of such improvement in the relative survival among type 2 diabetics after kidney transplant. Over an 18-year period, people with ESRD caused by type 2 diabetes who received a transplant were at least twice as likely to die as recipients without diabetes, with excess risk of death attributable to both cardiovascular disease and infection. Despite having a much higher likelihood of DGF, obese transplant recipients have only a slightly increased risk of graft loss and experience similar survival to recipients with normal BMI. Older kidney patients with chronic kidney disease benefit significantly from kidney transplantation. However, these older transplant recipients have greater mortality after transplantation than younger transplant recipients.

Answer: E

Hill CJ, Courtney AE, Cardwell CR, *et al*. Recipient obesity and outcomes after kidney transplantation: a systematic review and meta-analysis. *Nephrology, Dialysis, Transplantation* 2015; 30(8): 1403–1411.

Lim WH, Wong G, Pilmore HL, et al. Long term outcomes of kidney transplantation in people with type 2 diabetes: a population cohort study. *The Lancet* 2017; 5(1): 26–33.

Schaenman J, Liao D, Phonphok K, Bunnapradist S, Karlamangla A. Predictors of early and late mortality in older kidney transplant recipients. *Transplantation Proceedings* 2019: 51(3): 684–691.

Taber DJ, Gebregziabher M, Payne EH, *et al*. Overall graft loss versus death censored graft loss: Unmasking the magnitude of racial disparities in outcomes among U.S. kidney transplant recipients. *Transplantation* 2017; 101(2): 402–410.

8 *The patient in question 7 has done well over the past 5 years and is now following up for routine health check in clinic. Her immunosuppression regimen and renal function appear stable. She is reporting excellent compliance with all her medications including her statin. Long-term survival following renal transplant has steadily improved over the past 40 years. What is the most common cause of late deaths in patients following renal transplant?*

A *Infection*
B *Graft failure due to chronic rejection*
C *Cardiovascular disease*
D *Malignancy*
E *Stroke*

The survival following renal transplantation has improved significantly over the years and now approaches 95% at one year. While the mortality of post-transplant patients is higher than the general population, it is significantly better than patients with ESRD without transplantation. In the United States, the three leading causes of death after transplantation are cardiovascular disease, malignancy, and infections. Similar results were seen in Australia and New Zealand with the leading causes of long-term death following kidney transplant being cardiovascular disease, infection, and cancer. Despite a shift toward recipients who are older and have more comorbidities, mortality risk has declined for recipients at all time periods post-transplant, including the high-risk early post-transplant period (0–3 months), early maintenance phases (1–5 years), and into the longer-term (≥10 years) post-transplant.

Answer: C

Francis A, Johnson DW, Melk A, *et al.* Survival after kidney transplantation during childhood and adolescence. *Clinical Journal of the American Society of Nephrology* 2020; 15(3):392–400.

Ying T, Shi B, Kelly PJ, *et al.* Death after kidney transplantation: an analysis by era and time post-transplant. *Journal of the American Society of Nephrology* 2020; 31(12): 2887–2899.

9 *A 42-year-old renal transplant recipient is admitted to the ICU in respiratory failure with COVID-19. The usual isolation and supportive measures are started; however, the patient deteriorates and requires intubation and mechanical ventilation for acute hypoxic respiratory failure. A protease inhibitor is started. What changes need to be made to the patient's usual immunosuppressive medications?*

A *Increase the patient's usual dose of steroids to stress dose levels equivalent to 50–100 mg of hydrocortisone.*

B *Increase dose but not frequency of mycophenolate mofetil.*
C *Increase calcineurin inhibitor dose and frequency and check drug levels daily.*
D *Reduce calcineurin inhibitor dose and frequency and check drug levels daily 2 hours after administration of the calcineurin inhibitor.*
E *Reduce calcineurin inhibitor dose and frequency and check drug levels daily 4 hours after administration of the calcineurin inhibitor.*

Solid organ transplant recipients are perceived to be at increased risk of severe COVID-19 because of their chronic immunosuppressed status due to immunosuppressive drugs (ISDs). Many of the ISDs pharmacodynamics (PD) and pharmacokinetics (PK) can be affected by antivirals and other treatments for COVID-19. Furthermore, COVID-19 patients may exhibit features of systemic hyper-inflammation, which can be associated with so-called phenoconversion, a phenomenon whereby extensive metabolizers transiently exhibit drug metabolizing enzyme activity at a comparable level as that of poor metabolizers. Protease inhibitors (PIs) act by selectively inhibiting the HIV-1 protease, thereby preventing the post-translational processing of viral gag and gag-pol polyprotein products into smaller functional proteins, an essential step for the maturation of new virions. Drug–drug interactions with COVID-19 PI-based treatment can modify not only ISD concentrations but also the PK profile of the drug. One well-known interaction is that PIs significantly increase calcineurin inhibitor levels and flatten the drug concentration curves of calcineurin inhibitors (CNIs). Therefore, both the dose and frequency of CNIs should be reduced. Additionally, because of the flattened drug curves, optimal time for serum drug assays to be drawn should be moved from the usual 2 hours following administration to 4 hours following administration.

Answer: E

Elens L, Langman LJ, Hesselink DA, *et al.* Pharmacologic treatment of transplant recipients infeted with SARS-CoV-2: considerations regarding therapeutic drug monitoring and drug-drug interactions. *Therapeutic Drug Monitoring* 2020; 42(3): 360–368.

Laracy JC, Verna EC, Pereira MR. Antivirals for COVID-19 in solid organ transplant recipients. *Current Transplantation Reports* 2020: 1–11

10 *A 66-year-old man with a medical history significant for hypertension, diabetes, hepatitis C cirrhosis, and alcohol dependence is in the ICU with septic shock and acute-on-chronic liver failure due to spontaneous bacterial peritonitis (SBP). The patient is* *groggy but follows commands, his heart rate is 133 beats per minute in sinus rhythm, blood pressure is 75/33 mm Hg. He has an extremely distended abdomen with fluid wave. Labs demonstrate a leukocystosis, mild anemia with hemoglobin of 9 gm/dL, total bilirubin of 12 mg/dL, and albumin of 1.9 mg/dL. After obtaining adequate intravenous access and starting broad spectrum antibiotics, what is the next step in management of this patient?*

A *Bolus with albumin*

B *Bolus with normal saline*

C *Bolus with lactated ringer*

D *Bolus with hydroxyethyl starch*

E *Start an infusion of epinephrine*

Acute liver failure (ALF) and acute-on-chronic liver failure (ACLF) are conditions frequently encountered in the ICU and are associated with high mortality. Although the average patient with septic shock should be resuscitated with a balanced crystalloid solution as there is no mortality benefit to colloids and a significantly increased cost, ACLF patients, particularly those with albumin levels < 3 mg/dL, with shock, may benefit from albumin resuscitation. The rationale for this is threefold. First, in ACLF patients not only is the quantity of the albumin low, but the function may also be impaired and albumin resuscitation may restore some of the antioxidant, immunoregulatory, and endothelial regulatory effects in addition to providing increased intravascular oncotic pressure. Second, albumin administration in ACLF patients with terlipressin may reduce the impact of hepatorenal syndrome. Lastly, albumin replacement in patients with losses associated with paracentesis has been shown to prevent circulatory dysfunction and reduce mortality. Meta-analyses of available trials in critically ill patients suggest no benefit of hydroxyethyl starch over crystalloids, and starches may also exacerbate coagulopathy in liver failure. The standard of care for patients with septic shock is to institute fluid challenge and to consider vasopressors only if there is a failure or inadequate response to volume resuscitation. Additionally, epinephrine may cause splanchnic vasoconstriction and increase the risk of mesenteric and hepatic ischemia in the setting of liver failure. Administration of albumin in conjunction with high-volume paracentesis in patients with ascites has been shown by meta-analysis to prevent paracentesis-induced circulatory dysfunction. On review of recent literature, meta-analysis did not show benefits of albumin compared with crystalloids in patients with sepsis. Additionally, the ALBIOS trial did not show decreased mortality with albumin replacement targeted to a serum level greater than 3 mg/dL for the first 28 days. However,

the septic shock data are indirect for liver failure, costs may be prohibitive in resource poor settings and the paracentesis data may not be directly applicable to resuscitation for shock; nonetheless, the pathophysiologic rationale in liver failure suggest that albumin administration over crystalloid should be considered in this population. Albumin bolus is the current recommendation from the critical care medicine management guidelines for patients with ALF and ACLF (2020).

Answer: A

Karvellas CJ, Bagshaw SM. Advances in management and prognostication in critically ill cirrhotic patients. *Current Opinion in Critical Care* 2014; 20(2): 210–217.

Nachal R, Subramanian R, Karvellas CJ, *et al.* Guidelines for the management of adult acute and acute-on-chronic liver failure in the ICU: cardiovascular, endocrine, hematologic, pulmonary and renal considerations: executive summary. *Critical Care Medicine* 2020; 48(3): 415–419.

11 *The patient above in question 10 remains hypotensive after adequate fluid resuscitation, you have placed an arterial line and central venous catheter and sent cultures and repeated labs. What is the next step in management of his septic shock?*

A *Transfuse packed red blood cells until hemoglobin is over 11 gm/dL.*

B *Start dopamine infusion and maintain at 3 mcg/kg/minute for renal perfusion.*

C *Start dopamine infusion and titrate to achieve a goal mean arterial pressure > 65 mm Hg.*

D *Start a vasopressin infusion and titrate to achieve a goal mean arterial pressure > 65 mm Hg.*

E *Start norepinephrine infusion and titrate to achieve a goal mean arterial pressure > 65 mm Hg.*

Acute liver failure (ALF) and acute-on-chronic liver failure (ACLF) are conditions frequently encountered in the ICU and are associated with high mortality. Patients with liver failure exhibit hyperdynamic circulation, and shock states in these patients are typically characterized by distributive physiology. Despite the paucity of studies directly related to liver failure, indirect evidence from trials in other distributive shock states such as septic shock suggest norepinephrine is superior compared with dopamine in reversing hypotension and is associated with lower mortality and lower risk of arrhythmias. While there is significant data to support the use of vasopressin as a second-line agent demonstrating a reduction in catecholamine requirements and mortality when vasopressin is added to norepinephrine, studies comparing vasopressin as a first-line agent to other vasoactive agents are not available. There is significant data to support a restrictive transfusion threshold across multiple ICU populations including patients with liver failure. Villanueva et al. demonstrated that in cirrhotic patients with bleeding esophageal varices, a restricted transfusion strategy (transfusion cutoff of 7 g/dL vs. 9 g/dL) was associated with a trend toward improved survival. Red blood cell transfusion has also been associated with increased mortality after OLT.

Answer: E

Amin A, Mookerjee RP. Acute-on-chronic liver failure: definition, prognosis and management. *Frontline Gasteroenterology* 2020; 11: 458–467.

Karvellas CJ, Bagshaw SM. Advances in management and prognostication in critically ill cirrhotic patients. *Current Opinion in Critical Care* 2014; 20(2): 210–217.

Nachal R, Subramanian R, Karvellas CJ, *et al.* Guidelines for the management of adult acute and acute-on-chronic liver failure in the ICU: cardiovascular, endocrine, hematologic, pulmonary and renal considerations: executive summary. *Critical Care Medicine* 2020; 48(3): 415–419.

12 *A 65-year-old man is 2 years status-post heart transplant. He was admitted to the ICU with a small subarachnoid hemorrhage after a syncopal fall. He reports that he had been in his usual state of health but did experience some mild stomach upset over the holidays. He denies chest pain, dyspnea on exertion, or reduced overall tolerance to activity. Electrocardiogram done as part of his syncope workup does not reveal any ST segment changes. What is the next step?*
   A *Myocardial biopsy*
   B *Echocardiogram with tissue-doppler and strain imaging*
   C *Cardiac MRI*
   D *Coronary angiogram*
   E *Immediately list for re-transplantation*

Cardiac allograft vasculopathy (CAV) is caused by progressive thickening of the coronary vascular wall with narrowing of the vessel lumen after heart transplantation, which leads to blood flow impairment and ischemic consequences such as graft failure, arrhythmias, and sudden death. In contrast to coronary artery disease (CAD), which tends to affect proximal coronary arteries, CAV is diffused and affects all cardiac vessels including intra-myocardial arteries and, in some cases, coronary veins. Coronary angiography was the key diagnostic imaging for CAV before the development of intra-coronary imaging. However, coronary angiography has several drawbacks; it is invasive, requires specialized

personnel, exposure to ionizing radiation, and intravenous contrast. Additionally, it can only visualize the vessel lumen, but not the vessel wall, and thus cannot assess several CAV-associated features such as vascular remodeling and vasodilation. In a study by Colvin-Adams et al., perfusion magnetic resonance imaging (MRI) was used to detect CAV but yielded a sensitivity of only 41% and specificity of 74%. Echocardiography has emerged as one of the most promising tools for screening, especially after the addition of tissue Doppler (TDI) and strain imaging for ventricular wall motion and myocardial deformation analysis, allowing quantification of minor myocardial dysfunction not detectable by standard echocardiography. TDI and strain imaging can reveal subclinical acute rejection. Echocardiography also has the benefit of being less invasive and more easily tolerated by patients than angiography and endomyocardial biopsy, with few major risks and easy repeatability.

Answer: B

Dandel M, Hetzer R. Post-transplant surveillance for acute rejection and allograft vasculopathy by echocardiography: Usefullness of myocardial velocity and deformation imaging. *The Journal of Heart and Lung Transplantation* 2017; 36(2):117–131.

Habibi S, Ghaffarpasand E, Shojaei F, *et al.* Prognostic value of biomarkers in cardiac allograft vasculopathy following heart transplantation: a literature review. *Cardiology* 2020; 145(11):693–702.

Ramzy D, Rao V, Brahm J, *et al.* Cardiac allograft vasculopathy: a review. *Canadian Journal of Surgery* 2005; 48(4):319–327.

13 *A 57-year-old man with a medical history significant for hypertension and chronic obstructive pulmonary disease (COPD) due to previous heavy tobacco presents for lung transplantation. Fourteen hours after returning from surgery the patient develops acute respiratory deterioration. Chest x-ray reveals diffuse patchy infiltrates and arterial blood gas demonstrates a decreased PaO2/FiO2 ratio. The patient has increased airway pressures and reduced tidal volumes on the ventilator. What is the most likely diagnosis?*
   A *Transfusion-related acute lung injury (TRALI)*
   B *Ischemia-reperfusion lung injury (IR)*
   C *Pulmonary embolism (PE)*
   D *Obliterative bronchiolitis (OB)*
   E *Ventilator-associated pneumonia (VAP)*

Respiratory failure following lung transplantation is common, and the most common cause in the early period is ischemia-reperfusion injury (IR). IR leads to acute, sterile inflammation after transplant and is a cause for significant concern because it can lead to primary graft dysfunction (PGD), which is the major source of both short- and long-term morbidity and mortality after lung transplantation. Clinically, IR presents very early, within the first 72 hours following transplant. It manifests as increased pulmonary vascular resistance, reduced lung compliance, increased permeability causing acute pulmonary edema, ventilation/perfusion mismatch, and varying degrees of hypoxia. In contrast to IR, OB is most prominent in the late postoperative period with a median time to diagnosis of 16–20 months. Bacterial and fungal pneumonias are also common in the early postoperative period, but generally present later than IR. Pulmonary embolus may be an under-diagnosed cause of post-lung transplant respiratory failure in the first month. However, it usually presents later, does not result in infiltrate on chest x-ray, and is not associated with reduced airway compliance. TRALI can be difficult to differentiate from IR and PGD following lung transplantation as both occur in the acute setting immediately following surgery, and in the case of TRALI, within 6 hours of blood product transfusion and have similar clinical manifestations. However, TRALI is less likely in this clinical scenario and its overall incidence remains quite low ~0.1% of all transfused patients, and as low as 0.0008–0.001% in prospective studies, while IR can effect up to 15% of transplant patients.

Answer: B

Laubach VE, Sharma AK. Mechanisms of lung ischemia-reperfusion injury. *Current Opinion in Organ Transplantation* 2016; 21(3):246–252.

Nareg R. TACO and TRALI: biology, risk factors, and prevention strategies. *Hematology. American Society of Hematology. Education Program* 2018; 2018(1): 585–594.

Pena JJ, Bottiger BA, Miltiades AN. Perioperative management of bleeding and transfusion for lung transplantation. *Seminars in Cardiothoracic and Vascular Anesthesia* 2020; 24(1):74–83.

14 *A 37-year-old G3P3 woman with ESRD secondary to polycystic kidney disease is undergoing kidney transplantation. During the operation, the surgeon notes the transplanted organ acutely begins to appear dusky. Arterial and venous anastomosis are evaluated, which are both widely patent. What is the most likely cause of this intraoperative finding?*

A *Severe sepsis*
B *Ischemia-reperfusion injury*
C *Chronic rejection*
D *Acute rejection*
E *Hyperacute rejection*

There are several types of rejection: hyperacute, acute, and chronic. The types are defined by the timing of their occurrence and the underlying immunological cause. Hyperacute rejection occurs within minutes to hours of reperfusion and is caused by activation of complement by preformed antibodies to antigens present on the donor vascular endothelial cells that results in rapid agglutination, small vessel thrombosis, and graft loss. Acute rejection occurs within weeks to months of transplant and is thought to result from T-cell-mediated cellular rejection and B-cell-mediated humoral rejection. Chronic rejection occurs in a more delayed fashion and is the leading cause of graft loss. It can be mediated by either humoral or cellular responses. With the introduction of modern antibody-detection techniques, such as the L-SAB technology, acute and hyperacute antibody-mediated rejection of the kidney is seen infrequently. Exposure of an individual to foreign major histocompatibility antigens (MHC or HLA for human leukocyte antigens) can promote activation of the immune system and its memory components, resulting in sensitization. Such an exposure occurs, after prior transplantations, blood transfusions, and pregnancies. The graft itself will become soft, mottled, and cyanotic in appearance. Biopsy will demonstrate vascular wall edema and capillary microthrombi. The only treatment of hyperacute rejection is graft removal and emergent re-transplantation.

Answer: E

Becker LE, Morath C, Suesal C. Immune mechanisms of acute and chronic rejection. *Clinical Biochemistry* 2016; 49(4–5):320–323.

Moreau A, Varey E, Anegon I, *et al.* Effector mechanisms of rejection. *Cold Spring Harbor Perspectives in Medicine* 2013; 3(11):a015461. https://doi.org/10.1101/cshperspect.a015461

15 *A 57-year-old man presents to the ED for evaluation of progressive shortness of breath. Medical history is significant for cardiac transplant 7 years ago. On further questioning, the patient reports exertional dyspnea, intermittent diaphoresis, and an episode of syncope. On workup in the ED, the patient is found to have Q-waves on ECG. He is admitted to the cardiac service for further evaluation. Echocardiography is performed demonstrating loss of contractile function. Cardiac catheterization is performed demonstrating arterial main vessel disease with a diffuse and concentric pattern, with typical vessel pruning. Of the following medications, which one has been shown to decrease the arterial disease process seen in this patient?*

A *Tacrolimus*
B *Hydrocortisone*
C *Aldactone*

D *Pravastatin*

E *Metoprolol*

Cardiac allograft vasculopathy (CAV) is a progressive inflammatory vasculopathy that is a significant cause of death after cardiac transplant. Concentric fibrous intimal hyperplasia develops that appears along the entire length of the affected arteries. The graft endothelium represents the borderline between the donor's and recipient's immune systems and plays a critical role in the pathophysiology of CAV. The increased expression of major histocompatibility complex (MHC) class I alloantigens on coronary endothelial cells of the transplant heart are directly recognized by CD8+ T-cells, resulting in the secretion of cytokines with further activation of endothelial cells. CAV is a major determinant of long-term survival among cardiac transplantation recipients. CAV can be seen in 7–8% of patients at one year, but increases to approximately 40% at 8 years post-transplant. Because CAV has a substantially poor prognosis when it becomes symptomatic, the primary effort is directed to early prevention, detection, and initiation of treatment. Statins are considered mandatory in transplant patients because they improve patient survival, reduce both the incidence, and severity of vasculopathy, as well as the incidence of graft rejection. They are typically instituted by the end of the first week or during the second week after heart transplantation. Short-term enhancement of immunosuppressive therapy may slow down the progression of CAV (three days of methylprednisolone plus anti-thymocite globulin). This effect is more pronounced if applied early, i.e. within the first post-transplant year. However, due to significant risk of infections and malignant diseases, this approach is not adopted in routine practice. The remaining choices have not been studied and play no role in the treatment or prevention of CAV.

Answer: D

Chih S, Chong AY, Mielniczuk LM, *et al*. Allograft vasculopathy: the Achilles' heel of heart transplantation. *Journal of the American College of Cardiology* 2016; 68:80–91.

Skorić B, Čikeš M, Ljubas Maček J, *et al*. Cardiac allograft vasculopathy: diagnosis, therapy, and prognosis. *Croatian Medical Journal* 2014; 55(6):562–576. https://doi.org/10.3325/cmj.2014.55.562

Spartalis M, Spartalis E, Tzatzaki E, *et al*. Cardiac allograft vasculopathy after heart transplantation: current prevention and treatment strategies. *European Review for Medical and Pharmacological Sciences* 2019; 23(1): 303–311.

16 *A 29-year-old man with type 1 diabetes and ESRD presents for combined simultaneous pancreas-kidney (SPK) transplant. The patient has been dialysis-dependent for 3 years and has had frequent hospitalizations due to hypoglycemic events and diabetic ketoacidosis. Regarding the state of pancreas transplant which of the following is TRUE?*

A *SPK is not an option for type 2 diabetics with ESRD.*

B *Compared to pancreas transplantation alone (PTA), patients undergoing SPK have higher rates of technical graft loss and worse outcomes.*

C *Due to technical challenges and donor availability, SPK transplants are much less common than PTA or pancreas after kidney (PAK) transplants.*

D *SPK transplant outcomes have improved over time with good 5-year mortality, graft survival, and comparable renal graft survival compared to kidney transplant alone.*

E *While SPK results in good insulin independence, it does not address diabetic complications such as nephropathy, neuropathy, and gastroparesis*

Outcomes following pancreatic transplant have improved significantly over time. Five-year survival is 93% in the US and 88% in the United Kingdom. Graft survival is also high at 73% at 5 years. Both mortality and graft survival are better after SPK when compared to PAK and PTA. SPK patients also have lower rates of technical graft loss and acute rejection compared to PTA recipients. SPK transplants are the most common mode of pancreas transplant with total numbers of SPK recipients far exceeding those of PAK and PTA combined. While the total number of pancreas transplants in the US has been decreasing over the past decade, the number of patients undergoing pancreas transplant for type 2 diabetes with ESRD has increased. Highly selected individuals with type 2 diabetes are candidates for SPK and outcomes for these patients have been improving over time and are now comparable to SPK outcomes in type 1 diabetics. In addition to insulin-independence, pancreas transplantation can stabilize diabetic retinopathy and can reverse neuropathy, gastroparesis, orthostatic hypotension, and nephropathy in the native kidneys. SPK transplantation is also associated with improved quality of life in most patients and with theoretical cost benefits when compared to dialysis alone and kidney transplant alone.

Answer: D

Al-Qaoud TM, Odorico JS, Redfield RR. Pancreas transplantation in type 2 diabetes: expanding the criteria. *Current Opinion in Organ Transplantation* 2018; 23(4): 454–460.

Dean PG, Kukla A, Stegall MD, Kudva YC. Pancreas transplantation. *BMJ* 2017; 357:1321–1332.

Hau HM, Jahn N, Brunotte M, *et al.* Short and long-term metabolic outcomes in patients with type 1 and type 2 diabetes receiving a simultaneous pancreas kidney allograft. *BMC Endocrine Disorders* 2020; 20(30):30. doi; https://doi.org/10.1186/s12902-020-0506-9.

17 *A 23-year-old woman was found hanging in her garage in cardiac arrest after a suicide attempt. Return of spontaneous circulation was achieved but despite aggressive care apnea test confirms brain death due to anoxic injury. Her driver's license designates her as a registered organ donor. Which of the following have been associated with increased donor conversion rates and organs transplanted per donor?*

A *Early recognition and treatment of diabetes insipidus*

B *Hormonal replacement therapy in hemodynamically unstable donors*

C *Early involvement of Organ Procurement Organizations (OPO)*

D *Lung-protective ventilation and recruitment maneuvers*

E *All of the above*

Cerebral injury due to hemorrhage, trauma, or other causes of anoxia is a common diagnosis in potential organ donors. Cerebral injury has been shown to be associated with significant hemodynamic, metabolic, and hormonal changes. These result in a progressive and profound systemic inflammatory response, affecting function and viability of donor organs before retrieval and transplantation. Donor optimization is an essential active process in organ donation that switches the focus from treatments that are directed toward recovery of the injured brain to those that are focused on the cardiopulmonary and metabolic resuscitation of potentially transplantable solid organs, after the diagnosis of death by neurological criteria. The immediate objectives of donor optimization include correction of hypovolemia, commencement of vasopressin and weaning of catecholamine infusions, prompt diagnosis and management of diabetes insipidus, high-dose methylprednisolone, and application of lung-protective ventilation strategies. Additionally, observational data report an independent association between thyroid replacement therapy and higher numbers of procured organs, but these findings have not been replicated in randomized controlled trials.

Answer: E

Bera KD, Shah A, English MR, *et al.* Optimization of the organ donor and effects on transplanted organs: a narrative review on current practice and future directions. *Anaesthesia* 2020; 75(9): 1191–1204.

Meyfroidt G, Gunst J, Martin-Loeches I, *et al.* Management of the brain-dead donor in the ICU: general and specific therapy to improve transplantable organ quality. *Intensive Care Medicine* 2019; 45(3): 343–353.

Patel MS, Abt PL. Current practices in deceased organ donor management. *Current Opinion in Organ Transplantation* 2019; 24(3): 343–350.

18 *A 67-year-old man is admitted to the ICU with upper gastrointestinal bleeding. The patient has a medical history significant for cirrhosis due to hepatitis C, chronic alcoholism, diabetes, and coronary artery disease. The patient was intubated for airway protection, central venous, and arterial catheters were placed, and labs were sent. Upper endoscopy reveals the source of hemorrhage is esophageal varices. What is the optimal target hemoglobin in this patient?*

A *7–8 gm/dL*

B *8–9 gm/dL*

C *9–10 gm/dL*

D *10–11 gm/dL*

E *>11 gm/dL*

Recently, an overview was performed of all systematic reviews investigating hemoglobin transfusion threshold. The effect on mortality of restrictive (7–9 gm/dL) and liberal (10–12 gm/dL) transfusion strategies identified 19 systematic reviews and 33 meta-analyses that used data from 53 RCTs. Of the 33 meta-analyses, one was graded as high quality, 15 were moderate, and 17 were low. The 16 meta-analyses of mortality graded as high-to-moderate quality demonstrate no difference in mortality between these two transfusion strategies. Additionally, a study performed by Villanueva et al. examined cirrhotic patients with actively bleeding varices. In the study, a restricted transfusion strategy (transfusion cutoff of 7 gm/dL vs. 9 gm/dL) was associated with a trend toward improved survival.

Answer: A

Carson JL, Stanworth SJ, Roubinian N, *et al.* Transfusion thresholds and other strategies for guiding allogeneic red blood cell transfusion. *Cochrane Database of Systematic Reviews* 2016; 10(10): CD002042.

Odutayo A, Desborough MJ, Trivella M, *et al.* Restrictive versus liberal blood transfusion for gastrointestinal bleeding; a systematic review and meta-analysis of randomized controlled trials. *The Lancet Gastroenterology & Hepatology* 2017; 2(5): 354–360.

Trentino KM, Farmer SL, Leahy MF, *et al.* Systematic reviews and meta-analyses comparing mortality in restrictive and liberal haemoglobin thresholds for red cell transfusion: an overview of systematic reviews. *BMC Medicine* 2020; 18(1): 154.

19 *A 78-year-old man is admitted to the ICU with acute-on-chronic liver failure. His medical history includes heart failure, COPD, diabetes, hepatocellular carcinoma, and ESLD due to hepatitis C. This is his third ICU admission in the last year for complications of his ESLD. The patient is not a transplant candidate due to severe comorbid medical conditions. Regarding palliative care consultation in patients with ESLD, which of the following is true?*

A *Palliative care consult increases overall mortality.*

B *Palliative care consult increases reduces patient and family satisfaction.*

C *Palliative care consult increases quality of life.*

D *Palliative care consult increases clinical and depressive symptoms.*

E *Palliative care consult increases hospital and ICU resource utilization.*

In the US over 600 000 patients have cirrhosis, and it is one of the leading causes of death in the United States in adults older than the age of 25 years. Patients with decompensated cirrhosis (DC) with ascites, hepatic encephalopathy, variceal bleeding, jaundice, or hepatocellular carcinoma (HCC) are in the final stages of disease, termed end-stage liver disease (ESLD), with a 1-year survival of ~50%. These patients have the greatest palliative care (PC) needs for symptom management and advanced care planning for end-of-life care (EOLC). Early, concurrent involvement of PC versus usual care in chronic illnesses has been shown to lead to a better quality of life and overall patient satisfaction. In these patients, PC and hospice interventions in patients with DC/HCC reduce healthcare utilization, influenced EOLC, and also significantly improved patient symptoms. Early PC involvement has not been shown to increase overall mortality.

Answer: C

Bhanji RA, Carey EJ, Watt KD. Review article: maximizing quality of life while aspiring for quantity of life in end-stage liver disease. *Alimentary Pharmacology & Therapeutics* 2017; 46(1): 16–25.

Mudumbi SK, Bourgeois CE, Hoppman NA, *et al.* Palliative care and hospice interventions in decompensated cirrhosis and hepatocellular carcinoma: a rapid review of the literature. *Journal of Palliative Medicine* 2018; 21(8): 1177–1184.

20 *A 67-year-old man with a medical history significant for hypertension, diabetes, and Child-Pugh B NASH cirrhosis is admitted to the surgical intensive care unit with a working diagnosis of urosepsis. Despite IV antibiotics and fluid resuscitation, on hospital day 3, the urine output decreases to 5 mL/hr. Workup is consistent with hepatorenal syndrome. Which of the following have been most associated with higher rates of recovery from hepatorenal syndrome in a patient with liver failure?*

A *Albumin plus terlipressin*

B *Albumin alone*

C *Albumin plus epinephrine*

D *Albumin plus octreotide*

E *Albumin plus midodrine plus octreotide*

Hepatorenal syndrome (HRS) is a severe and frequent complication in advanced cirrhosis. HRS refers to acute kidney injury within the setting of severe liver failure. Hepatorenal syndrome is defined as renal failure in people with cirrhosis in the absence of other causes. In addition to supportive treatment such as albumin to restore fluid balance, the other potential treatments include systemic vasoconstrictor drugs (such as vasopressin analogues or noradrenaline), renal vasodilator drugs (such as dopamine), trans-jugular intrahepatic portosystemic shunt (TIPS), and liver support with molecular-adsorbent recirculating system (MARS). A recent Cochrane review citing low-certainty evidence suggests that albumin plus noradrenaline had fewer 'any adverse events per participant' than albumin plus terlipressin. Low- or very-low-certainty evidence also found that albumin plus midodrine plus octreotide and albumin alone had lower recovery from hepatorenal syndrome compared with albumin plus terlipressin. There have been 7 studies performed comparing albumin plus terlipressin vs albumin plus noradrenaline. While the quality of evidence is very low and the studies include both type 1 and type 2 HRS, both groups appear similar with respect to response rate and adverse events; however, one study found that terlipressin had better response and survival than noradrenaline in patients with acute on chronic liver failure.

Answer: A

Best LMJ, Freeman SC, Sutton AJ, *et al.* Treatment for hepatorenal syndrome in people with decompensated liver cirrhosis: a network meta-analysis. *Cochrane Database of Systematic Reviews* 2019; 9(9): CD013103.

Zhang J, Rossle M, Zhou X, *et al.* Terlipressin for the treatment of hepatorenal syndrome: an overview of current evidence. *Current Medical Research and Opinion* 2019; 35(5): 859–868.

23

Obstetric Critical Care

Gary Lombardo, MD

Division of Trauma and Acute Care Surgery, New York Medical College, Westchester Medical Center, Valhalla, NY

1 *Of the following statements, which correctly describes the physiologic changes of pregnancy that will impact resuscitation efforts in a critically ill obstetric patient?*

A *Plasma volume will increase 40–50%, but erythrocyte volume will only increase by 20% resulting in a dilutional anemia.*

B *Heart rate will decrease due to dextrorotation of the heart resulting in a functional outflow obstruction.*

C *Supine blood pressure will be increased due to increased venous return as a result of increased plasma volume and aortocaval compression.*

D *Respiratory rate will be decreased due to a decrease in minute ventilation and as a compensation for physiologic metabolic alkalosis.*

E *Functional residual capacity will increase more than 25% preventing atelectasis that may result from the gravid uterus.*

Physiologic changes of pregnancy are extensive and can be observed in many of the organ systems. The altered physiology results from various hormonal and anatomic alterations that affect the woman body during pregnancy. Clinicians in an ICU setting must be aware of such alterations as these physiologic changes of pregnancy can have a significant impact on resuscitative efforts. Plasma volume will increase by 40–50%, but erythrocyte volume by only 20% resulting in a dilutional anemia leading to a decreased oxygen carrying capacity; therefore, answer A is correct. As a result, heart rate will increase by 15–20 beats per minute and cardiac output will increase by 40%, which can result in increased CPR circulation demands (Answer B). An increase in dextrorotation of the heart may occur and will be noted with increased EKG left axis deviation. Blood pressure and venous return will be decreased in the supine position as a result of aortocaval compression, which will result in a decreased cardiac output by up to 30% (Choice

C). As such, care should be taken in positioning with left uterine displacement. Minute ventilation will be increased noted by an increased respiratory rate (progesterone-mediated), as well as an increased tidal volume (progesterone-mediated) resulting from an increased oxygen demand and increased oxygen consumption by up to 20% (Choice D). These changes may affect resuscitative efforts as a result of a baseline compensated respiratory alkalosis (decreased arterial PCO_2 and decreased serum bicarbonate) with a decreased buffering capacity and a rapid decrease of PaO_2 in hypoxia. Anatomic changes will additionally result in a decreased functional residual capacity by 25%, thus decreasing ventilatory capacity (Choice E). Resuscitative efforts may be aided by electronic fetal heart rate monitoring. Electronic fetal heart rate monitoring reflects uteroplacental perfusion and fetal acid-base status; therefore, changes in fetal heart rate monitoring (changes in baseline variability or new decelerations) should prompt reassessment of maternal blood pressure, oxygenation, ventilation, acid–base balance, or cardiac output.

Answer: A

American College of Obstetricians and Gynecologists' Committee on Practice Bulletins- Obstetrics. ACOG Practice Bulletin No. 211: Critical care in pregnancy. *Obstetrics and Gynecology* 2019 May;133(5):e303–e319.

2 *A 32-year-old woman is admitted to the ICU in her third trimester of pregnancy after testing positive for COVID 19 and is hypoxic requiring mechanical ventilation. Which of the following correctly describes the normal changes noted in arterial blood gas evaluation in pregnancy?*

A *pH in the third trimester will be altered by anatomical effect of the gravid uterus reflecting a decreased minute ventilation and therefore a respiratory acidosis.*

B *PaCO$_2$ cannot be used as a marker of increased work of breathing in the obstetric patient as it will not change due to required compensation of a baseline metabolic acidosis.*

C *PaCO$_2$ of 40 mm Hg is concerning for progressive respiratory failure in this patient.*

D *PaO$_2$ is irrelevant in the pregnant patient and is expected to decrease explained by a decrease in the minute ventilation associated with the third trimester of pregnancy.*

E *Serum bicarbonate levels will be increased on laboratory evaluation in the third trimester of pregnancy due to increased buffering required to compensate for the respiratory acidosis associated with the decreased minute ventilation.*

Respiratory insufficiency can naturally occur in the critically ill obstetric patient, and vigilance is warranted as pulmonary symptoms can rapidly progress to respiratory failure. Minute ventilation in pregnancy is increased reflected by an increased respiratory rate (progesterone-mediated), as well as an increased tidal volume (progesterone-mediated). This results from an increased oxygen demand and increased oxygen consumption due to the fetus, which may be increased by 20%. PaO$_2$ will not vary significant from the nonpregnant state through the third trimester, and most of the changes are due to increased minute ventilation. The obstetric patient will demonstrate a baseline-compensated respiratory alkalosis (decreased arterial PCO$_2$ and decreased serum bicarbonate) on ABG interpretation. Anatomic changes will additionally result in a decreased functional residual capacity by 25%, thus decreasing ventilatory capacity. The pH is normal, and there is a compensated respiratory alkalosis and not acidosis. An increasing PaCO$_2$ implies that the work of breathing is increasing and a PaCO$_2$ of 40 mm Hg in a pregnant patient, although normal in the nonpregnant state, is concerning for progressive respiratory failure (Choice B). The PaO$_2$ is normal or higher than in the nonpregnant state. Typically, the serum bicarbonate will be decreased due to compensated respiratory alkalosis and not increased (Choice E).

	Pregnancy State		
ABG measurement	Nonpregnant state	First trimester	Third trimester
pH	7.40	7.42–7.46	7.43
PaO$_2$ (mm Hg)	93	105–106	101–106
PaCO$_2$ (mm Hg)	37	28–29	26–30
Serum HCO$_3$ (mEq/L)	23	18	17

Answer: C

Hegewald MJ, Crapo RO. Respiratory physiology in pregnancy. *Clinics in Chest Medicine* 2011;32:1–13.

Mighty HE. Acute resp failure pregnancy. *Clinical Obstetrics and Gynecology* 2010;53(2):360–368.

3 *A healthy 32-year-old woman is in the obstetrics recovery room after a reported "difficult delivery." The obstetrician reports the patient was noted to be hypotensive immediately postpartum with mental status changes requiring transfusion of packed red blood cells, vasopressors, intubation, and mechanical ventilation. You are called to assess her for ICU admission after successful resuscitation. Which of the following is true regarding indications for ICU admission in the postpartum patient population?*

A *The most common admission diagnosis requiring ICU care for the obstetric patient is multisystem organ failure resulting from sepsis.*

B *Recently, maternal mortality rates in the United States have been reported to be rising while maternal morbidity is decreasing, thus ICU evaluation postpartum is recommended.*

C *Postpartum hemorrhage and preeclampsia-related complications are the most common reasons for ICU admission in the obstetric patient.*

D *Hemorrhage postpartum is a rare event as physiologic changes in pregnancy include a decrease in total blood volume and a decreased cardiac output due to increased uterine perfusion requirements.*

E *Obstetric patient ICU admission is common and is reported at over 25/1,000 deliveries.*

Sepsis and multisystem organ failure are not the most common diagnoses for ICU admission as it is only approximately 5% of obstetric-related ICU admissions (Choice A). The most common reasons for an obstetric patient to require admission to an ICU are preeclampsia-related complications and postpartum hemorrhage. The percentage of ICU admissions in the obstetric patient has been reported at 21.5% for postpartum hemorrhage and 32.5% for maternal hypertension. Complications related to preeclampsia include eclampsia, intracerebral hemorrhage, pulmonary edema, renal insufficiency, liver injury, and placental abruption (Choice C). Global maternal mortality rates are reported to be decreasing, but maternal morbidity has been reported to be increasing currently at 2.5% of hospital deliveries in the United States (Choice B). Pregnancy results in multiple physiologic changes including an increase in total blood volume, cardiac output and uterine blood flow, hemorrhage may result from placenta previa, placental abruption, uterine atony, and secondary coagulopathies (Choice D).

Additional reasons obstetric patients may require ICU admission are related to obstetric sepsis, obstetric heart disease, and complications related to anesthesia. Obstetric patient admission to an ICU has been reported in approximately 2–4/1000 deliveries in developed countries (Choice E).

Answer: C

Einav S, Leone M. Epidemiology of obstetric critical illness. *International Journal of Obstetric Anesthesia* 2019 Nov;40:128–139.

Intensive Care National Audit and Research Centre. Female admissions (aged 16–50 years) to adult, general critical care units in England, Wales and Northern Ireland reported as "currently pregnant" or "recently pregnant". London (UK): ICNARC; 2013.

Pollock W, Rose L, Dennis CL. Pregnant and postpartum admissions to the intensive care unit: a systematic review. *Intensive Care Medicine* 2010;36:1465–1474.

Zeeman GG. Obstetric critical care: a blueprint for improved outcomes. *Critical Care Medicine* 2006 Sep;34(9 Suppl):S208–S214.

4   *A 26-year-old G1 P0 woman at 20-week gestation is admitted from the ER to the ICU with presumed septic shock. The patient is intubated for respiratory failure with hypoxia, altered mental status, tachycardia (HR 130 beats per minute), and hypotension (SBP 85 mmHg). The patient is noted to have diffuse abdominal tenderness, greatest in the right lower quadrant of the abdomen. Subsequently, the patient is placed on broad-spectrum antibiotics and resuscitation initiated with crystalloid solution. Which of the following applies to the management priorities of the ICU team in the management of this critically ill obstetric patient?*

   A *Lifesaving medical interventions in a critically ill obstetric patient must be reviewed by the obstetrics team to avoid teratogenic complications.*

   B *Care of the critically ill obstetric patient in the ICU involves the care of two patients (mother and fetus) simultaneously with no priority in optimization.*

   C *Diagnostic imaging in the obstetric ICU patient is contraindicated due to teratogenic effects to the fetus.*

   D *Clinical status of the fetus has the highest priority in the management of the critically ill obstetric patient.*

   E *When caring for obstetric ICU patients, the mother is the primary priority as fetal status is predicted on optimization of the maternal condition.*

Management principles of obstetric patients admitted to the ICU follow similar principles as compared to nonpregnant patients. Therefore, many patient care

decisions might be impacted by the patient's status (antepartum vs postpartum) and should therefore be made in a multidisciplinary fashion collaboratively between the critical care, obstetrics/gynecology, and neonatology teams. However, all critical care intensivists should be aware of the basic management of teratogenic complications and reliance of others (Choice A). While it has been generally accepted that care of the obstetric patient in the ICU involves the care of two patients (mother and fetus) simultaneously, the principle follows that the woman's interest is paramount, and fetal status is predicted on optimization of the maternal condition (Choice C). Maternal stabilization is therefore the first priority when taking care of an obstetric ICU patient (Choices B and D). Medical interventions and diagnostic imaging may be modified to an extent but should not be withheld due to fetal concern (Choice C). Imaging will depend on the study but is not always contraindicated if needed to treat the mother.

Answer: E

American College of Obstetricians and Gynecologists' Committee on PracticeBulletins—Obstetrics. ACOG Practice Bulletin No. 211: critical care in pregnancy. *Obstetrics and Gynecology* 2019 May;133(5):e303–e319.

Guidelines for diagnostic imaging during pregnancy and lactation. Committee Opinion No. 723. American College of Obstetricians and Gynecologists [published erratum appears in Obstet Gynecol 2018;132:786]. *Obstetrics and Gynecology* 2017;130:e210–e2106.

5   *A 29-year-old woman G2P1 at 36-week gestation with a medical history of chronic liver disease, and morbid obesity was being treated for 5 days with oral antibiotics for urinary tract infection. The patient now comes to the Emergency Department with complaints of malaise and subjective fever. Her vitals are BP 120/85 mmHg, heart rate 125 beats per minute despite a 1-liter fluid administration, and administration of broad spectrum IV antibiotics. She now has shortness of breath without associated hypoxia (oxygen saturation 97%) and is agitated. Labs have been ordered. Which of the following is most correct regarding the management of this patient?*

   A *Based on the patient's symptoms and lack of documented organ failure, ICU admission is not required.*

   B *The patient should not be admitted to an ICU setting as the physiological criteria used to diagnose sepsis in the nonpregnant population often overlap in normal pregnant women.*

   C *Pregnancy has been associated with immunologic changes resulting in an increased protection and immunity to infection, and therefore ICU care is not warranted in the obstetric patient with signs of infection.*

D *Clinical parameters that should prompt ICU evaluation in pregnant women include heart rate > 120 bpm, oxygen saturation <95%, and maternal agitation.*

E *Pre-existing medical problems such as chronic liver disease, obesity, and congestive heart failure have no association with increased risk for sepsis during pregnancy.*

Maternal ICU admission has been classified to result from etiologies directly related to pregnancy (obstetric hemorrhage, hypertensive disease of pregnancy, puerperal sepsis, thrombo-embolic phenomena, fatty liver), those indirectly related to pregnancy (pre-existing disease exacerbation) and those coincidental to pregnancy (trauma, non-puerperal sepsis). It has been reported that sepsis is responsible for approximately 5% of obstetric-related ICU admissions. The most common cause for ICU involves complications related to preeclampsia (32.5%), and the second most common cause for ICU admission is related to postpartum hemorrhage (21.5%). While the symptoms the patient is presenting with may be the result of infection and may not meet traditional ICU admission criteria as there is no evidence of organ failure and/or the requirement for a life-saving intervention, clinical deterioration in an obstetric patient may be masked by multiple physiologic changes that occur normally in pregnancy. Additionally, the physiological criteria conventionally used to diagnose sepsis in the nonpregnant population often overlap both in normal pregnant women and in those with sepsis/infection. In response, the National Partnership for Maternal Safety developed a list of clinical parameters termed "maternal early warning criteria" that should prompt ICU evaluation.

These include systolic BP (mm Hg) < 90 or > 160, diastolic BP (mm Hg) > 100, heart rate (beats per minute) < 50 or > 120, respiratory rate (breaths per minute) <10 or >30, Oxygen saturation on room air at sea level <95%, Oliguria (ml/hr) <35 for > or equal to 2 hrs, maternal agitation, confusion or unresponsiveness, patient with preeclampsia reporting non-remitting headache or shortness of breath (Choices A and B). Additionally, pregnancy has been associated with immunologic changes resulting in an increased susceptibility to infection (Choice C). Pre-existing medical problems such as chronic liver disease, obesity, and congestive heart failure are associated with increased risk for sepsis during pregnancy (Choice E). Treatment for maternal sepsis follows the same recommendations as for the nonpregnant patient with timely diagnosis, fluid resuscitation, and early antibiotic therapy. Early antibiotic therapy (within the first hour) is recommended to reduce mortality, and each hour of delay is associated with an increase in mortality.

Answer: D

Carcopino X, Raoult D, Bretelle F, Boubli L, Stein AQ. Fever during pregnancy: a cause of poor fetal and maternal outcome. *Annals of the New York Academy of Sciences* 2009;1166:79–89.

Einav S, Leone M. Epidemiology of obstetric critical illness. *International Journal of Obstetric Anesthesia* 2019 Nov;40:128–139.

Lazariu V, Nguyen T, McNutt LA, Jeffrey J, Kacica M. Severe maternal morbidity: a population-based study of an expanded measure and associated factors. *PLoS One* 2017;12:e0182343.

Mhyre JM, D'Oria R, Hameed AB, Lappen JR, Holley SL, Hunter SK, et al. The maternal early warning criteria: a proposal from the national partnership for maternal safety. *Obstetrics and Gynecology* 2014;124:782–786.

Oud L, Watkins P. Evolving trends in the epidemiology, resource utilization, and outcomes of pregnancy-associated severe sepsis: a population-based cohort study. *Journal of Clinical Medical Research* 2015;7:400–416.

6 *A 27-year-old woman is in labor for several hours. The patient develops an increased work of breathing, hypotension, and hypoxia requiring intubation and mechanical ventilation. An ABG is obtained and reveals a PaO_2/FiO_2 ratio of 210. Rapid delivery of the fetus is performed via Cesarean delivery, and the patient remains hemodynamically unstable requiring vasopressor support. The patient is resuscitated with colloid and crystalloid fluid and currently has a CVP of 8 mm Hg and a mean arterial blood pressure of 70 mm Hg. A chest x-ray is obtained and reveals bilateral interstitial and alveolar infiltrates. Which of the following applies to this patient?*

A *Pregnant women are at decreased risk of developing ARDS and needing mechanical ventilation when compared with nonpregnant women.*

B *ARDS in pregnancy could be from the development of amniotic fluid embolism.*

C *In contrast to the nonpregnant patient, the lungs of the obstetric patient with ARDS demonstrate increased compliance with a decreased work of breathing yet with an associated hypoxemia.*

D *The management of ARDS currently involves low-tidal-volume ventilation with the priority placed on normalizing arterial blood gases and PaO_2/FiO_2 ratios.*

E *ARDS in pregnancy is rarely seen and due to increased lung compliance, low tidal volume ventilation strategies are not recommended.*

Acute respiratory distress syndrome may result as a response to a variety of insults. It is characterized by diffuse inflammation, increased fluid in the lung (noncardiogenic pulmonary edema) due to increased vascular permeability, bilateral lung infiltrates, severe progressive hypoxemia with loss of aerated lung units and increased shunt fraction, and decreased lung compliance. Pregnant women are at **increased** risk of developing ARDS and needing mechanical ventilation compared with nonpregnant women (Choice A). ARDS in pregnancy is seen most commonly in the setting of sepsis with infections such as influenza and pyelonephritis. It can also be seen as a complication of obstetric diagnoses such as preeclampsia, amniotic fluid embolism, and infections of pregnancy such as chorioamnionitis and endometritis (Choice B). As defined by the ARDS Definition Task Force, the onset of respiratory failure must be within 1 week of a known clinical event with evidence of bilateral opacities on chest imaging and no other identifiable etiology such as cardiac failure or fluid overload. The degree of ARDS severity (mild, moderate, severe) is based on oxygenation as measured by the partial pressure of arterial oxygen to fraction of inspired oxygen **(PaO_2/FiO_2) ratio of less than 300**. It is further subclassified into mild (PaO_2/FiO_2 200–300), moderate (PaO_2/FiO_2 100–200), and severe (PaO_2/FiO_2 less than 100). The lungs of the obstetric patient with ARDS demonstrate **decreased** compliance with an increased work of breathing and hypoxemia (Choice C). Although mechanical ventilation will be required, high concentrations of oxygen and the physical effects of positive pressure ventilation often required can result in damage to the lungs. The management of ARDS currently involves low-tidal-volume ventilation limiting inflation pressures rather than trying to normalize arterial blood gases. To reduce iatrogenic ventilator-associated injuries, hypercapnea and some degree of hypoxia are acceptable (Choice D). All patients with ARDS including pregnant patients should target a lower tidal volume 4–6 mL/kg predicted body weight and maintenance of plateau pressure between 25 and 30 cm H_2O. Although no studies have evaluated the efficacy of low tidal volume strategy in pregnant and postpartum women, similar to the nonpregnant patient (Choice E). Additionally, management concentrates on elucidating the etiology, minimizing ongoing injury and supportive therapy. Maternal mortality may be as high as 35–60%, and most often results from multiple organ dysfunction syndrome.

Answer: B

The Acute Respiratory Distress Syndrome Network (ARDSNet). Ventilation with lower tidal volumes as compared with traditional tidal volumes for acute lung injury and the acute respiratory distress syndrome. *The New England Journal of Medicine* 2000;342:1301–1308.

Catanzarite V, Willms D, Wong D, Landers C, Cousins L, Schrimmer D. Acute respiratory distress syndrome in pregnancy and the puerperium: causes, courses, and outcomes. *Obstetrics and Gynecology* 2001;97:760–764.

Cole DE, Taylor TL, McCullough DM, et al. Acute respiratory distress syndrome in pregnancy. *Critical Care Medicine* 2005;33(10 Suppl):S269–S278.

Fanelli V, Vlachou A, Ghannadian S, Simonetti U, Slutsky AS, Zhang H. Acute respiratory distress syndrome: new definition, current and future therapeutic options. *Journal of Thoracic Disease* 2013 Jun; 5(3): 326–334.

Ranieri VM, Rubenfeld GD, Thompson BT, Ferguson ND, Caldwell E, Fan E, et al. Acute respiratory distress syndrome: the Berlin definition. ARDS definition task force. *JAMA* 2012;307:2526–2533.

7 *A 34-year-old woman at 30-week gestation is admitted to the labor and delivery suite of a local community hospital without neonatal or ICU capabilities. She has premature contractions and subsequently develops slowly progressing hypoxia requiring intubation and mechanical ventilation. The obstetrics team is uncomfortable managing this and requests transfer to a tertiary referral hospital with both neonatal and ICU services available. Which of the following is correct regarding the appropriate transfer process in the obstetric patient?*

A *The minimum required transport monitoring for a critically ill pregnant woman includes continuous central venous pressure monitoring, cardiac rhythm, and pulse oximetry monitoring.*

B *Fetal monitoring and tocodynamometry during the transport process may be feasible, but its utility is unknown and it is not mandated for transfer.*

C *Transport with fetal monitoring is mandatory or the sending facility would be liable.*

D *Patient should be transported in a position maximizing right uterine displacement to allow venous return to the heart.*

E *Fetal monitoring is required as interventions based on fetal heart rate decelerations during transportation may be required.*

The care of any pregnant woman requiring ICU services ideally should be managed in a facility with obstetrics, adult ICU, and neonatal ICU capability. Transfer of a patient should occur prior to clinical deterioration and strongly encouraged if a patient is clinically unstable (hypotensive or hypoxemic), at high risk of deterioration (increasing work of breathing) or needs specialized ICU care such as mechanical ventilation. Necessary transport monitoring for a critically ill pregnant woman or for a woman during the postpartum period includes continuous cardiac rhythm and pulse oximetry monitoring and regular assessment of vital signs. Venous access must be established before transport but central line and CVP pressure monitoring is not a requirement (Choice A), and care should be taken in positioning with left uterine displacement to lessen inferior vena cava compression from the uterus (Choice D). Fetal monitoring and tocodynamometry during the transport process may be feasible and is a luxury. However, since interventions are seldom feasible during transport, it is not mandatory and its utility is unknown (Choice B). Transport should not be delayed by the inability to provide fetal monitoring in a critically ill pregnant woman as optimization of maternal status will optimize fetal status. Fetal monitoring is not mandated and the sending facility would not be liable for sending the patient with fetal monitoring in order to facilitate the transfer (Choice C). When fetal monitoring is possible, heart rate decelerations may signal the need for maternal resuscitative measures or alert the receiving team of the need to prepare for delivery soon after arrival.

Answer: B

American Academy of Pediatrics, *American College of Obstetricians and Gynecologists. Guidelines for perinatal care.* 8th ed. Elk Grove Village (IL): AAP; Washington, DC: American College of Obstetricians and Gynecologists;2017.

Donnelly JA, Smith EA, Runcie CJ. Transfer of the critically ill obstetric patient: experience of a specialist team and guidelines for the non-specialist. *International Journal of Obstetric Anesthesia* 1995;4:145–149.

8   *A 26-year-old woman presumed to be approximately 20-week gestation is admitted to the ICU after sustaining severe traumatic brain injury (GCS 6T) and lower extremity fractures following motor vehicle collision. The patient was intubated by prehospital providers. No previous medical/obstetric history is available. Which of the following is true concerning pharmacologic therapy in the care of this patient?*

   A *Medications with potential benefits may warrant use of the drug in pregnant women despite potential risks to the fetus.*

   B *When caring for a critically ill obstetric patient, determination of the fetal gestational age is mandatory to ensure harmful drugs to the fetus are avoided.*

   C *Diagnostic imaging in the care of the critically ill obstetric patient cannot be utilized until after accurate fetal age is determined.*

   D *Narcotics such as hydromorphone should be avoided as they are FDA pharmaceutical class D.*

   E *Cisatracurium is contraindicated in the care of the critically ill obstetric patient.*

Maternal stabilization is the priority when caring for a critically ill obstetric patient as fetal status is predicted on optimization of the maternal condition. Lifesaving medications and interventions should not be withheld from the mother due to fetal concern. However, if the patient is stable, determination of the fetal gestational age is obviously important as pregnancy often modifies drug effects or serum levels. Additionally, drugs that cross the placenta may effect fetal development. Prenatal care records should be reviewed, and if gestational age remains uncertain, bedside ultrasound evaluation can establish an estimated gestational age and is typically available. Medications commonly used in critical care settings may have adverse effects on the pregnancy such as decreased placental perfusion or increased risk of malformations. Conversely, many common obstetric medications may pose a particular challenge such as the negative inotropic effect on cardiac function with magnesium. When pharmacologic therapy is required in the obstetric ICU patient, adverse effects on the woman and the fetus must be monitored, potential drug interactions considered, and risk–benefit ratio assessed (Choice A). Knowing fetal age, while useful, is not mandated (Choice B). Necessary medications and required diagnostic imaging should not be withheld from a pregnant woman, although attempts should be made to limit fetal exposure to ionizing radiation and teratogenic medications when feasible (Choice C). Narcotic medications such as hydromorphone are FDA category C in pregnancy. There are no available data in pregnant women to inform a drug-associated risk for major birth defects and miscarriage although animal studies have shown adverse effects on the fetus (Choice D).

Cisatracurium is classified as FDA category B in pregnancy as there are no adequate and well-controlled studies in pregnant women and animal studies administered cisatracurium during organogenesis found no evidence of fetal harm (Choice E).

FDA Pharmaceutical Pregnancy Categories:

Category A

Adequate and well-controlled studies have failed to demonstrate a risk to the fetus in the first trimester of pregnancy (and there is no evidence of risk in later trimesters).

Examples of medications in this class are vitamins and levothyroxine.

Category B

Animal reproduction studies have failed to demonstrate a risk to the fetus and there are no adequate and well-controlled studies in pregnant women.

Examples of medications in this class are acetaminophen, cephalosporin antibiotics, and cisatracurium.

Category C

Animal reproduction studies have shown an adverse effect on the fetus, and there are no adequate and well-controlled studies in humans, but potential benefits may warrant use of the drug in pregnant women despite potential risks.

Examples of medications in this class are diltiazem, levetiracetam, fluoroquinolone antibiotics and hydromorphone.

Category D

There is positive evidence of human fetal risk based on adverse reaction data from investigational or marketing experience or studies in humans, but potential benefits may warrant use of the drug in pregnant women despite potential risks.

Examples of medications in this class are phenytoin and aminoglycoside antibiotics.

Category X

Studies in animals or humans have demonstrated fetal abnormalities, and/or there is positive evidence of human fetal risk based on adverse reaction data from investigational or marketing experience, and the risks involved in use of the drug in pregnant women clearly outweigh potential benefits.

Examples of medications in this class are thalidomide, metronidazole (1st trimester), and warfarin.

Answer: A

American College of Obstetricians and Gynecologists' Committee on Practice Bulletins—Obstetrics. ACOG Practice Bulletin No. 211: critical care in pregnancy. *Obstetrics and Gynecology* 2019 May;133(5):e303–e319.

Content and Format of Labeling for Human Prescription Drug and Biological Products; Requirements for Pregnancy and Lactation Labeling (Federal Register/Vol. 73, No. 104/Thursday, May 29, 2008)

Yazdy MM, Desai RJ, Brogly SB. Prescription opioids in pregnancy and birth outcomes: a review of the Literature. *J Pediatr Genet.* 2015;4(2):58–70.

9 *For critically ill obstetric patients admitted to the ICU in the preterm period, the administration of antenatal steroids should be:*

   A *Administered to all critically ill obstetric patients regardless of the documented week of gestation.*

   B *Not administered to the critically ill obstetric patient as the risk to the fetus far outweighs any perceived benefit of avoiding complications of prematurity.*

   C *Administered at any stage of gestation as studies have demonstrated significant benefit to the maternal critical illness.*

   D *Completed to avoid potential fetal complications and thus late-term delivery should be delayed whenever possible.*

   E *Considered in the critically ill obstetric patient in the preterm period between 24 and 37 weeks of gestation.*

In an attempt at reducing neonatal mortality and potential complications associated with prematurity, steroids for fetal benefit should be considered in the obstetric patient admitted to an ICU in the preterm period. Betamethasone or dexamethasone is recommended for pregnant women between 24 0/7 weeks of gestation and 33 6/7 weeks of gestation who are at risk of preterm birth within 1 week. There may be neonatal benefit as early as 23 weeks of gestation and steroids could be offered depending on the decision regarding neonatal resuscitation in this preterm period. The Maternal–Fetal Medicine Units Network Antenatal Late Preterm Steroids trial demonstrated reduced risk of neonatal respiratory morbidity with steroids administered between 34 0/7 weeks of gestation and 36 6/7 weeks of gestation. Answer B is incorrect as there is a benefit to the fetus, and answer C is incorrect because it is dependent upon the age of the fetus. Antenatal corticosteroids have not been evaluated in terms of benefit to the critical maternal illness exposing the patient to the known risk of steroid administration including hyperglycemia, hypokalemia, leukocytosis, and impaired wound healing. The risks and benefits of steroid administration should be weighed against the likelihood of delivery within 7 days. Answer D is incorrect as indicated delivery should not be delayed for administration of steroids in the late preterm period.

Answer: E

Antenatal corticosteroid therapy for fetal maturation. Committee Opinion No. 713. American College of Obstetricians and Gynecologists. *Obstetrics and Gynecology* 2017;130:e102–e109.

Gyamfi-Bannerman C, Thom EA, Blackwell SC, Tita AT, Reddy UM, Saade GR, et al. Antenatal betamethasone for women at risk for late preterm delivery. NICHD Maternal-Fetal Medicine Units Network. *The New England Journal of Medicine* 2016;374:1311–1320.

Periviable birth. Obstetric Care Consensus No. 6. American College of Obstetricians and Gynecologists. *Obstetrics and Gynecology* 2017;130:e187–e199.

10 *A 29-year-old obese woman with a 20-week old fetus is admitted for suspected acute cholecystitis to the ICU for hemodynamic and fetal monitoring with the diagnosis of sepsis related to suspected acute cholecystitis. The gravid uterus is palpated just above the umbilical region and the patient is noted to*

significantly tender in the right side of the abdomen. Ultrasound examination of the gallbladder in the ED prior was inconclusive due to body habitus. You recommend diagnostic laparoscopy and possible cholecystectomy, but the family and patient inquire about additional imaging prior to surgical intervention. Which of the following is the best answer concerning diagnostic radiation and fetal teratogenesis?

A *Fetal side effects to the ionizing radiation require all diagnostic radiation be withheld from a pregnant woman to avoid fetal side effects.*

B *Radiation dosage and fetal age at the time of exposure are important considerations in terms of fetal teratogenesis.*

C *No single diagnostic test should exceed 20 rad of ionizing radiation.*

D *CT scanning of the abdomen and pelvis is contraindicated due to teratogenic risk to the fetus regardless of the weeks of gestation.*

E *Intraoperative cholangiography should be avoided in the pregnancy as the ionizing radiation exposure to the fetus is above detrimental levels.*

Radiographic imaging is often indicated in the management of the obstetric patient. The fetal side effects to the ionizing radiation have significant impact on the plan of care and imaging utilized but depends upon the radiation dosage and fetal age. Necessary diagnostic imaging should not be withheld from a pregnant woman because of fetal concerns, although attempts should be made to limit fetal exposure to ionizing radiation (Choice A). Radiation dosage and fetal age at the time of exposure are important considerations in terms of fetal teratogenesis (Choice B). No single diagnostic test should exceed **5 rad** of ionizing radiation and particularly of concern is exposure during the first month post conception (Choice C). Common procedures, such as those listed, are all below the accepted accumulated dose of 4–10 rad of ionizing radiation during a pregnancy; cholangiography is estimated to expose the fetus to 0.2–0.5 rad, plain abdominal radiograph 0.1–0.3 rad, and CT scan of the abdomen and pelvis 2–4 rad of exposure to a fetus (Choices D and E).

Answer: B

Guidelines for diagnostic imaging during pregnancy and lactation. Committee Opinion No. 723. American College of Obstetricians and Gynecologists [published erratum appears in Obstet Gynecol 2018;132:786]. *Obstetrics and Gynecology* 2017;130:e210–e216.

Pearl J, Price R, Richardson W, Fanelli R. Society of American gastrointestinal endoscopic surgeons. Guidelines for diagnosis, treatment and use of laparoscopy for surgical problems during pregnancy. *Surgical Endoscopy* 2011;(11):3479–3492.

11 *Which of the following statements is correct when applied to airway and ventilation issues in critically ill obstetric patients?*

A *Intubation of the obstetric patient is no different when compared to the general population other than utilization of FDA Pharmaceutical Pregnancy Category A medications.*

B *It should be assumed to be significantly more difficult in terms of mask ventilation and subsequent endotracheal tube placement compared with the general population.*

C *The increased minute ventilation associated with pregnancy is protective and results in a prolonged period until hypoxemia occurs after the onset of apnea.*

D *The airway is easier by at least 1 class from the start to end of labor as the airway becomes more flexible due to hormonal changes.*

E *Intermittent mandatory volume controlled ventilation has been shown to confer benefit when utilized for respiratory failure.*

The normal physiologic changes to the respiratory system that occur in pregnancy resulting from hormonal changes, as well as from anatomic changes can make airway management in pregnancy challenging. The increased minute ventilation and decreased functional residual capacity, as well as an increased oxygen consumption, decrease the amount of time from onset of apnea to significant oxygen desaturation as hypoxemia occurs quickly (Choices A and C). Additionally, if a pregnant patient requires intubation, the likelihood of difficult mask ventilation and subsequent endotracheal tube placement is significantly increased compared with the general population (Choice B). Difficulty in direct laryngeal visualization has been reported with increased breast size associated with pregnancy. The risk of failed intubation in obstetrics is as high as 1 in 224 attempts (95% CI, 179–281), a rate eight times higher than in the general population. The percentage of women with Mallampati class IV airway examination, indicating potential difficulty with endotracheal tube insertion, has been shown to increase by 34% between 12 and 38 weeks gestational age, and 33% of women demonstrate a worsened airway classification by at least 1 class from the start to end of labor (Choice D). Airway edema as a result of preeclampsia, respiratory infections, or prolonged second stage of labor can further exacerbate these baseline changes. Prolonged periods of apnea as can occur with difficult intubation are less tolerated in pregnancy and can lead to clinically significant hypoxia and even cardiac arrest. While the etiologies of hypoxic respiratory failure are varied, the mainstay of treatment for all is the provision of supplemental oxygen, and no mode has been shown to confer benefit when utilized for respiratory failure in the obstetric critical care patient (Choice E).

Answer: B

Ende H, Varelmann D. Respiratory considerations including airway and ventilation issues in critical care obstetric patients. *Obstetrics and Gynecology Clinics of North America* 2016 Dec;43(4):699–708.

Kodali BS, Chandrasekhar S, Bulich LN, et al. Airway changes during labor and delivery. *Anesthesiology* 2008;108(3):357–362.

Quinn AC, Milne D, Columb M, Gorton H, Knight M. Failed tracheal intubation in obstetric anaesthesia: 2 year national case-control study in the UK. *British Journal of Anaesthesia* 2013;110:74–80.

12 *A 35-year-old woman who is suspected to be in her first trimester of pregnancy is admitted to the ICU with respiratory distress requiring intubation and mechanical ventilation. The patient has vaginal bleeding and is becoming hypotensive and tachycardic. Regarding Point of Care Ultrasonography (POCUS), it:*

   A *Has no role in the management of the critically ill obstetric patient.*

   B *Will be of limited utility in the obstetric patient due to the physiologic changes that accompany the pregnant state altering normal physiology.*

   C *Should be delayed in the care of this pending formal fetal monitoring and assessment to determine exact gestational dating.*

   D *Has limited utility in guiding fluid resuscitation in pregnancy as fluids can be provided without concern for pulmonary edema due to increased pulmonary compliance associated with the pregnant state.*

   E *Allows for rapid, noninvasive, and easily repeatable assessments of hemodynamics in addition to detecting fetal heart rate, assessing gestational age, and placenta position.*

Point-of-care ultrasonography (POCUS) has become increasingly important in critical care medicine and is rapidly replacing many of the previously utilized invasive monitoring tools. POCUS in critically ill patients allows for rapid, noninvasive, and easily repeatable assessments of hemodynamics. It has been used to guide procedures (vascular access, paracentesis, and thoracentesis); establish, confirm, or exclude diagnoses (ascites, mechanical reasons for acute renal failure, and lower extremity deep venous thrombosis); and direct therapies. It has been used to predict fluid responsiveness by measuring the diameter or collapsibility of the inferior vena cava, assess left ventricular systolic and diastolic function, and as an adjunct

to resuscitation in conditions such as pulseless electrical activity. During pregnancy, cardiac output rises resulting from increased stroke volume and heart rate with a parallel decrease in peripheral vascular resistance (Choice D). Additionally, the enlarged uterus may cause inferior vena cava compression, thereby decreasing venous return. These physiological changes associated with pregnancy predispose the patient to pulmonary edema exemplifying the necessity of guided i.v. fluid resuscitation. Point-of-care ultrasound is a noninvasive, nonionizing diagnostic tool that is available at the bed-side and has been applied specifically to aid in the diagnosis of ectopic pregnancy, detection of a nonviable pregnancy, gestational trophoblastic disease, as well as placental disorders such as placenta previa and abruption.

Answer: E

Frankel HL, Kirkpatrick AW, Elbarbary M, Blaivas M, Desai H, Evans D, et al. Guidelines for the appropriate use of bedside general and cardiac ultrasonography in the evaluation of critically ill patients-part I: general ultrasonography. *Critical Care Medicine* 2015;43:2479–502.

Levitov A, Frankel HL, Blaivas M, Kirkpatrick AW, Su E, Evans D, et al. Guidelines for the appropriate use of bedside general and cardiac ultrasonography in the evaluation of critically ill patients-part II: cardiac ultrasonography. *Critical Care Medicine* 2016;44:1206–1227.

Stein JC, Wang R, Adler N, Boscardin J, Jacoby VL, Won G, Goldstein R, Kohn MA. Emergency physician ultrasonography for evaluating patients at risk for ectopic pregnancy: a meta-analysis. *Annals of Emergency Medicine* 2010 Dec 1;56(6):674–683.

Zieleskiewicz L, Bouvet L, Einav S, Duclos G, Leone M. Diagnostic point-of-care ultrasound: applications in obstetric anaesthetic management. *Anaesthesia* 2018 Oct;73(10):1265–1279. doi: 10.1111/anae.14354. Epub 2018 Jul 26.

13 *A 19-year-old G1P0 woman has been in protracted labor. Due to progressive desaturation and hemodynamic instability, the patient required intubation and mechanical intubation and is currently requiring vasopressor therapy to support her blood pressure. The working diagnosis is amniotic fluid embolus. Which of the following statements best applies to the management of amniotic fluid embolus?*

   A *Amniotic fluid embolus is a common obstetric complication resulting from entry of fetal debris or amniotic fluid into the circulation of the mother during the peripartum period and patients are usually asymptomatic.*

B *The clinical picture of amniotic fluid embolus is usually dominated by respiratory manifestations.*

C *Treatment for amniotic fluid embolus includes aggressive volume resuscitation, inotropic support, and blood component therapy with early consideration for open pulmonary or catheter-assisted embolectomy.*

D *Amniotic fluid embolism rarely associated with cardiovascular collapse.*

E *Amniotic fluid embolus is a rare but serious obstetric complication with treatment being mainly supportive and often times requires early intubation and mechanical ventilation.*

Amniotic fluid embolus is a rare and serious obstetric complication caused by entry of fetal debris or amniotic fluid into the circulation of the mother during the peripartum period and is associated with protracted labor. Hypoxemia results from the ventilation-to-perfusion mismatch as a result of the embolus (Choice A). Hypoxia is thought to be an important finding predictive of the subsequent cardiovascular and coagulation alterations. The clinical picture of amniotic fluid embolus is usually dominated by cardiovascular collapse but respiratory manifestations are common (Choices B and D). The embolus is microscopic (Choice C). Cardiogenic pulmonary edema subsequently arises as a result of left ventricular failure. Capillary leak results in non-cardiogenic edema and the progression to ARDS. ARDS is one of the major causes of mortality in this patient population. Treatment is supportive, with aggressive volume resuscitation, inotropic support, and blood component therapy, and maintaining oxygenation often times requires early intubation and mechanical ventilation. Extracorporeal membrane oxygenation has been successfully used when mechanical ventilation is insufficient to provide adequate oxygenation. Rapid delivery of the fetus is indicated for an amniotic fluid embolism in a viable fetus.

Answer: E

Conde-Agudelo A, Romero R. Amniotic fluid embolism: an evidence-based review. *American Journal of Obstetrics and Gynecology* 2009;201(5):445.e1–3.

Hsieh YY, Chang CC, Li PC, et al. Successful application of extracorporeal membrane oxygenation and intra-aortic balloon counterpulsation as lifesaving therapy for a patient with amniotic fluid embolism. *American Journal of Obstetrics and Gynecology* 2000;183(2): 496–497.

O'Shea A, Eappen S. Amniotic fluid embolism. *International Anesthesiology Clinics* 2007;45(1): 17–28.

14 *A 30-year-old woman 28 weeks pregnant presents to the ED with a severe exacerbation of asthma. She is noted with inspiratory and expiratory wheezing, and* using accessory muscles of respiration. The patient stated symptoms began 2 days prior in which she continued utilizing her prescribed nebulizer at home until symptoms worsened this am. Her vital signs are HR 119 beats per minute, RR 32 breaths per minute with a BP of 120/80 mm Hg. ABG on nasal cannula supplemental oxygen at 4 liters per minute reveals pH 7.35, $PaCO_2$ 44 mm Hg and PaO_2 68 mm Hg. Which of the following is the correct management?

A *Nebulized albuterol only*

B *IV epinephrine with face mask oxygenation*

C *Noninvasive ventilation and nebulized albuterol*

D *Intubation, mechanical ventilation, and nebulized albuterol with IV epinephrine*

E *Nebulized albuterol, IV corticosteroids, and chest percussion to assist in clearing mucus plugging*

Asthma is a common respiratory comorbidity encountered in pregnant patients, and one-third of patients will experience an exacerbation during pregnancy. Most cases are mild and will not require ICU admission or intubation. In those cases, initial management includes administration of supplemental oxygen and inhaled beta-agonists to relieve bronchospasm. This patient, however, has a severe exacerbation of asthma and is progressing to respiratory failure as noted on the ABG with hypercapnia and hypoxia. A $PaCO_2$ of 44 mm Hg is abnormal in pregnancy due to the physiologic increased minute ventilation with an expected $PaCO_2$ of 28–30 mm Hg. While a pH of 7.35 would be considered normal in the nonpregnant state, this signifies a non-compensated respiratory acidosis as the pH expected in pregnancy should be 7.42–7.43. In addition, in severe cases, intravenous epinephrine may be required to treat refractory bronchospasm. This case represents a severe episode of asthma. The best option for this patient would be for intubation and treatment with nebulized B-2 agonist and IV administration of epinephrine. Thus, answer D is the best option.

Answer: D

Hanania NA, Belfort MA. Acute asthma in pregnancy. *Critical Care Medicine* 2005; 33:S319–S324.

Stenius-Aarniala BS, Hedman J, Teramo KA. Acute asthma during pregnancy. *Thorax* 1996;51(4):411–414.

Wendel P, Ramin S, Barnett-Hamm C, et al. Asthma treatment in pregnancy: a randomized controlled study. *American Journal of Obstetrics and Gynecology* 1996;175(1):150–154.

15 *A 28-year-old 26-week pregnant woman is admitted to the ICU post motor vehicle crash. The patient is noted with extensive pelvic and lower extremity fractures and received a massive transfusion in the*

trauma resuscitation area. The patient develops cardiopulmonary arrest 10 minutes after arrival in the ICU and CPR is initiated. Which of the following is most true concerning resuscitative hysterotomy (perimortem cesarean delivery)?

A *Resuscitative hysterotomy is not currently recommended for a pregnant woman in cardiac arrest in a woman at 20 weeks of gestation or more.*

B *Resuscitative hysterotomy should occur immediately post arrest as longer lengths of time are associated with significant fetal morbidity.*

C *Emptying the uterus and alleviating aortocaval compression during a resuscitative hysterotomy has been shown to increase maternal-fetal complications.*

D *Resuscitative hysterotomy should occur after 4–5 minutes of arrest without return of spontaneous circulation.*

E *There is a progressive decrease in the likelihood of injury free survival for women, but survival remains >95% for fetuses with lengthening time post arrest.*

Resuscitative hysterotomy (perimortem cesarean delivery) is recommended for a pregnant woman in cardiac arrest if efforts at resuscitation have been unsuccessful in a woman at 20 weeks of gestation or more (Choice A). By emptying the uterus and alleviating aortocaval compression, resuscitative hysterotomy may help permit the return of spontaneous circulation (Choice C). Consideration of resuscitative hysterotomy should occur as soon as there is a maternal cardiac arrest. The conventional teaching is that resuscitative hysterotomy should occur after 4–5 minutes of arrest without return of spontaneous circulation as there is a progressive decrease in the likelihood of injury free survival for women and fetuses with lengthening time post arrest (Choices B and D). In a review of 74 third-trimester cases of resuscitative hysterotomy, 45% of women died despite perimortem cesarean delivery, 45% survived without obvious sequelae, and 10% survived with significant morbidity. Of the involved fetuses, 23% died, 57% survived without obvious sequelae, and 19% survived with significant morbidity (Choice E).

Answer: D

Beckett VA, Knight M, Sharpe P. The CAPS Study: incidence, management and outcomes of cardiac arrest in pregnancy in the UK: a prospective, descriptive study. *BJOG: An International Journal of Obstetrics and Gynaecology* 2017;124:1374–1381.

Benson MD, Padovano A, Bourjeily G, Zhou Y. Maternal collapse: challenging the four-minute rule. *eBioMedicine* 2016;6:253–257.

Jeejeebhoy FM, Zelop CM, Lipman S, Carvalho B, Joglar J, Mhyre JM, et al. Cardiac arrest in pregnancy: a scientific statement from the American Heart Association. American Heart Association Emergency Cardiovascular Care Committee, Council on Cardiopulmonary, Critical Care, Perioperative and Resuscitation, Council on Cardiovascular Diseases in the Young, and Council on Clinical Cardiology. *Circulation* 2015;132:1747–1773.

Katz V, Balderston K, DeFreest M. Perimortem cesarean delivery: were our assumptions correct? *American Journal of Obstetrics and Gynecology* 2005;192:1916–1920.

Katz VL. Perimortem cesarean delivery: its role in maternal mortality. *Seminars in Perinatology* 2012;36:68–72.

16 *Which of the following statements regarding preeclampsia, eclampsia, and/or HELLP syndrome is correct?*

A *Preeclampsia is a multiple-system disorder, and it develops in patients with history of hypertension in women postpartum.*

B *Preeclampsia is characterized by hypertension and proteinuria and is very uncommon.*

C *Blood pressure control is important in preeclampsia and commonly used antihypertensive agents are hydralazine, labetalol, and nifedipine.*

D *Eclampsia is defined as the occurrence of tonic–clonic convulsions in pregnant women only, and thus the treatment is delivery of the fetus as soon as possible.*

E *HELLP syndrome is characterized by hemolysis, elevated liver enzymes, and a low platelet count, and the cause is preecampsia.*

Preeclampsia is a multiple-system disorder, it develops in previously normotensive women after 20 weeks of gestation (Choice A). Preeclampsia is characterized by hypertension and proteinuria and is relatively common with the average rate of preeclampsia in the United States estimated to be 26/1000 deliveries (Choice B). Answer C is correct as blood pressure control is important in the treatment to prevent cerebral hemorrhage and hypertensive encephalopathy. The most commonly used antihypertensive agents are hydralazine, labetalol, and nifedipine administered by continuous or bolus infusion. Eclampsia is defined as the occurrence of tonic–clonic convulsions in pregnant or puerperal women with preeclampsia (Choice D). The prevalence of eclampsia in the United States ranges from 0.6 to 3/1000 live births. Other neurologic presentations in eclampsia include blindness, altered state of consciousness, and coma. Convulsions occur antenatally in 38%, intrapartum in 18%, and postpartum in 44%, usually in the first 24–48 hours after delivery.

Intracerebral hemorrhage is a well-known complication of eclampsia, frequently leading to maternal death or permanent disability. Therapy is directed at lowering blood pressure to limit the development of vasogenic cerebral edema and subsequent ischemia. Magnesium sulfate ($MgSO_4$) is the anticonvulsant drug of choice as it is effective for prevention and treatment of seizures. In case of overdose, ensure adequate ventilation and administer 1 mg of 10% calcium gluconate over a 10-min period. HELLP is a syndrome comprising **h**emolysis, **e**levated **l**iver enzymes, and **l**ow **p**latelets and occurs in 4–12% of patients with severe preeclampsia. Hypertension may or may not be present and presents with vague symptoms of nausea and vomiting and right upper quadrant or epigastric discomfort. It can sometimes develop even after the bay is born (Choice E). The cause is unknown.

Answer: C

Einav S, Leone M. Epidemiology of obstetric critical illness. *International Journal of Obstetric Anesthesia* 2019 Nov;40:128–139.

Zeeman GG. Obstetric critical care: a blueprint for improved outcomes. *Critical Care Medicine* 2006 Sep;34(9 Suppl):S208–S214.

17 *Regarding massive obstetric hemorrhage, which of the following statements is true?*

A *Massive obstetric hemorrhage is an extremely rare event in modern medicine as medications can treat uterine atony.*

B *Massive obstetric hemorrhage usually results from undiagnosed inherited coagulopathies.*

C *Uterotonic agents such as oxytocin are the mainstay of therapy for massive obstetric hemorrhage but have a limited role in the treatment of uterine atony.*

D *Blood loss resuscitation with blood products and uterine atony drugs are the mainstay of treatment.*

E *Hysterectomy is the only surgical procedure utilized to assist with hemorrhage control in refractory massive obstetric hemorrhage.*

Massive obstetric hemorrhage, defined as the loss of > 2500 ml of blood, is ranked among the top three causes of maternal death and usually occurs intrapartum or within the first hour after delivery. It most commonly results from uterine atony complicating 5% of deliveries (Choice A). Most with obstetrical hemorrhage do not have inherent pre-hemorrhage coagulopathy (Choice B). The mainstay of management is centered on the restoration of the circulating blood volume, correction of coagulation, and the surgical control of bleeding. Uterotonic agents, such as oxytocin, are used in the management of uterine atony (Choice C). Injectable prostaglandins may also be used if oxytocin fails. Prostaglandin E2 and prostaglandin F2 stimulate myometrial contractions and have been used for refractory hemorrhage due to uterine atony. Methylergonovine, an ergot alkaloid, is used as a second-line uterotonic agent in the setting of massive obstetric hemorrhage due to atony. The use of a hydrostatic balloon has been advocated as an alternative to uterine packing for controlling hemorrhage. The inflated balloon can conform to the contour of the uterine cavity and provides tamponade. Life-threatening hemorrhage can also be treated by arterial embolization. In cases of refractory hemorrhage, surgical techniques such as bilateral uterine artery or internal iliac artery ligation or the use of a B-Lynch brace suture, which compresses the uterus without compromise of the major vessels, can be used to avoid a hysterectomy (Choice E).

Answer: D

B-Lynch C, Coker A, Lawal AH, et al: The B-Lynch surgical technique for the control of massive postpartum haemorrhage: an alternative to hysterectomy? Five cases reported. *British Journal of Obstetrics and Gynaecology* 1997; 104:372–375.

Dildy GA: Postpartum hemorrhage: new management options. *Clinical Obstetrics and Gynecology* 2002;45:2:330–344.

Einav S, Leone M. Epidemiology of obstetric critical illness. *International Journal of Obstetric Anesthesia* 2019 Nov;40:128–139.

Johanson R, Kumar M, Obhrai M, et al. Management of massive postpartum haemorrhage: use of a hydrostatic balloon catheter to avoid laparotomy. *BJOG* 2001; 108:420–422.

Pelage JP, Le Dref O, Mateo J, et al. Life threatening primary postpartum hemorrhage: Treatment with emergency selective arterial embolization. *Radiology* 1998; 208: 359–362.

Zeeman GG. Obstetric critical care: a blueprint for improved outcomes. *Critical Care Medicine* 2006 Sep;34(9 Suppl):S208–S214. doi: 10.1097/01.CCM. 0000231884.99763.69.

18 *A 26-year-old, 30-week pregnant patient is admitted to the ICU hypotensive, bradycardic, and cool extremities. The diagnosis of a massive pulmonary embolism is made on echocardiogram. Which of the following is correct regarding the diagnosis and/or management of a pregnant patient with a massive pulmonary embolism?*

A *A massive pulmonary embolism will present with dyspnea, chest pain, and associated tachycardia and hypoxia with preserved cardiac function.*

B *Echocardiography in a massive pulmonary embolism will demonstrate normal right ventricular size as compared to a dilated left ventricle due to the clot burden.*

C *Goals of treatment in the obstetric patient differ from the nonpregnant population as heparin therapy is contraindicated in pregnancy.*

D *Catheter-directed thrombolysis, surgical embolectomy, and extracorporeal membrane oxygenation (ECMO) are all contraindicated in pregnancy due to concerns of anesthetic-derived teratogenic effects to the fetus.*

E *It should be considered in pregnant patients presenting with pulselessness in cardiac arrest.*

The clot burden associated with a massive pulmonary embolism occludes the pulmonary vasculature to the extent that forward flow through the heart is insufficient to achieve systemic perfusion. As such, a massive pulmonary embolism will present with obstructive shock. Patients with a massive pulmonary embolism may present with sustained hypotension (systolic blood pressure <90 mm Hg), persistent profound bradycardia (heart rate < 40 beats per minute), and cool extremities (Choice A). Additionally, the initial clinical picture may be that of pulselessness, and in otherwise healthy pregnant patients presenting in cardiac arrest, massive pulmonary embolism should be considered (Choice E). Echocardiogram in these patients may demonstrate:

1) Decreased right ventricular (RV) function or right ventricular free wall dysfunction with preserved apical function (McConnel sign) (Choice B)
2) Dilated RV, either by 2-D or 3-D calculations or by RV/LV ratio
3) Decreased tricuspid annular plan systolic excursion (TAPSE)

Goals of treatment are the same in the pregnant as the nonpregnant patient (Choices C, D) and include:

1) Cardiopulmonary support
2) Anticoagulation
3) Reperfusion of the pulmonary circulation

Treatment options for massive pulmonary embolism in pregnancy include:

1) Intravenous unfractionated heparin (IV UFH): initiated with a loading dose of 80 units/kg followed by a continuous intravenous infusion of 18 units/kg/hour and adjusted using a weight-based nomogram following the activated partial thromboplastin time (APTT) level.
2) Thrombolytic therapy: anticoagulant therapy alone will likely fail at reducing the circulatory obstruction caused by the embolus. Following thrombolytic therapy, an infusion of unfractionated heparin at 18 units/kg/hour without a loading dose is initiated.
3) Catheter-directed thrombolysis
4) Catheter-directed embolectomy
5) Surgical embolectomy
6) Extracorporeal membrane oxygenation (ECMO) may be considered

Answer: E

Handal-Orefice RC, Moroz LA. Pulmonary embolism management in the critical care setting. *Seminars in Perinatology* 2019 Jun;43(4):205–212.

19 *A 26-year-old G1P0 woman who is 21 weeks pregnant presents to the emergency department with a two-day history of periumbilical abdominal pain that has since moved to her right abdomen. She is tachycardic with a HR: 110 beats/min and BP: 110/70 mm Hg. Her labs are significant for a WBC of 18,300 cells/μL. On exam, the patient has tenderness to palpation in the right mid and lower abdomen and exhibits guarding with deep palpation. The most appropriate initial study to confirm the diagnosis of appendicitis is:*

A *Computed tomography abdomen and pelvis with PO and IV contrast*

B *Abdominal ultrasound with compression*

C *Transvaginal ultrasound*

D *Hepatobiliary iminodiacetic acid scan (HIDA)*

E *Hysteroscopy*

Appendectomy is the most common non-obstetric surgical procedure performed on pregnant patients. Ultrasonography is useful as an initial imaging modality due to its low cost and ability to provide real-time imaging. Findings supportive of appendicitis include a noncompressible tubular structure, dilated appendix (>6 mm), periappendiceal fluid collection, and prominence of periappendiceal fat. In pregnant patients for which ultrasound does not visualize the appendix, further imaging with MRI can be obtained if clinical suspicion exists. Transvaginal ultrasound is more useful in identifying disorders of the pelvis, as well as for fetal evaluation during early pregnancy (Choice C). CT and HIDA scans expose the fetus to radiation and should not be utilized as initial treatment modalities (Choices A and D). Hysteroscopy allows for visualization of the inside of uterus and has no role in the diagnosis of acute appendicitis (Choice E).

Answer: B

Kave M, Parooie F, Salarzaei M. Pregnancy and appendicitis: a systematic review and meta-analysis on the clinical use of MRI in diagnosis of appendicitis in pregnant women. *World Journal of Emergency Surgery* 2019 July; 14:37.

Schwulst S, Son M. Diagnostic imaging in pregnant patients with suspected appendicitis. *Journal of the American Medical Association* 2019;322(5):455–456.

20 *A 31-year-old woman is diagnosed with symptomatic cholelithiasis at 21 weeks gestation and given a referral to a general surgeon. She has had three other episodes of abdominal pain related to gallstones over the past six months. Concerning the risk to her and her fetus, which of the following is the most true.*

A *Laparoscopy is contraindicated in the third trimester.*

B *Nonoperative management is associated with a higher rate of recurrent hospitalizations and preterm deliveries.*

C *Prophylactic antibiotics should be prescribed during acute episodes of biliary colic in order to prevent cholecystitis.*

D *Insufflation pressure should be maintained at less than 12 mm Hg to prevent adverse outcomes to fetus.*

E *Recurrent gallbladder symptoms occur in less than 10% of patients managed non-operatively during their first trimester.*

Symptomatic cholelithiasis during pregnancy can be safely managed with laparoscopic cholecystectomy. While nonoperative management followed by cholecystectomy postpartum was previously advocated, studies have shown that delaying cholecystectomy leads to higher rates of rehospitalization, as well as increased rates of preterm delivery and spontaneous abortion. Laparoscopic cholecystectomy during pregnancy is associated with shorter length of stay and fewer complications compared to open cholecystectomy, and laparoscopy can be performed safely during any trimester without an increase in risk to mother or fetus (Choice A). Prophylactic antibiotics are not indicated for biliary colic during pregnancy (Choice C). Pressures of 15 mm Hg have been used during laparoscopy in pregnant patients without increasing adverse outcomes to the patient or fetus (Choice D). Recurrent gallbladder symptoms develop in over 90% of patients managed non-operatively who presented with symptoms during their first trimester (Choice E). For patients greater than 36 weeks gestation, the goal would be to delay surgery if possible and if not, then inducing the labor and delivering the baby to perform the surgery later would be a viable option. Surgery then can be done with more ease. Laparoscopic surgery is an option but robotic surgery is not advised as the loss of haptics with the robotic instruments could jeopardize the fetus.

Answer: B

Date RS, Kaushal M, Ramesh A. A review of the management of gallstone disease and its complications in pregnancy. *American Journal of Surgery* 2008; 196:599–608.

Dhupar R, Smaldone GM, Hamad GG. Is there a benefit to delaying cholecystectomy for symptomatic gallbladder disease during pregnancy? *Surgical Endoscopy* 2010; 24:108–112.

Pearl J, Price R. *Guidelines for the use of laparoscopy during pregnancy*- A SAGES Publication. 2017.

24

Pediatric Critical Care
Juan P. Gurria, MD and J. Craig Egan, MD

Phoenix Children's Hospital, Phoenix, AZ, USA

1 *A 5-year-old boy is admitted to the PICU with fever, lethargy, cool extremities, sluggish capillary refill, narrowed pulse pressure, and weak peripheral pulses. The type of shock and initial vasoactive medications selected for this patient should be:*
  A *Cold shock, treat with inotropes.*
  B *Warm shock, treat with pressors.*
  C *Cold shock, treat with pressors.*
  D *Warm shock, treat with inotropes.*
  E *Clinical signs should not be used in isolation to categorize shock type.*

Despite common use of bedside clinical signs to categorize type of pediatric septic shock, there is inconsistent agreement between these signs. Extremity temperature, capillary refill, and pulse strength exhibited fair-to-good agreement with each other, while diastolic blood pressure and pulse pressure exhibited poor agreement. Prior studies have demonstrated that direct measurement of cardiac index and systemic vascular resistance can be used to categorize shock type and guide vasoactive therapy in children with septic shock. For patients treated with vasoactive medications as part of the sepsis pathway, neither shock type nor any of the clinical signs of shock type were strongly matched with vasoactive selection, and the resulting shock type-vasoactive mismatch was not associated with complicated course or worse clinical outcomes. These data support recent Surviving Sepsis campaign recommendations that clinical signs should not be used in isolation to categorize shock type.

Answer: E

Walker, S.B., et al., Clinical signs to categorize shock and target vasoactive medications in warm versus cold pediatric septic shock. *Pediatric Critical Care Medicine*, 2020. **21**(12): pp. 1051–1058.

2 *During ECMO in PICU patients, which condition is associated with more bleeding?*
  A *Peripheral cannulation*
  B *Central cannulation*
  C *Younger age*
  D *Low lactate*
  E *Veno-venous ECMO*

By 4 days of ECMO, 50% of ECMO users experience a "bleeding day." The proportion of patients bleeding on each day of ECMO run does not vary significantly as duration increases. Bleeding days occurred more frequently in older patients, patients with congenital cardiac diagnosis, patients who had a bleeding event before ECMO initiation, had surgery before ECMO, were centrally rather than peripherally cannulated, had ECMO initiated with crystalloid solution rather than blood primed circuit, and those who received veno-arterial ECMO compared with veno-venous ECMO. Laboratory values on bleeding days were notable for higher lactate levels and prothrombin times, as well as lower platelet counts, compared with nonbleeding days.

Bleeding patients, those who were over the 75% percentile with regards to bleeding frequency, resulted in patients who met study criteria for "bleeding day," recognized as frequent bleeding in 26% of their ECMO run. These patients compared with the remainder of the cohort, had fewer ventilator-free and hospital-free days in the 2 months after cannulation, and higher in-hospital mortality rate.

Answer: B

O'Halloran, C.P., et al., Mortality and factors associated with hemorrhage during pediatric extracorporeal membrane oxygenation. *Pediatric Critical Care Medicine*, 2020. **21**(1): pp. 75–81.
Walker, S.B., et al., Clinical signs to categorize shock and target vasoactive medications in warm versus cold

pediatric septic shock. *Pediatric Critical Care Medicine*, 2020. **21**(12): pp. 1051–1058.

3   *Risk factor in a pediatric patient, at the time of admission to the PICU, that predict acute kidney injury include:*
    A *Post-cardiopulmonary bypass*
    B *Preexisting pulmonary disease*
    C *Presence of infection*
    D *Weight*
    E *Male gender*

Up to 37% of critically ill children admitted to the PICU develop acute kidney injury (AKI). AKI is strongly associated with prolonged ICU and hospital length of stay (LOS). Recent studies reported a mortality from severe AKI in PICU between 11 and 64%. Those who underwent cardiopulmonary bypass had an adjusted odds ratio of 2.5. Even those who survive to discharge have an increased risk of repeat hospitalizations and physician visits. Furthermore, AKI in PICU is independently associated with long-term mortality beyond 5 years after PICU discharge. A proportion of the children who survive develop hypertension, and/or are dependent on renal support after discharge.

Answer: A

Raman, S., et al., Prediction of acute kidney injury on admission to pediatric intensive care. *Pediatric Critical Care Medicine*, 2020. **21**(9): pp. 811–819.

4   *In pediatric cardiac ICU patients, risk of catheter-related thrombosis is highest with:*
    A *Tunneled catheters, internal jugular vein*
    B *Percutaneous central catheters, femoral vein*
    C *PICC, upper extremity*
    D *PICC, lower extremity*
    E *Intracardiac catheters*

The most common location for a thrombus to occur was femoral (44%). Thrombosis was most commonly associated with percutaneous CVCs (51%). On univariate analysis, those factors associated with risk of thrombosis are as follows: age, STAT placement, total catheter days, multiple catheters concurrently in situ, history of a cardiac catheter intervention, cardiac arrest, use of mechanical circulatory support, chylothorax, prior infection, open chest, unplanned reintervention, and history of CLABSI. In multivariable analysis, independent predictors of thrombosis were younger age, STAT placement, 4–5 total catheter days, history of mechanical circulatory support, and unplanned reintervention. Patients with

PICC line associated thrombosis do not require immediate removal provided that the patient continues to require the line, the line is functional, and anticoagulation is started.

Answer: B

DiPietro, L.M., et al., Central venous catheter utilization and complications in the pediatric cardiac ICU: a report from the pediatric cardiac critical care consortium (PC4). *Pediatric Critical Care Medicine*, 2020. **21**(8): pp. 729–737.

5   *Regarding the use of REBOA catheters in pediatric patients with exsanguinating hemorrhage:*
    A *Length of insertion should be determined by holding the catheter over patient's abdomen.*
    B *Use has been well studied in all age groups.*
    C *Survival rates in older teenagers is similar to adults.*
    D *The 12 Fr catheter can be used for all sizes of children.*
    E *Only pediatric interventional radiologists should insert REBOA catheters into pediatric patients.*

One study (Norii et al.) evaluated the mortality and characteristics of children with severe traumatic injury who received REBOA. This study retrospectively reviewed 54 patients less than or equal to 18 years of age using the Japan Trauma Data Bank from 2004 to 2015. Patients had high anatomic injury severity scores (ISS) (median 41.2) with a survival rate of approximately 43%, similar to those found in adult patients who receive REBOA. However, it should be noted that most [n = 39, (72%)] children in this retrospective study were between 16 and 18 years of age, and only one child less than 10 years of age received REBOA. They concluded that both young children and adolescents who underwent REBOA were seriously injured with high ISS and had equivalent survival rates compared to reported survival rates from studies in adults. These results and conclusions are supported by an unpublished study performed in the United States that indicates REBOA is safe for use in adolescents despite their smaller caliber vasculature.

A 12 Fr sheath has an outer diameter of 4.67 mm and is often too large for very young pediatric patients. The 12 Fr-compatible REBOA catheter was the only commercially available catheter in the United States until 2016, when the 7 Fr sheath, whose outer diameter is only 3 mm, was introduced.

Carrillo et al. used the approximate aortic diameters from CT scans of 289 patients to create artificial aortas using a three-dimensional (3D) printer. The aortas were then inserted into a circulatory system model that both

Table 24.1 Recommended initial REBOA inflation volumes and zone distances (cm) for the five largest Broselow categories.[a]

Broselow Category	Average age (years)	Average weight (kg)	Inflation at zone 1: Aorta at the xyphoid process (ml)	Inflation at zone 3: Aorta at the umbilicus (ml)	Zone I-zone 3 distance (cm)
Black	12.3	49.1	7.5	5.5	21.8
Green	9.4	33.5	6	3.5	14.5
Orange	7.3	26.3	5.5	3	13.0
Blue	5.5	21.2	5	2	12.8
White	3.6	18.3	3	1.5	11.8

[a] Inflation volume based on occlusion of flow by approx. 75%. REBOA-resuscitative endovascular balloon occlusion of the aorta. Adapted from Carrillo et al.

simulated abdominal and upper body perfusion. Sonographic flow meters and pressure transducers were placed along the circuit, and measurements were recorded as REBOA device was inflated in the aortic segment. Zone 1 and 3 aortic diameters were measured and grouped according to pediatric Broselow category. Recommendations were then made for REBOA inflation volumes according to the results (Table 24.1).

Pediatric trauma surgeons should become familiar with the indications and technique for REBOA, and establishing institutional protocols in conjunction with vascular surgery or interventional radiology may be a consideration at free-standing pediatric trauma centers. Inserting the commercially available catheters requires minimal training that most pediatric surgeons skilled in vascular access should be comfortable with if interventional radiologists or vascular surgeons are not rapidly available.

Answer: C

Campagna, G.A., et al., The utility and promise of Resuscitative Endovascular Balloon Occlusion of the Aorta (REBOA) in the pediatric population: an evidence-based review. *Journal of Pediatric Surgery*, 2020. 55(10): pp. 2128–2133.

6 *A 1-year-old girl has been in the PICU for a week after sustaining a severe traumatic brain injury. Which of the following statements applies to her fluid management?*
   A *The rate of fluid overload in the pediatric severe TBI population is low, especially in infants under 1-year old.*
   B *The brisk diuresis that occurs with mannitol in pediatric patients does not lead to hypotension and an overall decrease in cerebral perfusion pressure.*
   C *Hypertonic saline lowers the ICP but is ineffective as an intravascular volume expander.*
   D *AKI has been associated with the use of hypertonic saline, regardless of serum sodium level.*

   E *There is no significant difference in clinical outcomes for the fluid overloaded group when compared with the group without fluid overload.*

The rate of fluid overload in the pediatric severe TBI population is high, especially in infants under 1-year old. However, unlike other PICU cohorts, fluid overload does not appear to be associated with worse clinical outcomes in the severe TBI patients. Hypertonic saline does not appear to be a contributing factor to the high rate of fluid overload in severe TBI.

Intracranial hypertension is a common sequela of severe TBI. Evidence-based guidelines recommend treatment of increased intracranial pressure (ICP) using a multisystem approach, including the use of hyperosmolar therapy. Hyperosmolar therapy creates an osmotic gradient that draws water from the interstitium into the vascular space. Mannitol and hypertonic saline represent two of the most commonly used hyperosmolar therapies. Mannitol is a sugar alcohol that works as an osmotic diuretic to raise serum osmolarity. Although very effective in lowering ICP, the brisk diuresis that occurs with mannitol in pediatric patients can lead to hypotension and an overall decrease in cerebral perfusion pressure. In contrast, hypertonic saline lowers the ICP without the diuretic effect seen with mannitol and acts as an intravascular volume expander, thus supporting the blood pressure. These hemodynamic differences have led to an increased use of hypertonic saline for the treatment of pediatric TBI.

There was no significant difference in clinical outcomes for the fluid overloaded group when compared with the group without fluid overload. After adjusting for differences in clinical and demographic variables, there was no increase in odds of mortality when comparing fluid overloaded versus children without fluid overload. There was also no significant increase in odds of AKI. There was no change in the mean PICU LOS (8.5 vs 9.3 days in non-fluid overload vs fluid overloaded children, respectively) ,and there was also no change in the mean ventilator-free days

(14.6 vs 13.0 days in non-fluid overload vs fluid overloaded children, respectively).

AKI has been associated with the use of hypertonic saline, but this was seen with sustained sodium greater than 170 mmol/L.

Answer: E

Stulce, C., et al., Fluid overload in pediatric severe traumatic brain injury. *Pediatric Critical Care Medicine*, 2020. **21**(2): pp. 164–169.

7 *Regarding antibiotic administration for presumed septic shock:*

  A *Do not obtain blood cultures before initiating antimicrobial therapy.*

  B *Start antimicrobial therapy as soon as possible, within 1 hour of recognition despite not having cultures drawn.*

  C *If no pathogen is identified, do not narrow or stop empiric antimicrobial therapy.*

  D *Remove intravascular access devices that are confirmed to be the source of sepsis or septic shock, without waiting until other vascular access has been established.*

  E *In children with immune compromise and/or at high risk for multidrug-resistant pathogens, use empiric monotherapy when septic shock or other sepsis-associated organ dysfunction is present/suspected.*

If collection of the blood cultures is likely to delay administration of antimicrobial therapy to the patient, then administration of antimicrobials should take precedence, in view of the impact of delayed antimicrobial administration on patient outcomes. However, because blood cultures may be the only source of information identifying bacterial antibiotic susceptibility, it is important to make all reasonable efforts to collect blood cultures before timely antimicrobial administration. The collection of other biological specimens to identify pathogens from non-blood sites (e.g. urine, cerebrospinal fluid, tracheal aspirate, bronchoalveolar lavage, drainage from collections) should also happen as soon as possible.

Many QI initiatives have shown improved pediatric sepsis outcomes with implementation of a bundle that includes rapid delivery of IV antimicrobials. Two retrospective observational studies have also demonstrated an association of faster time to antimicrobial therapy with reduced mortality for children with sepsis. If no pathogen is identified *and* bacterial/fungal infection is deemed unlikely, clinicians should stop empiric antimicrobial therapy to reduce unnecessary exposure. However, many children with a clinical diagnosis of septic shock do not have a pathogen isolated. Patients with

negative bacterial microbiological results may have false-negative tests due to antibiotic pretreatment, absence of bacteremia, or sepsis-related to viral infections. Thus, the decision to continue, narrow, or stop antimicrobial therapy must often be made on the basis of clinician judgment and indirect clinical information, taking into account the clinical presentation, site and type of infection, host risk factors, and adequacy of clinical improvement.

A common, but potentially preventable source of infection, is central-line-associated bloodstream infections. Delayed removal of a CVC in neonates and in patients with fungemia or Enterobacteriaceae bacteremia increases the risk of death or slows recovery. Removal of a CVC that is the source of infection is therefore generally warranted. Fungal infection dictates immediate removal, while in case of coagulase-negative *Staphylococcus* species or clinically stable patients with infection caused by gram-negative bacilli, infections can often be initially treated through the CVC as a temporizing measure. The decision to remove the CVC, or not, should ultimately be made based on the pathogen suspected/recovered and host factors, such as immune status. Add a second gram-negative agent and/or a glycopeptide when resistant organisms were suspected for patients who are clinically unstable (i.e. septic shock) and in centers with a high rate of resistant pathogens. Therefore, for children with septic shock or other sepsis-associated organ dysfunction who have immune compromise and/or are at high risk for multidrug-resistant pathogens, treat with empiric multidrug therapy.

Answer: B

Weiss, S.L., et al., Surviving sepsis campaign international guidelines for the management of septic shock and sepsis-associated organ dysfunction in children. *Pediatric Critical Care Medicine*, 2020. **21**(2): pp. e52–e106.

8 *Fluid management of the septic child:*

  A *In healthcare systems with no availability of intensive care and in the absence of hypotension, initiate bolus fluid administration while starting maintenance fluids.*

  B *In healthcare systems with no availability of intensive care, if hypotension is present, do not administering up to 40 mL/kg in bolus fluid (10–20 mL/kg per bolus) over the first hour with titration to clinical markers of cardiac output and discontinued if signs of fluid overload develop.*

  C *In healthcare systems with availability of intensive care, administer up to 40–60 mL/kg in bolus fluid (10–20 mL/kg per bolus) over the first hour,* titrated to clinical markers of cardiac output and discontinued if signs of fluid overload develop, for the initial resuscitation of children with septic shock or other sepsis-associated organ dysfunction.

D *Use albumin, rather than crystalloids, for the initial resuscitation of children with septic shock or other sepsis-associated organ dysfunction.*

E *Use 0.9% saline, rather than balanced/buffered crystalloids, for the initial resuscitation of children with septic shock or other sepsis-associated organ dysfunction.*

The Fluid Expansion as Supportive Therapy (FEAST) RCT demonstrated a lower mortality after 48 hours in children receiving conservative fluid therapy (i.e. no bolus fluid, maintenance fluid only) than among those given liberal initial fluid therapy (i.e. 20 mL/kg fluid bolus with maintenance fluid). For the subset of children with septic shock and *hypotension*, use cautious administration of fluid bolus therapy in low-resource settings. In the FEAST study, all children with "severe" hypotension were treated with 40 mL/kg of bolus fluid.

For children with septic shock diagnosed by abnormal perfusion or hypotension in healthcare systems with availability of advanced supportive and intensive care, and in the absence of signs of fluid overload, the panel suggests administering up to 40–60 mL/kg fluid bolus therapy in the first hour of resuscitation. Fluid resuscitation should be titrated to clinical markers of cardiac output and discontinued if signs of fluid overload develop. In the absence of any clear benefit of albumin administration in children with sepsis, and in view of the additional costs in comparison to crystalloids, problems of availability, and the potential risk of blood-borne infection, the routine use of albumin for initial fluid resuscitation in children with sepsis is not recommended. Although no pediatric RCTs compare balanced/buffered crystalloids (e.g. lactated Ringer's, Plasma-Lyte) to 0.9% saline, there are two large observational studies in children with sepsis. These studies showed that use of balanced/buffered crystalloids was associated with lower mortality but not AKI. Do not use starches in the acute resuscitation of children with septic shock or other sepsis-associated organ dysfunction.

Answer: C

Weiss, S.L., et al., Surviving sepsis campaign international guidelines for the management of septic shock and sepsis-associated organ dysfunction in children. *Pediatric Critical Care Medicine*, 2020. **21**(2): pp. e52–e106.

9 Vasoactive medications in septic shock:

A *Dopamine is preferred over epinephrine as the first-line agent in children with septic shock.*

B *Do not use epinephrine or norepinephrine in children with septic shock.*

C *There is no recommendation for a specific first-line vasoactive infusion for children with septic shock.*

D *Vasopressors should be started through peripheral intravenous access in order to avoid the complications of central venous access in small children.*

E *Add vasopressin or further titrate catecholamines in children with septic shock who require high-dose catecholamines.*

It is reasonable to begin vasoactive infusions after 40–60 mL/kg of fluid resuscitation if the patient continues to have evidence of decreased end-organ perfusion. Either epinephrine or norepinephrine may be administered through a peripheral vein (or intraosseous) if central venous access is not readily accessible. Dopamine may be substituted as the first-line vasoactive infusion, administered either peripherally or centrally. Epinephrine and norepinephrine both have vasopressor and inotropic effects, are widely used, and are effective in treating children with fluid-resistant septic shock. Epinephrine is associated with a lower risk of mortality and more organ failure-free days among survivors by day 28. Evidence is insufficient to recommend either epinephrine or norepinephrine as the initial vasoactive agent for children with fluid-resistant septic shock. Once cardiac echocardiography or other advanced monitoring is available, selection of vasoactive therapy should be driven by individual patient physiology. Until further data are available, it is reasonable to begin vasoactive infusions after 40–60 mL/kg of fluid resuscitation if the patient continues to have evidence of abnormal perfusion. All vasoactive agents, including norepinephrine, may be initiated through peripheral venous (or intraosseous) access if central venous access is not readily available to avoid delays in therapy. However, central venous access should be obtained as soon as reasonably practicable. Although epinephrine or norepinephrine is the preferred first-line medication, dopamine may be substituted as the first-line vasoactive infusion, administered either peripherally or centrally, if neither epinephrine nor norepinephrine is readily available.

No consensus was achieved on the optimal threshold for initiating vasopressin. Therefore, this decision should be made according to individual clinician preference. Weighing the benefit of avoiding renal replacement therapy against the potential harm from ischemic events and the nonsignificant difference in mortality, vasopressin may be added or catecholamines may be further titrated in children with refractory shock. There are no RCTs using inodilators (including milrinone, dobutamine, or levosimendan) in children with septic shock with persistent hypoperfusion and cardiac dysfunction.

Answer: E

Weiss, S.L., et al., Surviving sepsis campaign international guidelines for the management of septic shock and sepsis-associated organ dysfunction in children. *Pediatric Critical Care Medicine*, 2020. **21**(2): pp. e52–e106.

10 *Which is correct regarding ventilation in septic pediatric patient with ARDS?*
   A *Children with fluid-refractory, catecholamine-resistant septic shock may benefit from early invasive mechanical ventilation.*
   B *Etomidate should always be used when intubating children with septic shock or other sepsis-associated organ dysfunction.*
   C *Noninvasive ventilation is discouraged.*
   D *Prone positioning is only recommended for adults.*
   E *Inhaled NO and high-frequency oscillatory ventilation should be used early in all cases.*

A high metabolic demand from refractory shock typically indicated by progressive lactic acidemia and end-organ dysfunction can be, at least in part, mitigated by early invasive mechanical ventilation even without clinical symptoms of acute pulmonary edema or respiratory failure. It is well known that chest radiograph findings can "lag" behind clinical deterioration. Etomidate should be avoided when intubating children in septic shock. Studies have reported higher mortality after use of etomidate in septic shock. Noninvasive mechanical ventilation with continuous positive airway pressure ventilation or bi-level positive airway pressure ventilation may allow for decreased work of breathing and improved oxygenation in the face of sepsis-induced pediatric ARDS (PARDS). Prone positioning almost uniformly improves oxygenation in children with PARDS. Although the exact mechanisms continue to be elucidated, prone position has been shown to recruit areas of collapsed, de-recruited lung with resultant improved elastance, decreased lung stress and strain, and improved functional residual capacity. Given that pulmonary perfusion is thought to be consistent both dorsally and ventrally, an improvement in lung aeration can be met with continued perfusion, thereby reducing ventilation-perfusion mismatching.

The presumptive mechanism of sepsis-induced PARDS involves alveolar epithelial injury, vascular endothelial injury, and activation of inflammatory, fibrosis, and coagulation cascades. As such, PARDS is not a disease process primarily of pulmonary arterial hypertension, the therapeutic target of iNO therapy, and so it is not recommended for routine use in children with sepsis-associated PARDS. However, iNO therapy may be considered in children with documented pulmonary hypertension or severe right ventricular dysfunction confirmed by echocardiography. In regards to High Frequency Oscillatory Ventilation (HFOV), a large, multicenter, international RCT of HFOV compared with conventional mechanical ventilation in severe PARDS patients, including children with and without sepsis, is underway.

Answer: A

Weiss, S.L., et al., Surviving sepsis campaign international guidelines for the management of septic shock and sepsis-associated organ dysfunction in children. *Pediatric Critical Care Medicine*, 2020. **21**(2): pp. e52–e106.

11 *In which of these scenarios are these medications recommended?*
   A *IV hydrocortisone to treat children with septic shock if fluid resuscitation and vasopressor therapy are able to restore hemodynamic stability.*
   B *Insulin therapy to maintain a blood glucose target at or below 140 mg/dL (7.8 mmol/L).*
   C *Calcium is crucial to maintain a normal serum calcium level, with septic shock requiring vasoactive infusion support.*
   D *Levothyroxine in children with septic shock and other sepsis-associated organ dysfunction in a sick euthyroid state.*
   E *Antipyretics can be used in certain clinical scenarios (e.g. refractory shock, pulmonary hypertension), and to reduce extreme body temperatures.*

The use of random cortisol or stimulation tests to guide corticosteroid prescription in children with septic shock cannot be recommended at this time. No high-quality investigations currently support or refute the routine use of adjunctive corticosteroids for pediatric septic shock or other sepsis-associated organ dysfunction.

Although hyperglycemia has been associated with poor outcomes in numerous studies of critically ill children and adults, three prospective multicenter RCTs of glucose control to a low target range (including 50–80, 70–100, 72–126, 80–110 mg/dL or 2.8–4.4, 3.9–5.6, 4.0–7.0, 4.4–6.1 mmol/L) have not demonstrated clinical benefit in children. Treating hyperglycemia greater than or equal to 180 mg/dL ($\geq$10 mmol/L) may be desirable as incidence of insulin-induced hypoglycemia in the studied pediatric cohorts with targets of 140–180 mg/dL (7.8–10.0 mmol/L) is extremely low. Therefore, evidence cannot definitively guide this therapeutic target.

During septic shock, derangements in calcium regulation frequently occur in critically ill adults and children. However, a systematic review of adult literature found no evidence to support treating hypocalcemia of critical illness. Calcium supplementation may actually worsen organ dysfunction and is correlated with adverse outcomes in critically ill adult patients receiving PN. Although the prevalence of hypocalcemia in critically ill children has been reported to be up to 75% and is associated with organ dysfunction, no studies in children with septic shock have investigated the effect of calcium supplementation to treat hypocalcemia. This recommendation should not overlap with the recommended treatment of hypocalcemia mediated by blood product transfusions or during PALS/ACLS protocols.

Although of theoretical benefit, few trials of thyroid hormone replacement have been conducted in critically ill children and none in children with sepsis. Two prospective RCTs in children undergoing cardiac surgery (without sepsis) showed no difference in mortality, vasoactive days, or PICU LOS. One open-label study in premature neonates also showed no difference in clinical outcomes. Taken together, there are no direct data to inform a recommendation for children with sepsis, and no indirect data from other critically ill children to support a recommendation for the routine use of levothyroxine in children with septic shock and other sepsis-associated organ dysfunction in a sick euthyroid state.

No direct evidence for or against the use of antipyretics in febrile children with sepsis-associated organ dysfunction exists. At this time, we are not able to recommend the optimal approach to fever in children with sepsis. Antipyretics can optimize patient comfort, reduce metabolic demand under certain clinical scenarios (e.g. refractory shock, pulmonary hypertension), and reduce extreme body temperatures.

Answer: E

Weiss, S.L., et al., Surviving sepsis campaign international guidelines for the management of septic shock and sepsis-associated organ dysfunction in children. *Pediatric Critical Care Medicine*, 2020. **21**(2): pp. e52–e106.

12 *To optimize nutrition in the pediatric patient in septic shock:*

    A *Feeding should be held for septic children on vasoactive or inotropic medications.*

    B *Enteral nutrition is the preferred method of feeding and parenteral nutrition may be withheld in the first 7 days of PICU admission.*

    C *Gastric residual volumes should be checked to guide what rate feeds should be administered.*

    D *Feeding tube should be placed post-pyloric in order to reduce risk of aspiration pneumonia.*

    E *Prokinetics, as well as zinc, selenium, glutamine supplements, improve feeding tolerance.*

Enteral feeding is not contraindicated in children with septic shock after adequate hemodynamic resuscitation who no longer require escalating doses of vasoactive agents or in whom weaning of vasoactive agents has started. Studies have shown that enteral feeding was tolerated in patients on nonescalating/weaning doses of vasoactive agents without increased adverse effects or gastrointestinal complications such as vomiting, diarrhea, abdominal distension, bleeding, necrotizing enterocolitis, or perforation.

Withholding parenteral nutrition during the first week in PICU when enteral nutrition was less than 80% of prescribed goal is clinically superior to providing supplemental parental nutrition within 24 hours of admission. Withholding PN was also beneficial in term neonates and children who were undernourished at admission, although withholding parenteral nutrition in term neonates was also associated with increased risk of severe hypoglycemia. A long-term follow-up 2 years after PICU admission showed that withholding parenteral nutrition for 1 week did not affect survival, anthropometrics, or health status, but did improve certain domains of neurocognitive development.

In three small RCTs, gastric versus post-pyloric enteral feeding were compared in mechanically ventilated children with a variety of diagnoses. No significant difference was found in the incidence of ventilator-associated pneumonia between gastric and post-pyloric feeding. On the basis of these studies, there is no clear evidence that post-pyloric feeding is beneficial, and there is concern for potential harm through delayed optimization of enteral nutrition. Therefore, the preferred method is enteral nutrition.

Prokinetic agents, such as metoclopramide and erythromycin, are often used in the PICU in an effort to reduce feeding intolerance. A study looked at a combined intervention of enteral zinc, selenium, glutamine, and IV metoclopramide. In critically ill children, this combined intervention failed to reduce the development of sepsis or incidence of hospital-acquired infection in immunocompetent children, although the intervention including metoclopramide did reduce the rate of hospital-acquired infection and sepsis in immunocompromised children.

Prokinetic agents are also not without risk as they have been associated with prolongation of the QT interval and ventricular arrhythmias.

Answer: B

Weiss, S.L., et al., Surviving sepsis campaign international guidelines for the management of septic shock and sepsis-associated organ dysfunction in children. *Pediatric Critical Care Medicine*, 2020. **21**(2): pp. e52–e106.

13 *Transfusion goals for septic patients in the PICU include:*
   A *Transfuse PRBC's if hemoglobin <5 g/dL*
   B *Transfuse PRBC's to keep hemoglobin >9.5 g/dL*
   C *Transfuse platelets to maintain a level of 50,000, whether bleeding or not*
   D *Transfuse FFP to maintain normal PT/INR whether bleeding or not*

In critically ill children or those at risk for critical illness, a PRBC transfusion is recommended if the Hb concentration is <5 g/dL. Many descriptive studies have reported that the risk of adverse outcomes of hospitalized children is significantly higher if their Hb level is below 5 g/dL. Mortality was similar in children with Hb level <5 g/dL who were transfused and in children with Hb level ≥ 5 g/dL who were not transfused.

Patients were randomized to receive RBCs if hemoglobin decreased to either less than 7.0 g/dL (restrictive group) or 9.5 g/dL (liberal group). No differences were found between the restrictive versus liberal group in the primary endpoint of new or progressive multiple-organ dysfunction syndrome or mortality. There is no need for transfusion if hemoglobin is greater than 7 g/dL in hemodynamically stable children with sepsis.

One observational study demonstrated an association between the administration of platelet transfusions to critically ill children and worse clinical outcomes including longer ICU LOS, progressive organ dysfunction, and increased mortality. A study compared a platelet transfusion threshold of 50 000/mm³ (high threshold) with 25 000/mm³ (low threshold). More adverse events, including new major bleeding or death, were also seen in the high threshold group.

No direct data exist to inform a recommendation about plasma transfusion in pediatric sepsis. One RCT evaluates prophylactic plasma transfusion in critically ill children without sepsis. There is no difference in packed RBC transfusion requirements or blood loss between prophylactic or reactive FFP transfusion.

Answer: A

Doctor, A., et al., Recommendations on RBC transfusion in general critically ill children based on hemoglobin and/or physiologic thresholds from the pediatric critical care transfusion and anemia expertise initiative. *Pediatric Critical Care Medicine*, 2018. **19**(9S Suppl 1): pp. S98–S113.
Weiss, S.L., et al., Surviving sepsis campaign international guidelines for the management of septic shock and sepsis-associated organ dysfunction in children. *Pediatric Critical Care Medicine*, 2020. **21**(2): pp. e52–e106.

14 *Compared to pediatric trauma patients without PARDS, those who develop PARDS:*
   A *Are more likely to develop MODS*
   B *Experienced longer hospitalization in survivors*
   C *Had fewer PICU- and mechanical ventilator-free days at day 28*
   D *More than five-fold higher mortality*
   E *All of the above*

In a recent study, patients with trauma-related PARDS were more likely to have new or progressive MODS. Increases in age, ISS, as well as presence of trauma-related PARDS were all independent statistical predictors of MODS. Patients with trauma-related PARDS also experienced longer hospitalization in survivors, and fewer PICU- and mechanical ventilator-free days at day 28. There was no difference in readmission within 30 days of discharge between the two groups.

Twenty-nine patients (4.5%) died in the analyzed cohort. This was higher than the 1.2% mortality for the entire 7382-patient study population. Patients with trauma-related PARDS had a more than fivefold higher mortality than those without trauma-related PARDS. When comparing within ISS groups, those with trauma-related PARDS had a higher mortality at mild and moderate injury severity but not at severe injury severity. When comparing across ISS, mortality in patients without trauma-related PARDS increased with increasing injury severity, whereas mortality in patients with trauma-related PARDS was the same regardless of injury severity.

On multivariate logistic regression, both age and ISS were independently associated with mortality, whereas the presence of trauma-related PARDS did not reach statistical significance as an independent predictor of mortality.

Answer: E

Nair, A.B., M.J. Cohen, and H.R. Flori, Clinical characteristics, major morbidity, and mortality in trauma-related pediatric acute respiratory distress syndrome. *Pediatric Critical Care Medicine*, 2020. **21**(2): pp. 122–128.

15 *In pediatric trauma patients who require early transfusion, which of the following is associated with increased mortality?*
   A *RBC:FFP transfusion ratio at 24 hours*
   B *Abnormal fibrinogen within the first 2 hours*
   C *Abnormal PT or PTT within the first 2 hours*
   D *Abnormal platelets within the first 2 hours*
   E *ISS*

An abnormal PT or PTT taken within 2 hours of arrival was significantly associated with mortality, but no significant associations were seen for abnormal fibrinogen or platelet values. There was a significant difference between mean values for PT between transfused and non-transfused patients, but not for PTT, platelet count, or fibrinogen.

In univariate linear regression models, there were no associations between RBC to plasma ratios at 24 hours in all transfused patients and length of stay or ventilator days.

Several regression models were calculated for the odds of transfusion of any blood product in the first 24 hours, as well as for total transfusion volume. Multivariate logistic regression for the association between PT, ISS, and transfusion within 24 hours of admission showed a significant association between increasing ISS and transfusion of any blood product but no significant association between PT and any transfusion. Multivariate linear regression also showed no significant correlation between ISS and PT with total amount of blood products transfused at 24 hours. In univariate logistic regression, penetrating injury was significantly associated with increased likelihood of transfusion, and in a multivariate logistic regression model of any transfusion in the first 24 hours based on injury type and ISS, both retained significant positive associations with any transfusion in the first 24 hours.

Answer: E

Murphy, C.H., D.A. Spain, and H. Shan, Coagulopathy and transfusion ratios in pediatric trauma. *Journal of Trauma and Acute Care Surgery*, 2020. **88**(5): pp. 648–653.

16 *A 6-year-old girl in the PICU with severe TBI is receiving IV vasopressors and sedation. She rapidly develops fever, metabolic acidosis, and rhabdomyolysis. Of the following medications, which should be immediately discontinued?*
   A *Epinephrine drip*
   B *Norepinephrine drip*
   C *TPN*
   D *Propofol drip*
   E *Steroids*

In a recent literature review, 44 pediatric cases and 124 adult cases of propofol infusion syndrome (PIS) have been reported. Of these cases, 21 pediatric and 65 adult patients survived. The most common clinical feature affecting almost 80% of both children and adults was metabolic acidosis, with ECG changes the second most common feature (75% of children and almost 63% of adults). Lipidemia, fever, and hepatomegaly occurred more frequently in children than in adults, while rhabdomyolysis and hyperkalemia were more frequent in adults compared with children. The overall mortality was 52% in children and 48% in adults. Upon univariate analysis, fever, hepatomegaly, and cumulative dose of propofol > 240 mg/kg were associated with an increased risk of mortality in children. The administration of steroids in the ICU has also been linked to the development of propofol infusion syndrome (PIS). Previous data have shown that patients with traumatic brain injury have an increased risk of developing PIS, and the risk in these patients is doubled when receiving 5 mg/k propofol compared with those receiving lower doses. Low-carbohydrate intake has also been implicated, with some evidence suggesting that the risk of PIS could possibly be lowered by supplementary carbohydrate infusion. There are currently no established guidelines for the treatment for PIS. Once the diagnosis is made, there is the simultaneous imperative to eliminate propofol from the body and treat the effects of PIS. There is no antidote, but an infusion of dextrose may have some benefit if PIS has a mitochondrial etiology. Although acidosis itself was not a feature shown to be directly associated with mortality, it may be the cause of an arrhythmia and will obtund responses to catecholamines in the treatment of hypotension. Patients are likely to benefit from increased minute ventilation to compensate for metabolic acidosis. Extracorporeal membrane oxygenation has also been reported to be beneficial in some cases, where response to vascular compartment filling and vasopressors/inotropes was inadequate. Should hyperkalemia, acidosis, or fever not respond adequately or in a sustained way to simpler conventional measures, we urge the early consideration of the application of hemofiltration before the development of hypotension severe enough to preclude it.

Answer: D

Hemphill, S., et al., Propofol infusion syndrome: a structured literature review and analysis of published case reports. *British Journal of Anaesthesia*, 2019. **122**(4): pp. 448–459.

17 *Pediatric trauma patients who receive tranexamic acid have an increased risk of:*
   A *Thromboembolism*
   B *Seizure*
   C *Renal dysfunction*
   D *In-hospital mortality*
   E *Stroke*

One study created 1914 pairs of patients with and without TXA administration on the day of admission. The proportion of seizures was significantly higher in the TXA group than in the non-TXA group. No other outcomes were significantly different between the groups, including death. This may imply that TXA is associated with seizures, but not with mortality, in the pediatric trauma population.

Answer: B

Maeda, T., et al., Safety of tranexamic acid during pediatric trauma: a nationwide database study. *Pediatric Critical Care Medicine*, 2018. **19**(12): pp. e637–e642.

18 *Which statement applies to the use of ECMO in pediatric trauma patients?*
   A *Trauma patients are not ECMO candidates due to high risk of bleeding.*
   B *Trauma patients have a higher mortality risk than those put on ECMO for isolated pulmonary or cardiac failure.*
   C *The group with the highest rate of survival was for patients suffering an airway injury (85.7%), while that with the lowest survival rate was for patients with intracranial injuries (25.0%).*
   D *Trauma victims always require heparin anticoagulation when started on ECMO.*
   E *Hemorrhagic and overall complication rates are higher for trauma patients than for non-trauma patients.*

Extracorporeal life support has been used to support reversible causes of cardiac and respiratory failure in pediatric patients for more than 40 years. But while ECMO has been used with increasing efficiency and frequency since its inception, its use in trauma patients has long been viewed with caution. This is due in part to the perceived risks of hemorrhage from both pre-existing injuries such as intracranial trauma, long bone fractures, and solid organ injuries, and also from possible operative procedures (laparotomy, craniotomy, etc.), potentially needed to control and manage the sequela of traumatic injuries. But recent studies have shown that these long-held concerns may not be as significant as previously thought. The top three primary trauma diagnoses were drowning/non-fatal submersion, burn injuries, and thoracic injuries. Collectively, these three diagnosis groups made up 76% of total overall injury types. Overall survival was 55.3%, which is comparable to reported overall survival rates from ELSO in both cardiac (52%) and pulmonary (59%) modes for the most recent year of 2019. The group with the highest rate of survival was for patients suffering an airway injury (85.7%), while that with the lowest survival rate was for patients with intracranial injuries (25.0%) A recent systematic review summarized the results of four different studies examining ECMO in pediatric trauma patients that met inclusion criteria. They noted that overall survival was 60% and that the majority of patients (77%) underwent veno-arterial cannulation. Anton-Martin et al. demonstrated that pre-ECMO coagulopathy does not increase the incidence of hemorrhage. Furthermore, it has been shown that it is possible to place trauma patients on ECMO with no anticoagulation initially, followed by low-dose heparin with a low therapeutic target. This study showed that hemorrhagic complications were very much in line with ELSO historical rates, as were overall complications. ECMO should be considered a valid and safe treatment strategy for the management of traumatic injuries in the appropriate setting. Although there are limited data on functional and neurological outcomes, overall survival and complication rates of pediatric trauma patients on ECMO are comparable to those reported for other indications. Trauma should not be considered a contraindication for ECMO in pediatric trauma patients.

Answer: C

Behr, C.A., et al., Characteristics and outcomes of extracorporeal life support in pediatric trauma patients. *Journal of Trauma and Acute Care Surgery*, 2020. **89**(4): pp. 631–635.

25

Envenomation, Poisoning, and Toxicology

Michelle Strong, MD, PhD[1] and Elaine Cleveland, MD[2]

[1] Trauma and Acute Care Surgeon, Austin, TX, USA
[2] William Beaumont Army Medical Center, El Paso, TX, USA

1 *Regarding opioid overdose, which statement is correct?*
   A *Oral opioids have standard pharmacokinetics and elimination that is unrelated to dosage.*
   B *Chronic opioid users develop tolerance and have less risk of developing respiratory failure.*
   C *Co-ingestion with alcohol or benzodiazepines is common and increases risk of death.*
   D *Concomitant use of cytochrome P450 inhibitors and oxycodone decreases plasma levels of oxycodone.*
   E *Intravenous hydromorphone has the shortest half-life compared to intravenous morphine or fentanyl.*

Co-ingestion is common and alcohol is involved in 1 of 5 opioid-related deaths. Ninety-one percent of co-ingestions (often suicide attempts) required mechanical ventilation and ICU admission. Oral opioids have variable pharmacokinetics. At low dosage, they are eliminated through first-order kinetics, and therefore elimination is exponential. At high doses, opioids are eliminated via zero-order kinetics, which means there is fixed elimination per unit time and the rate of elimination is independent of concentration. This can lead to late-onset opioid toxicity. While chronic opioid users develop tolerance, the tolerance to respiratory depression is less than the tolerance to the analgesic effects of opioids and are at greater risk for respiratory failure. Concomitant use of cytochrome P450 inhibitors such as macrolides increase plasma levels of oxycodone. The most common cytochrome P450 involved in drug metabolism is 3A. Intravenous hydromorphone has a half-life of 4 hours, while intravenous morphine and fentanyl have half-lives of 2–3 hours.

Answer: C

Parthvi R, Agrawal A, Khanijo S, Tsegaye A, Talwar A, Parthvi R, et al. Acute opiate overdose: an update on management strategies in emergency department and critical care unit. *American Journal of Therapeutics* 2019May/Jun; **26**(3):e380–e387.

2 *A 24-year-old woman was assaulted several hours ago and is found down in a park. She has a Glasgow Coma Scale (GCS) score of 5, ecchymosis to the right side of her face, a right scalp laceration, pinpoint pupils, and track marks down both arms. There are needles found near her. Her vitals are HR 60 beats/minute, BP 90/40 mm Hg, RR 6 breaths/minute, and pulse oximetry of 82% on room air. EMS personnel intubate the patient and give her 0.4 mg of naloxone. Which statement is true regarding the management of this patient?*
   A *She should have gastrointestinal decontamination with charcoal.*
   B *She can receive one more dose of 0.4 mg of naloxone, and then alternative reversal agents should be used.*
   C *The most common arrhythmia is a narrow complex atrial fibrillation.*
   D *Patients typically develop respiratory alkalosis and metabolic acidosis.*
   E *Alpha-agonists can be used to assist with symptoms of opioid withdrawal.*

After giving naloxone, patients can experience severe opiate withdrawal symptoms to include fever, tachycardia, restlessness, insomnia, diaphoresis, rhinorrhea, nausea, vomiting, and myalgias. Clonidine and dexmedetomidine (both alpha agonists) may help manage some of these symptoms but should be given in a monitored setting. This patient likely took intravenous opioids, i.e. heroin. Gastrointestinal decontamination is only indicated if within 1 hour of oral opioid ingestion. In patients who develop cardiac arrest due to opioids, patients should receive 2 mg of naloxone initially. Naloxone can be repeated every 2–3 minutes as needed, up to 10 mg. If a long-acting opioid is suspected, patients may require additional dosing or IV infusion, as naloxone only lasts about 20–90 minutes. The most common arrhythmia is wide complex bradycardia, which can be managed with a bolus of 1–2 mEq/kg of sodium bicarbonate. Patients typically develop respiratory acidosis due to CO_2 retention. They can develop either metabolic acidosis if they are experiencing diarrhea, or metabolic alkalosis if they have emesis.

Answer: E

Donroe JH, Tetrault JM, Donroe JH, et al. Substance use, intoxication, and withdrawal in the critical care setting. *Critical Care Clinics* 2017 Jul; **33**(3):543–558.

Parthvi R, Agrawal A, Khanijo S, Tsegaye A, Talwar A, Parthvi R, et al. Acute opiate overdose: an update on management strategies in emergency department and critical care unit. *American Journal of Therapeutics* 2019May/Jun; **26**(3):e380–e387.

3   A 26-year-old man, with long-standing depression, ingests a large quantity of lorazepam and alcohol and walks into traffic on a busy highway. When EMS arrives, the patient has a GCS score of 10, obvious facial fractures, bruising to the left chest, and an open left tibia fracture. What should be the initial management of this patient in the trauma bay?
   A   Supplemental oxygen, continuous cardiac monitoring, and intubation if needed for hypoventilation or mental status decline
   B   Intubation followed by gastrointestinal decontamination with activated charcoal
   C   Whole bowel irrigation with polyethylene glycol electrolyte solution via nasogastric tube
   D   Flumazenil 0.2 mg with repeat dosing as needed, up to 1 mg
   E   Naloxone 0.4 mg and repeat dosing as needed until mental status improves

Benzodiazepine overdose in isolation has a low morbidity and mortality rate. However, when combined with alcohol or opioids, profound respiratory depression can result. The typical management for benzodiazepine overdose is supportive care and intubation as needed. There is no role for either activated charcoal or whole bowel irrigation in isolated benzodiazepine overdose.

Whole bowel irrigation is typically used for iron, lithium, illicit drug packets, or sustained-released medications (such as diltiazem). Flumazenil, a competitive antagonist of the benzodiazepine receptor, is controversial since it can lower the seizure threshold, especially in someone who is chronically taking benzodiazepines. Flumazenil is typically used to reverse procedural sedation when a known quantity of benzodiazepines has been given. While opioids and benzodiazepines are often co-ingested, there is no history that this patient also consuming opioids. Naloxone would be used for opioid overdose.

Answer: A

Donroe JH, Tetrault JM, Donroe JH, et al. Substance use, intoxication, and withdrawal in the critical care setting. *Critical Care Clinics* 2017 Jul; **33**(3):543–558.

Weinbroum AA, Flaishon R, Sorkine P, Szold O, Rudick V. A risk-benefit assessment of flumazenil in the management of benzodiazepine overdose. *Drug Safety* 1997; **17**(3):181.

4   A 37-year-old man used cocaine and drank alcohol earlier in the evening and then drove home. The patient was involved in a motor vehicle collision versus a tree, with airbag deployment. He is complaining of severe chest pain and is anxious. His vital signs are HR 145 beats/minute, BP 185/100 mm Hg, RR 20 breaths/minute, pulse oximetry 92% on room air, and temperature 38° C. A chest x-ray, FAST exam, and CT scan imaging are only notable for a small 4-mm subdural hematoma and a grade 3 splenic laceration without extravasation. Electrocardiogram shows ST elevation and his troponin I is elevated as well. What should be the initial management of this patient?
   A   Dual antiplatelet therapy
   B   Beta-blockers to decrease heart rate and blood pressure, with goal SBP 120 mm Hg and HR <100 beats/minute
   C   Benzodiazepines followed by nitroglycerin if patient is still hypertensive
   D   Morphine, oxygen, nitroglycerin, and aspirin
   E   Percutaneous coronary intervention

Management of cocaine-induced myocardial infarction is focused on decreasing platelet aggregation with aspirin (if appropriate), decreasing vasoconstriction and hypertension with either nitrates or calcium channel blockers, and decreasing overall sympathetic tone with benzodiazepines. Unfortunately, due to the concurrent injuries of a subdural hematoma and grade 3 splenic laceration, this patient will not be able to start aspirin or undergo percutaneous coronary intervention for at least 24–48 hours after repeat imaging is stable. Beta-blockers are contraindicated in the initial management because they theoretically increase vasoconstriction due to unopposed alpha-receptor stimulation. However, multiple patients have inadvertently received beta-blockers before disclosing cocaine usage and have had no adverse effects. The 2012 American College of Cardiology guidelines state that non-selective beta-blockers (such as propranolol) may be considered in persistently hypertensive and tachycardic patients after cocaine use, provided they received a vasodilator prior to treatment with beta-blocker.

Answer: C

Donroe JH, Tetrault JM, Donroe JH, et al. Substance use, intoxication, and withdrawal in the critical care setting. *Critical Care Clinics* 2017 Jul; **33**(3):543–558.

Havakuk O, Rezkalla SH, Kloner RA, et al. The cardiovascular effects of cocaine. *Journal of the American College of Cardiology* 2017 Jul 4; **70**(1):101–113.

5 *A 27-year-old man presents to the emergency room after an altercation with another party goer. He admits to taking multiple pills of ecstasy. His vitals are HR 125 beats/minute, BP 100/70 mmHg, RR 12 breaths/minute, and temperature is 40 °C. Which of these complications is paired with its appropriate treatment?*

   A *Hyperthermia: slow cooling with ice packs ± dantrolene*

   B *Rhabdomyolysis: addressing hyperthermia and aggressive IV fluid resuscitation*

   C *Serotonin syndrome: diphenhydramine and IV fluid resuscitation*

   D *Hypernatremia: rapid correction of sodium*

   E *MDMA withdrawal: haloperidol*

Ecstasy or methylenedioxy-methylamphetamine (MDMA) intoxication is associated with hyperthermia, rhabdomyolysis, and multi-organ failure. The hyperthermia must be managed with rapid (not slow) cooling and dantrolene, though dantrolene has not been subject to randomized controlled trials. Rhabdomyolysis requires hyperthermia management and aggressive IV fluid hydration. Serotonin syndrome is more common with co-ingestion of other drugs, especially selective serotonin reuptake inhibitors (SSRIs) and monoamine oxidase inhibitors (MAOIs) and results in altered mental status, increased muscle tone, clonus, and hyperreflexia. The treatment of serotonin syndrome is benzodiazepines ± cyproheptadine. Severe serotonin syndrome may require intubation. Hyponatremia, not hypernatremia, is due to MDMA-induced antidiuretic hormone release, as well as aggressive crystalloid fluid resuscitation. With any sodium imbalance, you never want to rapidly correct sodium. Management is fluid

restriction for mild cases and careful administration of hypertonic saline, not to exceed a 10 mEq increase in 24 hours for severe cases. MDMA has also been associated with acute renal failure and acute liver failure. MDMA withdrawal is relatively mild and usually presents with depression or fatigue for up to 5 days; management is supportive. Haloperidol is contraindicated in the acute setting since it can interfere with heat dissipation, prolongs the QTc interval, and reduces the seizure threshold.

Answer: B

Donroe JH, Tetrault JM, Donroe JH, et al. Substance use, intoxication, and withdrawal in the critical care setting. *Critical Care Clinics* 2017 Jul; **33**(3):543–558.

Kalant H. The pharmacology and toxicology of "ecstasy" (MDMA) and related drugs. *CMAJ* 2001; **165**(7):917.

6 *A 75-year-old man with a history of hypertension, atrial fibrillation, hyperlipidemia, and gout is admitted to the ICU for a small bowel obstruction and severe hypertension managed with a nicardipine drip. Unfortunately, his oral diltiazem is still on his medication list, and the extended-release diltiazem is crushed and given to the patient via nasogastric tube. The patient subsequently becomes hypotensive with a BP 70/40 mm Hg and bradycardic with a HR 35 beats/minute. The nicardipine drip is stopped. What is the next step in treatment?*

   A *Whole bowel irrigation with polyethylene glycol electrolyte mix*

   B *A bolus 3–4 L of crystalloid immediately until blood pressure improves*

   C *Atropine and cardioversion if indicated*

   D *Epinephrine 2–10 mcg/min followed by an epinephrine IV infusion*

   E *Milrinone 0.5 mcg/kg/min IV infusion*

For both beta-blocker and calcium channel blocker overdose, the two basic tenets of management are high-dose insulin euglycemia therapy (HIET) and catecholamine infusions. The best choice above is epinephrine, as it will provide positive inotrope and chronotrope effects. This patient would also benefit from high-dose insulin and calcium infusion, with goal calcium 2 times the reference range. For extended-release medications, whole bowel irrigation can be used, though small bowel obstruction is a contraindication for this therapy. Additionally, once a patient becomes hypotensive and bradycardic, whole bowel irrigation should not be initiated. While fluid bolus can be beneficial, judicious fluid administration is recommended as patients are usually euvolemic and 3–4 L can lead to pulmonary edema. Atropine is rarely effective in calcium channel blocker toxicity. Finally, milrinone might be needed if the patient remains

Suspected cardiogenic shock in beta-blocker or calcium channel blocker intoxication

Treatment	Dosing	Desired clinical effect	Adverse events
High-dose insulin euglycemia	Loading dose 1U/kg; infusion 1–10 U/kg/hr with 50% glucose infusion	Positive inotrope, increased CO, increased BP, reduced catecholamine infusion	Hypoglycemia, hypokalemia, mild vasodilation, no effect on heart rate
Epinephrine	2–10 mcg/min	Increased contractility and heart rate	Hyperglycemia lactic acidemia, limb ischemia
Isoproterenol	0.5–5 mcg/min	Positive inotrope and chronotropic	Ventricular arrhythmias, worsening of hypotension secondary to B2
Calcium infusion	Loading dose 0.6 mL/kg of 10% calcium gluconate; infusion 0.6–1.6 mL/kg/hr Aim for serum Ca 2× reference range	Increased BP from improved CA and SVR	Transient effect. No effect on heart rate

bradycardic; however, this patient is hypotensive as well, and milrinone could exacerbate hypotension.

Answer: D

Graudins A, Lee HM, Druda D, Graudins A, et al. Calcium channel antagonist and beta-blocker overdose: antidotes and adjunct therapies. *British Journal of Clinical Pharmacology* 2016 Mar; **81**(3):453–461. https://doi.org/10.1111/bcp.12763. Epub 2015Oct 30.

7 *A 44-year-old man who works as a park ranger was bit by a rattlesnake just above the right ankle about 2 hours ago and just arrived in the emergency room. His right calf is swollen, firm, and he has pain to passive movement. There does not appear to be any neurovascular compromise. What should be the next step in management?*

 A *Surgical exploration of the wound with excision of all visibly envenomated tissue.*
 B *Apply tourniquet above the knee and irrigation of the site of the bite.*
 C *Incision over the bite and venom extraction.*
 D *Emergent four compartment fasciotomies of the right lower leg.*
 E *Antivenom administration and check compartment pressures.*

The current recommendation is prompt administration of antivenom (Anavip® or Crofab®). Crotalidae immune F(ab)^2 is an equine-derived antivenin and Crotalidae polyvalent immune F(ab) (Crofab®) consists of the purified Fab fragments of sheep immunoglobulin (IgG) raised against the antivenom of four snakes. These F(ab) fragments bind venom in the intravascular space and are renally excreted. Both agents are indicated for the management of adult and pediatric patients with North American pit viper envenomation. Anavip® was recently approved and has significantly longer plasma persistence than Crofab®, and this is associated with a slower decline in platelet count and fibrinogen following hospital discharge. Excision of tissue to remove venom is not recommended because it has not been shown to improve outcomes and can be disfiguring. Placing a tourniquet has been found to worsen tissue outcomes and is currently not recommended. Incision is often ineffective and can be damaging based on location. While snake envenomation can mimic compartment syndrome, the diagnosis of compartment syndrome should not be made on soft signs (firm compartments, pain out of proportion, or pain with passive stretch). Measuring compartment pressures should be performed when possible. Fasciotomies should only be considered if antivenom is given without improvement in symptoms, neurovascular compromise after antivenom is given, or if compartment pressures are greater than 30–40 mmHg following antivenom administration.

Answer: E

Toschlog EA, Bauer CR, Hall EL, et al. Surgical considerations in the management of pit viper snake envenomation. *Journal of the American College of Surgeons* 2013 Oct; **217**(4):726–735. https://doi.org/10.1016/j.jamcollsurg.2013.05.004

8 *An 18-year-old otherwise healthy man is camping in New Mexico when he is stung by a scorpion on the left foot when he was putting on his hiking boots. His vital signs are HR 135 beats/minute, BP 165/85 mm Hg, RR 20 breaths/minute, temperature 37.5°C, and pulse oximetry is 99% on 2L oxygen/nasal cannula. He has some edema, erythema, and pain to the left foot. Calf compartments are soft and the patient is able to move*

his ankle and toes normally, however, he does report some numbness at the site of the bite. He is calm and able to follow instructions. What is the best treatment?

A *Admission to ICU, mechanical ventilation if needed*

B *Oral opioids, oral benzodiazepines, and IV fluid*

C *Antivenom, NSAIDs, prazosin*

D *Antivenom, mechanical ventilation, and dobutamine infusion*

E *Antivenom, mechanical ventilation, and benzodiazepine infusion*

Most scorpion bites only cause localized pain, however, about 10% of stings result in severe systemic envenomation. This patient has both local effects and autonomic excitation with resultant tachycardia and hypertension, giving him a clinical classification of grade 2 (see chart below). For this patient, he should receive antivenom (Anascorp®), NSAIDs, and prazosin to help lower his blood pressure. His current vital signs do not suggest cardiogenic shock, pulmonary edema, or multi-organ failure that would necessitate ICU care. As he is currently calm without severe neuromuscular excitation, there is no role for benzodiazepines. The use of antivenom for scorpion stings remains controversial; however, current recommendations are for its use. There is also concern that once a patient develops severe envenomation symptoms, antivenom may be less effective.

Treatment of Scorpion Stings According to Clinical Grade

Clinical grade	Clinical effects	Treatment
1	Local effects only	Analgesia, local anesthesia
2	Autonomic excitation	Antivenom, prazosin
	Agitation and anxiety	PO benzodiazepines
3	Pulmonary edema	ICU, mechanical ventilation, antivenom, prazosin, nitroglycerin,
	Hypotension and cardiogenic shock	
	Severe neuromuscular excitation	antivenom, dobutamine
		Antivenom, IV benzodiazepines
4	Multi-organ failure	Supportive care, mechanical ventilation, inotropes

Answer: C

Isbister GK, Bawaskar HS. Scorpion envenomation. *The New England Journal of Medicine* 2014 Jul 31; **371**(5):457–463. https://doi.org/10.1056/NEJMra1401108.

Rodrigo C, Gnanathasan A. Management of scorpion envenoming: a systematic review and meta-analysis of controlled clinical trials. *Systematic Reviews* 2017 Apr 8;6(1):74. https://doi.org/10.1186/s13643-017-0469-8

9 *A 54-year-old man who works as a farmer accidentally spilled a large container of pesticide on himself. He arrives to the hospital ten minutes after exposure. He is vomiting, drooling, sweating, and both eyes are tearing. He is becoming more agitated and trying to rip off his clothes. Which statement below is true regarding organophosphate poisoning management?*

A *Rarely do patients require intubation.*

B *Atropine IV bolus followed by 2 g IV pralidoxime.*

C *Maximum dosage of atropine in 48 hours is 70 mg regardless of symptoms.*

D *Haloperidol is the main treatment for agitation.*

E *Patient may need to be restrained if uncontrolled agitation.*

The classic cholinergic overdose symptoms for organophosphate poisoning can be remembered with the mnemonic DUMBBELLS – d̲iarrhea, u̲rination, m̲iosis and m̲uscle weakness, b̲ronchorrhea and b̲radycardia, e̲mesis, l̲acrimation, l̲ethargy, s̲alivation and s̲weating. Basic management includes airway monitoring (patients may need intubation if unable to protect their airway due to salvation and vomiting), starting normal saline with a goal SBP>80 mm Hg, and assessing the patient's level of consciousness. If organophosphate poisoning is suspected, atropine IV bolus is given followed by pralidoxime. Atropine can be dosed every 5 minutes with the aim of attaining the target endpoints of atropine therapy by evaluating the improvement in cardiovascular function (SBP >80 mm Hg, HR >80 bpm) and respiratory function (no bronchorrhea and bronchospasms). The regimen will allow for as much as 70 mg of atropine to be given in stages to a patient in <30 minutes, resulting in stabilization and a low risk of atropine toxicity. Once the patient achieves the target, an atropine infusion is started to maintain therapeutic effects of atropine. The guidelines suggest an infusion giving 20% of the total dose needed to initially stabilize the patient hourly for 48 hours. Pralidoxime reactivates cholinesterase (mainly outside the central nervous system) that has been inactivated by the phosphorylation due to the organophosphate pesticides. If the patient is agitated, diazepam can be used. Restraints should be avoided in these patients as struggling or muscle tension can lead to hyperthermia. If the patient develops seizures, diazepam is first-line therapy, followed by propofol or midazolam. One should avoid haloperidol in organophosphate poisoning because it can lower the seizure threshold and prolongs the QT interval.

Answer: B

Bajracharya SR, Prasad PN, Ghimire R. Management of organophosphorus poisoning. *Journal of Nepal Health Research Council* 2016 Sep; **14**(34):131–138.

10 *A 27-year-old woman ingests the remainder of her grandmother's metoprolol tartrate (about 20 pills) in a suicide attempt. Her vitals are HR 30 beats/minute and BP 60/20 mm Hg. She is intubated, central venous access is obtained, IV fluids are administered, and an epinephrine infusion is initiated. What is the first-line treatment for beta-blocker overdose?*

A *Whole bowel irrigation with polyethylene glycol electrolyte mix*

B *High-dose insulin euglycemia therapy*

C *Calcium infusion with ionized calcium two times reference range*

D *Glucagon infusion with loading dose followed by glucagon drip*

E *Intravenous lipid emulsion*

High-dose insulin euglycemia therapy (HIET) increases the intracellular transport of glucose, lactate, and oxygen into myocardial cells. HIET increases contractility, cardiac output, and blood pressure. In animal models, HIET provided greater hemodynamic stability compared to epinephrine or glucagon alone. Whole bowel irrigation can be utilized with extended-release or long-acting medications, but given she took a short-acting beta-blocker formulation, whole bowel irrigation likely will not be effective and is not considered the mainstay of therapy. Calcium infusion can be used with calcium channel blocker overdose, but likely would not have a significant effect with beta-blocker overdose. Glucagon can be considered a second-line treatment in beta-blocker overdose for refractory hypotension and bradycardia. Due to transient effects of glucagon, a glucagon infusion is needed, and hospitals may not have an adequate supply of glucagon to sustain an infusion. Intravenous lipid emulsion can be used in refractory cardiogenic or vasodilatory shock; however, they are considered a rescue therapy and other agents should be utilized first.

Answer: B

Graudins A, Lee HM, Druda D, et al. Calcium channel antagonist and beta-blocker overdose: antidotes and adjunct therapies. *British Journal of Clinical Pharmacology* 2016 Mar; **81**(3):453–461. https://doi.org/10.1111/bcp.12763.

11 *Which patient would most likely benefit from single-dose activated charcoal (SDAC)?*

A *A 15-year-old woman who ingested 2 gm of acetaminophen about 8 hours ago; she is currently protecting her airway and refusing anything orally.*

B *A 22-year-old woman ingested 400 mg of citalopram about 4 hours ago; she is currently protecting her airway, and has a normal QT interval.*

C *A 65-year-old man ingested 2 gm of quetiapine about 6 hours ago; he is currently protecting his airway, and has a normal QT interval.*

D *A 25-year-old man ingested 5 gm of acetaminophen about 2 hours ago; he is intubated and has a nasogastric tube in place.*

E *A 30-year-old man ingested 700 mg of citalopram about 8 hours ago; he is intubated, has a nasogastric tube in place, and has a normal QT interval.*

Although single-dose activated charcoal (SDAC) is unlikely to be beneficial in many overdose patients, there is a subgroup of severe poisoning that may benefit if administered within 4 hours of ingestion. The decision to give activated charcoal should be based on the ingested drug's toxicity, potential benefit, and willingness of the patient to take charcoal. Two large, randomized trials did not demonstrate an improvement with SDAC compared to supportive care. Thus, the use of activated charcoal is somewhat controversial. The risk of aspiration pneumonitis needs to be balanced with perceived benefits. Also, in the uncooperative or delirious patient, the care team needs to weigh the need for intubation for airway protection over the benefit of SDAC. There is more benefit for high-dose drugs with a long half-life than drugs with a short half-life. For acetaminophen toxicity, two studies showed there might be some benefit in ingestions >5 g and if given with 2 hours. For citalopram, if prolonged QT interval and within 4 hours of ingestion, SDAC might be beneficial. For normal QT interval and ingestion <4 hours, citalopram dosages <600 mg do not need SDAC, dosages 600–1000 mg may benefit from SDAC, and dosages >1000 mg should receive SDAC and at least 13 hours of cardiac monitoring post-ingestion.

Answer A is incorrect because the patient took a relatively low dose, it has been 8 hours since ingestion, and this is an uncooperative patient. N-acetylcysteine given within 8 hours of acetaminophen and supportive care is reasonable management for patient A. Answer B is incorrect because the patient took a relatively low dose and does not have any QT interval abnormalities. Answer C is incorrect because quetiapine has a rather short half-life of 6 hours and SDAC is less effective in drugs with a short half-life. Answer D is correct because the patient had a large dose of acetaminophen and it was consumed about 2 hours ago. For patient E, the ingestion was moderate; however, it has been longer than 4 hours and with a normal QT interval, the patient would not benefit from SDAC.

Answer: D

Isbister GK, Kumar VV. Indications for single-dose activated charcoal administration in acute overdose. *Current Opinion in Critical Care* 2011 Aug; **17**(4):351–357.

Juurlink, D. Activated charcoal for acute overdose: a reappraisal. *British Journal of Clinical Pharmacology* 2016 Mar; 81(3):482–487.

12 *A 19-year-old woman ingests 20 tablets of 500 mg acetaminophen about 5 hours ago. The patient currently has nausea, vomiting, and abdominal pain. Her vitals are HR 105 beats/minute, BP 100/70 mm Hg, RR 20 breaths/minute, pulse oximetry is 93% on room air. Which of the following statements is true regarding acetaminophen toxicity?*

A *It is important to get initial acetaminophen levels and the time since ingestion to guide N-acetylcysteine treatment.*

B *For oral N-acetylcysteine regimen, treat for 20 hours or until liver function tests normalize.*

C *For IV N-acetylcysteine regimen, treat every 4 hours for 18 doses.*

D *If patient presents <8 hours since ingestion, liver function tests, basic metabolic panel, and international normalized ratio are of little benefit.*

E *The Rumack-Matthew nomogram is useful 4–72 hours after ingestion.*

N-acetylcysteine (NAC) is an effective antidote for acetaminophen (APAP) overdose. NAC provides cysteine for the replenishment and maintenance of hepatic glutathione stores, enhances the sulfation pathway of elimination, and reduces the progression to fulminant liver failure if administered within 8 hours of ingestion. On presentation, acetaminophen concentration and the time since ingestion should be obtained (answer A). The Rumack-Matthew nomogram uses acetaminophen levels to determine the need for NAC administration, and it is only useful for single acute ingestions. NAC therapy is most effective when initiated in the first 8 hours following ingestion, but is recommended to be initiated no later than 24 hours (Answer E is incorrect). The Rumack-Matthews nomogram should not be used for chronic ingestions and is inaccurate in sustained-release products. Recommended dosing for oral NAC is 140 mg/kg loading dose followed by 70 mg/kg every 4 hours for 18 doses, which will take 72 hours (not 20 hours as in answer B). Dosing for IV NAC is a loading dose 150 mg/kg over 1 hour, then 50 mg/kg over 4 hours, then 100 mg/kg for 16 hours (answer C is incorrect). While liver function tests (LFTs), basic metabolic panel (BMP), and international normalized ratio (INR) are more important

for those patients presenting after 8 hours, it is important to get these laboratory tests as soon as the patient presents, since NAC may need to be started in those patients with significant liver derangements.

Answer: A

Fisher ES, Curry SC. Evaluation and treatment of acetaminophen toxicity. *Advances in Pharmacology* 2019; **85**:263–272.

Hodgman MJ, Garrard AR. A review of acetaminophen poisoning. *Critical Care Clinics* 2012 Oct; **28**(4):499–516.

Rumack BH, Matthew H. Acetaminophen poisoning and toxicology. *Pediatrics* 1975; **55**(6): 871–876.

13 *A 73-year-old woman with a medical history of chronic kidney disease and diabetes for which she takes glipizide was recently discharged from the hospital after treatment for a urinary tract infection. EMS was called because she was obtunded and slumped in her chair. Her finger stick glucose by paramedics was 42 mg/dL. She is given 50% dextrose intravenous and arouses. In the emergency department, she is initially alert and answering questions with the following vital signs: BP 115/68 mm Hg, HR 74 beats/minute, RR 16 breaths/minute, and her temperature is 36.8 °C. Her physical exam is unremarkable. During evaluation, the patient becomes confused, lethargic, and diaphoretic, and repeat finger stick glucose is 32 mg/dL. She again responds to 50% dextrose but becomes unresponsive 30 minutes later. She is started on an IV infusion of 10% dextrose, but still requires several boluses of 50% dextrose for hypoglycemia. Which is the most appropriate intervention for this patient?*

A *Thiamine 100 mg intravenous*

B *Dextrose 20% via nasogastric tube*

C *Octreotide subcutaneous*

D *Sodium bicarbonate infusion*

E *Glucagon intramuscular*

Severe, prolonged hypoglycemia is characteristic of ingestion of large doses of sulfonylureas. Sulfonylurea agents stimulate insulin release from the pancreas, resulting in hypoglycemia. Risk factors for hypoglycemia from supratherapeutic ingestion include age >65 years, multiple medications, frequent hospitalizations, use of agents with longer durations of action (e.g. chlorpropamide and glyburide) and impaired drug clearance; renal insufficiency can increase the risk of hypoglycemia fourfold. Patients with a sulfonylurea overdose and symptomatic hypoglycemia are immediately treated with IV dextrose. However, IV dextrose should not be used as monotherapy because it may cause hyperglycemia that triggers increased insulin release, leading to recurrent episodes of hypoglycemia. Octreotide is a somatostatin analogue that inhibits release of insulin from the pancreas and has been found to be effective in treating hypoglycemia and shortening the period of hypoglycemia. The most important mechanism of action is G-protein-mediated decrease in calcium influx through voltage-gated channels in pancreatic beta islet cells, which diminishes calcium-mediated insulin release. The dose of octreotide is 50–150 μg administered either intramuscular or subcutaneous as an injection every six hours. If thiamine deficiency (from alcoholism or other forms of malnutrition) is suspected, IV thiamine 100 mg is given in conjunction with glucose but will not treat symptomatic hypoglycemia. Glucagon given IM stimulates hepatic glycogenolysis and raises serum glucose levels slightly. The efficacy of glucagon is dependent upon hepatic glycogen stores, which may be depleted in the setting of prolonged hypoglycemia. The short duration of action of glucagon further limits its effectiveness. In addition, glucagon is not recommended for sulfonylurea exposure. Oral administration of dextrose in a severely ill patient is unreliable. Sodium bicarbonate is indicated only for metformin-induced metabolic acidosis.

Answer: C

Carr R, Zed PJ. Octreotide for sulfonylurea-induced hypoglycemia following overdose. *Annals of Pharmacotherapy* 2002; **36**:1727–1732.

Fasano CJ, O'Malley G, Dominici P, et al. Comparison of octreotide and standard therapy versus standard therapy alone for the treatment of sulfonylurea-induced hypoglycemia. *Annals of Emergency Medicine* 2008; **51**:400–406.

Green RS, Palatnik W. Effectiveness of octreotide in a case of refractory sulfonylurea-induced hypoglycemia. *Journal of Emergency Medicine* 2003; **25**:283–287.

Klein-Schwartz W, Stassinos GL, Ibister GK. Treatment of sulfonylurea and insulin overdose. *British Journal of Clinical Pharmacology* 2016 Mar; 81(3):496–504.

Shorr RI, Ray WA, Daugherty JR, et al. Incidence and risk factors for serious hypoglycemia in older persons using insulin or sulfonylureas. *Archives of Internal Medicine* 1997; **157**:1681–1686.

14   *A 27-year-old otherwise healthy man underwent multiple surgeries for gunshot wounds to the chest, abdomen, and lower extremity. On discharge, he is prescribed acetaminophen/oxycodone 2 tablets every 4 hours as needed for pain and has been taking additional acetaminophen at home. He presents to the emergency department with abdominal pain, nausea, and vomiting. Lab work is notable for an aspartate aminotransferase activity (AST) of 2000 U/L, alanine aminotransferase (ALT) of 2700 U/L, and an international normalized ratio (INR) of 2.3. Imaging, to include ultrasound and computed tomography of the abdomen, has no explanation for his elevated laboratory values. How should this patient be managed?*

   A *Patient can be discharged from the emergency department as imaging is unremarkable.*
   B *Patient should be admitted for IV hydration and pain control.*
   C *Patient should be admitted for IV hydration, and all acetaminophen products should be discontinued.*
   D *Serum acetaminophen (APAP) should be checked, and N-acetylcysteine (NAC) should be started if APAP level elevated.*
   E *Serum acetaminophen should be checked, but patient is outside the window for N-acetylcysteine treatment.*

This patient likely has had multiple supratherapeutic ingestions of acetaminophen. As this patient is demonstrating elevated liver enzymes, acetaminophen levels should be checked, and NAC should be started if the acetaminophen level is >10 μg/mL. Studies from the 1990s suggest improved transplant-free survival in APAP-induced fulminant liver failure with starting NAC therapy as early as possible. NAC improves hepatic perfusion, improves oxygenation, improves mitochondrial function, and improves scavenging of free oxygen radicals. Patients who present with liver failure have a less favorable prognosis, but it is still clear that NAC treatment improves their chance of surviving. Answer A, B, and C are incorrect as APAP should be checked and treatment initiated if elevated levels. Answer E is incorrect since the patient may still benefit from NAC therapy even if greater than 24 hours, especially given his elevated liver enzymes.

Answer: D

Fisher ES, Curry SC. Evaluation and treatment of acetaminophen toxicity. *Advances in Pharmacology* 2019;**85**:263–272.

Hodgman MJ, Garrard AR. A review of acetaminophen poisoning. *Critical Care Clinics* 2012 Oct; **28**(4):499–516.

15   *In a patient with acute salicylate poisoning, what acid–base status would you expect?*
   A *Metabolic acidosis followed by respiratory alkalosis*
   B *Respiratory acidosis followed by metabolic alkalosis*

C *Metabolic alkalosis followed by respiratory acidosis*

D *Respiratory alkalosis followed by metabolic acidosis*

E *Metabolic acidosis followed by respiratory acidosis*

The triad of salicylate poisoning consists of hyperventilation, tinnitus, and gastrointestinal irritation. Initially, salicylate poisoning will present with hyperventilation resulting in respiratory alkalosis due to low CO_2. As the poisoning progresses and more salicylate acid is incorporated into the mitochondria, lactic acidosis results and causes an anion gap metabolic acidosis. At the final stage, the ability to compensate for acidosis is overwhelmed and a profound metabolic acidosis results, which can lead to end-organ injury. With salicylate poisoning, patients should have laboratory evaluations to include salicylate levels, blood gas levels, and a basic metabolic panel. Serial laboratory levels should be checked until there is a clear downward trend. The most important first-line treatment is intravascular volume and alkalinization of the serum and urine. A good initial fluid is D_5W plus 3 ampules of bicarbonate plus 40 mEq of potassium chloride. This should be infused at a rate of 2–3 mL/kg/hr to maintain urine output of 1–2 mL/kg/hr. Patients may require intubation if pulmonary edema develops or they are unable to protect their airway. Hemodialysis is definitive treatment and is indicated in severe acidosis refractory to supportive care or with end-organ injury such as seizures, rhabdomyolysis, or renal failure.

Answer: D

O'Malley GF. Emergency department management of the salicylate-poisoned patient. *Emergency Medicine Clinics of North America* 2007 May; 25(2):333–346.
Palmer BF, Clegg DJ. Salicylate toxicity. *The New England Journal of Medicine* 2020 Jun 25;382(26):2544–2555.

16 *A 35-year-old man is brought to the emergency department by his roommates appearing quite intoxicated. His roommates state that he has been depressed recently and was working on his car this afternoon. He is alert, but oriented only to self. His vital signs are 122/70 mm Hg, HR 81 beats/minute, RR 26 breaths/minute. His serum ethanol concentration is 20 mg/dL and his serum ethylene glycol level is 98 mg/dL. Which is the most appropriate therapy?*

A *Thiamine intravenous*

B *Ethanol infusion*

C *Fomepizole*

D *Activated charcoal*

E *Observation in the ED and discharge when sober*

Toxicity due to non-ethanol alcohol ingestions are infrequent but can result in significant morbidity and mortality. Ethylene glycol is metabolized by alcohol dehydrogenase to glycoaldehyde and glycolic acid and then eventually to glyoxylic acid and oxalic acid. Methanol is metabolized by alcohol dehydrogenase to formaldehyde, which is then converted to formic acid. Accumulation and precipitation of calcium oxalate crystals in the renal tubules that leads to the development of acute tubular necrosis occurs after *ethylene glycol* ingestion. Fomepizole and ethanol are *inhibitors* of alcohol dehydrogenase (not inducers) and thus inhibit the formation of toxic metabolites of both substances. Fomepizole is the preferred agent because it does not exacerbate the inebriated state. Ethanol infusions can be difficult to dose. Metabolic acidosis with an elevated anion gap and an elevated osmolar gap are classic features of non-ethanol intoxication. The equation to calculate osmolality is [2xNa (mmol/L) + Glucose/18(mg/dL) +BUN/2.8(mg/dL) + Ethanol/3.7(mg/dL)]. A normal osmol gap is <10. Thiamine is a cofactor in the metabolism of ethylene glycol, but it would not be preferred to administer thiamine before fomepizole. Activated charcoal is not an option for gastric decontamination because it is not effective for alcohols.

Answer: C

Ammar KA, Heckerling PS. Ethylene glycol poisoning with a normal anion gap caused by concurrent ethanol ingestion: Importance of the osmolar gap. *American Journal of Kidney Diseases* 1996; 27:130–133.
Barceloux DG, Bond GR, Krenzelok EP, et al. American Academy of Clinical Toxicology practice guidelines on the treatment of ethylene glycol poisoning. *Journal of Toxicology. Clinical Toxicology* 1999; 37:537–560.
Kruse JA. Methanol poisoning. *Intensive Care Medicine* 1992; 18:391–397.
Mokhlesi B, Leiken JB, Murray P, et al. Adult toxicology in critical care: Part II: specific poisonings. *Chest* 2003; 123:897–922.
Rietjens AJ, deLange DW, Meulenbelt J. Ethylene glycol or methanol intoxication: which antidote should be used, fomepizole or ethanol? *The Netherlands Journal of Medicine* 2014 Feb;72(2):73–79.
Zimmerman JL (2003) Poisonings and overdoses in the intensive care unit: general and specific management issues. *Critical Care Medicine*; 31:2794–2801.

17 *A 26-year-old man, otherwise healthy and weighing 70 kg, thought he had 200 mg tablets rather than 800 mg tablets of ibuprofen and accidentally ingested 4000 mg of ibuprofen about 3 hours ago. He presents to the emergency department with mild epigastric pain and his vital signs are HR 75 beats/minute,*

BP 110/70 mm Hg, RR 18 breaths/minute, temperature 98.0° F, and pulse oximetry is 98% on room air.
What is the best course of action?

A The patient can be discharged immediately.

B The patient should be observed for 4–6 hours and
   can be discharged if vital signs remain normal.

C The patient should be observed for 4–6 hours,
   receive 2–3 L of crystalloid, and can be discharged
   if vital signs remain normal.

D The patient should be admitted with IV resuscitation and serial laboratory work.

E The patient should receive gastrointestinal decontamination with activated charcoal.

Most patients have no symptoms, or mild symptoms,
after ibuprofen toxicity. Asymptomatic patients with
mild GI symptoms can be observed for 4–6 hours and
can be discharged if vital signs remain normal (answer
B). Usually symptoms do not present unless someone
has ingested >100 mg/kg of ibuprofen. Ibuprofen is rapidly metabolized with a half-life of 2 hours and is usually
completely metabolized by 24 hours. Young children are
the most common group to present with ibuprofen toxicity. The most common symptoms following ibuprofen
toxicity are mostly gastrointestinal in nature and include
abdominal pain, nausea, vomiting, and mucosal hemorrhage. Renal toxicity has also been seen in <5% of ibuprofen toxicity, but typically the creatinine will normalize by
72 hours. In massive ibuprofen toxicity of >400 mg/kg,
CNS depression can result. Children after massive ingestions may have seizures and apnea. Patients may develop
metabolic acidosis and thrombocytopenia after ibuprofen toxicity. Mechanical ventilation, aggressive crystalloid resuscitation, cardiac monitoring, and frequent
laboratory testing should be considered in patients with
respiratory depression, hypotension, seizures, or metabolic acidosis. Since the half-life of ibuprofen is short and
this patient presents >2 hours after ingestion, there is no
role for single-dose activated charcoal administration
(answer E).

Answer: B

Ershad M, Ameer MA, Vearrier D. Ibuprofen toxicity. 2020
   Oct 5. In: *StatPearls* [Internet]. Treasure Island (FL):
   StatPearls Publishing; 2020 Jan.

18 A 45-year-old woman has been receiving a nitro-
    prusside infusion for severe hypertension for 3 days.
    When the nurse checks on her, she is unresponsive,
    hypoxic, hypotensive, and an arterial blood gas
    shows an anion gap metabolic acidosis with an ele-
    vated lactate. The nurse notes that when drawing
    labs from her previously placed IV, the blood is bright
    red and appears arterial even though it is a venous
    draw. What is the treatment for this patient?

A Methylene blue
B High-dose insulin euglycemic therapy
C Sodium thiosulfate
D Epinephrine
E N-acetylcysteine

This patient is likely suffering from cyanide poisoning.
When nitroprusside is administered at high doses for an
extended period, cyanide accumulates. Other sources of
cyanide toxicity come from industrial solvents, insecti-
cides in farming, electroplating, tanning, metal work,
jewelry cleaning, solvents for nail and glue removal,
combustion of synthetic polymers, and some foods such
as apricot pits and cherry pits. The hallmark presentation is hypoxia and metabolic acidosis with high lactate
levels. Other symptoms include dizziness, headache,
weakness, flushing, diaphoresis, dyspnea, and hyperventilation. The classic "bitter almond smell" is rarely recognized and the "cherry red flush" is more often seen
postmortem rather than in acute poisoning. Patients
sometimes have bright red venous blood. The treatment
is supportive and includes oxygen therapy and a cyanide
antidote kit, which consists of amyl nitrite, sodium
nitrite, and sodium thiosulfate. Sodium thiosulfate
enhances clearance of cyanide by acting as a sulfhydryl
donor. Thiosulfate combines with cyanide extracellularly
and forms thiocyanate, which is renally eliminated.
Methylene blue is the antidote for methemoglobinemia.
High-dose insulin euglycemic therapy is the antidote for
beta-blockers. Epinephrine can be used for shock.
N-acetylcysteine is used for acetaminophen toxicity.

Answer: C

Gracia R, Shepherd G. Cyanide poisoning and its
   treatment. *Pharmacotherapy* 2004 Oct;
   24(10):1358–1365.
Parker-Cote JL, Rizer J, Vakkalanka JP, et al. Challenges in
   the diagnosis of acute cyanide poisoning. *Clinical
   Toxicology (Philadelphia, Pa.)* 2018 Jul;56(7):609–617.
Udeh CI, Ting M, Arango M, et al. Delayed presentation of
   nitroprusside-induced cyanide toxicity. *The Annals of
   Thoracic Surgery* 2015 Apr;99(4):1432–1434.

19 A 23-year-old woman presents to the emergency
    department after taking 30 citalopram 20 mg tablets
    about 2 hours ago. Her vital signs are as follows:
    BP 130/82 mmHg, HR 74 beats/minute, RR
    16 breaths/minute, and temperature 98.1° F. Which
    is the best intervention for this patient?

A Recommend a cooling blanket to prevent serotonin
   syndrome-related hypothermia.

B Administer diazepam 5mg IV to prevent seizure
   activity.

C Discharge the patient home without therapy since
   her vitals are normal.

D *Administer 20% lipid emulsion bolus.*

E *Order a 12-lead electrocardiogram to monitor for cardiac conduction disturbances.*

Citalopram is a serotonin reuptake inhibitor (SSRI). Most SSRIs are relatively safe, and many patients will present asymptomatic after an overdose. However, there is a potential for patient's developing serious adverse effects such as serotonin syndrome, seizures, and cardiac toxicity. It is recommended that the patient be observed for at least 6–8 hours. Measures should be performed to reduce hyperthermia (not hypothermia) if a serotonergic syndrome develops; this should be treated with measures to reduce muscle activity, such as cypoheptadine, not by applying measures to enhance surface cooling. Although this patient is stable and has no specific concerns, it is recommended to check a 12-lead electrocardiogram (ECG) to measure QT-interval prolongation and treat with sodium bicarbonate, if necessary. A benzodiazepine should be administered if muscle rigidity develops, but it is not used prophylactically. Lipid emulsion can be used for cardiovascular collapse in SSRI overdose.

Answer: E

Alapat PM, Zimmerman JL. Toxicology in the intensive care unit. *Chest* 2008; **133**:1006–1013.

Cooke MJ, Waring WS. Citalopram and cardiac toxicity. *European Journal of Clinical Pharmacology* 2013 Apr;69(4):755–760.

Dunkley EJ, Isbister GK, Sibbritt D, et al. The Hunter Serotonin Toxicity Criteria: simple and accurate diagnostic rules for serotonin toxicity. *QJM* 2003; **96**:635–642.

20 *A 65-year-old man has MRSA bacteremia secondary to pneumonia. He undergoes an awake transesophageal echocardiogram (TEE) to look for vegetations and received 20% benzocaine spray (topical anesthetic) for the exam. The cardiologist is having trouble viewing the mitral valve and the procedure takes longer than anticipated. Shortly after the procedure, he develops central cyanosis, anxiety, and tachypnea. What is true about his condition?*

A *Textbooks describe cherry red flush and bright red venous blood.*

B *There is a discrepancy between oxygen saturation on pulse oximetry and oxygen saturation on arterial blood gas.*

C *Diagnosis is made clinically as laboratory values are often inaccurate.*

D *The treatment is supplemental oxygen and sodium thiosulfate.*

E *Patients with end-stage renal disease and liver failure are more prone to this condition.*

This patient has methemoglobinemia (MetHb) secondary to benzocaine given during the transesophageal echocardiogram (TEE) procedure. The two most common medications that cause methemoglobinemia are dapsone and benzocaine. Methemoglobinemia can also be hereditary, caused by a deficiency in cytochrome B5 reductase. Symptoms tend to correlate with MetHb levels. Answer C is incorrect because the symptoms are nonspecific and the laboratory test for MetHb confirms diagnosis. Cyanosis occurs with MetHb > 15%; anxiety, headache, and dizziness occur with MetHb > 20%; fatigue, confusion, and tachypnea occur with MetHb >30%; and arrhythmias, acidosis, seizures, and coma occur with MetHb > 50%. A unique feature of methemoglobinemia is chocolate brown color blood, not bright red blood (answer A), which is associated with cyanide poisoning. The pulse oximeter measures light absorbance at 660 and 940 nm wavelengths. MetHb absorbs light at both wavelengths, distorting the ratio. The pulse oximetry may read 85%; however, the arterial oxygen on a blood gas is usually much lower (answer B). Treatment is supplemental oxygen, withdrawal of the offending agent, and methylene blue given at a dose of 1–2 mg/kg for 5 minutes. Methylene blue accelerates the reduction of MetHb via the NADPH reductase pathway. Sodium thiosulfate is used for cyanide poisoning (answer D). Patients with anemia, underlying pulmonary conditions such as COPD or pneumonia, and cardiac disease, are more prone to symptoms at lower MetHb because there is less oxygen circulating from fewer boxcars transporting oxygen (anemia), poor gas exchange (pulmonary), or inability to circulate blood (cardiac). End-stage renal and hepatic diseases do not seem to influence the development of methemoglobinemia (answer E).

Answer: B

Cefalu JN, Joshi TV, Spalitta MJ, et al. Methemoglobinemia in the operating room and intensive care unit: early recognition, pathophysiology, and management. *Advances in Therapy* 2020; 37(5):1714–1723.

Skold A, Cosco DL, Klein R. Methemoglobinemia: pathogenesis, diagnosis, and management. *Southern Medical Journal* 2011 Nov; **104**(11):757–761.

21 *A 74-year-old man with atrial fibrillation, congestive heart failure, hypertension, and chronic kidney dysfunction confuses his medications and ingests 4 pills of 250 mcg digoxin. He presents to the emergency room with a wide complex bradycardia with multiple missed beats and hyperkalemia. What is the treatment of choice?*

A *High-dose insulin euglycemia therapy*

B *Calcium gluconate*

C *Fructose diphosphate*

D *Digoxin-specific antibody*

E *Glucagon*

Digoxin is a cardiac glycoside that works as a weakly positive inotrope that acts via inhibition of Na^+/K^+-ATPase. It induces an increase in intracellular sodium that will drive an accumulation of intracellular calcium via the Na^+-Ca^{++} exchange system. In the heart, increased intracellular calcium causes more calcium to be released by the sarcoplasmic reticulum, thereby more calcium can bind to troponin-C and increase contractility. Inhibition of the Na^+/K^+-ATPase in vascular smooth muscle causes depolarization that causes smooth muscle contraction and vasoconstriction. Digoxin increases vagal efferent activity of the heart. This parasympathomimetic action reduces the sinoatrial (SA) firing rate (decreases heart rate) and reduces conduction velocity of electrical impulses through the atrioventricular node (AV). Digoxin works in a narrow therapeutic window and toxicity can be profound. Digoxin-specific antibody (Fab) is a monovalent immunoglobin that binds to digoxin and is eventually renally excreted. High-dose insulin euglycemia therapy (Answer A) is used for beta-blocker or calcium channel overdose. Calcium gluconate (Answer B) would be used for calcium channel blocker overdose. Fructose diphosphate (Answer C) has some limited efficacy for digoxin toxicity, but it is not mainstay of treatment. Glucagon (answer E) is second line for refractory bradycardia or hypotension in beta-blocker toxicity.

Answer: D

Bauman JL, Didomenico RJ, Galanter WL. Mechanisms, manifestations, and management of digoxin in the modern era. *American Journal of Cardiovascular Drugs* 2006; **6**(2):77–86.

Chan BSH, Buckley NA. Digoxin-specific antibody fragments in the treatment of digoxin toxicity. *Clinical Toxicology (Philadelphia, Pa.)* 2014;52(8):824–836.

Haptman PJ, Blume SW, Lewis EF, et al. Digoxin toxicity and use of digoxin immune fab: Insights from a national hospital database. *JACC Heart Fail.* 2016 May;4(5):357–364.

22 *A 65-year-old man was involved in a motor vehicle crash and sustained multiple right rib fractures with a flail segment from ribs 6 to 10 with a pulmonary contusion and hemothorax. The patient was admitted to the trauma ICU. On post-trauma day 2, he has a rib stabilization procedure and an intercostal peripheral nerve block is performed using bupivacaine at the end of the case. The patient is extubated and brought back to the ICU to recover. Thirty minutes later, the patient complains of tongue numbness and blurred vision. The nurse notes the patient is becoming more confused and has not received any pain medication. His vital signs are BP 185/90 mm Hg and HR 125 beats/minute. He subsequently becomes unresponsive and unarousable and his blood pressure and HR both drop significantly (BP 100/60 mm Hg, HR 52 beats/minute). Following airway control and ACLS protocol to initially stabilize the patient, what is the next step in treatment for this patient?*

A *Propofol intravenous bolus to prevent seizures*

B *Vasopressin intravenous bolus followed by an infusion*

C *Nicardipine infusion*

D *Lipid emulsion 20% bolus followed by infusion*

E *Procainamide intravenous to treat arrhythmias*

This is likely an accidental intravascular injection of local anesthetic during administration causing local anesthetic systemic toxicity (LAST). The mechanism has been difficult to establish. Local anesthetics inhibit many components of the oxidative phosphorylation pathway. Thus, LAST affects the 2 organs that are inherently less tolerant of anaerobic metabolism: the heart and the brain. Lipid emulsion therapy is the treatment of choice after ACLS protocols and stabilization. A bolus of 1.5 ml/kg of 20% lipid emulsion followed by 0.25 ml/kg/min for 10 minutes. This therapy forms a "lipid sink" by expanding the intravascular lipid phase that acts to absorb the offending circulating lipophilic toxin. Thus, reducing the unbound free toxin available to bind. Propofol can be used to treat seizures; however, it may worsen associated hypotension or cardiac depression. If seizures develop, benzodiazepines are the treatment of choice. Epinephrine is recommended to restore cardiac output. Small doses (<1 mcg/kg) should be used to avoid impaired pulmonary gas exchange and increases in afterload. Vasopressin should be avoided as it can result in pulmonary hemorrhage. Calcium channel and beta blockers are not recommended. Patients may be hyperdynamic initially, then have cardiac depression later in the toxicity. These agents could exacerbate this condition. Ventricular arrhythmias are the potential result of the cardiac dysfunction. Procainamide can exacerbate the existing toxicity.

Answer: D

El-Boghdadly K, Pawa A, Chin KJ. Local anesthetics systemic toxicity: current perspectives. *Local and Regional Anesthesia* 2018; **11**:35–44.

Ok SH, Hong JM, Lee SH, et al. Lipid emulsion for treating local anesthetic systemic toxicity. *International Journal of Medical Sciences* 2018; **15**(7):713–722.

26

Common Procedures in the ICU

Fariha Sheikh, MD and Adam D. Fox, DO, DPM

Division of Trauma and Critical Care Surgery, Rutgers New Jersey Medical School, University Hospital, Newark, NJ, USA

1 *When preparing to intubate a patient with a difficult airway, which of the following is true?*
   A *An assistant is unnecessary*
   B *Having a variety of laryngoscopes is unnecessary*
   C *You do not need videolaryngoscopy as back up*
   D *Single person mask ventilation is ideal*
   E *Preoxygenating the patient is recommended*

Per the American Society of Anesthesiology guidelines for difficult intubations, the initial assessment for identifying a potentially difficult airway begins with history and physical exam. Physical characteristics that might indicate a difficult airway include, but are not limited to, a short and thick neck, overbite, thyromental distance less than 3 fingerbreadths, inability to extend the neck, and stiff or non-resilient mandible.

If a difficult airway is suspected, recommendations include having an assistant to help with adequate bag mask ventilation and preparing alternate tools and methods of intubation. A portable airway equipment kit is recommended and should include various types and sizes of laryngoscopes, various sizes of endotracheal and supraglottic tubes, and a device to assess for end-tidal CO2. If available, a videolaryngoscope is recommended to aid in visualization of the cords and safe intubation. A laryngeal mask airway or other supraglottic tube may also be useful in the event of a failed attempt at endotracheal intubation. Although data vary on the exact duration of preoxygenation, studies recommend at least one minute of preoxygenation prior to intubation. Additionally, attempts to oxygenate during intubation, such as through nasal cannula or a blow by mask, should be attempted.

Answer: E

American Society of Anesthesiologists (2013) Practice guidelines for management of the difficult airway: an updated report by the American Society of Anesthesiologists Task Force on Management of the Difficult Airway. *Anesthesiology*, 118 (2): 1–20.

Higgs, A., McGrath, B. A., Goddard, C. (2018) Guidelines for the management of tracheal intubation in critically ill adults. *British Journal of Anesthesia*, 120 (2): 323–352.

2 *Which of the following is true regarding arterial line catheters for hemodynamic monitoring?*
   A *The most common complication is permanent arterial occlusion.*
   B *The most common artery catheterized is the femoral artery.*
   C *A risk factor for line infection includes arterial catheters that have been in place for greater than 96 hours.*
   D *Sepsis occurs in up to 5% of all arterial line infections.*
   E *Axillary artery catheterization has a known risk of potential brain emboli.*

Arterial catheters are often placed for hemodynamic monitoring and frequent evaluation of arterial blood gas. The most common location for arterial line placement is the radial artery, though other commonly used sites include the femoral and axillary arteries. Potential complications from arterial catheterization include occlusion, line infection, sepsis, hemorrhage, pseudoaneurysm, and hematoma. The most common complication is temporary occlusion of the artery which has been reported at 1.5% to 35%, rather than permanent occlusion which occurs in <1% of cases. However, the risk of occlusion does increase when larger catheters are utilized.

Although infections associated with arterial lines are relatively rare, risk factors include an indwelling catheter for >96 hours, pseudoaneurysm, and lack of aseptic technique. Additionally rare is the rate of sepsis which has been reported to be <1%; however, this again can be linked to pseudoaneurysm.

Surgical Critical Care and Emergency Surgery: Clinical Questions and Answers, Third Edition.
Edited by Forrest "Dell" Moore, Peter M. Rhee, and Carlos J. Rodriguez.
© 2022 John Wiley & Sons Ltd. Published 2022 by John Wiley & Sons Ltd.
Companion website: www.wiley.com/go/surgicalcriticalcare3e

Answer: C

Bedford, R. F. (1977) Radial arterial function following percutaneous cannulation with 18- and 20-gauge catheters. *Anesthesiology*, 47: 37–39.

Brzezinski M, Luisetti T, London MJ. Radial artery cannulation: a comprehensive review of recent anatomic and physiologic investigations. *Anesthesia and Analgesia* 2009 Dec; 109(6): 1763–1781.

Scheer, B. V., Perel, A., Pfeiffer, U. J. (2002) Clinical review: complications and risk factors of peripheral arterial catheters used for haemodynamic monitoring in anaesthesia and critical care medicine. *Critical Care*, 6 (3): 199–204.

Wolf, S., Mangano, D. T. (1980) Pseudoaneurysm, a late complication of radial-artery catheterization. *Anesthesiology*, 52 (1): 80–81.

3 *A 60-year-old woman underwent a pelvic exenteration with significant blood loss. She is noted to be hypotensive and oliguric. After some time trying to resuscitate the patient through 2 large-bore peripheral intravenous lines without improvement, you have decided to place a central line. In terms of preventing central venous catheter line infections:*

A *Aseptic technique is only needed for immunocompromised patients.*

B *Maximum barrier precautions should be utilized.*

C *Antibiotic-coated catheters do not offer any benefit in preventing infections.*

D *Catheter insertion sites should be checked every 3 days for signs of infection.*

E *Catheters can remain in place for any number of days as long as the insertion site does not demonstrate signs of erythema.*

Aseptic technique, including maximum barrier precautions, is recommended for all patients when placing central venous access. The possible exception is for when the line is placed in an emergent fashion for the patient in extremis; however, central lines not performed under sterile technique must be removed as soon as possible and new lines placed using sterile technique. Antibiotic-coated catheters do decrease the risk of catheter-related blood infections. All catheters should have the dressing and insertion site assessed at least once per day to ensure it remains protected and clean in order to minimize risk of infection. Catheters should be removed once the catheter is no longer needed and they should not stay in longer than a maximum of 7 days.

Answer: B

Apfelbaum, J. L. (2020) Anesthesiologists task force on central venous access. *Anesthesiology*, 132: 8–43.

Ikusika, O., Waxman, M., Asher, S. (2013) Recommended site for central venous catheter placement: a review of current practice guidelines. *Critical Care Medicine*, 41 (12): A275.

4 *Which of the following are true when considering using ultrasound guidance for central line placement as opposed to landmark techniques?*

A *The landmark techniques allow for visualization of thrombus within the vein.*

B *Inadvertent puncture of the adjacent artery is always prevented when using ultrasound guidance.*

C *Ultrasound guidance for placing a central line in the subclavian vein has not shown any benefit in outcomes and less complications.*

D *There is a higher rate of success with the landmark technique.*

E *Ultrasound aids in identifying abnormal vascular anatomy prior to puncture.*

Use of ultrasound guidance for central line placement has increased due to numerous studies demonstrating decreased complication rates in terms of arterial puncture, hemothorax, pneumothorax, and hematoma formation. Furthermore, the number of puncture attempts is fewer when utilizing ultrasound guidance and overall success in line placement is higher with the use of ultrasound, including for access to the subclavian vein. Additional benefits to ultrasound use include visualization of thrombi or in identifying abnormal anatomy.

Answer: E

Fragou, M., Gravvanis, A., Dimitriou, V. (2011) Real-time ultrasound-guided subclavian vein cannulation versus the landmark method in critical care patients: a prospective randomized study. *Critical Care Medicine*, 39 (7): 1607–1612.

Saugel, B., Scheeren, T. W. L., Teboul, JL. (2017) Ultrasound-guided central venous catheter placement: a structured review and recommendations for clinical practice. *Critical Care*, 21: 225.

5 *A 63-year-old woman is being cared for in the ICU and undergoes a chest x-ray which demonstrates a large right pleural effusion. The decision was made to proceed with chest tube placement. Which of the following is true regarding tube thoracostomy?*

A *The trochar puncture technique is not associated with a higher risk of complications.*

B *Special consideration should be made when considering placing a drain in a patient with previous thoracic or cardiac surgery or previous tube placement.*

C *The chest tube should be placed along the inferior border of the rib.*

D *There is a risk of injuring the lung and cardiac ventricles when placing a chest tube, but the esophagus is far too medial to be at risk for injury.*

E *The borders of the triangle of safety for chest tube placement include the axillary fold of pectoralis major, serratus anterior, and the line along the 5ᵗʰ intercostal space or nipple.*

Chest tube placement in the ICU may be required for various diagnoses including pneumothorax, effusion, or hemothorax. A number of techniques are available for insertion of chest tubes. The trochar method, which is sometimes used for emergent placement, is associated with a higher risk of complications due to its sharp tip. In patients with prior chest surgery, adhesions may be present which can cause the lung or heart to be adhered to the chest wall, thus increasing the risk of injuring vital structures with placement of a tube. In such cases, CT-guided or ultrasound-guided tube placement might be safer. The neurovascular bundle runs along the inferior border of the rib and should be avoided due to risk of injury to these structures. Despite the esophagus lying relatively posterior and medial, there have been reports of injury to the esophagus with chest tube placement. The triangle of safety for chest tube placement is bordered by the axillary fold of pectoralis major, latissimus dorsi, and the line along the 5ᵗʰ intercostal space or the upper border of the nipple line.

Answer: B

Filosso, P. L., Guerrera, F., Sandri, A. (2017) Errors and complications in chest tube placement. *Thoracic Surgery Clinics*, 27 (1): 57–67.

Hernandez, M. C., Laan, D. V., Zimmerman, S. L. (2016) Tube thoracostomy: increased angle of insertion is associated with complications. *Journal of Trauma and Acute Care Surgery*, 81 (2): 366–370.

Meisel, S., Ram, Z., Priel, I. (1990) Another complication of tube thoracostomy: perforation of the right atrium. *Chest*, 98: 772–773.

6 *A 74-year-old man being cared for in the ICU is desaturating and now has evidence of mucus plugging of the right upper lobe on chest x-ray. He does not respond to suctioning and the decision to perform a bronchoscopy is made. Which of the following is true regarding bronchoscopy?*

A *Post-procedural problems can include fever and prolonged hypoxia.*

B *Pneumothorax is a frequent complication of bronchoscopy.*

C *Hypoxia is an absolute contraindication to bronchoscopy.*

D *There is no benefit in increasing the FiO2 during bronchoscopy.*

E *Vasovagal reaction is not a potential complication of bronchoscopy.*

Bronchoscopy is a procedure performed in the ICU setting for a multitude of reasons including diagnosis and treatment of ventilator-associated pneumonia, airway clearance, percutaneous tracheostomy, assistance with difficult intubations, and evaluation of inhalational injuries. Patients are often medicated for the procedure with benzodiazepines or propofol in addition to pain medication. Studies have evaluated the concurrent use of anticholinergics to decrease secretions during the procedure, but despite less secretions, no benefit has been shown with their use. Post-procedural complications include fevers, prolonged hypoxia, and pneumothorax which are relatively rare. Additional potential complications include vasovagal reactions, arrhythmia, bronchospasm, hypertension, and increase in intracranial pressure. Hypoxia is not an absolute contraindication and in certain cases such as the patient described above, bronchoscopy can be used to clear the bronchial tree for optimal ventilation and gas exchange. Oxygenation should be maximized by increasing the FiO2 to 100% for all bronchoscopic procedures to aid in limiting hypoxemia.

Answer: A

Cowl, C. T., Prakash, U. B., Kruger, B. R. (2000) The role of anticholinergics in bronchoscopy. A randomized clinical trial. *Chest*, 118 (1): 188–192.

Gorman, S. R., Beamis, J. (1988) Complications of flexible bronchoscopy. *Clinical Pulmonary Medicine*, 12: 177–183.

7 *A 56-year-old woman fell down stairs and sustains an intracranial hemorrhage and is now in the ICU. She is found to be in ventricular fibrillation and CPR is started. Which of the following is true regarding CPR in this patient?*

A *She has less chance of survival being in ventricular fibrillation compared to being in asystole.*

B *She does not have a better chance of survival being in a monitored ICU bed when compared to CPR being started in a non-monitored bed.*

C *If compressions are being performed slowly, the chance of achieving return of spontaneous circulation increases.*

D *There is no role for the use of an arterial line during CPR.*

E *Intubation can be performed during compressions and should not prolong pauses between chest compressions.*

Patients who arrest and undergo CPR in a monitored bed such as in the ICU have a higher chance of survival compared to those who require CPR in an unmonitored setting due to delay in diagnosis and initiation of CPR. Ventricular tachycardia and ventricular fibrillation have a higher chance of survival compared to asystole and pulseless electrical activity. Compressions that are not performed at a rate of approximately 100 to 120 per minute will lead to a low chance of achieving return of spontaneous circulation, falling from 72% to 42%. Arterial lines that are in place can aid in quickly assessing for intact flow and limiting the time spent on pulse checks. Pauses for intubation should be avoided. Intubations can be attempted during compressions and even a supraglottic airway or bagging will suffice if adequate ventilation is being achieved.

Answer: E

Karetzky, M., Zubair, M., Parikh, J. (1995) Cardiopulmonary resuscitation in intensive care unit and non-intensive care unit patients. Immediate and long-term survival. *Archives of Internal Medicine*, 155 (12): 1277–1280.

Meaney, P. A., Bobrow, B. J., Mancini, M. E. (2013) Cardiopulmonary quality: improving cardiac resuscitation outcomes both inside and outside the hospital: a consensus statement from the American Heart Association. *Circulation*, 128 (4): 417–435.

8 *An 83-year-old man is in need of nutritional access following a stroke. When placing a percutaneous endoscopic gastrostomy tube, which of the following is correct?*

A *Prior abdominal surgery is a contraindication to percutaneous endoscopic gastrostomy placement.*

B *1:1 visualization of ballottement does not aid in safe placement.*

C *Visualization of transillumination does not aid in safe placement.*

D *Preprocedural antibiotics is indicated to reduce the risk of infection.*

E *Visualization of succus when inserting the needle toward the stomach is expected.*

Placement of percutaneous endoscopic gastrostomy tube for nutritional access is indicated for patients who are in need of long-term feeding access. However, complications can occur such as tube dislodgement, infection, bleeding, and injury to adjacent organs such as liver

and colon. Safety steps have been delineated in order to minimize the risk of complications and aid in safe placement of the feeding tube. Although prior abdominal surgery is not an absolute contraindication, it should indicate to the proceduralist that endoscopic placement might carry with it increased risk and the patient might need an open procedure. Steps for safe placement include transillumination (visualizing the endoscopic light through the abdominal wall) in the area of intended placement, 1:1 ballottement (visualizing direct movement in the area of stomach that directly correlates to the area pressed on the abdominal wall), and aspiration of air upon visualization of the guide needle in the stomach. If any of these items are not seen, one should question going forward with the procedure. Preprocedural antibiotics is routine for coverage of gram-positive organisms to minimize the risk of infection.

Answer: D

Rahnemai-Azar, A. A., Rahnemaiazar, A. A., Naghshizadian, R. (2014) Percutaneous endoscopic gastrostomy: indications, technique, complications and management. *World Journal of Gastroenterology*, 20 (24): 7739–7751.

Schrag, S. P., Sharma, R., Jaik, N. P. (2007) Complications related to percutaneous endoscopic gastrostomy (PEG) tubes. A comprehensive clinical review *Journal of Gastrointestinal and Liver Diseases*, 16 (4): 407–418.

9 *Which of the following is correct regarding pulmonary artery catheters?*

A *Right-sided endocarditis is not an absolute contraindication to placement of pulmonary artery catheters.*

B *The left internal jugular and subclavian veins are the ideal insertion points.*

C *Pulmonary artery perforation is a common complication.*

D *The balloon on the tip of the catheter should remain inflated at all times.*

E *Insertion should take place under sterile technique just as with insertion of central lines.*

Although no longer routinely used in many ICU's, pulmonary artery catheters are able to provide information on volume status, cardiac function, and shunting in states of shock. Placement of pulmonary artery catheters in patients with right-sided endocarditis, tumor, or thrombi is contraindicated. Although very rare, perforation of the pulmonary artery is a potential and very serious complication. A risk factor for perforation is prolonged inflation of the balloon that sits at the tip of the catheter. This balloon should remain deflated at all times except when floating the catheter or when obtaining a wedge pressure. Insertion of a pulmonary artery catheter is done under sterile technique and is inserted through an inducer that should ideally be placed into the right internal jugular or subclavian veins due to ease of floating the balloon toward the pulmonary artery.

Answer: E

Kelly, C. R., Rabbani, L. E. (2013) Pulmonary-artery catheterization. *New England Journal of Medicine*, 369: e35.1–e35.7.

Kumar, A., Anel, R., Bunnell, E. (2004) Pulmonary artery occlusion pressure and central venous pressure fail to predict ventricular filling volume, cardiac performance, or the response to volume infusion in normal subjects. *Critical Care Medicine*, 32 (3): 691–699.

10 *A 35-year-old man with liver failure due to alcohol abuse is being monitored in the ICU for delirium tremens and now has evidence of melena. Which of the follow is true?*
   A *Melena is always considered a sign of lower GI bleed*
   B *NGT placement is indicated to assess for upper GI bleed*
   C *A bowel prep is always required prior to colonoscopy*
   D *Hypotension is a contraindication to EGD*
   E *Intubation is required for all EGD and colonoscopies*

It is difficult to discern an upper from lower gastrointestinal hemorrhage source based solely on the presence of melena. The first step to evaluate for an upper GI bleed is to place a nasogastric tube and evaluate for sanguinous drainage. If there is no evidence of sanguinous drainage, then evaluation for a more distal bleed is indicated. Despite a bowel preps potential to help with increased visibility, it is not necessary in a patient who needs an emergent colonoscopy. Hypotension is not an absolute contraindication to EGD and in fact can help with stabilization if bleeding is controlled. Intubation is not required for all EGDs or colonoscopies, but it is advised for patients who are hemodynamically unstable.

Answer: B

Chak, A., Cooper, G. S., Lloyd, L. E. (2001) Effectiveness of endoscopy in patients admitted to the intensive care unit with upper GI hemorrhage. *Gastrointestinal Endoscopy*, 53 (1): 6–13.

Mujtaba, S., Chawla, S., Massaad, J. F. (2020) Diagnosis and management of non-variceal gastrointestinal

hemorrhage: a review of current guidelines and future perspectives. *Journal of Clinical Medicine*, 9 (2): 402.

11 *A cirrhotic patient is admitted to the ICU after a ventral hernia repair and is found to have marked abdominal distention indicative of ascites. Which of the following is true regarding paracentesis?*
   A *Imaging should not be used to guide catheter placement.*
   B *Ideal placement is the lateral lower abdomen at the level of the bladder.*
   C *Bladder decompression is unnecessary.*
   D *Administration of crystalloid will minimize paracentesis-induced circulatory dysfunction.*
   E *Greater than 50 PMNs/mL in ascitic fluid is indicative of spontaneous bacterial peritonitis.*

Paracentesis is a procedure performed by a range of specialists and ultrasound use is recommended to aid in safe catheter placement. The ideal location is along the lower abdominal quadrants lateral to the epigastric vessels at the level of the bladder. Placing a needle in the right upper quadrant risks injury to the liver and in patient who may also have an enlarged liver. Because insertion typically occurs relatively close to the bladder, drainage is recommended prior to the procedure to avoid bladder injury. Because releasing large volumes of ascites from the abdominal cavity can lead to swift fluid shifts and intravascular depletion, albumin is recommended to maintain intravascular volume. Spontaneous bacterial peritonitis is diagnosed with greater than 250 to 500 PMNs/mL within the ascites that is drained.

Answer: B

Lindsay, A. J., Burton, J., Ray, C. E. Jr. (2014) Paracentesis-induced circulatory dysfunction: a primer for the interventional radiologist. *Seminars in Interventional Radiology*, 31 (3): 276–278.

Nazeer, S. R., Dewbre, H., Miller, A. H. (2005) Ultrasound-assisted paracentesis performed by emergency physicians vs. the traditional technique: a prospective, randomize stud. *American Journal of Emergency Medicine*, 23 (3): 363–367.

12 *A 45-year-old woman with a severe traumatic brain injury following a motorcycle crash remains ventilator-dependent and the family has consented to a percutaneous tracheostomy. Which of the following is true regarding this procedure?*
   A *Placement of tracheostomy does not facilitate weaning from the ventilator.*

B *Tracheostomy placement has been shown to decrease mortality compared to leaving an endotracheal tube in place.*

C *Percutaneous tracheostomy is not the ideal procedure if there is an inability to extend the neck for the procedure.*

D *There is no role for the use of ultrasound in the placement of a percutaneous tracheostomy.*

E *Bronchoscopy is indicated for all percutaneous tracheostomy procedures.*

Transition to tracheostomy is helpful in weaning patients from the ventilator, decreasing the risk of aspiration, decreasing hospital stay due to prolonged ventilator dependence, and minimizing sedation requirements. However, tracheostomy placement does not decrease overall mortality. Patients with difficult anatomy or inability to extend the neck are not ideal candidates for percutaneous tracheostomy and should be considered for open surgical tracheostomy. Although bronchoscopic assistance carries some advantages such as real-time confirmation of needle placement and avoidance of posterior tracheal wall injury, there is insufficient data to call for its use in every procedure. In addition to bronchoscopy, ultrasound is another adjunct that can be used for visualization assistance during percutaneous tracheostomy placement.

Answer: C

Mehta C., Mehta,Y. (2017) Percutaneous tracheostomy. *Annals of Cardiac Anaesthesia*, 20 (Suppl 1): S19–S25.

13 *Which of the following is true of echocardiography in the ICU?*
   A *Its accuracy is not affected by chest pathology or recent chest surgery.*
   B *It cannot be used to provide continuous information.*
   C *It can be used to assess for right heart strain.*
   D *It should not be used to assess volume status.*
   E *It cannot be used to assess volume responsiveness.*

The use of ultrasound has expanded a great deal in intensive care units and can be utilized for both invasive and noninvasive procedures. Echocardiography has traditionally been a noninvasive means of evaluating the patients in real-time and can be performed by a single practitioner. There are now possibilities allowing indwelling, continuous, transesophageal echocardiography. Echocardiography can be used to evaluate for cardiac output, right heart function, pericardial fluid, valvular disease, volume status, and response to volume resuscitation.

Answer: C

Marum, S., Price, S. (2011) The use of echocardiography in the critical ill; the role of FADE (Fast Assessment Diagnostic Echocardiography) training. *Current Cardiology Reviews*, 7 (3): 197–200.

14 *A patient is undergoing a lumbar puncture in the ICU. What is correct regarding lumbar puncture?*
   A *Aseptic technique should be utilized when performing a lumbar puncture and only iodine may be used.*
   B *Prolonged bed rest will prevent post-lumbar puncture headache.*
   C *Ultrasound use during the procedure will increase the success rate in identifying the inter-spinal space.*
   D *The L2 spinous process is the landmark that is utilized for lumbar puncture.*
   E *Ultrasound use does not change the risk of complication.*

As with any procedure that violates the skin, a lumbar puncture requires aseptic technique. Historically, it was felt that only iodine could be utilized for skin prep; however, Chloroprep has been shown to be safe. Although being placed in the supine position after a lumbar puncture will aid in easing symptoms from a lumbar puncture, it will not prevent post-lumbar puncture headache from occurring. Patients who have anatomic abnormalities or previous spinal surgery may benefit from fluoroscopic guidance of the lumbar needle. Additionally, ultrasound guidance may also be used and has been shown to decrease the risk of complications and increase success rate of retrieving a CSF sample. The bony landmark that is utilized for lumbar puncture is the spinous process of L4 which is where Tuffier's line can be found, and is essentially the intersection of the line at the top of the iliac crests and the lumbar spine midline. However, in women and obese patients, Tuffier's line is often above the level of L4.

Answer: C

Doherty, C. M., Forbes, R. B. (2014) Diagnostic lumbar puncture. *The Ulster Medical Journal*, 83 (2): 93–102.

Nomura, J. T., Leech, S. J., Shenbagamurthi, S. (2007) A randomized controlled trial of ultrasound-assisted lumbar puncture. *Journal of Ultrasound in Medicine*, 26 (10): 1341–1348.

Roos, K. (2003) Lumbar puncture. *Seminars in Neurology*, 23 (1): 105–114.

15 *A 21-year-old woman is injured during a diving accident and sustains a cervical spine injury. She*

has developed symptomatic bradycardia and the decision is made to place a transvenous pacemaker. Which of the following statements about transvenous pacemakers is true?

A Ideal placement is through the femoral vein
B They are placed solely in the emergent setting
C Complications can include pneumothorax
D Prophylactic antibiotics is recommended
E They are not used to treat tachyarrhythmias

Temporary transvenous pacing can be used to assist with management of both tachy- and brady- arrhythmias. The ideal insertion is through the internal jugular vein or subclavian vein, but the femoral and brachial arteries are also used. Pacers can be considered in the emergent or elective setting. Sometimes, they are placed prior to surgery to help regulate the rate in anticipation of anesthesia and surgical stimulation. Complications can include infection (though prophylactic antibiotics are not recommended), pneumothorax, bleeding, and patient discomfort.

Answer: C

Gammage, M. D. (2000) Temporary cardiac pacing. *Heart*, 83: 715–720.

Harrigan, R. A., Chan, T. C., Moonblatt, S. (2007) Temporary transvenous pacemaker placement in the emergency department. *Journal of Emergency Medicine*, 32 (1): 105–111.

Sullivan, B. L., Bartels, K., Hamilton, N. (2016) Insertion and management of temporary pacemakers. *Seminars in Cardiothoracic and Vascular Anesthesia*, 20 (1): 52–62.

16 When performing a bronchoalveolar lavage (BAL), all the following will produce a technically superior sample except:

A The bronchoscope should be advanced to wedge the tip in the lumen of the airway.
B At least 100 mL of lavage fluid should be utilized.
C The first 20 mL of fluid should be discarded.
D The sampling should be in the area of highest clinical concern.
E Only 2% of instilled lavage fluid return is needed.

Although large variability has traditionally existed in BAL techniques, this variability has led to hard-to-interpret results. Several consensus statements and studies have demonstrated that the yield for BAL will be increased when the bronchoscope is advanced and wedged into the airway to help prevent mixing of fluid from the proximal airways. Although variably reported, the minimum amount of lavage fluid should be 100 ml and the first aliquot of 20 or so ml should be discarded. Lastly, one should suction back at least 5–20% of instilled lavage fluid.

Answer: E

Baughman, R. P. (2007) Technical aspects of bronchoalveolar lavage: recommendations for a standard procedure. *Seminars in Respiratory and Critical Care Medicine*; 28 (5): 475–485.

Meduri, G. U., Chastre, J. (1992) The Standardization of Bronchoscopic technique for ventilator associated Penumonia. *Chest*, 102 (5, supplement 1): 557s–564s.

27

Diagnostic Imaging, Ultrasound and Interventional Radiology

Hang Ho, MD and Terence O'Keeffe, MB ChB

Augusta University Medical Center, Augusta, GA, USA

1 Which of the following patients is most likely to respond to intravenous fluid administration?
   A A patient with a 5% increase in aortic flow velocity after passive leg raise.
   B A patient with an IVC collapsibility index of (CI) 87%.
   C A patient with hyperechoic reverberation artifacts at the pleura on ultrasound evaluation of the lungs.
   D A patient whose right common carotid artery diameter did not significantly change with passive leg raise.
   E An increase in systolic blood pressure of < 10 points with passive leg raise.

Determining which patients will respond favorably to fluid resuscitation is a key skill required in the critical care setting, but has been notoriously difficult. Bedside ultrasound has become an increasingly useful tool for assessment. Measurements that have been studied include IVC collapsibility index, aortic flow velocity, evaluation for pulmonary edema, and evaluation of common carotid artery diameter.

An IVC CI close to 100% suggests that the patient will be highly likely to respond favorably to volume resuscitation. The IVC collapsibility index is one of the more frequently utilized measures and can be obtained with bedside ultrasound of the inferior vena cava. The IVC Collapsibility Index ranges from 0–100% and is described with the following equation:

$$\text{IVC CI} = \left[\left(\frac{\text{max vessel diameter} - \text{min vessel diameter}}{\text{/ mean vessel diameter}} \right) \right] \times 100$$

where the maximum and minimal vessel diameters are the diameters obtained during at least one full respiratory cycle. A IVC CI of 100% suggests high volume responsiveness, while an IVC CI approaching 0% suggests minimal/no volume responsiveness.

A is incorrect. Aortic flow velocity is based on the premise that the left ventricular outflow tract diameter is relatively constant, and therefore any increase in flow through this area correlates to a proportionate increase in stroke volume. Therefore, a measurement of aortic flow velocity at the aortic root can be correlated with an increase in stroke volume. An aortic flow velocity increase of >14% after passive leg raise is associated with volume responsiveness. An increase <10% is associated with a high negative predictive value of volume responsiveness.

B is the correct answer. An IVC CI approaching 0% suggests low volume responsiveness, while an IVC CI of 100% suggests minimal/no volume responsiveness.

C is incorrect. This is a description of B lines, which are an ultrasound finding consistent with pulmonary edema. This patient would likely not benefit from additional IV fluid administration.

D is incorrect. Significant carotid artery diameter increase with passive leg raise is correlated with volume responsiveness. No significant change would suggest that the patient is not intravascularly depleted.

E is incorrect. Passive leg raise will increase systolic blood pressure at least transiently in a hypovolemic patient. A patient with fairly minimal increase in systolic blood pressure is unlikely to benefit from additional intravascular fluid administration.

Answer: B

Feissel M, Michard F, Mangin O, et al. Respiratory changes in aortic blood velocity as an indicator of fluid responsiveness in ventilated patients with septic shock. *Chest* 2001 Mar;119(3):867–873.

Hilbert T, Klaschik S, Ellerkmann R, et al. Common carotid artery diameter responds to intravenous volume expansion: an ultrasound observation. *Springerplus* 2016 Jun;5(1):853.

Surgical Critical Care and Emergency Surgery: Clinical Questions and Answers, Third Edition.
Edited by Forrest "Dell" Moore, Peter M. Rhee, and Carlos R. Rodriguez.
© 2022 John Wiley & Sons Ltd. Published 2022 by John Wiley & Sons Ltd.
Companion website: www.wiley.com/go/surgicalcriticalcare3e

Pourmand A, Pyle M, Yamane D, et al. The utility of point-of-care ultrasound in the assessment of volume status in acute and critically ill patients. *World Journal of Emergency Medicine* 2019 Jul; 10(4):232–238.

2   *Which of the following findings on transcranial doppler ultrasound of the middle cerebral artery suggests a high risk of mortality and/or morbidity associated with traumatic brain injury?*
   A *High mean velocity, high diastolic velocity, high pulsatility index*
   B *Low mean velocity, high diastolic velocity, high pulsatility index*
   C *Low mean velocity, low diastolic velocity, high pulsatility index*
   D *High mean velocity, high diastolic velocity, low pulsatility index*
   E *Low mean velocity, high diastolic velocity, low pulsatility index*

Transcranial doppler (TCD) is a noninvasive ultrasound (US) study used to measure cerebral blood flow velocity (CBF-V) in the major intracranial arteries. It involves use of low-frequency (≤2 MHz) US waves to insonate the basal cerebral arteries through relatively thin bone windows. Transcranial doppler of the middle cerebral artery is a modality used to predict prognosis related to traumatic brain injury. Mean velocity, diastolic velocity, and pulsatility index are measured to identify hypoperfusion, which is correlated with increased morbidity and mortality. Hypoperfusion on transcranial doppler is defined as the presence of **two** of the following:

1) Mean velocity <35 cm/sec
2) Diastolic velocity <20cm/sec
3) Pulsatility index >1.4

Therefore, the correct answer is C. Answers A, B, D, and E do not meet these criteria.

Answer: C

Santbrink HV, Schouten JW, Steyerberg EW, et al. Serial transcranial doppler measurements in traumatic brain injury with special focus on the early post-traumatic period. *Acta Neurochirurgica* 2002 Nov; 144(11):1141–1149.
Ziegler D, Cravens G, Poche G, et al. Use of transcranial doppler in patients with severe traumatic brain injuries. *Journal of Neurotrauma* 2017 Jan; 34(1):122–127.

3   *The use of the IVC collapsibility index (CI) collapsibility index for assessment of intravascular volume status would be least useful in which of the following scenarios?*
   A *In a pregnant patient*
   B *To predict post-anesthesia hypotension*
   C *In a patient with positive pressure ventilation*
   D *In a septic patient*
   E *In a patient with suspected PE*

IVC collapsibility index is one of several measures that can be obtained to assess volume status in a critically ill patient. In a spontaneously breathing patient, inspiration generates negative intrathoracic pressure which subsequently is transmitted to the central venous system. The intra-abdominal inferior vena cava collapses on inspiration when the central venous pressure is lower than the intra-abdominal pressure. Positive pressure ventilation conversely increases intrathoracic pressure during inspiration. Therefore, patients who are on positive pressure ventilation may not demonstrate inspiratory IVC collapsibility indices which correlate accurately with volume status. It is not recommended to use IVC CI to guide therapy or intervention in mechanically ventilated patients.

Answers A, B, D, and E are all appropriate applications of the IVC collapsibility index.

Answer: C

Porter, TR, Shillcutt, SK, Adams MS, et al. Guidelines for use of echocardiography as a monitor for therapeutic intervention in adults: a report from the American Society of Echocardiography. *Journal of the American Society of Echocardiography* 2015; 28:40–56.

4   *A 63-year-old obese man is postoperative day 4 after exploratory laparotomy, sigmoidectomy, and end-colostomy for perforated diverticulitis. He has been minimally mobile due to his body habitus. He develops sudden onset of lightheadedness and shortness of breath. Vitals are significant for sinus tachycardia to 120 bpm, hypotension to 87/60 mmHg, and pulse oximeter shows hypoxia to 78%. Chest x-ray is unremarkable. Which of the following would confirm the diagnosis?*
   A *Anechoic layer between the heart and pericardium on TTE*
   B *IVC size <2.1 cm which collapses >50% during respiration*
   C *Troponin level of 7.6*
   D *CT of the chest with IV contrast*
   E *Diffuse ST elevation across the lateral leads*

The scenario presented above is consistent with a pulmonary embolus with right heart strain. Pulmonary embolism should always be suspected in patients with major surgery or trauma and/or prolonged immobility. Typical presentation involves acute onset hypoxia, sinus tachycardia. Severe cases will present with hypotension and evidence of right heart strain on echocardiography demonstrated by RVIDD/LVIDD > 0.9. The pathognomic echocardiogram finding is S1Q3T3 (prominent S wave in lead I, Q wave and inverted T wave in lead III).

A is not correct. This is a finding consistent with pericardial effusion. Pericardial effusion can present similarly but is unlikely to present with significant hypoxia.

B is not correct. These values suggest hypovolemia and are not consistent with pulmonary embolism.

C is not correct. While pulmonary emboli can present up to 50% of the time with elevated cardiac biomarkers, this finding is nonspecific and does not confirm a specific diagnosis without correlation with additional data.

E. This is found in pericarditis, which classically presents as chest pain alleviated by sitting up or leaning forward associated with shortness of breath. However, it is unlikely to cause significant hypotension or hypoxia. The more likely diagnosis is pulmonary embolism, which would be confirmed by CT of the chest with IV contrast.

Answer: D

Levis JT. ECG diagnosis: pulmonary embolism. The Permanente Journal 2011;15(4):75

Porter, TR, Shillcutt, SK, Adams MS, et al. Guidelines for use of echocardiography as a monitor for therapeutic intervention in adults: a report from the American Society of Echocardiography. *Journal of the American Society of Echocardiography* 2015; 28:40–56.

5   *A 32-year-old helmeted man presents after a downhill skiing accident where he fell and struck the left side of his neck. Under which of the following circumstances would he have an absolute indication for CTA?*
   A   *Leforte I fracture*
   B   *Closed head injury with diffuse axonal injury and GCS <6*
   C   *Fracture of the spinous process of T1*
   D   *Isolated first rib fracture*
   E   *Unremarkable neurologic exam with small nonexpanding Zone II neck hematoma*

The diagnosis of blunt cerebrovascular trauma is essential in the workup of a patient with blunt trauma to the head and neck. The following are risk factors for blunt cerebrovascular trauma:
High-energy transfer mechanism associated with:

- Displaced mid-face fracture (LeForte II or III)
- Basilar skull fracture with carotid canal involvement
- Closed head injury consistent with diffuse axonal injury and GCS < 6
- Cervical vertebral body or transverse foramen fracture, subluxation, or ligamentous injury at any level
- Any fracture at C1-C2
- Near hanging with anoxia
- Clothesline-type injury or seat belt abrasion with significant swelling, pain or altered mental status

A is incorrect. LeForte II and III are indications for CTA. A LeForte I fracture is a transverse fracture through the maxilla and pterygoid plates and therefore will not involve the carotid canals.

B is the correct answer. Closed head injury with GCS < 6 and concern for diffuse axonal injury on imaging should prompt a CTA neck.

C is incorrect. Thoracic spine injuries do not necessitate CTA of the neck. Furthermore, injuries such as spinous process fractures or transverse process fractures without ligamentous injury or involvement of the transverse foramen do not represent a high risk for BCVI. CTA is recommended in the setting of vertebral body fractures, fractures involving the transverse foramen, subluxation, or ligamentous injury at any cervical spine level.

D is incorrect. Isolated first rib fractures are a relative, not absolute, indication for CTA neck.

E is incorrect. A clothesline-type injury does not mandate a CTA neck in a patient who remains neurologically unremarkable with no significant pain or altered neurologic exam.

Answer: B

Geddes AE, Burlew CC, Wagenaar AE, et al. Expanded screening criteria for blunt cerebrovascular injury: a bigger impact than anticipated. *American Journal of Surgery* 2016 Dec;212(6):1167–1174.

Western Trauma Association. Screening for and Treatment of Blunt Cerebrovascular Injuries Algorithm (2020). https://www.westerntrauma.org/western-trauma-association-algorithms/screening-for-and-treatment-of-blunt-cerebrovascular-injuries-algorithm/references/

6   *An 18-year-old man who is hemodynamically normal presents after sustaining a gunshot wound to the posterior lower right thigh from a handgun. EMS reports brisk red bleeding on scene. On presentation, the patient has a nonpulsatile hematoma adjacent to the wound with palpable distal pulses bilaterally. ABI on the affected limb is 0.7. What is the next best step?*
   A   *Surgical exploration and vascular repair*
   B   *Interventional radiology consultation*
   C   *Observation and local wound care*
   D   *CTA of the affected extremity*
   E   *Vascular ultrasound*

Penetrating extremity trauma should always include assessment of the peripheral vasculature starting with pulse exam and ankle-brachial indices. Hard signs of vascular trauma should prompt surgical exploration. In the absence of hard signs of vascular injury, the presence of an abnormal ABI should prompt further diagnostic evaluation either in the form of CTA or vascular ultrasound. CTA is indicated in this patient, who demonstrates several soft signs of peripheral vascular injury in the setting of an abnormal ABI (defined as less than or equal to 0.9).

A is not correct. Immediate operative intervention is indicated in the setting of hard signs of vascular injury: (1) external arterial bleeding; (2) a rapidly expanding hematoma; (3) any of the classical signs of arterial occlusion (pulselessness, pallor, paresthesias, pain, paralysis = 5 "P"s); and (4) a palpable thrill/audible bruit.

B is not correct. Interventional radiology consultation for therapeutic intervention is indicated in the setting of active extravasation or arteriovenous fistula with an injury to the profunda femoris, anterior tibial, posterior tibial, or peroneal arteries.

C is not correct. Observation is only appropriate if no injury is demonstrated on imaging OR if the only injury identified is isolated occlusion of the profunda femoris, posterior tibial, anterior tibial, or peroneal artery.

D is the correct answer. In the absence of hard signs of vascular injury, the presence of an abnormal ABI should prompt further diagnostic evaluation either in the form of CTA or vascular ultrasound. CTA is indicated in this patient, who demonstrates several soft signs of peripheral vascular injury in the setting of an abnormal ABI (defined as less than or equal to 0.9).

E is not correct. While vascular ultrasound has been found to have excellent accuracy in identifying arterial injury with sensitivity ranging from 50–100% and specificity >95%, this modality's utility is limited to use in centers where vascular ultrasound technicians and/or ultrasound-experienced vascular surgeons are available. Therefore, in the practice setting described above, this would not be the best choice.

Answer: D

Biffl WL, Ray CE, Jr., Moore EE, Mestek M, Johnson JL, Burch JM. Noninvasive diagnosis of blunt cerebrovascular injuries: a preliminary report. *The Journal of Trauma* 2002;53:850–856.

Western Trauma Association. Evaluation and Management of Peripheral Vascular Injury Part 1 (2020). https://www. westerntrauma.org/western-trauma-association-algorithms/evaluation-and-management-of-peripheral-vascular-injury/note-m/

7 *A 23-year-old woman presents as a passenger in a high-speed rollover MVC. Her presenting vitals are a heart rate of 90 bpm, blood pressure 130/85 mm Hg, respiratory rate 24 breaths/minute, and SaO2 98%. She has moderate left upper abdominal pain on exam without peritonitis. Her fast is negative. She proceeds to CT, where she is found to have a distal pancreatic parenchymal laceration with moderate peripancreatic edema. What is the next best step in management?*

A *Distal pancreatectomy*
B *MRCP*
C *Exploratory laparotomy with drainage*
D *Expectant management*
E *ERCP*

Findings as described above of peripancreatic edema and pancreatic laceration in the setting of blunt abdominal trauma are concerning for pancreatic ductal injury. In an unstable patient with abnormal hemodynamics, operative exploration should be pursued. In a stable patient where nonoperative intervention is an option, MRCP is the appropriate modality to evaluate for ductal injury and is less invasive than ERCP.

A is not correct. Distal pancreatectomy is indicated for lacerations with high risk of ductal injury to the left of the SMV. However, in this stable patient with concerning findings for such an injury on CT, MRCP to better define the extent of the injury is preferable prior to proceeding to the OR.

C is not correct. It is best to further define the nature of the injury with MRCP in this stable patient. Laparotomy with drainage is indicated if the patient has indications for emergent laparotomy, such as refractory hemodynamic instability on presentation or peritonitis, and is subsequently found to have a low-risk laceration to the pancreas on exploration.

D is not correct. Expectant management is appropriate in the setting of normal pancreas or mid peripancreatic edema, but not in the setting of a parenchymal laceration. The presence of a parenchymal laceration necessitates further investigation.

E is not correct. The role for ERCP in the management of patients with traumatic pancreatic duct injuries is only in the setting of stable patients without ductal injury noted on MRCP who are subsequently noted to have a persistent pancreatic fistula during the course of expectant nonoperative management. MRCP is a better modality to evaluate for pancreatic ductal injury because it is less invasive and can usually be obtained more expeditiously.

Answer: B

Western Trauma Association. Management of Pancreatic Injuries (2020). https://www.westerntrauma.org/wp-content/uploads/2020/08/Management-of-Pancreatic-Injuries_FINAL.svg

8 *A 36-year-old man presents with a self-inflicted stab wound to the left neck that violates the platysma and the wound is below the level of the cricoid cartilage and above the sternal notch. His vitals are HR 90 beats/minute, BP 128/72 mm Hg, RR 26 breaths/minute, SaO₂ 97%. There is no active bleeding, significant*

hematoma, hematemesis, or air coming from the wound. What is the NEXT best step in management?

A *EGD and bronchoscopy*
B *Neck exploration*
C *Serial Exam*
D *CTA of the neck and chest*
E *Immediate intubation for airway protection*

A is not correct. Patients with penetrating neck wounds in Zone I–III with suspicion for injury should be evaluated with a CTA initially to rule out vascular injury prior to any evaluation for suspected aerodigestive tract injuries.

B is not correct. The patient is hemodynamically stable and therefore should be evaluated first with a CTA to determine the necessity of surgical intervention. Patients should proceed to surgical exploration if unstable or if the patient demonstrates hard signs of vascular or aerodigestive tract injury. Immediate neck exploration is not necessary in this case.

C is not correct. This patient described has a zone I penetrating neck injury. Although asymptomatic, a high index of suspicion needs to be maintained due to the fact that physical examination findings in this area can be anatomically obscured.

D is the correct answer. Given the drawback of this anatomical location mentioned above, the next best step would be to obtain a CTA. Structures at risk for injury in this area include both aerodigestive and vascular structures. CTA has also demonstrated high sensitivity and specificity for identifying aerodigestive tract injuries in addition to vascular injuries in this area.

E is not correct. The patient described is stable and protecting his own airway. Immediate intubation may exacerbate an injury if present and is not necessary in this setting.

There are some who advocate that with the advent of CTA that there is no need to categorize the injuries into different zones of the neck. They suggest that physical examination regardless of the zone of injury should be the primary guide to CTA or therapeutic neck exploration in patients with penetrating neck injury. Following traditional zone-based guidelines can result in unnecessary negative explorations in patients with soft signs and may need rethinking. Thus, the data support no evaluation and clinical observation for patients who are asymptomatic with no hard or soft signs.

Hard signs of vascular or aerodigestive injury include pulsatile bleeding, hemorrhagic shock, expanding or pulsatile hematoma, bruit, thrill, air bubbling from the wound, or active bleeding from the mouth. Soft signs include dysphagia, dyspnea, nonpulsatile wound, and non-expanding hematoma.

- Zone I: Clavicles/sternum to the **cricoid cartilage**.
- **Zone II: Cricoid cartilage** to the **angle of the mandible**.
- Zone III: Superior to the **angle of the mandible** to skull area.

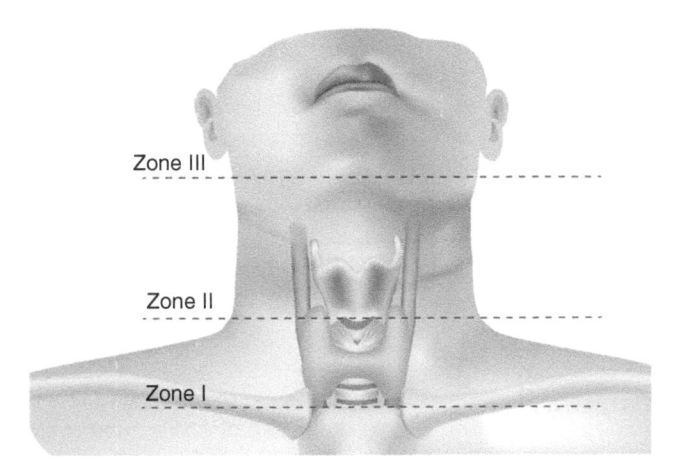

Answer: D

Inaba K, Branco BC, Menaker J, et al. Evaluation of multidetector computed tomography for penetrating neck injury: a prospective multicenter study. *Journal of Trauma and Acute Care Surgery* 2012;72:576–583.

Ibraheem K, Khan M, Rhee P, Azim A, O'Keeffe T, Tang A, Kulvatunyou N, Joseph B. "No zone" approach in penetrating neck trauma reduces unnecessary computed tomography angiography and negative explorations. *The Journal of Surgical Research* 2018 Jan;221:113–120. doi: https://doi.org/10.1016/j.jss.2017.08.033.

Western Trauma Association. Penetrating Neck Trauma. https://www.westerntrauma.org/wp-content/uploads/2020/08/Penetrating-Neck-Trauma_FINAL.svg

9 *A 19-year-old man presents after being shot in the chest at a house party with a handgun. On initial presentation, his vitals are HR 89 beats/minute, BP 128/79 mm Hg, RR 24 breaths/minute, and SaO$_2$ 97%. He has a wound on the left anterior axillary line at the nipple and a wound at the right mid-axillary line 8th intercostal space. A chest tube is placed for a right pneumothorax noted on chest XR. FAST demonstrates no remarkable cardiac injuries. What is the next best step in management?*

A *CT angiogram of the chest*
B *Observation*
C *VATS*
D *Thoracotomy*
E *EGD and bronchoscopy*

The scenario describes a transmediastinal penetrating thoracic injury in a hemodynamically normal and stable patient. The management depends highly upon the patient's presentation. Three scenarios exist. If the patient has no sign of life, an emergency resuscitative thoracotomy should be considered. In a patient with abnormal vital signs suggestive of blood loss who is considered to be unstable may need to be considered for bilateral chest tubes. For the patient with normal hemodynamics and stable vital signs, there is time for further evaluation to rule out mediastinal great vessels as well as the aerodigestive tract. Evaluation for vascular injury takes precedence in the case as it is more likely to cause rapid deterioration in the patient's clinical status. CTA should be obtained to determine the tract of the bullet. If there is a possibility of aerodigestive injuries, it should be followed by EGD and/or bronchoscopy or surgical exploration if concern for aerodigestive tract injury is demonstrated.

B is not correct. Observation alone is inadequate in the setting of a transmediastinal penetrating thoracic injury without first ruling out vascular and aerodigestive tract injuries.

C is not correct. VATS is indicated for concern for diaphragmatic injury, residual hemothorax, or persistent hemorrhage in the setting of trauma.

D is not correct. In a stable patient, CTA should be obtained first to evaluate for vascular and aerodigestive tract injuries; if these are identified on CTA, thoracotomy or sternotomy is indicated for surgical management afterward.

E is not correct. Identification of vascular injury takes precedence in this scenario. A CTA obtained to evaluate for vascular injury will also identify concerns for aerodigestive tract injuries.

Answer: A

Western Trauma Association. Penetrating Thoracic Injury: Stable (2020). https://www.nchima.org/westerntrauma. org/wp-content/uploads/2020/08/Stable-Penetrating-Chest-Trauma_FINAL.svg

10 *A 62-year-old woman involved in an MVA as the restrained driver presents with a grade IV renal laceration without extravasation on CT. Her vitals are normal and stable. She complains of moderate left flank pain. What is the NEXT best step in management?*
   A *Nephrectomy*
   B *Angiogram and embolization*
   C *Observation*
   D *Renal artery stent*
   E *Repeat CT scan in 48–72 hours*

High-grade renal lacerations are at increased risk of collecting system injury. All Grade IV/V renal injuries should undergo repeat delayed imaging to assess for urinary extravasation or urinoma.

A is not correct. Nephrectomy is indicated if a shattered kidney is encountered in the setting of laparotomy for other reasons, but otherwise is not necessary in a stable patient even with a high-grade injury.

B is not correct. Angiogram and embolization are indicated if there is evidence on CT of active extravasation of contrast, pseudoaneurysm, or AV fistula for all grades of kidney injuries. This patient does not have those findings.

C is incorrect. In a blunt renal injury graded IV–V, observation alone in inadequate. A repeat CT scan should be obtained to assess for collecting system injury.

D is incorrect. Renal artery stents are used in the setting of a grade IV–V injury with devascularization with desire for renal salvage. Not all grade IV–V renal injuries will require this intervention, though, so it is not the next best step in management.

E is the correct answer.

Answer: E

Western Trauma Association. Management of Renal Injury Found on CT Scan (2020). https://www.westerntrauma. org/wp-content/uploads/2020/07/Renal-CTscan.pdf

11 *Which of the following statements is true regarding measurement of optic nerve sheath diameters in the setting of traumatic brain injury?*
   A *Values greater than 5 mm suggest elevated ICP.*
   B *Increased ICP is transmitted through the dura to the optic nerve sheath, causing an increase in its diameter.*
   C *Optic nerve sheath measurements are performed via placement of an invasive catheter.*
   D *This method is neither sensitive nor specific.*
   E *This study requires specialists and equipment only available at major institutions.*

Traumatic brain injury and associated intracranial hypertension can cause significant morbidity and mortality if diagnosis is delayed. CT of the head is used commonly to assess for change in the acutely altered traumatic brain injury patient, but can be challenging and time-consuming to obtain in critically ill patients. ICP monitors and EVDs are also commonly used to obtain objective measurements of intracranial pressure, and EVDs have the additional benefit of allowing decompression of CSF; however, these procedures are also time-consuming and invasive. Bedside evaluation of intracranial pressures via ultrasonography of the optic nerve sheath diameter is emerging as an alternative modality to assess for elevated ICP. Diameters greater than 5mm suggest intracranial hypertension in the setting of traumatic brain injury.

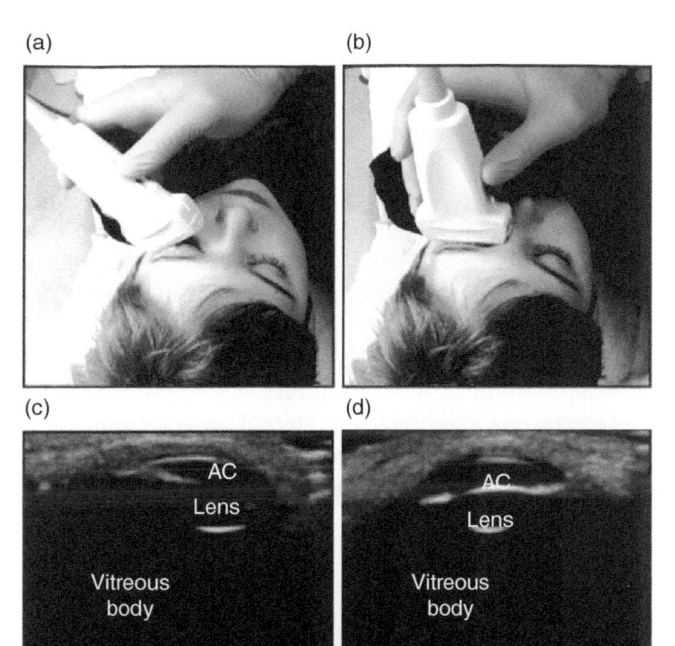

(a)   (b)

(c)   (d)

A *Pleural effusion*
B *Pulmonary edema*
C *Pneumothorax*
D *Mucus plugging*
E *Pulmonary embolism*

This image is representative of the "barcode sign" or lack of lung sliding and is indicative of pneumothorax. The "seashore sign" is the normal finding consistent with the presence of lung sliding.

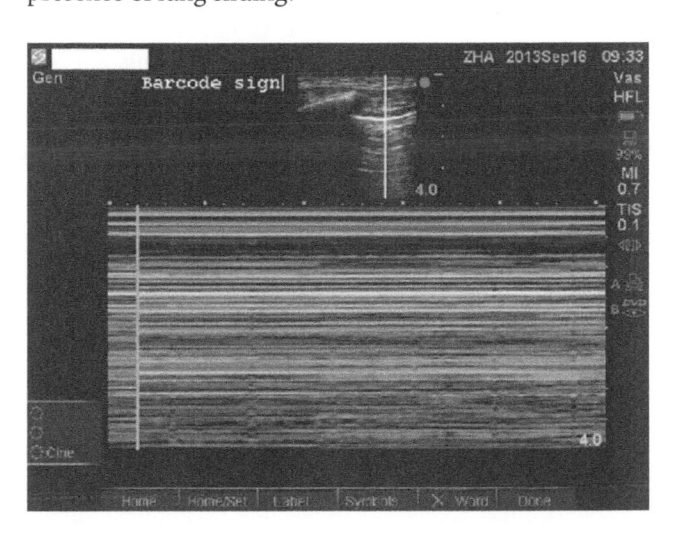

A is the correct answer. An optic nerve sheath diameter greater than 5mm suggests elevated intracranial pressure.

B is incorrect. Increased ICP is transmitted via the subarachnoid space to the optic nerve sheath, causing an increase in its diameter.

C is incorrect. The optic nerve sheath diameter is measured via bedside ultrasound and is a noninvasive way to monitor ICPs.

D is incorrect. This method demonstrates a sensitivity and specificity greater than 94% and 90%, respectively.

E is incorrect. Optic nerve sheath diameter measurements can be obtained at bedside with standard equipment available in most ICUs.

Answer: A

Kimberly H, Sahah S, Marill K, Noble V. Correlation of optic nerve sheath diameter with direct measurement of intracranial pressure. *Academic Emergency Medicine,* 2008; 15: 201–204.

Raffiz M, Abdullah J. Optic nerve sheath diameter measurement: a means of detecting raised ICP in adult traumatic and non-traumatic neurosurgical patients. *American Journal of Emergency Medicine* 2017 Jan;35(1):150–153.

12 *The following image is obtained while performing an ultrasound of a patient's lung. What is the correct diagnosis?*

A is incorrect. Pleural effusions appear as an anechoic, homogeneous signal in dependent portions of the pleural space.

B is incorrect. Pulmonary edema is suggested by "B lines" or "comet tails" on ultrasound. Lung sliding should still be present.

D is incorrect. Mucus plugging does not impair lung sliding and therefore will not give this finding on ultrasound.

E is incorrect. Pulmonary embolism is indicated by thrombus in the right heart or pulmonary artery, right ventricular dilation (>1:1 RV/LV ratio), or flattening or bowing of the intraventricular septum into the left ventricle. There would be few significant findings on ultrasound of the parenchyma itself.

Answer: C

Husain LF, Hagopian L, Wayman D, Baker W, Carmody KA. Sonographic diagnosis of pneumothorax. *Journal of Emergencies, Trauma, and Shock* 2012 Jan-Mar;5(1):76–81.

13 *Which of the following is **true** regarding the assessment of a pericardial effusion?*
  A *Pericardial effusions are not always present in dependent segments.*
  B *Diastolic collapse of both atriums in a significant pericardial effusion occurs in diastole.*

C *Peritoneal free fluid is easily discernible from a pericardial effusion on the subcostal view of the heart.*

D *A single view of a pericardial effusion via a trans-thoracic echocardiography (TTE) is adequate to identify its presence and amount.*

E *A pericardial effusion typically shows a simple echotexure on ultrasound.*

Pericardial effusion is often found in critically ill patients and can be life-threatening. It is characterized as a homogenously anechoic space visible during diastole located within the two layers of the pericardium via a TTE.

A. A pericardial effusion is always located along the posterior wall, lateral, and inferior wall in a supine patient. These are all dependent segments of the heart.

B. A significant pericardial effusion will cause diagnostic collapse of both atriums. The right atrium and right ventricular outflow tracts are the first to collapse. Once the effusion has become very severe, the left atrium and left ventricle will become collapsed as well. On TTE, the collapse of both atriums can be seen in atrial diastole or ventricular systole when a pericardial effusion is present.

C. Peritoneal free fluid or ascites can appear in the subcostal views, anterior to the right cardiac chambers, and may mimic a pericardial effusion. Viewing the falciform ligament within the fluid confirms the diagnosis. Additionally, examination of the rest of the abdomen will further assist in diagnosing ascites.

D. Pericardial effusions may be regional or circumferential, and may be irregularly distributed. Therefore, several views via transthoracic echocardiography TTE may be needed to identify its presence and amount.

E. The image of a pericardial effusion/fluid on ultrasound is typically anechoic. However, when the effusion contains purulence or clots, it can sometimes show a complex echotexture.

Answer: E

Blanco P, Volpicelli G. Common pitfalls in point-of-care ultrasound: a practical guide for emergency and critical care physicians. *Critical Ultrasound Journal* 2016;8:15.

14 *In patients with penetrating trauma to the neck, which of the following would be true regarding the use of CT angiography for diagnostic evaluation?*

A *Use of CT angiography does not reduce the negative operation exploration rate.*

B *Violation of the platysma is still an indication for mandatory operation.*

C *Most patients with hard signs should undergo CT scan if hemodynamically normal and stable.*

D *CT scanning should only be performed in hemodynamically normal and stable patients.*

E *Diagnosis of an injury by CTA always requires an operative intervention.*

A. The use of CT angiography as an initial screening modality in penetrating neck trauma has been well established. More than one study has shown that the negative exploration rate can be reduced by using this modality as an initial screening tool for the presence of injury.

B. Violation of the platysma is no longer regarded as a mandatory indication for exploration, as significant injuries can be effectively ruled out by CT angiography of the neck. CT scanning has greater than 90% sensitivity for injuries, including the aerodigestive tract.

C. Although there have been recent studies that have shown a reduced negative exploration rate when CT angiography is performed, even in the presence of hard signs, this remains controversial. The current recommendation is that patients with hard signs on physical examination should be explored in the operating room. It is imperative to protect the airway in these patients. Additionally, it is important to avoid bedside exploration in the emergency department as tamponaded bleeding may be disrupted.

D. CT Angiography of the neck is not appropriate in patients who are hemodynamically abnormal and unstable.

E. Not all injuries that are seen on CTA will require an intervention. Nonoperative management of internal jugular vein injuries, for example, has been safely performed in patients who were otherwise stable.

Answer: D

Osborn TM, Bell RB, Qaisi W, et al. Computed tomographic angiography as an aid to clinical decision making in the selective management of penetrating injuries to the neck: a reduction in the need for operative exploration. *The Journal of Trauma* 2008 Jun;64(6):1466–1471.

Schroll R, Fontenot T, Lipesey M, et al. Role of computed tomography angiography in the management of Zone II penetrating neck traumas in patients with clinical hard signs. *Journal of Trauma and Acute Care Surgery* 2015;79(6):943–950.

Sperry JL, Moore EE, Coimbra R, et al. Western trauma association critical decisions in trauma: penetrating neck trauma. *Journal of Trauma and Acute Care Surgery* 2013;75(6):936–940.

15 *A trauma patient is 12 weeks pregnant and presents after a rollover MVC with abdominal pain. Which of the following is TRUE regarding imaging of this patient?*

A *The patient should only undergo a FAST exam due to risk to the fetus.*

B *Ionizing radiation should be avoided at all costs.*

C *MRI imaging is the modality of choice to evaluate for intra-abdominal injuries.*

D *CT scan of the abdomen should only be done in the last trimester.*

E *It is acceptable to perform CT in patients with a high index of suspicion.*

While trauma in pregnancy is rare, it can be a complication in up to 5–7% of all pregnancies. Concern for fetal development and dosing of ionizing radiation has led to a major reluctance to perform necessary imaging on these patients. Although there are theoretical risks to the fetus from x-rays and CT scans, these are mostly less than the risk of misdiagnosis and delay in identifying significant injuries that could threaten the health of both the mother and the child. A CT scan of the abdomen (belly) and pelvis exposes a person to about 10 mGy. United States Nuclear Regulation Commission (USNRC) recommends total fetus exposure during pregnancy to be less than 5.0 mGy (500 mrem). The fetus radiation dose below 50 mGy is considered safe and will not cause any harm (Table 27.1).

A. While the FAST exam should certainly be the initial modality of choice to evaluate patients with blunt abdominal trauma, it carries all the usual problems with sensitivity and in fact may be less accurate in the pregnant trauma patient. It should certainly not be relied upon as the sole imaging study.

B. Given the choice of imaging that is potentially harmful but has the possibility of direct benefit to the mother and/or the fetus, any direct benefit should outweigh the potential risks of problems in the future, so it is NOT accurate to say that ionizing radiation should be completely avoided. We should image gently and appropriately but not hesitate where it is necessary (See EAST guidelines).

C. Many trauma centers currently have relatively easy access to MRI scanners, which makes it an attractive choice. While it is certainly an option, the length of time taken, lack of ability to provide direct care for the patient during the scan, and the need usually to transport the patient away from the trauma area makes this less than ideal, and only suitable for the completely stable patient.

D. If necessary, a CT scan can be done in ANY trimester. Clearly the risks to the fetus are lower in the last trimester, but again, a fetus in the first trimester will not be viable if the mother does not survive, and the focus should as always be on pregnant trauma patients, focus on care of the mother's injuries.

E. CT scans can and should be performed in pregnant trauma patients if the index of suspicion is high enough to warrant imaging. Intravenous contrast should be used as in a regular CT scan for trauma due to the need for evaluation of the perfused organs, as per the usual case in trauma, and there does not seem to be excessive risks to the fetus.

Answer: E

Barraco RD, Chiu WC, Clancy TV et al. Practice management guidelines for the diagnosis and management of injury in the pregnant patient: the EAST Practice Management Guidelines Work Group. *The Journal of Trauma* 2010 Jul;69(1):211–214.

Raptis CA, Mellnick VM, Raptis DA, et al. Imaging of trauma in the pregnant patient. Radiographics 2014 May-Jun;34(3):748–763.

Tirada N, Dreizin D, Khati NJ, et al. Imaging pregnant and lactating patients. *Radiographics* 2015 Oct;35(6):1751–1765.

Table 27.1 Typical Organ Radiation Doses from Various Radiologic Studies.

Study type	Relevant organ	Relevant organ dose[a] (mGy or mSv)
Dental radiography	Brain	0.005
Posterior–anterior chest radiography	Lung	0.01
Lateral chest radiography	Lung	0.15
Screening mammography	Breast	3
Adult abdominal CT	Stomach	10
Barium enema	Colon	15
Neonatal abdominal CT	Stomach	20

[a] The radiation dose, a measure of ionizing energy absorbed per unit of mass, is expressed in grays (Gy) or milligrays (mGy); 1 Gy = 1 joule per kilogram. The radiation dose is often expressed as an equivalent dose in sieverts (Sv) or millisieverts (mSv). For x-ray radiation, which is the type used in CT scanners, 1 mSv = 1 mGy.

16 *Which of the following is TRUE regarding the use of so-called "triple-contrast" CT scans, i.e., PO, IV, and rectal contrast for penetrating torso trauma?*

A *These studies should be reserved for the evaluation of patients with penetrating flank or back wounds.*

B *All trauma patients should receive triple-contrast CT scans.*

C *The addition of rectal contrast does not increase the sensitivity for the presence of bowel injuries.*

D *They should still be obtained in patients with an indication for immediate operative management as they will guide surgical intervention and decision-making.*

E *The use of oral contrast in patients with penetrating trauma is not safe.*

The use of triple-contrast CT scans to evaluate for penetrating torso trauma was described many years ago, as a way to evaluate the retroperitoneal organs and increase the sensitivity of this study in this population of trauma patients. The purported advantages are in helping to identify subtle injuries, trajectory of the wound, as well as helping to select patients who might be candidates for nonoperative management. The "added" benefit of rectal contrast may be effective in the diagnosis of extraperitoneal colonic injuries, where patients have sustained penetrating wounds to the flanks or back. These types of injuries are notoriously difficult to diagnose. The studies with triple-contrast studies have been criticized as being underpowered as extraperitoneal colonic injuries are rare. The benefit of oral contrast has also been questioned as it is not been shown to identify duodenal injuries in any studies.

A. The added benefit of rectal contrast is only really worthwhile for those retroperitoneal structures such as the ascending and descending colon. The pancreas, stomach, and solid organs can also be better imaged with the contrasting media in place. We would recommend the addition of rectal contrast only in this group of patients.

B. Although the use of rectal contrast in the trauma patient is by no means ideal, it is usually fairly well-tolerated in the stable patient, without other distracting injuries. Concern for patient tolerance should not be a consideration in ordering this study, although local protocols may have to be developed to provide clarity over who is responsible for the installation of the rectal contrast, e.g., physician, CT tech, nurse, etc. However, it is not required as a matter of routine.

C. The addition of rectal contrast does seem to confer a small advantage to the accuracy of the CT exam. Most studies have concluded that a negative triple-contrast helical CT scan has a negative predictive value of 98–100%. There have been no direct randomized trials comparing triple contrast versus IV contrast alone in trauma patients, so it is difficult to quantify the additional advantage, which is why we would specifically recommend it for those patients with penetrating back and flank injuries.

D. In patients who have clear indications for surgery (e.g., evisceration, peritonitis), CT scans should not be performed, and especially not a CT scan with PO contrast. These patients should proceed directly to the operating room.

E. Multiple studies have shown that the use of PO contrast in an awake and hemodynamically stable trauma patient is safe. Intoxicated patients, those with traumatic injuries or with indications for the OR, should not be given PO contrast. In those cases, a CT scan with IV contrast alone may have to suffice. Theoretical concerns over aspiration of oral contrast media due to gastric distention or ileus have not been borne out in clinical practice.

Answer: A

Chiu WC, Shanmuganathan K, Mirvis SE, et al. Determining the need for laparotomy in penetrating torso trauma: a prospective study using triple-contrast enhanced abdominopelvic computed tomography. *The Journal of Trauma* 2001 Nov;51(5):860–868.

Como JJ, Bokhari F, Chiu WC, et al. Practice management guidelines for selective nonoperative management of penetrating abdominal trauma. *The Journal of Trauma* 2010 Mar;68(3):721–33.

Lozano JD, Munera F, Anderson SW, et al. Penetrating wounds to the torso: evaluation with triple-contrast multidetector CT. *Radiographics* 2013 Mar-Apr;33(2):341–359.

17 *In which of the following patients could a pelvic x-ray be safely omitted?*
   A *23-year-old man following a motorcycle crash at high speed, hemodynamically stable but complaining of pain in the left hip.*
   B *78-year-old woman following a ground level fall.*
   C *47-year-old man who was ambulatory after a rear-end collision at 45 mph, with a normal clinical exam.*
   D *32-year-old woman, with a BP of 90/60 mm Hg and severe pain over the sacrum.*
   E *16-year-old man following a bicycle crash, with blood at the urinary meatus.*

Pelvic x-rays are notoriously inaccurate for the diagnosis of pelvic fractures, with a false-negative rate somewhere between 20 and 30%. However, there are a certain group of patients in which they provide useful information as a screening tool, particularly if those patients are not undergoing abdominal and/or pelvic CT scanning. More and more, pelvic x-rays are being omitted in neurologically normal, hemodynamically stable patients who are undergoing abdomen and pelvis CT scans as part of their workup.

A is not correct. This patient is at risk of either a femur fracture or pubic rami fractures and should therefore be imaged.

B is not correct. This patient requires imaging due to the increased fracture risk in the elderly because of osteoporosis.

C is correct answer. The 47-year-old man described here, who was ambulatory at the scene, is unlikely to have a clinically significant pelvic fracture and as long as a clinical exam is reliable (i.e., the patient is not intoxicated or has other distracting injuries), the x-ray could safely be emitted with a low risk for missed injury.

D is not correct. Any patient with significant mechanism for pelvic trauma that is hemodynamically unstable should have a pelvic x-ray performed to help assess for pelvic trauma which could be the etiology of the patient's hemodynamic instability and facilitate the initiation of appropriate intervention and resuscitative measures.

E is not correct. Any signs or symptoms of possible urethral trauma mandate a pelvic x-ray as part of the workup prior to placement of Foley catheter as a retrograde urethrogram may be necessary.

Answer: C

Guillamondegui OD, Pryor JP, Gracias VH, et al. Pelvic radiography in blunt trauma resuscitation: a diminishing role. *The Journal of Trauma* 2002 Dec;53(6):1043–1047.

Kessel B, Sevi R, Jeroukhimov I, et al. Is routine portable pelvic X-ray in stable multiple trauma patients always justified in a high technology era? *Injury* 2007 May;38(5):559–563.

Obaid AK, Barleben A, Porral D, et al. Utility of plain film pelvic radiographs in blunt trauma patients in the emergency department. *The American Surgeon* 2006 Oct;72(10):951–954.

Soto JR, Zhou C, Hu D, et al. Skip and save: utility of pelvic x-rays in the initial evaluation of blunt trauma patients. *American Journal of Surgery* 2015 Dec;210(6):1076–1079.

18 *Which of the following is correct regarding diagnostic imaging for pulmonary embolism?*

  A *Plain films of the chest will not demonstrate any significant findings.*

  B *VQ scanning should be avoided in women of childbearing age.*

  C *Chronic pulmonary emboli manifest on CT as wedge-shaped peripheral opacities with a "reverse halo" of consolidation around a central area of ground-glass opacification.*

  D *MRI of the pulmonary artery has a higher sensitivity for detecting pulmonary embolism than CTA.*

  E *The presence of right ventricular free wall hypokinesia/akinesia with preserved apical segment wall motion (McConnell Sign) is highly specific to pulmonary embolism even in the presence of cardiorespiratory disease.*

CTA of the chest is the gold standard for imaging to establish the diagnosis of pulmonary embolism. However, plain films, VQ scans, MRI, and ultrasonography are all modalities which can also help establish the diagnosis. It is important to note that findings consistent with PE on echocardiography are not usually specific to pulmonary embolism and can also be seen in many cardiorespiratory conditions causing elevated right ventricular and atrial pressures. The exception to this is the presence of right ventricular wall hypokinesia/akinesia with preserved apical segment wall motion (McConnell Sign), which is highly specific to pulmonary embolism.

A is not correct. Plain films of the chest can demonstrate an enlarged pulmonary artery (Fleischner sign), regional oligemia (Westermark sign), or the presence of a peripherally located wedge-shaped opacity consistent with pulmonary infarction (Hampton Hump) in the presence of PE.

B is not correct. VQ scans involve less radiation to the breast than CTA of the chest and therefore are a favorable alternative in young women of childbearing age where radiation exposure may be a concern.

C is not correct. This is a description of findings of acute pulmonary embolism. A chronic pulmonary embolism would manifest on CTA of the chest with intraluminal webs, calcifications, thrombus recanalization, and filling defects adherent to the wall of the vessel.

D is not correct. MRI of the pulmonary artery is less sensitive than CTA.

E is the correct answer.

Answer: E

Kurzyna M, Torbicki A, Pruszczyk P, et al. Disturbed right ventricular ejection pattern as a new Doppler echocardiographic sign of acute pulmonary embolism. *The American Journal of Cardiology* 2002;90:507–511.

Moore AJE, Wachsmann J, Chamarthy MR et al. Imaging of acute pulmonary embolism: an update. *Cardiovasc Diagn Ther.* 2018 Jun; 8(3):225–243.

McConnell MV, Solomon SD, Rayan ME, et al. Regional right ventricular dysfunction detected by echocardiography in acute pulmonary embolism. *The American Journal of Cardiology* 1996;78:469–473.

19 *A 22-year-old female G0P1 at 10w5d gestation develops sudden onset hypoxia, shortness of breath, and tachycardia. Pulmonary embolism is suspected. Which of the following is true regarding diagnostic imaging for this patient?*

  A *CTA delivers less radiation to the breast tissue than VQ scanning.*

  B *MRA does not pose a risk to the fetus.*

  C *Echo/ultrasound may be suggestive.*

  D *Both CTA and VQ scans should be avoided due to a high radiation dose.*

  E *There is more fetal radiation exposure with CTA than with VQ scanning.*

The pregnant patient poses a challenge in the workup of pulmonary embolism, especially in the first trimester. When possible, ultrasound is the best modality to establish the diagnosis as it does not convey the risk of ionizing radiation or gadolinium exposure.

A is not correct. CTA delivers more radiation to the breast tissue than VQ scanning, but exposes the fetus to less ionizing radiation.

B is not correct. MRA poses a risk to the fetus due to the use of gadolinium.

C is the correct answer. Ultrasound is a safe option for diagnostic imaging to establish the diagnosis of PE in a first trimester pregnant patient as it involves neither gadolinium nor ionizing radiation. However, its specificity is limited in settings where the patient has comorbid cardiorespiratory conditions that can cause elevated right ventricular or atrial pressures.

D is not correct. CTA and VQ scans have relatively low doses of ionizing radiation (<1mGy) and can be used if necessary. CTA delivers more radiation to the breast, while VQ scans expose the fetus to a higher total dose of radiation.

E is not correct. VQ scanning exposes the fetus to more radiation than CTA.

Answer: C

Moore AJE, Wachsmann J, Chamarthy MR et al. Imaging of acute pulmonary embolism: an update. *Cardiovascular Diagnosis & The*rapy 2018 Jun; 8(3):225–243.

Schembri GP, Miller AE, Smart R. Radiation dosimetry and safety issues in the investigation of pulmonary embolism. *Seminars in Nuclear Medicine* 2010;40:442–454.

20 *Which of the following patients with blunt pelvic fracture should proceed directly to pelvic angioembolization?*
   A *Hypotensive patient with a positive FAST.*
   B *Hypotensive patient with negative FAST and stable pelvis.*
   C *Normotensive stable patient without evidence of pelvic fracture on CT scan.*
   D *Normotensive stable patient with a pelvic fracture but no contrast blush on CT.*
   E *Normotensive stable patient with pelvic fracture and pelvic blush on CT.*

A is incorrect. A hypotensive unstable patient with a positive FAST should proceed directly to operative exploration as there is intraperitoneal hemorrhage that needs to be addressed. If the patient has a concurrent pelvic fracture contributing to the hemorrhagic shock, there are several alternatives to control hemorrhage including pelvic fixation, preperitoneal packing, internal iliac artery ligation or clipping, with subsequent angioembolization when available.

B is incorrect. A hypotensive unstable patient with a negative fast and a stable pelvis should be considered for diagnostic peritoneal aspiration to determine if the negative FAST was a false-negative test. If positive for gross blood, then the patient should be taken to the OR for exploration.

C is incorrect. A normotensive stable patient without a pelvic fracture or blush does not need pelvic angioembolization.

D is incorrect. A normotensive stable patient with a fracture without a blush on CT should not need angiography as the likelihood of arterial source of hemorrhage is low.

E is correct. A stable patient with a pelvic fracture with active blush should proceed to angioembolization as the next appropriate step in management prior to the patient becoming hypotensive from the hemorrhage.

Answer: E

Cullinane, DC, Shiller HJ, Zielinski MD, et al. Eastern Association for the Surgery of Trauma Practice Management Guidelines for Hemorrhage in Pelvic Fracture—Update and Systematic Review. *Eastern Trauma Association* (2011). www.east.org/pelvicPMG_Updated-Pub_Dec2011.

Western Trauma Association. Algorithm for management of pelvic fracture (2020). https://www.westerntrauma.org/wp-content/uploads/2020/10/2-image-from-jot.pdf

28

Neurotrauma

Bellal Joseph, MD[1] and Raul Reina Limon, MD[2]

[1] Division of Trauma, Surgical Critical Care, Burns and Acute Care Surgery, University of Arizona College of Medicine, Banner University Medical Center, Tucson, AZ, USA
[2] Division of Trauma, Critical Care, Burns, and Emergency Surgery, Department of Surgery, University of Arizona, Tucson, AZ, USA

The following vignette applies to questions 1 and 2:
A 72-year-old man presents to the emergency department with nausea, vomiting, and headaches for the last 36 hours. His wife says he has been irritable and forgetting to do routine errands for the last 2 weeks. He leads an active lifestyle but had a skiing accident 2 weeks ago. He has stable angina and moderately controlled hypertension. He has been drinking 2 glasses of whiskey every day for 30 years. He is not oriented to time, place, or person. His blood pressure is 170/100 mm Hg. Deep tendon reflexes are 4+ on the left and 2+ on the right. There is a positive Babinski sign on the left.

Question 1:

1 *A CT scan of the head without contrast is performed, which shows an extra-axial, isodense 17-mm crescent-shaped collection across the right hemisphere which crosses suture lines. No midline shift is noted. What is the most likely diagnosis?*
   A *Subarachnoid hemorrhage*
   B *Epidural hematoma*
   C *Intraventricular hemorrhage*
   D *Subacute subdural hematoma*
   E *Intracerebral hemorrhage*

Question 2:

2 *Which of the following is the most appropriate next step in the management of this patient?*
   A *Perform a lumbar puncture*
   B *Administer recombinant tissue plasminogen activator*
   C *Observe the patient for 24 hours*
   D *Administer low-molecular-weight heparin (LMWH)*
   E *Perform craniotomy and clot evacuation*

This patient has a history of recent blunt head injury and progressive neurological deterioration. He has sustained a subacute subdural hematoma (SDH) from a traumatic brain injury. Rapid acceleration and deceleration can lead to shearing of bridging veins of the cranium. These bridging veins are the connections between the intraparenchymal veins of the brain and the dural venous sinuses. This patient's advanced age and long-term alcohol consumption have likely contributed to brain parenchymal atrophy, leading to increased stretch on these bridging veins, placing him at high risk for subdural hematoma formation even with minimal trauma. First-line imaging indicated for the diagnosis of SDH is computed tomography (CT) of the head without IV contrast. Classic findings include a crescent-shaped, biconcave lesion that crosses suture lines but not the midline. There may or may not be a midline shift. The density of lesions depends on the timeframe of SDH. Acute SDH (symptom onset within 3 days of injury) will be hyperdense, subacute SDH (symptom onset within 4–20 days of injury) will be isodense to hyperdense, and chronic SDH (symptom onset beyond 21 days of injury) will be hypodense on imaging. An epidural hematoma would have a biconvex lens-shaped hyperdense lesion on head CT, that does not cross suture lines. A subarachnoid hemorrhage would reveal hyperdensities in the subarachnoid space, usually having a star-shaped appearance, on head CT. An intracerebral hemorrhage would reveal a hyperdensity within a lobe of the brain. An intraventricular hemorrhage would reveal hyperdensities within the third, fourth, or lateral ventricles on head CT.

All patients should receive supportive care, monitoring, and frequent neurological examinations, along with prevention of secondary bleeding or progression of existing bleed (immediate discontinuation or reversal of anticoagulant or antiplatelet medications), neuroprotective measures, and ICP management. Indications for neurosurgical intervention include hematoma size > 10 mm, midline shift > 5 mm, ICP > 20 mm Hg, signs of cerebral herniation, rapid neurological deterioration, and failure of conservative management. Options for neurosurgical intervention include decompressive craniectomy, craniotomy and clot evacuation, or emergency temporizing burr hole craniotomy.

Surgical Critical Care and Emergency Surgery: Clinical Questions and Answers, Third Edition.
Edited by Forrest "Dell" Moore, Peter M. Rhee, and Carlos J. Rodriguez.
© 2022 John Wiley & Sons Ltd. Published 2022 by John Wiley & Sons Ltd.
Companion website: www.wiley.com/go/surgicalcriticalcare3e

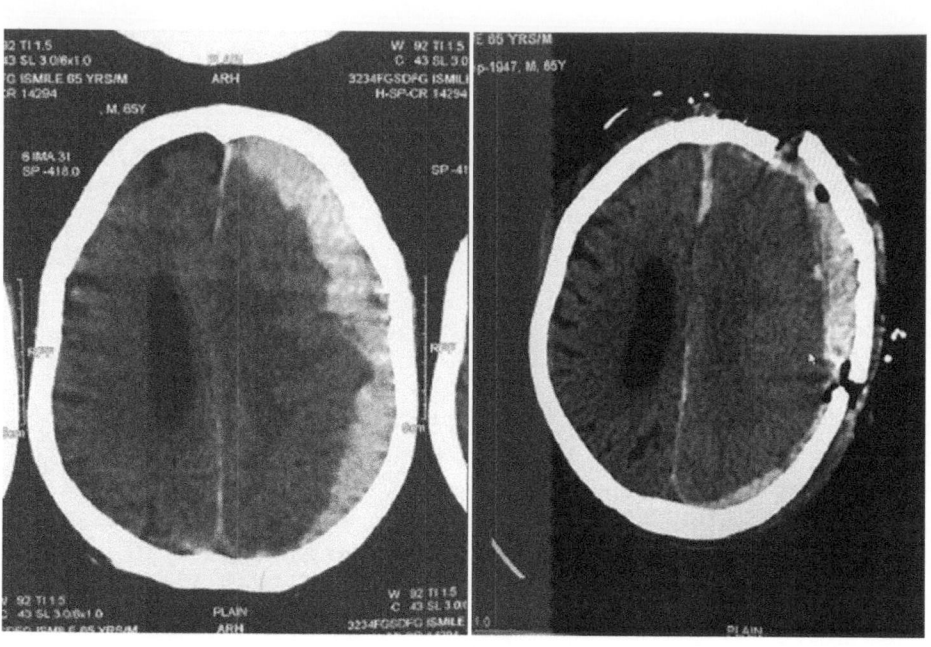

Left: Acute subdural hematoma. Right: Post-craniectomy

Fomchenko EI, Gilmore EJ, Matouk CC, Gerrard JL, Sheth KN. Management of subdural hematomas: part II. Surgical management of subdural hematomas. *Current Treatment Options in Neurology* 2018;20(8):34.

Mutch CA, Talbott JF, Gean A. Imaging evaluation of acute traumatic brain injury. *Neurosurgery Clinics.* 2016;27(4):409–439.

Wind JJ, Leiphart JW. Bilateral subacute subdural hematomas. *New England Journal of Medicine* 2009;360(17):e23.

Q1 Answer: D

Q2 Answer: E

The following vignette applies to questions 3 and 4:

A 40-year-old man is brought to the emergency department 30 minutes after crashing his car into a telephone pole. He has a history of alcohol abuse. On arrival his pulse is 63 beats/min, respiratory rate is 10 breaths/min, and blood pressure is 100/70 mm Hg. His pupils are sluggish. There are multiple bruises over the face, chest, abdomen, and upper extremities, a 5-cm laceration across his left cheek, and tactile crepitus over the left face. There are decreased breath sounds over the right lower lung field. His abdomen is soft but diffusely tender to palpation in all quadrants without guarding or rebound. Both wrists and elbows are swollen.

3   *He does not respond to commands but makes groaning sounds. Pinching his sternum tightly causes him to open his eyes and withdraw all his extremities. What is this patient's Glasgow Coma Scale (GCS)?*
   A *3*
   B *5*
   C *8*
   D *10*
   E *15*

4   *What is the next best step in the management of this patient?*
   A *CT scan of the head and neck*
   B *Insertion of an intercostal chest tube*
   C *Focused assessment sonography for trauma (FAST)*
   D *Intubation and mechanical ventilation*
   E *Bilateral x-rays of upper extremities*

The Glasgow Coma Scale (GCS) should be determined for all injured patients. It is calculated by adding the scores of the best motor response (1–6), best verbal response (1–5), and eye-opening (1–4). Scores range from 3 (the lowest) to 15 (normal). Scores of 13–15 indicate mild head injury, 9–12 moderate injury, and 8 or below severe injury. The GCS is useful for both triage and prognosis. The GCS score has been shown to have a significant correlation with outcome following severe TBI, both as the sum score or as just the motor component. A recent study has shown that pupil reactivity together with the GCS motor component correlates best with mortality. In patients with a different motor response between the left and right side, the best movement is used. This patient's GCS score is calculated as follows: groans = 2 (best verbal response); opens eyes to pain = 2 (best eye response); withdraws extremities to painful stimuli = 4 (best motor response); GCS score = 8.

Patients with a GCS score of 8 or below as a result of traumatic brain injury must be intubated and mechanically ventilated to protect their airway and ensure adequate respiratory function. These patients are most at risk of aspiration and hypoxia from the lack of gag reflex and decreased brainstem respiratory drive. Although the patient may eventually require all the other option choices listed (chest tube placement for possible hemothorax, head and neck CT to evaluate injuries, FAST to rule out abdominal or pericardial hemorrhage, x-rays to evaluate for extremity fractures), intubation and mechanical ventilation should be the next immediate step.

Score	Eyes	Verbal	Motor
1	Does not open eyes	Makes no sounds	Makes no movements
2	Opens eyes to painful stimuli only	Incomprehensible sounds	Extension response to pain (decerebrate posturing)
3	Opens eyes in response to voice command	Inappropriate words	Abnormal flexion response to pain (decorticate posturing)
4	Eyes are open spontaneously	Confused, disoriented	Flexion/ withdrawal from painful stimuli
5	N/A	Oriented, converses normally	Localizes painful stimuli
6	N/A	N/A	Obeys commands

Q3 Answer: C

Q4 Answer: D

Carney N, Totten AM, O'Reilly C, Ullman JS, Hawryluk GW, Bell MJ, et al. Guidelines for the management of severe traumatic brain injury. *Neurosurgery* 2017;80(1):6–15.

Hoffmann M, Lefering R, Rueger J, Kolb J, Izbicki J, Ruecker A, et al. Pupil evaluation in addition to Glasgow Coma Scale components in prediction of traumatic brain injury and mortality. *British Journal of Surgery* 2012;99(S1):122–130.

Mayglothling J, Duane TM, Gibbs M, McCunn M, Legome E, Eastman AL, et al. Emergency tracheal intubation immediately following traumatic injury: an Eastern Association for the Surgery of Trauma practice management guideline. *Journal of Trauma and Acute Care Surgery* 2012;73(5):S333–S340.

Teasdale G, Jennett B. Assessment of coma and impaired consciousness: a practical scale. *The Lancet.* 1974;304(7872):81–84.

The following vignette applies to questions 5 and 6:

A 40-year-old man presents after being thrown off his motorcycle and striking his head on the pavement. His breath smells of alcohol. He is unconscious. He has a 6 cm laceration across the right side of his head. Deep tendon reflexes are absent on the right side. His pupils are sluggish. His vitals are normal except for a respiratory rate of 8 breaths/min. He is immediately intubated and mechanically ventilated. Head CT is ordered, which reveals a depressed skull fracture, a 9 mm epidural hematoma and multiple 8 mm intraparenchymal hemorrhages of the right parietal and temporal lobes.

5 *The attending trauma surgeon declares the patient to be Brain Injury Guidelines (BIG) category 3. Which of the following additional findings would be most consistent with a BIG 3 categorization?*
  A *Trace subarachnoid hemorrhage found on head CT.*
  B *A 2 mm subdural hematoma on the right side found on head CT.*
  C *A normal neurological examination.*
  D *A 5 year history of taking aspirin for coronary artery disease.*
  E *No intraventricular hemorrhage found on head CT.*

6 *According to BIG, what should the management plan for this patient include?*
  A *Only observe the patient for 6 hours.*
  B *Admit the patient, but do not order a repeat head CT.*
  C *Admit the patient and order a repeat head CT, but do not consult neurosurgery.*
  D *Let the patient go home and return for follow-up the next day.*
  E *Admit the patient, request a neurosurgical consult, and order repeat head CT.*

Modern computed tomography (CT) technology has advanced to the point that even minor intracranial injuries are identified, often prompting reflex escalation of care. This has led to the over-utilization of valuable healthcare resources. The Brain Injury Guidelines (BIG) were developed and subsequently validated as a triage tool for acute care surgeons in the setting of traumatic brain injury (see figure below). Based on the patient's history, neurologic examination (an abnormal neurologic examination is defined as the presence of altered mental status, focal neurological deficits, or abnormal pupillary response), and initial head CT findings, BIG can help guide decisions on admission, repeat imaging, and neurosurgical consultation. Patients presenting with blunt TBI and positive initial head CT findings are stratified into one of three BIG categories. Failure to meet even one criterion of BIG category 1 or 2 (e.g., history of antiplatelet or anticoagulant use, displaced skull fracture, large or scattered intracranial hemorrhages, or abnormal neurologic examination) will immediately upgrade the patient to BIG category 3. Each BIG category then has a recommended therapeutic plan which will help decrease over- and under-triage of patients.

Brain Injury Guidelines

Variables	BIG 1	BIG 2	BIG 3
LOC	Yes/No	Yes/No	Yes/No
Neurologic examination	Normal	Normal	Abnormal
Intoxication	No	No/Yes	No/Yes
CAMP	No	No	Yes
Skull Fracture	No	Non-displaced	Displaced
SDH	≤4mm	5–7 mm	≥8 mm
EDH	≤4mm	5–7 mm	≥8 mm
IPH	≤4mm, 1 location	3–7 mm, 2 Locations	≥8 mm, multiple locations
SAH	Trace	Localized	Scattered
IVH	No	No	Yes

THERAPEUTIC PLAN

Hospitalization	No Observation (6hrs)	Yes	Yes
RHCT	No	No	Yes
NSC	No	No	Yes

BIG, brain injury guidelines; CAMP, Coumadin, Aspirin, Plavix; EDH, epidural hemorrhage; IVH, intraventricular hemorrhage; IPH, intraparenchymal hemorrhage; LOC, loss of consciousness; NSC, neurosurgical consultation; RHCT, repeat head computed tomography; SAH, subarachnoid hemorrhage; SDH, subdural hemorrhage

Q5 Answer: D

Q6 Answer: E

Joseph B, Friese RS, Sadoun M, Aziz H, Kulvatunyou N, Pandit V, et al. The BIG (brain injury guidelines) project: defining the management of traumatic brain injury by acute care surgeons. *Journal of Trauma and Acute Care Surgery* 2014;76(4):965–969.

Joseph B, Aziz H, Pandit V, Kulvatunyou N, Sadoun M, Tang A, et al. Prospective validation of the brain injury guidelines: managing traumatic brain injury without neurosurgical consultation. *Journal of Trauma and Acute Care Surgery* 2014;77(6):984–988.

Martin GE, Carroll CP, Plummer ZJ, Millar DA, Pritts TA, Makley AT, et al. Safety and efficacy of brain injury guidelines at a Level III trauma center. *Journal of Trauma and Acute Care Surgery* 2018;84(3):483–489.

The following vignette applies to questions 7–10:

A 45-year-old man is brought to the trauma bay after being an unrestrained passenger in a high-speed motor vehicle collision. He has a 7 cm laceration on the left side of his head, and multiple lacerations on his right upper and lower extremities. He is unresponsive, and is intubated and mechanically ventilated. His blood pressure is 140/90 mm Hg. Head CT reveals a depressed parietal bone fracture, multiple punctate hemorrhages at the gray-white junction, an 8 mm epidural hematoma, and 4 mm midline shift.

7   A decision is made to perform a craniotomy for clot evacuation. Afterward, the patient is admitted to the intensive care unit. According to the Brain Trauma Foundation guidelines, which of the following is an indication for ICP monitoring in this patient?
   A Severe head injury (GCS ≤ 8) and an abnormal head CT
   B Severe head injury, normal head CT, and age > 40 years
   C Severe head injury, normal head CT, and systolic blood pressure > 90 mm Hg
   D Severe head injury, irregular respiration, and > 5-cm head laceration
   E None of the above

The Brain Trauma Foundation guidelines recommend intracranial pressure (ICP) monitoring for patients with a severe head injury, defined as a GCS ≤ 8, and an abnormality on Head CT. In addition, ICP monitoring may be recommended for patients with a severe head injury and a normal Head CT if they also have 2 or more of the following: abnormal motor posturing; age > 40 years; systolic blood pressure < 90 mm Hg.

Answer: A

Bullock R, Chesnut R, Clifton G, Ghajar J, Marion D, Narayan R, et al. Guidelines for the management of severe head injury. *European Journal of Emergency Medicine* 1996;3:109–127.

Carney N, Totten AM, O'Reilly C, Ullman JS, Hawryluk GW, Bell MJ, et al. Guidelines for the management of severe traumatic brain injury. *Neurosurgery* 2017;80(1):6–15.

8 *Certain measures are undertaken to prevent secondary brain injury in this patient. Which of the following may prevent secondary brain injury?*

  A *Keeping the patient's core body temperature at or above 39 degrees Celsius.*

  B *Permissive hyperglycemia, not allowing the patient's blood glucose level to go below 180 mg/dL.*

  C *Seizure prophylaxis with anti-epileptic medications.*

  D *Keeping the patient's systolic blood pressure above 160 mm Hg.*

  E *Hypoventilation, to raise the $PaCO_2$*

The focus of attention during management of acute neurological injury must be on preventing secondary brain injury. There is a large and growing body of evidence on what factors can contribute to the development of secondary brain injury after the primary insult. Hyperthermia has been found to worsen outcomes and increase lengths of stay in the neurologic intensive care population. Hyperthermia is thought to cause harm by way of increased glutamate release and excitotoxicity, along with increased free radical production and worsening cerebral edema. In addition, both hyperglycemia and hypoglycemia have been shown to worsen outcomes for neuro-ICU patients. Although the ideal blood glucose target range for such patients has not been identified definitively and many studies advocate individualized blood glucose targets, a blood glucose level above 180 mg/dL is certainly contraindicated in all patients. Seizures frequently occur after neurologic injury and may contribute to secondary brain injury by increasing metabolic demands of brain tissue in the setting of reduced cerebral oxygen delivery. Anti-epileptic medications are recommended for the initial week after traumatic brain injury to prevent the development of post-traumatic epilepsy. Hypertension can frequently occur in severe head injury patients, either as an unmasking of underlying hypertension or as a compensatory response to the brain injury. In patients with traumatic brain injury, blood pressure is often kept between 110 and 140 mm Hg to prevent worsening cerebral edema or secondary hemorrhage. An overly aggressive blood pressure management strategy can also significantly worsen outcomes, as hypotension can lead to significant cerebral hypoperfusion. Finally, hyperventilation, not hypoventilation, is an initial management strategy employed in traumatic brain injury patients, to help induce cerebral arteriolar vasoconstriction and thus reduce cerebral edema formation, which helps prevent secondary brain injury.

Answer: C

Diringer MN, Reaven NL, Funk SE, Uman GC. Elevated body temperature independently contributes to increased length of stay in neurologic intensive care unit patients. *Critical Care Medicine* 2004;32(7):1489–1495.

Manno EM, Farmer JC. Acute brain injury: If hypothermia is good, then is hyperthermia bad? *Critical Care Medicine* 2004;32(7):1611–1612.

Temkin NR, Dikmen SS, Wilensky AJ, Keihm J, Chabal S, Winn HR. A randomized, double-blind study of phenytoin for the prevention of post-traumatic seizures. *New England Journal of Medicine* 1990;323(8):497–502.

9 *Which of the following central nervous system cell types is most susceptible to hypoxic ischemic injury?*

  A *Neurons*

  B *Oligodendrocytes*

  C *Astrocytes*

  D *Endothelial cells*

  E *Microglial cells*

In order of decreasing susceptibility to ischemia: neurons; oligodendrocytes; astrocytes; endothelial cells; microglial cells.

Answer: A

Lipton P. Ischemic cell death in brain neurons. *Physiological Reviews* 1999;79(4):1431–568.

Sugawara T, Lewén A, Noshita N, Gasche Y, Chan PH. Effects of global ischemia duration on neuronal, astroglial, oligodendroglial, and microglial reactions in the vulnerable hippocampal CA1 subregion in rats. *Journal of Neurotrauma* 2002;19(1):85–98.

Xu J, He L, Ahmed SH, Chen S-W, Goldberg MP, Beckman JS, et al. Oxygen-glucose deprivation induces inducible nitric oxide synthase and nitrotyrosine expression in cerebral endothelial cells. *Stroke* 2000;31(7):1744–1751.

10 *An overall strategy for treating intracranial hypertension following severe head injury usually includes attempts to maintain as high a cerebral perfusion pressure (CPP) and as low an ICP as possible. Which of the following is contraindicated considering such a strategy?*

  A *Barbiturate coma*

  B *Maintaining peak-end expiratory pressures (PEEP) less than 15–20 cm of H_2O*

  C *Hemicraniectomy with duraplasty for very refractory cases*

  D *Corticosteroids*

  E *Hypertonic saline administration*

Barbiturate coma and indeed other sedatives lead to reduced metabolic demands of the nervous tissue and subsequently reduce cerebral blood flow requirements via cerebral autoregulatory mechanisms. High PEEP pressures during mechanical ventilation can transmit high intrathoracic pressures to the valveless head and neck veins, reducing venous outflow from the brain and contributing to increased intracranial pressures. Thus, maintaining low PEEP would not be a contraindication. For very refractory cases, surgical procedures like craniectomy may be employed, where the cranial vault is opened to allow for the brain to expand outward and reduce intracranial pressure. Hypertonic saline administration can cause an osmotic shift of fluid from the cerebral interstitium and into the cerebral vasculature and subsequently drain out of the cranial vault, leading to reduced cerebral edema and thus reduced intracranial pressure. Although corticosteroids have shown utility in treating the vasogenic edema associated with brain tumors and infectious processes, they are not recommended for use in the head injury cohort. This patient has a severe head injury and thus corticosteroid use would not be indicated.

Answer: D

Cooper DJ, Rosenfeld JV, Murray L, Arabi YM, Davies AR, D'Urso P, et al. Decompressive craniectomy in diffuse traumatic brain injury. *New England Journal of Medicine* 2011;364(16):1493–1502.

Cooper PR, Moody S, Clark WK, Kirkpatrick J, Maravilla K, Gould AL, et al. Dexamethasone and severe head injury: a prospective double-blind study. *Journal of Neurosurgery* 1979;51(3):307–316.

Koenig M, Bryan M, Lewin J, Mirski MA, Geocadin R, Stevens RD. Reversal of transtentorial herniation with hypertonic saline. *Neurology* 2008;70(13):1023–1229.

Schalen W, Sonesson B, Messeter K, Nordström G, Nordström C-H. Clinical outcome and cognitive impairment in patients with severe head injuries treated with barbiturate coma. *Acta Neurochirurgica* 1992;117(3-4):153–159.

Tolias CM, Reinert M, Seiler R, Gilman C, Scharf A, Bullock MR. Normobaric hyperoxia – induced improvement in cerebral metabolism and reduction in intracranial pressure in patients with severe head injury: a prospective historical cohort – matched study. *Journal of Neurosurgery* 2004;101(3):435–444.

11 *In patients with a severe head injury who are intubated and cannot elicit a verbal response, the GCS score may be difficult to calculate. In place of the GCS, the FOUR score has been developed and validated to assess the coma status of patients, especially those who are intubated. Which of the following is taken into account during the assessment of the FOUR score?*

A *Brainstem reflexes (corneal and pupillary reflexes)*
B *Respiratory drive and breathing pattern*
C *Best motor response*
D *Best eye response*
E *All of the above*

The GCS score is frequently used as a quantitative assessment of neurologic function. However, in intubated patients, the Full Outline of UnResponsiveness (FOUR) score may be preferable to GCS, because a significant proportion of the GCS score becomes comprised in such situations. Moreover, the FOUR score takes into account brainstem injury, locked-in syndrome, uncal herniation, and includes an assessment of the respiratory drive. The FOUR score has been validated by multiple studies in different patient populations.

Score	Eye Response	Motor Response	Brainstem Reflexes	Respiration
4	Eyelids open or opened, tracking, or blinking to command	Thumbs-up, fist, or peace sign to command	Pupillary and corneal reflexes present	Not intubated, regular breathing pattern
3	Eyelids open but not tracking	Localizing to pain	One pupil wide and fixed	Not intubated, Cheyne-Stokes breathing pattern
2	Eyelids closed but open to a loud voice	Flexion response to pain	Pupillary *or* corneal reflex absent	Not intubated, irregular breathing pattern
1	Eyelids closed but open to pain	Extensor posturing	Pupillary *and* corneal reflexes absent	Intubated, breathes above ventilator rate
0	Eyelids remain closed with pain	No response to pain or generalized myoclonus status epilepticus	Absent pupillary, corneal, and cough reflexes	Intubated, breathes at ventilator rate or apnea

Answer: E

Almojuela A, Hasen M, Zeiler F. The Full Outline of UnResponsiveness (FOUR) Score and its use in outcome prediction: a scoping systematic review of the adult literature. *Neurocritical Care* 2019;31(1):162–175.

Foo CC, Loan JJ, Brennan PM. The relationship of the FOUR score to patient outcome: a systematic review. *Journal of Neurotrauma* 2019;36(17):2469–2483.

Wijdicks EF, Bamlet WR, Maramattom BV, Manno EM, McClelland RL. Validation of a new coma scale: the FOUR score. *Annals of Neurology: Official Journal of the American Neurological Association and the Child Neurology Society* 2005;58(4):585–593.

The following vignette applies to questions 12 and 13:

A 38-year-old man is admitted to the neuro ICU after he had been involved in a gang fight where he was beaten with baseball bats. CT scans showed a depressed skull fracture, an epidural hematoma, an intraparenchymal hemorrhage, 3 broken ribs, and a hemothorax. He was unconscious and thus was intubated and mechanically ventilated. He was managed promptly with a craniotomy and clot evacuation, and placement of a thoracostomy tube, but he is still unconscious and reliant on mechanical ventilation. He is also undergoing continuous ICP monitoring.

12 *The ICP monitor shows that his ICP has consistently been above 30 mm Hg. In addition, his blood pressure has been hard to correct and is consistently elevated at 160/100 mm Hg. Which of the following medications is indicated in this patient with traumatic brain injury who has consistently elevated ICP and blood pressure?*
   A *Propranolol*
   B *Atenolol*
   C *Aspirin*
   D *Low-molecular-weight heparin*
   E *Dabigatran*

13 *What is the mechanism of action by which this medication will achieve its intended effects?*
   A *Reduction in core body temperature, thus reducing the brain's metabolic activities.*
   B *Inhibit catecholamine surge-mediated inflammation and apoptosis in brain tissues, as well as reduce blood pressure.*
   C *Inhibition of hepatic gluconeogenesis and thus prevent hyperglycemia, which itself can cause secondary brain injury.*
   D *Prevent clot formation by inhibiting the intrinsic and extrinsic pathways.*
   E *Prevent clot formation and progression by irreversibly inhibiting cyclooxygenase.*

It has been well documented that catecholamine levels surge following traumatic brain injury in proportion to the severity of injury, and may remain elevated for up to 10 days following injury. The raised catecholamine levels contribute to brain tissue inflammation and apoptosis. In addition, they cause elevations in blood pressure that when transmitted to the cerebral vasculature and blood flow, cause significant elevations in ICP and lead to secondary brain injury. Beta-blockers can attenuate this catecholamine response by inhibiting beta-adrenergic receptors. Multiple studies have shown improved outcomes with beta-blocker use in critically ill traumatic brain injury patients with raised ICP levels. Among the beta-blockers, propranolol was found to be the most effective and is an effective blood pressure control agent in this patient. Atenolol, a cardioselective beta-blocker, is not as effective as propranolol. Aspirin, dabigatran, LMWH, or other antiplatelet or anticoagulant medications would be initially contraindicated in traumatic brain injury patients who are at risk of intracranial bleed progression if given such medications.

Q12 Answer: A

Q13 Answer: B

Alali AS, Mukherjee K, McCredie VA, Golan E, Shah PS, Bardes JM, et al. Beta-blockers and traumatic brain injury: a systematic review and meta-analysis. *Annals of Surgery* 2017;266(6):952.

Heffernan DS, Inaba K, Arbabi S, Cotton BA. Sympathetic hyperactivity after traumatic brain injury and the role of beta-blocker therapy. *Journal of Trauma and Acute Care Surgery* 2010;69(6):1602–1609.

Ley EJ, Leonard SD, Barmparas G, Dhillon NK, Inaba K, Salim A, et al. Beta blockers in critically ill patients with traumatic brain injury: results from a multicenter, prospective, observational American Association for the Surgery of Trauma study. *Journal of Trauma and Acute Care Surgery* 2018;84(2):234–244.

Lozano D, Gonzales-Portillo GS, Acosta S, de la Pena I, Tajiri N, Kaneko Y, et al. Neuroinflammatory responses to traumatic brain injury: etiology, clinical consequences, and therapeutic opportunities. *Neuropsychiatric Disease and Treatment* 2015;11:97.

14 *A 10-week-old boy is brought to the emergency department by his father because of a 6 hour history of decreased arousability, and two episodes of vomiting. His vital signs are within normal limits. His father says that the symptoms began after he rolled over and fell from the bed. Examination shows regions of skin discoloration on the chest bilaterally and tense fontanelles. Chest x-ray shows posterior rib fractures. Fundoscopy shows bilateral optic disc swelling with retinal hemorrhages. Which of the following is the most likely diagnosis?*
   A *Epidural hemorrhage*
   B *Base of skull fracture*
   C *Subdural hemorrhage*
   D *Meningitis*
   E *Periventricular hemorrhage*

A subdural hematoma is frequently seen in infants with shaken baby syndrome. Shaken baby syndrome is a serious brain injury caused by forcefully and violently shaking a baby. Whiplash and rapid rotational head movements can lead to tearing of the intracerebral bridging veins and diffuse axonal injury. It can result from as little as five seconds of shaking. It is more common in children under age 2, but it can affect children up to age 5. Most cases of shaken baby syndrome occur among infants that are 6–12 weeks old, which is when babies tend to cry the most. Characteristic physical exam findings of the shaken baby syndrome include irritability, difficulty staying awake, retinal hemorrhages (due to rupture of the retinal veins), and bulging fontanelles, all of which are seen in this patient. Other injuries indicative of child abuse include posterior rib fractures, fractures at multiple stages of healing, bruises to the upper torso caused by the forceful grip, and complex long bone fractures (e.g., spiral fractures of the humerus). Inconsistent history concerning patient age as in this case (10-week-old child is unable to roll) is an important clue to diagnose these patients.

Answer: C

Gabaeff SC. Challenging the pathophysiologic connection between subdural hematoma, retinal hemorrhage and shaken baby syndrome. *The Western Journal of Emergency Medicine* 2011;12(2):144.

Hung K-L. Pediatric abusive head trauma. *Biomedical Journal* 2020.

Mian M, Shah J, Dalpiaz A, Schwamb R, Miao Y, Warren K, et al. Shaken baby syndrome: a review. *Fetal and Pediatric Pathology* 2015;34(3):169–175.

15 *A 17-year-old man is brought to the emergency department after sustaining a fall from his skateboard and hitting his head on the sidewalk an hour ago. He had an initial loss of consciousness for 3 minutes. He is now complaining of a headache and has vomited twice during the last 30 minutes. His pulse is 50 beats/min. He is oriented to person, place, and time. There is a bruise on the right temporal side of the head. While performing the remainder of the physical examination, the patient has a seizure. Which of the following is the most likely diagnosis in this patient?*
   A *Epidural hematoma*
   B *Skull Base fracture*
   C *Subdural hemorrhage*
   D *Subarachnoidal hemorrhage*
   E *Periventricular hemorrhages*

An epidural hematoma should be suspected in any patient with severe head trauma and initial loss of consciousness followed by temporary recovery and a renewed decline in mental status with signs of elevated ICP. It is estimated that in 20–50% of cases of epidural hemorrhage, there is a "lucid interval" following a brief loss of consciousness or period of confusion before neurological deterioration. Epidural hemorrhage may occur secondary to tearing of a middle meningeal artery, middle meningeal vein, or dural sinus, and may be acute or subacute in presentation. The lucid interval represents the time required for the blood to accumulate in the epidural space to proportions great enough to compress the brain.

Answer: A

Kaoutzani L, Stippler M. Epidural Hematoma. *Neurotrauma*. 2019:35.

Khairat A, Waseem M. Epidural Hematoma. *StatPearls* [Internet]. 2020.

Kushner D. Mild traumatic brain injury: toward understanding manifestations and treatment. *Archives of Internal Medicine* 1998;158(15):1617–1624.

The following vignette applies to questions 16–18:

A 54-year-old man is brought to the emergency department 30 minutes after being hit by a car while crossing the street. He had a tonic-clonic seizure and one episode of vomiting while being transported to the hospital. A CT scan of the head shows subarachnoid hemorrhage. The patient undergoes an endovascular coiling procedure. After three days of ICU monitoring, the patient was discharged home without any residual neurological deficits.

16 *Two days later, he experiences weakness in his right leg. Neurologic examination shows 3/5 strength in the right lower extremity and 5/5 strength in the left lower extremity. What is the pathophysiology behind the deterioration of this patient?*
   A *Rebleeding of cerebral arteries*
   B *Vasospasm of cerebral arteries*
   C *Massive thromboembolism of the cerebral arteries*
   D *Carotid-cavernous fistula*
   E *Dissecting aneurysm of cerebral arteries*

17 *Treatment with which of the following drugs was most likely to have prevented the patient's current condition?*
   A *Fresh frozen plasma*
   B *Aspirin*
   C *Nitroglycerin*
   D *Nimodipine*
   E *Lorazepam*

18 *What is the optimal management for this patient now that he has developed this complication?*
   A *Vasopressor administration to increase mean arterial pressure*

B *Tissue plasminogen activator (tPA) administration*

C *Aspirin and clopidogrel administration*

D *Statin administration*

E *Emergent craniotomy*

Subarachnoid hemorrhage (SAH) is a devastating condition, and the most common causes include spontaneously ruptured saccular aneurysms, arteriovenous malformations, and trauma. The optimal initial management of an acute subarachnoid hemorrhage includes supportive care, management of blood pressure, careful management of ICP, seizure prevention, blood glucose management, and control of the bleeding vessel, either through endovascular or open neurosurgical procedures. Although there is a significant risk of rebleeding within the first 3 days, another complication potentially awaits the patient beyond this period: delayed cerebral ischemia (DCI) may occur due to the irritant effects of subarachnoid blood on the cerebral blood vessels, leading to vasospasm and ischemia. This patient's sudden-onset neurologic deficit 5 days after SAH is a common presentation of vasospasm and DCI, which is a complication in ~30% of SAH cases and is more common with aneurysms. Although microthrombosis of cerebral vessels has been implicated as a minor mechanism for the development of DCI in subarachnoid hemorrhage patients, massive thromboembolism of cerebral vessels is a different process and would be the incorrect answer here. Carotid-cavernous fistulae and dissecting aneurysms of cerebral arteries occur in different subsets of patients, are not associated with subarachnoid hemorrhages, and would present with a different timeline of symptoms.

Many studies have documented the neuroprotective effects of the calcium channel blocker nimodipine in this subset of patients. Nimodipine has been shown to reduce morbidity and mortality associated with SAH, but the exact mechanism of benefit of nimodipine beyond simply vasodilatation of cerebral blood vessels is not known clearly. It is recommended to give nimodipine for 21 days as prophylaxis against DCI in all patients with subarachnoid hemorrhage. Other medications that have been studied for neuroprotective effects in animal or human studies include statins, magnesium sulfate, other calcium channel blockers, tirilazad, antiplatelet agents (aspirin), nitric oxide donors (nitroglycerin), and endothelin-1 antagonists. However, their use is not recommended over nimodipine, and most have not demonstrated any benefit. Lorazepam and fresh frozen plasma have neither been studied for their prophylactic effects against DCI nor recommended for use.

Once vasospasm and DCI have developed, the Neurocritical Care Society recommends induced hypertension with the use of vasopressor agents, to increase the mean arterial pressure and cerebral perfusion pressure in the setting of vasospasm. Norepinephrine has shown better outcomes than phenylephrine. Further management may also include endovascular balloon angioplasty procedures. tPA, aspirin, or clopidogrel administration may prove harmful for these patients as there is a substantial risk of rebleeding with the use of such anticoagulant or antiplatelet medications. While the use of statins has been reported to be neuroprotective similar to the use of nimodipine, it would not be helpful in the acute management of vasospastic DCI. Finally, emergent craniotomy is a viable therapy option for patients with subarachnoid hemorrhage who develop refractory intracranial hypertension, but it would not be indicated in this patient who has developed DCI without any signs of refractory intracranial hypertension.

Q16 Answer: B

Q17 Answer: D

Q18 Answer: A

Athar MK, Levine JM. Treatment options for cerebral vasospasm in aneurysmal subarachnoid hemorrhage. *Neurotherapeutics* 2012;9(1):37–43.

Diringer MN, Bleck TP, Hemphill JC, Menon D, Shutter L, Vespa P, et al. Critical care management of patients following aneurysmal subarachnoid hemorrhage: recommendations from the Neurocritical Care Society's Multidisciplinary Consensus Conference. *Neurocritical Care* 2011;15(2):211.

Roy B, McCullough LD, Dhar R, Grady J, Wang Y-B, Brown RJ. Comparison of initial vasopressors used for delayed cerebral ischemia after aneurysmal subarachnoid hemorrhage. *Cerebrovascular Diseases* 2017;43(5-6):266–271.

Vergouwen MD, Vermeulen M, Coert BA, Stroes ES, Roos YB. Microthrombosis after aneurysmal subarachnoid hemorrhage: an additional explanation for delayed cerebral ischemia. *Journal of Cerebral Blood Flow & Metabolism* 2008;28(11):1761–1770.

19 *A 20-year-old man is brought to the emergency department after a motor vehicle accident where he hit his head on the sidewalk. On arrival his GCS is E2M3V3. His pulse is 68 beats/min and blood pressure is 148/87 mm Hg. A noncontrast CT scan of the head shows a skull fracture and subdural hematoma. A complete blood count and serum concentrations of electrolytes, urea nitrogen, and creatinine are all within reference ranges. A CT scan of the chest and abdomen is normal. He has some bruises on his thighs and back. His abdominal and pelvic examinations are normal. There is no blood at the urethral meatus, and a Foley catheter is passed successfully. The left pupil is*

6 mm in diameter and reacts minimally to light. He is intubated, undergoes a craniotomy, and is admitted to the neurointensive care unit. His urine output has been in the normal range. Repeat laboratory tests on day 2 shows a creatinine level of 4.1 mg/dL. The urine dipstick shows no blood. Which of the following is the most likely cause of deranged creatinine in this patient?

A *Obstructive uropathy*

B *Non-neurological organ dysfunction*

C *Rapidly progressive glomerulonephritis*

D *Contrast-induced nephropathy*

E *Rhabdomyolysis*

This patient has presented to the hospital with severe traumatic brain injury (TBI). He has developed an epidural hematoma which was promptly evacuated. Although his admission creatinine levels were normal, he has an acute rise in creatinine on day 2 of admission. Non-neurological organ dysfunction (NNOD) following severe head injuries has been described previously. Following the primary brian insult, secondary brain injury because of hypotension and hypoxia is further worsened by a robust catecholamine surge response. This leads to an inflammatory response not just in the brain but throughout the body and has been implicated in the development of multiple organ dysfunction in such patients. Nearly one in three patients with a severe isolated head injury will develop NNOD of another organ system. This patient has developed renal NNOD.

This patient's urine dipstick showed no blood, thus ruling out rapidly progressive glomerulonephritis and rhabdomyolysis as possible causes for the rise in creatinine. As his abdominal and pelvic examinations and chest and abdomen CT scans are normal, it effectively rules out obstructive uropathy as a cause. Finally, he did not receive contrast for his CT scans, thus contrast-induced nephropathy is not a possible cause.

Answer: B

Astarabadi M, Khurrum M, Asmar S, Bible L, Chehab M, Castanon L, et al. The impact of non-neurological organ dysfunction on outcomes in severe isolated traumatic brain injury. *Journal of Trauma and Acute Care Surgery* 2020;89(2):405–410.

Corral L, Javierre CF, Ventura JL, Marcos P, Herrero JI, Mañez R. Impact of non-neurological complications in severe traumatic brain injury outcome. *Critical Care* 2012;16(2):R44.

Hendrickson CM, Howard BM, Kornblith LZ, Conroy AS, Nelson MF, Zhuo H, et al. The acute respiratory distress syndrome following isolated severe traumatic brain injury. *The journal of trauma and acute care surgery.* 2016;80(6):989.

Zygun D, Berthiaume L, Laupland K, Kortbeek J, Doig C. SOFA is superior to MOD score for the determination of non-neurologic organ dysfunction in patients with severe traumatic brain injury: a cohort study. *Critical Care* 2006;10(4):R115.

The following vignette applies to questions 20 and 21:

A 25-year-old man was involved in a high-speed motorcycle collision and afterward experienced transient right upper extremity sensory changes. A computed tomography (CT) scan of the head was negative. CT scan of the cervical spine revealed a fracture into the foramen transversarium of the fourth cervical vertebra. CT angiography of the cervical spine revealed an intramural hematoma with ≥ 25% luminal narrowing and a raised intimal flap of the left vertebral artery. No other injuries were identified.

20 *What is the grade of blunt cerebrovascular injury (BCVI) in this patient?*

A *Grade I*

B *Grade II*

C *Grade III*

D *Grade IV*

E *Grade V*

21 *What would be the most appropriate next step in the management of this patient to minimize the risk of progression of stroke?*

A *Anticoagulation agents*

B *Antiplatelet agents*

C *Endovascular treatment*

D *Surgical intervention*

E *Repeat angiography*

Blunt vertebral artery injury is associated with complex cervical spine fractures involving subluxation, extension into the foramen transversarium, or upper cervical fractures. CT angiography (CTA) should be obtained after trauma in patients with neurologic signs and symptoms that are not explained by the CT scan or in blunt trauma patients presenting with epistaxis from a suspected arterial source. Routine screening should incorporate these findings to maximize yield while limiting the use of invasive procedures. The gold standard for the diagnosis of blunt cerebrovascular injury is cerebral digital subtraction arteriography and should only be performed if clinical suspicion remains high and the findings of other imaging are equivocal. The Biffl scale or grade illustrates the spectrum of blunt cerebrovascular injury (BCVI) seen on angiography (both CTA and digital subtraction angiography (DSA)). Figure 28.1 demonstrates the grading of BCVI.

Grade I: irregularity of the vessel wall or a dissection/intramural hematoma with <25% luminal stenosis

Grade II: intraluminal thrombus or raised intimal flap is visualized, or dissection/ intramural hematoma with 25% or more luminal narrowing

Grade III: pseudoaneurysm

Grade IV: vessel occlusion

Grade V: vessel transection/extravasation/carotid-cavernous fistula

Figure 28.1 Denver Grading Scale for BCVI.

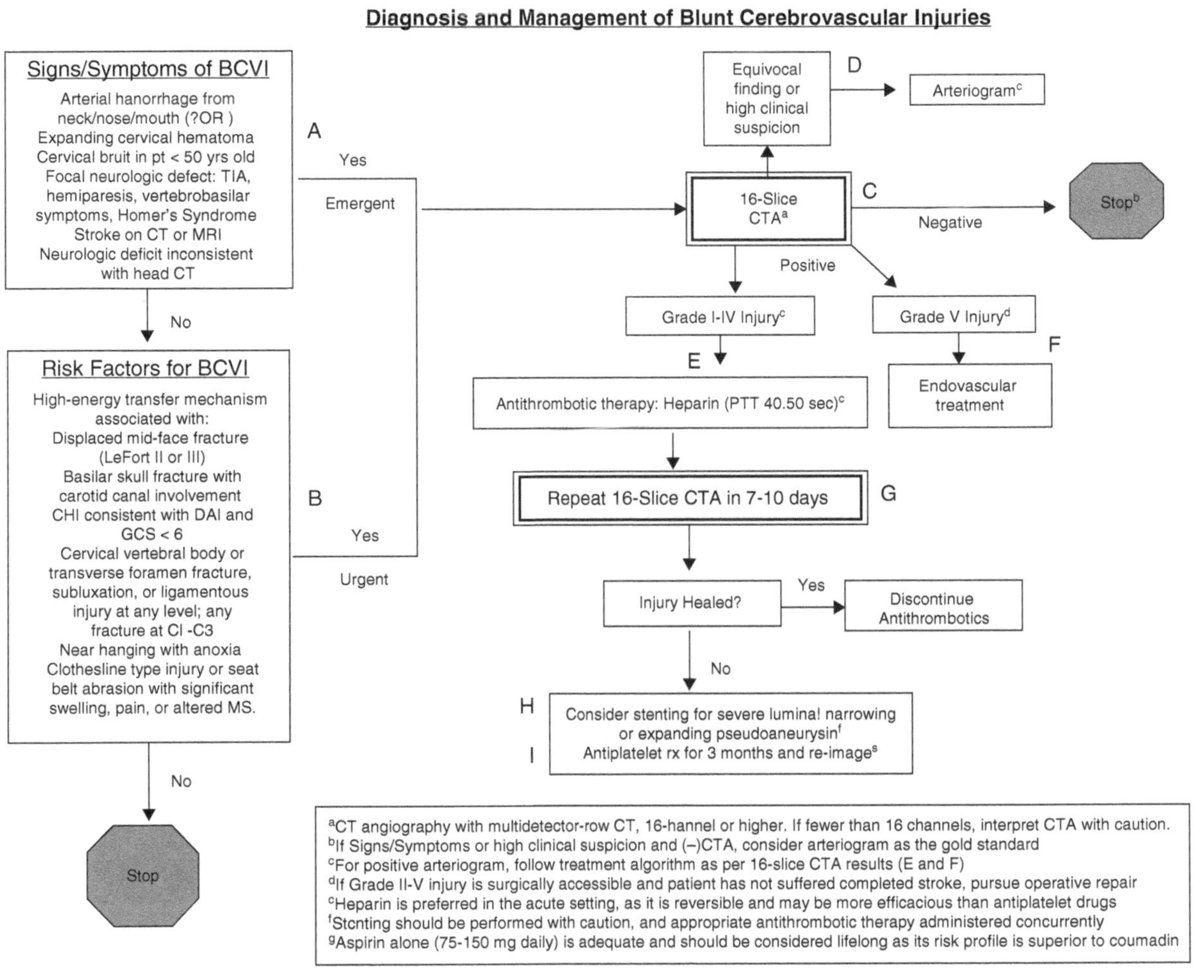

Diagnosis and Management of Blunt Cerebrovascular Injuries

[a]CT angiography with multidetector-row CT, 16-hannel or higher. If fewer than 16 channels, interpret CTA with caution.
[b]If Signs/Symptoms or high clinical suspicion and (−)CTA, consider arteriogram as the gold standard
[c]For positive arteriogram, follow treatment algorithm as per 16-slice CTA results (E and F)
[d]If Grade II-V injury is surgically accessible and patient has not suffered completed stroke, pursue operative repair
[c]Heparin is preferred in the acute setting, as it is reversible and may be more efficacious than antiplatelet drugs
[f]Stcnting should be performed with caution, and appropriate antithrombotic therapy administered concurrently
[g]Aspirin alone (75-150 mg daily) is adequate and should be considered lifelong as its risk profile is superior to coumadin

Figure 28.2 Algorithm for the diagnosis and management of blunt cerebrovascular injuries in adults.

The incidence of vertebral artery injury among total blunt trauma admissions ranged from 0.20 to 2.80%. The most appropriate initial treatment of this injury is systemic anticoagulation initially with heparin and subsequent conversion to warfarin. Endovascular treatment is an option when the lesion does not resolve with systemic anticoagulation; however, it should not be the initial treatment choice. Acute pseudoaneurysms are unstable lesions and the walls of these structures are weak, making stent deployment more dangerous in the acute setting. Repeat angiography should be performed. Antiplatelet agents should be reserved for patients who have undergone endovascular stent placement or those in whom systemic anticoagulation is contraindicated.

Figure 28.2 presents an algorithm for the diagnosis and management of blunt cerebrovascular injuries in adults.

Q20 Answer: B

Q21 Answer: A

Biffl WL, Cothren CC, Moore EE, Kozar R, Cocanour C, Davis JW, et al. Western Trauma Association critical decisions in trauma: screening for and treatment of blunt cerebrovascular injuries. *Journal of Trauma and Acute Care Surgery* 2009;67(6):1150–1153.

Cothren CC, Moore EE, Biffl WL, Ciesla DJ, Ray Jr CE, Johnson JL, et al. Cervical spine fracture patterns predictive of blunt vertebral artery injury. *Journal of Trauma and Acute Care Surgery* 2003;55(5):811–813.

Franz RW, Willette PA, Wood MJ, Wright ML, Hartman JF. A systematic review and meta-analysis of diagnostic screening criteria for blunt cerebrovascular injuries. *Journal of the American College of Surgeons* 2012;214(3):313–327.

Hanna K, Douglas M, Asmar S, Khurrum M, Bible L, Castanon L, et al. Treatment of blunt cerebrovascular injuries: Anticoagulants or antiplatelet agents? *Journal of Trauma and Acute Care Surgery* 2020;89(1):74–79.

29

Blunt and Penetrating Neck Trauma

Eric Raschke, DO[1] and Leslie Kobayashi, MD[2]

[1] *Madigan Army Medical Center, Tacoma, WA, USA*
[2] *Division of Trauma, Acute Care Surgery, Surgical Critical Care and Burns, University of California San Diego, San Diego, CA, USA*

1 *A 2-year-old sustains a fall from a second story window. There is significant facial trauma on the primary survey causing airway obstruction due to copious amounts of bloody secretions in the oropharynx. The patient is tachycardic and normotensive; oxygen saturation is 93% on 15 L by face mask but is difficult to mask ventilate. You have performed a jaw thrust and placed an oral airway. What is the next best step in management?*

   A *Supraglottic airway*
   B *Needle cricothyroidotomy*
   C *Open cricothyroidotomy*
   D *Open tracheostomy*
   E *Nasotracheal intubation*

Airway emergencies in pediatric patients are rare but lethal situations. The first attempt to secure the airway should be performed by the most senior operator under optimal conditions and can include advanced airway adjuncts such as bougies, fiberoptic or rigid bronchoscopy, and supraglottic devices such as laryngeal mask airways (LMAs). In contrast to adults, the preferred surgical airway for small children is open emergent tracheostomy. Cricothyroidotomy is not recommended for patients under 12 years of age as this is the narrowest portion of the pediatric airway and associated rates of subglottic stenosis are high. Instead, a percutaneous catheter or needle cricothyroidotomy and jet insufflation can be used to oxygenate the patient temporarily. Ventilation is necessarily restricted, and carbon dioxide levels will predictably rise over time. Conversion to an open tracheostomy or repeated attempt at intubation with advanced airway adjuncts or more experienced personnel should be performed rapidly to prevent carbon dioxide accumulation.

Answer: A

Krishna SG, Bryant JF, Tobias JD. Management of the difficult airway in the pediatric patient. *J Pediatr Intensive Care.* 2018; 7(3): 115–125.

Engelhardt T, Virag K, Veyckemans F, Habre W. Airway management in pediatric anaesthesia in Europe-insight from APRICOT (Anaesthesia Practice In Children Observation Trial): a prospective multicenter observational study in 261 hospitals in Europe. *British J Anaesthesia.* 2018; 121(1): 66–75.

2 *A patient who contracted viral pneumonia has been intubated in the intensive care unit (ICU) for 2 weeks; they have tested positive for COVID-19 on PCR; the patient failed initial attempt at extubation requiring immediate reintubation and now cannot be weaned from the ventilator. The decision is made to perform a tracheostomy. Which of the following maneuvers should be undertaken to decrease the risk of transmission during the procedure?*

   A *Use of N-95 mask or PAPR (powered air-purifying respirators).*
   B *Use of protective eyewear and full barrier precautions with gown and gloves.*
   C *Performance of procedure in an airborne infection isolation room.*
   D *Use of controlled apnea during the procedure.*
   E *All of the above.*

When dealing with aerosol-generating procedures in the face of SARS-type infection patients, it is essential to understand which measures need to be done to reduce transmission to the healthcare team. Any interaction should be performed using standard precautions, including handwashing and barrier precautions with gown, gloves, cap, mask, and eye protection. A higher risk of transmission is present during aerosol-generating procedures, and additional precautions should be taken. Aerosol-producing procedures include endotracheal intubation/extubation, bronchoscopy, mini-bronchoalveolar lavage, open suctioning of airways, manual ventilation, unintentional or intentional ventilator disconnections, bilevel positive airway pressure, continuous positive airway pressure, cardiopulmonary resuscitation, and high-flow oxygen. In these cases, additional use of N-95 masks and/or PAPR is recommended. In the particular case of tracheostomy placement, the use of controlled apnea during the airway maneuvers has been shown to be safe for the patient and efficacious in preventing transmission to the operating surgeon and staff.

Answer: E

Murphy P, Holler E, Lindroth H, *et al.* Short-term outcomes for patients and providers after elective tracheostomy in COVID-19 positive patients. *J Surg Res.* 2020; 260: 38–45.

Center for Disease Control and Prevention. Interim Infection Prevention and Control Recommendations for Healthcare Personnel During the Coronavirus Disease 2019 (COVID-19) Pandemic. 2020.

3 *A 33-year-old helmeted driver in a dune buggy crash is brought to the trauma bay. The patient is obtunded, requiring urgent intubation. Subsequent workup reveals a significant subdural hemorrhage and a fracture with a complete transection of the spinal cord at C3. The patient also has a flail chest on the right and hemopneumothorax. The patient is stabilized following intubation and chest tube placement, and the orthopedic spine service plans operative fixation of the spinal fracture the following day. Which of the following statements is true?*

A *Early use of high-dose steroids will significantly improve neurological outcomes in this patient.*

B *Early rib plating will significantly improve mortality in this patient.*

C *Early tracheostomy is safe even if anterior cervical spine fixation is required.*

D *Early tracheostomy should be avoided in this patient because of the risk of cross-contamination at the cervical spine fixation site.*

E *Percutaneous tracheostomy should be avoided because of the risk of surgical site infection after anterior spinal fixation.*

High cervical spinal cord injuries (SCI) have significant effects on patient respiratory status and carry a high risk of developing respiratory failure. Early tracheostomy has been shown to decrease hospital and ICU length of stay,

reduce sedation requirements, and lower rates of pneumonia and hospital costs. In this clinical scenario, not only does the patient have a high cervical SCI, there is also a concomitant flail chest wall injury, making short-term ventilator liberation unlikely. Early tracheostomy is recommended in these patients, and there has not been any associated increase in hardware infection rates with anterior approach cervical spine fixation or cross-contamination of surgical sites using either open or percutaneous approaches. While early rib plating may improve times to ventilator liberation, it has not been shown to reduce mortality. Additionally, the location of this patient's injury makes rib plating less impactful on time to ventilator liberation. While there are randomized controlled trials that demonstrate a modest improvement in ASIA grade with steroid administration following blunt SCI, more recent evidence to support their use is lacking and risks of infectious and metabolic complications likely outweigh the potential benefit for most patients, particularly those with complete injury.

Answer: C

Lozano CP, Chen KA, Marks JA, *et al.* Safety of early tracheostomy in trauma patients after anterior spinal fusion. *J Trauma Acute Care Surg.* 2018; 85(4): 741–746.

Kaczmarek C, Aach M, Hoffmann MF, *et al.* Early percutaneous dilational tracheostomy does not lead to an increased risk of surgical site infection following anterior spinal surgery. *J Trauma Acute Care Surg.* 2017; 82(2): 383–386.

4 *A 27-year-old restrained driver involved in a high-speed motor vehicle collision with rollover and significant passenger space intrusion presents to the emergency department (ED) reporting loss of consciousness and amnesia to the events following the accident. The primary survey is intact; the secondary survey demonstrates no external signs of injury. What diagnostic tests should be performed?*

A *CT scan of the head only*

B *CT scan of the head and cervical spine*

C *CT scan of the head, cervical spine and CT angiogram of the neck*

D *CT angiogram only*

E *CT scan of the cervical spine only*

This patient has several risk factors for a head injury, spinal injury, and blunt cerebrovascular injury (BCVI). Adjuncts to the secondary survey should evaluate for intracranial hemorrhage, spinal fracture, and BCVI. BCVI is present in up to 5% of blunt trauma admissions and can be devastating, associated with severe disability and even death. Early identification and treatment are paramount in modern trauma systems to reduce stroke risk and prevent poor outcomes associated with such injuries. CT angiography with multichannel (16–64) detectors has become the most commonly utilized screening modality. Screening criteria for BCVI have been a topic of evolution; however, the adoption of increasingly liberal criteria has been favored in many studies in an attempt to capture missed injuries. Commonly utilized screening criteria including the Denver criteria, Eastern Association for the Surgery of Trauma, Western Trauma Association, and the Scandinavian Neurotrauma Committee Guidelines have been associated with sensitivities as low as 57–84%, and missed injury rates of 20% including Denver grade 3 or higher injuries. While universal screening remains controversial, liberal criteria including screening for the mechanism of injury alone should be advocated to reduce the risk of missing significant injuries.

Answer: C

Muther M, Sporns PB, Hanning U, *et al*. Diagnostic accuracy of different clinical screening criteria for blunt cerebrovascular injuries compared with the liberal state of the art computed tomography angiography in major trauma. *J Trauma Acute Care Surg*. 2020; 88(6): 789–795.

Leichtle SW, Banerjee D, Schrader R, *et al*. Blunt cerebrovascular injury: The case for universal screening. *J Trauma Acute Care Surg*. 2020; 89(5): 880–886.

Geddes AE, Burlew CC, Wagenaar A E, *et al*. Expanded screening criteria for blunt cerebrovascular injury: a bigger impact than anticipated. *Am J Surg*. 2016; 212(6): 1167–1174.

5   *A 19-year-old marine was in a training exercise and fell from a 20 foot wall. Immediately after the fall, he reports that he cannot move his legs and only shrugs his shoulders. Glasgow Coma Scale (GCS) is 15. The primary survey is intact; on the secondary survey, you confirm there is no motor function in the bilateral lower extremities, and the patient can only shoulder shrug in the bilateral upper extremities. The patient is currently respiring comfortably on 2L nasal cannula and can speak in full sentences. Workup confirms cervical spine fracture with associated spinal cord injury. The patient is admitted to the ICU for observation while awaiting spinal decompression and fixation by Neurosurgery. Which of the following factors predict the need for intubation and mechanical ventilation?*
   A   *Decreasing vital capacity*
   B   *Young age*
   C   *Lower cervical spine (C5 and below) injury level*
   D   *Ability to cough*
   E   *GCS 15*

Cervical spinal cord injuries (SCI) have a high rate of morbidity and mortality from respiratory complica-

tions. Of hospitalized patients with cervical SCI, 4 out of 5 deaths are from pulmonary dysfunction and pneumonia. The phrenic nerve that innervates the diaphragm arises from the C3–C5 nerve roots; therefore, the injury's location plays a large role in the degree of pulmonary dysfunction, with higher injuries being associated with higher risks of respiratory complications. The diaphragm is responsible for generating approximately 65% of the normal respiratory tidal volume, with the remaining 35% attributed to the accessory muscles. Intact accessory muscle function and strong cough are associated with lower rates of respiratory complications. During the first 7 days post-injury, the patient should have frequent measurements of vital capacity (VC), and intubation should be considered with a decreasing VC or VC approaching < 10 mL/kg, which signifies fatigue and pending respiratory failure. Altered mental status with GCS ≤ 13, older age, and comorbid conditions also increase the risk of overall complications, respiratory complications, and death.

Answer: A

Berlly M and Shem K. Respiratory management during the first five days after spinal cord injury. *J Spinal Cord Med*. 2007; 30: 309–318.

Claxton AR, Wong DT, Chung F, Fehlings MG. Predictors of hospital mortality and mechanical ventilation in patients with cervical spinal cord injury. *Can J Anaesth*. 1998; 45(2): 144–149.

6   *A patient is brought into the trauma bay, the patient's eyes remain shut, there is no verbal response, and they exhibit extension with deep stimulation. Based on GCS, you decide to intubate for airway protection. Several attempts at endotracheal intubation via direct laryngoscopy have failed. What is the next step in airway management?*
   A   *Emergent cricothyroidotomy*
   B   *Percutaneous tracheostomy*
   C   *Open tracheostomy*
   D   *Blind nasotracheal intubation*
   E   *Extracorporeal membrane oxygenation*

This situation's goal is to not reach the point of "cannot intubate, cannot oxygenate" (CICO). Hypoxic brain injury occurs between 4 and 6 minutes of apnea and is irreversible after about 6 minutes. Studies have shown that hypoxemia in brain injury patients can significantly worsen the neurologic outcome. The first attempt to secure the airway should be for definitive tracheal access via direct laryngoscopy. Maneuvers to improve success at endotracheal intubation include appropriate positioning in patients without cervical spine precautions, use of video laryngoscopes, and use of a bougie. Attempts at tracheal intubation should be limited to 3–4 passes and should be halted immediately if any significant desaturations occur. Repeated attempts, even with experienced personnel, are associated with worse outcomes. Definitive surgical airway should be the next step in management; this is with a cricothyroidotomy in adults. Tracheostomy both open and percutaneous methods should only be utilized in controlled situations with a secure airway and are not emergent airway options in adult trauma patients.

Answer: A

Frerk, C, Mitchell, VS, McNarry, AF, *et al*. Difficult Airway Society 2015 guidelines for management of unanticipated difficult intubation in adults. *Br J. Anaesth*. 2015; *115*(6): 827–848.

Higgs A, McGrath BA, Goddard C, *et al*. Guidelines for the management of tracheal intubation in critically ill adults. *Br J Anaesth*. 2018; 120(2): 323–352.

7 *A 26-year-old polytrauma patient has been ventilator-dependent in the ICU for 7 days. The presence of traumatic brain injury and respiratory failure make long-term mechanical ventilation likely. Multiple studies have demonstrated the benefits of early tracheostomy. Regarding methods of tracheostomy placement, which of the following is correct?*
   A *Percutaneous tracheostomy is more expensive than open.*
   B *Mortality and bleeding rates are similar between open and percutaneous tracheostomy.*
   C *Percutaneous tracheostomy has higher rates of surgical site infection compared to open.*
   D *Technical difficulties are less likely in percutaneous compared to open tracheostomy.*
   E *Operative time is generally longer during percutaneous compared to open tracheostomy.*

The two techniques used for placement of a tracheostomy include open and percutaneous methods; both have been proven to be safe when performed in the operating room (OR) and in the ICU in the majority of patients. While these techniques have both been proven safe and effective, there are differences in the risks and benefits of implementing each approach. For example, significant benefits of performing a percutaneous tracheostomy include a decrease in operative times and reduced resource utilization, as well as an association with reduced infection rates. However, the percutaneous technique has been associated with more technical difficulties when compared to the open technique. Open tracheostomy has been advocated for particularly high-risk patients including the obese, patients with cervical spine injuries, traumatic brain injury with intracranial hypertension, and coagulopathy. Although

there are several retrospective studies of the percutaneous method being safe to perform in selected individual in each of these sub-populations. The open technique has fewer technical difficulties but requires more resources to perform and is associated with increased cost compared to percutaneous. There has been no proven difference in either mortality or intraoperative/postoperative hemorrhage when comparing the two techniques.

Answer: B

Johnson-Obaseki S, Veljkovic A, Javidnia H. Complication rates of open surgical versus percutaneous tracheostomy in critically ill patients. *Laryngoscope*. 2016; 126(11): 2459–2467.

Klotz R, Probst P, Deininger M, *et al*. Percutaneous versus surgical strategy for tracheostomy: A systematic review and meta-analysis of perioperative and postoperative complications. *Langenbecks Arch Surg*. 2017; 403: 137–149.

8 *A 9-year-old child ingests lye accidentally while visiting his grandmother's farm. The patient is hemodynamically stable and protecting their airway. What is the most reliable diagnostic modality for predicting the need for surgical intervention?*
   A *Flexible endoscopy*
   B *Clinical exam*
   C *Contrast-enhanced CT scan*
   D *Lactate level checked on admission and serially every 6 hours*
   E *Abdominal radiographs*

Ingestion of caustic agents such as alkalis and strong acids can cause severe injury to the gastrointestinal tract. While the ingestion of acids generally causes coagulative necrosis of the gastrointestinal tract, alkali agents are likely to cause a liquefactive type of necrosis. Full sequelae from the injury are likely to be delayed, and therefore laboratory and physical exam findings generally lag as markers for predicting the need for surgical intervention. While severe acidosis, elevated liver function tests, and leukocytosis are associated with transmural necrosis and poor outcomes, their absence does not necessarily preclude the need for surgical intervention. Multiple studies have demonstrated the sensitivity of contrast-enhanced CT scan to grade injury and predict the need for surgical intervention and risk of stricture. CT scan is more predictive than endoscopy, is less invasive, and more easily repeatable. Endoscopy should be reserved for when CT is unavailable, the patient has a contraindication to the use of IV contrast, and in the pediatric population.

Answer: C

Chirica M, Kelly MD, Siboni S, *et al.* Esophageal emergencies: WSES guidelines. *World J Emerg Surg.* 2019; 14;26 eCollection.

Chirica M, Bonavina L, Kelly MD, Sarfati E, Cattan P. Caustic ingestion. *Lancet.* 2017; 389(10083): 2041–2052.

9 *A helmeted construction worker was walking across the job site when a pallet of 4 × 4's was dropped directly on his head. The patient is brought to the ED in a cervical collar and backboard; he complains of pain in the back of his head and neck. He reports that he initially felt like they lost sensation in his arms and legs which resolved, but there are occasional feelings of "pins and needles" throughout. The primary survey is intact; the secondary survey reveals normal sensory and motor function but significant upper midline cervical spine pain. A representative slice of the CT scan of the cervical spine is seen below. What is the diagnosis and treatment of this injury?*

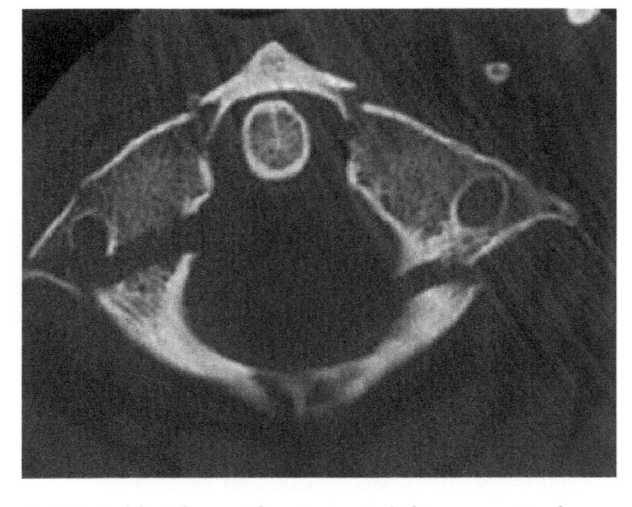

A *Unstable Chance fracture; stabilize operatively*
B *Stable type I dens fracture; stabilize with cervical collar*
C *Unstable type II dens fracture; stabilize operatively or with halo*
D *Stable type 1 Hangman's fracture; stabilize with collar*
E *Unstable Jefferson fracture; stabilize with halo traction or surgery*

Fractures of the atlas are generally caused by axial loading events such as shallow dives and falling objects striking the head. Even though fractures of C1 are treated most commonly with halo stabilization, they can be associated with vertebral artery injuries and atlantoaxial or atlanto-occipital instability. The fracture represented in the question is a C1 burst fracture, composed of bilateral posterior and anterior arch disruption, also known as a Jefferson type II fracture. This creates four separate osseous segments that typically do not cause neurologic symptoms secondary to fragments pushing away from the spinal cord. This is commonly treated with either halo traction or surgery, the latter being reserved depending on the degree of instability.

Answer: E

Mead LB, Millhouse PW, Krystal J, Vaccaro AR. C1 fractures: A review of diagnoses, management options, and outcomes. *Curr Rev Musculoskelet Med.* 2016; 9(3): 255–262.

Jackson RS, Banit DM, Rhyne AL, Darden BV. Upper cervical spine injuries. *J Am Acad Orthop Surg.* 2002; 10(4): 271–280.

10 *A 30-year-old man is brought in by ambulance after being found by family at home, hanging with an extension cord around his neck. The family reported that he was alone for about 5 minutes before he was found and cut down. Upon arrival, the patient is awake, alert, tearful, and denies pain or paresthesias. He does report loss of consciousness and dysphagia. The primary survey is intact; on the secondary survey, there is an abrasion on the anterior neck. What is the most appropriate management of this patient?*
A *Observation*
B *CT angiography of the neck with cervical spine reconstruction*
C *CT of the head, cervical spine and CT angiography of the neck*
D *CT of the head, cervical spine, chest with thoracic spine reconstruction, and CT angiography of the neck*
E *MRI of the brain and cervical spine*

The usual pattern of injuries in suicidal hangings without a fall from height is consistent with soft tissue compression causing jugular venous obstruction, hypoxia, and unconsciousness. As the body relaxes, the weight against the ligature leads to direct tracheal or carotid compression. The overall survival for nonlethal hangings that present to the hospital is favorable at about 90%. Patients with near-hangings and a normal GCS are unlikely to have significant injuries from the event; approximately 10% will have a clinically relevant injury. Diagnostic imaging workup is suggested to avoid missing a life-threatening and treatable injury. CT angiography of the neck is indicated in all hangings with suspected high energy (fall from height or complete suspension) mechanism and symptomatic (focal neurologic deficits, carotid bruit, expanding cervical hematoma, dysphagia, and dysphonia) low energy hangings. Low energy asymptomatic patients can be observed safely without further workup. During a hanging event, it is unlikely that the victim will sustain concomitant injuries outside of the neck, making CT scans of adjacent structures of limited diagnostic utility. It is important to look for external signs of trauma during the secondary survey to help guide additional imaging adjuncts, as victims are at risk of further blunt injuries when being released from the ligature device. While MRI's can be useful in determining the extent of anoxic injury sustained during a hanging, it is recommended they are deferred for at least 72 hours.

Answer: B

Berke DM, Helmer SD, Reyes J, Haan JM. Injury patterns in near-hanging patients: How much workup is really needed? *Am Surg.* 2019; 85(5): 549–555.

Subramanian M, Hranjec T, Lieu L, *et al.* (2016) A case for less workup in near hanging. *Injury*; 37(5): 435–439. *J Trauma Acute Care Surg.* 2016 Nov; 81(5); 925–930.

11 *An 18-year-old tourist presents to the trauma bay after falling off a barstool. After awaiting workup in the ED, the patient is no longer intoxicated, is awake, alert, and denies midline cervical tenderness. There are no neurological deficits on the physical exam. ED workup has so far only revealed a moderately painful left ankle sprain. The patient has requested to have his collar removed; which of the following is an acceptable response?*

   A *Further workup is not necessary, and you remove the collar.*

   B *Immediately sedate the patient and order a STAT MRI.*

   C *Politely inform the patient that further workup is needed and order a CT of the cervical spine while keeping the patient in a rigid collar and full spinal precautions.*

   D *Request regional anesthesia perform a nerve block to the left leg then repeat the physical examination.*

   E *Maintain the cervical collar but allow the patient to walk to radiology to obtain three-view plain film radiographs.*

Clinical clearance of the cervical spine can be performed in patients who are not intoxicated, have a normal neurological exam, deny spinal tenderness/pain, and do not have a high-risk mechanism of injury (e.g., high-speed MVC, fall from height). The two most commonly used protocols for cervical spine clearance are the NEXUS and Canadian C-spine criteria. Most studies have demonstrated a higher sensitivity using the Canadian

C-spine criteria, which includes age and mechanism of injury. Recently, challenges to excluding patients with distracting injuries from clinical cervical spine clearance have demonstrated that presence of a distracting injury in patients who are able to cooperate with a detailed physical exam should not remain a contraindication to clinical clearance of the cervical spine.

Answer: A

Khan AD, Lieebscher SC, Reiser HC, *et al.* Clearing the cervical spine in patients with distracting injuries: An AAST multi-institutional study. *J Trauma Acute Care Surg.* 2019; 86(1): 28–35.

Rose MK, Rosal LM, Gonzalez RP, *et al.* Clinical clearance of the cervical spine in patients with distracting injuries: It is time to dispel the myth. *J Trauma Acute Care Surg.* 2012; 73(2): 498–502.

Still IG, Wells GA, Vandemheen KL, *et al.* The Canadian C-spine rule for radiography in alert and stable trauma patients. *JAMA.* 2001; 286(15):1841–1848.

12 *An elderly bedbound nursing home resident is found down next to her bed. The patient was last seen in her usual state of health the previous night by the nursing home manager. Upon arrival, the patient has a GCS of 7, not protecting her airway; she is intubated using cervical spine precautions without incident. Upon examination, a subacute subdural hemorrhage was found, and neurosurgery was consulted. The initial trauma workup also included a CT of the cervical spine, which revealed mild degenerative changes appropriate for age, but no soft tissue swelling, loss of lordosis, or malalignment. The following day you are rounding in the ICU, the patient does not follow commands but localizes briskly in the bilateral arms and withdraws both legs briskly to stimuli; what is the next best step in managing the cervical spine?*

   A *Maintain full spinal precautions and obtain a fitted rigid cervical collar.*

   B *Order an MRI of the cervical spine to evaluate for ligamentous injury.*

   C *Request an emergent spine service consultation.*

   D *Remove the cervical collar and clear the patient of cervical spine precautions.*

   E *Obtain a CT angiogram of the neck.*

In the past, clearing cervical spine precautions in an obtunded patient presented a challenging issue in the ICU. Prolonged cervical collar placement has been associated with increased skin breakdown, increased intracranial pressure, agitation, more days on mechanical ventilation, and prolonged ICU and hospital stay. The goal of any cervical spine clearance protocol is to limit unnecessary imaging and prolonged cervical collar use without missing clinically significant injuries. With improved CT imaging, quality radiologists can more accurately identify fractures even in patients with severe degenerative disease. The negative predictive value of a high-quality multidetector (≥64 slice) CT scan approaches 100% and additional imaging with MRI provide little additional benefit and will increase cost and may significantly delay cervical spine clearance. With a negative high-quality cervical CT, it is highly unlikely that the patient will have a clinically significant unstable cervical injury, and removing the collar without further diagnostic workup is recommended by multiple trauma association guidelines.

Answer: D

Ciesla DJ, Shatz DV, Moore EE, *et al.* Western Trauma Association critical decisions in trauma: Cervical spine clearance in trauma patients. *J Trauma Acute Care Surg.* 2020; 88(2); 352–354.

Patel MB, Humble SS, Cullinane DC, *et al.* Cervical spine collar clearance in the obtunded adult blunt trauma patient: a systematic review and practice management guideline from the Eastern Association for the Surgery of Trauma. *J Trauma Acute Care Surg.* 2015; 78(2): 430–441.

13 *A 47-year-old trapeze artist presents after a 30-foot fall during a performance. The primary survey is intact; the secondary survey demonstrates midface instability and tenderness and midline cervical spine tenderness. Workup reveals a Le Forte 2 fracture on the left and an internal carotid artery dissection. The patient is placed into the ICU for serial neurological exams; what is the highest risk period for stroke development in this patient?*
   A *Within the first 72 hours*
   B *72–96 hours*
   C *96–120 hours*
   D *Greater than 1 week*
   E *Following hospital discharge*

The incidence of BCVI in trauma is low; however, the complications, if missed, can be devastating. Studies have shown a 20% risk of stroke in these patients if not treated with antithrombotic therapy. A large Western Trauma Association study demonstrated that 37% of strokes are present on admission. Among those that developed strokes after admission, it was found that 61% develop within the first 72 hours, with the median time to stroke diagnosis of 42 hours in asymptomatic and 54 hours in symptomatic patients. Other studies have

also demonstrated a high rate of stroke at admission ranging from 44 to 82% and the highest stroke rates after admission occurring within the first hours of hospitalization. The optimal type and duration of treatment for BCVI remains unknown; options include anticoagulation, antiplatelet therapy, surgical repair, and endovascular coils or stents. Antithrombotic therapy has been associated with a reduction in stroke rate.

Answer: A

Cothren Burlew C, Sumislawski JJ, Benfield CD, *et al.* Time to stroke: A Western Trauma Association multicenter study of blunt cerebrovascular injuries. *J Trauma Acute Care Surg.* 2018; 85(5): 858–866.

Griessenauer CJ, Fleming JB, Richards BF, *et al.* Timing and mechanism of ischemic stroke due to extracranial blunt traumatic cerebrovascular injury. *J Neurosurg.* 2013; 118(2): 397–404.

14 *A 34-year-old patient has a complete spinal cord injury (SCI) at C2-C3 after a motorcycle crash. Initially, the patient required the use of vasopressors and chronotropic medications for persistent neurogenic shock and bradycardia. After resuscitation and spinal fixation, the patient remains bradycardic to the 40s with occasional asystolic pauses. What pharmacologic therapy may improve the heart rate and reduce the need for pacemaker placement?*
   A *Atropine*
   B *Phenylephrine*
   C *Dopamine*
   D *Theophylline*
   E *Norepinephrine*

In high cervical spine injuries, unopposed vagal tone can also result in bradycardia and decreased cardiac output. Therapy for this complication needs to focus on efficacy and safety profile. Current treatments include atropine, dopamine, epinephrine, implanted pacemakers, and theophylline. Theophylline has multiple benefits for long-term management of SCI-induced bradycardia including enteral route administration and a low side effect profile. Theophylline directly antagonizes endogenous adenosine at the sinoatrial and AV nodes, and in patients with high SCI, it has the added benefit of increasing diaphragmatic muscle strength. Atropine can be quite efficacious in treating bradycardia, though its side effects can prohibit its long-term use. Phenylephrine is a strict alpha-1 agonist and would not provide the needed chronotropic effect. Norepinephrine may have some chronotropic effects; however, long-term administration is not recommended;

it requires a central venous catheter for administration and has significant ischemic and arrhythmogenic side effects.

Answer: D

Sadaka F, Naydenov SK, Ponzillo JJ. Theophylline for bradycardia secondary to cervical spine cord injury. *Neurocrit Care.* 2010; 13(3): 389–392.

Karim F, Chang P, Garrison C, Steiner M. Role of theophylline in management of bradycardia secondary to high cervical spinal cord injury in a seven-year-old child: Case report and a review of the literature. *Cureus.* 2020; 12(10): e10941.

15 *A 27-year-old jogger was stabbed in the neck while running on the boardwalk and was brought to the ED. The patient has a patent airway and is hemodynamically stable; however, there is a sizeable hematoma to the left of the thyroid cartilage that is visibly expanding. What is the next step in management?*

   A *Rapid sequence intubation in the ED, then transport to the OR for surgical neck exploration.*

   B *Observation in the ICU.*

   C *Place a nasal airway, apply supplemental oxygen, and go for CT angiography/esophagram.*

   D *Placement of Laryngeal Mask Airway (LMA) and CT angiography/esophagram.*

   E *Intubation in the operating room followed by surgical neck exploration.*

Penetrating neck injuries should be managed with the "no zone approach," with the clinical presentation being the primary determinant of management. Patients who are hemodynamically unstable, have hard signs of injury, or have impending airway collapse should be taken directly to the OR to secure the airway prior to emergent neck exploration. This patient, while hemodynamically stable now, has signs of impending airway collapse and hard signs of vascular injury. Further imaging or observation is not appropriate. Direct laryngoscopy is likely to be technically challenging due to distortion of the airway from the hematoma and bloody secretions. Risk for needing a surgical airway is high; therefore, the patient should be taken to the OR for any attempt to secure the airway. The OR has several advantages over the ED; it is a sterile environment, has anesthesia and extra nursing personnel, specialized surgical equipment, better positioning, and improved lighting. Patients that are hemodynamically stable and present with soft signs of injury should undergo screening CT angiogram regardless of the zone of injury. Stable patients without hard or soft signs of injury can be safely observed without further diagnostic tests.

Answer: E

Nowicki JL, Stew B, Ooi E. Penetrating neck injuries: A guide to evaluation and management. *Ann R Coll Surg Engl.* 2018; 100(1): 6–11.

Mandavia DP, Qualls S, Rokos I. Emergency airway management in penetrating neck injury. *Ann Emerg Med.* 2000; 35(3): 221–225.

16 *During a local protest, an individual was struck with a shard of shrapnel from a flash grenade in the left neck and was noted to have blood and saliva coming from the wound. The patient is taken to the OR for neck exploration, where a transected internal jugular vein and 1 cm full-thickness injury to the side of the esophagus is found. Which of the following statements regarding esophageal injury is true?*

   A *Women are more likely to have an esophageal injury than men.*

   B *Blunt mechanisms are much more common causes of esophageal injury than penetrating mechanisms.*

   C *Prompt open primary repair is associated with the best outcomes.*

   D *Esophageal stents have equivalent outcomes compared to open surgical repair for esophageal injury.*

   E *Cervical injuries have higher mortality than thoracic injuries.*

Traumatic esophageal injuries are rare and have a significant predilection for penetrating trauma, making them more common in men. The majority of injuries are treated with open surgical repair. Early primary repair remains the mainstay of treatment and is associated with the lowest rates of esophageal leak, morbidity, and mortality. Esophageal stents have higher rates of leak (80% vs. 22.6%) and a longer hospital length of stay compared to open repair. Injuries in the thoracic and abdominal esophagus can freely contaminate the peritoneal, mediastinal, and thoracic cavities leading rapidly to sepsis and death. Cervical location of injury has been associated with lower in-hospital, 30-day, and overall mortality as well as lower complication rates than the thoracic location of the injury.

Answer: C

Raff LA, Schinnerer EA, Maine RG, *et al.* Contemporary management of traumatic cervical and thoracic esophageal perforation: The results of an Eastern Association for the Surgery of Trauma multi-institutional study. *J Trauma Acute Care Surg.* 2020; 89(4): 691–697.

Aiolfi A, Inaba K, Recinos G, *et al.* Non-iatrogenic esophageal injury: a retrospective analysis from the

National Trauma Data Bank. *World J Emerg Surg.* 2017; 12: 19 published online.

17 *A high-school football player is injured in a vicious head-to-head tackle during the homecoming game. The primary survey is unremarkable. Secondary survey reveals significant bony tenderness in the mid-cervical spine without step off. CT reveals right-sided C4 pedicle and lamina fractures with transverse foramen involvement and a C5 vertebral body fracture. What is the most appropriate next step in diagnosis and management?*
   A *Diagnostic cerebral angiogram*
   B *Carotid ultrasound*
   C *MRI/MRA of the neck*
   D *CT angiography of the neck*
   E *Halo application*

The injury pattern described in this clinical vignette is an asymptomatic cervical spine fracture but is a high risk for blunt cerebrovascular injury (BCVI). Delay in diagnosis and treatment of BCVI is associated with increased stroke rates and can cause mortality and profound dysfunction. High-quality multidetector CT angiography is the screening modality of choice. Compared to traditional angiography, CT angiography has the benefit of being quick, widely available, and easy to perform and does not require the presence of a specially trained angiography team. It also avoids the morbidity associated with an arterial puncture and uses a lower contrast dose than traditional angiography. Sensitivity ranges from 83 to 100%, with negative predictive values of 92–98%. The sensitivity and specificity of ultrasound are low and can be limited due to associated soft tissue injuries, subcutaneous emphysema, and cervical collars; they have little to no role in diagnosis. MRI/MRA may have a role in further delineating injuries found on screening and in diagnosing associated strokes; however, they can be lengthy to perform, are not always available, and require prolonged time out of a monitored setting. MRI/MRA is not recommended for screening in the initial management of patients with suspected BCVI. Screening for associated BCVI should be performed before any spinal fixation to begin treatment to reduce the risk of associated strokes as soon as possible, and the presence of an injury can be taken into account in operative planning.

Answer: D

Kim DY, Biffl WL, Bokhari F, *et al*. Evaluation and management of blunt cerebrovascular injury: A practice management guideline from the Eastern Association for the Surgery of Trauma. *J Trauma Acute Care Surg* 2020; 88(6): 875–887.

Burlew CC, Biffl WL, Moore EE, Barnett CC, Johnson JL, Bensard DD. Blunt cerebrovascular injuries: redefining screening criteria in the era of non-invasive diagnosis. *J Trauma Acute Care Surg*; 2012; 72(2): 330–337.

18 *A 67-year-old inmate was assaulted in prison and sustained a penetrating wound to his neck immediately superior to the right clavicle. The patient denies pain, dysphagia, dysphonia, hemoptysis, hematemesis, or shortness of breath and denies any neurological symptoms. Examination reveals a 1 cm laceration in zone 1 of the neck without any hematoma, bleeding, or crepitus. Chest x-ray is unremarkable. What is the next best step?*
   A *CT angiogram*
   B *Esophagoscopy*
   C *Observation*
   D *Gastrografin esophagram*
   E *Awake fiberoptic bronchoscopy*

Historically, penetrating injuries to the neck were separated by anatomic zones, and management was determined by location, with zone I and III injuries undergoing angiography, endoscopy, and bronchoscopy; and zone II injuries undergoing mandatory operative exploration. However, this resulted in unacceptably high rates of negative explorations and exposure to radiation and invasive diagnostic tests. Currently, management has moved to a "no zone" approach, and the primary determinant of operative versus conservative management is clinical presentation. Patients with hard signs (active bleeding, instability, expanding/pulsatile hematoma, bruit/thrill, hematemesis, and air escaping from the wound) of injury should undergo exploration in the OR. Patients with soft signs (minor hemoptysis, hematemesis, dysphonia, dysphagia, subcutaneous or mediastinal air, nonexpanding hematoma) should be screened first with CT angiography. Use of invasive tests like endoscopy, bronchoscopy, and specialty examinations such as gastrografin or barium studies can then be obtained based on symptoms and trajectory of injury seen on screening CT angiogram. Asymptomatic penetrating neck injuries without any hard or soft signs of injury can be safely observed with a very low likelihood of a missed injury.

Answer: C

Inaba K, Branco BC, Menaker J, *et al*. Evaluation of multi-detector computed tomography for penetrating neck injury: a prospective multicenter study. *J Trauma Acute Care Surg.* 2012; 72(3): 576–584.

Ibraheem K, Wong S, Smith A, *et al*. Computed tomography angiography in the "no-zone" approach era for penetrating neck trauma: A systematic review. *J Trauma Acute Care Surg.* 2020; 89(6): 1233–1238.

Ibraheem K, Khan M, Rhee P, *et al.* "No zone" approach in penetrating neck trauma reduces unnecessary computed tomography angiography and negative explorations. *J Surg Res.* 2018; 221:113–120.

19 The 57-year-old helmeted driver of a motorcycle presents to the trauma bay after crashing into a wall. Workup reveals multiple injuries, including an open right femur fracture, grade 3 liver laceration, mandibular fracture, and an asymptomatic grade 2 internal carotid artery injury. What would be the best management of the blunt cerebrovascular injury?
   A Therapeutic heparin drip
   B Drug-eluting stent
   C Aspirin therapy
   D Neck exploration with repair
   E Silastic carotid shunt

BCVI has a relatively low incidence in approximately 0.1–3% of hospitalized trauma patients in the United States. When patients present with symptoms from BCVI, there is an associated morbidity rate of 80% and a mortality rate of 40%, illustrating the importance of screening and treatment. Once a BCVI has been identified on imaging, it must be graded and treated with the appropriate therapy in each clinical scenario. Antithrombotic therapy is recommended for grade 1 and 2 injuries. Choosing the appropriate therapy can be challenging in polytrauma patients, balancing the risk of hemorrhage and the risk of a cerebrovascular accident. Although ideal therapy needs to be tailored to individual patients, studies have shown a decrease in thrombotic events with the use of anticoagulant and antiplatelet medications. The patient detailed above is at high risk for hemorrhage from the liver laceration and is likely to require operative intervention for the multiple fractures; therefore, a heparin infusion would not be the ideal choice. An antiplatelet agent (answer C) is the most appropriate treatment in this case. Neck exploration, stents, and carotid shunts are only considered in the treatment of grade III and V injuries.

Answer: C

Burlew CC, Biffl WL. Blunt cerebrovascular trauma. *Curr Opin Crit Care.* 2010; 16(6): 587–595.

Kim DY, Biffl WL, Bokhari F, *et al.* Evaluation and management of blunt cerebrovascular injury: A practice management guideline from the Eastern Association for the Surgery of Trauma. *J Trauma Acute Care Surg.* 2020; 88(6): 875–887.

20 A 29-year-old bouncer is brought to the trauma bay after receiving multiple stab wounds to the neck and complaining of dysphagia and small volume hematemesis. The patient is hemodynamically stable, respiring comfortably on room air, and speaking in full sentences. There are two small lacerations to the right lateral zone 2 of the neck. There is no visible hematoma, nor is there any active bleeding from the wounds. There is minimal crepitus around the wounds and no bubbling or saliva coming from the wounds. What will you do next?
   A Proceed to the OR for neck exploration
   B CT angiography and CT esophagram
   C Rigid esophagoscopy and bronchoscopy
   D Flexible esophagoscopy and bronchoscopy
   E Gastrografin esophagram

Penetrating neck trauma should be managed with the "No zone approach." This patient is hemodynamically stable, without airway compromise but has multiple soft signs of injury, including dysphagia and subcutaneous emphysema concerning for possible aerodigestive injury and should undergo CT angiography as a first-line screening examination. Multichannel CT angiography is a rapid, easily performed, readily available diagnostic tool that gives meaningful information on bony and vascular structures and can easily demonstrate the trajectory of penetrating injuries. Given the small volume hematemesis, concern for esophageal is higher than average and CT esophagram is an excellent noninvasive option for screening with a sensitivity and specificity of 95% and 91%, respectively. CT esophagram is more sensitive than traditional gastrografin esophagram, which can miss 22–30% of injuries. Endoscopy and bronchoscopy are adjuncts to consider if the CT scan findings are equivocal. Surgical exploration should be reserved for hemodynamically unstable patients, those with hard signs of injury, or those with injuries identified on screening.

Answer: B

Chirica M, Kelly MD, Siboni S, *et al.* Esophageal emergencies: WSES guidelines. *World J Emerg Surg.* 2019; 14: 26 eCollection.

Biffl WL, Moore EE, Feliciano DV, Albrecht RA, Croce M, Karmy-Jones R, Brasel K. Western Trauma Association Critical Decisions in Trauma: Diagnosis and management of esophageal injuries. *J Trauma Acute Care Surg.* 2015; 79(6): 1089–1095.

21 During exploration for a left zone II neck stab wound, you find a laceration to the anterior trachea across the 1st and 2nd tracheal rings. The next step in her management would include:

A *Examination of the carotid sheath for injury to the vessels and vagus nerve.*

B *Examination of the posterior tracheal wall for injury.*

C *Examination of the esophagus for injury.*

D *Use of nonabsorbable sutures for tracheal repair with buttressing of the repair with healthy tissue if associated esophageal injury is present.*

E *All of the above.*

Neck exploration for trauma in this patient is performed via a longitudinal incision along the anterior border of the sternocleidomastoid. The presence of an anterior tracheal injury makes evaluation of the posterior wall of the trachea and the esophagus of paramount importance, as concomitant injuries are present in 10–15% of cases. Exploration of the ipsilateal carotid sheath and contents including the vagus nerve should be performed. Additional dissection to search for the superior or recurrent laryngeal nerves is not recommended, as this can increase the risk of iatrogenic injury. Most tracheal injuries can be closed primarily using an absorbable suture in a single layer. Associated injuries of the thyroid or cricoid cartilage can be closed with sutures or plates. Esophageal injuries should be explored to ensure the entire mucosal defect is addressed. Intraoperative esophagoscopy and insufflation of a nasogastric tube with air or dye can aid in the diagnosis of suspected esophageal injury. Once the injury has been identified, it can be repaired in one or two layers with absorbable suture. If there has been significant delay in treatment or there is severe tissue destruction, the repair can be protected with a T-tube; or diversion can be performed with a proximal cervical esophagostomy. All esophageal repairs should be buttressed with healthy tissue; this is of paramount importance if other suture lines are present. Buttressing can be done with one of the strap muscles, or the sternocleidomastoid. Wide drainage of all neck explorations is highly recommended.

Answer: E

Santiago-Rosado LM, Sigmon DF, Lewison CS. Tracheal Trauma. StatPearls [Internet] 2020 Jul 10. PMD 29763191.

Altinok T, Can A. Management of tracheobroncchial injuries. *Eurasion J Med.* 2014; 46(3): 209–215.

Zhao Z, Zhang T, Yin X, Zhao J, Li X, Zhou Y. Update on the diagnosis and treatment of tracheal and bronchial injury. *J Thorac Dis.* 2017; 9(1): E50–E56.

30

Cardiothoracic and Thoracic Vascular Injury

Charles J. Fox, MD[1] and Annalise Penikis, MD[2]

[1] R Adams Cowley Shock Trauma Center, Division of Vascular Surgery, University of Maryland School of Medicine, Baltimore, MD, USA
[2] University of Maryland Medical Center, Baltimore, MD, USA

1 *A 37-year-old woman sustained a stab wound to the left anterior chest. She is alert and hemodynamically stable with no neurologic deficits. On physical exam, there is a large supraclavicular wound with weak left upper extremity pulses. Which of the following statements regarding a left subclavian artery injury is true?*

A *Perform a chest radiograph followed by computed tomography angiography in stable patients.*

B *Proceed directly to the operating room for left posterolateral thoracotomy.*

C *A median sternotomy is preferred for obtaining proximal arterial control.*

D *A supraclavicular exploration is recommended for unstable patients.*

E *Covered stents have now completely replaced open repair techniques for left subclavian transections.*

A patient with a stab wound to the chest should first be evaluated with a chest radiograph to rule out pneumothorax. In a patient with a suspected left subclavian artery injury, a radiograph may also show a first rib fracture, widened mediastinum, apical pleural hematoma, or opacification along the expected course of the subclavian artery. In a hemodynamically stable patient or those without "hard signs" of vascular trauma, the next step in the evaluation would be a multi-slice computed tomography angiography (CTA) to diagnose the injury and aid the preoperative plan (choice A). There are no indications for a rush to the operating room in this case as the patient is stable (choice B). The safe approach to achieve proximal control for a left subclavian artery injury is a left anterolateral thoracotomy (choice C). Supraclavicular exploration is not advised particularly in unstable patients with hard signs of vascular injury because of the potential for uncontrolled surgical bleeding and the time to expose the artery with this approach is longer even in

the best of hands (choice D). The subclavian artery is easily visible through the chest and control is fast and simple. Right subclavian artery injuries, however, are best approached with a median sternotomy. Endovascular repairs are becoming more frequent but require a stable patient with suitable anatomy (choice E). Transactions are the most challenging to repair with an endovascular strategy and may require added challenges such as retrograde trans-brachial access and trans-femoral snaring for stent deployment. Preservation of the left vertebral artery remains an important consideration and may ultimately determine the best approach.

Hard signs	Soft signs
Active bleeding	Decreased pulse
Pulseless	Large nonexpanding hematoma
Ischemia	Nonpulsatile hematoma
Bruit or thrill	Nerve injury
Expanding pulsatile hematoma	History of active or pulsatile bleeding

Answer: A

Waller CJ, Cogbill TH, Kallies KJ, Ramirez LD, Cardenas JM, Todd SR, Chapman KJ, Beckman MA, Sperry JL, Anto VP, Eriksson EA, Leon SM, Anand RJ, Pearlstein M, Capano-Wehrle L, Cothren Burlew C, Fox CJ, Cullinane DC, Roberts JC, Harrison PB, Berg GM, Haan JM, Lightwine K. Contemporary management of subclavian and axillary artery injuries-A Western Trauma Association multicenter review. *J Trauma Acute Care Surg.* 2017; 83(6):1023–1031.

Ganapathy A, Khouqeer AF, Todd SR, Mills JL, Gilani R. Endovascular management for peripheral arterial trauma: The new norm? *Injury.* 2017; 48(5): 1025–1030.

Surgical Critical Care and Emergency Surgery: Clinical Questions and Answers, Third Edition.
Edited by Forrest "Dell" Moore, Peter M. Rhee, and Carlos J. Rodriguez.
© 2022 John Wiley & Sons Ltd. Published 2022 by John Wiley & Sons Ltd.
Companion website: www.wiley.com/go/surgicalcriticalcare3e

2   *A 45-year-old man is in MVC and found unrespon-*
    sive. His exam is notable for bruising over his anterior
    chest and a scalp laceration. A CTA confirms a blunt
    aortic intimal injury at the level of the aortic isthmus.
    Other injuries include subdural hematoma, pneumo-
    thorax, a 4 cm intraparenchymal splenic hematoma,
    and a right humerus fracture. His HR is 90/min,
    BP 115/65, and GCS is 15. What is the appropriate
    management for these injuries?

    A   *Place a chest tube followed by an open repair of the*
        aortic injury.
    B   *Place a chest tube and move to a hybrid room for*
        thoracic endovascular aortic repair.
    C   *Place a chest tube with nonoperative management*
        of the aortic and splenic injuries.
    D   *Place a chest tube followed by exploratory laparotomy.*
    E   *Systemic anticoagulation and nonoperative man-*
        agement for the aortic injury.

Several multicenter trials have demonstrated survival benefit for thoracic endovascular aortic repair (TEVAR) when compared to open aortic repair (choice A). An intimal flap is considered a mild blunt aortic injury and can be managed with medical therapies (blood pressure parameters and antiplatelet) and repeat imaging in several days to determine injury progression and the need for intervention (choice B). The pneumothorax is addressed early in accordance with advanced trauma life support (ATLS) guidelines (choice C). The splenic injury does not necessitate immediate exploration or intervention in a stable patient (choice D). Systemic anticoagulation is contraindicated in the setting of a traumatic brain injury and is not a good substitute for antiplatelet therapy that is recommended when the other injuries are stable, and the bleeding risk is lower (choice E).

Answer: C

Demetriades D, Velmahos GC, Scalea TM, Jurkovich GJ, Karmy-Jones R, Teixeira PG, Hemmila MR, O'Connor JV, McKenney MO, Moore FO, London J, Singh MJ, Lineen E, Spaniolas K, Keel M, Sugrue M, Wahl WL, Hill J, Wall MJ, Moore EE, Margulies D, Malka V, Chan LS; American Association for the Surgery of Trauma Thoracic Aortic Injury Study Group. Operative repair or endovascular stent graft in blunt traumatic thoracic aortic injuries: results of an American Association for the Surgery of Trauma Multicenter Study. *J Trauma.* 2008; 64(3):561–570; discussion 570-1.

Quiroga E, Starnes BW, Tran NT, Singh N. Implementation and results of a practical grading system for blunt thoracic aortic injury. *J Vasc Surg.* 2019; 70(4):1082–1088.

3   *A 65-year-old man suffers an isolated chest injury after*
    MVC. CTA demonstrates a hypoplastic right vertebral

artery and Grade III blunt aortic injury with intramural hematoma. Following TEVAR, the patient develops bilateral lower extremity numbness and weakness. What maneuver decreases the likelihood of this complication?

A   *Placement of a lumbar drain prior to endovascular*
    repair of the traumatic aortic injury.
B   *This is a known complication that cannot be*
    prevented.
C   *Preservation of the left subclavian artery.*
D   *Use of a larger diameter and longer covered stent*
    graft.
E   *Open repair.*

Placement of lumbar drain preoperatively is typically done for elective treatment of aneurysms in the setting of atherosclerosis but is not routinely recommended or performed for the trauma patient (choice A). Spinal cord ischemia is a dreaded complication but can be prevented with careful preoperative planning and precise TEVAR delivery (choice B). For example, intentional preservation of the left subclavian artery may reduce posterior circulation strokes and spinal cord ischemia (choice C). Limited subclavian artery coverage or revascularization strategies can be achieved with fenestration of the polyester thoracic graft, parallel stenting, or carotid subclavian artery bypass. Diameters are slightly oversized to the aortic wall and increased diameters risk dissection. Longer grafts sacrifice more intercostal arteries and therefore correlate with an increased risk of spinal cord ischemia (choice D). Open repair and endovascular repair continue to carry a measurable risk of spinal cord injury and paralysis (choice E).

Answer: C

Sobocinski J, Patterson BO, Karthikesalingam A, Thompson MM. The effect of left subclavian artery coverage in thoracic endovascular aortic repair. *Ann Thorac Surg.* 2016; 101(2):810–817.

Stafforini NA, Singh N, Hemingway J, Starnes B, Tran N, Quiroga E. Re-evaluating the need for routine coverage of the left subclavian artery in thoracic blunt aortic injury. *Ann Vasc Surg.* 2020; 31:S0890–5096(20) 31110-9.

4   *The patient with the least favorable prognosis is a:*
    A   *33-year-old with a stab wound to the right*
        ventricle.
    B   *23-year-old with a gunshot to the left atrium.*
    C   *42-year-old with a stab wound to the left atrium.*
    D   *36-year-old with stab wound to the left ventricle.*
    E   *27-year-old with a gunshot wound to the intra-*
        pericardial aorta.

In penetrating cardiac injuries, the mechanism of injury, physiologic status at presentation, and the anatomic site of injury can all determine the prognosis. For example, gunshot wounds carry higher mortality than stab wounds and left heart injuries are worse than right heart injuries due to higher pressure gradients (choices A–D). The thinner atrial myocardium may be a factor for a ventricular injury having a better prognosis. The intra-pericardial great vessel injuries have the worst prognosis of all injury patterns due to thin high-pressure walls (choice E). Multiple-chamber injuries, especially with great vessel involvement, were associated with the highest mortality rate. In addition to the location of injury, physiologic status and presence of tamponade impact outcome.

Answer: E

Morse BC, Mina MJ, Carr JS, Jhunjhunwala R, Dente CJ, Zink JU, Nicholas JM, Wyrzykowski AD, Salomone JP, Vercruysse GA, Rozycki GS, Feliciano DV. Penetrating cardiac injuries: A 36-year perspective at an urban, Level I trauma center. *J Trauma Acute Care Surg.* 2016; 81(4):623–631.

Tyburski JG, Astra L, Wilson RF, Dente C, Steffes C. Factors affecting prognosis with penetrating wounds of the heart. *J Trauma.* 2000; 48(4):587–590; discussion 590-1.

Rhee PM, Foy H, Kaufmann C, Areola C, Boyle E, Maier RV, Jurkovich G. Penetrating cardiac injuries: A population-based study. *J Trauma.* 1998; 45(20): 366–370.

5   A 45-year-old woman sustains blunt chest trauma. Her workup is notable for multiple rib fractures with flail chest and pulmonary contusions without hemothorax or pneumothorax. What would improve outcome in this patient?
   A *Surgical fixation of rib fracture after failure of medical management.*
   B *Multimodal therapy including the use of regional anesthesia to permit chest physiotherapy.*
   C *Mechanical ventilation to optimize tidal volumes.*
   D *Limiting narcotic pain medication to prevent depression of the respiratory drive.*
   E *Fluid restriction and steroids.*

Surgical stabilization of rib fractures are believed to improve chest wall stability leading to both better pain control and pulmonary mechanics. The sooner this stability is achieved, the less time the patient is exposed to secretion accumulation, atelectasis, and hypoventilation. Proponents of rib fixation suggest the greatest outcome is observed with early fixation by not allowing the patient the "opportunity" to fail medical management (choice A). Multimodal analgesia, including the use of narcotics and anti-inflammatory medications will permit chest physiotherapy and ensure the best outcome with improved pain control, pneumonia prevention, and a decreased need for mechanical ventilation (choice B). Mechanical ventilation is reserved for patients with respiratory failure and those who require mechanical ventilation have worse outcomes and higher mortality (choice C). The management of flail chest includes analgesia and aggressive chest physiotherapy but is not accomplished by limiting narcotic pain medication (choice D). Judicious fluid resuscitation is recommended in these patients to assure adequate tissue perfusion. However, steroids should be avoided in the management of pulmonary contusion (choice E).

Answer: B

Brasel KJ, Moore EE, Albrecht RA, deMoya M, Schreiber M, Karmy-Jones R, Rowell S, Namias N, Cohen M, Shatz DV, Biffl WL. Western Trauma Association Critical Decisions in Trauma: Management of rib fractures. *J Trauma Acute Care Surg.* 2017; 82(1): 200–203.

Pieracci FM, Coleman J, Ali-Osman F, Mangram A, Majercik S, White TW, Jeremitsky E, Doben AR. A multicenter evaluation of the optimal timing of surgical stabilization of rib fractures. *J Trauma Acute Care Surg.* 2018; 84(1):1–10.

6   A right-sided chest tube is placed in a hemodynamically stable patient after gunshot wound to the chest. After 4 hours, the chest tube has evacuated a steady rate of 1300 mL of sanguineous output. There is a persistent air leak and some subcutaneous emphysema noted around the chest tube and the BP is 90/60 mmHg. What is the next best step in management of this patient?
   A *Place another right-sided chest tube.*
   B *Obtain a supine chest radiograph.*
   C *Increase the wall suction on the right chest tube.*
   D *Proceed to the operating room for an emergent thoracotomy.*
   E *Correct coagulopathy and continue monitoring vital signs.*

Patient physiology rather than numbers should be the primary indication for thoracotomy after penetrating chest trauma. Regardless, an initial chest tube output >1500 mL or persistent bleeding of 200 mL/hour for 4 or more hours should prompt consideration for surgical intervention (choice D) versus continued monitoring in the setting of shock (choice E). The guidelines for thoracotomy in most textbooks are for when thoracotomy should be considered or when a trauma surgeon should be informed. When assessing and managing hemothorax, the two questions need to be answered. The first is how much has bled into the chest and the second is, are they still bleeding. Large amounts of blood out of the chest tube initially in a stable patient with no further bleeding may not need surgery. An unstable patient with bright red bleeding that continues may need surgery before a certain amount of blood has been collected. Chest tubes do not always reliably fully evacuate the hemothorax and the chest x-ray helps determine the effectiveness of the chest tube. A large amount of blood may be missed when viewing portable supine images and is not a reliable tool for managing this condition (choice B). A persistent air leak or retained hemothorax or when the bleeding seems to be "slowing" after chest tube placement can be managed with early video-assisted thoracoscopic surgery (VATS). Delays for further monitoring, extra suction (choice C), or placing additional tubes may increase the risk of complications. Blood in the chest always causes clotted residual blood to a relative degree. Blood clot in the chest does not come out of any sized chest tube but unclotted blood comes out of smaller bore chest tubes. Thus, although some trauma centers have advocated for second chest tubes if a certain amount comes out of the initial chest tube or if the diaphragm is not well visualized on chest X ray, this is no longer the standard (choice A). Retained clot is evaluated with CT scan and early VATS has become the standard.

Answer: D

Mowery NT, Gunter OL, Collier BR, Diaz JJ Jr, Haut E, Hildreth A, Holevar M, Mayberry J, Streib E. Practice management guidelines for management of hemothorax and occult pneumothorax. *J Trauma*. 2011; 70(2):510–518.

Karmy-Jones R, Namias N, Coimbra R, Moore EE, Schreiber M, McIntyre R Jr, Croce M, Livingston DH, Sperry JL, Malhotra AK, Biffl WL. Western trauma association critical decisions in trauma: Penetrating chest trauma. *J Trauma Acute Care Surg*. 2014; 77(6):994–1002.

Ahmed N, Jones D. Video-assisted thoracic surgery: State of the art in trauma care. *Injury*. 2004; 35(5):479–489.

7   After chest tube placement for a traumatic pneumothorax, a patient is noted to have a large air leak, subcutaneous emphysema, and hemoptysis. What should be ruled out and what is the appropriate next step in management?
   A *Retained hemothorax; video-assisted thoracoscopy surgery.*
   B *Intraparenchymal chest tube; upright chest radiographs.*
   C *Intraparenchymal chest tube; chest computed tomography (CT).*
   D *Tracheobronchial injury; thoracotomy.*
   E *Tracheobronchial injury; bronchoscopy.*

Air leaks are a common finding after traumatic injury to the chest and may be due to a leak in the drainage system or an intraparenchymal tube and can be excluded once serious injuries are ruled out (choices B, C). The associated severity of a missed tracheobronchial injury should prompt the diagnosis when a significant air leak, subcutaneous emphysema, hemoptysis, or pneumomediastinum is discovered. A CT scan is may be appropriate; however, a bronchoscopy will both diagnose and precisely localize the tracheobronchial injury for preoperative planning (choice E). Small injuries without leak can be managed nonoperatively. Most thoracic tracheal injures are approached via right posterolateral fourth intercostal thoracotomy and repaired with simple interrupted absorbable sutures although for trauma patients an anterior lateral thoracotomy is more commonly performed and is a viable option once the diagnosis is established (choice D). Distal air leaks will often seal with a tube thoracostomy, provided the suction is managed appropriately. VATS is appropriate for treating a retained hemothorax (choice A), but management of the tracheobronchial injury must take priority.

Answer: E

Karmy-Jones R, Wood DE. Traumatic injury to the trachea and bronchus. *Thorac Surg Clin*. 2007; 17(1):35–46.

Chouliaras K, Bench E, Talving P, Strumwasser A, Benjamin E, Lam L, Inaba K, Demetriades D. Pneumomediastinum following blunt trauma: Worth an exhaustive workup? *J Trauma Acute Care Surg*. 2015; 79(2):188–192; discussion 192-3.

8   Regarding blunt cardiac injury (BCI), which of the following is true?
   A *Electrocardiogram (ECG) is an appropriate screening tool in hemodynamically stable patients.*
   B *Males age older than 55 are the highest risk.*
   C *BCI can only be ruled out by transesophageal echocardiogram.*
   D *There is no role for cardiac enzyme testing in BCI.*
   E *Nuclear medicine studies can be useful and should be routinely used in suspected BCI.*

Blunt cardiac injury is rare. BCI is thought of in two ways. First is with power failure and this condition is very rare and more difficult to diagnose. The majority of BCI is stable and the main reason to identify this condition is to determine if arrhythmias are to occur and needs management. There are no specific injuries that predict the presence of a BCI, including a sternal fracture, but any patient who sustains significant blunt trauma to the anterior chest should be screened. There is no specific population that is most at risk for BCI (choice B). Patient in whom BCI is suspected should receive an ECG on admission to rule out any new abnormality such as an arrhythmia, ischemic change, or heart block (choice A). Recent EAST guidelines support the addition of a troponin I level to increase the negative predictive value of an ECG. A normal ECG and normal troponin I level rules out BCI. However, the difference in sensitivity of ECG alone versus troponins combined with ECG is minimal. The recommendation is that if the troponins are elevated, that ECG should be obtained. If normal, the chances of developing arrhythmia is extremely low, and the elevated troponins are insignificant. Troponins have been shown to be elevated in stressed blunt and penetrating trauma without cardiac injury. Diagnosis of BCI in stable patients without new arrhythmias is insignificant (choice D). An echocardiogram should be reserved for hemodynamic instability or new arrhythmias. Transesophageal echocardiogram is only recommended when a transthoracic echocardiogram is indeterminant (choice C). Nuclear medicine studies should not be routinely performed for this condition. This was done historically but it merely led to high utilization of resources and was found to be too sensitive (choice E).

Answer: A

Clancy K, Velopulos C, Bilaniku JW, Collier B, Crowley W, Kurek S, Lui F, Nayduch D, Sangosanya A, Tucker B, Haut ER. Screening for blunt cardiac injury: An Eastern Association for the Surgery of Trauma practice management guideline. *J Trauma Acute Care Surg*. 2012; 73(5 Suppl 4):S301–S306.

Joseph, B., Jokar, T.O., Khalil, M., Haider AA, Kulvatunyou N, Zangbar B, Tang A, Zeeshan M, O'Keeffe T, Abbas D, Latifi R Identifying the broken heart: Predictors of mortality and morbidity in suspected blunt cardiac injury. *Am J Sur*. 2016; 211(6):982–988.

Martin M, Mullenix P, Rhee P, Belzberg H, Demetriades D, Salim A. Troponin increases in the critically injured patient: mechanical trauma or physiologic stress? *J Trauma*. 2005; 59(5):1086–1091. doi: https://doi.org/10.1097/01.ta.0000190249.19668.37. PMID: 16385284.

9   *The most common site of aortic injury in blunt trauma is:*

  A *Intra-pericardial aorta.*

  B *Ascending aorta just proximal to the base of the innominate.*

  C *Aortic arch.*

  D *Aortic isthmus.*

  E *Descending aorta.*

In their extensive autopsy analysis published in 1958, Parmley et al. recognized that most blunt aortic trauma led to vessel rupture at the time of injury. For lesions that remained intact, the suggested natural history was progression and subsequent aortic rupture. Blunt aortic injury occurs most commonly at the aortic isthmus, just distal to the origin of the left subclavian artery (choice D). This location is the transition from mobile to fixed thoracic aorta. It is thought that these injuries are a result of deceleration injuries involving multiple forces including sheering, torsion, "water-hammer" effect (occlusion of artery with simultaneous increase in blood pressure), and an "osseous pinch" (compression between the anterior chest wall and the vertebral column). The other areas of the aorta that are injured is the ascending, aortic arch, and distal descending aorta but occur less commonly (choices A, B, C, E). The contemporary management includes computed tomography of the chest with intravenous contrast to diagnose clinically significant blunt thoracic aortic injury. Endovascular repair is strongly recommended for patients without contraindications. Delayed repair is permitted with the stipulation that effective blood pressure control must be used.

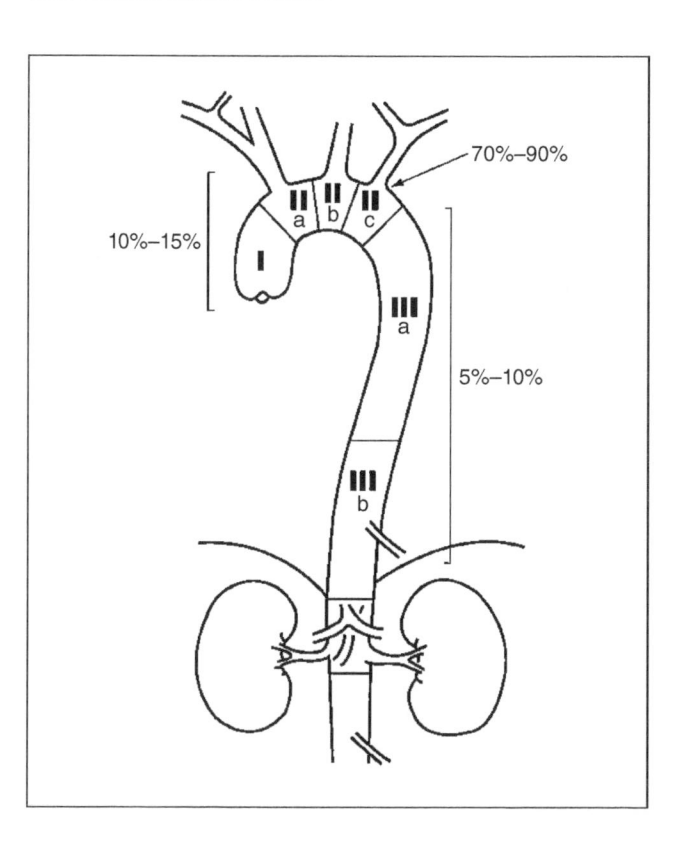

Answer: D

Parmley LF, Mattingly TW, Manion WC, Jahnke EJ Jr. Nonpenetrating traumatic injury of the aorta. *Circulation.* 1958; 17(6):1086–101.

Fox N, Schwartz D, Salazar JH, Haut ER, Dahm P, Black JH, Brakenridge SC, Como JJ, Hendershot K, King DR, Maung AA, Moorman ML, Nagy K, Petrey LB, Tesoriero R, Scalea TM, Fabian TC. Evaluation and management of blunt traumatic aortic injury: a practice management guideline from the Eastern Association for the Surgery of Trauma. *J Trauma Acute Care Surg.* 2015; 78(1):136–146.

10 *Which of the following statements regarding a traumatic widened mediastinum on chest radiograph (CXR) following blunt trauma is true?*
   A *Sternal fracture is not associated with mediastinal widening.*
   B *Upright posterior–anterior films are superior to portable supine anterior–posterior for accurately imaging the mediastinum.*
   C *Chest radiographs have a high sensitivity for detecting an aortic injury.*
   D *Chest radiographs alone are a reliable screening modality for an aortic injury.*
   E *Is defined by a width greater than 5 cm.*

A fractured sternum can produce a widening of the mediastinum even in the absence of an aortic injury (choice A). A widened mediastinum noted on CXR is defined by a mediastinal width greater than 6–8 cm (choice E). The mediastinal borders are composed of the right heart, ascending aorta, superior vena cava, aortic knob, descending aorta, and the left heart. The mediastinum contains the heart, thymus, trachea, esophagus, and vertebral column, and injury or disease of any of these structures (mediastinal masses, hilar lymphadenopathy, and thoracic aortic aneurysm) can cause a widened mediastinum. In trauma patients, the most common etiologies include sternal fracture, cardiac tamponade, thoracic spine fracture, and aortic disruption. Other factors such as poor technique associated with portable imaging will be improved with upright posterior anterior chest radiographs (choice B). In one study of 17 cases of confirmed blunt aortic injury, only 7 of 200 patients had a positive CXR for a mediastinal abnormality, for a sensitivity of 41% (95% CI: 19–67%). The remaining 59% had a normal mediastinum on CXR concluding that mediastinal abnormalities on CXR are not sufficiently sensitive to serve as the sole screening criteria for aortic injury (choices C, D). However, despite this low sensitivity, CXR cannot be eliminated altogether because of its utility in the diagnosis of other life-threatening injuries. In a stable patient, the next step in management would include CTA which would aid in diagnosing any traumatic causes, underlying aortic pathology, or masses.

Answer: B

Bruckner BA, DiBardino DJ, Cumbie TC, Trinh C, Blackmon SH, Fisher RG, Mattox KL, Wall MJ. Critical evaluation of chest computed tomography scans for blunt descending thoracic aortic injury. *Ann Thorac Surg.* 2006; 81(4):1339–1346.

Gutierrez A, Inaba K, Siboni S, Effron Z, Haltmeier T, Jaffray P, Reddy S, Lofthus A, Benjamin E, Dubose J, Demetriades D. The utility of chest x-ray as a screening tool for blunt thoracic aortic injury. *Injury.* 2016; 47(1):32–36.

11 *Most patients with traumatic thoracic aortic ruptures die before presentation or in the emergency department. A predictor of death from blunt aortic injury in the hospital is:*
   A *External aortic contour abnormality.*
   B *Pseudoaneurysm width measurement.*
   C *Size of periaortic hematoma.*
   D *Large intimal flaps with intramural hematoma.*
   E *Aortic diameter.*

Aortic Injury characteristics that predict death may persuade optimal timing and best mode of therapy. In a multivariate logistic regression, systolic blood pressure <90 mmHg was significantly associated with death from traumatic rupture. A retrospective review of various orthogonal measurements to the aortic flow channel showed that aortic diameter, large intimal flaps, pseudoaneurysm width, and external contour were not significantly correlated with death (choices A, B, D, E). Hematoma at the level of the aortic arch on computed tomography (CT) scan significantly correlated with death from blunt aortic injury with an average of 20.3 mm in those that died vs 7.7 mm in those that did not (P < 0.001) (choice C). A patient with an aortic pseudoaneurysm associated with a hematoma >15 mm was significantly more likely to die. This periaortic hematoma measurement may help to predict which injuries need urgent instead of semi-elective repair.

Answer: C

Starnes BW, Lundgren RS, Gunn M, Quade S, Hatsukami TS, Tran NT, Mokadam N, Aldea G. A new classification scheme for treating blunt aortic injury. *J Vasc Surg.* 2012; 55(1):47–54.

Harris DG, Rabin J, Starnes BW, Khoynezhad A, Conway RG, Taylor BS, Toursavadkohi S, Crawford RS. Evolution of lesion-specific management of blunt thoracic aortic injury. *J Vasc Surg.* 2016; 64(2):500–505.

12 *A hemodynamically stable 40-year-old construction worker fell 50 feet and suffered a small intimal tear to the descending thoracic aorta several centimeters below the left subclavian artery. Regarding the natural history of grade I-II blunt thoracic aortic (minimal) injury, the most likely conclusion regarding injury evolution is?*
   A *Repeat imaging is often stable, and a majority will have no interval change.*
   B *Risk of injury progression is high, and patients should be treated with pharmacotherapy.*
   C *Complete injury resolution is very rare.*
   D *When injury progression is noted, it occurs relatively late in surveillance imaging.*
   E *This is unknown as trauma patients do not return for follow-up examination.*

A growing body of literature on nonoperative management in blunt thoracic aortic injury (BTAI) has emerged since the 2011 publication of the Society for Vascular Surgery (SVS) practice guidelines. Injury progression in grade I-II BTAI is rare (5–7%) (choice B) and when injury progression was noted, it occurred relatively early (choice D). In one 10-year retrospective review of 49 patients and a subsequent metanalyses of 146 patients, injury resolution ranged from 40–55% (choices C, E). Pharmacotherapy remains a cornerstone of medical management in traumatic aortic injury as repeat imaging is often stable and the majority will have no interval change (choice A).

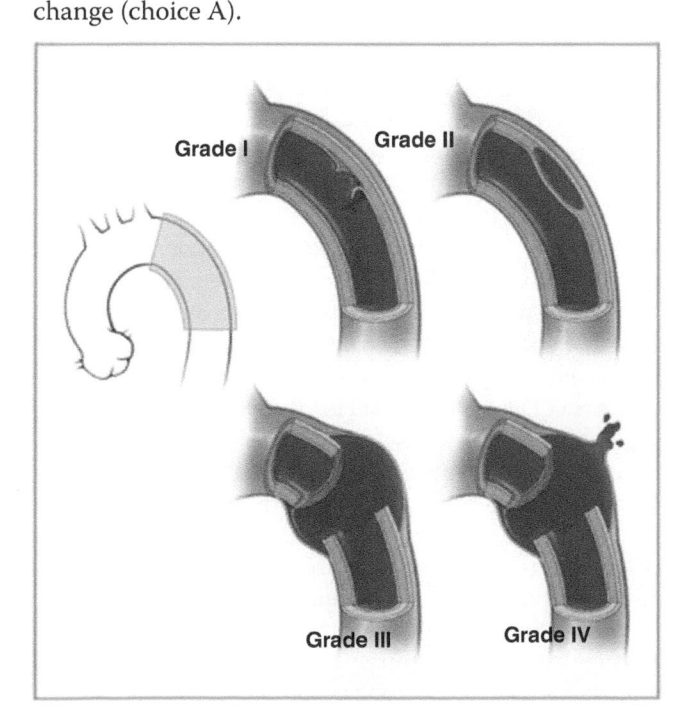

Grade I Intimal tear
Grade II Intramural hematoma
Grade III Pseudoaneurysm
Grade IV Rupture

Answer: A

Osgood MJ, Heck JM, Rellinger EJ, Doran SL, Garrard CL 3rd, Guzman RJ, Naslund TC, Dattilo JB. Natural history of grade I-II blunt traumatic aortic injury. *J Vasc Surg.* 2014; 59(2):334–341.

Jacob-Brassard J, Salata K, Kayssi A, Hussain MA, Forbes TL, Al-Omran M, de Mestral C. A systematic review of non-operative management in blunt thoracic aortic injury. *J Vasc Surg.* 2019; 70(5):1675–1681.

13 *Regarding emergency department thoracotomy (EDT), which of the following is the most important consideration for performing the procedure?*
   A *Potential for organ donation.*
   B *Signs of life on presentation.*
   C *Anatomic location of the traumatic injury.*
   D *Duration of prehospital cardiopulmonary resuscitation (CPR).*
   E *Asystole cardiac rhythm.*

The decision to perform resuscitative thoracotomy is usually based on information obtained at the time of patient arrival to the ED. Reported times of arrest are often "best estimates" (choice D) and the main deciding factor is the injury pattern (not location, choice C) and physiologic status with respect to achieving survival and neurologically intact survival (choice B). Regarding the duration of CPR, one multicenter trial done by the Western Trauma Association (WTA) reported no documented survivors of resuscitative thoracotomy for patients sustaining blunt trauma and requiring >10 minutes of prehospital CPR, and for patients with penetrating injuries undergoing >15 minutes of CPR and noted that asystole without pericardial tamponade is unlikely to yield a productive survival (choice E). Although procurement of organs is one of the tangible outcomes after EDT, the guidelines have been focused on survival and attempts to minimize futile care and not the issues surrounding organ donation (choice A).

Answer: B

Seamon MJ, Haut ER, Van Arendonk K, Barbosa RR, Chiu WC, Dente CJ, Fox N, Jawa RS, Khwaja K, Lee JK, Magnotti LJ, Mayglothling JA, McDonald AA, Rowell S, To KB, Falck-Ytter Y, Rhee P. An evidence-based approach to patient selection for emergency department thoracotomy: A practice management guideline from the Eastern Association for the Surgery of Trauma. *J Trauma Acute Care Surg.* 2015; 79(1):159–173.

Moore EE, Knudson MM, Burlew CC, Inaba K, Dicker RA, Biffl WL, Malhotra AK, Schreiber MA, Browder TD, Coimbra R, Gonzalez EA, Meredith JW, Livingston DH, Kaups KL; WTA Study Group. Defining the limits of resuscitative emergency department thoracotomy: a contemporary Western Trauma Association perspective. *J Trauma.* 2011; 70(2):334–339.

14 *Regarding emergency department thoracotomy (EDT), which of the following statements is NOT TRUE regarding pulseless patients presenting to the emergency department?*

   A *EDT is recommended for penetrating chest injury with signs of life.*

   B *EDT is recommended for non-penetrating chest injury without signs of life.*

   C *EDT is recommended for penetrating extra-thoracic injury without signs of life.*

   D *EDT is recommended for penetrating extra-thoracic injury with signs of life.*

   E *EDT is recommended for penetrating chest injury without signs of life.*

A practice management guideline was published by the Eastern Association for the Surgery of Trauma. They reported the data from 72 studies that evaluated 10 238 patients who underwent EDT. Patients presenting pulseless after penetrating thoracic injury had the most favorable EDT outcomes both with and without signs of life (choices A, E). In patients presenting pulseless after penetrating extra-thoracic injury, EDT outcomes were more favorable with signs of life (choice D) than without. Outcomes after EDT in pulseless blunt injury patients were limited with signs of life and dismal without signs of life (choice B). Therefore, the society conditionally recommended against EDT for blunt arrest without signs of life but strongly recommended EDT for penetrating thoracic injury with signs of life. Patients who present pulseless and have absent signs of life after penetrating thoracic injury, present or absent signs of life after penetrating extra-thoracic injury (choice C), or present signs of life after blunt injury received a conditional recommendation to perform an EDT.

Answer: B

Seamon MJ, Haut ER, Van Arendonk K, Barbosa RR, Chiu WC, Dente CJ, Fox N, Jawa RS, Khwaja K, Lee JK, Magnotti LJ, Mayglothling JA, McDonald AA, Rowell S, To KB, Falck-Ytter Y, Rhee P. An evidence-based approach to patient selection for emergency department thoracotomy: A practice management guideline from

the Eastern Association for the Surgery of Trauma. *J Trauma Acute Care Surg.* 2015; 79(1): 159–173.

Moore EE, Knudson MM, Burlew CC, Inaba K, Dicker RA, Biffl WL, Malhotra AK, Schreiber MA, Browder TD, Coimbra R, Gonzalez EA, Meredith JW, Livingston DH, Kaups KL; WTA Study Group. Defining the limits of resuscitative emergency department thoracotomy: a contemporary Western Trauma Association perspective. *J Trauma.* 2011; 70(2):334–339.

15 *Which of the following statements regarding pericardial tamponade (PT) is true?*

   A *Ultrasound is rapid screening test with limited sensitivity.*

   B *Acute PT is not associated with large amounts of clotted blood.*

   C *Pericardial drainage is commonly performed as a diagnostic maneuver.*

   D *In patients with stab wounds, PT is associated with a higher survival rate.*

   E *The phrenic nerve is located medially and should be avoided.*

One of the most significant advances in the management of cardiac injury was the advent of surgeon-performed ultrasound. A focused assessment for the sonographic evaluation of trauma (FAST) has been used for detection of hemopericardium in trauma patients. In a study of 247 patients, Rozycki and colleagues documented the use of surgeon-performed ultrasound in potential cardiac wounds and detected a hemopericardium with 100% sensitivity, specificity, and accuracy (choice A). Pericardiocentesis and pericardial window were historically the most commonly used techniques for diagnosis of hemopericardium; however, the use of pericardiocentesis has declined dramatically (choice C). Ivatury noted that PT resulting from penetrating cardiac injury (PCI) is frequently associated with large amounts of clotted blood rather than free fluid (choice B). In conditions with chronic pericardial blood, the blood clot may be liquefied over time due to the cardiac motion but in acute injury, there is almost always clot in the pericardium if the bleeding was acute. In a review of 100 consecutive patients at Denver General Hospital with acute penetrating cardiac injury (PCI), it found that the presence of tamponade was a critical independent factor for survival (choice D). The study by Rhee from Seattle in 1998 also confirmed the association of PT and higher survival. The authors concluded that pericardial tamponade may have a "protective" effect on outcome and is consistent with recent findings by Morse and colleagues. It may prevent exsanguination. The phrenic nerve is the lateral most structure on the pericardium and should be avoided by using a craniocaudal incision during resuscitative thoracotomy (choice E).

Answer: D

Morse BC, Mina MJ, Carr JS, Jhunjhunwala R, Dente CJ, Zink JU, Nicholas JM, Wyrzykowski AD, Salomone JP, Vercruysse GA, Rozycki GS, Feliciano DV. Penetrating cardiac injuries: A 36-year perspective at an urban, Level I trauma center. *J Trauma Acute Care Surg.* 2016; 81(4):623–631.

Rhee PM, Foy H, Kaufmann C, Areola C, Boyle E, Maier RV, Jurkovich G. Penetrating cardiac injuries: A population-based study. *J Trauma.* 1998; 45(20: 366–370.

Moreno C, Moore EE, Majure JA, Hopeman AR. Pericardial tamponade: A critical determinant for survival following penetrating cardiac wounds. *J Trauma.* 1986; 26(9):821–825.

16 *Which of the following statements regarding the management of a traumatic diaphragmatic injury (TDI) is true?*
  A *Laparoscopy when compared to computed tomography (CT) may decrease the incidence of a missed TDI in a hemodynamically stable patient with a left thoracoabdominal stab wound.*
  B *Nonoperative management is inappropriate for a stable patient with a penetrating thoracoabdominal wound in which a right diaphragm injury is suspected.*
  C *In hemodynamically stable trauma patients with acute diaphragm injuries, a thoracic approach to repair the diaphragm lowers the risk of procedural complications.*
  D *In patients with acute penetrating diaphragmatic injuries without concern for other intra-abdominal injuries, an open repair is strongly recommended.*
  E *A chronic diaphragmatic hernia repair from a missed TDI is usually approached from the chest.*

The superior diagnostic capability of laparoscopy to CT along with its relative safety and feasibility make it the preferred choice for most patients needing evaluation of a penetrating TDI (choice A). Laparoscopy may be a preferred surgical approach over open repair in stable patients without peritonitis for isolated TDI (choice D). For an acute injury, the abdominal approach is generally recommended (choice C) but is ultimately determined by the associated injuries and surgeon preference and no conclusions can be made regarding the superiority of one approach over the other. It is widely accepted that early recognition will reduce the incidence of late complications. Chronic diaphragmatic hernias from a missed

TDI can be approached through the chest or abdomen and the choice of approach will depend on patient factors and surgeon preference (choice E). Weighing the concern for procedural complications and a missed thoracoabdominal organ injury, nonoperative management is appropriate for a stable patient with a penetrating right-sided thoracoabdominal wound when a diaphragm injury is confirmed or suspected (choice B).

Answer: A

McDonald AA, Robinson BRH, Alarcon L, Bosarge PL, Dorion H, Haut ER, Juern J, Madbak F, Reddy S, Weiss P, Como JJ. Evaluation and management of traumatic diaphragmatic injuries: A practice management guideline from the Eastern Association for the Surgery of Trauma. *J Trauma Acute Care Surg.* 2018; 85(1):198–207.

Onat, S., Ulku, R., Avci, A., Ates G, Ozcelik C. Urgent thoracotomy for penetrating chest trauma: analysis of 158 patients of a single center. *Injury.* 2011; 42(9):900–904.

Ahmed N, Jones D. Video-assisted thoracic surgery: State of the art in trauma care. *Injury.* 2004; 35(5):479–489.

17 *Which of the following statements regarding retained hemothorax (RH) is most accurate?*
  A *A small (<300 cc) RH do not require observation. False*
  B *RH in trauma is associated with a poor predictor of empyema and pneumonia and prolonged hospitalization.*
  C *Observation, drainage, thoracostomy, intrapleural fibrinolytics, video-assisted thoracoscopy, and thoracotomy are all appropriate management options.*
  D *Larger initial hemothorax volumes are not independently associated with RH.*
  E *Thoracotomy provides incomplete visualization of the thorax compared to VATS.*

Traumatic hemothorax is common after thoracic injury and is associated with rib fractures, pneumothorax, pulmonary contusion, and diaphragmatic injury. Incomplete evacuation of blood results in a retained hemothorax and is an independent predictor of pneumonia, empyema, and prolonged hospitalization (choice B). Patients with computed tomography estimated volumes <300 cc were less likely to progress to RH and therefore observation is considered safe (choice A). Likewise, large initial hemothorax volumes were independently associated with RH (choice D) and when diagnosed are treated with a variety of management strategies. Treatment options range from observation, drainage, thoracostomy, intrapleural fibrinolytics, video-assisted thoracoscopy, and thoracotomy (choice C). Recognizing inherent risk, thoracotomy provides the best visualization of the thorax for and is the definitive intervention for RH that all newer therapies are compared (choice E). In modern management, VATS is a commonly used initial intervention. The optimal management after diagnosis remains a matter of debate.

Answer: C

Prakash PS, Moore SA, Rezende-Neto JB, Trpcic S, Dunn JA, Smoot B, Jenkins DH, Cardenas T, Mukherjee K, Farnsworth J, Wild J, Young K, Schroeppel TJ, Coimbra R, Lee J, Skarupa DJ, Sabra MJ, Carrick MM, Moore FO, Ward J, Geng T, Lapham D, Piccinini A, Inaba K, Dodgion C, Gooley B, Schwartz T, Shraga S, Haan JM, Lightwine K, Burris J, Agrawal V, Seamon MJ, Cannon JW. Predictors of retained hemothorax in trauma: Results of an Eastern Association for the Surgery of Trauma multi-institutional trial. *J Trauma Acute Care Surg.* 2020; 89(4):679–685.

DuBose J, Inaba K, Demetriades D, Scalea TM, O'Connor J, Menaker J, Morales C, Konstantinidis A, Shiflett A, Copwood B; AAST Retained Hemothorax Study Group. Management of post-traumatic retained hemothorax: A prospective, observational, multicenter AAST study. *J Trauma Acute Care Surg.* 2012; 72(1):11–22; discussion 22-4; quiz 316.

Meyer DM, Jessen ME, Wait MA, Estrera AS. Early evacuation of traumatic retained hemothoraces using thoracoscopy: A prospective, randomized trial. *Ann Thorac Surg.* 1997; 64(5):1396–1400; discussion 1400-1.

18 *Which of the following statements regarding repair of a penetrating cardiac injury is the most true?*

   A *Even in the absence of major cardiac compromise, an injury to the right coronary or circumflex should be repaired.*

   B *Electrocardiogram (ECG) is an appropriate screening tool to rule out septal or valve defects.*

   C *Sternotomy followed by splitting the pericardium anteriorly up to the origin of the ascending aorta and laterally along the diaphragmatic reflection will obtain maximal exposure.*

   D *Traumatic coronary fistulas or persistent myocardial ischemia detected on coronary angiography should not be stenting in the early postoperative period.*

   E *An intra-aortic balloon pump cannot temporize marginal cardiac dysfunction by reduced afterload, increased diastolic perfusion pressure, and increased cardiac output avoiding the need for cardiopulmonary bypass.*

Although anterior lateral thoracotomy is acceptable and maybe even preferable for posterior cardiac injuries, median sternotomy is the optimal approach to manage cardiac injuries if the patient is stable enough to allow the time to perform it. Opening the pericardium anteriorly, up to the origin of the ascending aorta, and dividing laterally along the diaphragmatic reflection obtain maximal exposure (choice C). If there are posterior wounds, a sponge can be packed along the diaphragmatic surface to elevate the posterior surface of the heart. Most cardiac injuries can be repaired with simple 3-0 mattress sutures with or without using felt or pericardial pledgets. If the injury is close to a major coronary artery, placing horizontal sutures deep to either side of the artery will reduce the chance of coronary occlusion. Direct injuries to the coronary artery can be repaired primarily with 6-0 or 7-0 sutures, usually in an interrupted fashion. As a rule, proximal left anterior descending coronary arteries require repair as do proximal right coronary artery. More distal injuries, right coronary, and/or circumflex injuries in the absence of obvious major cardiac compromise can sometime be managed by ligation (choice A). A formal transesophageal echocardiogram should be performed to rule out septal or valve defects (choice B). Persistent evidence of myocardial ischemia should prompt coronary angiogram when possible to exclude rare coronary fistula or occlusions that might be amenable to stenting (choice D). For marginal cardiac dysfunction after coronary ligation, an intra-aortic balloon pump is recommended as a temporizing maneuver (Choice E).

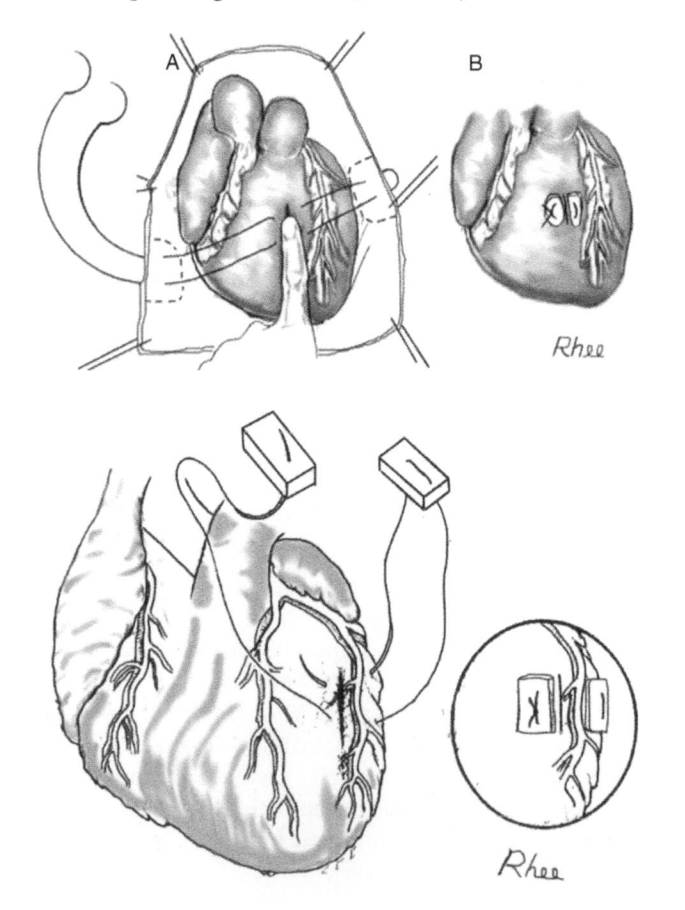

(a)

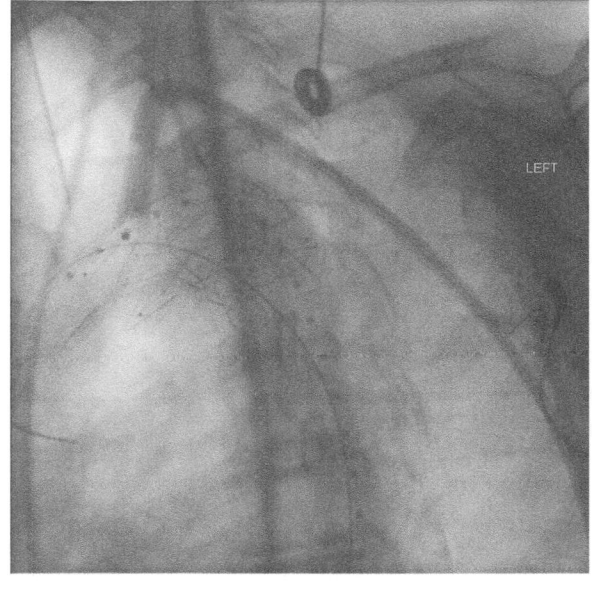

(b)

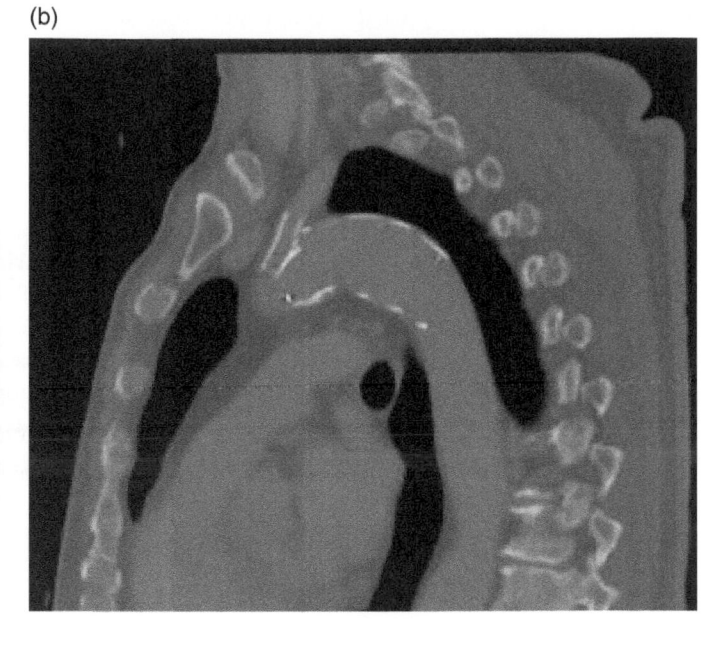

Answer: C

Karmy-Jones R, Namias N, Coimbra R, Moore EE, Schreiber M, McIntyre R Jr, Croce M, Livingston DH, Sperry JL, Malhotra AK, Biffl WL. Western Trauma Association critical decisions in trauma: Penetrating chest trauma. *J Trauma Acute Care Surg.* 2014; 77(6):994–1002.

Wall MJ Jr, Mattox KL, Chen CD, Baldwin JC. Acute management of complex cardiac injuries. *J Trauma.* 1997; 42(5):905–912.

19 *Which of the following statements regarding a trans-mediastinal gunshot wound is not true?*

A *Contrast-enhanced helical CT scanning is a safe, efficient, and cost-effective diagnostic tool for evaluating hemodynamically stable patients with mediastinal gunshot wounds.*

B *The diagnosis for stable patients is confirmed by finding at physical examination and on chest x-ray films in most cases.*

C *In the dying patient, bilateral chest tubes are inserted and the incision for the approach is based on the output.*

D *Detection of occult vascular, esophageal, or tracheobronchial injuries are indicated but the extent and order of the evaluation is debatable.*

E *Every patient should undergo bronchoscopy and esophagram to rule out injury to the trachea and esophagus.*

Trans-mediastinal gunshot injuries are associated with high mortality due to injuries to cardiac and other major vascular structures. Evaluation and management depends on whether the patient is dead, dying, or stable. In the dead patient, meaning that they do not have signs of life, EDT is a consideration. In the dying patient, bilateral chest tubes are inserted and the incision for the approach is based on the chest tube output (choice C). If the left chest has large output of blood and the right does not, then a left thoracotomy is considered. Right thoracotomy is for the patient with blood coming out of the right side predominantly. If the blood output is equivalent, then median sternotomy or clamshell thoracotomy is considered. In the absence of obvious bleeding, contrast-enhanced helical CT scanning is a safe, efficient, and cost-effective diagnostic tool for evaluating hemodynamically stable patients (choice A). The diagnosis for stable patients is confirmed by finding at physical examination and on chest x-ray films in most cases (choice B). Detection of occult vascular, esophageal, or tracheobronchial injuries are indicated but the extent and order of the evaluation is debatable (choice D). Not every patient that has a wide mediastinum on chest x-ray has a vascular injury that requires an operation and patients who do not have a vascular injury can be spared an unnecessary operation. In one study, only 7 of 200 trauma patients with a mediastinal abnormality on CXR were diagnosed with a BTAI yielding a positive predictive value of 3.5% (choice E). Although it was once taught that all trans-mediastinal gunshot wounds must undergo bronchoscopy to rule out tracheal injury and contrast esophagram, the recommended approach is to start with CT angiogram with particular attention to the trajectory to determine what further tests may be necessary. If the trajectory is not near the esophagus, vessels, or airway tract, no further evaluation is necessary. If the trajectory is worrisome for an injury to the esophagus, then an EGD or swallow may be useful. For thoracic vascular injury, CTA would be of use; therefore, for transmediastinal GSW, the initial scan should be a CTA. For the airway tract injury, bronchoscopy may be useful.

Answer: E

Okoye OT, Talving P, Teixeira PG, Chervonski M, Smith JA, Inaba K, Noguchi TT, Demetriades D. Transmediastinal gunshot wounds in a mature trauma centre: Changing perspectives. *Injury*. 2013; 44(9):1198–1203.

Stassen NA, Lukan JK, Spain DA, Miller FB, Carrillo EH, Richardson JD, Battistella FD. Reevaluation of diagnostic procedures for transmediastinal gunshot wounds. *J Trauma*. 2002; 53(4):635–638; discussion 638.

Renz BM, Cava RA, Feliciano DV, Rozycki GS. Transmediastinal gunshot wounds: A prospective study. *J Trauma*. 2000; 48(3):416–21; discussion 421-2.

Gutierrez A, Inaba K, Siboni S, Effron Z, Haltmeier T, Jaffray P, Reddy S, Lofthus A, Benjamin E, Dubose J, Demetriades D. The utility of chest x-ray as a screening tool for blunt thoracic aortic injury. *Injury*. 2016; 47(1):32–36.

20 Which of the following statements regarding resuscitative endovascular balloon occlusion of the aorta (REBOA) is not true?
   A Balloon rupture is reduced with careful inflation technique.
   B REBOA is a useful adjunct for noncompressible subdiaphragmatic hemorrhage.
   C Zone II is from the celiac artery to the highest renal artery.
   D Zone I is measured from the left subclavian to the celiac artery.
   E Is not advised for penetrating injury to the thorax.

REBOA has been promoted as an effective endovascular resuscitative device for noncompressible torso hemorrhage originating from the abdomen or pelvis (choice B). The aortic zones of occlusion include Zone 1 (origin of the left subclavian to the celiac artery), Zone II (celiac artery to the lowest renal artery), and Zone III (lowest renal artery to the aortic bifurcation) (choices C, D). Tactile sensitivity is required to recognize subtle changes in resistance during inflation. Selecting a goal volume in excess of the aortic diameter and ignoring tactile feedback can lead to balloon or vessel rupture (choice A). Patients with penetrating chest trauma should undergo exploration when hemodynamically unstable (choice E).

Answer: C

Moore LJ, Brenner M, Kozar RA, Pasley J, Wade CE, Baraniuk MS, Scalea T, Holcomb JB. Implementation of resuscitative endovascular balloon occlusion of the aorta as an alternative to resuscitative thoracotomy for non-compressible truncal hemorrhage. *J Trauma Acute Care Surg*. 2015; 79(4):523–530; discussion 530-2.

Davidson AJ, Russo RM, Reva VA, Brenner ML, Moore LJ, Ball C, Bulger E, Fox CJ, DuBose JJ, Moore EE, Rasmussen TE; BEST Study Group. The pitfalls of resuscitative endovascular balloon occlusion of the aorta: Risk factors and mitigation strategies. *J Trauma Acute Care Surg*. 2018; 84(1):192–202.

21 A 52-year-old man is brought in by EMS after sustaining a stab wound to the chest. The patient is awake and alert. Primary survey is notable for diminished breath sounds on the right. He is otherwise stable with HR 90 beats/min, BP 123/77 mm Hg, and SpO2 95%. eFAST performed in the trauma bay demonstrates a large anechoic area in the pleural space on the right. This condition is best managed with:
   A Supplemental oxygen and observation.
   B Emergent needle decompression followed by tube thoracostomy.
   C Tube thoracostomy with 36 French tube.
   D Percutaneous catheter placement.
   E VATs evacuation of hematoma.

The sonographic presence of a large anechoic area above the diaphragm following a penetrating injury should raise the suspicion of a traumatic hemothorax. Initial management of a large hematoma would include drainage to prevent the complications of a retained hemothorax (Answer A). Needle decompression is an unnecessary ineffective step that delays the ultimate treatment (Answer B). The traditional treatment of a traumatic hemothorax has been the insertion of a large bore 36-40 French chest tube; however, small caliber tubes as demonstrated in recent randomized trials are equally effective in the ability to drain the hemothorax (Answer C). Smaller percutaneous catheters have the added advantages of having the perception of less pain and discomfort (Answer D). VATS evacuation would be reserved for the management of a retained hemothorax (Answer E).

Answer: D

Staub LJ, Biscaro RRM, Kaszubowski E, Maurici R. Chest ultrasonography for the emergency diagnosis of traumatic pneumothorax and haemothorax: A systematic review and meta-analysis. *Injury*. 2018; 49(3):457–466.

Kulvatunyou N, Bauman ZM, Bou Zein Eddine S, de Moya M, Krause C, Mukherjee K, Gries L, Tang AL, Joseph B, Rhee P. (2021) The small 14-French (Fr) percutaneous catheter vs. large (28-32Fr) open chest tube for traumatic hemothorax (P-CAT): A multi-center randomized clinical trial. J Trauma Acute Care Surg. doi: https://doi.org/10.1097/TA.0000000000003180

22 *A 24-year-old man is brought in by EMS after a motor vehicle accident with blunt thoracic injury. Which of the following is TRUE regarding the extended focused assessment with sonography for trauma (eFAST) and other imaging modalities for the management of an occult or overt pneumothorax?*

 A *A stable patient with a positive thoracic ultra-sonography should have an immediate tube thoracostomy.*

 B *A stable patient with a positive thoracic ultra-sonography and positive supine chest radiography should proceed to computed tomography.*

 C *A stable patient with a positive thoracic ultra-sonography and negative chest radiography should proceed to computed tomography.*

 D *An unstable patient with a positive thoracic ultra-sonography should have a tube thoracostomy after confirmatory chest radiography.*

 E *A stable patient with a positive thoracic ultra-sonography and negative supine chest radiography can be observed to reduce the risk of radiation exposure with computed tomography.*

The supine plain chest radiograph (CXR) remains an insensitive test for the traumatic pneumothorax. However, computed tomography (CT) and eFAST are common imaging modalities in the modern era for the detection of pneumothoraces in blunt thoracoabdominal trauma. An occult pneumothorax was originally defined as a pneumothorax noted on CT that was not seen on a preceding radiograph. More recently, eFAST with a diagnostic sensitivity of 92–100% can easily detect the absence of lung sliding and has overcome some limitations of supine chest radiography (CXR) while promoting refinement of the indications for thoracic CT. Since the eFAST is a simple extension of the clinical exam, unstable patients with a pneumothorax should undergo tube thoracostomy without further delay (Answer D). For stable patients, a positive eFAST should be confirmed with a complimentary study and if an overt pneumothorax is detected, a chest tube is inserted (Answer A). Thoracic CT is best reserved for discovering false-negative chest radiographs (Answers C, E) but is preferable to avoid the risk of radiation exposure when both an eFAST and CXR are positive by placing a chest tube (Answers B).

Answer: C

Ball CG, Kirkpatrick AW, Feliciano DV. The occult pneumothorax: What have we learned? *Can J Surg*. 2009; 52(5):E173–E179.

Staub LJ, Biscaro RRM, Kaszubowski E, Maurici R. Chest ultrasonography for the emergency diagnosis of traumatic pneumothorax and haemothorax: A systematic review and meta-analysis. *Injury*. 2018; 49(3):457–466.

31

Abdominal and Abdominal Vascular Injury

Melike Harfouche, MD[1] and Joseph DuBose, MD[2]

[1] Division of Trauma and Acute Care Surgery, University of Maryland – Shock Trauma Center, Baltimore, MD, USA
[2] Department of Surgery, Dell School of Medicine, University of Texas Austin, Austin, TX, USA

1 *A 40-year-old man sustained a single gunshot wound to the left gluteal region. He is hemodynamically normal, with no abdominal pain nor tenderness. A digital rectal exam reveals gross blood. A CT scan of the pelvis confirms the trajectory, which is consistent with an extraperitoneal rectal injury. An intraoperative sigmoidoscopy reveals a nondestructive injury to the lower one third of the rectum. The best choice below for the management of this injury involves:*

A *Exploratory laparotomy with primary repair of the injury*

B *Presacral drains, sigmoid diversion, and distal rectal washout*

C *Laparoscopy or laparotomy and sigmoid loop colostomy for proximal diversion*

D *Trans anal primary repair of the injury without diversion*

E *Laparoscopy, resection of the injury, with primary anastomosis*

Hemodynamically stable patients with suspected rectal injuries should undergo a CT scan of the abdomen and pelvis with IV contrast to further define trajectory. This should be followed by an intraoperative flexible or rigid sigmoidoscopy to delineate the extent of injury and whether it involves the upper two thirds or lower one third of the rectum. Injuries to the upper two thirds of the rectum can be repaired primarily (choice A), whereas injuries to the lower one third are usually inaccessible and not amenable to primary repair. Injury to the lower one third should undergo proximal diversion with a sigmoid loop colostomy (choice C). Distal rectal washout has been associated with increased morbidity related to infectious complications and is now no longer

recommended (choice B). Presacral drains when performed routinely have also been associated with increased morbidity but can usually only offer benefit in the setting of destructive posterior rectal injuries. Prophylactic presacral drains for injuries to the anterior rectum or lateral wounds that do not traverse the posterior space may do more harm. Trans anal repair can be performed if the injury is easily visualized, or if edges can be approximated, but these repairs should prudently be combined with proximal diversion to offer the best chance for long-term healing and morbidity reduction.

Answer: C

Bosarge, Patrick L., John J. Como, Nicole Fox, Yngve Falck-Ytter, Elliott R. Haut, Heath A. Dorion, Nimitt J. Patel, et al. "Management of Penetrating Extraperitoneal Rectal Injuries: An Eastern Association for the Surgery of Trauma Practice Management Guideline." *Journal of Trauma and Acute Care Surgery* 80, no. 3 (2016): 546–51. https://doi.org/10.1097/TA.0000000000000953.

Weinberg, Jordan A., Timothy C. Fabian, Louis J. Magnotti, Gayle Minard, Tiffany K. Bee, Norma Edwards, Jeffery A. Claridge, and Martin A. Croce. "Penetrating Rectal Trauma: Management by Anatomic Distinction Improves Outcome." *The Journal of Trauma: Injury, Infection, and Critical Care* 60, no. 3 (2006): 508–14. https://doi.org/10.1097/01.ta.0000205808.46504.e9.

Brown, Carlos V.R., Pedro G. Teixeira, Elisa Furay, John P. Sharpe, Tashinga Musonza, John Holcomb, Eric Bui, et al. "Contemporary Management of Rectal Injuries at Level I Trauma Centers: The Results of an American Association for the Surgery of Trauma Multi-Institutional Study." *Journal of Trauma and Acute Care Surgery* 84, no. 2 (2018): 225–33. https://doi.org/10.1097/TA.0000000000001739.

2 *A 50-year-old woman sustained a single gunshot wound to the left lower quadrant. A plain film demonstrates a bullet in the right lower quadrant. She is hemodynamically normal but has peritonitis. The patient has been taken to the operating room right away for an exploratory laparotomy and several small bowel injuries, and a nondestructive injury to the sigmoid colon has been found. Which of the following intraoperative findings should be considered a contraindication to primary repair of the intraperitoneal colon injury?*

   A *Extensive fecal contamination*
   B *Intraoperative transfusion requirement of 2 units of packed red blood cells*
   C *Concomitant abdominal vascular injury*
   D *Involvement of greater than 25% of the bowel circumference of the sigmoid colon*
   E *None of the above*

Management of colon injuries has undergone significant evolution over the past several decades. Initially, it was mandated during World War I that all colon injuries should undergo colostomy creation for all penetrating colon injuries. However, over time several randomized studies have demonstrated low leak rates in the setting of primary repair or primary anastomosis. Whereas initially the recommendation was to perform a diversion in the setting of extensive fecal contamination, concomitant vascular injury or blood transfusion requirements, several studies have demonstrated improved outcomes when compared to colostomy or diversion even in these settings. In the modern era, attempts should be made to either repair colon injuries when less than 50% of the bowel circumference is involved or perform a resection and primary anastomosis if the injury is >50% of the bowel circumference in all hemodynamically stable patients. In the 2001 study by Demetriades et al., risk factors for abdominal complications in terms of abscess formation in the setting of penetrating colon injury were severe peritoneal contamination, ≥4 units of blood transfusion in the first 24 hours, and single-agent antibiotic prophylaxis. The type of repair performed (anastomosis vs. diversion) was not associated with increased complication risk. Since colostomy reversal with a second-stage elective operation later is also associated with complications, overall the best result is repair of colon at the first index operation without a colostomy.

Answer: E

Stone, H. Harlan, and Timothy C. Fabian. "Management of Perforating Colon Trauma: Randomization between Primary Closure and Exteriorization." *Annals of Surgery* 190, no. 4 (1979): 430–36. https://doi.org/10.1097/00000658-197910000-00002.

Gonzalez, Richard P., Gary J. Merlotti, and Michele R. Holevar. "Colostomy in Penetrating Colon Injury: Is It Necessary?" *Journal of Trauma and Acute Care Surgery* 41, no. 2 (1996): 271–5.

Demetriades, D., J. A. Murray, L. Chan, C. Ordoñez, D. Bowley, K. K. Nagy, E. E. Cornwell, et al. "Penetrating Colon Injuries Requiring Resection: Diversion or Primary Anastomosis? An AAST Prospective Multicenter Study." *The Journal of Trauma* 50, no. 5 (2001): 765–75. https://doi.org/10.1097/00005373-200105000-00001.

3 *In which of the following scenarios would nonoperative management of a gunshot wound with a defined tract through the right upper quadrant be considered an appropriate management option?*

   A *Hemodynamically normal, no peritonitis but has a positive Focused Assessment with Sonography in Trauma (FAST) exam at Morrison's Pouch*
   B *Hemodynamically unstable with a positive FAST exam at Morrison's Pouch*
   C *Hemodynamically normal with negative FAST but has peritonitis*
   D *Hemodynamically normal with a right hemothorax requiring a chest tube*
   E *None of the above*

Literature has shown that selective nonoperative management of abdominal gunshot wounds resulting in solid organ injury is an acceptable practice associated with success rates nearing 100% in certain circumstances. Contraindications to nonoperative management are hemodynamic instability (Answer B) and peritonitis (Answer C). It is crucial that patients undergo CT scan of the abdomen and pelvis with IV contrast followed by serial abdominal examinations if the nonoperative approach is selected. If a hollow viscus injury is suspected, operative intervention should not be delayed. A positive FAST (Answer A) and/or high-grade solid organ injury on CT imaging alone are not contraindications to nonoperative management in appropriate settings with close monitoring capabilities. Patients who sustain a right hemothorax from a gunshot wound to the right upper quadrant do not necessarily need operative intervention. Aside from chest tube placement, close observation is warranted as these patients are at risk for developing a thoracic biloma or biliary fistula, at which point chest exploration and drainage is indicated with diaphragm repair.

Answer: A

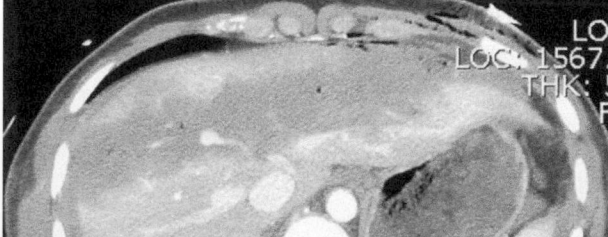

DuBose, Joseph, Kenji Inaba, Pedro G.R. Teixeira, Antonio Pepe, Michael B. Dunham, and Mark McKenney. "Selective Non-Operative Management of Solid Organ Injury Following Abdominal Gunshot Wounds." *Injury* 38, no. 9 (2007): 1084–90. https://doi.org/10.1016/j.injury.2007.02.030.

Schellenberg, Morgan, Elizabeth Benjamin, Alice Piccinini, Kenji Inaba, and Demetrios Demetriades. "Gunshot Wounds to the Liver: No Longer a Mandatory Operation." *Journal of Trauma and Acute Care Surgery* 87, no. 2 (2019): 350–55. https://doi.org/10.1097/TA.0000000000002356.

4   *A 30-year-old-man suffered multiple thoracoabdominal gunshot wounds. He has a thready pulse, with a systolic blood pressure of 60 mm Hg, and a positive FAST in the right upper quadrant. He is immediately taken to the operating room for an exploratory laparotomy. A large, nonpulsatile hematoma is identified in Zone 1, inferior to the transverse colon mesentery. You suspect an inferior vena cava injury. Which of the operative maneuver provides the optimal exposure to the infrarenal inferior vena cava?*

A   *Right medial visceral rotation (Cattell-Braasch maneuver)*

B   *left medial visceral rotation (Mattox maneuver)*

C   *Direct exposure at the base of the transverse colon mesentery*

D   *Extraperitoneal approach via a Gibson incision*

E   *Kocher maneuver*

Exposure of the infrarenal IVC for trauma is best done with a right medial visceral rotation, which is sometimes referred as the Cattell-Braasch maneuver. This involves medial mobilization of the right colon in conjunction with medal mobilization of the C-loop of the duodenum. The kidney is usually left in situ unless there is a posterior IVC injury, or an injury at the junction of the renal vein and IVC, which is better visualized if the kidney is also rotated medially. A left medial visceral rotation is often referred as the Mattox maneuver even though he was not the first to describe it. Dr. Mattox did, however, popularize it in the field of trauma. It is best for exposure of the supraceliac aorta (choice B). Although the IVC can be visualized through a midline retroperitoneal incision at the base of the mesentery, this approach is usually less familiar to the trauma surgeon and precious time may be lost if the surgeon is not experienced in this approach (choice C). Medial mobilization of the C loop of the duodenum alone, also known as a Kocher maneuver, is not optimal for exposure of the infrarenal IVC (choice C). Although an extraperitoneal exposure may allow adequate visualization of the infrarenal IVC, it will not allow for

identification and repair of intraperitoneal injuries. The Gibson incision is right or left lower quadrant incision that is curvilinear and is commonly used for renal transplantation or as extra peritoneal approach to the distal ureter.

Answer: A

Burch, Jon M, David V Feliciano, Kenneth L Mattox, and Mark Edelman. "Injuries of the Inferior Vena Cava." *The American Journal of Surgery* 156 (1988): 548–52.

Graham, Joseph M., Kenneth L. Mattox, Arthur C. Beall, and Michael E. DeBakey. "Traumatic Injuries of the Inferior Vena Cava." *Archives of Surgery (Chicago, Ill.: 1960)* 113, no. 4 (1978): 413–18. https://doi.org/10.1001/archsurg.1978.01370160071011.

5   *A 22-year-old woman with a gunshot wound to the right upper quadrant. She is hemodynamically unstable and has a positive FAST. Exploratory laparotomy reveals >50% transection of the infrarenal IVC. She remains hemodynamically unstable, with a temperature of 33 °C, lactate of 12 and base deficit of -13 from too much crystalloid infusion. Given this clinical presentation, what is the best approach to management and its most common associated complication?*

A   *Interposition graft with ringed PTFE and graft infection*

B   *IVC ligation and lower extremity compartment syndrome*

C   *Primary repair of IVC and pneumonia*

D   *Patch angioplasty of the IVC and acute renal failure*

E   *Interposition graft with common femoral vein and lower extremity deep vein thrombosis*

IVC injuries carry a high mortality rate, with an in-hospital mortality ranging between 38 and 66% due to uncontrolled bleeding. When on-scene deaths are included, the mortality rate is much higher. Expedient hemorrhage control offers the patient the best chance for survival. Suprarenal IVC ligation should be avoided, as few will survive the morbidity of that operation. However, infrarenal IVC ligation is an acceptable approach for the moribund patient. Patients can avoid the lethal triad of acidosis, coagulopathy, and hypothermia with massive transfusion protocols, which will transfuse warm PRBC, FFP, and platelets. If room temperature crystalloid fluids are used, the lethal triad can occur more frequently. The most common complication associated with IVC ligation is lower extremity compartment syndrome, for which the patient should be closely monitored and undergo four-compartment fasciotomies if needed. Some will apply ace wraps and elevate the legs after ligation of the IVC. Several series have shown IVC ligation to be associated with higher complication rates when compared to repair. However, there may be a selection bias as patients with more severe injury and bleeding may undergo ligation and the lesser injured vessels may undergo repair. If the uncontrolled hemorrhage has been controlled and the patient is stabilizing, venorrhaphy or interposition with ringed PTFE depending on the amount of destruction should be considered and performed. Graft infection and lower extremity DVT are also potential complications of IVC repair. The common femoral vein is usually too small in diameter to be used as an interposition graft for IVC injuries.

Answer: B

Matsumoto, Shokei, Kyoungwon Jung, Alan Smith, and Raul Coimbra. "Management of IVC Injury: Repair or Ligation? A Propensity Score Matching Analysis Using the National Trauma Data Bank." *Journal of the American College of Surgeons* 226, no. 5 (2018): 752–759.e2. https://doi.org/10.1016/j.jamcollsurg.2018.01.043.

Sullivan, Patrick S., Christopher J. Dente, Snehal Patel, Matthew Carmichael, Jahnavi K. Srinivasan, Amy D. Wyrzykowski, Jeffrey M. Nicholas, et al. "Outcome of Ligation of the Inferior Vena Cava in the Modern Era." *The American Journal of Surgery* 199, no. 4 (2010): 500–6. https://doi.org/10.1016/j.amjsurg.2009.05.013.

6 *A 50-year-old man arrives to the emergency room having sustained a single stable wound to the left lower quadrant. He is alert, oriented, and cooperative, hemodynamically normal, with no signs of peritonitis nor abdominal tenderness on exam. The stab wound is 2 cm in length with no underlying hematoma or active bleeding. Which of the following options is the most appropriate management?*

A *Immediate exploratory laparotomy.*

B *Serial abdominal examinations for 4 hours, followed by discharge if no clinical changes.*

C *CT of the abdomen and pelvis with IV contrast followed by diagnostic laparoscopy if fascial penetration is suspected.*

D *Local wound exploration followed by exploratory laparotomy if penetration of Scarpa's fascia.*

E *Diagnostic peritoneal aspirate followed by exploratory laparotomy if blood or succus aspirated.*

There are several options for the management of anterior abdominal stab wounds. The anterior abdominal area is defined by the costal margin, anterior axillary lines, and groin creases bilaterally. Stab wounds between the umbilicus and costal margins can also injure the diaphragm and cardiothoracic structures, which should be taken into consideration when evaluating these patients. Immediate laparotomy should be performed in patients who are hemodynamically unstable due to hemorrhage and/or have peritonitis, which is indicative of hollow viscous injury (choice A). Serial abdominal examinations is a valid option if the patient is examinable. Patients are not examinable if they are altered by drugs/alcohol, do not have distracting injuries and are not intubated. Serial exam is typically 8–24 hours in most practice guidelines and 4 hours is inadequate (choice B). CT imaging is highly sensitive and specific for intrabdominal injury, with several studies reporting numbers >90%, and can be performed in stable patients but should be done with IV contrast (choice C). A prospective study by Demetriades et al. found CT scan to have a negative predictive value of 100% for intraabdominal injuries requiring laparotomy. Depending on resources, diagnostic imaging can be the first step in assessment. If no injuries are identified, the patient can be observed or discharged based on clinician judgment. Depending on the surgeon's skill set, this can be followed by exploratory laparotomy or diagnostic laparoscopy if fascial penetration is identified on CT. If the stab wound is amenable to local wound exploration (nonobese patient, sizeable stab wound, non-tangential in appearance) and the patient is cooperative, this is an alternative approach to initial evaluation. If there is penetration of the anterior rectus fascia (not Scarpa's), either serial abdominal exams or diagnostic imaging can be performed (choice D). Local exploration is most helpful when it definitively demonstrates that the anterior fascia has not been penetrated, and in these patients the wound can be irrigated and closed. Laparotomy is not mandatory, as a large proportion of these patients will not have intraabdominal injuries. Diagnostic peritoneal aspiration is not a commonly employed part of the algorithm for management of anterior abdominal stab wounds. Historically, it has been done and studied. Lavage showing microscopic red cell counts of 1000–100 000 has been used as the determining factor for the need for surgery. Using 1000 rbc results in unacceptably high number of nontherapeutic laparotomies and using 100 000 rbc results in unacceptably high missed injuries. Although serial examinations can be done to rule out hollow viscous injuries with high sensitivity, it does not always address facial injuries, which may need surgical repair.

Answer: C

Salim, Ali, Burapat Sangthong, Matthew Martin, Carlos Brown, David Plurad, Kenji Inaba, Peter Rhee, and Demetrios Demetriades. "Use of Computed Tomography in Anterior Abdominal Stab Wounds:

Results of a Prospective Study." *Archives of Surgery (Chicago, Ill.: 1960)* 141, no. 8 (2006): 745–50; discussion 750-752. https://doi.org/10.1001/archsurg.141.8.745.

Martin, Matthew J., Carlos V.R. Brown, David V. Shatz, Hasan B. Alam, Karen J. Brasel, Carl J. Hauser, Marc de Moya, et al. "Evaluation and Management of Abdominal Stab Wounds: A Western Trauma Association Critical Decisions Algorithm." *Journal of Trauma and Acute Care Surgery* 85, no. 5 (2018): 1007–15. https://doi.org/10.1097/TA.0000000000001930.

7   *A 65-year-old woman involved in a motor vehicle collision is hemodynamically unstable with a positive FAST at Morrison's pouch. She has been taken emergently to the operating room, where a splenectomy and non-anatomic wedge resection of a liver injury is performed, followed by fascial closure. Throughout the operation, she undergoes massive transfusion of blood products. Over the subsequent 12 hours, her hematocrit stabilizes, but she develops decreased urine output, increased peak airway pressures, and hypotension. What is the next step in management?*

   A   *Check bladder pressure*

   B   *Bedside ultrasound and therapeutic aspiration of intraperitoneal fluid*

   C   *Stat ultrasound of the liver to evaluate for portal vein thrombosis*

   D   *Stat CT scan of the abdomen and pelvis to assess for missed injuries*

   E   *Crystalloid fluids and lasix*

Intraabdominal hypertension, defined as a sustained intraabdominal pressure (IAP) > 10 mm Hg, can be concerning. Abdominal compartment syndrome (ACS) is defined as an IAP > 20 mm Hg associated with new organ dysfunction. The most common manifestations of organ dysfunction are kidneys manifesting as oliguria and lungs manifesting as elevated peak airway pressures. Severely injured trauma patients are at high risk for developing ACS if they receive large volumes of crystalloids or pelvic fractures resulting in retroperitoneal hematomas. Delayed diagnosis of ACS can be lethal, and intervention should not be delayed for further imaging (choice C). The most common and cost-effective way to measure IAP is by measuring bladder pressure by instilling 25 mL of saline into the bladder through a foley catheter and connecting the catheter to a pressure transducer. ACS can be managed in a variety of methods including decompressive laparotomy. In some cases, laparotomy can be avoided by placement of an indwelling percutaneous drainage catheter although this is usually done for non-trauma patients who may have medical etiologies for their ACS. Simple aspiration may provide temporary relief

if there is fluid, and it can be accessed. While this is useful approach to ACS, it is not typically useful nor recommended for the immediate postoperative period. Using ultrasound is useful in certain circumstances to find fluid but in the immediate postoperative period, ACS is typically from bowel edema and not fluid accumulation (choice B). Patients can still develop ACS with an open abdomen, usually secondary to abdominal packing. In these cases, the patients should be taken to the operating room and have the number of packs reduced until symptoms resolve. Crystalloids do not remain in the intravascular space, and it has been shown that less than 200 cc out of 1000 cc remains in the intravascular space in 1 hour. Diuresis may increase urine output, but infusing crystalloids and giving Lasix would make the patient more depleted in the intravascular space and can lead to acute kidney injury. It would also miss the diagnosis and make matters worse (choice E).

Answer: A

Meldrum, Daniel R., Frederick A. Moore, Ernest E. Moore, Reginald Franciose, Angela Sauaia, and Jon M. Burch. "Prospective Characterization and Selective Management of the Abdominal Compartment Syndrome." *The American Journal of Surgery* 174, no. 6 (1997): 667–73. https://doi.org/10.1016/S0002-9610(97)00201-8.

Kirkpatrick, Andrew W., Derek J. Roberts, Jan De Waele, Roman Jaeschke, Manu L. N. G. Malbrain, Bart De Keulenaer, Juan Duchesne, et al. "Intra-Abdominal Hypertension and the Abdominal Compartment Syndrome: Updated Consensus Definitions and Clinical Practice Guidelines from the World Society of the Abdominal Compartment Syndrome." *Intensive Care Medicine* 39, no. 7 (2013): 1190–1206. https://doi.org/10.1007/s00134-013-2906-z.

8   *A 12-year-old boy in a bicycle accident resulted in a handlebar injury to his epigastrium. He is hemodynamically normal but complaining of severe abdominal pain. He has no guarding or rigidity on abdominal exam. A CT of the abdomen demonstrates lack of enhancement of the second portion of the duodenum with thickening of the bowel wall and evidence of retroperitoneal extraluminal air. He is taken emergently to the operating room where you identify a near-complete transection of the 2nd portion of the duodenum. In which of the following scenarios is a pyloric exclusion with gastrojejunostomy most likely to be indicated?*

   A   *Delayed diagnosis of duodenal rupture with extensive peripancreatic inflammation*

B *Near-complete transection of the 2nd portion of the duodenum*

C *25% transection of the duodenum with associated pancreatic injury*

D *Combined duodenum and superior mesenteric artery injury*

E *Combined duodenal and inferior vena cava injury*

Blunt duodenal trauma is usually caused by a direct blow (handlebars, seatbelt, steering wheel, etc.) that causes increased intraluminal pressure in the duodenum that stretches along fixed points (the pyloroduodenal and duodenojejunal junctions). This often results in hematoma development in the duodenal wall that can be managed conservatively with nasogastric decompression and total parenteral nutrition. Rarely, it can result in duodenal perforation that requires operative intervention. Traditionally, this was diagnosed with a Gastrografin swallow study but in the modern era is diagnosed with a CT scan that demonstrates extraluminal retroperitoneal air. Several studies have demonstrated that pyloric exclusion adds little benefit in the acute management of duodenal injuries and can increase morbidity by prolonging the procedure and permanently altering anatomy through the addition of a gastrojejunostomy. A high-grade duodenal injury, associated pancreatic injury, and concomitant vascular injury are not indications for pyloric exclusion. A delayed diagnosis of duodenal rupture with extensive peripancreatic inflammation is associated with high duodenal repair leak rates and represents the scenario most likely to benefit from the utilization of pyloric exclusion.

Answer: A

Seamon, Mark J., Paola G. Pieri, Carol A. Fisher, John Gaughan, Thomas A. Santora, Abhijit S. Pathak, Kevin M. Bradley, and Amy J. Goldberg. "A Ten-Year Retrospective Review: Does Pyloric Exclusion Improve Clinical Outcome after Penetrating Duodenal and Combined Pancreaticoduodenal Injuries?" *The Journal of Trauma* 62, no. 4 (2007): 829–33. https://doi.org/10.1097/TA.0b013e318033a790.

DuBose, Joseph J., Kenji Inaba, Pedro G. R. Teixeira, Anthony Shiflett, Bradley Putty, D. J. Green, David Plurad, and Demetrios Demetriades. "Pyloric Exclusion in the Treatment of Severe Duodenal Injuries: Results from the National Trauma Data Bank." *The American Surgeon* 74, no. 10 (2008): 925–29. https://doi.org/10.1177/000313480807401009.

9 *A 48-year-old woman is involved in a motor vehicle collision. She is hypotensive, with a negative FAST exam and an open-book pelvic fracture identified on x-ray. Massive transfusion protocol is initiated, and she is placed in a pelvic binder centered over the greater trochanters. Despite adequate binder positioning, she remains hypotensive with ongoing resuscitation. Diagnostic peritoneal aspiration shows no gross blood in the abdomen. Which of the following is the best option in this patient?*

A *Zone 1 Resuscitative Endovascular Balloon Occlusion of the Aorta (REBOA) placement*

B *Intraperitoneal pelvic packing*

C *Internal fixation of the pelvis*

D *Angioembolization of the external iliac artery*

E *Preperitoneal pelvic packing while waiting for interventional radiologist*

The management of severe pelvic fractures, defined as hemodynamic instability resulting from pelvic fracture-associated hemorrhage, varies by center based on resource availability. Universally, all centers will initiate transfusion and apply a pelvic binder when the fracture pattern is consistent with anteroposterior compression (APC). Open book fracture can have their pelvic space volume reduced effectively with commercial pelvic binders, and this has now become standard of care. While effective in reducing pelvic volume and whether this decreases bleeding, is not yet been shown. Potential additional interventions include preperitoneal pelvic packing, angioembolization of the internal iliac artery or of its branch vessels, external fixation of the pelvis, and Zone 3 REBOA placement. The benefit of each intervention or combination of interventions over another remains unknown and is highly dependent on institutional guidelines and resource availability. Some centers perform preperitoneal packing due to the delay associated with waiting for an Interventional Radiologist to perform angioembolization. In contrast, centers who have access to a hybrid room with endovascular capabilities can expediently proceed with angioembolization. Pelvic fracture patterns associated with need for a hemorrhage-control intervention are APC III and open pelvic fracture subtypes. Choice A is not optimal as placement of REBOA for pelvic bleeding is in Zone 3. Intraperitoneal packing was tried many decades ago and is not effective as the packs will slide out of position (choice B). Internal fixation of the pelvis is rarely available immediately and is typically done electively later after stabilization (choice C).

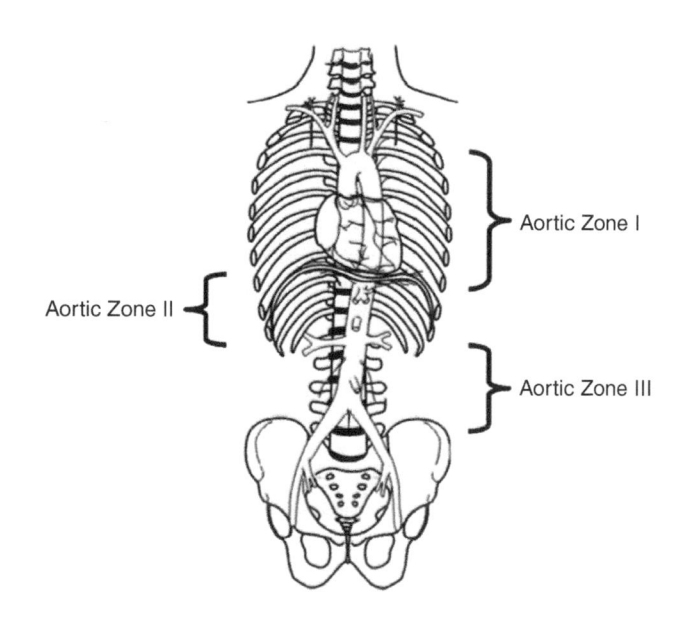

Aortic Zone I

Aortic Zone II

Aortic Zone III

B *A 30-year-old man who was involved in a motor vehicle collision with a widened mediastinum on chest x-ray*

C *A 22-year-old man with multiple gunshot wounds to the thoracoabdominal region who arrives in cardiac arrest*

D *A 50-year-old woman pedestrian struck arriving with pressure of 50 mm Hg over palp and an APC III pelvic fracture on x-ray*

E *A 62-year-old man who fell from 30 feet, with bilateral lower extremity deformities, who has CPR initiated in the trauma bay*

REBOA is a device that provides temporary aortic occlusion through endovascular means, avoiding the morbidity associated with a resuscitative thoracotomy and open aortic cross clamping. If femoral arterial access is obtained expediently, then REBOA placement can occur faster than the open technique in some hands. The exact patient population for which REBOA offers a survival benefit is currently unknown, due to the heterogeneity of the patients for which REBOA is used, and the lack of a suitable control group in several retrospective series that have been published to date. The current contraindications to REBOA use are the presence of a blunt thoracic aortic injury (BTAI) as evidenced by a widened mediastinum on chest x-ray or penetrating trauma to the chest, as increased thoracic aortic pressures can worsen BTAI and sources of thoracic hemorrhage (choices A, B, C). Pelvic fractures causing life-threatening hemorrhage with deployment in zone 3 may offer benefit to resuscitative thoracotomy and aortic cross clamping as the blood loss from the thoracotomy is significant if the patient regains ROSC. Although there are conflicting studies on which patient population would benefit from REBOA, existing data does not support an increase in survival over resuscitative thoracotomy among patients who arrive in cardiac arrest or have CPR initiated in the trauma bay.

Answer: D

Brenner, Megan, Kenji Inaba, Alberto Aiolfi, Joseph DuBose, Timothy Fabian, Tiffany Bee, John B. Holcomb, et al. "Resuscitative Endovascular Balloon Occlusion of the Aorta and Resuscitative Thoracotomy in Select Patients with Hemorrhagic Shock: Early Results from the American Association for the Surgery of Trauma's Aortic Occlusion in Resuscitation for Trauma and Acute Care Surgery Registry." *Journal of the American College of Surgeons* 226, no. 5 (2018): 730–40. https://doi.org/10.1016/j.jamcollsurg.2018.01.044.

Yamamoto, Ryo, Ramon F. Cestero, Masaru Suzuki, Tomohiro Funabiki, and Junichi Sasaki. "Resuscitative Endovascular Balloon Occlusion of the Aorta (REBOA)

Answer: E

Costantini, Todd W., Raul Coimbra, John B. Holcomb, Jeanette M. Podbielski, Richard D. Catalano, Allie Blackburn, Thomas M. Scalea, et al. "Pelvic Fracture Pattern Predicts the Need for Hemorrhage Control Intervention—Results of an AAST Multi-Institutional Study." *Journal of Trauma and Acute Care Surgery* 82, no. 6 (2017): 1030–38. https://doi.org/ 10.1097/ TA.0000000000001465.

Burlew, Clay Cothren, Ernest E. Moore, Wade R. Smith, Jeffrey L. Johnson, Walter L. Biffl, Carlton C. Barnett, and Philip F. Stahel. "Preperitoneal Pelvic Packing/ External Fixation with Secondary Angioembolization: Optimal Care for Life-Threatening Hemorrhage from Unstable Pelvic Fractures." *Journal of the American College of Surgeons* 212, no. 4 (2011): 628–35. https:// doi.org/10.1016/j.jamcollsurg.2010.12.020.

Frassini, Simone, Shailvi Gupta, Stefano Granieri, Stefania Cimbanassi, Fabrizio Sammartano, Thomas M. Scalea, and Osvaldo Chiara. "Extraperitoneal Packing in Unstable Blunt Pelvic Trauma: A Single-Center Study." *Journal of Trauma and Acute Care Surgery* 88, no. 5 (2020): 597–606. https://doi.org/ 10.1097/TA.0000000000002618.

10 *In which of the following patient scenarios is Resuscitative Endovascular Balloon Occlusion of the Aorta (REBOA), most likely to offer a survival benefit when compared with resuscitative thoracotomy for aortic occlusion?*

A *A 42-year-old woman who sustained a single gunshot wound to the left chest with a systolic blood pressure of 80 mm Hg*

Is Associated with Improved Survival in Severely Injured Patients: A Propensity Score Matching Analysis." *The American Journal of Surgery* 218, no. 6 (2019): 1162–68. https://doi.org/10.1016/j.amjsurg.2019.09.007.

11 *A 50 year-old-woman who was injured after an MVC is complaining of left thoracoabdominal rib pain but is otherwise hemodynamically normal. She is taken for a CT scan of the abdomen and pelvis, which shows a grade IV splenic injury, with a large intraparenchymal pseudoaneurysm and some surrounding hemoperitoneum in the left upper quadrant. She remains hemodynamically normal without peritonitis. What is the best management of this patient?*

A *Observation with serial abdominal exams alone*
B *Immediate exploratory laparotomy and splenectomy*
C *Repeat CT evaluation in 24–48 hours*
D *Diagnostic laparoscopy and splenorrhaphy*
E *Proximal angioembolization of the splenic artery*

An injured spleen is the most common solid organ injury requiring laparotomy in trauma. However, there has been a significant paradigm shift over the last several decades away from immediate splenectomy to selective nonoperative management (NOM). Management of splenic injury is no longer simple as there are many options. In general, splenic injuries stop bleeding spontaneously. However, some continue to bleed or can bleed again later. Concomitant injuries such as traumatic brain injury also play a role in the management of the splenic injury. Neither grade of injury nor degree of hemoperitoneum are indications for immediate operative intervention, but they do increase the rate of failure of NOM. The only absolute indication for splenectomy is ongoing hemodynamic instability with delay to interventional angiography. Recent changes in the Organ Injury Scale by the American Association for The Surgery of Trauma have upgraded any vascular injury (pseudoaneurysm, arteriovenous fistula, contrast blush) from Grade III to Grade IV, indicating higher rates of failure of NOM in the setting of vascular injury. Although there are no strict guidelines on when to perform splenic angioembolization, higher-grade injuries and the presence of a vascular lesion are indications for angiography. A meta-analysis comparing splenic angioembolization to observation found statistically higher splenic salvage rates for Grade IV and V injuries that underwent angioembolization. Even the resuscitation management of hypotensive patients with splenic injury is evolving. Management is highly dependent on concomitant injuries. For isolated injuries, permissive hypotension and restriction of fluids, along with when to use blood products, are all being considered and studied.

Grade	Type of injury	Description of injury
I	Hematoma	Subcapsular, <10%
	Laceration	Capsular tear, <1 cm in depth
11	Hematoma	Subcapsular, 10–50%; intraparenchymal, <5 cm in diameter
	Laceration	Capsular tear, 1–3 cm in parenchymal depth, not involving trabecular vessel
III	Hematoma	Subcapsular, >50% surface area or expanding, ruptured sub-capsular or parenchymal hematoma; intraparenchymal hematoma, ≥5 cm or expanding
	Laceration	>3 cm in parenchymal depth or involving trabecular vessel
IV	Laceration	Segmental or hilar vessels, major devascularization (>25%)
V	Laceration	Completely shattered spleen
	Vascular	Hilar vascular injury that devascularizes the spleen

Note: Advance one grade for multiple injuries, up to Grade III.

Answer: E

Requarth, Jay A., Ralph B. D'Agostino, and Preston R. Miller. "Nonoperative Management of Adult Blunt Splenic Injury with and without Splenic Artery Embolotherapy: A Meta-Analysis." *The Journal of Trauma* 71, no. 4 (2011): 898–903; discussion 903. https://doi.org/10.1097/TA.0b013e318227ea50.

Kozar, Rosemary A., Marie Crandall, Kathirkamanthan Shanmuganathan, Ben L. Zarzaur, Mike Coburn, Chris Cribari, Krista Kaups, Kevin Schuster, and Gail T. Tominaga. "Organ Injury Scaling 2018 Update: Spleen, Liver, and Kidney." *Journal of Trauma and Acute Care Surgery* 85, no. 6 (2018): 1119–22. https://doi.org/10.1097/TA.0000000000002058.

12 *A 70 year-old-man on coumadin for atrial fibrillation is involved in a fall down 8 steps. He is hemodynamically normal but complaining of severe back pain. A CT scan of the abdomen and pelvis with IV contrast demonstrate a T12 vertebral body fracture, right-sided 9th–12th rib fractures, and a perinephric hematoma with a small area of active extravasation from within the parenchyma. Which of the following findings have the greatest association with need for operative intervention?*

A *Evidence of urine leak*

B *Renal artery thrombosis*
C *>1 cm laceration*
D *Vascular contrast extravasation*
E *Large perinephric hematoma*

According to a multi-institutional study conducted by Keihani et al., vascular contrast extravasation has the strongest association with need for operative intervention (choice D). Despite risks, most cases of vascular contrast extravasation can be managed with selective angioembolization. Size of perinephric hematoma and laceration depth also increase need for operative management, but less so (choices C and E). In fact, the majority of hemodynamically stable patients with both penetrating and blunt renal injures can be managed nonoperatively. Complications such as urine leak and renal artery thrombosis are also usually managed with percutaneous and endovascular techniques and rarely require operative intervention (choices A and B). Hemodynamic instability and hilar avulsion are two absolute indications for operative intervention. Other findings such as those listed above, as well as high-grade injury (IV or V) and renal parenchymal devascularization, are relative indications for operative intervention that vary based on clinician judgment and center practice patterns.

Answer: D

Keihani, Sorena, Bryn E Putbrese, Douglas M Rogers, Chong Zhang, Raminder Nirula, Xian Luo-Owen, Kaushik Mukherjee, et al. "The Associations between Initial Radiographic Findings and Interventions for Renal Hemorrhage after High-Grade Renal Trauma: Results from the Multi-Institutional Genitourinary Trauma Study" *Journal of Trauma and Acute Care Surgery* 86, no. 6 (2019): 974–982.

Coccolini, Federico, Ernest E. Moore, Yoram Kluger, Walter Biffl, Ari Leppaniemi, Yosuke Matsumura, Fernando Kim, et al. "Kidney and Uro-Trauma: WSES-AAST Guidelines." *World Journal of Emergency Surgery: WJES* 14 (2019): 54. https://doi.org/ 10.1186/ s13017-019-0274-x.

13 *A 19-year-old man presents after being shot in his right flank. He is hemodynamically unstable with a positive FAST exam in the right upper quadrant and is rushed to the operating room. At laparotomy, he is found to have a Grade V renal injury for which a nephrectomy is performed and a central liver injury through the right hepatic lobe that is actively bleeding from the tract of the gunshot wound. Pringle maneuver and packing fail to control hemorrhage. What option can be first attempted to control exsanguination?*

A *Right hepatic lobectomy*
B *Balloon tamponade of the gunshot wound tract*
C *Argon beam laser utilization*
D *Non-anatomic wedge resection*
E *Finger fracture with direct suture ligation*

Although all of the answer choices listed are options for operative management of liver trauma, balloon tamponade can be an effective method for temporary hemorrhage control in this situation. Also known as the Poggetti Balloon, balloon tamponade to control central penetrating liver injury was described by Renato Poggetti in 1992. It is constructed by placing a 12 French red rubber catheter inside 12 by 1 inch Penrose drain and tying both ends closed (see Figure 31.1 below). It is then placed through the abdominal wall, inside the liver tract and inflated with saline. Keeping it inflated if there is a slow leak can be challenging. It can be left in place for 24–48 hours and then deflated and removed during a separate trip to the operating room. After that period of tamponade, usually all bleeding has ceased. There are premade balloons specifically for this purpose, but most trauma centers do not stock it. Thus, the simple and quick approach for managing penetrating central liver injuries that are challenging to expose can be this device. The Pringle Maneuver is temporary and can usually be left in place for no more than 30 minutes while other methods for hemorrhage control are used. Perihepatic packing would not address the arterial bleeding coming from the injury tract. A wedge resection is more appropriate for peripheral injuries, and finger fracture would not be feasible with such a deep injury.

Answer: B

Ball, Chad G., Amy D. Wyrzykowski, Jeffrey M. Nicholas, Grace S. Rozycki, and David V. Feliciano. "A Decade's Experience With Balloon Catheter Tamponade for the Emergency Control of Hemorrhage." *The Journal of Trauma: Injury, Infection, and Critical Care* 70, no. 2 (2011): 330–33. https://doi.org/10.1097/TA.0b013e318203285c.

Kodadek, Lisa M., David T. Efron, and Elliott R. Haut. "Intrahepatic Balloon Tamponade for Penetrating Liver Injury: Rarely Needed but Highly Effective." *World Journal of Surgery* 43, no. 2 (2019): 486–89. https://doi.org/10.1007/s00268-018-4812-6.

14 *A 22-year-old woman sustains a single gunshot wound to the lower abdomen. She is hypotensive and has signs of peritonitis. She is immediately taken to the operating room and a laparotomy reveals several small bowel injuries, a colon injury, and partial right common iliac artery and vein transection. She remains critically ill with persistent acidosis, coagulopathy, and hypothermia, and is undergoing massive transfusion. Of the available choices, what is the*

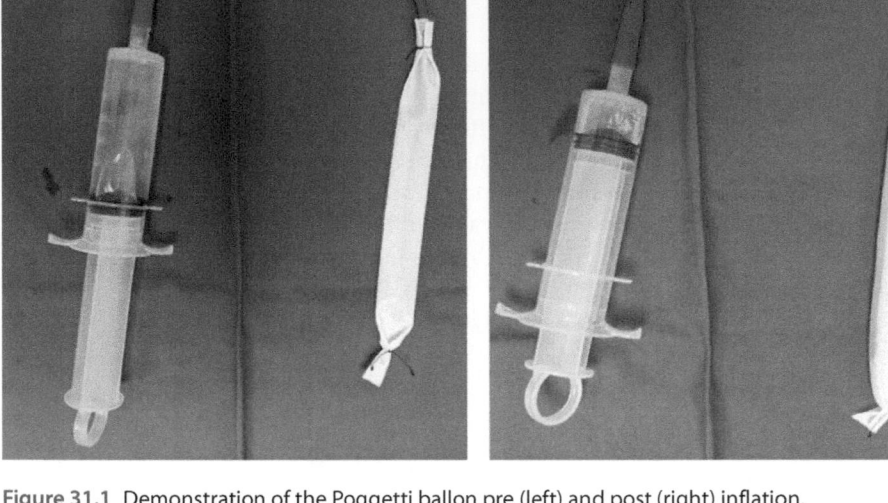

Figure 31.1 Demonstration of the Poggetti ballon pre (left) and post (right) inflation.

optimal management of the vascular injuries in this scenario?

A *Placement of arterial and venous Argyle shunts*
B *Placement of an arterial Argyle shunt and venous ligation*
C *Interposition graft of the iliac artery and venous ligation*
D *Interposition graft of the iliac artery and lateral venorrhaphy*
E *Primary repair of both artery and vein*

This patient is critically ill and likely suffering from the lethal triad of coagulopathy, acidosis, and hypothermia. A damage control operation may be an option but at the vascular injury can be temporized by utilizing shunts. A vascular repair would be rushed and even in the best of circumstances may take considerable time. Patients with combined penetrating iliac arterial and venous injuries have mortality rates higher than 50%, as they often present in severe hemorrhagic shock. Placement of both arterial and venous iliac shunts would be expedient and give the patient the best chance for long-term limb salvage. The venous shunt may be difficult, however, as proximal control with various branches makes proximal isolation sometime difficult to do the venous plexus closer to the bifurcation. Although the data is not definitive, preservation of venous outflow in the setting of combined arterial and venous injuries is recommended by most surgeons experienced with this type of injury. It will aid in preserving the arteria shunt. Even if the decision is made to ligate the iliac vein at the return operation, placement of a shunt still leaves the opportunity for a future

repair if conditions are suitable. However, there may be scenarios when shunting the vein is technically difficult and ligation of the vein may be necessary. Primary repair for stab wounds are feasible, but gunshot wounds often require debridement and mobilization of the vessels in the pelvis to be able to perform a tension-free vascular repair, and this scenario is uncommon (choice E), especially if there are numerous concomitant injuries.

Answer: A

Lauerman, Margaret H., Denis Rybin, Gheorghe Doros, Jeffrey Kalish, Naomi Hamburg, Robert T. Eberhardt, and Alik Farber. "Characterization and Outcomes of Iliac Vessel Injury in the 21st Century: A Review of the National Trauma Data Bank." *Vascular and Endovascular Surgery* (2013). https://doi.org/10.1177/1538574413487260.

Guice, Jordan L., Shaun M. Gifford, Kai Hata, Xiaoming Shi, Brandon W. Propper, and David S. Kauvar. "Analysis of Limb Outcomes by Management of Concomitant Vein Injury in Military Popliteal Artery Trauma." *Annals of Vascular Surgery* 62 (2020): 51–56. https://doi.org/10.1016/j.avsg.2019.05.007.

15 *A 34 year-old-woman was the front passenger in an MVC. She is hemodynamically normal and is only complaining of mild upper abdominal pain, where she is noted to have a seat belt sign. A CT scan of the abdomen and pelvis with intravenous contrast demonstrates a grade IV injury to the head of the pancreas. No other injuries are noted. What is the best approach to management?*

A *Observation with serial serum amylase and abdominal examination*
B *Exploratory laparotomy and pancreaticoduodenectomy*
C *Endoscopic retrograde cholangiopancreatography and pancreatic stent placement*
D *Exploratory laparotomy and closed suction drainage*
E *Distal pancreatectomy and splenectomy*

Blunt pancreatic trauma results from direct force to the upper abdominal region resulting in compression of the pancreas against the vertebral column. This injury is fortunately rare but certainly possible. Patients often have few, if any, symptoms specifically from the pancreatic injury, which makes the diagnosis of pancreatic injury particularly challenging. Serum amylase is no longer used to diagnose or monitor pancreatic injury, as it lacks both sensitivity and specificity. Rather, the best method of diagnosis is computed tomography. CT scan of the abdomen is not sensitive in identifying pancreatic injury but is very specific if the injury is demonstrated. If the CT is equivocal, magnetic resonance cholangiopancreatography (MRCP) can be helpful. Injuries are graded by the American Association for the Surgery of Trauma Organ Injury Scale from I to V, with I–III reserved for injuries to the left of the superior mesenteric vein and IV–V reserved for major injuries to the pancreatic head (to the right of the superior mesenteric vein). Grade I–II injuries do not involve the main duct of Wirsung and can be observed. Grade III injuries should be managed with a distal pancreatectomy and splenectomy. Spleen preserving distal pancreatectomy has been reported, but this procedure can make the surgery much longer, and the benefits have not been shown. Grade IV injuries should be managed with closed suction drainage, and Grade V injuries require a pancreaticoduodenectomy versus closed suction drainage based on the extent of injury. The role of ERCP in the management of pancreatic duct injuries is growing, but there is limited data on when they should be used. Current recommendations are for the management of late complications of pancreatic duct injury, such as pseudocyst and pancreatic fistula formation.

Grade	Type of injury	Injury description
I	Hematoma	Minor contusion without ductal injury
	Laceration	Superficial laceration without ductal injury
II	Hematoma	Major contusion without ductal injury or tissue loss
	Laceration	Major laceration without ductal injury or tissue loss

Grade	Type of injury	Injury description
III	Laceration	Distal transection or pancreatic parenchymal injury with ductal injury
IV	Laceration	Proximal transection or pancreatic parenchymal injury involving the ampulla
V	Laceration	Massive disruption of the pancreatic head

Answer: D

Biffl, Walter L., Ernest E. Moore, Martin Croce, James W. Davis, Raul Coimbra, Riyad Karmy-Jones, Robert C. McIntyre, et al. "Western Trauma Association Critical Decisions in Trauma: Management of Pancreatic Injuries." *The Journal of Trauma and Acute Care Surgery* 75, no. 6 (2013): 941–46. https://doi.org/10.1097/TA.0b013e3182a96572.

Siboni, Stefano, Edward Kwon, Elizabeth Benjamin, Kenji Inaba, and Demetrios Demetriades. "Isolated Blunt Pancreatic Trauma: A Benign Injury?" *The Journal of Trauma and Acute Care Surgery* 81, no. 5 (2016): 855–59. https://doi.org/10.1097/TA.0000000000001224.

16 *What is the most appropriate initial diagnostic modality to evaluate for blunt bladder injury in a stable patient without other operative indications?*
A *Plain film cystogram*
B *Retrograde urethrogram*
C *CT cystogram*
D *IV pyelogram*
E *Triple-phase CT scan*

Blunt trauma patients with pelvic fractures and/or gross hematuria should be evaluated for bladder injury. The most appropriate diagnostic modality to evaluate for blunt bladder injury is a computed tomography cystogram. In this case, the bladder is filled with approximately 300 mL of diluted contrast through a foley catheter and clamped. A CT scan is obtained and evaluated for evidence of contrast extravasation. Traditionally, this assessment was performed with a standard cystogram, during which the bladder was filled with non-diluted contrast and x-ray images of the bladder while filled and after emptying were obtained. Any residual contrast that remained outside the confines of the bladder after emptying was consistent with a bladder injury. Although sensitivity and specificity rates for detection of blunt bladder injury for traditional cystography and CT cystography are both >95%, the latter can be performed concurrently with other CT imaging and provide expedient results. A triple-phase CT scan with delayed-phase imaging demonstrating urinary excretion is not adequate to identify bladder injury but may help identify ureteral injuries. A retrograde urethrogram is used to identify urethral injuries. An IV pyelogram was traditionally used to evaluate for renal injuries but has been replaced by CT imaging.

Answer: C

Quagliano, Peter V., Sean M. Delair, and Ajai K. Malhotra. "Diagnosis of Blunt Bladder Injury: A Prospective Comparative Study of Computed Tomography Cystography and Conventional Retrograde Cystography." *The Journal of Trauma* 61, no. 2 (2006): 410–21; discussion 421-422. https://doi.org/10.1097/01.ta.0000229940.36556.bf.

Yeung, Lawrence L., Amy A. McDonald, John J. Como, Bryce Robinson, Jennifer Knight, Michael A. Person, Jane K. Lee, and Philipp Dahm. "Management of Blunt Force Bladder Injuries: A Practice Management Guideline from the Eastern Association for the Surgery of Trauma." *Journal of Trauma and Acute Care Surgery* 86, no. 2 (2019): 326–336. https://doi.org/ 10.1097/ TA.0000000000002132.

17 *A 22-year-old man who sustained multiple gunshot wounds to the torso is severely hypotensive. CXR is normal and during laparotomy there is extensive fecal contamination secondary to colon injury, a distal pancreatic injury, and a splenic injury. Patient is now stable in the operating room after 10 units of PRBC, 10 units of FFP, and 2 units of platelets. Regarding damage control surgery, which of the following is true?*
    A *It should be done on all trauma laparotomies.*
    B *It should never be done as the morbidity is too high.*
    C *It should definitely be done on patients receiving more than 6 units of PRBC no matter how stable the patient is.*
    D *It should always be done if there is colon injury.*
    E *It can lead to higher rate of open abdomens and their complications.*

Damage control surgery (DCS) was recommended for patients who are approaching physiologic exhaustion as evidenced by hypothermia (<34C), coagulopathy (INR/PT/PTT > 1.5x normal), and acidosis (pH < 7.2). Similarly, a patient who has received >10 units of packed red blood cells, who remain in severe hemorrhagic shock and used to be a guideline for the need for DCS. DCS was initially applied to the management of abdominal trauma with control of hemorrhage and contamination, intra-abdominal packing, and temporary closure with delay of definitive surgery until physiologic parameters improve. Since the changes in resuscitation with early blood product usage and minimization of crystalloid use, the need

for DCS has been questioned. Although it was initially adopted with enthusiasm, the proof of benefit has yet not been shown. DCS in certain circumstances may be encouraged such as the patients that required concomitant emergency resuscitative thoracotomy. Enthusiasm regarding DCS has led to overuse of the procedure resulting in unnecessary morbidity. The most common complications are increased hospital length of stays, abdominal wall hernias, open abdomen, and entero-atomospheric fistulas. There was an associated evolution of abdominal wall complications since the adoption of DCS. An elevated lactate and tachycardia are potentially correctible physiologic parameters and are not indications for DCS. Although altered mental status could be an indication of shock, it is not an indication for DCS. If the patient has had hemorrhage control and has stabilized, most advocate definitive surgery.

Answer: E

Rotondo, Michael F., C. William Schwab, Michael D. McGonigal, G. R. Phillips, Todd M. Fruchterman, Donald R. Kauder, Barbara A. Latenser, and Peter A. Angood. "'Damage Control': An Approach for Improved Survival in Exsanguinating Penetrating Abdominal Injury." *The Journal of Trauma* 35, no. 3 (1993): 375–82; discussion 382-383.

Higa, Guillermo, Randall Friese, Terence O'Keeffe, Julie Wynne, Paul Bowlby, Michelle Ziemba, Rifat Latifi, Narong Kulvatunyou, and Peter Rhee. "Damage Control Laparotomy: A Vital Tool Once Over Utilized." *Journal Trauma* 69, no. (1) (2010): 53–9. doi: 10.1097/TA.0b 013e3181e293b4.

Harvin, John A., Lillian S. Kao, Mike K. Liang, Sasha D. Adams, Michelle K. McNutt, Joseph D. Love, Laura J. Moore, Charles E. Wade, Bryan A. Cotton, and John B. Holcomb. "Decreasing the Use of Damage Control Laparotomy in Trauma: A Quality Improvement Project." *Journal of the American College of Surgeons* 225, no. 2 (2017): 200–9. https://doi.org/ 10.1016/ j.jamcollsurg.2017.04.010.

Cirocchi, Roberto, Iosief Abraha, Alessandro Montedori, Eriberto Farinella, Isabella Bonacini, Ludovica Tagliabue, and Francesco Sciannameo. Damage Control Surgery for Abdominal Trauma. *Cochrane Database of Systematic Review*. 2013 2013, no. (3): CD007438. doi: 10.1002/14651858.CD007438.pub3. PMID: **23543551,** PMCID: PMC7202128, DOI: 10.1002/14651858. CD007438.pub3.

18 *Which of the following factors is associated with failure to achieve primary closure after damage control laparotomy?*
    A *Blunt mechanism*
    B *ISS > 15*

C *Female gender*
D *Use of vacuum closure device*
E *Obesity*

The importance of early fascial closure after open abdomen (OA) cannot be overstated. Prolonged periods of OA lead to the development of enteroatmospheric fistulae and loss of abdominal domain that compromise further attempts at fascial closure. Of the answer choices, only greater injury severity is associated with failure of primary fascial closure (PFC) after OA. Increased number of abdominal re-explorations, greater blood product transfusions, and elevated lactate are also associated with failure of PFC. Mechanism of injury and obesity are not associated with PFC after OA. In the results published by the AAST Open Abdomen study group, male gender was associated with failure of PFC. There is some data to support improved fascial closure after use of a vacuum closure device for management of the open abdomen. Most centers will use a commercial vacuum closure device or fashion one out of a sterile polyethylene sheet and flat silicone drains as originally described by Donald E. Barker in 1999. Minimizing crystalloid resuscitation and adhering to the principles of damage control resuscitation reduce edema formation and improve rates of PFC.

Answer: B

Barker, Donald E., Henry J. Kaufman, Lisa A. Smith, David L. Ciraulo, Charles L. Richart, and R. Phillip Burns. "Vacuum Pack Technique of Temporary Abdominal Closure: A 7-Year Experience with 112 Patients." *The Journal of Trauma* 48, no. 2 (2000): 201–6; discussion 206-207. https://doi.org/10.1097/00005373-200002000-00001.

Dubose, Joseph J., Thomas M. Scalea, John B. Holcomb, Binod Shrestha, Obi Okoye, Kenji Inaba, Tiffany K. Bee, et al. "Open Abdominal Management after Damage-Control Laparotomy for Trauma: A Prospective Observational American Association for the Surgery of Trauma Multicenter Study." *The Journal of Trauma and Acute Care Surgery* 74, no. 1 (2013): 113–20; discussion 1120-1122. https://doi.org/10.1097/TA.0b013e31827891ce.

19 *A 45-year-old-man arrives having been struck by a vehicle at low speed while walking across the street. He is intoxicated upon arrival, but hemodynamically normal and has no complaints. His physical exam is only significant for an abrasion and mild ecchymosis in the left lower quadrant. A CT scan of the abdomen and pelvis with IV contrast is normal except for free fluid in the pelvis. Which of the following options is the most appropriate next step in management?*

A *Diagnostic laparoscopy*
B *Serial abdominal examination for 12 hours*
C *Repeat CT scan of the abdomen/pelvis in 12 hours*
D *Discharge home*
E *Diagnostic peritoneal aspiration*

The ability of computed tomography to identify hollow viscus injury (HVI) has improved as the technology has advanced, although the diagnosis relies heavily on secondary findings such as free fluid, mesenteric stranding, and bowel wall thickening rather than pneumoperitoneum or contrast extravasation. Abnormal quantities of free fluid is the most common radiographic finding associated with blunt bowel injury, and in many cases the only finding. Patients with abnormal CT findings who have sustained significant abdominal trauma should undergo further evaluation to rule out blunt bowel perforation. Thus, patients with free fluid that do not have solid organ injuries to the liver or spleen should have additional evaluation to rule out HVI. Depending on clinician expertise, this can be performed with a diagnostic laparoscopy or an exploratory laparotomy. Patients with abnormal CT findings but low clinical suspicion who can undergo reliable abdominal examinations (not altered by drugs/intoxication/brain injury, not intubated, etc.) can be observed for 24 hours, with early intervention if there is any clinical change (choice B). The reliability of serial CT scans of the abdomen has not been extensively done and is not the current standard. It is costly and does require the patient to receive large amounts of radiation (choice C). Patients rarely present with peritonitis, so any presence of abdominal tenderness in the presence of CT abnormalities should raise concern. Delay of intervention beyond 8 hours has been reported to increase mortality from 13% to 30%, underscoring the importance of early diagnosis and intervention. Diagnostic peritoneal aspiration has been largely replaced by CT imaging as a method of diagnosis of HVI (choice E). Discharging a patient that is intoxicated and thus does not have a reliable exam with abnormal CT findings is not standard and would not be supported (choice D). Free fluid without solid organ injuries is also more concerning in men than women.

Answer: A

Fakhry, Samir M., Michelle Brownstein, Dorraine D. Watts, Christopher C. Baker, and Dale Oller. "Relatively Short Diagnostic Delays (<8 Hours) Produce Morbidity and Mortality in Blunt Small Bowel Injury: An Analysis of Time to Operative Intervention in 198 Patients from a Multicenter Experience." *The Journal of Trauma: Injury, Infection, and Critical Care* 48, no. 3 (2000): 408–15. https://doi.org/10.1097/00005373-200003000-00007.

Fakhry, Samir M., Ahmed Allawi, Pamela L. Ferguson, Christopher P. Michetti, Anna B. Newcomb, Chang Liu, and Michelle R. Brownstein. "Blunt Small Bowel Perforation (SBP): An Eastern Association for the Surgery of Trauma Multicenter Update 15 Years Later." *Journal of Trauma and Acute Care Surgery* 86, no. 4 (2019): 642–50. https://doi.org/10.1097/TA.0000000000002176.

20 *A 54-year-old man is stabbed at the left anterior axillary line, 8th intercostal space. He is hemodynamically normal. His chest x-ray is normal. Which of the following tools or approaches is recommended as most appropriate for the diagnosis of penetrating diaphragm injury in this patient?*

    A *CT scan of the chest*
    B *Exploratory laparotomy*
    C *Diagnostic laparoscopy*
    D *Video-assisted thoracoscopic surgery*
    E *Left posterolateral thoracotomy*

The thoracoabdominal region is defined by the nipple line down to the costal margins anteriorly and the posterior axillary lines laterally. A stab wound to this region could injure structures in the chest and/or the intraabdominal cavities. Initial management of a patient with a stab wound to the left thoracoabdominal region should include a chest x-ray. Hemodynamically stable patients should proceed either to CT imaging or to diagnostic laparoscopy to evaluate for intraabdominal injury. Although CT imaging can be helpful in the diagnosis of most intra-abdominal pathology, it can miss up to 32% of penetrating diaphragm injuries. Given the low risk associated with diagnostic laparoscopy, the latest Eastern Association for the Surgery of Trauma guidelines recommend laparoscopy to rule out traumatic diaphragm injury in the setting of left thoracoabdominal stab wounds. A laparoscopic approach would be favored over the other approaches listed due to lower morbidity than thoracotomy or laparotomy and the versatility to convert to laparotomy if other intra-abdominal injuries are identified. Occult injury to the left diaphragm is associated with latent complication as hernia and incarceration can be lethal. Due to the negative pressure in the chest and positive pressure in the abdomen, it has a tendency to suck abdominal contents into the chest. Thus, although this injury is often silent, it needs to be ruled out and repaired if found. The right chest is considered different. Due to the liver under the diaphragm, the hernia rate is much less but has been reported. Most surgeons would not necessarily repair all the right diaphragm injuries on the right side. Experienced surgeons would recommend identification of right diaphragm injuries to repair if it is anterior. In addition, if the right diaphragm

injuries results in right hemo/pneumothorax with liver injury, these patients are high risk for developing right biliary pleural fistula in over 30% of the time. Thus, diagnosing and repairing these injuries are recommended.

Answer: C

Berg, Regan J., Efstathios Karamanos, Kenji Inaba, Obi Okoye, Pedro G. Teixeira, and Demetrios Demetriades. "The Persistent Diagnostic Challenge of Thoracoabdominal Stab Wounds." *The Journal of Trauma and Acute Care Surgery* 76, no. 2 (2014): 418–23. https://doi.org/10.1097/TA.0000000000000120.

McDonald, Amy A., Bryce R. H. Robinson, Louis Alarcon, Patrick L. Bosarge, Heath Dorion, Elliott R. Haut, Jeremy Juern, et al. "Evaluation and Management of Traumatic Diaphragmatic Injuries: A Practice Management Guideline from the Eastern Association for the Surgery of Trauma." *The Journal of Trauma and Acute Care Surgery* 85, no. 1 (2018): 198–207. https://doi.org/10.1097/TA.0000000000001924.

21 *A 46-year-old man injured in an MVC has a seatbelt sign and is intubated for GCS of 8. Patient is stable and undergoes CT of abdomen and pelvis. He has a L2 chance fracture and free fluid in the abdomen without solid organ injuries. In the operating room, you resect and anastomose a bucket handle tear and you note a Zone I retroperitoneal hematoma. Which of the following is most true?*

    A *Explore all Zone I hematoma no matter the size or stability.*
    B *Do not explore the hematoma as it is most likely due to lumbar fracture.*
    C *Never explore the hematoma in blunt trauma as vascular injuries are rare.*
    D *Perform damage control surgery and perform computerized tomographic angiogram.*
    E *Place a REBOA catheter in Zone I and then explore the hematoma.*

22 *A 46-year-old man is shot and has a GSW to the right side of the umbilicus and another GSW to his right back. He responds to two units of PRBC. In the operating room, you see a Zone I retroperitoneal hematoma. Which of the following is most true?*

    A *Explore the hematoma to determine vascular or urinary system injury.*
    B *Do not explore the hematoma as it is most likely due to psoas muscle bleeding and this is very difficult to repair.*
    C *Never explore the hematoma in penetrating trauma if it is not expanding.*

D *Perform damage control surgery and perform computerize tomographic angiogram.*

E *Place a REBOA catheter in Zone I and then explore the hematoma.*

The retroperitoneal space lies directly posterior to the peritoneal cavity and is divided into three different "zones." The central-medial zone (Zone I) falls between the two psoas muscles and contains midline structures such as the abdominal aorta, inferior vena cava, pancreas, and duodenum. The perirenal zone (Zone II) begins lateral to the psoas muscles on either side and contains the kidneys, ureters, and portions of the colon. The pelvic zone (Zone III) includes the bladder, as well as a multitude of vascular structures, including a robust network for presacral veins. Also, the retroperitoneum contains vital musculoskeletal structures such as the psoas muscles, vertebra, quadratus lumborum, and iliacus muscles. It houses connections to the diaphragm and bony pelvis. The management of retroperitoneal hematomas differ considerably based on three factors, and those are mechanism and hemodynamic status of the patient and extent of risk-associated injuries. After blunt trauma, most of the hematoma was should not be opened if the patient is stable and if the hematoma is not expanding. Vascular injuries requiring treatment will typically result in large hematomas, expanding hematomas or hemodynamic instability. In stable patient's with spine fractures if the hematoma is at the level of the spine fracture exploring these hematomas are more likely to cause harm then to help. If the hematoma is midline and at the root of the mesenteric vessels with hemodynamic instability, they can be explored if the visceral distribution is at risk but proximal vascular control should probably be obtained first. Retrohepatic hematomas can be quite difficult and unless actively hemorrhaging should not be open. After penetrating trauma, the rule of thumb is to open all hematomas as the gunshot wound track should be followed and injuries diagnosed. The patient has a perirenal hematoma that is not expanding, and there is preoperative imaging by CT, then these can be drained and not opened. The rationale is that exploring these hematomas typically may result in higher rates of nephrectomies as opening Gerota's fascia may cause more bleeding in a stable scenario. Typically, most textbooks recommend exploring all Zone I injuries in blunt trauma. They also recommend exploring all penetrating violation of retroperitoneal area. Following the tract of the gunshot wound to ensure that there are no ureteral injuries or vascular injuries is advised.

Question 21. Answer: B

Question 22. Answer: A

Manzini N, and Madiba T. E. The Management of Retroperitoneal Haematoma Discovered at Laparotomy for Trauma. *Injury* 45, no. 9 (2014): 1378–83. doi:10.1016/j.injury.2014.01.026. Epub 2014 Feb 3. PMID:24606980 DOI: 10.1016/j.injury.2014.01.026.

Kamber, Harth Mohamed, Tawfiq Jasim Mohammed Al-Marzooq, Haider Raheem Neamah, and Qays Ahmed Hassan. "Outcomes of Operative Management of 96 Cases with Traumatic Retroperitoneal Hematoma: A Single-Institution Experience." *Open Access Macedonian Journal of Medical Sciences* 6, no. 11 2018: 2128–2132. PMID: 30559874, PMCID: PMC6290419. DOI: 10.3889/oamjms.2018.437.

Wang, Fengbiao, and Fang Wang. "The Diagnosis and Treatment of Traumatic Retroperitoneal Hematoma." *Pakistan Journal of Medical Sciences* 29, no. 2 (2013): 573–6. PMID: 24353579. PMCID: PMC3809226. DOI: 10.12669/pjms.292.3168.

32

Orthopedic and Hand Trauma
Brett D. Crist, MD and Gregory J. Della Rocca, MD, PhD

Department of Orthopaedic Surgery, University of Missouri, Columbia, MO, USA

1 *A 30-year-old woman fell 6 feet off a ladder at home. She sustained a Gustilo and Anderson type IIIA open tibia fracture. Which of the following has been associated with the lowest risk of infection?*
   A *Operative debridement within 18 hours of injury*
   B *Operative debridement within 6 hours of injury*
   C *Oral antibiotic administration within 24 hours of injury*
   D *Intravenous antibiotic administration within 3 hours of injury*
   E *Intramedullary nailing of the tibia within 12 hours*

Several factors have been evaluated to look at risk of infection after open fractures. Of the factors listed, early antibiotic administration is the most appropriate answer. Antibiotic administration within 3 hours of injury significantly reduced the rate of infection in a series of 1104 open fractures compared to patients receiving antibiotics greater than 3 hours from injury or no antibiotics at all. Patients should receive intravenous antibiotics within 3 hours from injury and within 1 hour from hospital admission. Timing of surgical debridement as long as it is within 24 hours from injury has not been associated with a significant difference in infection rates of open fractures.

Answer: D

Pollak AN, Jones AL, Castillo RC, *et al.* The relationship between time to surgical debridement and incidence of infection after open high-energy lower extremity trauma. *J Bone Joint Surg Am* (2010);92(1):7–15.

2 *The same 30-year-old woman received cefazolin for her type IIIA open tibia fracture upon arrival to the emergency room. She goes to the operating room within 6 hours for formal debridement, definitive fixation with an intramedullary nail of her tibia, and closure of her open fracture wound. How long should intravenous cefazolin be continued postoperatively?*
   A *16 hours*
   B *48 hours*
   C *72 hours*
   D *24 hours*
   E *6 hours*

Based on the best available data, most open fractures should receive intravenous antibiotics for 24 hours after each operative debridement and then 24 hours after definitive soft tissue management (closure for this patient). Exceptions could be those with significant gross contamination like a type IIIB tibia fracture where 72 hours may be indicated.

Answer: D

Halawi MJ, Morwood MP. Acute management of open fractures: an evidence-based review. *Orthopedics* (2015);38(11):e1025–e1033.

Hoff WS, Bonadies JA, Cachecho R, Dorlac WC. East Practice Management Guidelines Work Group: update to practice management guidelines for prophylactic antibiotic use in open fractures. *J Trauma*. 2011;70(3):751–754.

3 *A 27-year-old man sustains a tibia fracture and develops compartment syndrome after intramedullary nailing of his tibia. The attending orthopedic surgeon is eventually sued because the patient undergoes a below-knee amputation 1 week after the initial surgery. The factor most likely associated with the surgeon losing the lawsuit is a/an:*

   A *Tibia fracture*
   B *Open fracture*
   C *Eventual amputation*
   D *Delay in fasciotomy*
   E *Associated vascular injury*

Compartment syndrome can have devastating complications that can be avoided with early diagnosis and fasciotomy. Bhattacharyya *et al.* reviewed medical malpractice claims and identified these risk factors associated with unsuccessful defense and increased liability:

1 Physician documentation of abnormal findings on neurological exam but no action taken
2 Poor physician communication
3 Increased number of cardinal signs (pain, pallor, pulselessness, paralysis, pain with passive stretch)
4 Increased time to fasciotomy

Answer: D

Bhattacharyya T, Vrahas MS The medical-legal aspects of compartment syndrome. *J Bone Joint Surg Am*. 2004;86-A(4):864–868.

4 *A 53-year-old woman was involved in a motorcycle accident. She sustained the Anterior-Posterior Compression (APC) type 3 pelvic fracture seen below. When she arrives in the trauma bay, her blood pressure is 90/50 mm Hg, and her heart rate is 140 beats/min. A pelvic binder is applied. She is found to have a splenic injury on her abdominal computed tomography (CT) and goes to the operating room. The pelvic binder is positioned over the greater trochanters during surgery to close down her pelvic volume. However, she remains hemodynamically unstable intraoperatively after splenectomy; 3 units of packed red blood cells (PRBC) and 3 units of fresh frozen plasma (FFP) are given. There are no other known sources of uncontrolled bleeding. The next step in resuscitating this patient should include:*

   A *Repeat head CT.*
   B *Transfer to angiography for pelvic arterial embolization.*
   C *Transfuse 3 more units PRBC and 3 FFP and reassess.*
   D *Repeat her chest-abdomen-pelvis CT.*
   E *Perform retroperitoneal packing.*

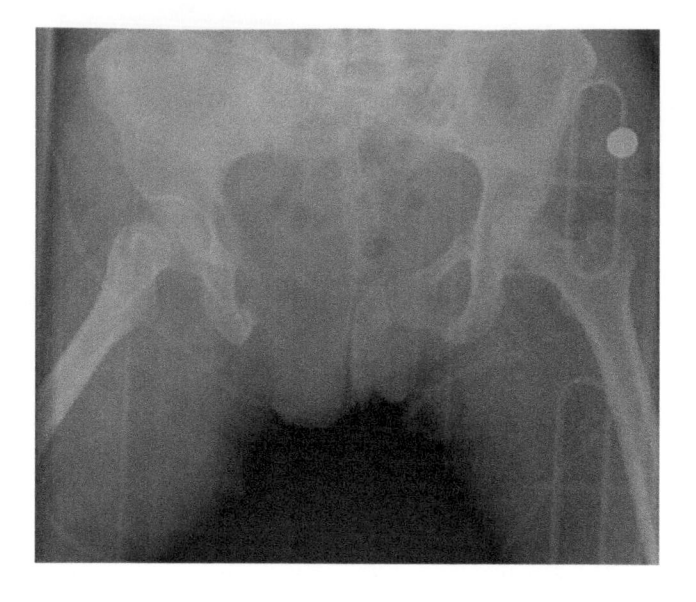

The most common causes of bleeding associated with pelvic fractures are injury to the posterior venous plexus and cancellous fracture surfaces (85–90%). Approximately 10–15% of bleeding is associated with injures to branches of the internal iliac system (superior gluteal or pudendal arteries). Although decreasing the pelvic volume is an important first step, patients that are in the operating room and continue to be hemodynamically unstable after all other known sources of bleeding are addressed should undergo retroperitoneal packing to address the venous and bony bleeding that occurs. Hemodynamically unstable patients should not be transferred to the CT scanner. The patient has already received adequate fluid resuscitation; another source of bleeding must be identified and addressed. Since the patient is already in the operating room and the most likely cause of pelvic bleeding is venous or fracture surfaces, pre- or retroperitoneal packing should be performed prior to going to angiography. If the patient remains hypotensive after retroperitoneal packing and external fixation, then angiography should be performed to address the probable arterial injury. Following this protocol, only 16.7% of hemodynamically unstable patients required subsequent embolization, and there were no mortalities.

Answer: E

Langford JR, Burgess AR, Liporace FA, Haidukewych GJ. Pelvic fractures: part 1. Evaluation, classification, and resuscitation. *J Am Acad Orthop Surg*. 2013;21(8):448–457.

Cothren CC, Osborn PM, Moore EE, Morgan SJ, Johnson JL, Smith WR. Preperitonal pelvic packing for hemodynamically unstable pelvic fractures: a paradigm shift. *J Trauma*. 2007;62(4):834–839; discussion 839-842.

5 *The above 53-year-old woman with the APC 3 pelvic ring injury is significantly more likely to complain of which of the following when compared to a man with the same injury:*
A *Leg length discrepancy*
B *Genitourinary dysfunction*
C *Low back pain*
D *Posterior pelvic pain*
E *Dyspareunia*

Although patients that sustain pelvic ring injuries complain of pelvic and low back pain, women are at significant risk for dyspareunia—pain/discomfort with sexual intercourse. Dyspareunia may occur in up to 91% of women and most likely occurs with anteroposterior compression (APC) type fractures. Furthermore, women also have a high incidence of genitourinary complaints (49%). It is critical to ask patients about these complaints during follow-up, so they may be addressed. Of note, a woman with a pelvic fracture is more than twice as likely to give birth by cesarean section. The rate of low back pain, posterior pelvic pain, and leg length discrepancy is not different from men.

Answer: E

Vallier HA, Cureton BA, Schubeck D. Pelvic ring injury is associated with sexual dysfunction in women. *J Orthop Trauma*. 2012;26(5):308–313.
Cannada LK, Barr J. Pelvic fractures in women of childbearing age. *Clin Orthop Relat Res*. 2010;468(7):1781–1789.

6 *A 22-year-old man falls off of a roof and sustains a Gustilo and Anderson type 1 open tibia and fibula fractures with a 1 cm anteromedial tibial wound. There's no gross contamination and minimal periosteal stripping. His wound is irrigated with saline, and a saline-soaked gauze dressing is applied. He is placed in a splint, and there is no neurovascular compromise or concern for compartment syndrome. His Glasgow Coma Scale (GCS) score is 7 and is noted to have a left-sided intraparenchymal cerebral hemorrhage. Formal operative irrigation and debridement and stabilization of his open tibia fracture should occur:*
A *Within 24 hours*
B *As soon as the OR is ready*
C *Within 6 hours*
D *When his head injury allows*
E *Within 12 hours*

The "6-hour" rule for debridement of open fractures originated from an 1898 presentation by Paul Leopold Frederich where he contaminated guinea pigs with garden mold and stair dust to illustrate the importance of surgical debridement. In this antiquated animal study, debridement of the contaminated wound was less likely to be effective after 6–8 hours. Several studies have shown no association between timing of debridement and infection when debridement occurs within 24 hours. Others have shown a difference between debridement within 6 hours and less than 24 hours. However, all of these studies either have flawed study designs or too small a sample size to gain statistical significance. Therefore, emergent debridement is not necessarily supported, but neither is elective debridement. Current practice is based upon the current best evidence and includes debridement of open fractures urgently when the life-threatening emergencies have been addressed, patient's medical condition is stabilized and when the appropriate surgical resources are available.

Answer: D

Werner CM, Pierpont Y, Pollak AN The urgency of surgical debridement in the management of open fractures. *J Am Acad Orthop Surg*. 2008; 16(7):369–375.
Halawi MJ, Morwood MP. Acute management of open fractures: an evidence-based review. *Orthopedics*. 2015;38(11):e1025–e1033.

7 *A 32-year-old man sustains a distal one third Gustilo and Anderson type IIIB open tibia fracture with an associated segmental fibula fracture from a motorcycle accident. Which finding should you consider performing a below-knee amputation?*
A *5.5 cm of tibial bone loss after debridement*
B *Absent plantar foot sensation*
C *Absent dorsalis pedis pulse*
D *Transected tibial nerve*
E *Inability to actively dorsiflex the ankle*

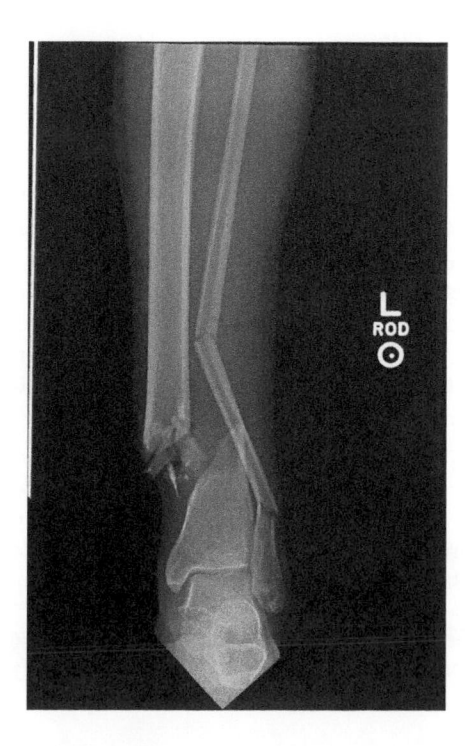

A visibly documented transected tibial nerve is the only answer that should have a patient consider an amputation. Inability to actively dorsiflex the ankle could be related to the fracture and associate pain, or a peroneal nerve palsy. As long as there is an identifiable posterior tibialis pulse, the absence of a dorsalis pedis pulse does not indicate an amputation; 5.5 cm of tibial bone loss can be reconstructed with a variety of bone-grafting techniques. The lack of plantar foot sensation alone no longer indicates amputation. The Lower Extremity Assessment Project (LEAP) was a multicenter prospective outcome study that involved 601 patients with severe, limb-threatening lower extremity patients that compared limb salvage versus amputation; 67% of patients in the limb salvage group with lack of plantar sensation upon admission had complete return of plantar sensation within 24-months. There were no significant outcomes differences found between the insensate salvage, insensate amputation, and the sensate control groups. The presence or absence of plantar sensation should not be used to direct treatment.

Answer: D

Bosse MJ, McCarthy ML, Jones AL, *et al*. The insensate foot following severe lower extremity trauma: an indication for amputation? *J Bone Joint Surg Am*. 2005;87:2601–2608.

8   *The surgeon taking care of the same man with the Gustilo and Anderson type IIIB open tibia fracture is trying to determine the best antibiotic prophylaxis. He has no medical allergies. The most appropriate antibiotic(s) to start include:*

   A   *Vancomycin*
   B   *Penicillin*
   C   *Gentamicin and penicillin*
   D   *Ancef and gentamicin*
   E   *Vancomycin and gentamicin*

Antibiotic prophylaxis has been based on the type of open fracture. Gustilo and Anderson type I, II, and IIIA fractures are covered by a third-generation cephalosporin, whereas type IIIB and C should receive a third-generation cephalosporin and an aminoglycoside to enhance gram-negative bacterial coverage. Penicillin is added if there is concern for anaerobes with soil contamination.

Answer: D

Halawi MJ, Morwood MP. Acute management of open fractures: an evidence-based review. *Orthopedics*. 2015;38(11):e1025–e1033.

9   *A 16-year-old boy falls off of his roof. He is complaining of right wrist pain. He has significantly limited*

range of wrist motion and an obvious deformity. Wrist radiographs are below. The injury that must be ruled out to avoid a poor outcome if diagnosed in a delayed fashion is:

   A   *Scapholunate ligament injury*
   B   *Minimally displaced distal radius fracture*
   C   *Scaphoid fracture*
   D   *Perilunate dislocation*
   E   *Hamate fracture*

The lateral wrist x-ray shows a volarly dislocated lunate (white arrow) indicating a perilunate dislocation.

Although any of the listed diagnoses may cause pain and minor deformity in the wrist/carpal area, only a perilunate dislocation will lead to limited wrist range of motion. Up to 25% of perilunate injuries are missed on initial evaluation. A high-quality lateral wrist radiograph is required for diagnosis. To avoid missing these injuries, a normal lateral wrist radiograph will show the lunate and capitate bones located in their fossa and in line with each other. Delayed diagnosis and management leads to poor outcomes and are more likely to require salvage procedures like a proximal row carpectomy.

Answer: D

Muppavarapu RC, Capo JT. Perilunate dislocations and fracture dislocations. *Hand Clin*. 2015;31(3):399–408.

10   *A 20-year-old man sustains an isolated lateral compression (LC) type 1 pelvic fracture after a fall from a retaining wall. It involves his left hemipelvis, and he is hemodynamically stable. After his imaging is reviewed, it is decided that he will be admitted for pain control and mobilization*

with physical therapy, and the fracture will be treated nonoperatively with limited weightbearing on the left leg for 6 weeks. Upon admission, deep vein thrombosis (DVT) prophylaxis should consist of:

A *Mechanical prophylaxis and 325 mg aspirin daily*

B *Low-molecular-weight heparin within 24 hours*

C *Mechanical prophylaxis alone*

D *Subcutaneous heparin 5000 units twice daily*

E *Low-molecular-weight heparin started after 48 hours*

Although it is universal to use DVT prophylaxis in patients with pelvic fractures, the exact protocol may differ significantly. A systematic review of DVT prophylaxis for pelvis and acetabular fractures evaluated 11 studies involving 1760 patients. Due to the limited and poorly controlled data available, no consistent protocol could be recommended except for following published guidelines for the general trauma population. However, low-molecular-weight heparin (LMWH) started within 24 hours of admission or within 24 hours of hemodynamic stability in patients with pelvic and acetabular fractures had a significantly lower DVT and pulmonary embolism (PE) rates when compared to patients started after 24 hours. The 2008 CHEST guidelines do not recommend post-hospital discharge chemoprophylaxis in pelvic fracture patients that are able to ambulate (although it may be limited), have no other DVT risk factors, and are not undergoing inpatient rehabilitation. This was not specifically mentioned in the 2012 CHEST guidelines update.

Answer: B

Slobogean GP, Lefaivre KA, Nicolaou S, *et al*. A systematic review of thromboprophylaxis for pelvic and acetabular fractures. *J Orthop Trauma*. 2009;**23**(5):379–384.

Geerts WH, Bergqvist D, Pineo GF, *et al*. Prevention of venous thromboembolism: American College of Chest Physicians evidence-based clinical practice guidelines (8th edition). *Chest*. 2008;133(6 Suppl):381S–453S.

11 *A 30-year-old man is involved in an unrestrained rollover motor vehicle accident. He sustains a pelvic fracture and bladder injury. What Young and Burgess fracture type is most commonly associated with a bladder injury?*

A *Lateral compression (LC) mechanism*

B *Combined mechanism*

C *Antero-posterior compression (APC) mechanism*

D *Transverse mechanism*

E *Vertical shear (VS) mechanism*

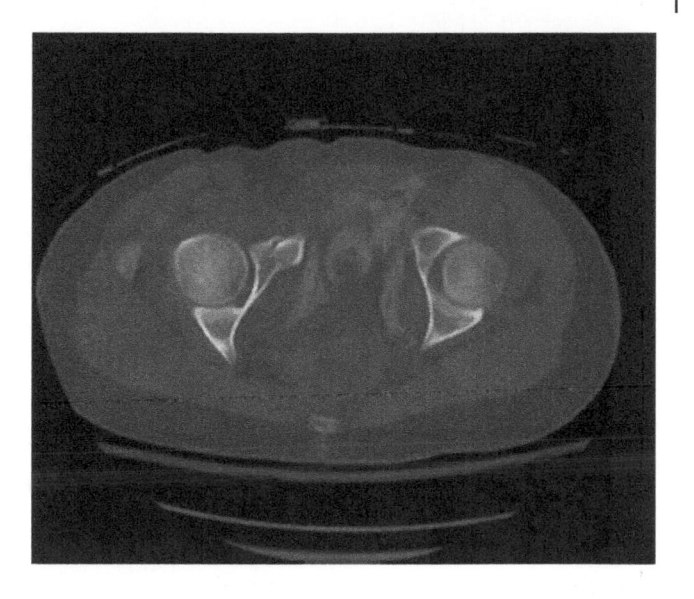

Injuries to the bladder and urethra occur in ~15–20% of patients with pelvic fractures. Bladder injuries are more commonly associated with lateral compression (LC) fractures. The fractured rami are forced into the bladder with the lateral compression mechanism. Urethral injuries are more commonly seen in patients with anterior-posterior compression (APC) fractures. Vertical and combined mechanisms are less common causes. Transverse mechanism is not part of the Young and Burgess classification. Mortality may be as high as 34% in pelvic fracture patients with bladder ruptures. Gross hematuria is identified in 95% of pelvic fracture patients with bladder injury, while microscopic hematuria is seen in the remaining 5% of those with bladder injury.

Answer: A

Durkin A, Sagi HC, Durham R, *et al*. Contemporary management of pelvic fractures. *Am J Surg*. 2006;192(2):211–223.

Fallon B, Wendt JC, Hawtrey CE Urological injury and assessment in patients with fractured pelvis. *J Urol*. 1984;**131**(4):712–714.

12 *A 50-year-old morbidly obese (BMI = 50) woman sustains a knee dislocation after tripping over a curb. Compared to a 20-year-old man with a BMI of 28 that sustains a knee dislocation during a motorcycle crash, the morbidly obese patient is more likely to:*

A *Require an above-knee amputation*

B *Have a lower complication rate*

C *Require vascular repair*

D *Require a formal reduction maneuver*

E *Have an associated femur fracture*

Knee dislocations occur from both high- and low-energy mechanisms. They are four times more likely to occur in males; ~50% of knee dislocations spontaneously reduce in both patient groups, so vigilence is needed and thorough history and physical should be done. If the knee is swollen, a ligamentous stability exam should be performed in addition to the normal physical exam including a very careful neurovascular exam. Patients with a BMI greater than 40 are more likely to sustain a dislocation after activities of daily living. When compared to knee dislocations related to high energy trauma, obese patients with low-energy dislocations are more likely to be a woman, sustain a vascular injury, sustain both a combined nerve and vascular injury, require a vascular repair, more likely to have a postoperative complication, and higher associated hospital costs. However, obese and morbidly obese patients are not at a higher risk of amputation when the vascular injury is controlled.

Answer: C

Johnson JP, Kleiner J, Klinge SA, McClure PK, Hayda RA, Born CT. Increased incidence of vascular injury in obese patients with knee dislocations. *J Orthop Trauma*. 2018;32(2):82–87. doi: https://doi.org/10.1097/BOT.0000000000001027. PMID: 29065033.

Werner BC, Gwathmey FW Jr, Higgins ST, Hart JM, Miller MD. Ultra-low velocity knee dislocations: patient characteristics, complications, and outcomes. *Am J Sports Med*. 2014;42(2):358–63. doi: https://doi.org/10.1177/0363546513508375. Epub 2013 Nov 8. PMID: 24214926.

13 *A 36-year-old man was struck by a motor vehicle while walking. He has a large right-knee effusion and has a positive Lachman test (anterior knee laxity at 30° of flexion), posterior drawer test (posterior knee laxity at 90°), and unstable to varus and valgus stress at 30° of flexion. His knee radiograph is below. His right lower extremity posterior tibialis pulse is 1+/4 and is asymmetric. After attempting a closed reduction and stabilizing the knee with a well-padded knee immobilizer, his posterior tibialis pulse is still 1+/4. What is the next step in managing this patient:*

A *Arteriogram*
B *Re-evaluation in 1 hour*
C *Ankle-brachial index determination*
D *Duplex ultrasound*
E *Emergent surgery for revascularization of the extremity and external fixation of the knee*

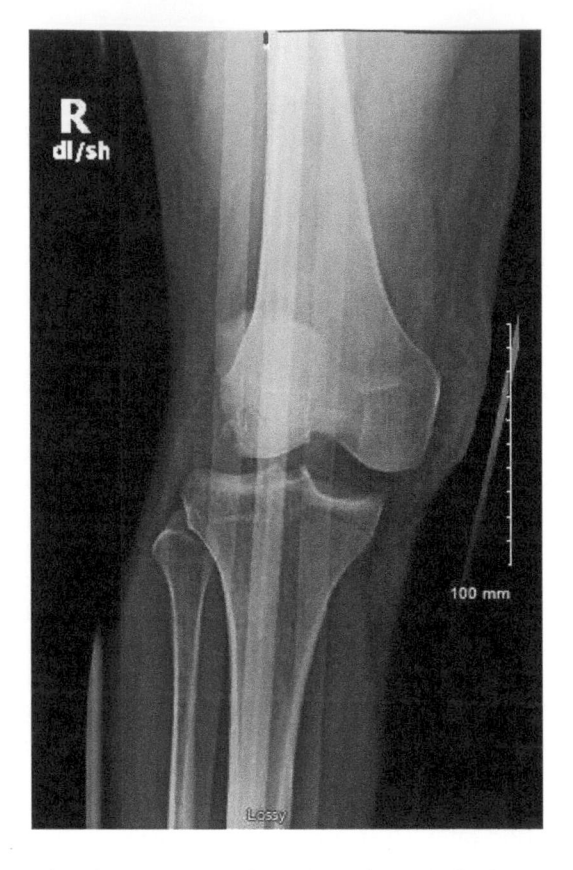

The above patient has clinical exam findings consistent with a multiligamentous knee injury (knee dislocation). Numerous studies have shown that **routine** angiography in all patients with a knee dislocation is unnecessary. Multiple studies, including two prospective trials, evaluated 543 patients with knee dislocations and showed that physical exam alone was sufficient to identify clinically significant vascular injuries. Furthermore, many of the vascular injuries associated with knee dislocations are non-flow-limiting arterial intimal tears. Current management of intimal tears in patients with a normal vascular examination includes observation and serial examinations. An arteriogram is indicated in any patient with an abnormal vascular exam. Since this patient had an asymmetric pulse, arteriogram is indicated. The asymmetric pulse also precludes the need for ankle-brachial index evaluation. Ultrasound is not indicated in a patient with an acute arterial injury. Arteriogram is indicated prior to surgery as long as getting the arteriogram doesn't lead to significant delay. Ideally, the arteriogram could be done in the operating room prior to revascularization if resources are available rather than going to radiology to have the procedure performed.

Answer: A

Boyce RH, Singh K, Obremskey WT. Acute management of traumatic knee dislocations for the generalist. *J Am Acad Orthop Surg*. 2015;23(12):761–768.

Levy BA, Fanelli GC, Whelan DB, *et al.* Controversies in the treatment of knee dislocations and multiligament reconstruction. *J Am Acad Orthop Surg.* 2009;17(4):197–206.

14 *A 45-year-old right hand dominant man fell 8 feet from a ladder and complains of right radial-sided right wrist pain. There's no obvious deformity. He has pain with ulnar deviation of his wrist and is tender to palpation just distal to the radial styloid. He did have loss of consciousness and has a forehead abrasion; however, he is currently alert and oriented with no facial asymmetry, or any vision changes. Head and cervical spine computed tomography (CT) scans are negative. Radiographs of the wrist show no obvious fracture. What is the next step in managing this patient in the emergency room (ER):*

A *CT scan of the wrist*

B *Magnetic resonance imaging (MRI) of the wrist*

C *Re-evaluate in 10–14 days*

D *Orthopaedic surgery consult*

E *Activities as tolerated*

Wrist pain without acute radiographic findings occur. Radial-sided wrist pain may indicate an occult scaphoid fracture. These can be initially missed up to 60% of the time. If a patient has radial-sided wrist pain, referral to an orthopedic surgeon is appropriate. Splinting the patient or placing them in a wrist brace for comfort is also appropriate but immobilizing them for 14 days leads to overtreatment. Recent studies have shown that only 4–20% of these patients have a fracture; therefore, immobilizing them for 14 days may not allow them to return to work or increase the risk of wrist and hand stiffness. Generally, advanced imaging is not indicated in the ER; however, getting an MRI (preferably) within 3–5 days of injury expedites appropriate care and limits overtreatment. If MRI isn't available, CT scan can be performed. Activities as tolerated may cause displacement if a fracture is present or at least leads to poor pain control.

Answer: D

Clementson M, Björkman A, Thomsen NOB. Acute scaphoid fractures: guidelines for diagnosis and treatment. *EFORT Open Rev.* 2020;5(2):96–103. Published 2020 Feb 26. doi: https://doi.org/10.1302/2058-5241.5.190025.

15 *A 17-year-old right hand dominant man sustains a table saw injury to his right hand. He presents with right thumb, index, and middle finger amputations through the proximal phalanges. He brought his amputated digits with him in a plastic bag on ice. The injury occurred 10 hours ago because he was transferred from another facility 2 hours away. The most appropriate definitive management includes:*

A *Replantation of the middle finger and revision amputation of the index finger and thumb*

B *Replantation of all digits*

C *Replantation of the index finger only with revision amputation of the thumb and middle finger*

D *Revision amputation of all digits through the metacarpophalangeal joints*

E *Replantation of the thumb only with revision amputation of the index and middle fingers*

Thumb amputation, multiple digit amputations, and pediatric digit amputations are indications for replantation. Single-digit replantation is always indicated for the thumb; however, it is also considered for other digits if the amputation is distal to the insertion of flexor digitorum superficialis and results from a sharp mechanism of injury. A sharp mechanism of injury, like being amputated with a knife, indicates a smaller zone of injury and structures that are more likely to be primarily repaired without tissue loss. Amputations secondary to significant crush or avulsion injuries are typically not replantable because of the increased zone of injury. Sharp-cut amputations in young and healthy patients are ideal. Maximum ischemia time for digits includes 12 hours warm and 24 hours cold. However, up to 96 hours cold ischemia time has been reported for digits.

Answer: B

Wolfe VM, Wang AA. Replantation of the upper extremity: current concepts. *J Am Acad Orthop Surg.* 2015;23(6):373–381.

Waikakul S, Sakkarnkosol S, Vanadurongwan V, Unnanuntana A Results of 1018 digital replantations in 552 patients. *Injury.* 2000;31(1):33–40.

16 *An intoxicated 22-year-old woman was involved in a rollover motor vehicle accident. She presents to the trauma bay with a Glasgow Coma Scale (GCS) score of 14, hemodynamically stable, and complains of right hip pain. Her right hip is flexed and internally rotated. Her right lower extremity is shortened compared to the left, and she is not able to dorsiflex her ankle or extend her great toe. Her posterior tibialis pulse is +2/4. Sensory exam is difficult due to the amount of pain she has. The most appropriate next step is:*

A *Consult orthopedic surgery*

B *Computed tomography (CT) scan of the pelvis*

C *Attempted closed reduction of his right hip*

D *Anteroposterior (AP) right hip radiograph*

E *Anteroposterior (AP) pelvis radiograph*

The most likely diagnosis is a dislocated right hip; however, closed reduction should not be performed without radiographic evaluation because the acetabulum or femoral head/neck may be fractured as well. Attempted closed reduction prior to imaging could increase the likelihood of damaging the femoral head or neck. The hip should be reduced as quickly as possible after the AP pelvis radiograph is completed. In a stable patient, the hip should be reduced prior to CT scan to decrease the incidence of avascular necrosis. An AP hip radiograph would show the hip dislocation but would not show an associated pelvic or opposite hip injury that may be present. Orthopedic surgery should be consulted but obtaining an AP pelvis is the first step in making the correct diagnosis.

Answer: E

Foulk DM, Mullis BH. Hip dislocation: evaluation and management. *J Am Acad Orthop Surg.* 2010;18(4):199–209.

17 *A 65-year-old woman fell down three stairs in her home and sustains a dorsally displaced left distal radius fracture with associated volar index and middle finger numbness. She also has right periorbital ecchymosis and a subarachnoid hemorrhage identified on her head computed tomography (CT) scan. She undergoes a two closed reduction attempts and splinting of her left distal radius by orthopedic surgery. Her volar index and middle finger numbness progresses after closed reduction and splinting. The symptoms do not improve with loosening the splint and icing and elevating the wrist. To minimize the risk of permanent neurological deficits, a carpal tunnel release should be performed:*

A *Within 24 hours*
B *Within 6 hours*
C *Within 48 hours*
D *Within 2 hours*
E *Within 12 hours*

Nerve injury occurs in ~17% of distal radius fractures with the median nerve most commonly involved. Acute carpal tunnel syndrome occurs most frequently in patients with higher energy and comminuted distal radius fractures. It can also occur in patients that undergo multiple closed reductions. If carpal tunnel symptoms progress after elevation, loosening of the splint and minimizing flexion of the wrist, a carpal tunnel release should be performed **emergently**. Patients undergoing early release have better long-term outcomes.

Answer: D

Gillig JD, White SD, Rachel JN. Acute carpal tunnel syndrome: a review of current literature. *Orthop Clin North Am.* 2016;47(3):599–607.

18 *A 30-year-old woman is thrown from a motor vehicle going 45 miles/hour. She has a Glasgow Coma Scale (GCS) score of 8 secondary to a closed head injury and is intubated. She has a closed right tibia fracture with significant swelling after closed reduction and splinting. Her dorsalis pedis pulse is +2/4 and symmetric to the other side. You are concerned about compartment syndrome. His blood pressure is 110/80 mm Hg. Orthopedic surgery performs compartment pressure monitoring. Her anterior leg compartment pressure is 75 mm Hg and her lateral compartment measures 55 mm Hg. Emergent fasciotomies are indicated. When undergoing fasciotomies, what is the minimum length of the fasciotomy that the compartment should be released in centimeters (cm) to adequately decompress the involved leg compartment?*

A *5 cm*
B *8 cm*
C *10 cm*
D *12 cm*
E *16 cm*

When using dual incision fasciotomies for acute traumatic leg compartment syndrome, at least 16 cm long incisions are required to adequately decompress the leg compartments. Pressures continue to decrease until the incision reached is 16 cm. Although several different compartment pressure thresholds have been used, the current recommendation is to proceed to fasciotomy when there is less than a 30 mm Hg difference between the compartment pressure and the diastolic blood pressure (compartment pressure – diastolic blood pressure). A differential pressure of 30 mm Hg led to no missed cases of acute compartment syndrome and avoided unnecessary fasciotomies. The indication to use invasive compartment pressure monitoring in this patient is the fact that she is obtunded and intubated. If the patient is alert and awake, clinical exam is usually sufficient, but compartment pressure monitoring can be used to verify clinical findings.

Answer: E

Frink M, Hildebrand F, Krettek C, *et al.* Compartment syndrome of the lower leg and foot. *Clin Orthop Relat Res.* 2010;468(4):940–950.

McQueen MM, Court-Brown CM Compartment monitoring in tibial fractures. The pressure threshold for decompression. *J Bone Joint Surg British.* 1996;78(1):99–104.

19 *A 32-year-old female is runover by a motor vehicle and sustains a pelvic fracture. Her blood pressure is 85/40 mm Hg, and her heart rate is 150 beats/min. She receives 2 units of packed red blood cells (RBCs) but is still hypotensive. You are considering placing a pelvic binder to help with her hypotension. What Young and Burgess pelvic fracture type would most benefit from applying a pelvic binder or circumferential sheet to significantly reduce pelvic volume:*

A *Anterior–posterior compression (APC) fracture type 3*

B *Lateral compression (LC) fracture type 1*

C *Vertical shear fracture*

D *Lateral compression (LC) fracture type 2*

E *Anterior–posterior compression (APC) fracture type 1*

Commercially available pelvic binders or standard bed sheets have been incorporated into the acute management of pelvic fractures to aid in patient transport and resuscitation. They should be applied at the level of the greater trochanters. The primary function of these pelvic compression devices is to reduce pelvic volume; therefore, fractures that do not have increased pelvic volume (lateral compression injuries and vertical shear injuries) should not have these devices placed. APC 1 injuries do not have significant increase in pelvic volume either. APC 3 injuries have a significant increase in pelvic volume and benefit from external compression devices.

Pelvic binders have been shown to generate more compression than sheets and have been thought to more effectively reduce the pelvic volume to an amount similar to the reduction obtained with definitive surgical management. Pelvic binders reduce transfusion requirements, length of hospital stay, and mortality in patients with APC injuries. It's important to remember that sheets can be used in lieu of commercial binders. Prolonged use of binders or sheets may lead to pressure ulcers and nerve palsies. Regular skin checks should be performed to minimize this risk, particularly in patients that are having large fluid shifts. Furthermore, definitive management of the pelvic ring injury should be performed as early as the patient status allows in order to minimize the risk of skin and neurological issues.

Answer: A

Spanjersberg WR, Knops SP, Schep NW, van Lieshout EM, Patka P, Schipper IB. Effectiveness and complications of pelvic circumferential compression devices in patients with unstable pelvic fractures: a systematic review of literature. *Injury.* 2009;40(10):1031–1035.

Langford JR, Burgess AR, Liporace FA, Haidukewych GJ. Pelvic fractures: part 1. Evaluation, classification, and resuscitation. *J Am Acad Orthop Surg.* 2013;21(8):448–457.

20 *A 40-year-old man sustains a closed tibial and fibular shaft fracture after a fall from a ladder. He has a Glasgow Coma Scale (GCS) score of 14. His Visual Analog Scale (VAS) is 9 and he complains of numbness in his leg. He undergoes closed reduction and splinting of his leg. His leg pain does not improve after splinting. He receives intravenous (IV) morphine, his splint is loosened, his leg elevated to heart level, and ice is applied. His VAS is still 9 and has increased leg pain with passive flexion and extension of his great toe. His posterior tibialis pulse is 2+/4 and capillary refill is 3 seconds. The next step in this patient's management should include:*

A *Consult anesthesia for a regional nerve block*

B *Compartment pressure evaluation*

C *Perform ankle-brachial index (ABI)*

D *IV toradol and re-examine in 1 hour*

E *Emergent fasciotomies*

In an awake and alert patient, pain is the earliest and most sensitive clinical sign of compartment syndrome. After the fracture is immobilized in a splint, passive motion of the muscles within the involved compartments (i.e. moving the great toe involves stretching the anterior and deep posterior leg compartments) has been used to correlate with diagnosis of compartment syndrome. Paresthesia is also an early clinical sign. If these signs develop after splinting, the first step should be loosening any constrictive splint/dressing and elevation of the extremity up to the level of the heart. The limb can be elevated, and ice applied to help with pain, but elevation above the heart should be avoided in order to maximize limb perfusion. Since outcomes associated with compartment syndrome are associated with time to fasciotomy, if clinical signs indicate a high likelihood that the patient has a compartment syndrome, compartment pressure monitoring should be bypassed, and emergent fasciotomies should be performed. Ankle-brachial indices are indicated in knee dislocations and would be too difficult to do in someone with a tibia fracture. A regional nerve block would mask an evolving compartment syndrome since pain is the best early indicator. Continued IV pain medication is not indicated if his symptoms and signs are progressing.

Answer: E

Frink M, Hildebrand F, Krettek C, *et al.* Compartment syndrome of the lower leg and foot. *Clin Orthop Relat Res.* 2010;468(4):940–950.

Schmidt AH. Acute compartment syndrome. *Orthop Clin North Am* 2016;47(3):517–525.

33

Peripheral Vascular Trauma

Yousef Abuhakmeh, DO[1] and Jonathan Swisher, MD[2]

[1] MAJ, MC US Army, Banner University Medical Center, University of Arizona College of Medicine, Tucson, AZ, USA
[2] LTC, MC US Army, William Beaumont Army Medical Center, El Paso, TX, USA

1   *A 27-year-old man presents with an inflamed groin mass. It is swollen, tender to palpation, and the patient is febrile. He admits to a history of frequent intravenous drug abuse with injection at various sites. The best initial diagnostic study paired with the likely diagnosis is:*

   A *Duplex ultrasound/subcutaneous abscess*
   B *Duplex ultrasound/lymphoma*
   C *Incision and drainage/subcutaneous abscess*
   D *Duplex ultrasound/infected pseudoaneurysm*
   E *Incision and drainage/infected pseudoaneurysm*

Infected pseudoaneurysms are common in younger patients who are addicted to illicit IV drugs and should be suspected if there is concern for abscess near any major vessel used as an injection site. Trauma is also a well-known cause of pseudoaneurysms that may become infected by hematogenous seeding or direct inoculation. Initial imaging workup should include duplex ultrasound for evaluation of the underlying fluid collection or pseudoaneurysm. Incision and drainage should not be performed for presumed abscess without imaging to rule out pseudoaneurysm in the region of major vessels. Malignancy such as lymphoma would likely present with palpable lymphadenopathy in multiple nodal basins, likely not isolated with focal signs of infection.

Answer: D

Jacobowitz G, Cayne NS. Lower Extremity Aneurysms. *Rutherford's Vascular Surgery and Endovascular Therapy*, 9th ed., (ed. Anton N Sidawy and Bruce A Perler) Elsevier, 2019, pp. 1080–1083.

2   *A patient arrives to the trauma bay with report from EMS that he sustained a stab wound to the right lower extremity. He has had continuous bleeding of bright red blood throughout his ambulance transport, with a tourniquet in place. During the primary survey, the tourniquet is loosened, revealing pulsatile blood from the wound. You find no other injuries. The initial management goals should be:*

   A *Fluid resuscitation and CT imaging with contrast*
   B *Blood product resuscitation and immediate operative exploration*
   C *Tetanus administration, intravenous gentamycin and bedside ankle-brachial index*
   D *Fluid resuscitation and bedside ankle-brachial index*
   E *Intravenous antibiotics and orthopedic trauma consultation*

This patient is presenting with an isolated penetrating trauma with hard signs of bleeding. Immediate blood product resuscitation and operative intervention are warranted with the goal of hemorrhage control and repair of the vessels. Hard signs of arterial extremity injury include active bleeding, expanding hematoma, signs of distal ischemia, lack of distal pulses, and palpable thrill or audible bruit. Any patient presenting with these signs/symptoms should forego any further workup (CT imaging and ankle-brachial index) and proceed directly to immediate operative exploration and repair. While intravenous antibiotics and orthopedic consultation may be appropriate, it should not take priority over immediate operative exploration and resuscitation.

Answer: B

Callcut RA, Mell MW. Modern advances in vascular trauma. *Surg Clin North Am.* 2013;93(4):941–961. doi: 10.1016/j.suc.2013.04.010. Epub 2013 Jun 13. Review. PubMed [citation] PMID: 23885939.
Feliciano DV. Pitfalls in the management of peripheral vascular injuries. *Trauma Surg Acute Care Open.* 2017;2(1):e000110. doi: 10.1136/tsaco-2017-000110.

Surgical Critical Care and Emergency Surgery: Clinical Questions and Answers, Third Edition.
Edited by Forrest "Dell" Moore, Peter M. Rhee, and Carlos J. Rodriguez.
© 2022 John Wiley & Sons Ltd. Published 2022 by John Wiley & Sons Ltd.
Companion website: www.wiley.com/go/surgicalcriticalcare3e

eCollection 2017. Review. PubMed [citation] PMID: 29766105, PMCID: PMC5877918.

Fox N, Rajani RR, Bokhari F, Chiu WC, Kerwin A, Seamon MJ, Skarupa D, Frykberg E, Eastern Association for the Surgery of Trauma. Evaluation and management of penetrating lower extremity arterial trauma: an Eastern Association for the Surgery of Trauma practice management guideline. *J Trauma Acute Care Surg.* 2012;73(5 Suppl 4):S315–S320. doi: 10.1097/TA.0b013e31827018e4. PubMed [citation] PMID: 23114487.

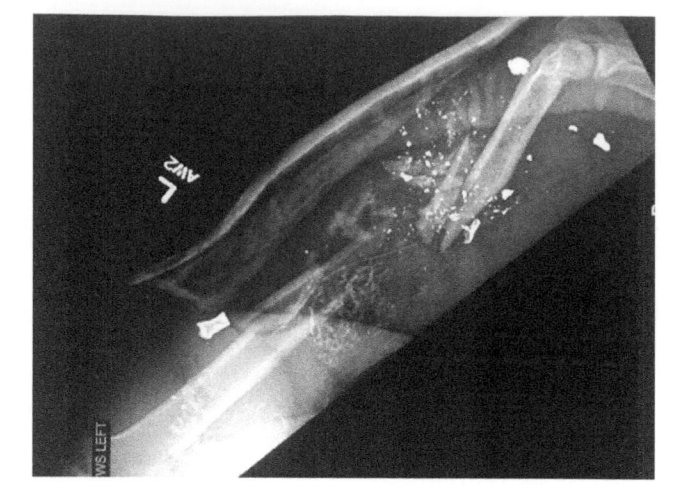

3 *A 25-year-old man sustains a gunshot wound to the left upper leg (pictured below). The patient is hypotensive, acidotic, and hypothermic, with absent pulses below the level of the injury. The massive transfusion protocol is initiated in the trauma bay and the patient is taken immediately to the operating room. The patient remains unstable. What is the appropriate operative sequence?*

   A *Open reduction internal fixation of the femur followed by definitive vascular repair with reverse saphenous vein graft*

   B *External fixator placement followed by definitive artery repair with prosthetic graft*

   C *Temporary shunting of injured artery followed by external fixator placement and delayed vascular and bone repairs*

   D *Open reduction internal fixation of the femur followed by definitive vascular repair with prosthetic graft*

   E *External fixator placement, definitive artery repair, and delayed bone repairs*

Temporary intravascular shunting is now widely accepted as a bridge to definitive vessel repair, such as in combined orthopedic and vascular injuries. The indications for temporary shunting include open extremity fractures with extensive soft tissue injury and concurrent arterial injury, need for perfusion during complex vascular reconstruction, damage control for patients in extremis, perfusion prior to limb replantation, truncal vascular control, and complex repair of zone III neck injuries. As this patient is in extremis, damage-control vascular (shunt) and orthopedic (external fixator) surgery techniques should be performed, and the patient returned to the intensive care unit for ongoing and aggressive resuscitation. The patient should return to the operating room as soon as endpoints of resuscitation have been met for definitive vascular and bone repairs. Answers A, B, D, and E are not damage-control techniques and will potentially result in limb loss and death should the patient spend several hours in the operating room undergoing definitive procedures.

Answer: C

Abou Ali AN, Salem KM, Alarcon LH, Bauza G, Pikoulis E, Chaer RA, Avgerinos ED. Vascular shunts in civilian trauma. *Front Surg.* 2017;4:39. doi: 10.3389/fsurg.2017.00039. eCollection 2017. Review. PubMed [citation] PMID: 28775985, PMCID: PMC5517780.

Liang NL, Alarcon LH, Jeyabalan G, Avgerinos ED, Makaroun MS, Chaer RA. Contemporary outcomes of civilian lower extremity arterial trauma. *J Vasc Surg.* 2016;64(3):731–736. doi: 10.1016/j.jvs.2016.04.052. Epub 2016 Jul 18. PubMed [citation] PMID: 27444360, PMCID: PMC5002387.

Woodward EB, Clouse WD, Eliason JL, Peck MA, Bowser AN, Cox MW, Jones WT, Rasmussen TE. Penetrating femoropopliteal injury during modern warfare: experience of the balad vascular registry. *J Vasc Surg.* 2008;47(6):1259–1264; discussion 1264-5. doi: 10.1016/j.jvs.2008.01.052. Epub 2008 Apr 14. PubMed [citation] PMID: 18407450.

4 *EMS brings a patient to the emergency department who has been stabbed in the left upper chest, just below the lateral portion of the clavicle. The patient is anxious, tachycardic, and has no other wounds. The wound is bleeding briskly once manual pressure is removed. At exploration, the axillary artery is found to be transected cleanly without tension from the ends. He is stable after initial resuscitation, with normal parameters on his ABG. The most appropriate method of repair is:*

   A *Endovascular repair with stent graft*

   B *Repair with interposition vein graft*

   C *Repair with interposition prosthetic graft*

   D *Primary repair*

   E *Temporary shunting with delayed primary repair*

This patient has hard signs of bleeding and should be explored immediately. In addition, complete vessel transection has been shown to have high failure rates with endovascular repair. Caution is advised with primary repair, as tension with an end-to-end anastomosis increases the risk of suture line/anastomotic failure and thrombosis. In this patient with a sharp transection (and no undue tension) of the axillary artery from a penetrating knife injury, primary repair is most expeditious. Interposition graft is not necessary unless there is undue tension on the vessel ends. Shunting prior to repair is not necessary in this case as the patient is stable and adequately resuscitated in the operating room. Shunting would be appropriate if the patient was unstable, had ongoing resuscitation requirements, or had other life-threatening injuries at the time of exploration.

Answer: D

Feliciano DV. Pitfalls in the management of peripheral vascular injuries. *Trauma Surg Acute Care Open.* 2017;2(1):e000110. doi: 10.1136/tsaco-2017-000110. eCollection 2017. Review. PubMed [citation] PMID: 29766105, PMCID: PMC5877918.

Klocker J, Bertoldi A, Benda B, Pellegrini L, Gorny O, Fraedrich G. Outcome after interposition of vein grafts for arterial repair of extremity injuries in civilians. *J Vasc Surg.* 2014;59(6):1633–1637. doi: 10.1016/j.jvs.2014.01.006. Epub 2014 Feb 19. PubMed [citation] PMID: 24560243.

Shalhub S, Starnes BW, Tran NT. Endovascular treatment of axillosubclavian arterial transection in patients with blunt traumatic injury. *J Vasc Surg.* 2011;53(4):1141–1144. doi: 10.1016/j.jvs.2010.10.129. Epub 2011 Jan 26. PubMed [citation] PMID: 21276694.

5   *A middle-aged man presents to the trauma bay after sustaining multiple gunshot wounds. He is hemodynamically unstable and massive transfusion is initiated. FAST exam is positive, and he has active bleeding from a proximal left thigh wound as well. In the operating room, his leg is explored simultaneously during laparotomy. In addition to a liver laceration and multiple bowel injuries, the proximal superficial femoral artery is transected. He is hypothermic. The most prudent course of action regarding the arterial injury is:*
    A *Interposition graft with reversed contralateral saphenous vein*
    B *Ligation*
    C *Temporary shunt placement with systemic heparinization*
    D *Interposition graft with PTFE prosthetic*
    E *Temporary shunt placement*

Damage control surgery is a widely accepted method of management for patients in extremis. Patients with vascular injuries who are in extremis (hypothermia, acidosis, hemodynamic instability) should undergo temporary intravascular shunt placement rather than ligation, if possible, as ligation of major inflow vessels may lead to irreversible ischemia and subsequent limb amputation. Interposition repair would be time consuming in this case, making temporary shunt placement a better option for the patient overall until they are stabilized. Definitive vascular repair should be performed in a situation where the patient has a more normal and stable physiology. Although civilian trauma centers have reported higher rates of shunting in blunt trauma patients with concomitant orthopedic injuries, penetrating and blast injuries in patients who are unstable may warrant shunt placement as part of the index damage control operation. Studies have shown that shorter ischemic time (facilitated by shunt placement) may result in a lower incidences of fasciotomy, repeat operations, and shorter hospitalizations. Systemic heparinization in this patient is contraindicated in the setting of liver laceration and ongoing hemorrhage from penetrating trauma requiring massive transfusion.

Answer: E

Abou Ali AN, Salem KM, Alarcon LH, Bauza G, Pikoulis E, Chaer RA, Avgerinos ED. Vascular shunts in civilian trauma. *Front Surg.* 2017;4:39. doi: 10.3389/fsurg.2017.00039. eCollection 2017. Review. PubMed [citation] PMID: 28775985, PMCID: PMC5517780.

Hossny A. Blunt popliteal artery injury with complete lower limb ischemia: is routine use of temporary intraluminal arterial shunt justified? *J Vasc Surg.* 2004;40(1):61–66. PubMed [citation] PMID: 15218463.

Sharrock AE, Tai N, Perkins Z, White JM, Remick KN, Rickard RF, Rasmussen TE. Management and outcome of 597 wartime penetrating lower extremity arterial injuries from an international military cohort. *J Vasc Surg.* 2019;70(1):224–232. doi: 10.1016/j.jvs.2018.11.024. Epub 2019 Feb 18. PubMed [citation] PMID: 30786987.

Wahlgren CM, Riddez L. Penetrating vascular trauma of the upper and lower limbs. *Curr Trauma Rep.* (2016);2:11–20. https://doi.org/10.1007/s40719-016-0035-1.

6   *A patient presents to the emergency department with a shotgun injury to the left upper extremity. There is grossly devitalized soft tissue around the humerus, without active hemorrhage. The radial pulse is palpable, but clearly diminished when compared to the contralateral arm. What is the most appropriate imaging for accurate diagnosis of presumed vascular injury in this extremity?*
    A *Conventional angiography*
    B *Duplex ultrasound*
    C *CT angiogram*
    D *Wrist-to-brachial index measurement*
    E *Pulse volume recording (PVR)*

Arteriogram proves helpful in the setting of shotgun injuries and may offer better diagnostic capability than CTA. Although CT angiogram will likely be performed initially in most trauma centers, the imaging will often be negatively impacted by image artifact from the numerous bullet particles near the injury in question. Duplex ultrasound will not show the extent of vessel and tissue injury in this setting. Wrist-to-brachial index and PVRs will not give the detail needed to identify and repair focal vessel lesions, especially in the setting of a devastating trauma such as this. Shotgun injuries, particularly at close range, are more devastating than other low-velocity gunshot wounds. These patients will typically require more operations, and plastic surgery reconstruction may be warranted. Vascular injury from shotgun blasts may be direct, from bullet particles, or indirect, from nearby blast effect. Patients typically have injuries involving arteries, veins, bones and nerves of the affected limb.

Answer: A

Aydın H, Okçu O, Dural K, Sakıncı U. Management of community-based shotgun injuries of the extremities: impact of emergent vascular repair without angiography. *Ulus Travma Acil Cerrahi Derg.* 2011;17(2):152–158.

Dozier KC, Miranda MA, Kwan RO, Cureton EL, Sadjadi J, Victorino GP. Despite the increasing use of nonoperative management of firearm trauma, shotgun injuries still require aggressive operative management. *J Surg Res.* 2009;156(1):173–176. doi: 10.1016/j.jss.2009.04.019.

Fox N, Rajani RR, Bokhari F, Chiu WC, Kerwin A, Seamon MJ, Skarupa D, Frykberg E, Eastern Association for the Surgery of Trauma. Evaluation and management of penetrating lower extremity arterial trauma: an Eastern Association for the Surgery of Trauma practice management guideline. *J Trauma Acute Care Surg.* 2012;73(5 Suppl 4):S315–S320. doi: 10.1097/TA.0b013e31827018e4. PubMed [citation] PMID: 23114487.

Kauvar DS, Kraiss LW. Vascular Trauma: Extremity. *Rutherford's Vascular Surgery and Endovascular Therapy*, 9th ed. (ed. Anton N Sidawy and Bruce A Perler), Elsevier, 2019, pp. 2414–2415.

7 *Regarding the use of temporary intravascular shunts, which of the following is true?*

   A *Shunting, compared to ligation, has shown to result in similar rates of amputation, fasciotomy, and mortality.*

   B *The most commonly shunted vessel is the popliteal artery.*

   C *Venous shunting, compared to ligation, shows no improvement in rates of compartment syndrome, fasciotomies, or amputations.*

D *Thrombosis rates for arterial shunts has been reported to be as low as 4–5%.*

E *The most commonly shunted vessel is the external iliac artery.*

Among reports from both civilian and military vascular trauma populations, the superficial femoral artery is the most commonly shunted artery. The use of temporary intravascular shunting has been reliably proven to decrease the incidence of amputations, fasciotomies, and mortality after injury. Although lateral venorrhaphy is the best option for vein repair when possible, temporary venous shunting may also be performed. In patients with life-threatening injuries and hemodynamic instability, there is no indication for immediate vein repair, and ligation should be performed. With regards to shunting of injured veins, this has been shown to decrease rates of compartment syndrome, need for fasciotomies, and amputations. Injuries to the femoral and popliteal veins should be repaired for these same reasons. Venous ligation should be avoided if possible in extremities with arterial injuries requiring shunts, as the venous hypertension will also contribute to arterial shunt failure. Although there is no standard recommendation, systemic anticoagulation is typically not needed in patients with indwelling arterial shunts, and rates of thrombosis are reported to be as low as 4%.

Answer: D

Abou Ali AN, Salem KM, Alarcon LH, Bauza G, Pikoulis E, Chaer RA, Avgerinos ED. Vascular shunts in civilian trauma. *Front Surg.* 2017;4:39. doi: 10.3389/fsurg.2017.00039. eCollection 2017. Review. PubMed [citation] PMID: 28775985, PMCID: PMC5517780.

Feliciano DV. Pitfalls in the management of peripheral vascular injuries. *Trauma Surg Acute Care Open.* 2017;2(1):e000110. doi: 10.1136/tsaco-2017-000110. eCollection 2017. Review. PubMed [citation] PMID: 29766105, PMCID: PMC5877918.

Sharrock AE, Tai N, Perkins Z, White JM, Remick KN, Rickard RF, Rasmussen TE. Management and outcome of 597 wartime penetrating lower extremity arterial injuries from an international military cohort. *J Vasc Surg.* 2019;70(1):224–232. doi:10.1016/j.jvs.2018.11.024. Epub 2019 Feb 18. PubMed [citation] PMID: 30786987.

Wahlgren CM, Riddez L. Penetrating vascular trauma of the upper and lower limbs. *Curr Trauma Rep.* 2016;2:11–20. https://doi.org/10.1007/s40719-016-0035-1.

8 *A patient presents to the emergency department after sustaining a hyperextension injury of the left knee during a basketball game. He has palpable pedal pulses. Of the following, which is the most appropriate*

indication for obtaining advanced imaging such as CT angiogram or conventional arteriogram?

A *Mechanism of injury*
B *Suspected posterior cruciate ligament injury*
C *Inability to bear weight on the extremity*
D *Ankle-brachial index < 0.9 on physical exam*
E *Gross swelling of the knee*

Patients may not always have hard signs of arterial injury. The evaluation of patients with suspected arterial injuries should always include a bedside ankle-brachial index (ABI) at the time of pulse exam in stable patients. Normal ABI in a healthy individual is >0.9, and that a patient with this value is presumed to have an artery without occlusive lesions or traumatic disruption. If an ABI is found to be ≤0.9, advanced imaging of the artery in question is warranted, either with CT arteriography or conventional arteriogram. ABI ≤ 0.9 has been shown in one study to have a sensitivity of 87% and specificity of 97% for arterial injury. Answers A, B, C, and E are incorrect and have no specific data to support using them as risk factors or predictors of significant arterial injury.

Answer: D

Feliciano DV. Pitfalls in the management of peripheral vascular injuries. *Trauma Surg Acute Care Open.* 2017;2(1):e000110. doi: 10.1136/tsaco-2017-000110. eCollection 2017. Review. PubMed [citation] PMID: 29766105, PMCID: PMC5877918.

Fox N, Rajani RR, Bokhari F, Chiu WC, Kerwin A, Seamon MJ, Skarupa D, Frykberg E, Eastern Association for the Surgery of Trauma. Evaluation and management of penetrating lower extremity arterial trauma: an Eastern Association for the Surgery of Trauma practice management guideline. *J Trauma Acute Care Surg.* 2012;73(5 Suppl 4):S315–S320. doi: 10.1097/TA.0b013e31827018e4. PubMed [citation] PMID: 23114487.

9 *A 59-year-old woman is brought to the emergency department after a motor vehicle collision. She was unrestrained and reportedly ejected >25 feet from the car. Her right arm has a proximal tourniquet in place and is visibly deformed and de-gloved below the mid-portion of the upper arm. After removing the tourniquet, she is found to have no sensation below the elbow, and no bleeding. The forearm is de-gloved >50% with dirty, exposed muscle and bone. Plain radiographs show fractures of the proximal radius, mid- and distal humerus. There is no capillary refill of the fingertips. She is hypotensive and transiently responsive to IV fluid boluses. Of the following surgical options, which should be most strongly considered in this patient?*

A *Primary amputation of the extremity*
B *External fixation and synthetic bypass grafting of the inflow artery*
C *Arteriogram with planning for upper extremity bypass graft and complex reconstruction*
D *Washout and external fixation followed by CT angiogram*
E *Washout, fixation, and wound vac placement*

Components of the Mangled Extremity Severity Score (MESS) include skeletal/soft tissue injury (low, medium, high, or very high energy mechanism), limb ischemia (normal perfusion, diminished perfusion with paresthesia and lack of pulse, insensate and paralyzed), shock (systolic <90 mm Hg, transient hypotension, persistent hypotension), and patient age (<30 years old, 30–50 years old, >50 years old). Ray et al. have shown that patients with a MESS ≥ 11 should be considered for primary amputation. This patient in the question has a calculated MESS of 10. Poor outcomes are likely with a MESS ≥ 9, and MESS ≥ 7 predicts worse outcomes for patients undergoing bypass grafting for lower extremity arterial extremity injuries. Keeping these factors in mind can guide decision-making for patients with mangled extremities. In addition to the MESS, other known factors that ultimately contribute to delayed amputations are blunt trauma mechanisms and a pulseless exam on presentation.

Answer: A

Liang NL, Alarcon LH, Jeyabalan G, Avgerinos ED, Makaroun MS, Chaer RA. Contemporary outcomes of civilian lower extremity arterial trauma. *J Vasc Surg.* 2016;64(3):731–736. doi: 10.1016/j.jvs.2016.04.052. Epub 2016 Jul 18. PubMed [citation] PMID: 27444360, PMCID: PMC5002387.

Ray HM, Sandhu HK, Meyer DE, Miller CC 3rd, Vowels TJ, Afifi RO, Azizzadeh A, Charlton-Ouw KM. Predictors of poor outcome in infrainguinal bypass for trauma. *J Vasc Surg.* 2019;70(6):1816–1822. doi: 10.1016/j.jvs.2019.03.056. Epub 2019 Jun 24. PubMed [citation] PMID: 31248764.

10 *Compared to open repair, endovascular repair of traumatic arterial injuries is associated with which of the following?*
A *Lower mortality rates*
B *Higher mortality rates*
C *Higher overall rates of major amputation*
D *More blood transfusions*
E *Lower patient satisfaction*

Over the past two decades, there has been a substantial increase in the use of endovascular surgical management of both truncal and extremity vascular injuries. Outside of thoracoabdominal injuries, common/external iliac artery injuries are among the most commonly repaired with endovascular stent grafts. One analysis of the National Trauma Data Bank has shown trends toward lower extremity amputation rates in patients who underwent endovascular repair (compared to those undergoing open repair). The overall mortality rates also significantly decreased for patients with penetrating trauma during the studied time period. Studies have also demonstrated lower mortality, lower hospital costs, and fewer blood transfusions for patients who underwent endovascular repairs.

Answer: A

Branco BC, DuBose JJ, Zhan LX, Hughes JD, Goshima KR, Rhee P, Mills JL Sr. Trends and outcomes of endovascular therapy in the management of civilian vascular injuries. *J Vasc Surg*. 2014;60(5):1297–1307.e1. doi: 10.1016/j.jvs.2014.05.028. Epub 2014 Jun 26. PubMed [citation] PMID: 24974784a.

11 *At exploration of a gunshot wound to the distal thigh, you identify a devastating transection of the above-knee popliteal artery, with no distal artery clearly identified until below-knee exploration is performed. With regards to patency of the repair, which repair is the best option based on this injury pattern and location?*

   A *Prosthetic interposition graft with polytetrafluoroethylene (PTFE)*

   B *Primary anastomosis with running 5-0 prolene suture*

   C *Reversed saphenous vein graft harvested from the contralateral leg*

   D *Reversed cephalic vein graft*

   E *Primary amputation, above knee*

Studies have shown worse outcomes with regards to graft patency at or below the knee, with prosthetic graft such as PTFE, compared to vein grafts which have been shown to have lower failure rates. In general, saphenous vein graft should be harvested from the contralateral leg, especially if there is venous damage to the injured extremity. Saphenous vein is a better size match for a popliteal anastomosis than cephalic vein. Primary anastomosis in this scenario is not possible. Above-knee amputation is not indicated in this scenario, as the limb is salvageable with arterial repair.

Answer: C

Klocker J, Bertoldi A, Benda B, Pellegrini L, Gorny O, Fraedrich G. Outcome after interposition of vein grafts for arterial repair of extremity injuries in civilians. *J Vasc Surg*. 2014;59(6):1633–1637. doi: 10.1016/
j.jvs.2014.01.006. Epub 2014 Feb 19. PubMed [citation] PMID: 24560243.

Martin LC, McKenney MG, Sosa JL, Ginzburg E, Puente I, Sleeman D, Zeppa R. Management of lower extremity arterial trauma. *J Trauma*. 1994;37(4):591–598; discussion 598-9. doi: 10.1097/00005373-199410000-00012. PMID: 7932890.

12 *You care consulted by the emergency department for a 22-year-old man who was stabbed in the lower leg with a steak knife. He has normal vital signs and no active hemorrhage. He has symmetric palpable dorsalis pedis and posterior tibial pulses. You calculate an ABI, which is 0.94 on the injured leg. What is the next most reasonable step in management?*

   A *CT angiogram of the injured leg*

   B *Arterial duplex ultrasound*

   C *Conventional angiogram of the injured leg*

   D *Local wound care and discharge home with planned outpatient follow-up*

   E *Immediate operative exploration*

Not all patients with penetrating trauma need imaging as part of the workup. It is now well established that there is a select group of patients that may forego imaging and operative exploration. The patient in this scenario is stable, has no hard signs of injury, has an ABI > 0.9, a normal physical exam (pulses), and no other injuries. It has been shown that an ABI > 0.9 has a sensitivity of >87% and specificity of 97% for arterial injury. A patient with an ABI > 0.9 is presumed to have a normal artery or one with a small, nonocclusive lesion.

Answer: D

Feliciano DV. Pitfalls in the management of peripheral vascular injuries. *Trauma Surg Acute Care Open*. 2017;2(1):e000110. doi: 10.1136/tsaco-2017-000110. eCollection 2017. Review. PubMed [citation] PMID: 29766105, PMCID: PMC5877918.

Fox N, Rajani RR, Bokhari F, Chiu WC, Kerwin A, Seamon MJ, Skarupa D, Frykberg E, Eastern Association for the Surgery of Trauma. Evaluation and management of penetrating lower extremity arterial trauma: an Eastern Association for the Surgery of Trauma practice management guideline. *J Trauma Acute Care Surg*. 2012;73(5 Suppl 4):S315–S320. doi: 10.1097/TA.0b013e31827018e4. PubMed [citation] PMID: 23114487.

13 *You are called to the trauma operating room for assistance managing a patient with a common femoral vein injury in whom an intraluminal shunt was placed by your colleague. The venous defect is approximately 2 cm and you are inclined to repair*

the vein. Which of the following is the best option with regards to expected patency?

A *Interposition graft with ring-supported PTFE graft*

B *Interposition graft with autogenous vein from the contralateral greater saphenous vein*

C *End-to-end primary repair*

D *Primary repair with lateral venorrhaphy*

E *A and B are both viable options for repair in this scenario*

One study has shown no significant difference in patency rates between primary and complex venous repairs for penetrating trauma. Options include primary repair with lateral venorrhaphy, vein patch repair, autogenous interposition vein grafts, or interposition repair with ring-supported PTFE graft. For the most part, early patency rates appear similar (around 73%) across different studies, irrespective of the type of repair performed. Lateral venorrhaphy and primary end-to-end anastomosis are not reasonable options in this scenario as there is a complete defect in the vein with a gap and primary repair would be under too much tension. In the setting of arterial injury with a temporary shunt in place, vein repair will help mitigate shunt failure and compartment syndrome.

Answer: E

Pappas PJ, Haser PB, Teehan EP, Noel AA, Silva MB Jr, Jamil Z, Swan KG, Padberg FT Jr, Hobson RW 2nd. Outcome of complex venous reconstructions in patients with trauma. *J Vasc Surg.* 1997;25(2):398–404. doi: 10.1016/s0741-5214(97)70362-8. PMID: 9052575.

Parry NG, Feliciano DV, Burke RM, Cava RA, Nicholas JM, Dente CJ, Rozycki GS. Management and short-term patency of lower extremity venous injuries with various repairs. *Am J Surg.* 2003;186(6):631–635. doi: 10.1016/j.amjsurg.2003.08.006. PMID: 14672770.

14 *You have a patient who underwent primary repair of both popliteal artery and vein injuries after high-velocity gunshot wound to the knee. Orthopedics is planning delayed distal femur repair, and external fixator is in place now for stability. The operative time for your repair was 4 hours. Prior to leaving the operating room, what should you most strongly consider as your next step in management?*

A *Compressive bandage wrap to the thigh and lower extremity*

B *Ropivacaine infusion catheter placement for post-operative pain control*

C *Compartment pressure measurement of the anterior and lateral compartments*

D *Prophylactic lower extremity fasciotomy of all 4 compartments*

E *Systemic anticoagulation in the setting of arterial and venous repairs*

It is generally agreed upon that prophylactic fasciotomy in patients with high-risk injuries is preferable to therapeutic fasciotomy performed after the development of signs and symptoms of tissue loss. Well-known risk factors for lower leg compartment syndrome are as follows: popliteal artery injury, combined arterial and venous injury, prolonged ischemia (>4–6 hours), complex and multiple extremity fractures, combined vascular and bone or soft tissue injury, arterial or venous ligation, thrombosed repair, and elevated compartment pressures (>30 mm Hg).

Answer: D

Cooper N, Roshdy M, Sciarretta JD, Kaufmann C, Duncan S, Davis J, Macedo FI. Multidisciplinary team approach in the management of popliteal artery injury. *J Multidiscip Healthc.* 2018;11:399–403. doi: 10.2147/JMDH.S151498. PMID: 30214221; PMCID: PMC6118273.

Frykberg ER. Popliteal vascular injuries. *Surg Clin North Am.* 2002;82(1):67–89. doi: 10.1016/S0039-6109(03)00141-5. PMID: 11905952.

15 *You are consulted urgently by a practitioner who has just placed a right subclavian central venous catheter at the bedside and is concerned that the blood return from the catheter may be arterial, rather than venous. What would you recommend as the next courses of action in this scenario?*

A *Leave the catheter in place, attempt to transduce an arterial waveform, obtain CT angiogram of the chest and neck to identify catheter placement.*

B *Remove the catheter, apply direct manual compression, obtain chest radiograph.*

C *Remove the catheter, apply direct manual compression, obtain CT angiogram of the chest.*

D *Obtain blood gas analysis from the catheter blood, remove catheter, and apply direct manual compression.*

E *Proceed directly to the operating room for open surgical repair of presumed subclavian artery injury.*

Inadvertent arterial cannulation has the potential to cause devastating outcomes. Cannulation of an artery with a large bore catheter should be quickly diagnosed by the person performing the procedure. Well-described methods of diagnosing arterial cannulation include blood gas analysis, transduction of arterial waveforms, manometry, and radiologic studies such as CT imaging. With regards to treatment, a systematic review has identified manual compression as having the highest overall failure and complication rates. Common complications include stroke, pseudoaneurysm formation, arterial dissection, arteriovenous fistula formation, and hemodynamic instability. Options for repair of the arteriotomy include percutaneous closure devices, endovascular repair with covered stent placement, balloon tamponade, or open surgical repair. When an arterial cannulation is recognized, the catheter should be left in situ, placement confirmed by radiologic imaging if other techniques such as transduction or blood gas analysis are equivocal, and consultation with a vascular/endovascular surgeon should be obtained. Manual compression of subclavian, carotid, or brachiocephalic arteries or aortic arch vessels can be challenging or impossible, and immediate imaging should be performed to help determine the most appropriate treatment strategy. In scenarios when consultation is not possible, or resources are limited, open surgical repair should be considered, as it has been shown to have high success rates, with less morbidity and complications in select groups such as with carotid artery injury.

Answer: A

Dornbos DL 3rd, Nimjee SM, Smith TP. Inadvertent arterial placement of central venous catheters: systematic review and guidelines for treatment. *J Vasc Interv Radiol.* 2019;30(11):1785–1794. doi: 10.1016/j.jvir.2019.05.017. Epub 2019 Sep 14. PMID: 31530491.

Yoon DY, Annambhotla S, Resnick SA, Eskandari MK, Rodriguez HE. Inadvertent arterial placement of central venous catheters: diagnostic and therapeutic strategies. *Ann Vasc Surg.* 2015;29(8):1567–1574. doi: 10.1016/j. avsg.2015.05.030. Epub 2015 Aug 7. PMID: 26256713.

16 *A 23-year-old man presents with a stab wound to his right groin. Paramedics report pulsatile bleeding on the scene, controlled with pressure. Pressure is removed in the trauma bay and no active bleeding is present, but there is a large pulsatile mass with a bruit. Distal pulses in the ipsilateral extremity are palpable. No other injuries are discovered. The patient is hemodynamically stable, and CT scan shows an 8 cm pseudoaneurysm arising from the common femoral artery 5 mm proximal to the femoral bifurcation. What is the best approach for repair?*

A *Covered stent of the injured artery via percutaneous contralateral access*

B *Proximal control via midline laparotomy*

C *Direct exposure of the injured vessel via groin incision*

D *Proximal control via extraperitoneal exposure of the external iliac artery, arterial repair via groin incision*

E *Proximal control with balloon occlusion from contralateral percutaneous access, arterial repair via groin incision*

Covered stenting of vascular injuries is well-described and sometimes the best choice, especially in anatomically difficult areas to access. In this location, surgical repair is preferred, especially with the injury being close to the femoral bifurcation. A laparotomy would provide adequate possibilities for proximal control but is unnecessarily invasive with no intraperitoneal injures identified. Direct groin cutdown with a large pseudoaneurysm present risks entering the pseudoaneurysm and having uncontrolled hemorrhage prior to proximal control. Endovascular methods using balloon proximal occlusion are possible but more appropriate for areas difficult to expose. In this case, a simple extraperitoneal exposure would be the quickest and simplest approach to the external iliac for proximal control.

Answer: D

Radowsky JS, Rodriguez CJ, Wind GG, Elster EA. A surgeon's guide to obtaining hemorrhage control in combat-related dismounted lower extremity blast injuries. *Mil Med.* 2016;181(10):1300–1304. doi: 10.7205/MILMED-D-15-00324. PMID: 27753567.

Wahlgren CM, Riddez L. Penetrating vascular trauma of the upper and lower limbs. *Curr Trauma Rep.* 2016;2:11–20. 10.1007/s40719-016-0035-1.

17 *A 75-year-old woman poly-trauma patient from a motor-vehicle accident underwent urgent placement of a right femoral arterial line during initial resuscitation. She is in hospital day #2 and has stabilized significantly. Injuries include bilateral hemopneumothoraces and multiple rib fractures with bilateral chest tubes in place, multiple long-bone fractures s/p external fixation, and a mild traumatic brain injury. Once a radial arterial line is placed, the femoral arterial line is removed and no bleeding from the site is noted after a 10 minute pressure hold. Twenty minutes later, the patient is severely hypotensive and tachycardic. The right groin is soft without visible hematoma, and the bilateral chest tubes are functioning properly. What is the most likely cause of the patient's shock?*

A *Missed intra-abdominal injury*

B *Massive pulmonary embolism*

C *Hemorrhagic shock from retroperitoneal hematoma*

D *Decompensation due to pulmonary contusions*
E *Cerebral herniation*

A missed intra-abdominal injury or massive pulmonary embolism are both possibilities in this patient, but given the timing of decompensation shortly after femoral arterial line removal, a retroperitoneal hematoma is most likely. Femoral arterial access holds the possibility of a high/proximal puncture leading to a retroperitoneal hematoma, and an urgently placed line is likely to have been placed with less than ideal conditions, possibly making a high-stick more likely. Access site complications have several known risk factors and include female gender, advanced age, prior anemia, heart failure, low creatinine clearance, rest pain, heparin use, and non-use of a closure device. Blossoming pulmonary contusions are a possibility, but the patient would have progressive hypoxia. Cerebral herniation is unlikely in a patient with mild traumatic brain injury and would manifest with bradycardia.

Answer: C

Ortiz D, Jahangir A, Singh M, Allaqaband S, Bajwa TK, Mewissen MW. Access site complications after peripheral vascular interventions: incidence, predictors, and outcomes. *Circ Cardiovasc Interv.* 2014;7(6):821–828. doi: 10.1161/CIRCINTERVENTIONS.114.001306. Epub 2014 Nov 11. PMID: 25389345; PMCID: PMC4529288.

18 *With 4-compartment fasciotomy, what deficit will be present if the nerve in the proximal lateral compartment is injured?*
    A *Weakened plantar flexion*
    B *Weakened knee extension*
    C *Weakened thigh adduction*
    D *Loss of patellar reflex*
    E *Foot drop*

The lateral fasciotomy incision is used to approach the anterior and lateral compartments of the lower leg. One cadaver study demonstrated that the superficial peroneal nerve was anatomically located within the lateral compartment of the lower leg in 71% of the cases. The second most common anatomical finding was that the nerve penetrated the intermuscular septum usually around 12 cm distal to the fibular head prior to completing its course in the anterior compartment. This nerve courses around the fibular head and ultimately innervated the muscles responsible for ankle eversion and dorsiflexion of the foot and toes. Weakened plantar flexion would be due to injury of the tibial nerve. Knee extension is a function of the femoral nerve. Thigh adduction is performed by the medial thigh muscle group, innervated by the obturator nerve.

Answer: E

Apaydin N, Basarir K, Loukas M, Tubbs RS, Uz A, Kinik H. Compartmental anatomy of the superficial fibular nerve with an emphasis on fascial release operations of the leg. *Surg Radiol Anat.* 2008;30(1):47–52. doi: 10.1007/s00276-007-0284-3. Epub 2007 Dec 11. PMID: 18071623.

Kashuk JL, Moore EE, Pinski S, Johnson JL, Moore JB, Morgan S, Cothren CC, Smith W.. Lower extremity compartment syndrome in the acute care surgery paradigm: safety lessons learned. *Patient Saf Surg.* 2009;3(1):11. doi: 10.1186/1754-9493-3-11. PMID: 19527510; PMCID: PMC2704180.

19 *A 50-year-old obese man is in the SICU after blunt trauma with a liver laceration, managed successfully with selective arterial embolization. He has been hemodynamically stable, with a rising hemoglobin. Some ecchymosis was noted surrounding the right femoral access site with a palpable mass. There is no skin breakdown, and duplex ultrasound shows a 1.5 cm pseudoaneurysm with an area of active swirling blood flow seen on color duplex. The most appropriate management of this pseudoaneurysm is:*
    A *Duplex-directed thrombin injection*
    B *Open repair via groin incision*
    C *Observation*
    D *Covered stenting via contralateral femoral access*
    E *IV antibiotics*

Multiple studies have shown the safety and efficacy of observation with small pseudoaneurysms from percutaneous access, some even showing safety of observation with a size up to 6 cm. Intervention is recommended when there are side effects from compression (such as pain), skin changes/breakdown, or failure after observation and continued growth. Pseudoaneurysms smaller than 2 cm can usually be managed without any intervention at all. One predictor of failure is systemic anticoagulation. For ultrasound-guided compression and/or thrombin injection, information such as size, complexity, duration, and anticoagulation status should be considered when deciding if a pseudoaneurysm will benefit from thrombin injection or not. Open repair is effective but unnecessary unless there is a failure of observation, compression, or thrombin injection. Covered stenting could be effective if intervention was needed but would be least preferred, given the high cost and need for additional contralateral access (with its own potential complications).

Answer: C

Kent KC, McArdle CR, Kennedy B, Baim DS, Anninos E, Skillman JJ. A prospective study of the clinical outcome of femoral pseudoaneurysms and arteriovenous fistulas induced by arterial puncture. *J Vasc Surg.* 1993;17(1): 125–131; discussion 131-3. doi: 10.1067/mva.1993. 41707. PMID: 8421328.

Toursarkissian B, Allen BT, Petrinec D, Thompson RW, Rubin BG, Reilly JM, Anderson CB, Flye MW, Sicard GA. Spontaneous closure of selected iatrogenic pseudoaneurysms and arteriovenous fistulae. *J Vasc Surg.* 1997;25(5):803–808; discussion 808-9. doi: 10.1016/ s0741-5214(97)70209-x. PMID: 9152307.

Vlachou PA, Karkos CD, Bains S, McCarthy MJ, Fishwick G, Bolia A. Percutaneous ultrasound-guided thrombin injection for the treatment of iatrogenic femoral artery pseudoaneurysms. *Eur J Radiol.* 2011;77(1):172–174. doi: 10.1016/j.ejrad.2009.06.032. Epub 2009 Aug 5. PMID: 19660885.

20   *A 30-year-old man is stabbed in the left shoulder. Paramedics report pulsatile bleeding on the scene. A military-style tourniquet is applied directly over the wound along with a gauze packing within and around the wound. The wound is in the mid-axilla, and the tourniquet is wrapped over the shoulder to achieve hemostasis. With any loosening of the tourniquet pulsatile bleeding is encountered, which stops with forceful manual pressure around the clavicle only. Resuscitation is ongoing, chest radiograph is normal, and blood pressure has improved from 90/50 mm Hg on presentation. What is the appropriate intervention?*

A   *OR for exploration, supraclavicular incision for proximal control*

B   *OR for exploration, sub-clavicular incision for initial proximal control*

C   *Angiography suite for covered stenting*

D   *OR for exploration, pneumatic tourniquet for proximal control*

E   *OR for exploration, left thoracotomy for proximal control*

Based on the described location and control with compression/tourniquet, the injury is most likely distal enough for proximal control at the distal subclavian or axillary artery via a sub-clavicular incision. This incision is easily extended medially to include division of the clavicle or distally to the deltopectoral groove if necessary. An arterial injury more proximal than this would be expected to be non-compressible. Stab wounds with unknown trajectory could yield a more proximal injury, appearing controlled with the tourniquet, but with uncontrolled bleeding elsewhere such as into the ipsilateral hemithorax. Supra-clavicular exposure would be appropriate for a more proximal injury, and a high left thoracotomy would be appropriate for control of the proximal left subclavian artery. Angiography with endovascular repair is more likely to be successful for focal lesions and are most appropriate for stable patients. It should be performed in a combined endovascular/surgical hybrid suite with a surgeon immediately available. A pneumatic tourniquet is an excellent option for more distal injuries of the circumferential arm or leg, but in this case, the injury is at a very proximal compressible area (by digital manual pressure only), making a tourniquet ineffective at a location such as the axilla or peri-clavicular where only deep, directed manual compression is effective.

Answer: B

Carrick MM, Morrison CA, Pham HQ, Norman MA, Marvin B, Lee J, Wall MJ Jr, Mattox KL. Modern management of traumatic subclavian artery injuries: a single institution's experience in the evolution of endovascular repair. *Am J Surg.* 2010;199(1):28–34. doi: 10.1016/j.amjsurg.2008.11.031. Epub 2009 Jun 11. PMID: 19520356.

Graham JM, Mattox KL, Feliciano DV, DeBakey ME. Vascular injuries of the axilla. *Ann Surg.* 1982;195(2):232–238. doi: 10.1097/00000658-198202000 -00020. PMID: 7055402; PMCID: PMC1352449.

Mazzini FN, Vu T, Prichayudh S, Sciarretta JD, Chandler J, Lieberman H, Marini C, Asensio JA. Operative exposure and management of axillary vessel injuries. *Eur J Trauma Emerg Surg.* 2011;37(5):451. doi: 10.1007/ s00068-011-0134-1. Epub 2011 Jul 29. PMID: 26815415.

34

Urologic Trauma and Disorders

Daniel Roubik, MD[1] and Luke Hofmann, DO[1,2]

[1] Brooke Army Medical Center, San Antonio, TX, USA
[2] F. Edward Hebert School of Medicine, Uniformed Services University, Bethesda, MD, USA

The following clinical scenario applies to questions 1–2

A 48-year-old man presents to the emergency department after falling from a tree while intoxicated. He is hemodynamically stable. Physical exam is notable for some abrasions on his extremities, as well as some bruising to his left side. As part of his workup, a urinary drug screen is ordered. The urine is dilute but has a pink tinge. Portable chest x-ray, pelvic x-ray, and Focused Assessment with Sonography in Trauma (FAST) scan are all negative.

1 *What is the next best step in management?*
   A *Discharge from the emergency department once sober if a repeat FAST is normal at 2 hours*
   B *Retrograde cystourethrogram*
   C *Computed tomography scan (CT) abdomen and pelvis without contrast*
   D *CT abdomen and pelvis with intravenous (IV) contrast and delayed images*
   E *Renal angiogram*

Per the 2020 American Urological Association (AUA) guidelines for urotrauma, "Clinicians should perform diagnostic imaging with IV contrast-enhanced CT in stable blunt trauma patients with gross hematuria or microscopic hematuria and systolic blood pressure < 90 mm Hg. (Standard; Evidence Strength: Grade B)." This patient's mechanism has potential for renal injury, so when combined with gross hematuria, further assessment for renal injury is required. A renal arterial phase is typically obtained 20–30 seconds after administration of intravenous contrast, which the venous phase is seen on delays of 70–80 seconds. Urinary extravasation is best visualized on furthered delayed imaging, after about 5 minutes. Because you may not always know when to obtain delayed imaging on initial presentation, a provider who is proficient in reading CT scans should be available for immediate review of the images prior to the patient leaving the CT scanner. The results of a CT scan will guide management in regards to disposition and whether interventions are warranted.

A normal FAST scan (Choice A) is inadequate to rule out renal injury since FAST scans will classically miss retroperitoneal blood. A retrograde cystourethrogram (Choice B) would be considered if there was specific concern for urethral trauma, such as blood at the urethral meatus or a high-riding prostate on digital rectal exam. A CT scan without contrast (Choice C) may be the image of choice if the patient has a known anaphylactic reaction to IV contrast but provide much less information than a high-quality contrasted study. Finally, going straight to a renal angiogram (Choice E) would be premature prior to determining the presence and/or extent of imaging on CT scan.

Answer: D

Morey, A. F., Brandes, S., Dugi, D. D., Armstrong, J. H., Breyer, B. N., Broghammer, J. A., . . . & Reston, J. T. (2014). Urotrauma: AUA guideline. *The Journal of Urology*, *192*(2), 327–335.

Erlich, T., & Kitrey, N. D. (2018). Renal trauma: the current best practice. *Therapeutic Advances in Urology*, *10*(10), 295–303.

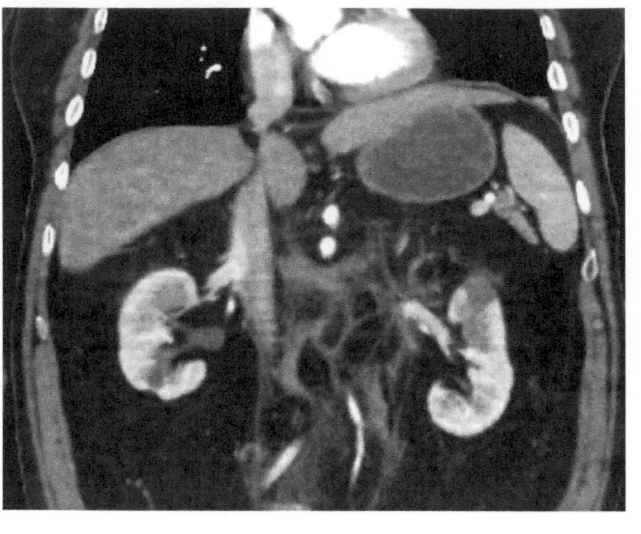

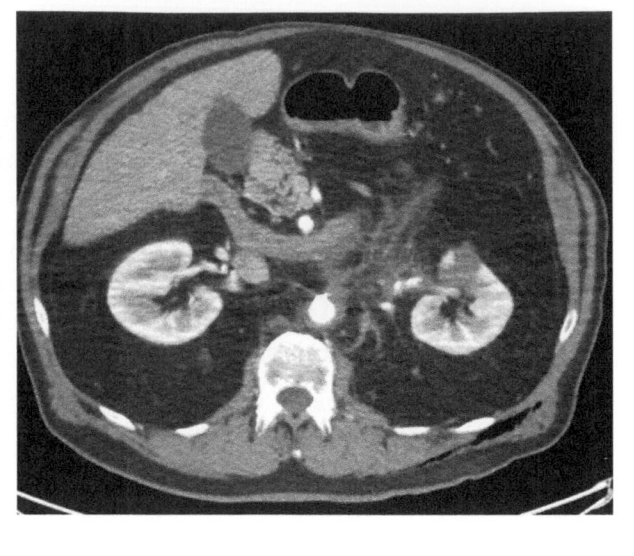

2 *A CT scan is performed and demonstrates a parenchymal laceration that is 1.5 cm deep in the superior pole with no urinary extravasation or vascular injury. After CT scan, his heart rate is 75 beats/min with a blood pressure of 118/72 mm Hg. He's breathing comfortably on room air with oxygen saturation of 99%. He received 50 mcg of fentanyl and 1 L of LR in the trauma bay with tolerable pain. What is the next best step in management?*

A *Discharge home once sober with outpatient follow-up in 1 week*

B *Admit to an intermediate care unit with serial labs*

C *Admit to the ICU for q2h CBC and continuous bladder irrigation*

D *Immediate angioembolization and prophylactic ureteral stenting*

E *Operative exploration for attempted renorrhaphy*

This injury is consistent with an AAST grade III renal laceration in a hemodynamically stable patient. Nonoperative management, including angioembolization and/or stenting, should be the mainstay for renal trauma in a stable patient. Operative exploration decreases rates of renal salvage and should be reserved for refractory cases, so answer E in incorrect. Likewise this patient has no target (active extravasation) or indication for angioembolization given his hemodynamic stability (answer D). While many institutions will monitor patients with grade III renal lacerations in the ICU, recent literature suggests that very few (<5%) ever result in operative management, so more recent societal guideline suggest these patients can be monitored on the floor. Regardless, answer C is incorrect since there is no role for routine continuous bladder irrigation. Finally, due to potential for ongoing bleeding, some period of inpatient observation is warranted for grade III renal lacerations (answer A).

Grade	Type	Description
I	Contusion	Microscopic or gross hematuria. Normal urologic studies
	Hematoma	Subcapsular, non-expanding hematoma without parenchymal laceration
II	Hematoma	Non-expanding perirenal hematoma confined to the renal retroperitoneum
	Laceration	<1.0 cm parenchymal depth of renal cortex without urinary extravagation
III	Laceration	>1.0 cm parenchymal depth of renal cortex without urinary extravagation or collecting system rupture
IV	Laceration	Parenchymal laceration extending through the renal cortex, medulla, and collecting system
	Vascular	Main renal artery or vein injury with contained hemorrhage
V	Laceration	Completely shattered kidney
	Vascular	Avulsion of renal hilum that devascularizes kidney

American Association for Surgery of Trauma Renal Injury Scale.

Answer: B

Buckley, J. C., & McAninch, J. W. (2011). Revision of current American Association for the Surgery of Trauma Renal Injury grading system. *Journal of Trauma and Acute Care Surgery, 70*(1), 35–37.

Erlich, T., & Kitrey, N. D. (2018). Renal trauma: the current best practice. *Therapeutic Advances in Urology, 10*(10), 295–303.

Keihani, S., Xu, Y., Presson, A. P., Hotaling, J. M., Nirula, R., Piotrowski, J., . . . & Majercik, S. (2018). Contemporary management of high-grade renal trauma:

results from the American Association for the Surgery of Trauma Genitourinary Trauma study. *Journal of Trauma and Acute Care Surgery, 84*(3), 418–425.

3 *Which of the following is true regarding high-grade (grades IV and V) renal injury?*

A *A grade V renal injury is a contraindication for minimally invasive interventions, such as embolization or drainage procedures.*

B *High-grade renal injuries from blunt mechanisms are more likely to result in nephrectomy than penetrating mechanisms.*

C *Early renal exploration results in higher rates of renal salvage.*

D *Renal salvage is successful in 70–80% of patients with high-grade renal injury.*

E *Due to the confined location in the retroperitoneum, renal injuries, rarely if ever, result in morbidity and mortality.*

According to a 2018 study including 14 level 1 trauma centers, 431 cases of penetrating and blunt high-grade renal injury were identified. They noted that around 80% of cases could be managed with conservative or minimally invasive approaches (embolization, percutaneous nephrostomy or drainage, or ureteral stenting); therefore, answer A is incorrect. Their reported nephrectomy rates were 0.4% for grade III, 15% for grade IV, and 62% for grade V (overall 28% for grade IV/V). The New England Trauma Consortium reported nephrectomy rates of 21% for grade IV/V, but they excluded penetrating trauma. Penetrating trauma has a much higher incidence of nephrectomy compared to blunt trauma; therefore, answer B is incorrect. One of the most important means of renal salvage is avoiding renal exploration unless it is absolutely necessary (answer C is incorrect). When intact, Gerota's fascia will contain and tamponade most renal hematomas, but renal exploration alleviates the tamponade, which leads to more bleeding, and nephrectomy follows in many cases. This is seen when looking at National Trauma Data Bank studies that found that 30% of patients with grades I–III renal injuries who required laparotomy underwent nephrectomy. Finally, high-grade renal lacerations can lead to many complications, including urinoma, urinary fistulae, infection, continued hemorrhage, and death (answer E), so nonoperative management is not always appropriate.

Answer: D

Erlich, T., & Kitrey, N. D. (2018). Renal trauma: the current best practice. *Therapeutic Advances in Urology, 10*(10), 295–303.

Keihani, S., Xu, Y., Presson, A. P., Hotaling, J. M., Nirula, R., Piotrowski, J., . . . & Majercik, S. (2018). Contemporary management of high-grade renal trauma: results from the American Association for the Surgery of Trauma Genitourinary Trauma study. *Journal of Trauma and Acute Care Surgery, 84*(3), 418–425.

McClung CD, Hotaling JM, Wang J, Wessells H, & Voelzke BB. (2013). Contemporary trends in the immediate surgical management of renal trauma using a national database. *The Journal of Trauma and Acute Care Surgery, 75*(4), 602–606.

4 *A 55-year-old woman is involved in a motorcycle collision. She is hemodynamically stable upon presentation and has a negative FAST scan. Secondary survey reveals bruising to the right flank and diffuse tenderness but no significant injuries. Trauma labs are sent, and a CT abdomen/pelvis with IV contrast is normal. A plan is made to discharge the patient from the ER. Prior to discharge, the ER provider calls to inform you the urinalysis demonstrated 4+ blood with >50 red blood cells per high power field (RBC/HPF), although the urine sample was clear. What is the next best step in management?*

A *Proceed with discharge with close interval outpatient follow-up with a urologist or primary care doctor*

B *Send a creatinine kinase*

C *Repeat a CT abdomen/pelvis with and without IV contrast and delayed images*

D *Admit the patient for observation overnight with q4 hour labs*

E *Perform an MRI of the kidneys*

Microscopic hematuria is defined as three or more RBC/HPF in adults and over 50 RBC/HPF in pediatric patients with no visible blood in the urine sample. Visible hematuria is seen in 35–77% of renal trauma cases. It is important to note there is no correlation between the degree of hematuria with the renal injury. The above case has a stable patient with microscopic hematuria. In the absence of renal injury on imaging, this would be classified as a renal contusion or grade I injury, of which no immediate intervention is warranted. In the absence of other findings, the patient can be discharged home with close interval follow-up with either a primary care provider or urologist to ensure the microscopic hematuria clears and doesn't represent another pathology, such as an undiagnosed genitourinary malignancy. While myoglobinuria can interfere with the urinalysis dipstick, the visualization of RBC under microscope definitively diagnoses true hematuria, so a creatinine kinase is not needed (answer B). A repeat CT scan would subject the patient to an additional contrast dose with limited diagnostic benefit, especially in light of normal vitals on presentation, so answer C is incorrect. Admission for microscopic hematuria alone is unnecessary (answer D). Finally, renal MRI has no role in the initial trauma evaluation in the presence of a normal CT scan, so answer E is incorrect.

Answer: A

Erlich, T., & Kitrey, N. D. (2018). Renal trauma: the current best practice. *Therapeutic Advances in Urology*, 10(10), 295–303.

Morey, A. F., Brandes, S., Dugi, D. D., Armstrong, J. H., Breyer, B. N., Broghammer, J. A., . . . & Reston, J. T. (2014). Urotrauma: AUA guideline. *The Journal of Urology*, 192(2), 327–335.

The following scenario applies to questions 5 and 6

A 25-year-old man was riding a bicycle when he hit a car that pulled out in front of him, resulting in him sliding forward and forcefully straddling his bike. He presents to the ER where he is found to have perineal bruising and blood at the urethral meatus. Chest x-ray is normal, but the pelvic x-ray shows a pelvic fracture. FAST is negative.

5   What is the best next step to workup the urethral finding?
   A *Insert a small-bore Foley catheter*
   B *Place a condom catheter*
   C *Do nothing*
   D *Perform a retrograde urethrogram*
   E *Cystoscopy in the operating room*

Blood at the urethral meatus is highly suspicious for a urethral injury. A retrograde urethrogram (RUG) should be performed before attempting placement of a Foley catheter. A RUG is performed by inserting a 12 Fr Foley catheter into the fossa navicularis (distal part of penile urethra) and either secured with manual pressure or 1–2 mL of fluid/air into the balloon. Undilute contrast material is instilled through the catheter, and radiographs or fluoroscopic images are taken. Inserting a Foley catheter (answer A) is dangerous because it could make the urethral injury worse. At times, it may be appropriate for an expert (urologist or experienced trauma surgeon) to attempt one pass, and one pass only, of a Foley catheter into the bladder. A large diameter catheter is typically used to decrease the likelihood of cannulating a false tract. Placing a condom catheter (answer B) will not guarantee the flow of urine out of the bladder; it might be blocked by the urethral injury. If nothing is done (answer C), the patient has a high risk of urinary retention and/or urethral stricture. Cystoscopy (answer E) may be needed to place a catheter into the bladder, but it is not the best next step.

   The image below shows a urethral disruption at the junction of the bulbar urethra and the membranous portion of the urethra.

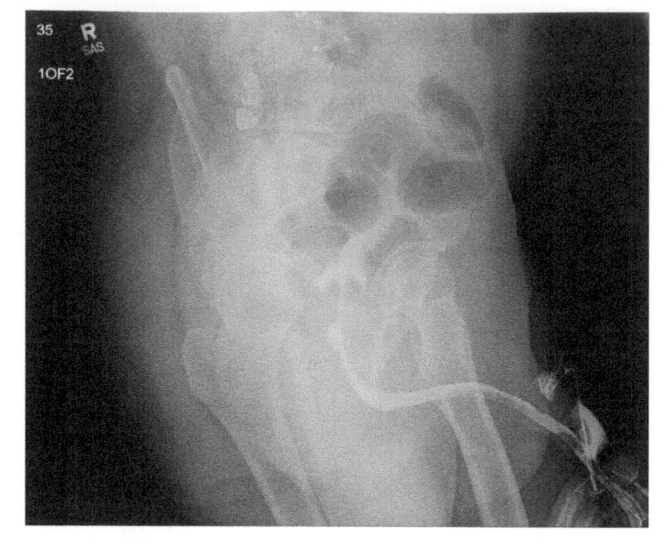

Answer: D

Stein, D. M., & Santucci, R. A. (2015). An update on urotrauma. *Current Opinion in Urology*. 25(4), 323–330.

Doiron, R. C., & Rourke, K. F. (2019). An overview of urethral injury. *Canadian Urological Association Journal*, 13(6 Suppl4), S61.

6   *A radiologist reviewed the imaging and believes there is a posterior urethral injury. The patient remains hemodynamically stable and has a fairly distended bladder. Urology was consulted, but they are in another emergency case and will be unavailable for several hours. What is the next best step in management?*
   A *Do nothing until urology is available*
   B *Attempt to pass the smallest Foley available*
   C *Perform suprapubic catheterization*
   D *Request the trauma staff attempt immediate primary repair*
   E *Consult IR to place bilateral percutaneous nephrostomy tubes*

When urethral disruption is diagnosed, suprapubic catheterization is usually the treatment of choice. Delaying bladder decompression for an undefined period of time is not a reasonable treatment option (answer A). As mentioned before, an experienced provider may attempt a single pass with a Foley, but it is typically recommended to use a large-bore catheter to decrease the likelihood of the catheter going into a false tract and exacerbating the injury (answer B). In the absence of concomitant bladder neck or rectal injuries, repair should be delayed. Immediate open urethroplasty of posterior injuries is complicated by poor visualization and difficulty assessing the injury due to acute swelling and bruising.

Furthermore, incontinence (21%) and impotence (56%) rates are higher when compared to delayed repair, which should always be done by a specialist (answer D). The gold standard for treatment is a delayed urethroplasty, which usually occurs after 3 months, when all orthopedic injuries have healed, and swelling has resolved. Patients will usually maintain suprapubic catheterization during this time. Nephrostomy drains will not decompress the bladder (answer E).

Answer: C

Cooperberg, M. R., McAninch, J. W., Alsikafi, N. F., & Elliott, S. P. (2007). Urethral reconstruction for traumatic posterior urethral disruption: outcomes of a 25-year experience. *The Journal of Urology, 178*(5), 2006–2010.

Martínez-Piñeiro, L., Djakovic, N., Plas, E., Mor, Y., Santucci, R. A., Serafetinidis, E., . . . & Hohenfellner, M. (2010). EAU guidelines on urethral trauma. *European Urology, 57*(5), 791–803.

Mundy, A. R. (1991). The role of delayed primary repair in the acute management of pelvic fracture injuries of the urethra. *British Journal of Urology, 68*(3), 273–276.

7   Which of the following strategies is most reliably proven to reduce the risk of contrast-associated acute kidney injury (CA-AKI)?
   A   Limit contrast administration to those with a glomerular filtration rate (GFR) of greater than 90 mL/min
   B   Initiate early renal replacement therapy to clear contrast in patients with baseline renal compromise
   C   Utilize high-osmolar contrast over low-osmolar contrast when able
   D   Start a bicarbonate drip and give N-acetylcysteine before and after the contrast dose
   E   Pre-hydrate patient prior to contrast dose with isotonic crystalloid

There are several proposed mechanisms that are felt to be associated with AKI after contrast administration. Contrast may lead to increased blood viscosity and cause vasoconstriction, thus leading to decreased blood flow to the renal medulla. Another proposed mechanism is direct cellular damage to the endothelial and tubular cells that's compounded by increased urine viscosity. A rise in creatinine is typically not seen until 2–6 days after exposure to contrast. Rates of CA-AKI have been reported to occur between 1.3 and 15.8% of the time after contrast administration. Risk factors include GFR < 45 (answer A), advanced age, women, malignancy, anemia, and cardiovascular disease, among others.

Multiple preventative strategies have been proposed. Many protocols advocate the use of N-acetylcysteine and bicarbonate (answer D). Bicarbonate is thought to be a scavenger for free radicals, while N-acetylcysteine is associated with decreased creatinine production. Diuretics have been used in an effort to increase tubular flow and mitigate the effects of the contrast on the renal tubules. The PRESERVE and AMACING trials found no interventions superior to pre-hydration with isotonic crystalloid (answer E) in preventing death, need for dialysis, or persistent renal dysfunction at 90 days. Renal replacement therapy has not been shown to decrease CA-AKI (answer B). Although dialysis can remove up to 70–80% of contrast, it's thought that the fluid shifts that occur during a dialysis session offset the benefits.

Some interventions have shown promise in reducing CA-AKI rates but are not commonly adopted. Vitamins C and E have antioxidant scavenging effects and have shown promise in limited trails in reducing CA-AKI. Also, statins have anti-inflammatory, antioxidant, and antithrombotic properties and have been shown in several studies to decrease AKI in patients undergoing coronary angiography. An expert panel of the European Society of Intensive Care Medicine now suggests the use of rosuvastatin or atorvastatin in patients undergoing coronary angiography to decrease rates of CA-AKI. Further studies are needed prior to widespread application.

Answer: E

Chalikias, G, Drosos, I., Tziakas, D. N. (2016). Contrast-induced acute kidney injury: an update. *Cardiovascular Drugs and Therapy, 30*(2), 215–228.

Nijssen, E. C., Rennenberg, R. J., Nelemans, P. J., Essers, B. A., Janssen, M. M., Vermeeren, M. A., . . . & Wildberger, J. E. (2017). Prophylactic hydration to protect renal function from intravascular iodinated contrast material in patients at high risk of contrast-induced nephropathy (AMACING): a prospective, randomised, phase 3, controlled, open-label, non-inferiority trial. *Lancet, 389*(10076), 1312–1322.

Weisbord, S. D., Gallagher, M., Jneid, H., Garcia, S., Cass, A., Thwin, S. S., . . . & Parikh, C. R. (2018). Outcomes after angiography with sodium bicarbonate and acetylcysteine. *New England Journal of Medicine, 378*(7), 603–614.

8   23-year-old man who was performing skateboard tricks on camera presents to the hospital after slipping during a stunt. On review of the video, you see the skateboard slip out from under him resulting in blunt trauma to his genitalia from a metal hand rail. What is the best means to assess for blunt testicular trauma?

A *Physical exam alone*
B *Testicular ultrasound*
C *CT scan of the pelvis*
D *MRI pelvis with contrast*
E *Operative exploration*

Testicular ultrasound with a linear-array transducer is the imaging modality of choice in blunt testicular trauma. It is nonionizing, reliably depicts the tunica albuginea to indicate rupture, and can visualize hematomas. When coupled with color flow, testicular perfusion can further be assessed. Testicular rupture requires operative exploration and removal of any nonviable tissue. Salvage with prompt intervention within 72 hours of injury results in a >80% testicular salvage rate. Testicular rupture can occur with a normal overlying scrotum, so physical exam alone is not adequate (answer A). Ultrasound also has superior sensitivity and specificity for scrotal rupture when compared to CT and MRI (answers C and D respectively). Imaging should be conducted prior to operative intervention for a blunt testicular mechanism unless there is clear evidence of testicular trauma on exam (answer E).

Answer: B

Bhatt, S., & Dogra, V. S. (2008). Role of US in testicular and scrotal trauma. *Radiographics, 28*(6), 1617–1629.

Deurdulian, C., Mittelstaedt, C. A., Chong, W. K., & Fielding, J. R. (2007). US of acute scrotal trauma: optimal technique, imaging findings, and management. *Radiographics, 27*, 357–369.

Holliday, T. L., Robinson, K. S., Dorinzi, N., Vucelik, A. W., Setzer, E. L., Williams, D. L., . . . & Minardi, J. J. (2017). Testicular rupture: a tough nut to crack. *Clinical Practice and Cases in Emergency Medicine, 1*(3), 221.

9 *Which imaging technique has the highest sensitivity and specificity for detecting bladder rupture?*
   A *A retrograde plain film cystogram with filling of the bladder to no more than 100 mL*
   B *Ultrasound with power color Doppler*
   C *CT scan with IV contrast and delayed images and a clamped Foley*
   D *CT cystogram with filling the bladder to at least 350 mL using water-soluble contrast*
   E *CT cystogram with filling the bladder to at least 350 mL using barium*

An appropriately performed CT cystogram has a very high sensitivity and specificity for bladder rupture (95–99% and 95–100%, respectively). A CT cystogram involves retrograde filling of the bladder with dilute water-soluble contrast to a volume of at least 350 mL. In the case of intraperitoneal rupture, water-soluble contrast is inert, while barium can provoke a profound peritonitis (answer E). Conventional CT scan of the abdomen and pelvis, even with delayed images, can miss up to 40% of bladder ruptures, even with clamping a Foley catheter, as there is typically inadequate intravesicular volume to distend the bladder (answer C). While power Doppler is an ultrasound adjunct to traditional color Doppler that can provide better assessment of low-flow fluids, such as a ureteral jet, it has no described role in the detection of bladder injuries (answer B). Finally, while a retrograde plain film cystogram has a reported sensitivity of nearly 100% in some trials, a CT scan provides better resolution of the injury and has a higher specificity (answer A). In times where the patient is being taken emergently to the operating room and bladder rupture is suspected, a plain film cystogram can be performed rapidly. The study is performed by placing a Foley catheter and performing a pelvic x-ray. The bladder is then filled with 350 mL of dilute contrast, the Foley is clamped, and another anterior-posterior pelvic film is performed. Finally, the bladder is allowed to drain and a final plain film is obtained to look for extravasated contrast that was initially obscured by the radio-opaque bladder. Extraperitoneal bladder injury is noted by a "flame sign," while intraperitoneal bladder injury may show outlining of loops of bowel.

Answer: D

Doyle, S. M., Master, V. A., & McAninch, J. W. (2005). Appropriate use of CT in the diagnosis of bladder rupture. *Journal of the American College of Surgeons, 200*(6), 973.

Quagliano, P. V., Delair, S. M., & Malhotra, A. K. (2006). Diagnosis of blunt bladder injury: a prospective comparative study of computed tomography cystography and conventional retrograde cystography. *Journal of Trauma and Acute Care Surgery, 61*(2), 410–422.

Stern, N., Pignanelli, M., & Welk, B. (2019). The management of an extraperitoneal bladder injury associated with a pelvic fracture. *Canadian Urological Association Journal, 13*(6 Suppl4), S56.

10 *A 52-year-old man with history of diabetes presents to the emergency department with a 3-day history of progressively increasing painful cellulitis involving the scrotum and perineum. Which of the following laboratory findings is most suggestive of Fournier's gangrene?*
   A *CRP of 21 mg/dL*
   B *WBC count of 22 000/mm³*
   C *Hemoglobin of 11.5 g/dL*
   D *Blood glucose of 325 mg/dL*
   E *Sodium of 129 mmol/L*

Fournier's gangrene refers to a rapidly-progressive necrotizing soft tissue infection (NSTI) of the external genitalia, perianal region, and/or perineum. It's named after Jean-Alfred Fournier, a Parisian venereologist, who described a patient with the disease bearing his name in a lecture in 1883. Despite incredible medical advances since that time, mortality remains around 20–40% in some case series; therefore, a high index of suspicion and early treatment is required. When clinical concern is high, the diagnosis is made clinically and should prompt immediate surgical debridement. In cases where there is debate, one common adjunct used is the Laboratory Risk Indicator for Necrotizing Fasciitis (LRINEC) score. In the initial study, 10% of patients with a LRINEC score < 6 has necrotizing fasciitis, while a score of ≥ 6 had a positive predictive value of 92% and negative predictive value of 96%. In subsequent validation studies, these numbers have not been reproduced, but it remains a popular scoring system. Of all the components, a CRP ≥ 15 mg/dL is the most predictive of an NSTI. The components with their relative point assignments are as follows:

- CRP (mg/dL)
  - <15: 0 points
  - ≥15: 4 points
- WBC count ($\times 10^3$/mm^3)
  - <15: 0 points
  - 15–25: 1 point
  - >25: 2 points
- Hemoglobin (g/dL)
  - >13.5: 0 points
  - 11–13.5: 1 point
  - <11: 2 points
- Sodium (mmol/L)
  - ≥135: 0 points
  - <135: 2 points
- Creatinine (mg/dL)
  - ≤1.6: 0 points
  - >1.6: 2 points
- Glucose (mg/dL)
  - ≤180: 0 points
  - >180: 1 point

Answer: A

Hagedorn, J. C., & Wessells, H. (2017). A contemporary update on Fournier's gangrene. *Nature Reviews Urology*, 14(4), 205–214.

Mallikarjuna, M. N., Vijayakumar, A., Patil, V. S., & Shivswamy, B. S. (2012). Fournier's gangrene: current practices. *International Scholarly Research Notices*, 2012, 942437.

Wong, C. (2004). The LRINEC (Laboratory Risk Indicator for Necrotizing Fasciitis) score: a tool for distinguishing necrotizing fasciitis from other soft tissue infections. *Critical Care Medicine*. 32(7):1535–1541.

11 *A 54-year-old man presents to the trauma bay after a motor vehicle collision. He is found to have a pelvic fracture and urinary retention. Due to concern for a urethral injury, urology successfully placed an 18-French Foley catheter without any urethral imaging. Microscopic hematuria is noted. CT scan demonstrates no renal, ureteral, or bladder injury. In order to guide how soon the catheter can be removed, the trauma team requests urethral imaging. Which option provides the most reliable data with the least risk to the patient?*

A *Remove the catheter most of the way, inflate 1–3 mL of saline in the balloon, and inject contrast through the Foley*

B *Insert an angiocath or 5-Fr sheath into the urethra and inject contrast around the Foley*

C *Perform a CT scan of the pelvis with the Foley balloon down and delayed imaging to allow contrast to leak around the Foley*

D *Place a wire through the Foley and perform a traditional urethrogram*

E *Just leave the Foley in place for 2 weeks*

The presence of a pelvic fracture with urinary retention and hematuria are all concerning for urethral injury. Prior to placement of a catheter, urethral injuries should be evaluated by performing a retrograde urethrogram (RUG). This would be a reliable means to assess for injury, but if an injury was discovered in this patient, there would be risk of causing an injury by replacing the Foley again (not A). A peri-catheter RUG is a technique most commonly used by urologists after urethroplasty to ensure the catheter can safely be removed. Most papers describe inserting a 5-Fr sheath in the urethra next to the catheter and then using manual pressure or a special clamp to hold the sheath in place while the contrast is instilled. In the image below, an 18-Ga angiocath was used on the above-listed patient to confirm the absence of a urethral injury, allowing the Foley to be removed shortly thereafter. Performing a delayed IV contrasted CT scan would be an unreliable way to achieve complete opacification of the urethra (not C). While placing a wire through the catheter would help maintain access to the true lumen in the case of an injury, it would require fluoroscopy and more resources than a simple peri-catheter RUG (not D). Since catheters should be removed as early as possible, it's not appropriate to leave a catheter in place for an injury that has not been definitively diagnosed (Not E)

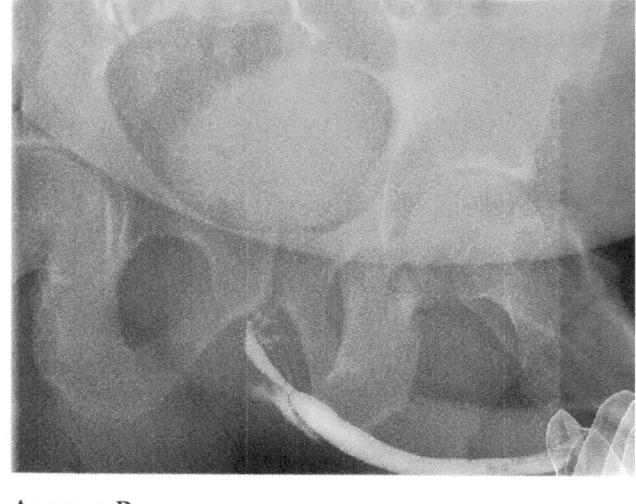

Answer: B

Balogun, B. O., Ikuerowo, S. O., Akintomide, T. E., & Esho, J. O. (2009). Retrograde peri-catheter urethrogram for the post-operative evaluation of the urethra. *African Journal of Medicine and Medical Sciences*, *38*(2), 131–134.

Sussman, R. D., Hill, F. C., Koch, G. E., Patel, V., & Venkatesan, K. (2017). Novel peri-catheter retrograde urethrogram technique is a viable method for postoperative urethroplasty imaging. *International Urology and Nephrology*, *49*(12), 2157–2165.

12 *A 21-year-old man was standing on the sidewalk at night when a stranger shot him multiple times in the abdomen and assaulted him. He was taken immediately to the operating room, where he underwent a small bowel resection, sigmoidectomy, diverting loop ileostomy, and abdominal closure. Postoperatively he underwent a CT scan to assess for any other injuries. On delayed imaging, he was noted to have disruption of the pelvic portion of the left ureter. What is the next best step in management?*

A *Reimage in 72 hours and place a percutaneous drain in a uroma if present*

B *Percutaneous nephrostomy tube placement*

C *Cystoscopy with attempted stenting*

D *Return to the operating room for primary ureteroureterostomy*

E *Return to the operating room for direct reimplantation into the bladder (ureteroneocystostomy)*

Ureteral injuries are an uncommon direct consequence of trauma, occurring in <1% of blunt and <4% of penetrating injuries. Ureteral injuries should be classified by location: ureteropelvic junction (UPJ), abdominal ureter (UPJ to the iliac vessels), and pelvic ureter (iliac vessels to the bladder). When ureteral injuries are discovered in

the operating room, immediate repair should be considered in hemodynamically stable patients. Injuries that are diagnosed post-operatively should undergo repair if diagnosed within 72 hours. After that point, ureteral stenting and/or nephrostomy tube placement should be considered with repair at 6 weeks.

To perform ureteral repair, first debride any devitalized tissue. For transection of the abdominal ureter, primary ureteroureterostomy may be performed if there is no tension after debridement. The ureteral ends should be spatulated, and a water-tight, tension-free, mucosa-to-mucosa anastomosis with interrupted absorbable suture (approx. 5-0) may be performed over a stent. If tension exists, the proximal ureter is anastomosed to the contralateral ureter via a window in the mesocolon (transureteroureterostomy) or to the bladder with a psoas hitch or Boari flap.

When the pelvic ureter is transected, the proximal ureter should be reimplanted into the bladder (ureteroneocystostomy), so answer E is correct. This may be facilitated with a psoas hitch or Boari flap. A psoas hitch involves pulling the bladder dome cephalad and suturing it to the psoas tendon to offload tension. A Boari flap involves using a tubularized portion of the bladder as an anastomotic conduit.

There is no role for watchful waiting with ureteral transections (not A). Since the injury was detected within 72 hours, immediate repair is warranted as long as the patient is otherwise stable (not B). A stent, if able to traverse the injury, would be a temporizing maneuver for delayed repair. Again, given the temporal proximity of the injury, immediate repair is warranted (not C). Finally, implantation into the bladder is widely preferred over ureteroureterostomy for distal injuries, as the blood supply to the distal injury may have been disrupted during the inciting trauma (not D).

Answer: E

Engelsgjerd, J. S., & LaGrange, C. A. Ureteral Injury. [Updated 2020 Jul 10]. In: *StatPearls [Internet]*. Treasure Island (FL): StatPearls Publishing; 2020. https://www. ncbi.nlm.nih.gov/books/NBK507817/.

Martínez-Piñeiro, L., Djakovic, N., Plas, E., Mor, Y., Santucci, R. A., Serafetinidis, E., . . . & Hohenfellner, M. (2010). EAU guidelines on urethral trauma. *European Urology*, *57*(5), 791–803.

Morey, A. F., Brandes, S., Dugi, D. D., Armstrong, J. H., Breyer, B. N., Broghammer, J. A., . . . & Reston, J. T. (2014). Urotrauma: AUA guideline. *The Journal of Urology*, *192*(2), 327–335.

13 *A 32-year-old woman presents to the hospital after multiple gunshot wounds to the abdomen. She is* *unstable on arrival and is taken immediately to the operating room, where she undergoes splenectomy, descending colectomy, and small bowel resection. During your exploration, you note a transected left ureter with a large defect around the mid-portion. She remains acidotic and hypotensive. What is the best option for immediate management of her ureteral injury?*

A *Ligation with percutaneous nephrostomy*

B *Spatulated primary ureteroureterostomy*

C *Trans-ureteroureterostomy*

D *Reimplantation into the bladder with a psoas hitch or Boari flap*

E *Call urology to perform cystoscopy with retrograde stenting*

For patients with ureteral transections who are unlikely to tolerate a formal repair, the most expeditious treatment option is ligation to prevent a uroma and percutaneous nephrostomy tube placement is appropriate with plans for delayed repair after 6 weeks. Any attempt at surgical repair would be time-consuming and be at high risk for stricture and leak complications related to poor perfusion (not B, C, or D). If immediate expertise and supplies are available for stenting, that is an option, but waiting for another service to arrive and get supplies for cystoscopy and stenting adds unnecessary delays in getting the patient to the ICU for further resuscitation (not E).

Answer: A

Engelsgjerd, J. S., & LaGrange, C. A. Ureteral Injury. [Updated 2020 Jul 10]. In: *StatPearls [Internet]*. Treasure Island (FL): StatPearls Publishing; 2020. https://www.ncbi.nlm.nih.gov/books/NBK507817/.

Martínez-Piñeiro, L., Djakovic, N., Plas, E., Mor, Y., Santucci, R. A., Serafetinidis, E., . . . & Hohenfellner, M. (2010). EAU guidelines on urethral trauma. *European Urology*, *57*(5), 791–803.

Morey, A. F., Brandes, S., Dugi, D. D., Armstrong, J. H., Breyer, B. N., Broghammer, J. A., . . . & Reston, J. T. (2014). Urotrauma: AUA guideline. *The Journal of Urology*, *192*(2), 327–335.

14 *A 55-year-old obese woman presents to the trauma bay after a motor vehicle collision. She is hemodynamically stable with an elevated heart rate to 119 beats/min.*

Her FAST exam is positive only in the suprapubic region. Chest x-ray and pelvic x-ray are unremarkable. On physical exam, she has an abdominal seatbelt sign. A Foley catheter is placed with blood and scant urine returned. CT scan is obtained, which identifies a grade 2 intraparenchymal liver injury and free fluid around the Foley catheter with associated stranding of small bowel mesentery suspicious for either bladder rupture or bowel injury. Which of the following is the next best option?

A *Exploratory laparotomy, EndoGIA for repair of all injuries*

B *Exploratory laparotomy, double-layer repair of all injuries*

C *Exploratory laparoscopy with intrabdominal drains and continued Foley drainage*

D *Cystogram and push endoscopy*

E *Admission with repeat CT scan in 6 hours*

Most blunt bladder injuries occur at the dome of the bladder. Patients with full bladders prior to high-speed motor vehicle collisions are at especially high risk of rupture. The majority of intraperitoneal ruptures will require operative repair. The bladder should be inspected to ensure the ureteral orifices are uninvolved. Rarely, an anterior cystotomy will be required to ensure adequate efflux of urine. Intraperitoneal bladder injuries should not be delayed (not E). As there is a risk of concomitant bowel and bladder injury with an associated liver injury, exploratory laparotomy is warranted with repair at that time (not C or D). Bladder repair should be in two or more layers using absorbable suture. Multiple studies have demonstrated an increased risk of infection and stone formation with nonabsorbable stapling of the bladder (not A).

Answer: B

Leslie, S. W., Sajjad, H., & Murphy, P. B. Bladder Stones. [Updated 2020 Jun 12]; 2020. Available from: https://www.ncbi.nlm.nih.gov/books/NBK441944/.

Morey, A. F., Brandes, S., Dugi, D. D., Armstrong, J. H., Breyer, B. N., Broghammer, J. A., . . . & Reston, J. T. (2014). Urotrauma: AUA guideline. *The Journal of Urology*, *192*(2), 327–335.

Rödder, K., Olianas, R., & Fisch, M. (2005). [Bladder injury. Diagnostics and treatment]. *Urologe A*, *44*(8), 878–882.

35

Care of the Pregnant Trauma Patient

Navdeep Samra, MD[1] and Jaideep Sandhu, MBBS, MPH[2]

[1] LSU Health, Shreveport, LA, USA
[2] City of Hope National Medical Center, Duarte, CA, USA

1 *What is the leading cause of trauma in pregnant women?*
   A *Motor vehicle collisions*
   B *Intimate partner violence*
   C *Falls*
   D *Poisoning/overdoses*
   E *Penetrating trauma*

MVC is the leading mechanism of maternal injury, which causes non-obstetric maternal deaths. MVC is one of the prominent causes of fetal and maternal mortality. It is estimated that maternal and fetal mortality rates are 3.7 and 1.4 per 10 000 pregnancies, respectively. Prevention strategies such as usage of proper seat belt reduces the risk of adverse outcomes for both mother and fetus.

Answer: A

Weiss HB, Sauber-Schatz EK, Cook LJ. The epidemiology of pregnancy-associated emergency department injury visits and their impact on birth outcomes. *Accid Anal Prev.* 2008;40(3):1088–1095.

Mendez-Figueroa H, Dahlke JD, Vrees RA, Rouse DJ. Trauma in pregnancy: an updated systematic review. *Am J Obstet Gynecol.* 2013;209(1):1–10.

2 *A physician was educating a pregnant woman about trauma in pregnancy. At the end of the counseling session, she posed a question about if she is at increased risk for falls related trauma. The risk for fall in pregnancy increases the most during:*
   A *1st, 2nd, and 3rd months of pregnancy*
   B *6th, 7th, 8th months of pregnancy*
   C *9th month of pregnancy*
   D *Equal throughout the pregnancy*
   E *Pregnancy does not increase the risk of fall*

Falls are one of the leading cause of injury during the pregnancy, second in number to motor vehicle crashes. Falls during the pregnancy can lead to multiple injuries with varying severity: sprains, fractures, head injury, abruptio placentae, rupture of uterus and membranes, and sometimes fetal or maternal death. Almost 2/3 (61%) of the fall occur during 6th through 8th gestational months. The anatomical and physiologic changes that occur during the pregnancy increases the risk for falls. The center of gravity shifts forward with the fetus and the hormonal changes causes loosening of joints causes hypermobility, putting the stability of pregnant women at risk of fall. Furthermore, studies show that there is an increase in postural sway during second and third trimesters, adding further instability to the pregnant women.

Answer: B

Dunning K, LeMasters G, Bhattacharya A. A major public health issue: the high incidence of falls during pregnancy. *Matern Child Health J.* 2010;14(5):720–725.

Harland KK, Saftlas AF, Yankowitz J, Peek-Asa C. Risk factors for maternal injuries in a population-based sample of pregnant women. *J Womens Health.* 2014;23(12):1033–1038.

3 *A 24-year-old woman was involved in a minor motor vehicle accident. A pregnancy test was performed and she was at 27 weeks of gestation. The patient was wearing a seat belt when the car slipped into the telephone pole. Her blood pressure is 112/83 mm Hg, pulse 116 beats/min, respiration 23 breaths/min, and SaO_2 is 96%. Emergency physician completed the*

Surgical Critical Care and Emergency Surgery: Clinical Questions and Answers, Third Edition.
Edited by Forrest "Dell" Moore, Peter M. Rhee, and Carlos J. Rodriguez.
© 2022 John Wiley & Sons Ltd. Published 2022 by John Wiley & Sons Ltd.
Companion website: www.wiley.com/go/surgicalcriticalcare3e

primary assessment. After completing the primary assessment (ABC), what is the next best step?

A *Wait and watch for any hemodynamic changes*

B *Transfer the patient to the radiology department for a CT imaging*

C *Place an indwelling urinary catheter and reassess the patient after 6 hours*

D *Initiate fetal heart monitoring*

E *Call obstetric consultation*

While noting the vital signs in the event of trauma to the pregnant woman, it is helpful to keep in mind that the heart rate increases in the pregnancy by 15%. Typical signs of hypovolemic shock, tachycardia, and hypotension can be masked by normal physiologic changes in the pregnancy. Signs of hypovolemic shocks can appear late in pregnant trauma patients due to increased plasma volume. Maternal perfusion and vital signs are preserved in the pregnant trauma patient at the expense of uteroplacental perfusion. It is not uncommon in the pregnant trauma patients to note significant loss of blood without any signs of hemodynamic instability, which in turn may have already reduced uteroplacental perfusion. Therefore, in the pregnant patients who are ≥ 23 weeks of gestation age, fetal heart monitoring should be initiated as earlytas possible. Abnormal or atypical fetal heart rate pattern may be the first indicator of significant blood loss or maternal hypovolemia, which is putting fetus at elevated risk of shock.

Answer: D

Jain V, Chari R, Maslovitz S, et al. Guidelines for the management of a pregnant trauma patient. *J Obstet Gynaecol Can.* 2015;37(6):553–574.

Murphy NJ, Quinlan JD. Trauma in pregnancy: assessment, management, and prevention. *Am Fam Physician.* 2014;90(10):717–722.

4 *A 26-year-old G1P0 woman at 35 weeks of pregnancy was in an MVC. She was wearing her seatbelt when a truck hit her car from the back. Her blood pressure is 109/70 mm Hg, pulse 120 beats/min, respirations are 28 breaths/min, and SaO_2 is 92%. One liter of normal saline is given through large-bore IV. Fetal heart monitoring is initiated and the nurse asks if you want the Kleihauer-Betke test ordered. What is Kleihauer-Betke test used for?*

A *The presence of disseminated intravascular coagulopathy (DIC)*

B *Assessing fetal maturity*

C *Identifying Rh status of the mother*

D *Identifying fetal blood group*

E *Identifying fetal blood cells in the maternal circulation*

The Kleihauer-Betke (KB) test is conducted on the maternal blood to determine the amount of fetal hemoglobin (HgF) in the maternal circulation that may have leaked due to the break in placental barrier. Multiple reasons can lead to this placental disruption, including trauma. Trauma is a leading cause of pregnancy-associated maternal deaths in America. When fetomaternal hemorrhage occurs, HgF get mixed with maternal blood, which in turn triggers maternal immune system. Activation of maternal immune system can lead to isoimmunization if the mother is RhD negative and fetus blood type is RhD positive. RhoGAM is indicated to prevent isoimmunization (formation of Anti-RhD antibodies).

RhoGAM (rho(d) immune globulin) is used to prevent antibodies from forming when a mother has Rh-negative blood and the fetus is Rh-positive or presumed to be positive, therefore answers A, B, C, and D are incorrect.

A single 300 microgram dose contains sufficient anti-D to suppress the immune response to 15 mL of D-positive red cells (or 30 mL fetal D-positive whole blood). A single 50 microgram dose contains sufficient anti-D to suppress the immune response to 2.5 mL of D-positive red cells (or 5 mL fetal whole blood).

Fetomaternal bleeding has been reported in 2.6–30% of pregnant trauma patients.

Answer: E

Murphy NJ, Quinlan JD. Trauma in pregnancy: assessment, management, and prevention. *Am Fam Physician.* 2014;90(10):717–722.

Krywko DM, Yarrarapu SNS, Shunkwiler SM. *Kleihauer Betke Test. StatPearls.* Treasure Island (FL), 2020.

Muench MV, Baschat AA, Reddy UM, et al. Kleihauer-betke testing is important in all cases of maternal trauma. *J Trauma.* 2004;57(5):1094–1098.

Committee on practice bulletins-obstetrics. Practice bulletin no. 181: Prevention of Rh D alloimmunization. *Obstet Gynecol* 2017; 130:e57. Reaffirmed 2019.

Wylie BJ, D'Alton ME. Fetomaternal hemorrhage. *Obstet Gynecol* 2010; 115:1039.

5 *A 27-year-old G1P0 woman at 34 weeks of gestation was involved in a MVC. Her blood pressure is 95/65 mm Hg, pulse 125 beats/min, respirations are 28 breaths/min, equal bilaterally, and SaO_2 is 92%. Her Glasgow Coma Scale score is 10. IV access was obtained. What is the next best step?*

A *Transfer the patient to the radiology for CT imaging*

B *Call obstetric consultation*

C *Chest X ray*

D *Tilt the backboard or use left lateral decubitus positioning*

E *Observe as hypotension could be transient*

After the primary assessment (ABC), the next best step is to use left lateral decubitus positioning. Patient is hypotensive on primary survey and a quick and the relatively easy maneuver can be attempted to treat the abnormality found in the primary survey. This is done to reduce inferior vena cava compression by the uterus and increase venous return to the heart when the blood pressure is low. Aortocaval compression is also called supine hypotension. This pathophysiologic state is usually seen after 20 weeks of gestation when patient is placed straight supine position. The uterus compresses the inferior vena cava and impede the blood flow from lower extremities to the central circulation thereby cause hypotension in pregnant patients. Subsequently, this compression and resulting hypotension limit the blood flow to the placenta and increases the risk of both morbidity and mortality to both mother and fetus. Physiologic changes in pregnancy results in peripheral vasodilation, which is mediated through endothelium-dependent factors and vasodilatory prostaglandins (PGI2); 25–30% decrease in systemic vascular resistance is attributed to peripheral vasodilation, which is compensated by increase in cardiac output. It is stated that turning the pregnant woman from lateral position to the supine may lead to the reduction of cardiac output by 25%, which in turn decrease the blood flow of the uterus and interfere in placental perfusion, thereby compromise the health status of the fetus. Transferring a patient to the CT scan would not be appropriate in a hypotensive patient (choice A). Obtaining a consultation may be useful, but it is not the next step (choice B). The chest X-ray is also a high priority, but one should do what is known (treating hypotension) before looking for the unknown to treat (Choice C). Observing a hypotensive patient is obviously incorrect (choice E).

Answer: D

Krywko DM, King KC. *Aortocaval Compression Syndrome. StatPearls.* Treasure Island (FL), 2020.

Kinsella SM, Lohmann G. Supine hypotensive syndrome. *Obstet Gynecol.* 1994;83(5):774–788.

Soma-Pillay P, Nelson-Piercy C, Tolppanen H, Mebazaa A. Physiological changes in pregnancy. *Cardiovasc J Afr.* 2016;27(2):89–94. doi:10.5830/CVJA-2016-021.

6 *A 19-year-old G2P1 woman came to her obstetrician's office to discuss end her pregnancy at the gestational age of 29 weeks. She has not initiated prenatal care until now. Her gestational weight gain is inadequate. Her vitals are within normal limits. Physical exam shows injuries at her back and breasts at different stages of healing. The physician screened the patient for intimate partner violence. What are the most significant risk factor for intimate partner violence in pregnant woman?*

A *Young age, poverty, and relationship status-single*

B *High educational level and employment*

C *Relationship status – married and employment*

D *High socioeconomic status*

E *Planned pregnancy*

Intimate Partner Violence (IPV) is a serious public health challenge, which results in adverse health outcomes for both mother and fetus. It is potentially a preventable problem. Data shows that 3–9% of women experience IPV during the pregnancy. Literature indicates that there are well-known risk factors, which are associated with high rates of abuse; these risk factors includes poverty, young age, single relationship status, low educational level, and minority race. IPV can lead to multiple negative outcomes, which include low weight gain, 1st/2nd trimester bleeding, preterm birth, hemorrhage, uterine rupture, hospitalization, and death. Placenta abruption, which contributes to 12% of all perinatal deaths, is also linked to IPV. Physical violence such as blunt force to abdomen by their partner is one of the top leading cause on list of pregnancy trauma. The types of violence can be physical, sexual, psychological, emotional, spiritual, cultural, verbal, and even financial.

Answer: A

Alhusen JL, Ray E, Sharps P, Bullock L. Intimate partner violence during pregnancy: maternal and neonatal outcomes. *J Womens Health (Larchmt).* 2015;24(1):100–106.

Leone JM, Lane SD, Koumans EH, et al. Effects of intimate partner violence on pregnancy trauma and placental abruption. *J Womens Health (Larchmt).* 2010;19(8):1501–1509.

Centers for Disease Control and Prevention (2020). Risk Factors for Intimate Partner Violence Perpetration. https://www.cdc.gov/violenceprevention/intimatepartnerviolence/riskprotectivefactors.html (accesses 27 July 2021).

7 *A 29-year-old who is 32 weeks pregnant was involved in an MVC. Her blood pressure is 85/60 mm Hg, pulse 120 beats/min, and SaO₂ was 93%. You are concerned*

about hemorrhagic shock. Hemorrhagic shock may also lead to:

A *Fetal bradycardia*

B *Fetal demise*

C *Pituitary insufficiency*

D *Late or variable decelerations on fetal heart rate monitoring*

E *All of the above*

Hemorrhagic shock contributes to approximately 40% of total trauma mortality. Traumatic hemorrhagic shock accounts for about 6–7% of total deaths in pregnancy. Hypotension, as marked below ≤90 mm Hg, is commonly used to identify patients who are experiencing hemorrhagic shock. Hemorrhagic shock in pregnancy may lead to fetal bradycardia, fetal demise, and pituitary insufficiency. Shock index was found to be highly associated with early blood product transfusions compared to systolic blood pressure in injured pregnant trauma patients. Shock index is calculated by dividing your heart rate by your systolic blood pressure. While this may seem difficult to calculate during a crisis, a simple rule of thumb is that if your heart rate is greater than your systolic blood pressure, your shock index is greater than 1. Shock index of greater than 1 has been associated with the need for blood transfusions, higher injury severity, and need for intervention.

Answer: E

Jenkins PC, Stokes SM, Fakoyeho S, Bell TM, Zarzaur BL. Clinical indicators of hemorrhagic shock in pregnancy. *Trauma Surg Acute Care Open*. 2017;2(1):e000112.

Joseph B, Haider AA, Pandit V, et al. Impact of hemorrhagic shock on pituitary function. *J Am Coll Surg*. 2015;221(2):502–508.

Pillarisetty LS, Bragg BN. *Late Decelerations. StatPearls*. Treasure Island (FL), 2020.

8 *A 24-year-old who was 20 weeks pregnant fell down a flight of stairs. She has left chest pain and her breathing is splinted. You ordered a chest X-ray. What is radiation dose of chest X-ray?*

A *0.001 mSv*

B *0.1 mSv*

C *1.5 mSv*

D *2.0 mSv*

E *7 mSv*

The approximate effective radiation dose for chest X-ray is 0.1 mSv. The approximate radiation dose for extremity (hand, foot, etc.) X-ray and chest CT is 0.001 mSv and 7 mSv, respectively.

Radiology procedure	Effective radiation dose (approximate)
X-ray extremity (hand, foot, etc.)	0.001 mSv
X-ray dental	0.005 mSv
X-ray chest	0.1 mSv
X-ray spine	1.5 mSv
CT Head	2 mSv
CT Chest	7 mSv
CT Abdomen and pelvis	10 mSv

Answer: B

Radiation Dose in X-Ray and CT Exams (2019). https://www.radiologyinfo.org/en/info.cfm?pg=safety-xray. Cited in U.S. Food & Drug Administration. Medical X-ray Imaging. https://www.fda.gov/radiation-emitting-products/medical-imaging/medical-x-ray-imaging (accessed 27 July 2021).

Ratnapalan S, Bentur Y, Koren G. "Doctor, will that x-ray harm my unborn child?" (vol 179, pg 1293, 2008). *Can Med Assoc J*. 2009;180(9):952–952.

9 *A 23-year-old G2P1 who is 32 weeks pregnant has severe abdominal pain after tripping and falling down a flight of stairs. Her blood pressure was 105/67 mm Hg, pulse 125 beats/min, respirations are 25 breaths/min and SaO$_2$ is 94%. She has abdominal pain and vaginal discharge. Which of the following is the highest risk factor for placenta abruption?*

A *Young age*

B *Nulliparous*

C *Hypotension*

D *Hypothyroid*

E *Trauma*

The premature separation of placenta from the uterus is placental abruption. It can decrease the supply of oxygen and nutrients to the fetus. Placental abruption occurs frequently in the last trimester of pregnancy, especially close to time of birth. The presentation of placental abruption includes abdominal pain, vaginal bleeding, uterine tenderness, and frequent uterine contractions. Often, placenta abruption starts with sudden onset of back or abdominal pain. The severity of vaginal bleeding depends on amount of separation of placenta from uterus. Risk factors for placental abruption include increased maternal age, chronic hypertension, cocaine use, history of previous abruption, and trauma. Placental abruption can result in health consequences of both maternal (couvelaire uterus, hemorrhagic shock, DIC) and fetal (preterm, low birth weight, birth asphyxia); 50–70% of fetal death following trauma is attributed to placenta abruption. It is worth noting that major abruptions have been seen even after relatively minor injuries.

Answer: E

Talley CL, Edwards A, Wallace P. et al. Epidemiology of Trauma in Pregnancy. *Curr Trauma Rep.* 2018;4:205–210.

Ghaheh HS, Feizi A, Mousavi M, Sohrabi D, Mesghari L, Hosseini Z. Risk factors of placental abruption. *J Res Med Sci.* 2013;18(5):422–426.

Pitaphrom A, Sukcharoen N. Pregnancy outcomes in placental abruption. *J Med Assoc Thai.* 2006;89(10):1572–8. PMID: 17128829.

Tikkanen M, Nuutila M, Hiilesmaa V, Paavonen J, Ylikorkala O. Clinical presentation and risk factors of placental abruption. *Acta Obstet Gynecol Scand.* 2006;85(6):700–5. doi: 10.1080/00016340500449915. PMID: 16752262.

10 *A 22-year-old G1P0 pregnant woman was in a rollover MVC. She was ejected and suffered a severe traumatic brain injury. She was not wearing a seatbelt and her older sister states that she never wore a seatbelt when she was pregnant. You inform her that:*
   A *She should not wear seat belt as it can cause uterine rupture if in an MVC*
   B *Do not need it if driving within speed limits*
   C *Only need it when driving at high speed*
   D *It will kill the child if she is in an MVC*
   E *Wear a lap and shoulder belt every time while traveling*

The U.S. Department of Transportation (National Highway Traffic Safety Administration) and the American College of Obstetricians and Gynecologists (ACOG) recommend that during pregnancy, women should wear seat belts properly. It is recommended that everyone including pregnant woman should wear seat belt while riding the vehicle. Motor collisions or traffic accidents are one of the leading cause of deaths worldwide. The number increases when we add injured patients, injuries that lead to permanent disabilities. Road traffic accidents and trauma are often preventable. The most important innovation for vehicle crash safety which led to the reduction of mortality rates is the proper usage of seat belts. The scientific literature indicates significant negative correlation between seat belt compliance and traffic accident mortality rates. Approximately 2% of the pregnant woman are involved in motor accidents during the term of pregnancy. Over 50% of all trauma during pregnancy is attributed to motor vehicle accidents, and this accounts for 82% of fetal deaths. The use of seat belt decreases during the pregnancy because the pregnant woman fears that seat belt will hurt their fetus. However, it is estimated that if women wear seat belts properly, there would be about 84% reduction in the risk of adverse outcomes for fetus. For proper use, the lap belt needs to be placed under the dome of the abdomen and across the pelvis to reduce pressure on the uterus during a motor vehicle collision. The shoulder harness should lay across the clavicle and between the breasts.

Answer: E

Vladutiu CJ, Weiss HB. Motor vehicle safety during pregnancy. *Am J Lifestyle Med.* 2012;6(3):241–249.

The American College of Obstetricians and Gynecologists. ACOG (2018). Car Safety for Pregnant Women, Babies, and Children (accessed 27 July 27 2021).

Murphy NJ, Quinlan JD. Trauma in pregnancy: assessment, management, and prevention. *Am Fam Physician.* 2014;90(10):717–724.

Abbas AK, Hefny AF, Abu-Zidan FM. Seatbelts and road traffic collision injuries. *World J Emerg Surg.* 2011;6(18). https://doi.org/10.1186/1749-7922-6-18.

11 *A 21-year-old woman was a pedestrian struck by a car while she was crossing the road. She has severe chest pain and vaginal bleeding. She says she thinks she is pregnant and the nurse says she needs to be tested for possible pregnancy. The nurse also states that her blood pressure is <80/40 mm Hg by manual cuff pressure. What should be the primary focus of emergency physician while treating traumatized women who may be pregnant?*
   A *Continuous monitoring for any hemodynamic changes*
   B *Ultrasound her uterus*
   C *Radiologic imaging to identify injuries*
   D *Call for obstetric consultation*
   E *Assess airway, breathing, and circulation*

In the case of major trauma to the pregnant patient, primary focus of the primary assessment should be on the airway, breathing, and circulation (A, B, C). After securing the ABC, focus of assessment should move on to other obstetric/non-obstetric injuries and well-being of the fetus. Changes in pregnancy – both anatomical and physiological – influence the evaluation and treatment process for trauma in pregnancy. Physiologically, blood volume increases 30–50% and respiratory rate goes up by 40–50% in the pregnancy. Anatomically, as the pregnancy grows the uterus becomes prominent and is exposed to abdominal trauma whether it is blunt or penetrating. Severity of injuries and gestational age are the two main factors that are considered while managing the pregnant patient with trauma. Best outcome is when maternal health and well-being takes priority over the treatment strategies tailored toward fetus health. Determining gestational age is of use as the fetus is not viable if delivered at an age less than 23 weeks. If the gestational age is greater than 23 weeks, the patient may be transferred to the maternity unit for monitoring if the patient does not have any limb or life-threatening injury.

Answer: E

Murphy NJ, Quinlan JD. Trauma in pregnancy: assessment, management, and prevention. *Am Fam Physician*. 2014;90(10):717–722.

Krywko DM, Toy FK, Mahan ME, et al. Pregnancy Trauma. [Updated 2020 Dec 12]. In: *StatPearls [Internet]*. Treasure Island (FL): StatPearls Publishing; 2020. Available from: https://www.ncbi.nlm.nih.gov/books/NBK430926/.

12 *A 24-year-old woman who is 27 weeks pregnant was in a minor motor vehicle collision. The patient was the driver and wearing a seat belt when the car hits a telephone pole while distracted when texting. Airbags did not deploy. Her blood pressure is 112/83 mm Hg, pulse 80 beats/min, respiration 18 breaths/min, and SaO$_2$ is 99%. The patient wants to go home before her husband arrives. Fetal monitor is placed and the childs' heart rate is 80 beats/min. Which of the following is the most appropriate?*

A *Mandatory monitoring for next 24 hours*

B *Patient is stable and can be observed*

C *Assume that there is fetal distress*

D *Thank her for wearing a seat belt*

E *Obtain a MRI and not a CT scan*

At approximate 12th week of gestation, fetal heart tones can be detected. Normally fetal heart rate ranges between 110 and 160 beats/min. At the initial stage of distress, fetal hypoxia can exhibit as tachycardia. However, as the distress continues and arterial oxygen content goes down with passing time, fetal heart tones ultimately display bradycardia. To conclude, if pregnant women experience trauma even minor, sustained fetal heart rate below 120 should be considered as distress signal and maternal blood loss should be suspected. If the fetal heart rate is the same as the mother's, you must assume that it is not a correct assessment.

Answer: C

Krywko DM, Toy FK, Mahan ME, et al. Pregnancy Trauma. [Updated 2020 Dec 12]. In: *StatPearls [Internet]*. Treasure Island (FL): StatPearls Publishing;

2020. Available from: https://www.ncbi.nlm.nih.gov/books/NBK430926/.

Pillarisetty LS, Bragg BN. Late Decelerations. [Updated 2020 Jul 19]. In: *StatPearls [Internet]*. Treasure Island (FL): StatPearls Publishing; 2020. Available from: https://www.ncbi.nlm.nih.gov/books/NBK539820/.

13 *A 25-year-old is 33 weeks pregnant when she tripped and fell down the steps in front of her house. She is complaining of severe pain in her right knee. Her blood pressure and respiratory rate are normal, but her heart rate is 100 beats/min. Her physical examination was normal except small bruise on her right knee. She does not have any vaginal bleeding. What are the commonest causes of fetal death in descending order of their frequency?*

A *Uterine rupture, direct fetal injury, placental abruption, maternal shock*

B *Direct fetal injury, uterine rupture, placental abruption, maternal shock*

C *Placental abruption, uterine rupture, direct fetal injury, maternal shock*

D *Maternal shock, placental abruption, direct fetal injury, uterine rupture*

E *Frequency of all the causes of fetal death are same*

Causes of fetal death in decreasing order of frequency include maternal shock (30.7~36%), placental abruption (32%), direct fetal injury (20%), and uterine rupture (<1%). Trauma is sustained in 8% of all pregnancies. Although MVC is the single largest cause of fetal death, regardless of mechanism, trauma can be life threatening for both the mother and fetus. Rapid evaluation and treatment of the mother in trauma should be even further heightened, as maternal shock is associated with an 80% fetal mortality. Pelvic fracture is the most common maternal injury that results in fetal death. The most devastating injuries following direct blunt trauma include placental abruption and uterine rupture. Abruption is thought to complicate 1–6% of minor injuries and up to 50% of major injuries. Uterine rupture is overall rare, occurring in less than 1% of pregnant trauma patients, and is most commonly associated with direct impact with sustained force to a previously scarred uterus. In contrast to blunt trauma, maternal mortality is more favorable following penetrating injury as the gravid uterus serves as protection to the maternal internal organs. Conversely, fetal mortality following penetrating injury has been reported to be as high as 73%.

Answer: D

Krywko DM, Toy FK, Mahan ME, et al. Pregnancy Trauma. [Updated 2020 Dec 12]. In: *StatPearls*

[Internet]. Treasure Island (FL): StatPearls Publishing; 2020. Available from: https://www.ncbi.nlm.nih.gov/books/NBK430926/.

Corsi PR, Rasslan S, de Oliveira LB, Kronfly FS, Marinho VP. Trauma in pregnant women: analysis of maternal and fetal mortality. *Injury*. 1999;30(4):239–43. doi: 10.1016/s0020-1383(98)00250-2. PMID: 10476291.

14 *What is the most common injury associated with falls in the third trimester of pregnancy?*

A *Right arm fracture*

B *Rib fracture*

C *Shoulder dislocation*

D *Lower extremity fracture*

E *None of the above*

Increase in joint laxity and weight gain during the pregnancy predisposes pregnant patients to fall-related trauma. Particularly in the third trimester, the decline in dynamic postural stability is seen. This is evident through decrease in initial and total sway along with reduction in the velocity of sway. According to one of the population studies, more than 75% of women who experienced fall and got hospitalized were in their 3rd trimester of pregnancy. The percentage of pregnant woman hospitalized for fall were 79.3% in third trimester, 11.3% in the second, and 9.4% in the first trimester of the pregnancy. Among the hospitalized pregnant women, the most common injury was lower extremity fracture. In addition, pregnant woman hospitalized for fall were at the elevated risk of placental abruption (8 folds), preterm labor (4.4 folds), labor induction (90%), and caesarean section (30%). Risk of fetal distress and hypoxia increased by 2.1 and 2.9 folds, respectively.

Answer: D

Schiff MA. Pregnancy outcomes following hospitalisation for a fall in Washington State from 1987 to 2004. *BJOG*. 2008;115(13):1648–1654. doi: 10.1111/j.1471-0528. 2008.01905.x. Epub 2008 Oct 8. PMID: 18947341.

Figueroa-Mendez H, Dahlke JD, Vrees RA, Rouse DJ. Trauma in pregnancy: an updated systematic review. 2013;209(1):1–10. https://doi.org/10.1016/j.ajog.2013.01.021.

15 *In the pregnant trauma patient, what are the factors that increase the risk of aspiration during intubation?*

A *Pregnancy*

B *Diabetes*

C *Morbid obesity*

D *Full stomach*

E *All of the above*

Aspiration is inhalation of gastric or oropharyngeal contents into larynx and lower respiratory tract. Depending on the amount, frequency, and nature of aspirated contents, aspiration may result in several pulmonary complications, which includes airway obstruction, aspiration pneumonitis, aspiration pneumonia, and lung abscess. Multiple factors can elevate the risk of aspiration of gastric contents. These factors include:

- Full stomach
- Delayed gastric emptying, which can be seen in systemic diseases such as diabetes and opioid use
- Incompetent lower esophageal sphincter (Hx of gastrointestinal surgery, pregnancy, morbid obesity, hiatus hernia)
- Reduced level of consciousness (Interrupt cough reflux and glottic closure)

The normal physiology of pregnancy predisposes pregnant woman to the aspiration. Increased intra-abdominal pressure due to gravid uterus, delayed gastric emptying and relaxed lower esophageal sphincter due to pregnancy hormones, all of these contribute to elevated risk for aspiration of gastric contents.

Answer: E

Robinson M, Davidson A. Aspiration under anaesthesia: risk assessment and decision-making, *Contin Educ Anaesth Crit Care Pain*. 2014;14(4): 171–175. https://doi.org/10.1093/bjaceaccp/mkt053

Froio S, Valenza F. Aspiration of Gastric Contents in the Critically Ill. In: Andrew Webb, Derek Angus, Simon Finfer, Luciano Gattinoni, and Mervyn Singer, *Oxford Textbook of Critical Care*. 2 ed.. Oxford, UK: Oxford University Press; 2016. https://oxfordmedicine.com/view/10.1093/med/9780199600830.001.0001/med-9780199600830-chapter-106.

Wu JCY, Mui LM, Cheung CMY, Chan Y, Sung JJY. Obesity is associated with increased transient lower esophageal sphincter relaxation. *Clinical-Alimentary Tract*. 2007;132(3):P883–P889. https://doi.org/10.1053/j.gastro.2006.12.032.

16 *A 24-year-old G2 P1 woman who is 24 weeks pregnant was seatbelted passenger in a front-end MVC. Airbags were deployed. Her primary assessment showed intact airway, breath sounds equal, blood pressure was 95/65 mm Hg, pulse 120 beats/min. Her Glasgow Coma Scale Score is 7, so you ask for intubation. Which of the following is the preferred position to reduce the risk of aspiration during intubation?*

A *Supine position*

B *Prone position*

C *Lateral position with angle ≤ 50°*

D *Lateral position with angle ≤ 25°*

E *Lateral position with angle ≥ 70°*

Aspiration during tracheal intubation can cause life-threatening complications. Even with rapid sequence intubation, aspiration is not totally avoidable, especially in pregnant women. During vomiting and regurgitation, gastric contents flow back from esophagus to pharynx and enter larynx/trachea or thrown out of the mouth. In the supine position, head-down tilt is done so that the mouth is placed inferiorly than the larynx, which in turn avoid gastric content to enter trachea. However, in supine patient head neck position, which is frequently used for tracheal intubation, head-down tilt required to protect pulmonary system from aspiration do not fall within a clinical relevant range. Therefore, preventing aspiration in the supine position is difficult. Contrary, in the lateral position, aspiration can be prevented due to similar height of the larynx and mouth. The scientific literature recommends this position for tracheal intubation in patients with heightened risk of aspiration. Furthermore, research suggests that aspiration can be prevented at lateral or excessive lateral position ($\geq 70\sim90°$) in head neck positions frequently used for tracheal intubation.

Answer: E

Kirchner E. Emergencies and aspiration. Can the usual methods for the prophylaxis of aspiration be further developed? *Anaesthesist.* 1978;27:119–126.

Takenaka I, Aoyama K. Prevention of aspiration of gastric contents during attempt in tracheal intubation in the semi-lateral and lateral positions. *World J Emerg Med.* 2016;7(4):285–289. doi:10.5847/wjem.j.1920-8642.2016.04.008.

17 *Which of the following is the most true regarding complete rupture of uterine wall in pregnant patient?*
   A *Fetal heart rate abnormalities are in the most frequent sign.*
   B *Hematuria is frequently present.*
   C *The triad of abdominal pain, vaginal bleeding, and abnormal fetal heart rate is very common.*
   D *Delivery should be done through a Pfannenstiel incision.*
   E *If identified, bedrest remains the best option.*

Uterine rupture is full thickness separation of the uterine wall. It can lead to serious health consequences for both mother and her child. Although most uterine rupture is found in pregnant woman, there are reports of uterine rupture in nonpregnant woman with malignancy, infections, or trauma. Falls and motor vehicle accidents account for most abdominal trauma in pregnancy in the United States. Delay in definitive diagnosis and treatment

can be devastating for the patient and fetus. Signs and symptoms that point toward uterine rupture after blunt abdominal trauma included abnormal fetal heart rate (FHR –82%). Fetal bradycardia is the most frequent abnormality related with uterine rupture (choice A). Absent tracing of fetal heart is pathognomonic for uterine rupture and demands urgent radiologic imaging. Hematuria is not frequently associated with uterine rupture (choice B) Abdominal pain and vaginal bleeding are other signs of uterine rupture. However, the classic triad of abdominal pain, vaginal bleeding, and FHR abnormalities is only found in 9% of cases of complete uterine rupture (choice C). Fetal heart rate provides valuable information on the health status of both mother and fetus. It indicates end-organ perfusion status of mother. Late decelerations, reduced variability in heart rate, and fetal bradycardia represent reduced blood flow and fetal hypoxia. In trauma, a midline incision is preferred over the Pfannenstiel incision as maternal hemorrhage control is paramount, and limiting the incision assumes that the fetal well-being is the highest and only priority (choice D). C-section is often needed if uterine rupture is diagnosed (choice E).

Answer: A

Guiliano M, Closset E, Therby D, LeGoueff F, Deruelle P, Subtil D. Signs, symptoms and complications of complete and partial uterine ruptures during pregnancy and delivery. *Eur J Obstet Gynecol Reprod Biol.* 2014;179:130–4. doi:10.1016/j.ejogrb.2014.05.004. Epub 2014 May 22. PMID: 24965993.

American College of Obstetricians and Gynecologists. ACOG practice bulletin no. 205: vaginal birth after cesarean delivery. *Obstet Gynecol.* 2019;133(2):e110–e127.

Ozdemir I, Yucel N, Yucel O. Rupture of the pregnant uterus: a 9-year review. *Arch Gynecol Obstet.* 2005;272(3):229–231.

Togioka BM, Tonismae T. Uterine Rupture. [Updated 2021 Jan 5]. In: *StatPearls [Internet].* Treasure Island (FL): StatPearls Publishing; 2021. Available from: https://www.ncbi.nlm.nih.gov/books/NBK559209/.

18 *A 25-year-old G2P1 woman presents with 20% TBSA partial-thickness burns following a motor vehicle collision. The patient develops burn wound sepsis during her ICU course. Which of the following antibiotics is a grade B drug?*
   A *Quinolones*
   B *Itraconazole*

C *Fluconazole*
D *Cephalosporins*
E *None of the above*

The treatment for burns in pregnancy is challenging not only for mother but also influences the health status of the fetus. If the burn patient is at the late stage of pregnancy, literature suggest terminating the pregnancy early in time to prevent fetal distress and improve the chances of survival for fetus. Early termination of pregnancy will also help in simplifying treatment for mother with burns. Therefore, knowledge of exact gestational week/age is important. On the other side, if the fetus is immature, pregnancy could be continued with close monitoring and supervision with various treatment strategies. This comes at the cost of risk to the health of fetus. Septicemia is the prominent reason for maternal mortality in pregnant patients with burns, thus necessitate the use of antibiotics. Based on the potential side effects for the fetus, the Food and Drug Administration categorized antibiotics into five grades: A, B, C, D, X. Grade B drugs such as cephalosporins, clindamycin, macrolides, and penicillins are considered safe during the pregnancy. Grade C drugs such as fluconazole and quinolones have shown negative influence on fetus in animal experiments and are only considered when benefits outweigh the potential risks.

A	No risk in human studies; adequate and well-controlled human studies have failed to demonstrate a risk to the fetus in the first trimester of pregnancy (and there is no evidence of risk in later trimesters)	None
B	No risk in other studies; animal reproduction studies have failed to demonstrate a risk to the fetus, and there are no adequate and well-controlled studies in pregnant women	Nevertheless, because the studies in humans cannot rule out the possibility of harm, [name of drug] should be used during pregnancy only if clearly needed
C	Risk not ruled out; animal reproduction studies have shown an adverse effect on the fetus, and there are no adequate and well-controlled studies in humans, but potential benefits may warrant use of the drug in pregnant women despite potential risks	[Name of drug] should be given to a pregnant woman only if clearly needed
D	Positive evidence of risk; there is positive evidence of human fetal risk based on adverse reaction data from investigational or marketing experience or studies in humans, but potential benefits may warrant use of the drug in pregnant women despite potential risks	If this drug is used during pregnancy, or if the patient becomes pregnant while taking this drug, the patient should be apprised of the potential hazard to the fetus
X	Contraindicated in pregnancy; studies in animals or humans have demonstrated fetal abnormalities and/or there is positive evidence of human fetal risk based on adverse reaction data from investigational or marketing experience, and the risks involved in use of the drug in pregnant women clearly outweigh potential benefits	[Name of drug] is contraindicated in women who are or may become pregnant. If this drug is used during pregnancy, or if the patient becomes pregnant while taking this drug, the patient should be apprised of the potential hazard to the fetus

Bookstaver PB, Bland CM, Griffin B, Stover KR, Eiland LS, McLaughlin M. A review of antibiotic use in pregnancy. *Pharmacotherapy*. 2015;35(11):1052–62. doi:10.1002/phar.1649. PMID: 26598097.

Rezavand N, Seyedzadeh A, Soleymani A. Evaluation of maternal and fetal outcomes in pregnant women hospitalized in Kermanshah Hospitals, Iran, owing to burn injury, 2003-2008. *Ann Burns Fire Disasters*. 2012;**25**:196–199.

Rayburn W, Smith B, Feller I, Varner M, Cruikshank D. Major burns during pregnancy: effects on fetal well-being. *Obstet Gynecol*. 1984;**63**:392–395.

Shi Y, Zhang X, Huang BG, Wang WK, Liu Y. Severe burn injury in late pregnancy: a case report and literature review. *Burns Trauma*. 2015; 3:2. Published 2015 May 28. doi:10.1186/s41038-015-0002-z.

19 *A 27-year-old G2P1 pregnant woman was involved in a MVC. She was intubated in the field. You palpate the top of the womb and it is two fingers above the umbilicus. The estimated gestational age is?*
A *3½–4 months*
B *4½–5 months*

C *5½–6 months*
D *6½–7 months*
E *None of the above*

Accurate week of gestation is important in decision-making for trauma patients with pregnancy. Fetus with more than 23 weeks of gestation may be viable. Therefore, fetal heart monitoring is initiated as early as possible as delivery may be needed. In case, the pregnant woman is unconscious and cannot communicate gestational age, then fundal height measurement may give rough idea of gestational age. Injuries causing abdominal distention may interfere with measurement. Also, it should be documented here that there is conflicting literature about the accuracy of measurement.

Answer: C

36–38 weeks
fundus usually
right up under
sternum

36–38
32
26
24
20
14–16
12

40 weeks (term)
fundus drops below
38-week level as
presenting part
drops down into
pelvis

12 weeks
fundus just
above pubic
bone

Jain V, Chari R, Maslovitz S, et al. Guidelines for the management of a pregnant trauma patient. *J Obstet Gynaecol Can.* 2015;37(6):553–574.
Engstrom JL. Measurement of fundal height. *J Obstet Gynecol Neonatal Nurs.* 1988;17(3):172–8. doi:10.1111/j.1552-6909.1988.tb00422.x. PMID: 3292729.

20 *A 27-year-old pregnant woman comes in with multiple gunshot wounds. She had GSW to (1) right breast above her nipple, (2) right lateral thoraco-abdominal GSW xyphoid level, (3) left lateral abdomen GSW above the iliac crest, and (4) right back at tip of the scapula. Top of the fundus is at the subxyphoid level. Her blood pressure is 90/60 and heart rate is 119/min. FAST shows normal pericardium. She is rushed to the operating room where she was intubated and a right chest tube placed, and you note blood from her vagina. Midline laparotomy showed through and through liver injury, multiple small bowel injuries*

and two through and through gunshot wounds to the uterus. The bleeding from the liver is minor and mesenteric bleeding controlled. Your next step is:
A *Call the obstetrician on call and have them take over the surgery*
B *Nonoperative management of the fetus*
C *Plain film chest and abdominal X ray to see if there are retained bullets*
D *Damage control surgery, pack her up and take her to the CT scanner*
E *C-section and examine the fetus*

In the gravid state, the visceral organs are displaced upwards and are less likely to be injured. Upper abdominal stab or gunshot wounds can result in complex bowel injury. Depending on the gestational age and the size of the uterus, the fetus is much more likely than the mother to sustain significant injury (and to die) after a penetrating abdominal trauma. In general, the fetus sustains injury in 60–70% of cases, while visceral maternal injuries are seen only in 20% of penetrating abdominal trauma. If the fetus is injured, 40–65% of these fetuses die. Penetrating injuries in pregnant trauma patients are managed in essentially the same way as in nonpregnant patients. The standard of care is to prioritize the mother above that of her fetus. The hemodynamically stable patient can be assessed by noninvasive diagnostic methods such as ultrasound and triple contrast CT scan. The same indications for surgical exploration apply as in the nonpregnant patient (positive findings on lavage, free air under the diaphragm before lavage, progressive abdominal distention with a declining hematocrit, or abdominal wall disruption or perforation). In cases of exploration, the decision to proceed with Caesarean section should be weighed against the likelihood for fetal survival and long-term complications of prematurity. Factors that can influence the decision to proceed with Caesarean section are gestational age, extent and severity of fetal injury, degree of uteroplacental compromise, parameters of fetal well-being, and the need for hysterectomy with extensive uterine injury. If the bullet has penetrated the uterus and the fetus is viable, then Caesarean section should be done to evaluate if the fetus has been injured. The management of the gunshot wound of the fetus would again generally follow basic trauma principles. If intraoperative ultrasound can determine that the fetus is dead, this may be an indication for nonoperative management of the fetus. A dead or injured fetus is not considered an indication for exploration, as the fetus will usually spontaneously abort or can be delivered vaginally. If the fetus is alive and the mother is stable, c section and examination of the fetus to determine injury and treat the injury would be indicated.

Answer: E

Jain V, Chari R, Maslovitz S, Farine D, et al. Guidelines for the management of a pregnant trauma patient. *J Obstet Gynaecol Can*. 2015;37(6):553–574.

Salim A, Velmahos GC. When to operate on abdominal gunshot wounds. *Scand J Surg*. 2002;91(1):62–66. doi:10.1177/145749690209100110. PMID: 12075838 DOI: 10.1177/145749690209100110.

36

Esophagus, Stomach, and Duodenum

Collin Stewart, MD and Andrew Tang, MD

Banner University Medical Center, University of Arizona College of Medicine, Tucson, AZ, USA

1 *Which of the following is true about the esophagus?*
   A *The middle third of the esophagus is accessed through the left chest.*
   B *The esophagus has two layers of muscle surrounded by serosa.*
   C *The recurrent laryngeal nerve runs posterior to the esophagus.*
   D *The cricopharyngeus functions as the upper esophageal sphincter.*
   E *The lower esophagus courses to the right of the spine to pass through the diaphragm.*

The esophagus begins at the 6th cervical vertebrae and travels down to the 11th thoracic vertebra, approximately 25 cm in distance. It has 2 layers. The inner mucosal layer is lined proximally with squamous epithelium that transitions to columnar epithelium near the gastroesophageal junction. The outer muscular layer is composed of an inner circular muscle layer and an outer longitudinal muscle layer. There is no serosal layer to the esophagus. There are four anatomic segments of the esophagus.

The cervical esophagus is located between the hypopharynx and the thoracic inlet. The recurrent laryngeal nerve can be found in tracheoesophageal groove. The location of the nerve is more consistent in the left neck. Therefore, the cervical esophagus is approached through a left neck incision. The cricopharyngeus is located in this segment and acts, along with the inferior constrictor, as the upper esophageal sphincter.

The upper thoracic esophagus is located between the thoracic inlet and the lower border of the azygous vein. The middle thoracic esophagus then begins and extends to the inferior pulmonary veins. Finally, the lower thoracic esophagus begins and extends inferiorly to the stomach. As the esophagus approaches the thoracic inlet, it deviates to the left before returning to a midline

position at approximately the T5 vertebrae. It again courses to the left as it approaches the diaphragmatic hiatus. The middle third of the esophagus is approached typically through the right chest while the distal esophagus is exposed with a left thoracotomy.

Besides the upper esophageal sphincter, there are two other areas of increased pressure and narrowing. There is an area of increase pressure as the esophagus passes posterior to the left mainstem bronchus. The last area is the lower esophageal sphincter, which is a physiologic sphincter contributed to by multiple components, including abdominal esophageal length and pressure, the diaphragmatic hiatus, and the Angle of His.

Answer: D

Patti, M., Gantert, W., Way, L. (1997) Surgery of the esophagus: anatomy and physiology. *The Surgical Clinics of North America*, **77**, 959–970.

2 *A 35-year-old man presents with chest pain and dysphagia following an esophagogastroduodenoscopy. Which of the following is true about esophageal perforations?*
   A *The most common cause of perforation is malignancy.*
   B *Esophagogastroduodenoscopy is the diagnostic test of choice.*
   C *Early, broad-spectrum antibiotics is the mainstay of treatment.*
   D *The most common site of perforation is cervical near the cricopharyngeus.*
   E *There is no role for conservative, nonoperative management of perforation.*

Iatrogenic injury is the most common cause of esophageal perforation. The most common site of perforation is at the narrowing caused by the cricopharyngeus. Patients should be asked about recent instrumentation of the esophagus.

Surgical Critical Care and Emergency Surgery: Clinical Questions and Answers, Third Edition.
Edited by Forrest "Dell" Moore, Peter M. Rhee, and Carlos J. Rodriguez.
© 2022 John Wiley & Sons Ltd. Published 2022 by John Wiley & Sons Ltd.
Companion website: www.wiley.com/go/surgicalcriticalcare3e

Patients will often present with dysphagia, chest pain, back pain, or epigastric abdominal pain. Physical exam may reveal crepitus and diminished lung sounds. Chest radiographs may show a left pleural effusion for proximal or distal perforations or a right pleural effusion for midesophageal perforations. Saliva or food particle return after chest tube placement is diagnostic.

If esophageal perforation is suspected, upper endoscopy can be performed but is not the first test of choice as it may worsen the injury. Either CT scan with PO contrast or esophagography with water-soluble contrast followed by thin barium should be used to diagnose the injury.

Early operative management is the mainstay of treatment for esophageal perforation. Delay in treatment leads to a high incidence of morbidity and mortality. For some contained perforations without signs of sepsis, conservative management may be attempted. This may include endoscopic stenting or clipping. Obstructive pathology or malignancy is a contraindication to conservative management. Antibiotic coverage should include aerobe, anaerobe, and fungal coverage.

Answer: D

Chirica, M., Kelly, M.D., Siboni, S., *et al.* (2019) Esophageal emergencies: WSES guidelines. *World Journal of Emergency Surgery*, **14**, 26.

Nirula, R. (2014) Esophageal perforation. *Surgical Clinics of North America*, **94**, (1) 35–41.

3 *A 48-year-old man presents with large volume hematemesis. He has an extensive history of alcohol abuse and on physical exam, he is tachycardic and has an abdominal fluid wave. He is tachycardic to 135 and his blood pressure is 90/47 mmHg. Which of the following is true of the management of gastroesophageal varices?*

A *There is no role in postoperative antibiotic use.*

B *Band ligation is first-line therapy for bleeding esophageal varices.*

C *Tamponade with a Sengstaken–Blakemore tube is often successful for long-term control.*

D *Surgical portosystemic shunts should be pursued early to prevent bleeding.*

E *Upper endoscopy should be avoided to prevent provoked bleeding.*

Gastroesophageal varices are the result of portal hypertension, most often the result of cirrhosis. In patients with cirrhosis, varices form at a rate of approximately 8% per year. The most common acute presentation is gastrointestinal hemorrhage. If a patient presents with suspected bleeding varices, other signs of portal hypertension and cirrhosis, such as spider nevi, jaundice, and ascites, may be present.

Initial management of bleeding varices involves appropriate resuscitation. In patients with altered mental status, intubation may be necessary to prevent aspiration. Upper endoscopy is necessary for accurate diagnosis and treatment. Band ligation is the first-line treatment for bleeding esophageal varices. This treatment modality has a success rate of over 70% and can be repeated as necessary. Continuing antibiotics in the postprocedural period has been shown to decrease rates of rebleeding. Sengstaken–Blakemore tubes may be used to temporarily control bleeding not alleviated by initial endoscopic treatment. However, the treatment is only temporary and has a high rate of complications including aspiration and esophageal rupture. Portosystemic shunts may be considered for bleeding that does not resolve with primary or secondary treatments. Transjugular intrahepatic portosystemic shunt (TIPS) may be attempted, while surgical portosystemic shunts only be used when other modalities have failed.

Answer: B

Sharma, M., Singh, S., Desai, V., *et al.* (2019) Comparison of therapies for primary prevention of esophageal variceal bleeding: a systematic review and network meta-analysis. *Hepatology*, **69**, (4) 1657–1675.

Seo, Y.S. (2018) Prevention and management of gastroesophageal varices. *Clinical and Molecular Hepatology*, **24**, (1) 20–42.

Garcia-Tsao, G., Bosch, J. (2010) Management of varices and variceal hemorrhage in cirrhosis. *New England Journal of Medicine*, **362**, (9) 823–832.

4 *A 37-year-old woman presents via ambulance after ingesting an unknown household cleaner. The patient is complaining of nausea and dysphagia and is having difficulty controlling her secretions. She has mild tachycardia but is otherwise hemodynamically stable. Which of the following statements is false?*

A *Esophagogastroduodenoscopy is indicated in symptomatic patients without evidence of perforation.*

B *Acid ingestion causes deeper esophageal injury than alkali ingestion.*

C *Neutralizing agents are contraindicated in treatment.*

D *The most common late complication is esophageal stricture.*

E *Early enteral feeding is not contraindicated in low-grade injuries.*

Household cleaner ingestions are a common occurrence. While children with accidental exposure are likely to vomit and limit the amount of substance and contact time, purposeful ingestion for self-harm is associated with larger volume of substance and more serious injury. Acid ingestion is associated with coagulative necrosis, while alkali ingestions lead to liquefactive necrosis that causes a deeper injury. Therefore, alkali ingestions have a higher morbidity and mortality.

Patients with ingestions should be evaluated based on clinical symptoms. They should be resuscitated and evaluated for signs of perforation. If patients have no overt signs of perforation, upper endoscopy should be performed to evaluate the extent of injury. Grade 1 injuries only show edema and hyperemia. Grade 2A and 2B have superficial or deep ulceration, respectively. Grade 3A demonstrates focal necrosis while Grade 3B has extensive necrosis. Grade 1 and 2A have good prognosis, 2B and 3A have a high rate of stricture, and 3B has a high rate of mortality.

Emetics should not be used as they cause re-exposure of the esophagus to the agent upon regurgitation. Likewise, neutralizing agents should not be used as they cause an exothermic reaction that also can worsen the injury. In patients with low-grade injuries can be started on a liquid diet early and advanced as tolerated.

Answer: B

Hoffman, R.S., Burns, M.M., Gosselin, S. (2020) Ingestion of caustic substances. *New England Journal of Medicine*, **382**, (18) 1739–1748.

5 *Following a stab wound to the left neck, a 22-year-old man presents to the emergency department. He is complaining of dysphagia. There is no active bleeding, the patient is hemodynamically normal, and the patient has no dyspnea or hoarseness. Which of the following is most accurate about esophageal injury?*
   A *Blunt injuries are more common to the cervical esophagus than penetrating.*
   B *A negative physical exam is adequate to rule out an esophageal injury.*
   C *The injury to the mucosal layer is never larger than the injury to the muscular layer.*
   D *Full strength barium is the initial contrast of choice in evaluating for injury.*
   E *Esophagoscopy has a high negative predictive value.*

Diagnosis and management of esophageal injury is imperative as delay in diagnosis significantly worsens patient outcomes. Injuries to the esophagus are most often associated with penetrating wounds. Blunt cervical esophageal injuries are often associated with impact on a hyperextended neck. Rupture may also occur with rapidly increased pressure.

While hard signs such as saliva in the wound are indicative of injury, lack of physical exam signs of injury are not adequate to rule out injury. Diagnostic modalities include an upper GI study with water-soluble contrast. If this study is negative, it should be followed by a study with thin barium for confirmation. Full strength barium

should be avoided as it can cause mediastinitis and mediastinal fibrosis. Esophagoscopy is also a component of diagnosis and has a high negative predictive value.

Exposure of esophageal injury is dependent on the location. Cervical injuries are approached from the left neck, mid-esophageal injuries from the right chest, and distal injuries from the left chest. The muscle should be divided past the area of injury to expose the full extent of the mucosal injury as this often extends further than the muscular injury. The edges of the wound should be debrided of necrotic and nonviable tissue. The esophagus is repaired in two layers and should be buttressed with a muscle flap. Inspection for a through-and-through injury should also be done, either through the operative field or by intraoperative endoscopy.

Answer: E

Chirica, M., Kelly, M.D., Siboni, S., *et al.* (2019) Esophageal emergencies: WSES guidelines. *World Journal of Emergency Surgery*, **14**, 26.

Biffl, W.L., Moore, E.E., Feliciano, D.V., *et al.* (2015) Western Trauma Association critical decisions in trauma: diagnosis and management of esophageal injuries. *Journal of Trauma and Acute Care Surgery*, **79**, (6) 1089–1095.

6 *A 5-year-old boy presents to the emergency department after his mother reports seeing him swallow a flat, round object. The child has no difficulty breathing but is drooling and is complaining of dysphagia. A chest radiograph shows a round object in the mid-chest with a surrounding halo. There is no apparent pneumomediastinum. What is the next best step in management?*
   A *Monitor for passage of the foreign body*
   B *Emergent endoscopy*
   C *Administration of emetics to clear foreign body*
   D *CT scan of the chest*
   E *Emergent bronchoscopy*

Ingestions of foreign bodies are common occurrences in children. Most foreign body ingestions do not require treatment and will pass on their own. However, if the patient is symptomatic or the identity of the foreign body is unknown, further investigation is necessary. Ingestions of coin batteries represent an emergent situation and require prompt action to prevent further complications. Coin batteries, when in contact with surrounding tissue, produce hydrochloric acid and, if left untreated, will lead to ulcerating and perforation. Patients may present with dysphagia, drooling, or PO intolerance.

Plain films of the chest may show the presence of the foreign body if it is in the esophagus. While coins will show up as round objects on imaging, coin batteries have a classic double halo appearance when viewed en face and a step-off appearance on lateral views.

Suspected or known ingestion of a coin battery should prompt immediate removal. This is accomplished with upper endoscopy. When the diagnosis is made on plain film imaging, no further radiographic studies are needed.

Answer: B

Torrecillas, V., Meier, J.D. (2020) History and radiographic findings as predictors for esophageal coins versus button batteries. *International Journal of Pediatric Otorhinolaryngology*, **137**, 110208.

Wright, C.W., Closson, F.T. (2013) Updates in pediatric gastrointestinal foreign bodies. *Pediatric Clinics of North America*, **60**, (5) 1221–1239.

7 *Which of the following statements about the stomach is false?*
   A *The gastrosplenic ligament contains the short gastric arteries.*
   B *The pylorus receives its blood supply from the left gastric artery.*
   C *The stomach is acidified by hydrochloric acid production in the parietal cells.*
   D *Total gastrectomy places patients at risk for pernicious anemia.*
   E *The right gastric artery most often arises from the proper hepatic artery.*

The stomach is located in the left upper quadrant of the abdomen, although its exact location can vary based on patient positioning and the amount of gastric contents at the time. The stomach is attached to surrounding structures laterally by the gastrosplenic ligament, which contains the short gastric arteries, medially by the gastrohepatic ligament and retroperitoneal duodenum, and cephalad by the gastrophrenic ligament. The stomach is loosely attached to the transverse colon by the gastrocolic ligament.

The stomach receives its rich blood supply from the left and right gastric arteries, the left and right gastroepiploic arteries, and the short gastric arteries. The left gastric artery most often arises from the celiac axis, but variants may originate from the common hepatic artery, splenic artery, aorta, or superior mesenteric artery. The right gastric artery originates from the proper hepatic artery the majority of the time, but also can come from the left hepatic artery or common hepatic artery. The right gastroepiploic artery is a branch of the gastroduodenal artery, while the left gastroepiploic artery is most often a branch of the splenic artery. The pylorus receives arterial supply from the gastroduodenal artery.

The gastric mucosa is made up of columnar cells. Parietal cells produce hydrochloric acid to acidify the stomach. Parietal cells also produce intrinsic factor, which is necessary for the absorption of vitamin B_{12}.

Following gastrectomy patients are at risk for pernicious anemia secondary to intrinsic factor deficiency. Gastrin, which is produced by G cells in the antrum, stimulates acid secretion.

Answer: B

Soybel, D.I. (2005) Anatomy and physiology of the stomach. *Surgical Clinics of North America*, **85**, (5) 875–894.

8 *A 47-year-old man presents with mid-epigastric pain and hematemesis. On esophagogastroduodenoscopy, the patient is noted to have a 2 cm ulceration in the antrum without evidence of active bleeding. Which of the following about gastric ulcers is true?*
   A *Type V gastric ulcers are associated with anticoagulant use.*
   B *Acid lowering medications will treat type II and III ulcers.*
   C *Cushing's ulcers are associated with burn patients.*
   D *Most ulcers are located along the greater curve.*
   E *Patients with head trauma may develop Curling's ulcers.*

Gastric ulcers are divided into five types based on anatomic location and causality. Type I ulcers are located in the lower part of the lesser curvature of the stomach. They are associated with decreased mucosal protection. Type II ulcers are located on the lesser curve of the stomach along with a duodenal ulcer. They are caused by acid hypersecretion. Prepyloric ulcers are classified as type III, and they are also associated with acid hypersecretion. Type IV ulcers are located in the cardia of the stomach and are associated with decreased mucosal protection. Nonsteroidal anti-inflammatory drug use causes type V ulcers, which may be located throughout the stomach. Because of these causes, acid lowering medications will only prove effective in the treatment of type II and III ulcers.

Cushing's ulcers are ulcerations in the stomach that occur in patients following head trauma. They are believed to be caused by stimulation of the vagal nuclei in the head from increased intracranial pressure. Curling's ulcers are associated with major burn patients. They are caused by mucosal necrosis and sloughing secondary to hypovolemia. They have a high rate of bleeding and perforation.

Answer: B

Kavitt, R.T., Lipowska, A.M., Anyane-Yeboa, A., Gralnek, I.M. (2019) Diagnosis and treatment of peptic ulcer disease. *American Journal of Medicine*, **132**, (4) 447–456.

Kempenich, J.W., Sirinek, K.R. (2018) Acid peptic disease. *Surgical Clinics of North America*, **98**, (5) 933–944.

9 *Which of the following is true about Helicobacter pylori?*
   A *The best test for eradication is serologic testing.*
   B *Histologic biopsies for diagnosis should be taken from the fundus.*
   C *Patients should stop taking proton pump inhibitors before undergoing a urea breath test.*
   D *Amoxicillin monotherapy has high rates of H. pylori eradication.*
   E *The majority of patients with H. pylori infection are symptomatic.*

Helicobacter pylori is a gram-negative helical bacterium. It is found predominantly in the stomach. Some projections have estimated that over 50% of the world's population is infected with *H. pylori*. However, the majority of patients infected are asymptomatic.

Multiple testing modalities are available for diagnosis. Serologic testing is widely available and low cost. This exam detects IgG antibodies to *H. pylori*. However, because of the longevity of IgG antibodies, the test cannot be used to confirm a positive response to eradication treatment. *H. pylori* has intrinsic urease which is utilized in the urea breath test. The bacteria convert radiolabeled oral urea into detectable carbon dioxide. This test is the best choice for evaluating successful eradication. Stool tests utilize antibodies to detect *H. pylori* specific antigens. The fecal test and urea breath test can be affected by proton pump inhibitor or H2 blocker use as well as antimicrobial use. These medications should be stopped prior to the administration of the test as they may cause a false-negative result.

Endoscopic diagnosis involves biopsies taken from the antrum of the stomach. This allows for histologic diagnosis of the bacteria as well as gastritis. Culture may be undertaken although is not widely available. Biopsy specimens may also be tested with urea. If present, the specimen will convert the urea to ammonia.

Treatment for *H. pylori* consists of triple therapy with dual antibiotics and a proton pump inhibitor. An example includes clarithromycin, amoxicillin, and a proton pump inhibitor. Single antibiotic therapy is inadequate treatment for eradication.

Answer: C

Crowe, S.E. (2019) Helicobacter pylori infection. *New England Journal of Medicine*, **380**, (12) 1158–1165.

10 *A 65-year-old woman presents with worsening dysphagia and gastroesophageal reflux. Esophagogastroduodenoscopy shows a large hiatal hernia. Which of the following statements is true?*
   A *Inability to vomit and failure to advance a nasogastric tube are evidence of a surgical emergency.*
   B *Type II hiatal hernias have an abnormal location of the gastroesophageal junction.*
   C *Mesh placement during hiatal hernia repair reduces long-term recurrence.*
   D *Upper GI with gastrografin is the study of choice to evaluate gastric volvulus.*
   E *Adjacent organ displacement is a feature of a type III hiatal hernia.*

There are four types of hiatal hernias. These are defined by the location of the gastroesophageal junction. Type I hiatal hernias, or a sliding hernia, are defined as upward displacement of the gastroesophageal junction into the mediastinum. Type II hernias, or paraesophageal hernias, have the GE junction in a normal anatomic location with herniation of the gastric fundus through the diaphragmatic hiatus. Type III hernias have the combined features of type I and type II hernias. Type IV hernias have herniation of the stomach as well as adjacent organs, such as the spleen or duodenum.

Elective repair of symptomatic hiatal hernias may be undertaken, but asymptomatic hernias do not necessitate surgical intervention. However, the complication of gastric volvulus does exist, albeit the risk is low. Gastric volvulus is a surgical emergency. Inability to vomit and failure to pass a nasogastric tube are clinical features of a volvulus and are sufficient to warrant surgical intervention without endoscopy. Gastrografin contrast studies should be avoided in patients with suspected gastric volvulus, given the risk of aspiration.

Hiatal hernias may be repaired through either an abdominal or thoracic approach. The abdominal approach is prudent in cases of volvulus with suspected strangulation. Repair involves returning the gastroesophageal junction to its normal anatomic location and reapproximation of the esophageal hiatus. Studies have shown that use of mesh in hiatal hernia repairs decreases short-term hernia recurrence but has no effect on long-term recurrence.

Answer: A

Watson, D.L., Thompson, S.K., Devitt, P.G., *et al.* (2020) Five year follow-up of a randomized controlled trial of laparoscopic repair of very large hiatus hernia with sutures versus absorbable versus nonabsorbable mesh. *Annals of Surgery*, **272**, (2) 241–247.

Zhang, C., Diangang, L., Li, F., *et al.* Systematic review and meta-analysis of laparoscopic mesh versus suture repair of hiatus hernia: objective and subjective outcomes. (2017) *Surgical Endoscopy*, **31**, (12) 4913–4922.

Siegal, S.R., Dolan, J.P., Hunter, J.G. (2017) Modern diagnosis and treatment of hiatal hernia. *Langenbeck's Archives of Surgery*, **402**, 1145–1151.

Tam, V., Winger, D.G., Nason, K.S. (2016) A systematic review and meta-analysis of mesh vs suture cruroplasty in laparoscopic large hiatal hernia repair. *American Journal of Surgery*, **211**, (1) 226–238.

11 *A 53-year-old man presents with two episodes of hematemesis. His blood pressure is 93/52 mmHg and he is tachycardic to 117 beats/min. A nasogastric tube is placed with return of bright red blood. The patient undergoes emergent esophagogastroduodenoscopy. Which of the following findings would place the patient at highest risk for rebleeding?*

A *1 cm prepyloric shallow ulcer with hemosiderin deposit at the base*

B *1 cm prepyloric shallow ulcer with no active bleeding*

C *1.5 cm ulcer on the lesser curve with visible, non-bleeding vessel*

D *2 cm antral ulcer with active bleeding*

E *2 cm antral ulcer with adherent clot at base*

Bleeding proximal to the ligament of Treitz is classified as upper gastrointestinal bleeding. Melena and hematemesis are more likely indicative of upper GI bleeding, while hematochezia is more often associated with lower GI bleeding. Esophagogastroduodenoscopy is the modality of choice for upper gastrointestinal bleeding as it can be both diagnostic and therapeutic.

The risk of rebleeding in a peptic ulcer can be assessed by the Forrest Score. The highest risk for rebleeding is an ulcer with active bleeding, which has a recurrence rate as high as 55%. This is followed by visualization of a non-bleeding vessel with a rebleeding rate of 43%. An ulcer with an adherent clot, an ulcer with hematin at the base, and clean-based ulcer have decreasing rates of recurrence, respectively.

Forrest score	Endoscopic appearance	Risk of rebleeding*
Ia	Ulcer with active pulsating bleeding	55%
Ib	Ulcer with active nonpulsating bleeding	
IIa	Ulcer with a visible nonbleeding vessel	43%
IIb	Ulcer with an adherent clot	22%
IIc	Ulcer with hematin on ulcer base	10%
III	Ulcer with a clean base without signs of recent bleeding	5%

*Risk of rebleeding if endoscopic therapy is not performed. *Source*: Adapted from Laine, L., Peterson, W. L. (1994) Bleeding peptic ulcer. *New England Journal of Medicine*, **331**, 717–727.

Answer: D

Laine, L., Jensen, D.M. (2012) Management of patients with ulcer bleeding. *American Journal of Gastroenterology*, **107**, (3) 345–360.

12 *A 37-year-old woman is seen in the emergency department for mid-epigastric abdominal pain as well as nausea and vomiting. The patient has a history of hypertension and diabetes mellitus type II. The patient is hemodynamically normal with no fever or leukocytosis. The patient underwent a gastric band placement 5 years ago with a 30-pound weight loss. Abdominal imaging shows a gastric band with an angle of 70° between the vertical axis along the spine and the long axis of the band. What is the best next step to prevent further complications in this patient?*

A *Deflation of the gastric band*

B *Emergent gastric band removal*

C *Conversion of gastric band to a Roux-en-Y gastric bypass*

D *Administration of proton pump inhibitors*

E *Esophagogastroduodenoscopy*

While the placement of gastric bands has fallen out of favor, providers will still encounter patients with previous placement. Early complications from band placement include dysphagia, band slippage, balloon rupture, or esophagogastric injury. Late complications include band slippage, erosion, band fracture, and band intolerance. Band slippage may be diagnosed on plain radiographs of the abdomen. The angle formed between the long axis of the band and the vertical axis of the spine is called the phi angle. A normal angle is approximately 45°, with any angle over 58° indicative of band slippage.

If untreated, band slippage can lead to erosion and gastric necrosis if left untreated. The initial step is deflation of the gastric band, which can be done at the bedside and will often alleviate the patient's symptoms. However, if patients are septic or unstable, emergent operative intervention is indicated. Upper endoscopy is not necessary for the diagnosis of gastric band slippage if imaging is diagnostic, although it can be useful in diagnosing gastric erosion. Definitive treatment is band removal but deflating the balloon often will alleviate the need for emergent operative intervention. Proton pump inhibitors are not a treatment for a slipped gastric band.

Answer: A

Abdelbaki, T.N., Abdelsalam, W.N., ElKayal, S. (2016) Management modalities in slipped gastric band. *Surgery for Obesity and Related Diseases*, **12**, (3) 714–716.

13 *A 45-year-old woman is postoperative day 2 from a laparoscopic Roux-en-Y gastric bypass. Overnight the patient has become tachycardic and febrile. Laboratory evaluation reveals leukocytosis of 16 000 WBCs per microliter. Physical exam reveals healing incisions and mild tenderness in the mid-epigastric region but no peritonitis. What is the next diagnostic step in this patient?*

A *Gastrografin upper gastrointestinal series*
B *Esophagogastroduodenoscopy*
C *Diagnostic laparoscopy*
D *CTA chest with PO and IV contrast*
E *Acute abdominal series radiographs*

Postoperative complications from weight loss operations are well within the purview of acute care surgeons. Early complications of gastric bypass and sleeve gastrectomy include leak, bleeding, and early obstruction. As bariatric patients often have multiple medical comorbidities, the presentation of an anastomotic leak may be subtle. Therefore, a high index of suspicion must be maintained for this potentially devastating complication.

Persistent tachycardia in the postoperative period should raise suspicion for anastomotic or staple line leak. However, bariatric patients are also high risk for other associated complications, such as pulmonary embolus, which must also be considered and ruled out prior to repeat operative intervention. An acute abdominal series may show free air under the diaphragm, but in the immediate postoperative period is difficult to interpret. In a hemodynamically unstable or septic patient, emergent operative intervention should be undertaken. However, if the patient is hemodynamically stable, further workup for a leak may be undertaken. An upper gastrointestinal series may be obtained with water-soluble contrast. However, CTA scan with PO and IV contrast will rule out a pulmonary embolism, has a higher sensitivity rate for anastomotic leak, and provides more detailed anatomic information when compared with fluoroscopy. The most sensitive and specific test for a leak is reexploration, either laparoscopically or open. However, conservative treatment of contained anastomotic leaks is acceptable in a stable patient and therefore initial imaging is more appropriate than immediate operative intervention in this patient.

Answer: D

Lim, R., Beeklye, A., Johnson, D.D., *et al.* (2018) Early and late complications of bariatric operation. *Trauma Surgery and Acute Care Open*, **3**, e219.

Kim, J., Azagury, D., Eiseberg, D., *et al.* (2015) ASMBS position statement on prevention, detection, and treatment of gastrointestinal leak after gastric bypass and sleeve gastrectomy, including the roles of imaging, surgical exploration, and nonoperative management. *Surgery for Obesity and Related Disorders*, **11**, (4) 739–148.

Jacobsen, H.J., Nergard, B.J., Leifsson, B.G. *et al.* (2014) Management of suspected anastomotic leak after bariatric laparoscopic Roux-en-y gastric bypass. *British Journal of Surgery*, **101**, (4) 417–423.

14 *Which of the following statements about the duodenum is false?*

A *The common bile duct enters the second portion of the duodenum.*
B *The first portion of the duodenum is retroperitoneal.*
C *The boundary between the duodenum and jejunum is the ligament of Treitz.*
D *The superior mesenteric artery and the gastroduodenal artery supply the duodenum.*
E *Up to 10 L of fluid pass through the duodenum per day.*

The duodenum is the first portion of the small bowel. It begins at the pylorus and ends at the ligament of Treitz, approximately 30 cm in length. It derives its names from the Latin word *duodeni* which means twelve. It was so named for the length of twelve digits. The duodenum is divided into four segments. The first portion of the duodenum extends from the pylorus to the common bile duct and is intraperitoneal. This is the location of the majority of duodenal ulcers. The second portion begins at the common bile duct to the ampulla of Vater. The third portion then extends to the superior mesenteric artery and vein. Both the second and third portions are retroperitoneal. The final portion then transitions back to the intraperitoneal space and ends at the ligament of Treitz.

The duodenum receives its blood supply from the superior and inferior pancreaticoduodenal arteries which branch from the gastroduodenal artery and the superior mesenteric artery, respectively. Histologically, the duodenal mucosa is lined with Brunner's glands which serve to secrete mucus and bicarbonate, thereby neutralizing the acidic contents from the stomach. Between pancreatic enzymes, bile, and gastric contents, as much as 10 L of fluid pass through the duodenum each day. This is important surgically as the consequences of a duodenal leak or fistula can lead to severe fluid shifts and electrolyte imbalances.

Answer: B

Androulakis, J., Colborn, G.L., Skandalakis, P.N., *et al.* (2000) Embryologic and anatomic basis of duodenal surgery. *Surgical Clinics of North America*, **80**, (1) 171–199.

15 A 57-year-old woman presents with sudden onset mid-epigastric abdominal pain. On physical exam, the patient has peritonitis and CT imaging shows free air and inflammation around the stomach and duodenum. On exploratory laparotomy, the patient is found to have a 1 cm perforation on the anterior wall of the post-pyloric duodenum. Which of the following is true about duodenal ulcer perforation?

A All patients should undergo an acid reduction operation as part of the treatment.

B Primary repair of the defect is the best initial operation.

C H. pylori treatment has no effect on ulcer healing.

D Omental patch closure without primary closure is an acceptable treatment.

E Laparoscopic repair is contraindicated in elderly patients.

Duodenal ulcers are the result of increased acid production and decreased mucosal protection. Perforation occurs most often with anterior duodenal ulcers. Patient will present with sudden onset mid-epigastric abdominal pain. Free intra-abdominal air may be present on upright plain films but is not always present. Further investigation with cross-sectional imaging can provide further information leading to the diagnosis.

Operative repair is dependent on patient history and ulcer causation. Non-acid-related ulcers, such as with NSAID use, may be primarily repaired with omental patch closure. Not all acid-related ulcers require an acid reduction component in addition to the repair. If a patient has not been on acid-reducing medications, then it is acceptable to only complete the primary omental patch repair and trial the patient on proton pump inhibitors. The patient should also be tested for *H. pylori* and undergo treatment if positive as eradication has been shown to improve ulcer healing rates. However, in patients with prior antacid treatment or those who are deemed high risk for medication noncompliance, an acid reduction procedure should be considered. Vagotomy alone has a higher recurrence rate but lower complication rate when compared to resective operations such as an antrectomy. Selective vagotomy preserves the hepatic and celiac branches while denervating the stomach. Because this includes the pylorus, a drainage procedure such as pyloroplasty is needed. A highly selective vagotomy only denervates the distal branches to the parietal cells and therefore does not require a drainage procedure. Laparoscopic repair has been shown to be safe in repairing perforated duodenal ulcers. Patient age is not a contraindication to laparoscopic repair.

Answer: D

Soreide, K., Thorsen, K., Harrison, E.M., *et al.* (2015) Perforated peptic ulcer. *Lancet*, **386**, (10000) 1288–1298.

16 A 37-year-old woman presents with hematemesis. Upper endoscopy reveals a 1.5 cm duodenal ulcer with active bleeding. Which of the following is true about bleeding duodenal ulcers?

A Operative intervention is initial mode of treatment.

B Bleeding is most often associated with anterior duodenal ulcers.

C Surgical treatment involves ligation of the gastroduodenal artery and the pancreatic branch.

D Bleeding is the second most common complication from duodenal ulceration.

E Angiography should only be attempted after failed surgical treatment.

Bleeding is the most common complication of duodenal ulcers. Bleeding occurs most often from erosion of a posterior gastric ulcer into the gastroduodenal artery. Patient may present with hematemesis or melena. Upper endoscopy is the initial test of choice as it is both diagnostic and therapeutic. If endoscopic management fails to control bleeding, angiographic embolization is considered secondary line therapy.

Following endoscopic and angiographic treatment, if patients have evidence of continued bleeding and hemodynamic instability, surgical intervention may be considered. Surgical control involves three-point ligation. Stitches are placed superior and inferior to ligate the gastroduodenal ulcer. A medial suture is placed to ligate the pancreatic branch of the gastroduodenal artery. As explained above with perforated duodenal ulcers, the need for an acid-reducing procedure should be evaluated based on prior medication use and ability to comply with medical therapy.

Answer: C

Laine, L., Jensen, D.M. (2012) Management of patients with ulcer bleeding. *American Journal of Gastroenterology*, **107**, (3) 345–360.

17 A 25-year-old construction worker falls and is impaled by rebar in the mid-epigastric region. He is emergently taken to the operating room where an isolated injury to the antimesenteric portion of the second portion of the duodenum is found. The patient remains hemodynamically stable. Which of the following is the most appropriate operative intervention?

A Primary longitudinal repair of an injury involving 75% of the wall circumference.

B Pancreaticoduodenectomy with injury involving 50% of the wall circumference.

C Transverse primary repair of injury involving 25% of the wall circumference.

D *Transverse primary repair of injury involving 25% of the wall circumference and ampulla.*

E *Duodenojejunostomy partial thickness laceration to anterior wall.*

Injuries to the duodenum are rare and usually occur from penetrating injury. Patients should be evaluated based on relative stability. Unstable patients should undergo immediate surgical intervention. Hemodynamically normal patients may undergo further workup with cross-sectional imaging to further elucidate their injury burden prior to treatment.

Repair of the duodenum is dictated by the overall status of the patient as well as the extent of the duodenal injury and associated injuries. Patients in extremis warrant damage control with closure and drainage. In stable patients, the injury should be assessed for suitability for repair. Injuries involving less than 50% of the wall circumference are amenable to primary repair. Primary repair should be performed in a transverse fashion to avoid narrowing the bowel lumen. However, an injury involving the ampulla is a contraindication to simple primary repair and requires either reimplantation of the bile duct if the duodenum can be repaired or a pancreaticoduodenectomy. More extensive injuries are less likely to be amenable to primary repair. Techniques to achieve closure include duodenal mobilization or Roux-en-Y duodenojejunostomy.

Pyloric exclusion may also be considered in the treatment of duodenal injuries. Studies have shown mixed results, with some showing increased mortality and others showing no difference. Large medial injuries to the second portion of the duodenum and combined duodenal and pancreatic injuries may warrant pyloric exclusion. This is performed with either a noncutting stapler or suture ligation of the pylorus followed by a drainage procedure such as a gastrojejunostomy.

Answer: C

Schroeppel, T.J., Saleem, K., Sharpe, J.P., *et al.* (2016) Penetrating duodenal trauma: a 19-year experience. *Journal of Trauma and Acute Care Surgery*, **80**, (3) 461–465.

Malhotra, A., Biffl, W.L., Moore, E.E., *et al.* (2015) Western Trauma Association critical decisions in trauma: diagnosis and management of duodenal injuries. *Journal of Trauma and Acute Care Surgery*, **79**, (6) 1096–1101.

Ferrada, P., Wolfe, L., Duchesne, J., *et al.* (2019) Management of duodenal trauma: a retrospective review from the Panamerican Trauma Society. *Journal of Trauma and Acute Care Surgery*, **86**, (3) 392–396.

18 *A 12-year-old man presents after a bicycle crash where the handlebars impacted his abdomen. He presents with nausea and vomiting. A CT scan of the abdomen reveals a duodenal hematoma. Which of the following statements about duodenal hematomas is true?*

A *Early operative intervention improves outcomes.*

B *The majority of hematomas resolve with conservative management.*

C *Stenosis is a common long-term complication.*

D *Feeding gastrostomy should be placed if patient has associated injuries requiring abdominal operation.*

E *CT-guided drainage has no role in conservative management.*

Duodenal hematomas are a rare occurrence, most often the result of blunt abdominal trauma. As a mostly retroperitoneal structure, the duodenum is somewhat protected from blunt injury. The management is largely conservative. Due to the rich blood supply of the duodenum, most hematomas will ultimately resolve with nonoperative management. Early operative intervention for duodenal hematomas is therefore not indicated and converts a closed injury into an open injury. Most patients will have resolution of symptoms from a duodenal hematoma in approximately 7–10 days as the hematoma liquifies and resorption begins. In the study by Peterson *et al.*, 19 patients were found to resolve with nonoperative treatment of their duodenal hematoma. 5 patients underwent laparotomy for suspected hollow viscus injury but without hematoma drainage and one patient underwent percutaneous hematoma drainage. Early operative feeding access placement is therefore not indicated. However, in a small number of cases prolonged total parenteral nutrition may be required before symptoms resolve. Stenosis is a rare complication following duodenal hematoma. Some reports have shown success with image-guided percutaneous drainage in promoting resolution of symptoms.

Answer: B

Peterson, M., Abbas, P., Fallon, S., *et al.* (2015) Management of traumatic duodenal hematomas in children. *Journal of Surgical Research*, **199**, (1) 126–129.

19 *A 65-year-old man with known history of peptic ulcer disease presents with 3 days of nausea and PO intolerance. On physical exam, he is tympanic in the mid-epigastric region and has mild tenderness to palpation. He is mildly tachycardic and hypotensive but improves with IV fluid resuscitation. Abdominal imaging shows a dilated stomach with a paucity of air in the rest of the gastrointestinal tract. He undergoes an upper endoscopy which shows an obstructive duodenal ulcer. Which of the following is true of gastric outlet obstruction from peptic ulcer disease?*

A *Early operative intervention is needed to relieve the obstruction.*

B *Endoscopic treatment is contraindicated.*

C *Most patients have resolution of symptoms with conservative management.*

D *Obstruction is a common complication of peptic ulcer disease.*

E *Medical therapy does not improve obstruction resolution rates.*

Gastric outlet obstruction is a rare complication from peptic ulcer disease. The incidence in developed countries ranges from 1–3 per 100 000. The vast majority of obstruction is caused by duodenal ulcers. In the acute setting, obstruction is caused by the inflammation and swelling surrounding the ulcer. A trial of conservative management with gastric decompression, proton pump inhibitors, and *H. pylori* eradication in positive patients yields favorable results the majority of the time. In patients that fail to resolve with conservative management, endoscopic stenting has shown good short- and long-term effects in the resolution of obstruction resulting from peptic ulcer disease.

Surgical intervention for obstruction in peptic ulcer disease is most often the result of stenosis or stricture. However, this indication is rare as the complications from peptic ulcer disease have decreased with improved medical management options. In addition, endoscopic balloon dilation is an acceptable alternative with favorable results.

Answer: C

Hasadia, R., Kopelman, Y., Oded, O., *et al.* (2018) Short- and long-term outcomes of surgical management of peptic ulcer complications in the era of proton pump inhibitors. *European Journal of Trauma and Emergency Surgery*, **44**, (5) 795–801.

Hamzaoui, L., Bouassida, M., Mansour, I., *et al.* (2015) Balloon dilation in patients with gastric outlet obstruction related to peptic ulcer disease. *Arab Journal of Gastroenterology*, **16**, (3) 121–124.

Cherian, P., Cherian, S., Sing, P. (2007) Long-term follow-up patients with gastric outlet obstruction related to peptic ulcer disease treated with endoscopic balloon dilation and drug therapy. *Gastrointestinal Endoscopy*, **66**, (3) 491–497.

20 *A 37-year-old man has a history of abdominal gunshot wound necessitating gastrectomy with Roux-en-Y reconstruction. The patient presents complaining of abdominal pain and diarrhea 30 minutes after eating. Which of the following is true about dumping syndrome?*

A *Dumping syndrome is caused by rapid transport of protein into the duodenum.*

B *Late dumping syndrome is more common than early dumping.*

C *Dietary modifications are the mainstay of treatment.*

D *Late dumping syndrome is characterized by hyperglycemia.*

E *Hypoosmotic loads cause fluid to shift into the bowel.*

Dumping syndrome can occur following gastrectomy or vagotomy with pyloroplasty, thereby causing rapid gastric emptying. The rapid transport of carbohydrates precipitates symptoms. Patients may present with abdominal pain, nausea, diarrhea, sweating, dizziness, or flushing following PO intake.

There are two phases of dumping syndrome. Early dumping syndrome is more common. It is causes by hyperosmotic fluid loads leading to fluid shifts in the small bowel. This leads to the aforementioned symptoms. Late dumping syndrome presents as hypoglycemia. The rapid influx of carbohydrates into the small intestines causes a transient rise in the blood glucose level. In response, there is an increase in insulin production, leading to rebound hypoglycemia.

Most patients with dumping syndrome are successfully treated with dietary modifications. Patients are encouraged to eat multiple, smaller meals throughout the day that are high in protein content and low in carbohydrates. Surgical intervention is reserved for patients who fail to respond to lifestyle modifications. However, surgical interventions have a poor success rate. Most data are based on low volume case series. Operations include pancreatic resection, gastric bypass reversal, and gastric pouch restriction. Of these, pancreatic resection has the worst outcomes. In addition to failure to alleviate symptoms, complications from surgical treatment include weight gain and diabetes.

Answer: C

Van Beek, A.P., Emous, M., Laville, M., *et al.* (2017) Dumping syndrome after esophageal, gastric or bariatric surgery: pathophysiology, diagnosis, and management. *Obesity Reviews*, **18**, (1) 68–85.

21 *A 63-year-old woman is admitted to the intensive care unit and requires intubation for respiratory failure. The patient is started on nasogastric tube feeds. Which of the following is true regarding gastrointestinal ulcer prophylaxis?*

A *Gastrointestinal stress ulcer prophylaxis is not beneficial in patients receiving enteral nutrition.*

B *Clostridium difficile infection is decreased with gastrointestinal stress ulcer prophylaxis.*

C *Pharmacologic stress ulcer prophylaxis has been shown to decrease mortality.*

D *Stress ulcer prophylaxis is protective against pneumonia.*

E *Proton pump inhibitors should be used in conjunction with H2 receptor antagonists.*

The choice of an appropriate patient for pharmacologic stress ulcer prophylaxis is an evolving question. Some studies have shown an increased incidence of pneumonia with pharmacologic stress ulcer prophylaxis as it may alter the microbiome of the stomach. In addition, studies have failed to show an improvement in mortality with pharmacologic prophylaxis, even in patients considered high risk, including those on mechanical ventilation or who have coagulopathy or renal failure. Studies on the effects of pharmacologic prophylaxis on *Clostridium difficile* infection have had mixed results, with some showing increased incidence with treatment and others showing no effect. Studies have also shown that the use of pharmacologic prophylaxis is not beneficial in patients who are also receiving enteral nutrition. The use of both a proton pump inhibitor and H2 receptor antagonist has historically not been advised as H2 receptor antagonists may interfere with the efficacy of proton pump inhibitors.

Answer: A

Huang, H.-B., Jiang, W., Wang, C.-Y. (2018) Stress ulcer prophylaxis in intensive care unit patients receiving enteral nutrition: a systematic review and meta-analysis. *Critical Care*, **22**, (1) 20.

Krag, M., Marker, S., Perner, A., *et al.* (2018) Pantoprazole in patients at risk for gastrointestinal bleeding in the ICU. *New England Journal of Medicine*, **379**, (22) 2199–2208.

37

Small Intestine, Appendix, and Colorectal

Elise Sienicki, MD[1], Vishal Bansal, MD[2], and Jay J. Doucet, MD, MSc[3]

[1] *Naval Medical Center, San Diego, CA, USA*
[2] *Scripps Mercy Hospital, San Diego, CA, USA*
[3] *Department of Surgery, University of California San Diego, San Diego, CA, USA*

Colon, Small Bowel, and Appendix

1 *A 21-year-old man is brought by ambulance to the trauma bay after sustaining a gunshot wound to the abdomen. He is alert and oriented with a heart rate of 130 beats/min and blood pressure 95/55 mm Hg. His FAST exam is positive and he is taken urgently for laparotomy. During surgery, there is extensive damage to the transverse colon. You notice an expanding hematoma at the base of the transverse mesocolon and suspect a superior mesenteric artery (SMA) injury. As you expose the SMA, you find a near-complete transection of the SMA just distal to the middle colic artery. Which of the following is true about this injury?*

   A *Ligation at the point of injury would most likely result in loss of significant portions of small bowel.*

   B *This is a zone 3 injury, which carries a mortality rate of 40%.*

   C *The preferred method of repair involves temporary shunting with a second-look operation.*

   D *This patient's greatest mortality risk is due to infection.*

   E *Most SMA injuries can be managed successfully with angioembolization.*

Injuries to the SMA carry significant morbidity and mortality. The incidence of these injuries is unknown; however, they generally account for less than 1% of cases at large trauma centers. Most laparotomy deaths for SMA injuries are due to exsanguination, not infection. Review of the literature reveals that those who undergo primary repair have a lower incidence of associated vascular and nonvascular injuries, and have improved survival, compared to those who undergo ligation (and have a higher

number of associated injuries). The SMA zones of injury were first described in the 1970s.

Zone of injury	Anatomic location	Mortality (%)
Zone 1	Aorta to inferior pancreato-duodenal artery	Close to 100
Zone 2	Inferior pancreato-duodenal artery to middle colic artery	43
Zone 3	Trunk distal to middle colic artery	25
Zone 4	Segmental branches	25

There are no definitive published guidelines for management of these injuries; however, there are various options that have been extensively reviewed. Ligation should be considered in unstable patients when bowel ischemia is present. Ligation in zones 1 and 2 carries a significant risk of bowel ischemia, unless sufficient collaterals are present. Ligation in zones 3 and 4 carry a lower risk of ischemia, but the risk may be increased if the patient has significant atherosclerotic disease. In a damage-control setting, shunting can be performed with a planned second-look operation, with later reconstruction with a saphenous vein graft or PTFE. Angioembolization has been successful in managing these injuries recently, although there is significant risk of ischemia and it is advised to only perform angioembolization in hemodynamically stable patients.

Answer: A

Asensio JA, Britt LD, Borzotta A, et al. Multi-institutional experience with the management of superior mesenteric artery injuries. *J Am Coll Surg.* 2001, 193(4):354–366. Erratum in Journal of the American College of Surgeons, 193 (6), 718.

Phillips B, Reiter S, Murray EP, et al. Trauma to the superior mesenteric artery and superior mesenteric vein: A narrative review of rare but lethal injuries. *World J Surg*. 2018;42(3):713–726.

2   *A 60-year-old woman presents to the trauma bay after a head-on motor vehicle collision. She is alert, oriented, and complaining of abdominal pain. Her vitals are normal on initial assessment. Bruising is present across her low abdomen and she has tenderness without peritoneal findings. Initial CT scan of the abdomen shows no solid organ injury but a small amount of free fluid in the right paracolic gutter and some mild small bowel wall thickening. Her abdominal pain improves in the trauma bay and she is admitted for observation. Six hours later, you are called to reassess her because her pain has returned. Her vitals remain within normal limits. She is tender in the right hemi-abdomen, but again without peritoneal signs. Her labs have since resulted and show a WBC count of 11 000. Which of the following is the next best course of action?*

   A   *Repeat CT scan of the abdomen with IV contrast only*
   B   *Repeat CT scan of the abdomen with IV and PO contrast*
   C   *Continued observation until she develops peritonitis*
   D   *Surgical exploration*
   E   *Acute abdominal series*

Answer: D

3   *Which of the above patient's signs or symptoms predict, with the greatest accuracy, the presence of blunt small bowel injury?*

   A   *Tenderness on physical exam*
   B   *Free fluid on CT scan*
   C   *Bowel wall thickening*
   D   *Lower abdominal bruising from seat belt*
   E   *Elevated WBC count*

Blunt small bowel perforation (SBP) remains a diagnostic challenge to this day, even though our diagnostic capabilities have improved. Rates of small bowel injury range from 5 to 15% of blunt abdominal trauma patients, and perforation occurring in 1%. These injuries are often found incidentally on laparotomy for other intra-abdominal injuries. The presence of abdominal free fluid in the trauma patient, in the absence of solid organ injury or other obvious source of bleeding, should prompt evaluation for small bowel injury.

Another mechanism of small bowel injury in trauma is mesenteric injury resulting from shearing forces that can tear the small bowel loose from its blood supply, which may result in delayed perforation, stricture, and internal hernia from bowel being trapped in the new mesenteric defect.

Blunt abdominal trauma patients can present a diagnostic challenge. Many recommend additional diagnostic/therapeutic intervention by 8 hours after arrival in these patients, as the mortality from blunt SBP increases to 30.8% from 13% in those who receive surgical therapy greater than 8 hours from injury. Repeat CT scans may provide some useful information; however, in this patient who has reasonable signs of small bowel injury on her initial scan, will only delay operative intervention. Continued observation in this patient who is high risk is also not the best course of action.

Recent studies show that the most accurate indicator of blunt SBP is the presence of free fluid on abdominal CT. Other signs including tenderness on physical exam, bowel wall thickening, seat belt sign, and elevated WBC count are less reliable.

Answer: B

Fakhry SM, Allawi A, Ferguson PL, et al. Blunt small bowel perforation (SBP): An Eastern Association for the Surgery of Trauma multicenter update 15 years later. *J Trauma Acute Care Surg*. 2019;86(4):642–650.

4   *A 38-year-old woman is horseback riding when she is thrown from the horse and lands on a wood pile. She is brought to the hospital for evaluation of rectal pain. She is hemodynamically normal. There is blood present on digital rectal exam and a small external wound is noted that is not bleeding. A CT scan with IV contrast shows evidence of a rectal injury 8 cm above the anal verge that is confirmed on rigid proctoscopy. What procedure should this patient undergo?*

   A   *Transanal repair without fecal diversion*
   B   *Transanal repair with sigmoid loop colostomy*
   C   *Transanal repair with end-sigmoid colostomy*
   D   *Primary repair, presacral drainage, and sigmoid loop colostomy*
   E   *Primary repair, distal limb washout, and sigmoid end colostomy*

In the 1970s, Vietnam-era surgeons taking care of combat casualties published the 4 "Ds" of rectal trauma, and advocated for their regular use when dealing with penetrating rectal injuries: direct repair, diversion, distal rectal washout, and presacral drain. Over time, however, these data have been challenged, and current guidelines and the data do not support the use of presacral drainage or distal limb washout. In traumatic injury to the anus, the concern for severe fecal incontinence as well as pelvic sepsis is paramount; therefore, aggressive surgical management is still a surgical mainstay. Careful examination of the anus under anesthesia will help ascertain the continuity and of the internal and external sphincter, as well as the integrity of the anal canal and distal rectum. Immediate repair of the sphincter and transanal repair of the rectum should combined with diversion by loop colostomy in those with extraperitoneal injuries to avoid the development of pelvic sepsis. End-colostomy is a surgical option, but the ease of colostomy takedown with a loop colostomy makes it preferred in this setting.

Answer: B

Brown CVR, Teixeira PG, Furay E, et al. The AAST contemporary management of rectal injuries study group contemporary management of rectal injuries at level I trauma centers: The results of an American Association for the Surgery of Trauma multi-institutional study. *J Trauma Acute Care Surg*. 2018;84(2):225–233

5 *A 57-year-old man is brought to your trauma bay after sustaining multiple stab wounds to the abdomen. He has a history of asthma but is otherwise healthy. He is tachycardic and hypotensive and is given two units of whole blood in the trauma bay and is transferred urgently to the operating room for exploration. During surgery, you encounter a significant splenic laceration with active hemorrhage, a full-thickness descending colon injury involving less than 50% of the circumference of the colon, as well as a serosal tear of the stomach. A splenectomy is successfully performed and the stomach thoroughly examined with no posterior injury identified and no pancreatic injury. At this point, the patient has received another two units of packed red blood cells, and is hemodynamically stable with an arterial pH of 7.34. How should the colon injury be addressed?*
   A *Resection, primary anastomosis, diverting transverse loop colostomy*
   B *Resection, primary anastomosis*
   C *Primary repair, diverting transverse loop colostomy*
   D *Primary repair*
   E *Transverse loop colostomy, drain placement*

The grade of injury in adult civilian patients with penetrating colon injuries is less important for determining the management of colon injuries than is the risk factors for anastomotic breakdown. Even destructive injuries (>50% of circumference) may be managed without diversion in low-risk patients. For high-risk penetrating colon injuries (delay >12 hours, shock, associated injuries, transfusion > 6 units of blood, contamination, or left-side colon injuries), colon repair or resection may be still be performed rather than mandatory colostomy. Colostomy may have a role in select patients with other injuries (pancreas). Low-risk patients with penetrating colon injury without signs of shock, significant hemorrhage, severe contamination, or delay to surgical intervention should preferentially undergo colon repair or resection and anastomosis versus colostomy. In cases of damage-control laparotomy, there is increased risk of anastomotic breakdown; however, colostomy is still not mandatory and clinical judgment is required.

Answer: D

Cullinane DC, Jawa RS, Como JJ, et al. Management of penetrating intraperitoneal colon injuries: A meta-analysis and practice management guideline from the Eastern Association for the Surgery of Trauma. *J Trauma Acute Care Surg*. 2019;86(3):505–515.

6 *An 89-year-old woman is brought to the ED by ambulance from a skilled nursing facility, where she has been recovering from hip replacement surgery, with a chief complaint of constipation for 7 days. She has a past medical history that includes diabetes, dementia, and hypertension. On exam, she is quite distended but nontender to palpation in her abdomen. Plain radiographs of the abdomen are obtained which show significant dilation of the entire colon without air in the sigmoid or rectum, and without free air. In addition to admission, electrolyte replacement and cessation of narcotics, what is the next best step in management?*
   A *Rectal tube placement*
   B *Anoscopy*
   C *Placement of an NG tube*
   D *Laparotomy*
   E *Upper GI contrast study*

Answer: C

7 *The above patient is admitted for conservative medical management, cessation of narcotics, and an NG tube but has not had relief of symptoms after 72 hours. What is the next best step to relieve her symptoms?*
   A *Decompressive rectal tube placed at bedside*
   B *Subcutaneous neostigmine in a monitored setting*
   C *Colonoscopic decompression*
   D *Exploratory laparotomy and subtotal colectomy*
   E *Loop sigmoid ostomy for colonic pseudo-obstruction*

Acute colonic pseudo-obstruction (ACPO), or Ogilvie's syndrome, almost exclusively occurs in hospitalized or immobilized patients. Risk factors include older age, recent major orthopedic procedure, narcotic use, and electrolyte disturbances. Despite the dramatic appearance of the colon on imaging, these patients rarely need surgery. The most serious adverse events of ACPO are ischemia and perforation, with an increased risk in patients with cecal diameters greater than 10–12 cm and in those with abdominal distention greater than 6 days. When evaluating these patients, a mechanical obstruction must be ruled out first. This can be done with either rigid proctoscopy or CT scan. CT imaging is not only highly sensitive and specific for detecting mechanical obstruction, but it can also show evidence of ischemia, perforation, and evaluate for extrinsic or intrinsic compression. Water-soluble contrast enema of the rectum and distal colon is another diagnostic option, although CT has largely replaced contrast enema studies. It is worth noting that mechanical obstruction rarely occurs in a patient admitted for unrelated illnesses (i.e., pneumonia, elective non-GI surgery). Rectal tube placement at the bedside rarely is helpful because the right colon is frequently adynamic. After maximal medical management with narcotic avoidance, electrolyte correction, and NG decompression (if needed), the next step is neostigmine administration which is 85–94% effective. Male gender, younger age, postsurgical status, and having electrolyte imbalance are risk factors for nonresponse to neostigmine. Daily administration of polyethylene glycol via nasogastric tube has also been shown to decrease recurrence. Continuous infusion or subcutaneous administration of neostigmine may reduce cardiovascular effects while remaining effective. Traditionally, endoscopic decompression with colonoscopy is second-line therapy after failure of medical management and neostigmine. There are no randomized controlled trials of pharmacologic versus endoscopic therapy for ACPO; however, two retrospective studies found colonoscopic decompression to be superior to neostigmine. The data are considered limited and the 2020 American Society for Gastrointestinal Endoscopy ACPO guidelines continue to recommend initial pharmacologic therapy.

Answer: B

Naveed M, Jamil LH, Fujii-Lau LL, et al. American Society for Gastrointestinal Endoscopy guideline on the role of endoscopy in the management of acute colonic pseudo-obstruction and colonic volvulus. *Gastrointest Endosc.* 2020;91(2):228–235. doi: 10.1016/j.gie.2019.09.007. Epub 2019 Nov 30. Erratum in: Gastrointest Endosc. 2020 Mar;91(3):721.

8 *A 65-year-old woman with a history of chronic constipation and rheumatoid arthritis, presents with a 12 hour history of severe right lower quadrant abdominal pain, nausea, and vomiting. She takes methotrexate for her arthritis as well as multiple laxatives for constipation. On examination, she is distended and has mild lower abdominal tenderness without peritoneal signs. Her labs are normal including WBC count and renal function. A coffee-bean sign is seen on an abdominal plain film taken in the ED. She is taken to surgery, where patchy ischemic bowel is found at the involved segment. What is the best management strategy for this patient?*

A *Detorsion and placement of a venting tube through the abdominal wall*

B *Detorsion and pexy of the non-ischemic portion of the involved bowel to the abdominal wall*

C *Resection and diverting ileostomy*

D *Resection and primary anastomosis*

E *Detorsion and observing the involved portion of bowel with resection only if it does not appear viable*

The figure shows cecal volvulus. Cecal volvulus affects a younger population than sigmoid volvulus, and is also relatively more common in females. Cecal volvulus should be considered a surgical emergency. Decompressive colonoscopy is rarely successful (30%) in cases of cecal volvulus, and should not be performed. The best management of this condition is a right hemicolectomy and primary anastomosis, to remove the mobile portion of bowel. Cecopexy is not favored as the recurrence rate is high, and recurrent volvulus would place the patient at risk for perforation. Cecostomy placement is a relatively easy procedure but is also not recommended for this patient as it is associated with a high risk of complications including missed intestinal ischemia. In the debilitated, frail patient who would not tolerate a resection, these procedures may be considered, with great caution. Detorsion and observation of the bowel (E) is not recommended due to high rate of recurrence without resection. Diverting ileostomy is rarely required for this condition unless hemodynamic instability or significant intra-abdominal contamination is present.

Answer: D

Vogel JD, Feingold DL, Stewart DB, et al. Clinical practice guidelines for colon volvulus and acute colonic pseudo-obstruction. *Dis Colon Rectum.* 2016;59(7):589–600.

Perrot L, Fohlen A, Alves A, Lubrano J. Management of the colonic volvulus in 2016. *J Visc Surg.* 2016;153(3): 183–192.

9 *You are asked to see a 91-year-old man who is admitted to the internal medicine service from a skilled nursing facility for dehydration and failure to thrive with significant weight loss over the past month. The medicine team reports the patient experienced an*

episode of severe abdominal distension, and plain radiographs showed a "bent inner tube" sign. On exam, he is still distended and has mild tenderness to palpation in the low abdomen. Rectal exam shows no stool in the vault. During colonoscopy, the colon appears viable except for a 7 cm segment of sigmoid with black mucosa. What is the next step in management?

A *Open detorsion and sigmoidpexy in the OR*

B *Sigmoidectomy, primary reanastomosis*

C *Continue colonoscopic detorsion and admit for observation*

D *Sigmoidectomy, end-colostomy*

E *Percutaneous endoscopic colostomy*

Volvulus of the sigmoid colon is the most common presentation of colonic volvulus. It is frequently present in those with significant comorbidities and in the institutionalized, so careful history, examination, and routine blood work are all indicated in the workup of this condition. Sigmoid volvulus can be diagnosed via plain radiographs only in 31–66% of patients. Contrast enema and CT scan also play a diagnostic role. Endoscopy is first-line therapy in the absence of peritonitis. During endoscopic detorsion, if there is evidence of ischemic bowel, sigmoid resection is mandated. Primary reanastomosis can be established in most cases; however, in patients who are significantly immunosuppressed or that have extremely poor nutritional status, it may be safer to perform a colostomy with resection. Percutaneous endoscopic colostomy is a minimally invasive procedure that is reserved only for the poorest of surgical candidates, and it contraindicated if ischemic bowel is present. Sigmoidpexy is not recommended as there is not only high rate of recurrence, but the redundant sigmoid makes the procedure technically unfeasible. A second attempt at endoscopic detorsion is not appropriate given the necrotic mucosa witnessed on initial endoscopy. Urgent sigmoid resection is the best next step in management.

Answer: D

Vogel JD, Feingold DL, Stewart DB, et al. Clinical practice guidelines for colon volvulus and acute colonic pseudo-obstruction. *Dis Colon Rectum.* 2016;59(7):589–600.

Naveed M, Jamil LH, Fujii-Lau LL, et al. American Society for Gastrointestinal Endoscopy guideline on the role of endoscopy in the management of acute colonic pseudo-obstruction and colonic volvulus. *Gastrointest Endosc.* 2020;91(2):228–235. doi: 10.1016/j.gie.2019.09.007. Epub 2019 Nov 30. Erratum in: Gastrointest Endosc. 2020 Mar;91(3):721.

10 *A 19-year-old man undergoes an uncomplicated laparoscopic appendectomy for acute appendicitis and is discharged the same day. Final pathology of the appendix shows a 2 cm carcinoid tumor at the midportion of the appendix. What do you recommend the patient undergo?*

A *Observation, no further therapy required*

B *Ileocecectomy*

C *Right hemicolectomy with lymph node sampling*

D *Right hemicolectomy, no lymph nodes required*

E *Octreotide and neoadjuvant chemotherapy, followed by right hemicolectomy*

Neuroendocrine tumors, commonly carcinoid tumors, are the most common neoplasm found in the appendix. Prognosis is based on size. For tumors less than 1 cm, appendectomy is sufficient. For tumors greater than 2 cm, or for tumors between 1 and 2 cm in the presence of deep meso-appendiceal invasion (>3 mm), positive or unclear margins, a higher proliferative rate (grade ≥2), lymphovascular invasion, and mixed histology (goblet cell adenocarcinoma), a right hemicolectomy with lymph node sampling (oncologic resection) is recommended by the North American Neuroendocrine Tumor Society (NANETS) and the European Neuroendocrine Tumor Society (ENETS). National Comprehensive Cancer Network (NCCN) guidelines currently recommends appendectomy for T1 tumors (<1 cm). For incomplete resection, re-exploration with right hemicolectomy should be considered. For T2-T4 lesions, staging by imaging and hemicolectomy is the treatment of choice. The risk of nodal metastases at diagnosis is 0, 7.5, and 33% for patients with appendiceal carcinoid < 1, 1 to 1.9, and > 2 cm, respectively. Octreotide and chemotherapy would be treatments for disseminated disease.

Answer: D

Kunz PL, Reidy-Lagunes D, Anthony LB, et al. North American Neuroendocrine Tumor Society. Consensus guidelines for the management and treatment of neuroendocrine tumors. *Pancreas.* 2013;42(4):557–577.

Landry CS, Woodall C, Scoggins CR, et al. Analysis of 900 appendiceal carcinoid tumors for a proposed predictive staging system. *Arch Surg.* 2008;143(7): 664–670.

11 *A 70-year-old woman with a history of COPD and current tobacco use is admitted to the MICU with severe pneumonia, and is intubated for respiratory failure. You are called to evaluate her several hours later for abdominal distension and for an abnormal CT finding. Her vitals are as follows: blood pressure 105/70 mm Hg, HR 105 beats/min, temp 99 °F.*

Although intubated, she is awake and can interact with you and indicates she is not having abdominal pain. Her abdomen is distended and tympanic, but soft and minimally tender. Her urine output has been 0.5 mL/kg/hr for the past 3 hours and she is not currently on pressors. A representative image from her CT scan is shown. She is on antibiotics for her pneumonia. What is the most appropriate management of her abdominal distension at this time?

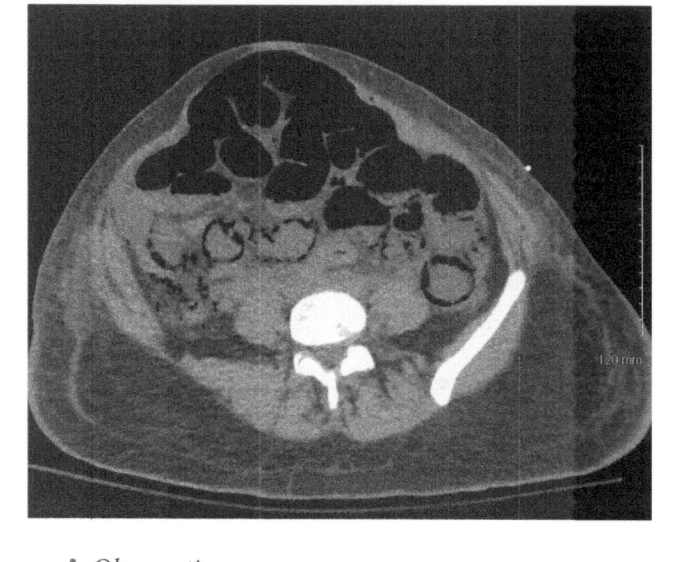

A *Observation*
B *Diagnostic laparoscopy*
C *Exploratory laparotomy with resection of involved bowel*
D *Splanchnic vasodilators*
E *IV fluid resuscitation*

Pneumatosis intestinalis are pockets of air within the bowel wall, typically in the submucosal or subserosal layers. Most cases are associated with COPD or an immunocompromised state, such as HIV or after transplantation. Other associated conditions include intestinal ischemia, inflammatory and obstructive conditions of the intestine, and iatrogenic causes including recent endoscopy or jejunostomy placement. If this patient had altered physiology, signs of sepsis, or had peritoneal findings on physical exam, surgical exploration would be warranted; however, she is hemodynamically stable with a relatively benign abdominal exam. Splanchnic vasodilators have no role to play in this condition, regardless of the underlying cause. She does not require further IV fluid resuscitation given her current urine output, and one should try to avoid fluid overload in those with tenuous pulmonary physiology. Risk factors for pathological PI are best defined in a 2013 study by the EAST Pneumatosis Study Group and include hypotension, vasopressor use, peritonitis, lactate > 2 mmol/L, and acute renal failure.

Answer: A

Braumann C, Menenakos C, Jacobi CA. Pneumatosis intestinalis - A pitfall for surgeons? *Scand J Surg.* 2005, 94(1):47–50. Published online.

DuBose JJ, Lissauer M, Maung AA, et al., EAST Pneumatosis Study Group. Pneumatosis Intestinalis Predictive Evaluation Study (PIPES): a multicenter epidemiologic study of the Eastern Association for the Surgery of Trauma. *J Trauma Acute Care Surg.* 2013;75(1):15–23.

Ferrada P, Callcut R, Bauza G, et al. Pneumatosis intestinalis predictive evaluation study: A multicenter epidemiologic study of the American Association for the Surgery of Trauma *J Trauma Acute Care Surg.* 2017;82(3):451–460.

12 *A 45-year-old man presents to the ED with 2 days of abdominal pain, nausea, and vomiting. He has a history of bloating/burping for several weeks but has not yet sought medical care. He is otherwise healthy and has never had abdominal surgery before. He is tachycardic and normotensive in the ED. A CT is performed which shows dilated loops of small bowel with a clear transition point. There are no abnormalities in the mesentery or other abdominal organs. You proceed to the operating room and perform an exploratory laparotomy. The cause of the obstruction is identified as a 6 cm extraluminal mass in the distal jejunum. The proximal bowel is dilated but appears viable. What is the recommended surgical procedure?*

A *Small bowel resection with peri-tumor margins proximally and distally, with reanastomosis.*
B *Small bowel resection with 10 cm margins proximally and distally, with regional lymphadenectomy, and reanastomosis.*
C *Small bowel resection to uninvolved small bowel proximally and distally, with reanastomosis.*
D *Small bowel resection to uninvolved small bowel proximally and distally, with regional lymphadenectomy and reanastomosis.*
E *Biopsy the mass and wait for pathologic diagnosis to proceed.*

Small bowel neoplasms are a rare but important cause of primary small bowel obstruction. The characteristics of this mass are most consistent with a gastrointestinal stromal tumor (GIST). These masses are commonly exophitic, and therefore cause obstruction when they have reached significant size. Adenocarcinomas and leiomyomas grow intraluminally and present earlier with obstructive symptoms. Biopsy of GISTs is not recommended, as tumor rupture portends a higher rate of peritoneal recurrence. There is no recommended margin length for resection. The goal is resection to normal-appearing bowel bilaterally, avoiding both an unnecessary long resection, as well as a peri-tumoral resection. Routine lymphadenectomy is unnecessary because the rate of nodal metastases is rare (1.1–3.4% of cases). Prognosis after resection is largely based on tumor size and mitotic rate.

Answer: C

Bamboat ZM, DeMatteo RP. Updates on the management of gastrointestinal stromal tumors. *Surg Oncol Clin N Am*. 2012;21(2):301–316.

Eisenberg BL, Pipas JM. Gastrointestinal stromal tumor-background, pathology, treatment. *Hematol Oncol Clin North Am*. Published online 2012, 26(6): 1239–1259.

13 *A 31-year-old man with a history of ulcerative colitis and an episode of otitis media treated with amoxicillin is admitted to the hospital for management of an acute flare of his colitis, with abdominal pain and bloody diarrhea. He is on adalimumab for maintenance of his disease, and is started on a course of prednisone while inpatient. His symptoms temporarily improve, but he develops watery diarrhea and worsening pain on hospital day 3. You are consulted for evaluation of his pain. His vitals on evaluation are temperature 38.0 °C, heart rate 110 beats/min, and blood pressure 130/68 mm Hg. On exam, he is distended, with diffuse tenderness to palpation with guarding throughout. His WBC count is 24 000/mm³ and his creatinine is 2.1 mg/dL, an increase from 0.9 mg/dL. A plain radiograph is obtained which shows dilated large bowel from the cecum to the sigmoid colon, with a transverse colon diameter of 11 cm. The next best step in management is:*

A *Colonoscopy to evaluate for colonic ischemia*

B *Exploratory laparotomy, diverting loop ileostomy, and colonic lavage*

C *Exploratory laparotomy, segmental resection of any abnormal appearing colon, and primary anastomosis*

D *Exploratory laparotomy, subtotal colectomy, end-ileostomy*

E *Exploratory laparotomy, subtotal colectomy, ileorectal anastomosis*

Clostridium difficile (*C. difficile*) colitis has increased in incidence and severity over the past 20 years. Severe *C. difficile* colitis is defined as WBC > 15 000 cells/mm³, albumin < 3 g/dL, and/or a creatinine level > 1.5 times the premorbid level. The initial treatment for severe disease is oral vancomycin, with IV metronidazole often being added in the setting of ileus. Fecal transplants do not have a defined role for severe disease at this time, but are effective in treating recurrent mild-to-moderate bouts of recurrent *C. difficile* colitis.

Toxic megacolon is a feared complication of severe *C. difficile* colitis. The most widely used criteria for clinical diagnosis are

- Radiographic evidence of colonic distension (>6 cm)
- Plus three of the following: Fever > 38 °C, HR > 120 bpm, neutrophilic leukocytosis > 10 500/mL, and anemia
- Plus at least one of the following: dehydration, altered mental status, electrolyte disturbances, hypotension

The recommended procedure for *C. difficile* colitis is subtotal colectomy. Removal of only grossly abnormal colon is not recommended, as there may be severe mucosal and submucosal disease not visible to the surgeon. Death rates are higher in those who receive partial colectomy, presumably due to residual disease as the ongoing source of sepsis. Reanastomosis should not be performed due to ongoing inflammation and risk of dehiscence.

Diverting loop ileostomy with colonic lavage with high-volume polyethylene glycol-based solution and postoperative antegrade colonic vancomycin treatment through the ileostomy has been described as a colon-preserving procedure. In one study, preservation of the colon was achieved in 93% of patients. Despite a possible less morbid operative approach, the patient in the question above has signs of peritonitis with possible necrotic colon secondary to toxic megacolon. The safest next step is subtotal colon resection and end ileostomy.

Answer: D

Koss K, Clark MA, Sanders DS, et al. The outcome of surgery in fulminant Clostridium difficile colitis. *Colorectal Dis*. 2006;8(2):149–154.

Neal MD, Alverdy JC, Hall DE, et al. (2011) Diverting loop ileostomy and colonic lavage: an alternative to total abdominal colectomy for the treatment of severe, complicated Clostridium difficile associated disease. *Ann Surg*;254(3):423–429.

Sartelli M, Di Bella S, McFarland LV, et al. 2019 update of the WSES guidelines for management of Clostridioides (Clostridium) difficile infection in surgical patients. *World J Emerg Surg*. 2019;14:8. doi: 10.1186/s13017-019-0228-3. PMID: 30858872; PMCID: PMC6394026.

14 *A 64-year-old obese man who has never had a colonoscopy before presents to the ED with left lower quadrant pain for 3 days. He has poorly controlled* diabetes, hypertension, and a history of a myocardial infarction 5 years prior. He is febrile to 38.4 °C and his heart rate is 110 beats/min, and his abdomen is tender to percussion in the left lower quadrant. His WBC count is 16 000/mm³. Abdominal CT imaging shows a thickened sigmoid with a 5 cm abscess, and free fluid in the pelvis without air. The next step in management should be:

A Resuscitation, IV antibiotics, and emergent colonoscopy to look for malignancy

B Resuscitation, IV antibiotics, and consultation to IR for percutaneous drainage

C Laparoscopic exploration and lavage, with drain placement

D Exploration with sigmoidectomy and colorectal anastomosis

E Exploration with sigmoidectomy and descending end colostomy (Hartmann's procedure)

Complicated diverticulitis often requires intervention, whether it be percutaneous drainage or a surgical procedure. Hinchey I is defined as colonic inflammation with associated pericolic abscess; stage II includes inflammation with pelvic abscess; stage III is purulent peritonitis; stage IV is feculent peritonitis. This patient has Hinchey III diverticular disease, as evidenced by the large abscess with free fluid. Percutaneous drainage is not viable in a patient with a ruptured abscess and free fluid. Laparoscopic lavage and drain placement is a newer procedure that has frequently been performed in an attempt to save the patient from an ostomy and staged procedure, which carries its own morbidity. Frail, septic patients, as well as those with major comorbidities like this patient, are not good candidates for lavage. Colorectal anastomosis can be performed in these patients depending on surgeon comfort and patient factors; however, it is recommended to also perform proximal fecal diversion.

Answer: E

Sartelli M, Catena F, Ansaloni L, et al. WSES guidelines for the management of acute left sided colonic diverticulitis in the emergency setting. *World J Emerg Surg.* 2016;11(1):1–15.

Biffl WL, Moore FA, Moore EE. What is the current role of laparoscopic lavage in perforated diverticulitis? *J Trauma Acute Care Surg.* Published online 2017, 82(4):810–813.

15 A 92-year-old woman with a history of urinary and fecal incontinence and severe COPD with supplemental oxygen requirement is brought to the ED via ambulance from her nursing home, with complaint of a protruding mass from the anus. She is bedbound and malnourished. The staff there did not know how long the mass had been protruding. On exam, you see a 5 cm mass with concentric rings protruding from the anus. It is firm to the touch and the edges are dusky in appearance. Attempted reduction of the mass in the ED is unsuccessful due to pain. You transfer her to the operating room for reduction under sedation. If unsuccessful, what is the next best step in management?

A Perineal rectosigmoidectomy (Altemeier procedure)

B Mucosal proctectomy

C Laparoscopic rectopexy

D Laparoscopic rectopexy and sigmoidectomy

E Open rectopexy and sigmoidectomy

Rectal prolapse is a circumferential full-thickness intussusception of the rectum out of the anus. It affects women more commonly than men, and has a higher prevalence in the institutionalized patient and those with neurological disorders. It is associated with pelvic floor dysfunction, but treatment of rectal prolapse does not treat the underlying pelvic floor abnormalities, and associated symptoms are therefore not resolved once the prolapse is treated. Prolonged prolapse can lead to congestion of the exposed rectum, which can make reduction impossible. To assist, applying topical osmotic agents (granulated sugar) can decrease the edema to facilitate reduction. If monitored sedation does not allow reduction, then general anesthesia may allow reduction.

Irreducible rectal prolapse is uncommon, but if it occurs, emergent surgical removal of the affected bowel is warranted. There are open and laparoscopic abdominal options, as well as perineal procedures. The Altemeier procedure is a perianal rectosigmoidectomy that can be done under local anesthesia, and is useful in the patient who would not be able to tolerate an abdominal surgery. This patient, who is severely debilitated, bedbound, and with severe lung disease, would not be able to tolerate a laparosopic procedure, and an open abdominal procedure would be highly morbid for her. A mucosal proctectomy can be performed if there is prolapse of the mucosa only, which is not applicable in this case. If able to tolerate, abdominal procedures have the lowest recurrence rate, especially when combined with resection of the redundant colon.

Answer: A

Bordeianou L, Hicks CW, Kaiser AM, Alavi K, Sudan R, Wise PE. Rectal prolapse: An overview of clinical features, diagnosis, and patient-specific management strategies. *J Gastrointest Surg.* 2014;18(5):1059–1069.

16 *A 24-year-old man presents to the ED complaining of rectal pain for 2 days. He states he is otherwise healthy and takes no medications. He has normal vital signs, but appears uncomfortable in the gurney. His abdomen is nontender, and on rectal exam, you palpate a smooth foreign body high in the rectum, which is later confirmed on plain x-ray of the abdomen. There is no free air seen. Attempted extraction with IV pain medication and mild sedation is unsuccessful in the ED. You take him to the operating room, where conscious sedation is achieved with the assistance of anesthesia. The object is removed after multiple difficult attempts. Rigid proctoscopy after the procedure reveals rectal lacerations with minor bleeding. The patient remains hemodynamically normal. What is the next step in management?*

A *Admit the patient for serial abdominal exams, and repeat rigid proctoscopy prior to discharge*

B *Operative exploration to evaluate for perforation*

C *Rectal contrast study*

D *Upright chest x-ray*

E *Flexible sigmoidoscopy with hemostatic treatments to the bleeding mucosa*

Rectal foreign bodies do not commonly need surgical consultation, as they are often removed by emergency room providers with the assistance of sedation and local anesthesia, which includes pudendal nerve block, perianal block, and/or spinal anesthesia. Other nonoperative methods of retrieval include using forceps to grasp the object, palpation of the left iliac fossa from above to facilitate downward movement of the object, and the use of a Foley catheter inserted past the object and inflated, to break the vacuum seal above the object and allow easier passage. If nonoperative methods are unsuccessful, laparotomy is warranted, to either "milk" the object down the rectum internally, or to perform a colotomy for object extraction. After object removal, rigid proctoscopy or flexible sigmoidoscopy is mandated to evaluate for transmural injury, as well as imaging to document the presence or absence of free air (answer D). If a transmural injury is present, management of the injury follows that of other penetrating rectal trauma, based on location of injury and presence of fecal contamination. Rectal lacerations can occur from foreign bodies or iatrogenically during the removal process. Most bleeding from these lacerations resolves spontaneously without the need for intervention. Rectal contrast studies are not required if the patient remains hemodynamically stable and asymptomatic. There is no need to repeat a rigid proctoscopy prior to discharge, if the patient does not otherwise show signs of perforation.

Answer: D

Goldberg JE, Steele SR. Rectal foreign bodies. *Surg Clin North Am.* 2010;90(1):173–184.

Lake JP, Essani R, Petrone P, Kaiser AM, Asensio J, Beart RW. Management of retained colorectal foreign bodies: Predictors of operative intervention. *Dis Colon Rectum* 2004;47(10):1694–1698.

17 *A 55-year-old woman who is receiving chemotherapy for leukemia presents to the ED complaining of right lower quadrant pain and bloody bowel movements. Her last chemotherapy session was 14 days ago; her next session was scheduled for today. Her vitals are T 38.2 °C and pulse 105 beats/min. She is tender in the right lower quadrant with mild guarding. Her WBC is 0.8/mm^3 with 30% neutrophils. What is the most appropriate next step in management?*

A *Colonoscopy to evaluate the source of her bleeding*

B *IV fluid resuscitation, C. difficile testing, start oral vancomycin*

C *Abdominal x-ray*

D *CT abdomen/pelvis*

E *Urgent exploratory laparotomy for ischemic colon*

Neutropenic enterocolitis, or typhlitis, is a well-described complication arising in immunosuppressed patients, including those with HIV, those receiving chemotherapy, and those status-post organ transplant. The pathophysiology is unclear. It typically affects the right colon; left-sided involvement is rare. The most common presenting symptoms are right-sided abdominal pain, fever, neutropenia, with or without peritonitis. It is a clinical diagnosis, but an important step in the diagnostic evaluation is an abdominal CT scan, which can evaluate both the extent of the disease as well as for indications to operate. Surgical exploration in these cases is reserved for those with perforation, uncontrolled sepsis, refractory bleeding despite correction of cytopenias and coagulopathy, or development of another indication for surgery (i.e., appendicitis). Abdominal imaging will typically show bowel wall edema and thickening of the terminal ileum and ascending colon. Colonoscopy in these patients is risky and can cause perforation easily. Testing for other infectious sources should be performed, but abdominal cross-sectional imaging should be prioritized.

Answer: D

Cloutier RL. Neutropenic enterocolitis. *Hematol Oncol Clin North Am.* 2010;24(3):577–584.

Rodrigues FG, Dasilva G, Wexner SD. Neutropenic enterocolitis. *World J Gastroenterol.* 2017;23(1):42–47.

Xia R, Zhang X. Neutropenic enterocolitis: A clinico-pathological review. *World J Gastrointest Pathophysiol.* Published online 2019, 10(3):36–41.

18 *A 52-year-old man presents to the emergency room complaining of bright red blood per rectum for 2 days. His vital signs are normal in the ED and his hematocrit is 32%. Nasogastric lavage in the ED shows bilious output. He is resuscitated and admitted. Colonoscopy shows sigmoid diverticulosis with stigmata of recent hemorrhage, but no obvious source. He continues to have intermittent bloody bowel movements requiring multiple transfusions, but has remained hemodynamically normal during his stay. What is the next step in management?*

   A *Mesenteric angiography*
   B *Tagged red blood cell scan*
   C *Sigmoid resection*
   D *Subtotal colectomy*
   E *Catheter-directed heparin to reveal the source*

Lower GI bleeding should first be managed with aggressive resuscitation and correction of coagulopathy as needed. Nearly 15% of lower GI bleeding is caused by an upper GI source; therefore, expeditious gastric lavage is important. The recommended procedure for unlocalized lower GI bleeding is a subtotal colectomy, and should only be performed if the patient is *in extremis* or if attempted localization through multiple avenues does not reveal a source. Segmental colectomy is not recommended for unlocalized lower GI bleeding as it carries significant risk of recurrent bleeding.

In hemodynamically normal patients, colonoscopy is the preferred procedure as it can also provide therapeutic intervention. If colonoscopy is unsuccessful, nuclear RBC scanning and angiography can be utilized. Angiography requires the offending vessel to be actively bleeding at the time of the procedure, and cannot detect very slow bleeds (less than 0.5 mL/min). Tagged RBC studies can detect bleeding as low as 0.1 mL/min, and if positive, can localize the bleeding area of colon and so a segmental resection or localized angiography can be performed if needed. For this patient, his rate of bleeding is unlikely to be fast enough to be detected by angiography, so tagged RBC is a reasonable option to attempt localization. Catheter-directed heparin, also known as provocative angiography, is a method of detecting a lower GI bleeding source. However, it is limited in availability and large trials proving its efficacy and safety have yet to be concluded.

Answer: B

Oakland K, Chadwick G, East J, et al, Diagnosis and management of acute lower gastrointestinal bleeding:

guidelines from the British Society of Gastroenterology. *Gut* 2019;68(5):776–789

Kim CY, Suhoki PA, Miller MJ, et al. Provocative mesenteric angiography for lower gastrointestinal hemorrhage: results from a single-institution study *J Vasc Interv Radiol.* 2010;21(4):477–83

19 *A 30-year-old man with von Willebrand disease presents with 4 days of right lower quadrant abdominal pain. He is febrile but normotensive with a pulse of 89 beats/min. He is tender to palpation with guarding, and has a WBC count of 16000/mm³. An abdominal CT scan shows no visualized appendix, but a 4 cm fluid collection with a radiopaque object near the edge. What is the next step in management?*

   A *Laparoscopic drainage of the abscess, drain placement, interval appendectomy in 6 weeks*
   B *Percutaneous drainage of abscess, interval appendectomy in 6 weeks*
   C *Percutaneous drainage of abscess, no follow up if feeling well at 2 weeks*
   D *IV broad-spectrum antibiotics and inpatient observation*
   E *Percutaneous drainage of abscess, colonoscopy prior to appendectomy in 6 weeks*

There is competing literature comparing medical therapy alone to surgical therapy for appendicitis. Data supporting antibiotic treatment for appendicitis must be taken with caution, since most studies exclude septic patients and patients with perforation. The recently completed CODA trial is the largest randomized controlled trial in the United States, comparing 10 days of antibiotic therapy with appendectomy in patients with confirmed appendicitis. Nonoperative management failed in 29% of those in the antibiotics group, including 41% with an appendicolith and 25% without. Complication rates are higher in those with fecoliths, so in this population, appendectomy is encouraged once feasible. In this case, percutaneous drainage should be pursued due to the fluid collection. Operative drainage can be considered if this fails. Intravenous antibiotics are unlikely to resolve an abscess of this size. He has no risk factors for colon cancer that would mandate colonoscopy prior to interval appendectomy.

Answer: B

The CODA Collaborative. A randomized trial comparing antibiotics with appendectomy for appendicitis. *N Engl J Med.* 2020;383(20):1907–1919.

Varadhan KK, Humes DJ, Neal KR, Lobo DN. Antibiotic therapy versus appendectomy for acute appendicitis: A meta-analysis. *World J Surg.* 2010;34(2):199–209.

20 *You are consulted to evaluate a 75-year-old man who is recovering in the ICU from an abdominal aortic aneurysm repair. He complains of left-sided abdominal pain that has now generalized, anorexia, and bloody bowel movements for the past 24 hours. The pain has been worsening and is now severe. His temperature is 39 °C and his pulse is 110 beats/min, but he has a normal blood pressure. He has peritonitis on exam. What is the next step in management?*

A *Mesenteric angiogram*

B *Flexible sigmoidoscopy to confirm diagnosis prior to treatment*

C *Exploration, segmental resection, end-colostomy*

D *Exploration, segmental resection, primary anastomosis*

E *Diagnostic laparoscopy*

This patient has ischemic colitis, which complicates about 2% of all abdominal aortic aneurysm repairs. Other etiologies of ischemic colitis include hypovolemia due to sepsis or cardiac failure, atherosclerosis, vasculitis, and emboli. Most mild-to-moderate cases can be treated with IV fluid resuscitation and antibiotics. If the patient fails to improve with medical management, or develops signs of sepsis or perforation, laparotomy is warranted. Angiogram is not indicated in a septic patient and may cause unnecessary delay. Sigmoidoscopy is not indicated in this case as it will not change management, but should be performed in mild-to-moderate cases to confirm diagnosis. Diagnostic laparoscopy is not typically performed in the management of ischemic colitis. Primary anastomosis can be performed in patients who have appropriate physiology, but should be avoided in those who have a prosthetic aortic graft, as an anastomotic leak risks graft contamination.

Answer: C

Halaweish I, Alam HB. Surgical management of severe colitis in the intensive carew unit *J Intensive Care Med.* 2015;30(8):451–461

Steele SR. Ischemic colitis complicating major vascular surgery. *Surg Clin North Am.* 2007;87(5):1099–1114. doi: 10.1016/j.suc.2007.07.007.

Sun MY, Maykel JA. Ischemic colitis. *Clin Colon Rectal Surg.* 2007;20(1):5–12.

21 *Two months ago, a 52-year-old man presented to the emergency department with a 3-day history of right lower quadrant pain. He had no significant medical or family history. At that time, he had rebound tenderness in the right lower quadrant of the abdomen. His initial white blood count was 15 000/mm³. A CT scan of the abdomen obtained by the emergency department at the initial admission demonstrated a dilated appendix with abscess and a surrounding inflammatory mass. The patient was started on intravenous antibiotics, and his symptoms markedly improved over 36 hours; he was discharged on oral antibiotics. He now presents for a follow-up visit and is asymptomatic. Which of the following is the best next step in his care?*

A *No further observation*

B *Abdominal MRI*

C *Interval appendectomy*

D *Screening colonoscopy*

E *Carcinoembyonic antigen (CEA) level*

The age of the patient dictates the management. Given that appendiceal neoplasm is overall a low possibility, the highest probability is in patients that have an acute inflammatory process coupled with advancing age. Therefore, the best answer in a 52-year-old man with successful nonoperative appendicitis management is an interval surgical appendectomy following colonoscopy. Lesions found at interval appendectomy include adenomas, polyps, neuroendocrine tumors, goblet cell carcinoids, and mucinous adenocarcinoma and mucinous neoplasms. CEA testing would not detect the presence of most of these tumor types. Further studies including MRI are not the best next step in management.

Answer: D

Mällinen J, Rautio T, Grönroos J, et al: 1-year outcomes of the peri-appendicitis acuta randomized clinical trial. *JAMA Surg.* 2019;154(3):200–207.

Son J, Park YJ, Lee SR, et al. Increased risk of neoplasms in adult patients undergoing interval appendectomy. *Ann Coloproctol.* 2020, 36(5):311–315.

Siddharthan RV, Byrne RM, Dewey E, et al. Appendiceal cancer masked as inflammatory appendicitis in the elderly, not an uncommon presentation (Surveillance Epidemiology and End Results (SEER)-medicare analysis). *J Surg Oncol.* 2019;120(4):736–739.

22 *A 32-year-old woman in her third trimester of pregnancy presents with internal hemorrhoids that have prolapsed out of the anal canal; these cannot be reduced with gentle manual pressure. What is the best therapy?*

A *Hemorrhoidectomy*

B *Infrared coagulation*

C *Rubber band ligation*

D *Phlebotonics*

E *Topical nifedipine*

This patient has grade III or IV internal hemorrhoids. Hemorrhoidectomy should typically be offered to patients whose symptoms result from external hemorrhoids or combined internal and external hemorrhoids with prolapse (grades III–IV). Infrared coagulation is typically an office-based procedure that involves the direct application of infrared light resulting in protein necrosis within the hemorrhoid. This is most commonly used for grade I and II hemorrhoids. A Cochrane review evaluated the efficacy of rubber band ligation (RBL) with respect to grade of hemorrhoids and found that excisional hemorrhoidectomy was superior to RBL for grade III hemorrhoids. Phlebotonics are a heterogeneous class of drugs used to treat both acute and chronic hemorrhoidal disease. While useful for medical management of symptoms of pruritis, bleeding and other chronic symptoms, they do not have a defined role in prolapsed internal hemorrhoids. Topical nifedipine has been described as a treatment for anal fissure, but does not have a defined role for hemorrhoids.

Answer: A

Davis BR, Lee-Kong SA, Migaly J, et al. The American society of colon and rectal surgeons clinical practice guidelines for the management of hemorrhoids. *Dis Colon Rectum*. 2018;61(3):284–292.

38

Gallbladder and Pancreas
Kirstie Jarrett, MD[1] and Andrew Tang, MD[2]

[1] Banner University Medical Center, Tucson, AZ, USA
[2] Banner University Medical Center, University of Arizona College of Medicine, Tucson, AZ, USA

1   Which of the following is true regarding the natural history of asymptomatic cholelithiasis?
   A Less than 10% of patients will develop complications requiring cholecystectomy during their lifetime.
   B 20–30% of patients will develop complications requiring cholecystectomy during their lifetime.
   C Cholecystectomy is indicated for asymptomatic gallstones > 1 cm in diameter.
   D It is common for patients to develop acute cholecystitis without any prior symptoms of biliary colic.
   E It is never appropriate to perform a prophylactic cholecystectomy for asymptomatic gallstones.

Cholelithiasis is extremely prevalent and affects approximately 10% of the United States population. Most patients never go on to develop symptoms that warrant surgical intervention. In fact, only about 30% of patients with asymptomatic gallstones will develop complications that require cholecystectomy during their lifetime. Further, it is quite rare for a patient to develop severe complications (cholecystitis, cholangitis, pancreatitis, gallbladder cancer) from gallstones if they have not previously had symptoms of biliary colic. For these reasons, the risks of prophylactic cholecystectomy do not outweigh the potential benefits for most patients.

That being said, some patients are at a higher risk of developing severe complications and so are likely to benefit from prophylactic cholecystectomy in the setting of asymptomatic cholelithiasis. This includes patients with large (>2 cm) gallstones, hemolytic anemias, porcelain gallbladder (calcified gallbladder wall), and/or a long common bile duct or pancreatic duct. These patients are more likely to benefit from prophylactic cholecystectomy to reduce risk of gallstone complications and/or gallbladder cancer.

Answer: B

Festi D, Reggiani ML, Attili AF, et al. Natural history of gallstone disease: expectant management or active treatment? Results from a population-based cohort study. *Journal of Gastroenterology and Hepatology.* 2010;25(4):719–24.

Lammert F, Gurusamy K, Ko CW, et al. Gallstones. *Nature Reviews Disease Primers.* 2016;2:16024.

2   A 50-year-old woman with a history of biliary colic presents to the emergency department with right upper quadrant pain and subjective fever that started 6 hours ago. Heart rate is 115 bpm, blood pressure is 110/70 mmHg, and she is febrile to 39.3 °C. On exam, she has mild jaundice, scleral icterus, and severe tenderness in the right upper quadrant. Which of the following is true regarding this constellation of signs when used as a diagnostic tool for acute cholangitis?
   A <5% of patients with acute cholecystitis are falsely diagnosed with acute cholangitis based on these findings.
   B Low sensitivity, high specificity.
   C High sensitivity, low specificity.
   D >50% of patients with acute cholecystitis are falsely diagnosed with acute cholangitis based on these findings.
   E Of these symptoms, abdominal pain is the most specific for acute cholangitis.

The 2007 Tokyo Guidelines (TG07) outlined data from a large, systematic review that compared Charcot's Triad (fever, right upper quadrant abdominal pain, jaundice) to the gold standard for diagnosis of cholangitis (purulent bile, clinical improvement after biliary drainage, and/or remission after antibiotic therapy alone). This review showed that Charcot's Triad had excellent specificity for diagnosing acute cholangitis (95.9%), but lacked sensitivity (26.4%). Based on these findings, a new set of diagnostic criteria were proposed. These criteria were revised in the 2013 Tokyo Guidelines (TG13) and were found to have significantly improved sensitivity (91.8%) with comparable specificity (77.7%) to Charcot's Triad.

These criteria are based on three categories: inflammation (leukocytosis/elevated inflammatory markers and/or fever/chills), cholestasis (elevated bilirubin and/or jaundice/icterus), and imaging findings (ductal dilatation and/or obstruction). Inflammation plus either cholestasis or imaging evidence qualifies as "suspected diagnosis," while patients who fulfill criteria in all three of the categories qualify for a "confirmed diagnosis." The TG13 diagnostic criteria also showed a lower false-positive rate in patients who were ultimately diagnosed with acute cholecystitis (5.9%) compared to Charcot's Triad (11.9%), presumably because the TG13 criteria excluded abdominal pain and prior history of biliary disease.

Answer: B

Kiriyama S, Takada T, Strasberg SM, et al.; Tokyo Guidelines Revision Committee. TG13 guidelines for diagnosis and severity grading of acute cholangitis. *Journal of Hepato-biliary-pancreatic Sciences.* 2013;20(1):24–34.

Wada K, Takada T, Kawarada Y, et al. Diagnostic criteria and severity assessment of acute cholangitis: Tokyo guidelines. *Journal of Hepato-biliary-pancreatic Surgery.* 2007;14(1):52–8.

3   Which of the following is false regarding pigmented gallstones?

   A They form when heme breakdown products become concentrated in the bile.

   B Black pigment stones predominantly occur in the gallbladder and not the biliary tree.

   C Brown pigment stones are associated with biliary dysmotility and stasis.

   D Dark pigmentation comes from the combination of calcium and cholesterol, as opposed to pure cholesterol stones which are lighter in color.

   E Biliary infection is a risk factor for brown stone formation.

Gallstone formation results when bile becomes concentrated, when stone components become supersaturated in the bile, and/or when gallbladder dysmotility/stasis is present. There are two major types of gallstones: cholesterol and pigment stones. Cholesterol stones are most commonly a combination of precipitated cholesterol and calcium, while pure cholesterol gallstones account for less than 10% of the gallstones identified in the United States. Risk factors for cholesterol stone formation include high-estrogen states, parenteral nutrition, advanced age, and rapid weight loss.

Pigment stones are further subclassified into black and brown stones. Black stones are more common and are formed when bile becomes super-saturated with bilirubin and its metabolic conjugates, all of which are formed in the breakdown of heme. As such, black stones are almost always associated with diseases that cause hyperbilirubinemia (i.e., hemoglobinopathies, hemolytic diseases, cirrhosis). Because the super-saturated bile is further concentrated in the gallbladder, black stones form nearly exclusively in the gallbladder. Brown pigment stones are made up of bilirubin as well, but also have a significant cholesterol content which makes them lighter in color. Brown stones can form anywhere along the biliary tract and arise when there is biliary stasis and/or infection.

Answer: D

Jackson PG, Evans SRT (2017). Biliary System. In Townsend CM, Beauchamp RD, Evers BM, Mattox KL (Ed.). *Sabiston Textbook of Surgery: The Biological Basis of Modern Surgical Practice* (20th edition). Philadelphia, PA: Elsevier Saunders.

Lammert F, Gurusamy K, Ko CW, et al. Gallstones. *Nature Reviews Disease Primers.* 2016;2:16024.

4   A 76-year-old man with COPD (baseline oxygen requirement of 2L) and heart failure with ejection fraction of 35% presents to the emergency department with clinical and radiographic evidence of acute cholecystitis. His blood pressure is 91/55 mmHg, heart rate is 118 bpm, and he is requiring 6 L via nasal cannula to maintain SpO2 in the high 80s. He is mildly confused. He is admitted to the ICU where appropriate antibiotics and resuscitative measures are initiated. By noon the following day, his hypotension worsens and pressors are started. Which of the following is the best plan to achieve source control in this patient?

   A Laparoscopic cholecystectomy within 72 hours of admission.

   B Continued antibiotics and supportive care, cholecystectomy as soon as the patient is optimized and deemed an acceptable surgical candidate.

   C Urgent percutaneous cholecystostomy tube placement, cholecystectomy as soon as the patient is optimized and deemed an acceptable surgical candidate.

   D Urgent percutaneous cholecystostomy tube placement, outpatient cholecystectomy only if cholangiogram at 3 weeks shows persistent blockage of the cystic duct.

This patient, who is a poor surgical candidate at baseline, meets criteria for grade III cholecystitis (Table 38.1) based on the 2013 and 2018 Tokyo Guidelines (TG13 and TG18). Per TG18, it is reasonable to try nonoperative management with IV antibiotics and supportive therapy first. The patient in this scenario did not respond and in fact worsened after this treatment. While there has been some debate as to the best step from this point, the general consensus is that source control and gallbladder decompression should be achieved via placement of a percutaneous cholecystostomy (PC) tube.

The next step is definitive treatment with cholecystectomy, though timing will depend on patient-specific factors. In patients with grade III cholecystitis who do not have significant baseline comorbidities, cholecystectomy should be completed as soon as the patient is stabilized from a sepsis standpoint. This patient, however, will also need to be medically optimized from a cardiopulmonary standpoint. The patient may be discharged home with the PC tube in place if he is suitable for discharge but not for major surgery. If he is discharged with the PC tube in place, the tube may be removed once the patient is asymptomatic and a cholangiogram demonstrates a

Table 38.1 TG13/18 severity grading for acute cholecystitis.

Grade III (severe) acute cholecystitis

"Grade III" acute cholecystitis is associated with dysfunction of any one of the following organs/systems:
1) Cardiovascular dysfunction: hypotension requiring treatment with dopamine ≥ 5 µg/kg per min, or any dose of norepinephrine
2) Neurological dysfunction: decreased level of consciousness
3) Respiratory dysfunction: PaO_2/FiO_2 ratio <300
4) Renal dysfunction: oliguria, creatinine >2.0 mg/dL
5) Hepatic dysfunction: PT-MR >1.5
6) Hematological dysfunction: platelet count <100 000/mm^3

Grade II (moderate) acute cholecystitis

"Grade II" acute cholecystitis is associated with any one of the following conditions:
1) Elevated WBC count (>18 000/mm^3)
2) Palpable tender mass in the right upper abdominal quadrant
3) Duration of complaints >72 h^a
4) Marked local inflammation (gangrenous cholecystitis, pericholecystic abscess, hepatic abscess, biliary peritonitis, emphysematous cholecystitis)

Grade I (mild) acute cholecystitis

"Grade I" acute cholecystitis does not meet the criteria of "Grade III" or "Grade II" acute cholecystitis. It can also he defined as acute cholecystitis in a healthy patient with no organ dysfunction and mild inflammatory changes in the gallbladder, making cholecystectomy a safe and low-risk operative procedure

---

Source: Reproduced from Yokoe et al. (2018); with permission from publisher John Wiley and Sons.

patent cystic duct. However, per the 2018 Tokyo Guidelines, the only definitive management for calculous cholecystitis is cholecystectomy when able.

Answer: C

Dimou FM, Riall TS. Proper use of cholecystostomy tubes. *Advances in Surgery*. 2018;52(1):57–71.

Okamoto K, Suzuki K, Takada T, et al. Tokyo Guidelines 2018: flowchart for the management of acute cholecystitis. *Journal of Hepato-biliary-pancreatic Sciences*. 2018;25(1):55–72.

5 *A 35-year-old woman with a history of obesity and biliary colic has been admitted to the trauma ICU for the last 5 days after a motor vehicle crash in which she sustained a femur fracture, pelvic fractures, and multiple left-sided rib fractures with an associated large left pneumothorax. On hospital day six, the patient develops fever to 39.5 °C, significant right-sided abdominal pain and right upper quadrant tenderness, jaundice with total bilirubin of 4 mg/dL, alkaline phosphatase of 300 U/L, mild transaminitis, and a white blood cell count of 20 000/µL. Imaging reveals choledocholithiasis. Which of the following antibiotic regimens would be inappropriate at this time?*
A *Ciprofloxacin and vancomycin*
B *Piperacillin/tazobactam and vancomycin*
C *Meropenem and linezolid*
D *Cefepime and linezolid*
E *Cefepime and daptomycin*

The most common organisms isolated from both community-acquired and healthcare-associated biliary infections include *E. coli*, Klebsiella species, Pseudomonas species, and Enterococcus species. This patient has been hospitalized for >48 hours prior to development of cholangitis, which by definition is a hospital-associated biliary infection. According to the 2018 Tokyo Guidelines, vancomycin should be added for all hospital-associated biliary infections due to the increased risk of multidrug-resistant Enterococcus species. If the patient has a history of vancomycin-resistant Enterococcus (VRE) infection, has a severe vancomycin allergy, has already failed vancomycin therapy, and/or there is a high local prevalence of VRE in the area, daptomycin or linezolid may be substituted for vancomycin. Piperacillin/tazobactam, meropenem, and cefepime-based regimens with the addition of vancomycin (or other Enterococcus-covering agent) would all be appropriate options. Ciprofloxacin-based therapy, however, would not be appropriate for hospital-associated or grade III community-acquired cholangitis due to high fluoroquinolone resistance in Gram-negative extended-spectrum beta-lactamase (ESBL) species.

Answer: A

Gomi H, Solomkin JS, Schlossberg D, et al. Tokyo guidelines 2018: antimicrobial therapy for acute cholangitis and cholecystitis. *Journal of Hepato-biliary-pancreatic Sciences*. 2018;25(1):3–16.

6 *Which vessel is most commonly injured during laparoscopic cholecystectomy?*
   A *Proper hepatic artery*
   B *Left hepatic artery*
   C *Portal vein*
   D *Branches of the superior pancreaticoduodenal artery*
   E *Right hepatic artery*

The right hepatic artery (RHA) is the most frequently injured vessel during laparoscopic cholecystectomy. This is likely related to its proximity to the common hepatic duct, which can be mistaken for an accessory duct or aberrant cystic duct during difficult dissections. Transection of the RHA typically results in brisk bleeding intraoperatively and may cause significant postoperative hemorrhage requiring reoperation or angioembolization. Occlusion of the RHA is often silent but can result in clinically relevant hepatic ischemia and/or abscess in about 10% of patients, some of whom go on to require partial hepatectomy.

Answer: E

Stewart L. Iatrogenic biliary injuries: identification, classification, and management. *Surgical Clinics of North America*. 2014;94(2):297–310.
Strasberg SM, Helton WS. An analytical review of vasculobiliary injury in laparoscopic and open cholecystectomy. *HPB (Oxford)*. 2011;13(1):1–14.

7 *A 32-year-old woman is currently admitted with grade II, community-acquired, acute cholangitis with choledocholithiasis on ultrasound. She was started on appropriate antibiotic therapy when she was admitted last night and underwent urgent ERCP with successful removal of a large stone from the common bile duct. She is no longer febrile and has remained hemodynamically normal. She is scheduled for laparoscopic cholecystectomy tomorrow morning. What is the most appropriate duration of antibiotic therapy for this patient?*
   A *Four to 7 days after source control (ERCP).*
   B *Seven to 14 days after source control (ERCP).*
   C *Discontinue antibiotics now that the patient is afebrile and source control has been achieved.*
   D *Total 14-day course of IV antibiotics to decrease the patient's risk of infective endocarditis.*
   E *Continue antibiotics perioperatively, then discontinue after successful completion of cholecystectomy.*

Per the 2018 Tokyo Guidelines, the appropriate treatment sequence for grade II (Table 38.2) acute cholangitis is: antibiotics and supportive care, urgent biliary drainage (ERCP vs. PTC), then subsequent definitive treatment of the cause of cholangitis (for this patient, cholecystectomy to decrease the risk of recurrent choledocholithiasis). Though source control has technically been achieved in this patient, continuation of antibiotics for an additional four to 7 days is recommended. It is also important to follow-up on the results of this patient's blood cultures. Gram-positive bacteremia would necessitate a full 2 weeks of IV antibiotics to reduce her risk of infective endocarditis. While the majority of biliary flora are Gram-negative, Enterococcus species are relatively common both in bile cultures and in blood cultures collected from cholangitis patients who developed bacteremia.

Table 38.2 TG13/18 severity grading for acute cholangitis.

Grade III (severe) acute cholangitis

"Grade III" acute cholangitis is defined as acute cholangitis that is associated with the onset of dysfunction at least in any one of the following organs/systems:
1) Cardiovascular dysfunction: hypotension requiring dopamine ≥5 μg/kg per min, or any dose of norepinephrine
2) Neurological dysfunction: disturbance of consciousness
3) Respiratory dysfunction: PaO_2/FiO_2 ratio <300
4) Renal dysfunction: oliguria, serum creatinine >2.0 mg/dL
5) Hepatic dysfunction: PT-INR >1.5
6) Hematological dysfunction: platelet count <l00 000/mm^3

Grade II (moderate) acute cholangitis

"Grade II" acute cholangitis is associated with any two of the following conditions:
1) Abnormal WBC count (>12 000/mm^3, <4000/mm^3)
2) High fever (≥39 °C)
3) Age (≥75 years old)
4) Hyperbilirubinemia (total bilirubin ≥5 mg/dL)
5) Hypoalbuminemia (<STD^a × 0.7)

Grade I (mild) acute cholangitis

"Grade I" acute cholangitis does not meet the criteria of "Grade III (severe)" or "Grade II (moderate)" acute cholangitis at initial diagnosis.

Source: Reproduced from Kiriyama et al. (2018); with permission from publisher, John Wiley and Sons.

Answer: A

Miura F, Okamoto K, Takada T, et al. Tokyo Guidelines 2018: initial management of acute biliary infection and flowchart for acute cholangitis. *Journal of Hepato-biliary-pancreatic Sciences.* 2018;25(1):31–40.

Gomi H, Solomkin JS, Schlossberg D, et al. Tokyo guidelines 2018: antimicrobial therapy for acute cholangitis and cholecystitis. *Journal of Hepato-biliary-pancreatic Sciences.* 2018;25(1):3–16.

8 *A 28-year-old woman who is 27 weeks pregnant with her first child presents to the emergency department with acute onset right upper quadrant pain, nausea, vomiting, and fever. She is hemodynamically normal and febrile to 39.2 °C. Labs and imaging suggest acute cholecystitis with low concern for choledocholithiasis. She is started on antibiotics and scheduled for same-admission cholecystectomy. Which of the following is the most appropriate operative plan?*

A *Prophylactic tocolytics, laparoscopic cholecystectomy with patient in partial left lateral decubitus position.*

B *Prophylactic tocolytics, open cholecystectomy with patient in partial left lateral decubitus position.*

C *Open cholecystectomy with patient in supine position, tocolytics only as needed if preterm labor occurs perioperatively.*

D *Laparoscopic cholecystectomy with patient in supine position, tocolytics only as needed if preterm labor occurs perioperatively.*

E *Laparoscopic cholecystectomy with patient in partial left lateral decubitus position, tocolytics only as needed if preterm labor occurs perioperatively.*

According to recent literature, laparoscopic surgery can be safely performed during any trimester of pregnancy without increased risk to the mother or fetus. Further, postponing necessary operations has been associated with higher rates of fetal loss during the first trimester, as well as preterm labor during the third trimester. A 2017 meta-analysis conducted by SAGES found that the benefits of laparoscopy over laparotomy in pregnant patients are similar to the benefits observed in nonpregnant patients. When patients have passed the first trimester, the gravid uterus can compress the vena cava while in supine position and lead to decreased cardiac preload. It is recommended that the patient be placed in partial left lateral decubitus position intraoperatively to alleviate this compression. There is no literature to support prophylactic use of tocolytics to prevent preterm labor. However, perioperative-threatened preterm labor can be successfully managed with tocolytics administered at the recommendation of an obstetrician.

Answer: E

Pearl JP, Price RR, Tonkin AE, et al. SAGES guidelines for the use of laparoscopy during pregnancy. *Surgical Endoscopy.* 2017;31(10):3767–82.

9 *A 60-year-old man undergoes outpatient laparoscopic cholecystectomy for biliary colic. Pathology reveals gallbladder carcinoma that invades the muscularis propria. The tumor does not extend to the cystic duct. CT of the chest, abdomen, and pelvis is negative for nodal involvement and metastases. What is the most appropriate recommendation for this patient?*

A *Close observation, no further surgical interventions*

B *Medical Oncology referral for chemotherapy, no further surgical interventions*

C *Gallbladder fossa wedge resection and portal lymphadenectomy*

D *Gallbladder fossa wedge resection, portal lymphadenectomy, CBD resection and reconstruction*

E *Neoadjuvant chemotherapy, gallbladder fossa wedge resection, portal lymphadenectomy*

This patient's tumor invades into the muscularis propria, making it T1b disease. T1a tumors are considered cured by cholecystectomy alone, while all tumors with higher T stages will require further surgery due to the high risk of residual disease. The recommended surgical management of gallbladder carcinoma is wedge resection of the gallbladder fossa and portal lymphadenectomy. Extrahepatic bile duct resections are only indicated when the tumor invades past the cystic duct and CBD resection is necessary to achieve negative margins. Neoadjuvant chemotherapy may be helpful for down-staging more advanced tumors to allow for a more limited resection. However, neoadjuvant chemotherapy has not been studied thoroughly enough to warrant routine use.

Answer: C

Cherkassky L, D'Angelica M. Gallbladder cancer: managing the incidental diagnosis. *Surgical Oncology Clinics of North America.* 2019;28(4):619–630.

10 *An otherwise healthy, 48-year-old woman presents to the emergency department with severe right upper quadrant pain. Vital signs are remarkable for a temperature of 39.5 °C, blood pressure 92/58 mmHg, and heart rate 122 bpm. Jaundice and mild scleral icterus are noted on exam, as well as severe tenderness in the right upper quadrant. She has a white blood cell count of 18 000/μL, total*

bilirubin of 3.5 mg/dL, mild transaminitis, and creatinine of 1.5 mg/dL. Abdominal ultrasound shows cholelithiasis, pericholecystic fluid, and common bile duct diameter of 7 mm, though no choledocholithiasis is noted. After starting antibiotics and IV fluids, what are the next best steps in management?

A Confirmatory MRCP, ERCP if choledocholithiasis is present, same-admission laparoscopic cholecystectomy

B Urgent ERCP, same-admission laparoscopic cholecystectomy

C Confirmatory MRCP, laparoscopic cholecystectomy, laparoscopic common bile duct exploration if MRCP was positive for choledocholithiasis

D Urgent laparoscopic cholecystectomy without intraoperative cholangiogram

E Urgent laparoscopic cholecystectomy with intraoperative cholangiogram

When considering further work-up and management of suspected choledocholithiasis, the American Society of Gastroenterology recommends stratifying patients based on likelihood of having choledocholithiasis. "Very strong" predictors of choledocholithiasis include clinical ascending cholangitis, choledocholithiasis noted on ultrasound, and total bilirubin > 4 mg/dL. "Strong" predictors include common bile duct (CBD) dilatation and total bilirubin level 1.8–4 mg/dL (Table 38.3). Patients have a high likelihood of choledocholithiasis if they have any one of the "very strong" predictors, or if they have both of the "strong" predictors.

Patients with a high likelihood of choledocholithiasis do not need further diagnostic evaluation and should proceed directly to ERCP for biliary decompression (Figure 38.1). Low likelihood patients may proceed to laparoscopic cholecystectomy for treatment of cholecystitis/symptomatic cholelithiasis. Patients with intermediate likelihood may proceed to laparoscopic cholecystectomy with intraoperative cholangiogram, or they may be further evaluated with MRCP prior to intervention.

Though this patient's ultrasound was negative for choledocholithiasis, she has clinical signs of ascending cholangitis. As such, she does not require confirmatory MRCP and should proceed directly to ERCP for biliary decompression.

Answer: B

Costi R, Gnocchi A, Di Mario F, Sarli L. Diagnosis and management of choledocholithiasis in the golden age of imaging, endoscopy and laparoscopy. *World Journal of Gastroenterology.* 2014;20(37):13382–401.

Table 38.3 American Society for Gastrointestinal Endoscopy estimation of risk for choledocholithiasis in patients with symptomatic cholelithiasis.

Predictors of choledocholithiasis	
"Very strong"	
CBD stone on transabdominal US	
Clinical ascending cholangitis	
Bilirubin > 4 mg/dL	
"Strong"	
Dilated CBD an US (>6 mm with gallbladder *in situ*)	
Bilirubin level 1.8–4 mg/dL	
"Moderate"	
Abnormal liver biochemical rest other than bilirubin	
Age older than 55 years	
Clinical gallstone pancreatitis	
Assigning a likelihood of choledocholithiasis based on clinical predictors	
Presence of any very strong predictor	High
Presence of both strong predictors	High
No predictors present	Low
All other patients	Intermediate

Source: Reproduced from ASGE Standards of Practice Committee: The Role of Endoscopy in the Management of Choledocholithiasis (2011); with permission from publisher, Elsevier.

ASGE Standards of Practice Committee, Maple JT, Ikenberry SO, Anderson MA, et al. The role of endoscopy in the management of choledocholithiasis. *Gastrointestinal Endoscopy.* 2011;74(4):731–44.

11 A 49-year-old man is currently on ICU day eight with severe acute pancreatitis. CT scan shows pancreatic necrosis without gas formation. The patient has been persistently febrile and his white blood cell count is currently 21 000/μL; up from 15 000/μL on admission. Fine needle aspiration confirms the diagnosis of infected pancreatic necrosis. What is the next best step?

A Antibiotics, open necrosectomy once patient is stable enough for surgery

B Antibiotics, aggressive fluid resuscitation, NPO, NJ tube placement for enteral nutrition

C Antibiotics, image-guided drain placement, video-assisted retroperitoneal debridement if needed

D Antibiotics, image-guided drain placement, open necrosectomy if needed

E Antibiotics, video-assisted retroperitoneal debridement once patient is stable enough for surgery

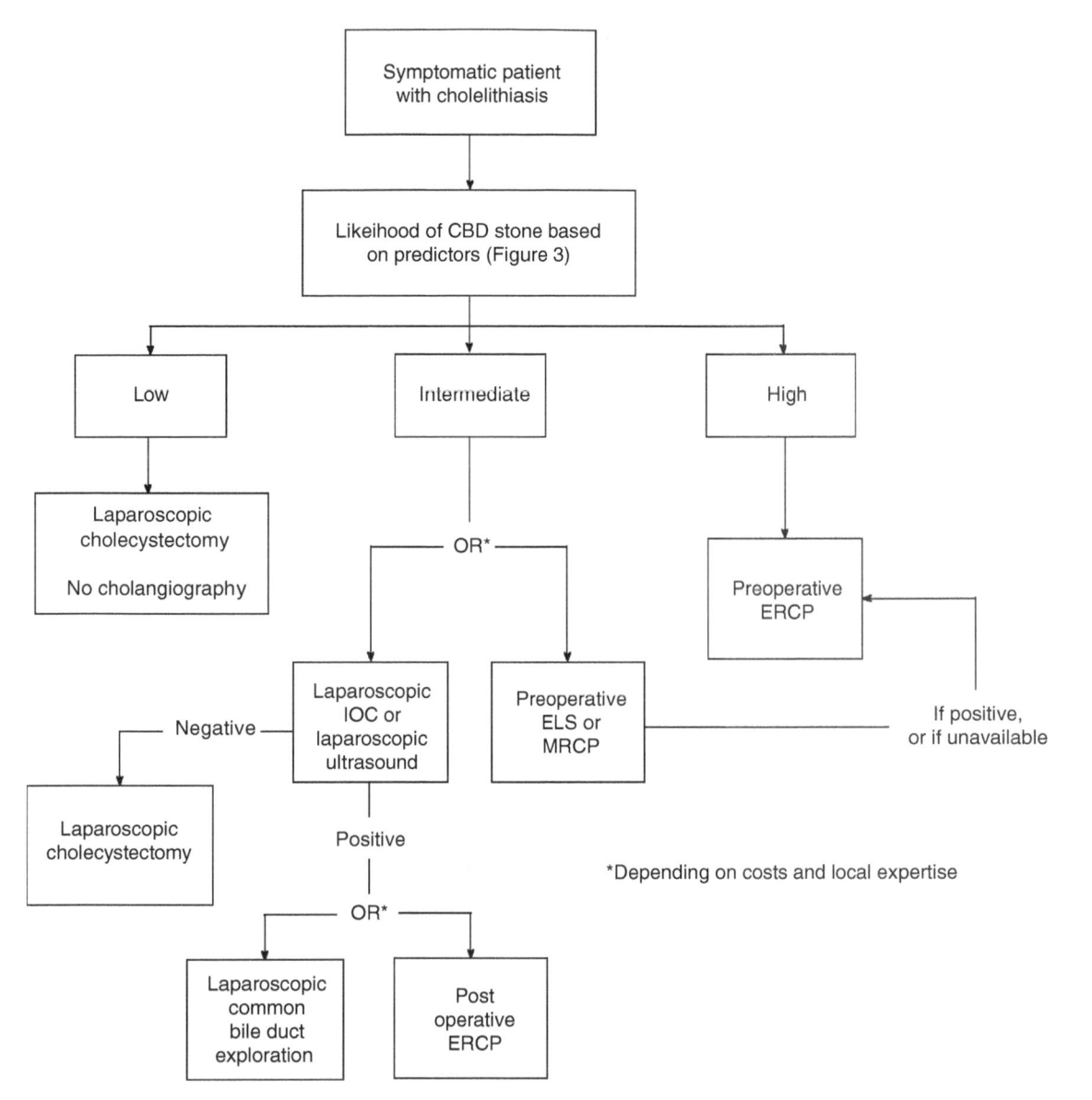

Figure 38.1 American Society for Gastrointestinal Endoscopy algorithm for management of symptomatic cholelithiasis based on likelihood of choledocholithiasis. *Source*: Reproduced from ASGE Standards of Practice Committee: The Role of Endoscopy in the Management of Choledocholithiasis (2011); with permission from publisher, Elsevier.

Infected pancreatic necrosis is a feared complication of necrotizing pancreatitis. The risk of infection is directly proportional to the extent of pancreatic necrosis, with over 40% risk in patients who have >70% pancreatic necrosis. Antibiotics do not prevent the infection of pancreatic necrosis; however, once infection is confirmed or at least strongly suspected, antibiotics need to be initiated. Previously, the standard of treatment for infected pancreatic necrosis was to perform a laparotomy and complete debridement of necrotic tissue. However, the 2010 PANTER Trial showed that the "step up" approach leads to decreased rates of mortality, major complications, and postoperative development of diabetes. In the "step up" approach, a percutaneous drain is placed near the pancreas first. In about 35% of patients, no further intervention is required. If the patient's clinical condition still requires further source control, video-assisted retroperitoneal debridement surgery (VARDS) is the procedure of choice.

Answer: C

van Santvoort HC, Besselink MG, Bakker OJ, et al.; Dutch Pancreatitis Study Group. A step-up approach or open necrosectomy for necrotizing pancreatitis. *New England Journal of Medicine.* 2010;362(16):1491–502.

Beger HG, Rau BM. Severe acute pancreatitis: clinical course and management. *World Journal of Gastroenterology.* 2007;13(38):5043–51.

12 *A 40-year-old woman with a history of type 2 diabetes and biliary colic presents to the emergency department with 6 hours of intense epigastric pain that radiates to the back, as well as nausea, vomiting, and anorexia. She is afebrile, blood pressure is 102/55 mmHg, and heart rate is 112 bpm. On exam she is non-distended and very tender to palpation of the epigastrium. There is no jaundice or scleral icterus present. Labs are remarkable for white blood cell count of 12 000/μL, creatinine of 0.8 mg/dL, lipase of 1025 U/L, amylase 465 U/L, total bilirubin of 0.9 mg/dL, and normal AST/ALT and alkaline phosphatase. RUQ ultrasound shows cholelithiasis without cholecystitis, no choledocholithiasis, and CBD measuring 5 mm. What are the next best steps after initial fluid resuscitation?*

A *Confirmatory MRCP, cholecystectomy at 6 weeks*

B *Urgent ERCP, same-admission cholecystectomy*

C *Same-admission cholecystectomy*

D *IV antibiotics, urgent ERCP, same-admission cholecystectomy*

E *IV antibiotics, same-admission cholecystectomy*

Acute pancreatitis (AP) is a common illness with more than 240 000 cases in the United States per year. By far, the two most common etiologies are gallstone disease and alcohol abuse. In this patient with characteristic abdominal pain and serum amylase and lipase greater than three times the upper limits of normal, the diagnosis of acute pancreatitis can be reasonably made without further investigation. There is no indication for confirmatory CT scan or MRCP unless the diagnosis is unclear or the patient fails to respond to treatment within 72 hours of presentation. The recommended treatment course for this patient with likely biliary pancreatitis is supportive care followed by same-admission cholecystectomy. When patients have concomitant cholangitis or evidence of biliary obstruction, ERCP is recommended within the first 24 hours. However, this patient has no evidence of cholangitis or biliary obstruction and so does not require ERCP. In fact, preoperative ERCP for patients with isolated, mild AP has been shown to increase length of stay and hospital cost without any significant benefit on mortality or local/systemic complications. This patient has mild AP (no evidence of organ dysfunction or local complications such as necrosis), so same-admission cholecystectomy is preferred over delayed cholecystectomy due to the high risk (~20%) of recurrent biliary events. There is no indication for antibiotics in AP unless infected necrosis is confirmed or at least strongly suspected, or unless there is a concomitant infection (cholangitis, pneumonia, UTI, etc.).

Answer: C

Tenner S, Baillie J, DeWitt J, Vege SS; American College of Gastroenterology. American college of gastroenterology guideline: management of acute pancreatitis. *American Journal of Gastroenterology.* 2013;108(9):1400–15; 1416.

Costi R, Gnocchi A, Di Mario F, Sarli L. Diagnosis and management of choledocholithiasis in the golden age of imaging, endoscopy and laparoscopy. *World Journal of Gastroenterology.* 2014;20(37):13382–401.

Chang L, Lo S, Stabile BE, et al. Preoperative versus postoperative endoscopic retrograde cholangiopancreatography in mild to moderate gallstone pancreatitis: a prospective randomized trial. *Annals of Surgery.* 2000;231(1):82–7.

13 *Which of the following is true regarding nutrition in a patient with severe acute pancreatitis?*

A *Nasojejunal and oral feeds are associated with similar rates of major infection and death.*

B *Nasojejunal feeds are favored over oral feeds.*

C *Oral feeds are associated with a greater risk of major infection than nasojejunal feeds.*

D *Parenteral feeding is favored over enteral feeding.*

E *Enteral feeds should not be started until amylase and lipase are down-trending.*

Previously, parenteral feeding was thought to be superior to enteral feeding because it avoided stimulation of the inflamed pancreas. However, pancreatic rest did not demonstrate a clear benefit and instead, likely contributes to bowel atrophy with increased risk of bacterial translocation. Multiple studies over the years have demonstrated a clear reduction in risk of peripancreatic infection and multiple organ failure with enteral feeding when compared to parental feeding. As such, enteral feeding, if tolerated, is the preferred route of nutrition in acute pancreatitis.

Nasojejunal feeds were previously considered superior to oral feeds. In 2014, the Dutch Pancreatitis Study Group conducted a randomized controlled trial in patients with severe AP (all patients had an APACHE II score >7). This landmark trial compared nasojejunal feeds started at 24 hours and oral feeds started at 72 hours. No significant differences were found in rates of major infection or death. The most current recommendation from the Dutch Pancreatitis Study Group is to start oral feeds once abdominal pain starts to resolve, and not to start nasojejunal feeds unless the patient is unable to tolerate oral feeds after three to 5 days. They do not recommend starting feeds based on trends in serum amylase or lipase levels.

Answer: A

Bakker OJ, van Brunschot S, van Santvoort HC, et al.; Dutch Pancreatitis Study Group. Early versus on-demand nasoenteric tube feeding in acute pancreatitis. *New England Journal of Medicine.* 2014;371(21):1983–93.

van Dijk SM, Hallensleben NDL, van Santvoort HC, et al.; Dutch Pancreatitis Study Group. Acute pancreatitis: recent advances through randomised trials. *Gut.* 2017;66(11):2024–32.

James TW, Crockett SD. Management of acute pancreatitis in the first 72 hours. *Current Opinion in Gastroenterology.* 2018;34(5):330–335.

14 *A 43-year-old man with alcoholism and a recent episode of acute pancreatitis 3 weeks ago is admitted following a motor vehicle crash. No acute injuries are identified on radiographic survey; however, CT of the abdomen notes a 7 cm × 3 cm × 5 cm, uncomplicated pseudocyst near the tail and body of the pancreas which was not present on his last CT scan 3 weeks ago. The patient denies abdominal pain, distension, early satiety, nausea, and emesis. Vital signs and labs are unremarkable. Which of the following is correct?*

A *Because the pseudocyst is large, endoscopic drainage should be performed during this admission.*

B *Because the pseudocyst is large, endoscopic intervention is unlikely to be successful and surgical drainage should be performed.*

C *Endoscopic drainage should be performed as this patient's alcoholism puts him at high risk of recurrent pancreatitis, which makes the pseudocyst unlikely to resolve on its own.*

D *No intervention is indicated at this time as the patient is asymptomatic and is only 3 weeks out from his episode of pancreatitis.*

E *Endoscopic drainage is associated with fewer complications than surgical cystogastrostomy, but is also significantly less effective.*

This patient has a large pseudocyst as a complication of a recent episode of acute pancreatitis. While the pseudocyst is large, the patient is completely asymptomatic and has no evidence of infection, so intervention is not indicated at this time. Though the patient's alcoholism puts him at risk of developing recurrent pancreatitis, that alone is not a reason to intervene on a pseudocyst. The large size (>4 cm) does decrease the likelihood of spontaneous resolution; however, the patient is asymptomatic and so it is still reasonable to allow time for spontaneous resolution. If the pseudocyst does not resolve on its own by 6 weeks, it is unlikely to do so and will likely require

intervention. Typically, endoscopic intervention is preferred over surgical intervention as it has been associated with similar success and recurrence rates but also with fewer complications and shorter length of stay.

Answer: D

Tenner S, Baillie J, DeWitt J, Vege SS; American College of Gastroenterology. American college of gastroenterology guideline: management of acute pancreatitis. *American Journal of Gastroenterology.* 2013;108(9):1400–15; 1416.

Andalib I, Dawod E, Kahaleh M. Modern management of pancreatic fluid collections. *Journal of Clinical Gastroenterology.* 2018;52(2):97–104.

15 *A 21-year-old man is riding a dirt bike and crashes head-on into a pole. Upon arrival in the trauma bay, he is mildly tachycardic, normotensive, and complains of severe abdominal pain. On exam, he is very tender in the epigastrium and has ecchymoses in that area, but he has no peritoneal signs. CT scan shows a moderate-size duodenal hematoma, as well as fat stranding near the pancreatic groove. It is unclear based on this scan whether or not a pancreatic injury is present. What is the best initial management strategy for this potential pancreatic injury?*

A *Exploratory laparotomy to evaluate for missed pancreatic injury.*

B *Consult to Interventional Radiology for percutaneous drain placement.*

C *Consult to Gastroenterology for ERCP with pancreatic duct stent placement.*

D *Serial abdominal exams, trend lipase and amylase every 6 hours, pancreatic protocol CT scan at 12–24 hours.*

E *Serial abdominal exams, pancreatic protocol CT scan at 12–24 hours.*

Traumatic pancreatic injuries are rare but can occur, especially in blunt mechanisms and with associated duodenal injuries. Up to 40% of pancreatic injuries can be missed on initial CT scan, and sensitivity for ductal injuries is only about 50% on initial CT. The sensitivity and specificity of CT scan for pancreatic injury increases significantly after the first 12–48 hours, especially when a pancreatic protocol (curved, multi-planar reconstruction with specific pancreatic phase contrast) is utilized.

Given this patient's hemodynamic stability and lack of obvious intra-abdominal injury, surgical intervention is not indicated at this time. In 2019, the World Society of Emergency Surgery (WSES) and American Association for the Surgery of Trauma (AAST) released a set of guidelines on management of pancreatic, biliary, and duodenal injuries. Their recommendation in unconfirmed pancreatic injuries is to trend lipase and amylase every three to 6 hours. Up-trending values would indicate the presence of a pancreatic injury and would warrant a repeat CT scan with pancreatic protocol. If a pancreatic injury were confirmed on repeat CT, management would depend on the severity of the pancreatic injury (see Table 38.4 and Figure 38.2). WSES class I injuries should receive nonoperative management first as this is successful in 96–100% of cases. If the patient were to fail nonoperative management, intervention should ideally occur within the first 24 hours to reduce the risk of complications. Depending on their location, WSES class II injuries would require percutaneous/endoscopic intervention or distal pancreatectomy. However, it would still be reasonable to confirm this diagnosis via labs and CT scan over a 12 to 24-hour period prior to intervention.

Table 38.4 WSES-AAST severity classification of traumatic pancreatic injuries.

Grade	WSES class	Organ	AAST	Description of injury
Minor	WSES class I	Pancreas	I–II	• Minor contusion without duct injury Superficial laceration without duct injury • Major contusion without duct injury or tissue loss Major laceration without duct injury or tissue loss
		Duodenum	I	• Hematoma involving a single portion of duodenum Laceration: partial thickness, no perforation
		Extrahepatic biliary three	I–II–III	• Gallbladder contusion/hematoma. Portal triad contusion • Partial gallbladder avulsion from liver bed; cystic duct intact Laceration or perforation of the gallbladder • Complete gallbladder avulsion from liver bed. Cystic duct laceration
Moderate	WSES class II	Pancreas	III	• Distal transection or parenchymal injury with duct injury
		Duodenum	II	• Hematoma involving more than one portion Laceration with disruption of less than 50% of circumference
		Extrahepatic biliary three	IV	Partial or complete right hepatic duct laceration Partial or complete left hepatic duct laceration Partial common hepatic duct laceration (<50%) Partial common bile duct laceration (<50%)
Severe	WSES class III	Pancreas	IV–V	• Proximal transection or parenchymal injury involving ampulla • Massive disruption of pancreatic head
		Duodenum	III–IV–V	• Disruption 50–75% of circumference of D2 • Disruption 50–100% of circumference of D1, D3, and D4 • Disruption >75% of circumference of D2 involving ampulla or distal common bile duct • Massive disruption of duodeno-pancreatic complex Devascularization of duodenum
		Extrahepatic biliary three	V	50% transection of common hepatic duct 50% transection of common bile duct Combined right and left hepatic duct injuries Intraduodenal or intrapancreatic bile duct injuries
	WSES class IV	Any	Any	Any degree of lesion with hemodynamic instability

Source: Reproduced from Coccolini et al. (2019); open-access article published by Springer Nature.

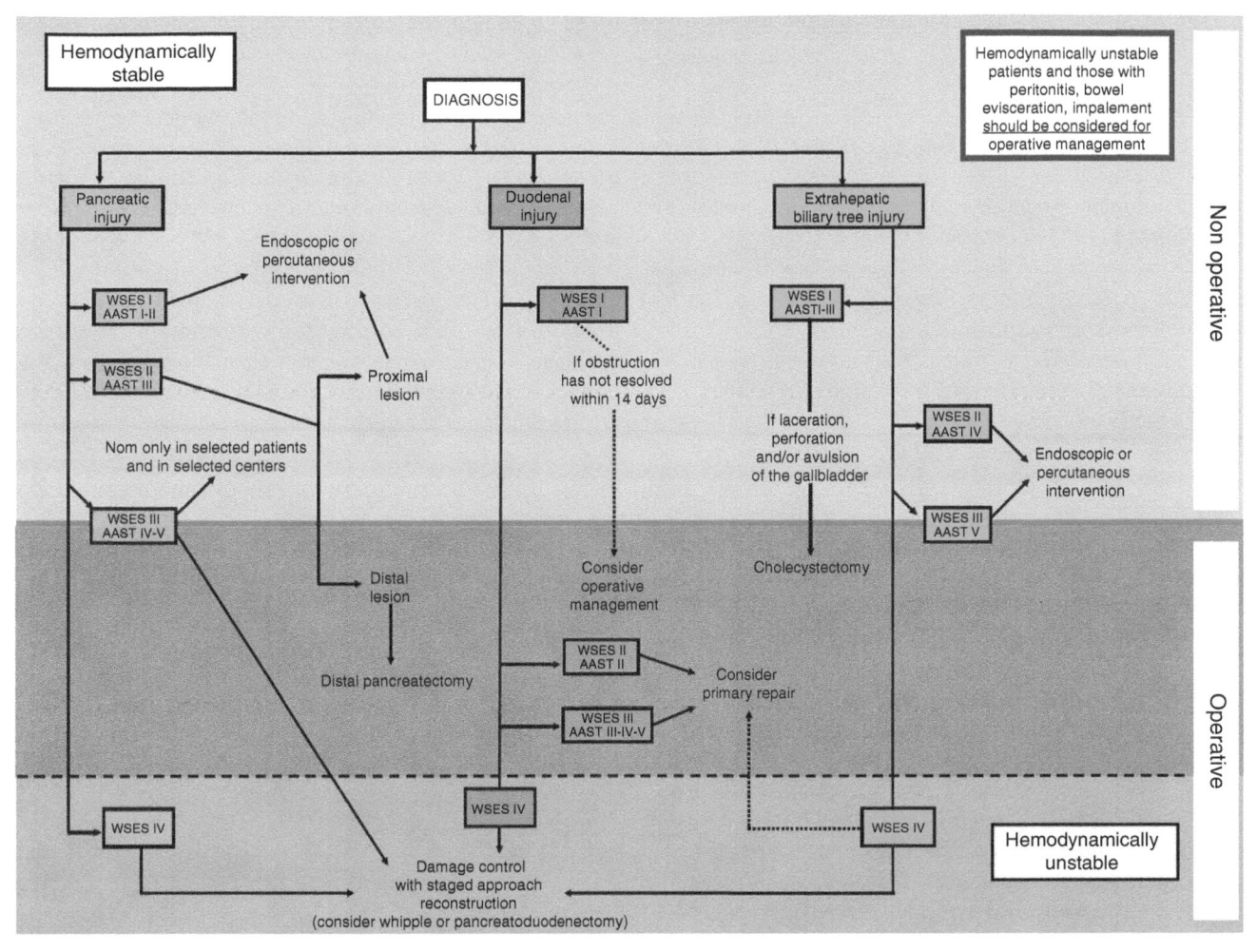

Figure 38.2 WSES-AAST algorithm for treatment of duodenal, pancreatic, and extrahepatic biliary injuries after trauma. *Source*: Reproduced from Coccolini et al. (2019); open-access article published by Springer Nature.

16 *A 47-year-old man presents with severe acute pancreatitis. Aggressive fluid resuscitation is initiated and the patient is admitted to the ICU. Which of the following is an appropriate strategy for determining the rate of fluid administration?*

A *Initial 30 mL/kg fluid bolus followed by goal-directed resuscitation with goal urine output of 1.0 mL/kg/hr.*

B *Rapid resuscitation with goal hematocrit <35% 48 hours after admission.*

C *Initial fluid bolus of 20 mL/kg followed by goal-directed resuscitation with goal heart rate < 120 bpm.*

D *Initial 10 mL/kg bolus followed by 1.5 mL/kg/hr and additional boluses as needed.*

E *10–15 mL/kg/hr continuously until mean arterial pressure is > 85 mmHg.*

While adequate fluid resuscitation is a cornerstone in the management of acute pancreatitis, specific resuscitation protocols remain under debate. Overly aggressive resuscitation

protocols (i.e., 10–15 mL/kg/hr continuously) have been associated with increased rates of abdominal compartment syndrome, need for mechanical ventilation, and mortality. Under-resuscitation has also been associated with poor outcomes. Most current recommendations involve early, goal-directed therapy. A review by the Dutch Pancreatitis Group in 2017 recommended goal-directed therapy with initial fluid bolus of 20 mL/kg, followed by continuous crystalloid infusion rates titrated according to clinical parameters of heart rate < 120 bpm, urine output >0.5 mL/kg/hr, and mean arterial pressure 64–85 mmHg. Dilutional anemia should be avoided and goal hematocrit should be 35–44% during resuscitation.

Answer: C

van Dijk SM, Hallensleben NDL, van Santvoort HC, et al.; Dutch Pancreatitis Study Group. Acute pancreatitis: recent advances through randomised trials. *Gut.* 2017;66(11):2024–32.

17 Which of the following is true regarding pancreatic pseudocysts that directly abut intra-abdominal vasculature?
   A *Pseudocyst-induced hemorrhage is usually caused by pseudocyst erosion into splenic and gastroduodenal veins.*
   B *Pseudocyst-induced hemorrhage most commonly involves the pancreaticoduodenal arteries.*
   C *Angiography is the most appropriate treatment for acute pseudocyst-induced hemorrhage with hemodynamic instability.*
   D *After hemorrhage control, the best definitive management of the pseudocyst is surgical resection.*
   E *After hemorrhage control, the best definitive management of the pseudocyst is cystoenterostomy.*

Pancreatic pseudocysts that abut the vasculature pose a significant risk of life-threatening arterial hemorrhage. Pseudocysts tend to compress adjacent veins, leading to thrombosis rather than hemorrhage. Arteries, however, are not as compressible and instead can develop inflammation-induced pseudoaneurysms, which then can rupture and hemorrhage. The most common source of pseudocyst-induced hemorrhage is the splenic artery, followed by the gastroduodenal and pancreaticoduodenal arteries. When hemorrhage is present but the patient is stable enough for interventional radiology, the preferred treatment is angiography and embolization. Due to the significant increase in associated complications and mortality, surgical intervention is typically reserved for patients who are hemodynamically unstable. Intraoperatively, once the hemorrhage has been controlled, preferred definitive management of the pseudocyst is resection rather than cystoenteric drainage. Resection of the cyst decreases the risk of further hemorrhagic complications. For hemorrhage associated with the splenic artery, this typically requires distal pancreatectomy and splenectomy. For hemorrhage associated with the gastroduodenal or pancreaticoduodenal arteries, pancreaticoduodenectomy is usually the operation of choice.

Answer: D

Matsuoka L, Alexopoulos SP. Surgical management of pancreatic pseudocysts. *Gastrointestinal Endoscopy Clinics of North America.* 2018;28(2):131–41.

18 Which of the following is the most common complication of nonoperative management for pancreatic injuries?
   A *Pancreatic fistula*
   B *Intra-abdominal abscess*
   C *Glucose intolerance*
   D *Pancreatic pseudocyst*
   E *Exocrine pancreatic insufficiency*

The most common complication following nonoperative management of pancreatic injury (PI) is a pancreatic pseudocyst. This occurs in about one-fifth of patients who succeed without operative intervention. Intra-abdominal abscess occurs in up to 25% of all patients with PI; however, it is more common in patients who undergo operative intervention. Pancreatic fistulae develop in 10–35% of patients who undergo operative drainage and/or pancreatic resection, but are rare for nonoperative patients. Endocrine and exocrine pancreatic insufficiency are very rare complications. When they do occur, they are typically transient and occur after pancreatic resection, not nonoperative management.

Answer: D

Coccolini F, Kobayashi L, Kluger Y, et al.; WSES-AAST Expert Panel. Duodeno-pancreatic and extrahepatic biliary tree trauma: WSES-AAST guidelines. *World Journal of Emergency Surgery.* 2019;14:56.
Ho VP, Patel NJ, Bokhari F, et al. Management of adult pancreatic injuries: a practice management guideline from the Eastern Association for the Surgery of Trauma. *Journal of Trauma and Acute Care Surgery.* 2017;82(1):185–99.

19 A 22-year-old woman is recovering in the ICU after she was struck by a car while crossing the street. She is currently on postoperative day three after exploratory laparotomy, splenectomy, and distal pancreatectomy. Drain amylase has been 300–500 U/L daily, suggesting pancreatic leak. She is afebrile and hemodynamically normal, and her white blood cell count is down-trending. What is the next best step?
   A *Obtain a stat CT scan of the abdomen and pelvis to evaluate for fluid collection.*
   B *Close observation and nutritional optimization.*
   C *Stat consult to Interventional Radiology for placement of a second percutaneous drain.*
   D *Initiate antibiotic therapy, obtain a CT scan of the abdomen and pelvis to evaluate for fluid collection.*
   E *Planned return to OR for exploratory laparotomy, washout, and wide drainage.*

According to the International Study Group on Pancreatic Fistula (ISGPF), this patient has a biochemical leak (Table 38.5). Since she has no evidence of infection, close observation and nutritional optimization (preferably enteral if tolerated) would be sufficient.

Table 38.5 2017 ISGPF definitions and grades of postoperative pancreatic fistula.

Event	Biochemical leak	Grade B POPF	Grade C POPF
Drain amylase concentration >3 × upper limit of normal serum value	Yes	Yes	Yes
Persisting peripancreatic drainage >3 weeks	No	Yes	Yes
Clinically relevant change in the management of POPF	No	Yes	Yes
Percutaneous or endoscopic drainage of POPF-associated collections	No	Yes	Yes
Angiographic procedures for POPF-associated bleeding	No	Yes	Yes
Reoperation for POPF	No	No	Yes
Signs of infection related to POPF	No	Yes (without organ failure)	Yes (with organ failure)
POPF-related organ failure	No	No	Yes
POPF-related death	No	No	Yes

Abbreviations: ISGPF, International Study Group on Pancreatic Fistula; POPF, postoperative pancreatic fistula.
Source: Reproduced from Bassi et al. (2017); with permission from publisher, Elsevier.

Somatostatin analogues have been evaluated for their role in expedited resolution of pancreatic fistulae, though no clear benefit has been demonstrated in the literature. If the patient were to develop signs of infection, a contrast-enhanced CT scan and initiation of broad-spectrum antibiotics would be appropriate. Additional percutaneous drainage and/or endoscopic drainage could also be considered if there were concern for infection. Re-exploration is typically reserved for hemodynamically unstable patients and patients in whom more conservative treatments have failed.

Answer: B

Nahm CB, Connor SJ, Samra JS, Mittal A. Postoperative pancreatic fistula: a review of traditional and emerging concepts. *Clinical and Experimental Gastroenterology*. 2018;11:105–118.

20 *Which of the following is true regarding amylase and lipase when diagnosing acute pancreatitis?*
   A *Elevated serum amylase is more specific for acute pancreatitis than serum lipase.*
   B *Serum lipase returns to normal levels more quickly than serum amylase.*
   C *Serum lipase may be artificially low in patients with diabetes mellitus.*
   D *Serum amylase may remain normal in patients with alcohol or triglyceride-induced acute pancreatitis.*
   E *Serum amylase and lipase have similar sensitivities for acute pancreatitis.*

According to the American College of Gastroenterology (ACG), the diagnosis of acute pancreatitis can be made if the patient has at least two of the following: characteristic abdominal pain, serum amylase and/or lipase greater than three-to-five times the upper limit of normal, and/or characteristic findings on abdominal imaging. While elevation in either serum amylase or lipase is sufficient based on these criteria, lipase is typically relied upon more heavily as it has better sensitivity, specificity, and positive and negative predictive values than amylase. Serum lipase also remains elevated longer than serum amylase, which typically normalizes as soon as 3–5 days after onset of pancreatitis. Importantly, serum amylase may remain within normal limits during episodes of alcohol or hypertriglyceridemia-induced acute pancreatitis. While lipase does appear to be the superior test for acute pancreatitis, patients with diabetes mellitus tend to have higher median levels of serum lipase at baseline compared to non-diabetics. This is why most guidelines recommend a serum lipase threshold of at least three times the upper limit of normal to support the diagnosis of acute pancreatitis.

Answer: D

Tenner S, Baillie J, DeWitt J, Vege SS; American College of Gastroenterology. American college of gastroenterology guideline: management of acute pancreatitis. *American Journal of Gastroenterology*. 2013;108(9):1400–15; 1416.

References

Bassi, C., Marchegiani, G., Dervenis, C. et al. (2017). The 2016 update of the International Study Group (ISGPS) definition and grading of postoperative pancreatic fistula: 11 years after. *Surgery* 161 (3): 584–591.

Coccolini, F., Kobayashi, L., Kluger, Y. et al. (2019). Duodeno-pancreatic and extrahepatic biliary tree trauma: WSES-AAST guidelines. *World Journal of Emergency Surgery* 14: 56.

Yokoe, M., Hata, J., Takada, T. et al. (2018). Tokyo Guidelines 2018: diagnostic criteria and severity grading of acute cholecystitis (with videos). *Journal of Hepato-biliary-pancreatic Sciences* 25 (1): 41–54.

Kiriyama, S., Kozaka, K., Takada, T. et al. (2018). Tokyo Guidelines 2018: diagnostic criteria and severity grading of acute cholangitis (with videos). *Journal of Hepato-biliary-pancreatic Sciences* 25 (1): 17–30.

39

Liver and Spleen
Narong Kulvatunyou, MD[1] and Peter M. Rhee, MD[2]

[1] Department of Surgery, University of Arizona School of Medicine, Banner University Medical Center, Tucson, AZ, USA
[2] Division of Trauma and Acute Care Surgery, New York Medical College, Westchester Medical Center, Valhalla, NY, USA

1 *Concerning the liver functional anatomy, the liver is divided into 8 segments based on the distribution of portal pedicles and hepatic veins. A lesion, detected on the left side gallbladder but medial and posterior to the ligament of teres with the left branch of the portal vein running transversely below, represents what Couinaud segment?*
   A *Segment 2*
   B *Segment 3*
   C *Segment 4*
   D *Segment 5*
   E *Segment 8*

The liver is morphologically divided into the right and left lobe by the line divided between gallbladder and inferior vena cava. Functionally, however, the liver is divided into 8 Couinaud segments based on the distribution of portal pedicles (hepatic artery, biliary, and portal vein) and hepatic veins. The left lobe of the liver is split into anterior (segments III, laterally and segment IV, medially) and posterior (segment II) sector by the left scissura which runs behind the ligament of teres and it contains left hepatic vein. The portal vein divides into main right and left branches at the hilum, and the left branch runs transversely at the base of segment IV and into the umbilical fissure, where it gives off branches to segments II & III and feedback branches to segment IV. The left portal vein also gives off posterior branches of the left side of caudate lobe (segment I). Therefore, the lesion appears to be in segment IV.

Answer: C

COUINAUDS SEGMENTS OF THE LIVER

Surgical Critical Care and Emergency Surgery: Clinical Questions and Answers, Third Edition.
Edited by Forrest "Dell" Moore, Peter M. Rhee, and Carlos J. Rodriguez.
© 2022 John Wiley & Sons Ltd. Published 2022 by John Wiley & Sons Ltd.
Companion website: www.wiley.com/go/surgicalcriticalcare3e

How a cholangiogram corresponds to liver segments

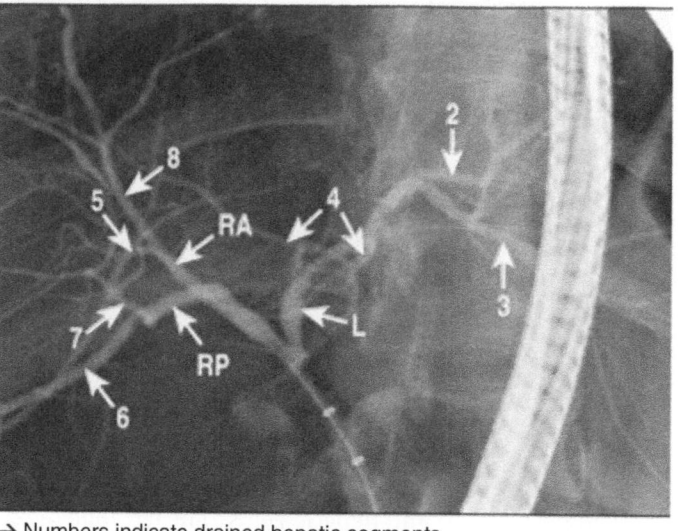

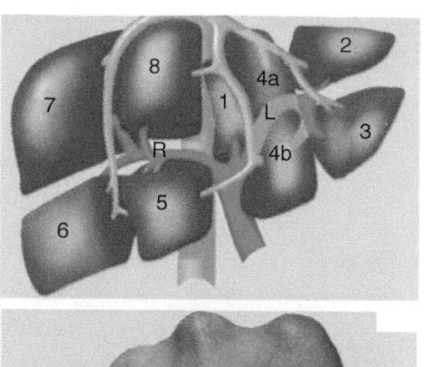

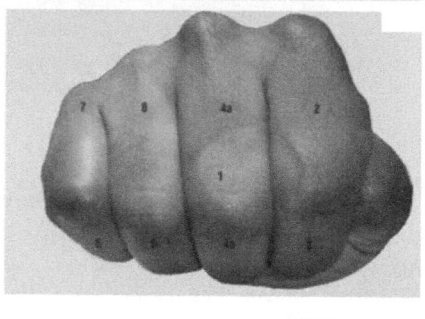

→ Numbers indicate drained hepatic segments
→ Right anterior duct has a relatively vertical and medial course
→ Right posterior duct has a more horizontal and lateral course

✔ Follow @tberzin

Source: Pauli et al. Arch Surg 2012 (Diagram), and abdominalkey.com (cholangiogram).

Sabiston Chapter 53: The Liver; Anatomy and Physiology. In: CM Townsend, RD Beauchamp, BM Evers and KL Mattox *Textbook of Surgery: The Biologic Basis of Modern Surgical Practice*, April 2016, Elsevier, 20th edition.

2 *A 45-year-old man presents to your institution, a level I trauma center, after a motorcycle crash. On arrival, he complains of right thoracoabdominal pain. Primary survey shows heart rate of 110 beats/min, blood pressure of 90/50 mm Hg. FAST exam is positive in all 3-quadrants. Abdominal exam is benign other than right upper quadrant tenderness. His BP improves after 2 units of packed RBC. He is then taken to*

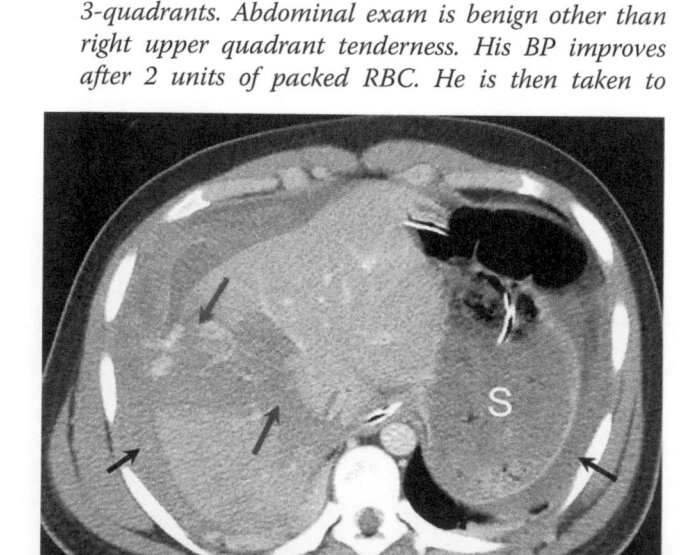

computed tomography (CT) scan which is shown below. What is the next appropriate step of management?

A *Exploratory laparotomy*
B *Give 2 L of crystalloid*
C *Admit to regular ward for observation*
D *Diagnostic laparoscopy*
E *Angioembolization*

This patient suffers a grade V blunt liver injury. Since he is a responder to 2 units of blood transfusion, he is a candidate for a nonoperative management which has 80–100% success rate. CT scan, however, demonstrates a contrast blush (red arrow) which makes him a candidate for angiogram and angioembolization. It also shows hemoperitoneum (black arrow) and liver injury (blue arrow). Angiographic embolization (AE) can be an adjunct to a nonoperative management and helps improve the success rate. Giving additional 2 L of crystalloid in this hemodynamically stable patient is not indicated and would hemodilute the patient (answer B). Admitting the patient to the ward for observation would be very risky as the patient may quickly become unstable and the blush indicates ongoing bleeding during the CT scan (answer C). Diagnostic laparoscopy is not needed as CT is an excellent method of diagnosis and diagnostic laparoscopy would not be therapeutic in terms of hemorrhage control (answer D). Taking the patient to operating room for either diagnostic laparoscopy or exploratory laparotomy is not yet indicated (answer D).

Grade	Injury type	Injury descriptor
I	Hematoma	Subcapsular < 10% surface
	Laceration	Capsular tear < 1 cm parenchymal depth
II	Hematoma	Subcapsular 10–50% surface area; intraparenchymal, <10 cm diameter
	Laceration	1–3 cm parenchymal depth, <10 cm in length
III	Hematoma	Subcapsular > 50% surface area or expanding, ruptured subcapsular or parenchymal hematoma, intraparenchymal hematoma > 10 cm
	Laceration	>3 cm parenchymal depth
IV	Laceration	Parenchymal disruption 25–75% of hepatic lobe
V	Laceration	Parenchymal disruption involving > 75% of hepatic lobe
	Vascular	Juxtavenous hepatic injuries, i.e., retrohepatic vena cav/central major hepatic veins
VI	Vascular	Hepatic avulsion

Advance one grade for multiple injuries up to grade III AAST liver injury scale (1994 revision).

Answer: E

Stassen NA, Bhullar I, Cheng JD, et al. Non-operative management of blunt hepatic injury: an eastern association for the surgery of trauma practice management guideline. *J Trauma & ACS* 2012; 73: S288–S293.

Polanco PM, Brown JB, Puyana JC, et al. The swinging pendulum: a national perspective of nonoperative management in severe blunt liver injury. *J Trauma & ACS* 2013; 75: 590–595.

3 *A 67-year-old woman presents to the emergency department with a 1 day history of acute right upper quadrant pain. She denies nausea, vomiting, change in appetite, or weight loss. Surgical history is significant for cholecystectomy. Vital signs are normal. Abdominal exam shows she is not jaundiced but has a mild nonspecific right upper quadrant tenderness. Laboratory results are within normal. A CT scan of the abdomen is shown below. Which of the following statement is the most correct regarding this condition?*

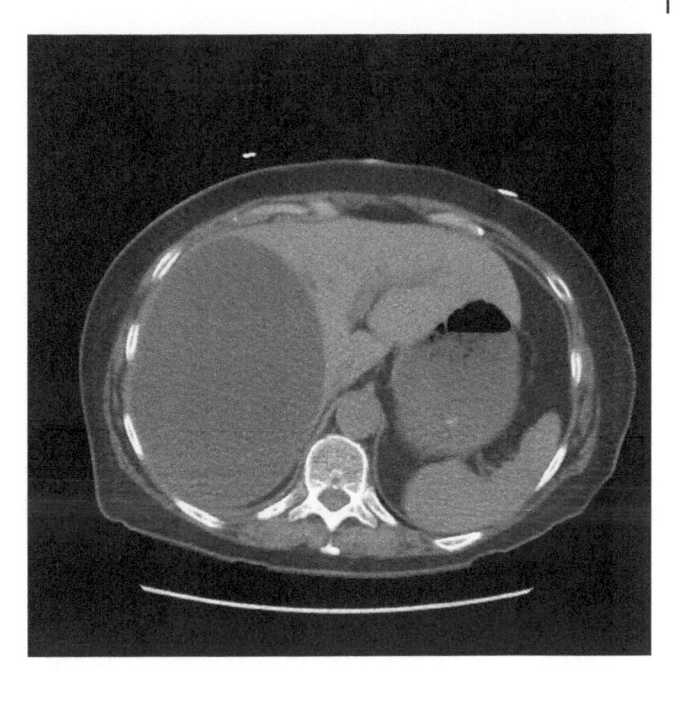

A *The majority (>90%) of patients with simple cysts are asymptomatic and do not need any intervention.*

B *Atypical wall characteristics (asymmetric, thickening, nodular, lobular) and non-homogeneous fluid are all benign changes and is not suspicious for malignancy.*

C *Magnetic Resonance Imaging (MRI) is more accurate than ultrasound or computerized tomography (CT) scan in terms of characterizing the wall and the fluid content.*

D *Sclerosing therapy is not appropriate for cyst that is easily accessible by surgery and has a high recurrence rate.*

E *Laparoscopic fenestration (unroofing) while simple is dangerous and has high recurrence rate.*

A simple liver cyst is the most common liver parenchymal imaging abnormality. The vast majority (>90%) of simple liver cysts are asymptomatic and do not need intervention. Increasing in size (stretching of the Gleason capsule), sudden hemorrhage, and/or communication with biliary system may cause patient to present with abdominal symptoms, early satiety, etc. Ultrasound and CT scan have classic characteristics of smooth wall without radiographic features of thickening, nodularity, or asymmetry; and the simple cyst contains homogenous fluid appearance. MRI has the advantage over the US/CT in its ability to characterize the fluid as well as identifying subtle mural nodules/projections that make one suspicious of something different than simple cyst. Interventional radiographic-guidance needle aspiration and sclerosing is very effective (>90%) in the management of simple liver cyst but is limited by the size and the volume, but it has the advantage over surgery where cyst is not easily accessible. Laparoscopic fenestration (unroofing) also has >90% success rate and more applicable to a very large size simple cyst that is easily accessible. Surgery is also appropriate if cyst communicates with biliary system which requires surgical closure.

Answer: C

Cameron JL, Cameron AL. (2017) Current Surgical Therapy, 13th Edition. In: John L. Cameron and Andrew M Cameron *Cystic Disease of the Liver*. Philadelphia, PA: Elsevier, p. 353–355.

Alshaikhli A, Al-Hillan A. (2021) Liver Cystic Disease. In: *StatPearls [Internet]*. Treasure Island (FL): StatPearls Publishing Jan–. PMID: 33620816.

Mavilia MG, Pakala T, Molina M, Wu GY. Differentiating cystic liver lesions: a review of imaging modalities, diagnosis and management. *J Clin Transl Hepatol*. 2018; 6(2): 208–216. doi: 10.14218/JCTH.2017.00069. Epub 2018 Jan 5. PMID: 29951366; PMCID: PMC6018306.

Moorthy K, Mihssin N, Houghton PW. The management of simple hepatic cysts: sclerotherapy or laparoscopic fenestration. *Ann R Coll Surg Engl*. 2001;83(6):409–14. PMID: 11777137; PMCID: PMC2503687.

4   *A 50-year-old woman presents with right upper quadrant pain. A CT scan of the abdomen is obtained which demonstrates a 5 cm hepatic adenoma. Which of the following statement is the most correct?*

A   *Hepatic adenoma is benign and never needs resection.*

B   *Hepatic adenoma is commonly seen in the elderly.*

C   *Hepatic adenoma is the most common benign lesion of the liver.*

D   *Focal nodular hyperplasia (FNH) is a benign liver tumor that seldom appears similar to hepatic adenoma.*

E   *This patient needs resection due to her pain, size and possible degeneration into hepatocellular carcinoma.*

Distinguishing hepatic tumors as benign or malignant is important in liver management. History and radiographic CT findings will help guide the diagnosis and management. Hepatic adenoma is a benign tumor that is seen in women of childbearing age and who are taking oral contraceptives. They often present with abdominal pain because of their size. They can require resection because of symptoms, and they can degenerate into hepatocellular carcinoma. Men and the beta-catenin history pathological hepatic adenoma subtype are risk factors for malignant transformation. In comparison, lesion size and number, exophytic nature, and recent hormonal use in women are associated with bleeding. However, they are not the most common benign hepatic tumor as hemangiomas are the most comment benign hepatic tumor. Hemangioma has the CT characteristic of early enhancement of periphery. Focal nodular hyperplasia (FNH) is another benign hepatic tumor that can be difficult to distinguish from hepatic adenoma but it has a CT characteristic of central scarring.

Answer: C

Cameron JL, Cameron AL. (2017) Current Surgical Therapy, 13th Edition. In: John L. Cameron and Andrew M Cameron *Management of Benign Liver Tumors*. Philadelphia, PA: Elsevier, p. 371–372.

Silva JP, Klooster B, Tsai S, Christians KK, Clarke CN, Mogal H, Clark GT. Elective regional therapy treatment for hepatic adenoma. *Ann Surg Oncol*. 2019; 26(1): 125–130. doi: 10.1245/s10434-018-6802-1. Epub 2018 Oct 23. PMID: 30353390.

Rodrigues BT, Mei SLCY, Fox A, Lubel JS, Nicoll AJ. A systematic review on the complications and management of hepatic adenomas: a call for a new approach. *Eur J Gastroenterol Hepatol*. 2020; 32(8): 923–930. doi: 10.1097/MEG.0000000000001766. PMID: 32433418.

5   *Which of the following statement regarding liver biliary cystadenoma (BCA) is the most true?*

A   *BCA is usually a multi-focal, non-septate lesion*

B   *BCA has no potential for malignant transformation*

C   *BCA has characteristics similar to biliary intraductal papillary mucinous neoplasm (IPMN)*

D   *BCA predominately affects men*

E   *Surgical resection is a recommended treatment*

Biliary cystadenoma (BCA) is a cystic neoplasm of the biliary ductular system that is thought to arise from ectopic clusters of embryonic bile ducts. BCA is typically a solitary multi-septate lesion, often occupies left lobe, and is more common among woman with a median age of diagnosis of 45. Although BCA is biliary in nature, it lacks the papillary pathologic projection and superficial spreading growth as seen in biliary intraductal papillary mucinous neoplasm (IPMN) which is considered a malignant form. BCA is a benign neoplasm, but it has the potential for malignant transformation (20%) to biliary cystadenocarcinoma and hence, surgical resection is currently recommended. Due to the difficulty in accurately diagnosing these biliary cystic lesions and the availability of different surgical approaches, patients with suspected BCA or BCAC should be treated in a center specializing in liver surgery with state-of-the-art imaging and all surgical techniques available to manage this rare disease.

Answer: E

Cameron JL, Cameron AL. (2017) Current Surgical Therapy, 13th Edition. In: John L. Cameron and Andrew M Cameron *Management of Benign Liver Tumors*. Philadelphia, PA: Elsevier, p. 371–372.

Klompenhouwer AJ, Ten Cate DWG, Willemssen FEJA, Bramer WM, Doukas M, de Man RA, Ijzermans JNM. The impact of imaging on the surgical management of biliary cystadenomas and cystadenocarcinomas; a systematic review. *HPB (Oxford)*. 2019; 21(10): 1257–1267. doi: 10.1016/j.hpb.2019.04.004. Epub 2019 May 10. PMID: 31085104.

6 *A 52-year-old woman presents with a newly diagnosed liver lesion. Which imaging finding indicates that the patient should undergo resection?*

   A *A 3 cm lesion with bright homogeneous enhancement in the arterial phase with a central scar.*

   B *A 3 cm lesion with a heterogeneous appearance and arterial-phase enhancement with a smooth surface.*

   C *A 3 cm lesion with centripetal enhancement on liver protocol CT.*

   D *A 3 cm asymmetric cystic lesion with no internal septation.*

   E *A 3 cm lesion with arterial enhancement and washout in the portal phase of CT.*

Hepatocellular carcinoma (HCC) demonstrates CT arterial enhancement and a washout in the portal phase; hence, a surgical resection is indicated. A homogeneous enhancement in the arterial phase with central scarring is a classic presentation of focal nodular hyperplasia (FNH) which is a benign liver lesion and does not require surgical resection. A heterogenous appearance and arterial-phase enhancement with a smooth surface suggests hepatic adenoma, again a benign liver lesion which does not require resection unless patient is symptomatic. A liver lesion with centripetal enhancement is a classic presentation of hemangioma, a cystic lesion with no internal septation suggests a simple cyst; both do not require surgical resection.

Answer: E

Cameron JL, Cameron AL. (2017) Current Surgical Therapy, 13th Edition. In: John L. Cameron and Andrew M Cameron *Management of Benign Liver Tumors*. Philadelphia, PA: Elsevier, p. 371–372.

Sabiston Chapter 53. The Liver. In: CM Townsend, RD Beauchamp, BM Evers and KL Mattox *Textbook of Surgery: The Biologic Basis of Modern Surgical Practice*, April 2016, Elsevier, 20th edition.

Gupta P, Bansal A, Das GC, Kumar MP, Chaluvashetty SB, Bhujade H, Gulati A, Kalra N. Diagnostic accuracy of liver imaging reporting and data system locoregional treatment response criteria: a systematic review and meta-analysis. *Eur Radiol*. 2021 Mar 30. doi: https://doi.org/10.1007/s00330-021-07837-6. Epub ahead of print. PMID: 33786656.

7 *Which of the following statements regarding hydatid cyst disease of the liver is INCORRECT?*

   A *Hydatid cyst disease of the liver is caused by a larvae form of Echinococcus, tapeworms found in the intestines of sheepdogs.*

   B *The cyst has the ultrasonographic/CT scan findings of hyperechoic ring with central septation and/or necrosis.*

   C *Chemotherapy treatment with benzimidazole agent offers a complete cure.*

   D *PAIR is recommended treatment which includes percutaneous needle aspiration and injection of protoscolicidal agent.*

   E *Surgery is reserved for more complicated disease like cyst with several septation, cyst that communicates with biliary tree, etc.*

Hydatid cyst of the liver is caused by a human echinococcosis, a zoonosis caused by a larval form of Echinococcus tapeworms found in the small intestines of a definitive host (a sheepdog or cat) but a sheep (or human) serves as an intermediate host. Echinococcus has two species, *E. granulosus* and *E. multilocularis,* both of which respond to the parasitostatic treatment of benzimidazole agents (mebendazole and albendazole) but only about one-third of patients respond to chemotherapy treatment alone. PAIR is a recommended initial treatment and it consists of a percutaneous drainage of the cyst, followed by an injection of protoscolicidal agent. Surgical treatment, open or laparoscopic, is reserved for a more complicated cyst such as large size cyst pending rupture, cyst with multiple septation, or cyst that communicates with biliary tree. However, the level of evidence is low, concerning the treatment of complicated cysts.

Answer: C

Cameron JL, Cameron AL. (2017) Current Surgical Therapy, 13th Edition. In John L. Cameron and Andrew M Cameron *Management of Echinococcal Cyst Disease of the Liver*. Philadelphia, PA: Elsevier, p. 361–365.

Gavara CG, Lopez-Andujar R, Ibanez TB, et al. Review of the treatment of liver hydatid cysts. *W J Gastro* 2015; 21(1): 124–131.

Sokouti M, Sadeghi R, Pashazadeh S, Abadi SEH, Sokouti M, Ghojazadeh M, Sokouti B. A systematic review and meta-analysis on the treatment of liver hydatid cyst using meta-MUMS tool: comparing PAIR and laparoscopic procedures. *Arch Med Sci*. 2019; 15(2): 284–308. doi: 10.5114/aoms.2018.73344. Epub 2018 Mar 2. PMID: 30899281; PMCID: PMC6425195.

Dziri C, Haouet K, Fingerhut A. Treatment of hydatid cyst of the liver: where is the evidence? *World J Surg*. 2004; 28(8): 731–736. doi: 10.1007/s00268-004-7516-z. Epub 2004 Aug 3. PMID: 15457348.

8 Which of the following statement is the most correct regarding hepatic abscess?
   A Liver abscess are mostly caused by parasites but can also be pyogenic or amebic
   B Amebic abscess is caused by Entamoeba granulosis
   C Pyogenic liver abscess (PLA) is commonly caused by appendicitis
   D PLA is treated with appropriate antibiotic and percutaneous drainage
   E Amebic liver abscess (ALA) rarely responds well to antibiotic treatment alone

Liver abscesses are uncommon but can be lethal if not properly recognized and adequately treated. A liver abscess is a pus-filled mass in the liver and can develop from injury to the liver or an intra-abdominal infection disseminated from the portal circulation. They can be from pyogenic or amebic but in a minority of cases can be from parasites and fungi. Pyogenic liver abscess (PLA) is more common in North America, but clinician must beware of the possible fungal cause in those with underlying malignancy or immunocompromised, and amebic cause in those who come from endemic area which is caused by *Entamoeba histolytic*. It affects the liver by first causing amebic colitis, then seen in the portal system and migrating to the liver and causing amebic liver abscess. This is rare in United States but can be found in immigrants or travels from other countries. Another rare but important parasitic organism is *Echinococcus granulosis*, which causes a hydatid cyst of the liver. It used to be true that, PLA was commonly caused by undiagnosed appendicitis, but now the common cause is biliary origin, particularly those with instrumentation or biliary-enteric anastomosis. Half of all bacterial cases are due to cholan-

gitis. The most common bacterial organisms are *E. coli*, *Klebsiella*, *Streptococcus*, *Staphylococcus*, and anaerobic organisms but are generally polymicrobial. PLA treatment is appropriate course of antibiotic of choice and source control with percutaneous drainage. Amoebic abscess is often diagnosed by serum serology and treatment is effective with 7–10 days course of metronidazole.

Answer: D

Cameron JL, Cameron AL. (2017) Current Surgical Therapy, 13th Edition. In: John L. Cameron and Andrew M Cameron *Management of Hepatic Abscess*. Philadelphia, PA: Elsevier, p. 368–393.

Lo JZ, Leow JJ, Ng PL et al. Predictors of therapy failure in a series of 741 adult pyogenic liver abscesses. *Hep Pancr Sci* 2015; 22:156–165.

Cai YL, Xiong XZ, Lu J, Cheng Y, Yang C, Lin YX, Zhang J, Cheng NS. Percutaneous needle aspiration versus catheter drainage in the management of liver abscess: a systematic review and meta-analysis. *HPB (Oxford)*. 2015; 17(3): 195–201. doi: 10.1111/hpb.12332. Epub 2014 Sep 10. PMID: 25209740; PMCID: PMC4333779.

9 A 50-year-old man suffers a golf cart-related accident in which he suffers a grade V liver injury, requiring a radiographic intervention (IR) embolization of liver segment VI & VII. Over the next few days in the hospital, he continues to be febrile, jaundiced, tachycardic, but BP remains normal. His abdominal exam was benign other than significantly distended. Hemoglobin remains unchanged, WBC slightly elevates 11 500/mm³. A repeated CT scan of the abdomen is obtained and shown below? What would be the next appropriate step of management?
   A Repeat angiography
   B Exploratory laparotomy
   C Endoscopic Retrograde Cholangiopancreaticography (ERCP)
   D Laparoscopy and abdominal washout
   E C and D

Nonoperative management of high-grade (grade IV & V) blunt liver injuries can be performed successfully but clinician must beware of its increased biliary-related complication. A biloma and a persistent bile leak are common and should be managed with CT-guided percutaneous drainage and/or an endoscopic retrograde cholangiography (ERCP) with possibly biliary stent. A few patients may continue to demonstrate a clinical systemic inflammatory syndrome (SIRS) with persistent fever, tachycardia, and jaundice due to bile (mixed with blood) peritonitis that deserve a diagnostic laparoscopy (DL) and abdominal washout. This patient underwent an ERCP which did not demonstrate any persistent bile leak but had a stent placed

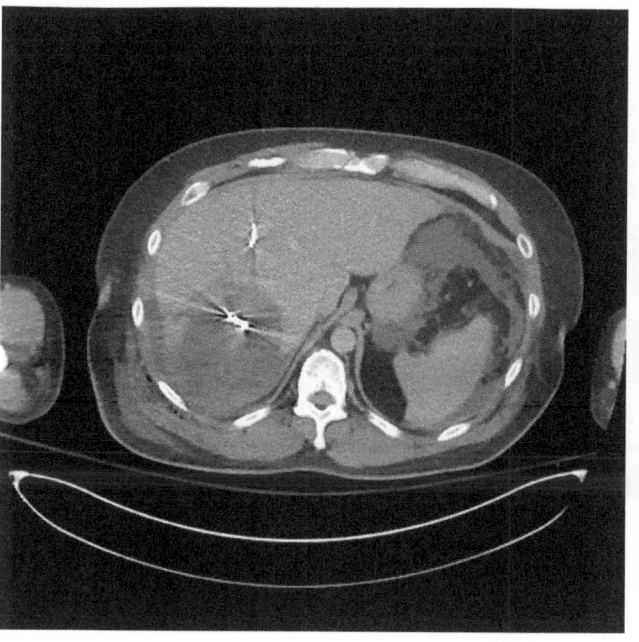

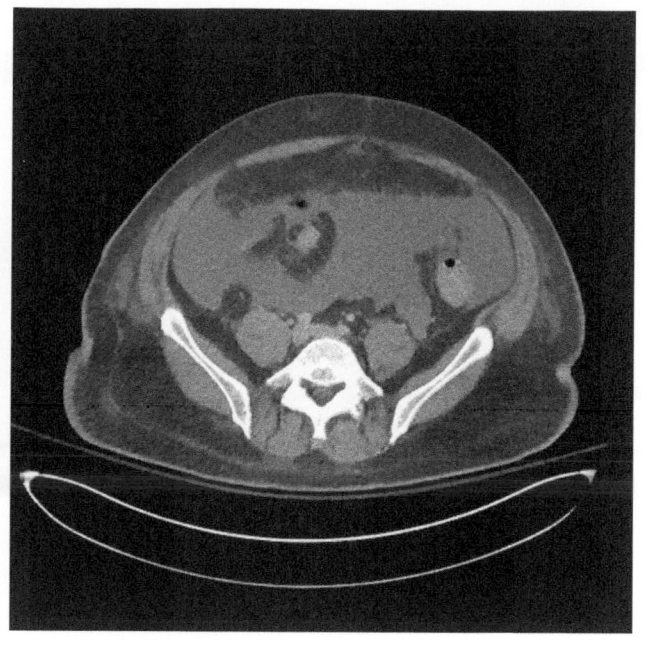

to reduce pressure backflow of the biliary system. Due to persistent jaundice and abdominal distension, he is subsequently taken to the operating room for a DL with abdominal washout. Total of 3.2 L of blood mixed with bile were evacuated from the abdomen and a drain placed. Patient showed a dramatic improvement after the DL procedure.

Answer: E

Kozar RA, Moore JB, Niles SE, et al. Complications of nonoperative management of high-grade blunt hepatic liver injuries. *J Trauma* 2005; 59 (5), 1066–1071.

Carrillo EH, Reed DN, Gordon L, et al. Delayed laparoscopy facilitates the management of biliary peritonitis in patients with complex liver injuries. *Surg Endosc.* 2011; 15: 319–322.

Hommes M, Nicol AJ, Navsaria PH, et al. Management of biliary complications in 412 patients with liver injuries. *J Trauma & ACS* 2014; 77: 448–451.

10 *A 24-year-old man presents to the emergency department with a vague right upper quadrant abdominal pain and hematemesis. He denies any fever, weight loss, or change in appetite. One month ago, he suffered a grade IV liver injury from a gunshot wound in which he was managed nonoperatively. His current vital signs are normal. His abdominal exam is benign. His upper endoscopy does not demonstrate any obvious sources of bleeding. What would be the most definitive next step in the management of this patient?*

A *Assure the patient that his symptoms will resolve*
B *Transfuse 2 units of blood*
C *Prescribe H2-blocker and ask him to see his primary care physician*
D *Exploratory laparotomy*
E *Angiography*

Fifty percent of high-grade (IV-V) liver injuries may develop delayed complications such as seen in this patient. The development of pseudoaneurysms is common if the grade of injury is high. Pseudoaneurysm which is a contained injury of the hepatic artery can sometimes bleed into the biliary tree and this is called hemobilia. It is a rare complication after hepatic trauma. This patient has hemobilia as he is vomiting blood. Although this patient will undoubtedly get a CT scan first, he will ultimately need an angiogram. Answer (A) is incorrect as this will typically not spontaneously heal and it can be a life-threatening hemorrhage. Answer (B) is an option but not a definitive treatment. This patient has had an upper endoscopy which did not show an ulcer disease and therefore answer (C) is incorrect. The diagnosis and definitive treatment of is (E) an angiography and embolization. Because angiography can be curative and is relatively less invasive than surgery, exploratory laparotomy is not yet indicated (answer D).

Below is a picture of blood coming out of the ampula.

(a)

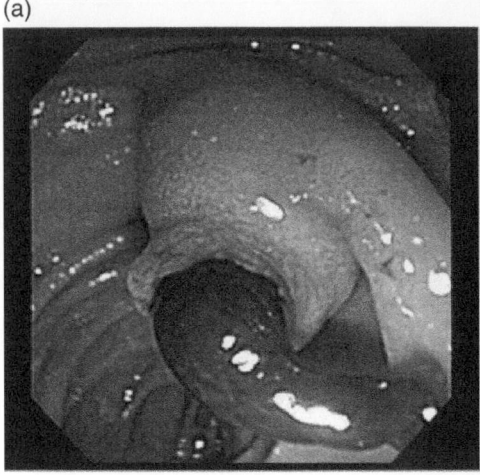

(b)

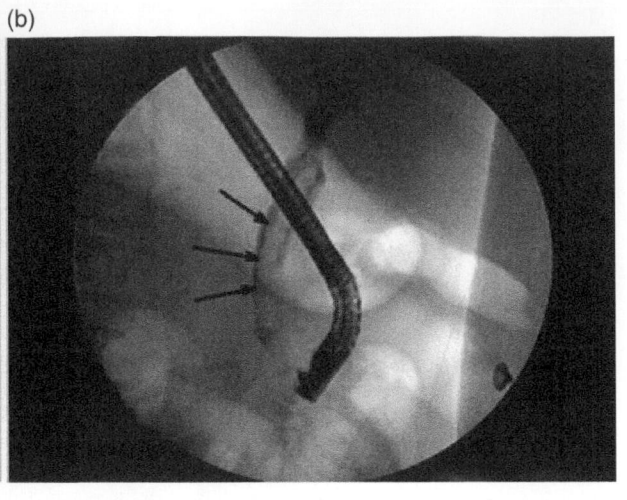

Answer: E

Schouten VD, Velden AP, De Ruijter WM, et al. Hemobilia as a late complication after blunt abdominal trauma: a case report and review of the literature. *J Emer Med* 2010; 39(5): 592–595.

Carillo EH, Wohltmann C, Richardson JD. Evolution in the treatment of complex blunt liver injuries. *Curr Prob Surg.* 2001; 38: 1–60.

11 *A 50-year-old man presents to the trauma bay after being hit by a car. He complains of left side thoraco-abdominal pain and left leg pain. On exam, his vital signs are normal, abdomen exam is notable for left upper quadrant tenderness without guarding or peritoneal signs. Imaging workup demonstrates two separate splenic lacerations of 0.5 and 0.9 cm with no evidence of active blush. What is the grading of this splenic injury and treatment plan?*

A *Grade I - observation*
B *Grade I - splenectomy*
C *Grade II - observation*
D *Grade II - angioembolization*
E *Grade III - observation*

Understanding solid organ injury grading (spleen or liver) helps one understand the natural tendency of progression including diagnosis, management, and grade-related complications.

Grade	Injury description	
I	Hematoma	Subcapsular, <10% surface area
	Laceration	Capsular tear, <1 cm parenchymal depth
II	Hematoma	Subcapsular, 10–50% surface area
		Intraparenchymal, <5 cm diameter
	Laceration	1–3 cm parenchymal depth not involving a parenchymal vessel
III	Hematoma	Subcapsular, >50% surface area or expanding
		Ruptured subcapsular or parenchymal hematoma
		Intraparenchymal hematoma >5 cm
	Laceration	>3 cm parenchymal depth or involving trabecular vessels
IV	Laceration	Laceration of segmental or hilar vessels producing major devascularization (>25% of spleen)
V	Laceration	Completely shatters spleen
	Vascular	Hilar vascular injury which devascularized spleen

This patient has a multiple grade I injuries which makes him a grade II. Since he is hemodynamically normal with CT imaging that shows no evidence of active blush, non-operative management with observation is recommended.

Answer: C

Coccolini F, Montori G, Catena F, et al. Splenic trauma: WSES classification and guidelines for adult and pediatric patients. *W J Emerg Surg* 2017; 12: 40.

McCray VW, Davis JW, Lemaster D, Parks SN. Observation for nonoperative management of the spleen: how long is long enough? *J Trauma*. 2008; 65(6): 1354–1358. doi: 10.1097/TA.0b013e31818e8fde. PMID: 19077626.

Moore EE, Cogbill T, Jurkovich GJ, et al. Organ injury scaling: spleen and liver (1994 revision). *J Trauma* 1995; 38(3): 323–324.

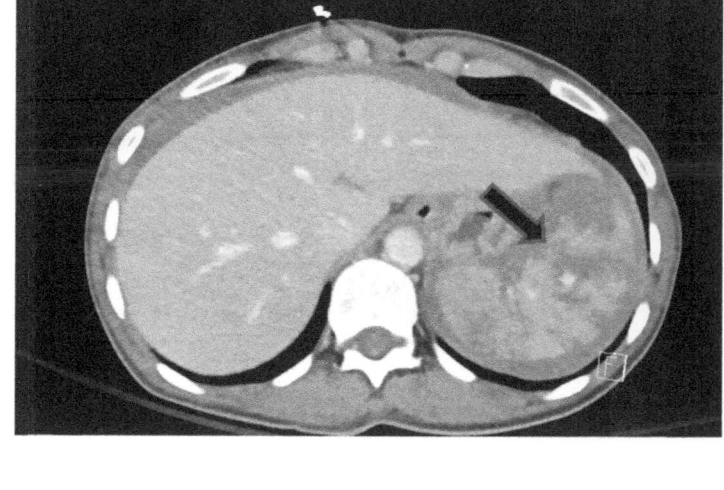

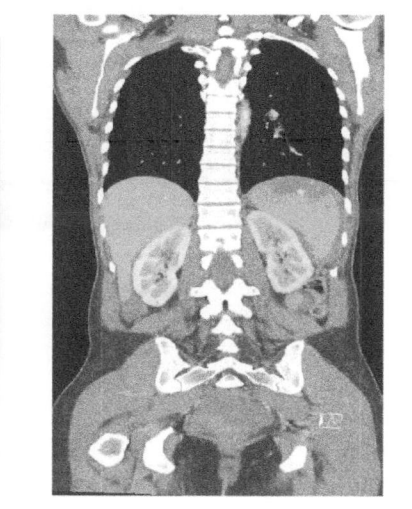

12 *A 31-year-old woman was an unrestrained passenger in a vehicle that hit a pole. On arrival to your facility, she complains of pain in her left upper quadrant. She is mildly tachycardia but blood pressure is normal. FAST exam is positive. An abdominal CT scan finding demonstrates below and no other injuries. What would be the least appropriate step in the management of this patient?*

A *Admit patient to the floor*

B *Administer 2 units of O positive blood*

C *Consult the interventional radiologist (IR) for a possible angiography*

D *Consider taking the patient for emergent laparotomy if indicated*

E *Activate massive transfusion protocol (MTP) if indicated*

This patient suffers a high-grade splenic injury (IV/V) with an active blush (arrow). With a class II hemorrhagic shock (tachycardia), the patient can be resuscitated with volume and volume of choice is blood (Answer B). If the patient responds to the blood transfusion and/or the facility has the capability of interventional radiography (IR) that can perform embolization in a timely fashion, patient should be considered for IR embolization (choice C). If IR, however, is not available, or cannot be activated, or delayed, and/or patient becomes hypotensive, then taking patient to the operating room for a splenectomy should be a consideration. With a positive FAST, tachycardia, patient met the criteria (ABCs) for MTP activation (choice E) and can be considered if clinically indicated.

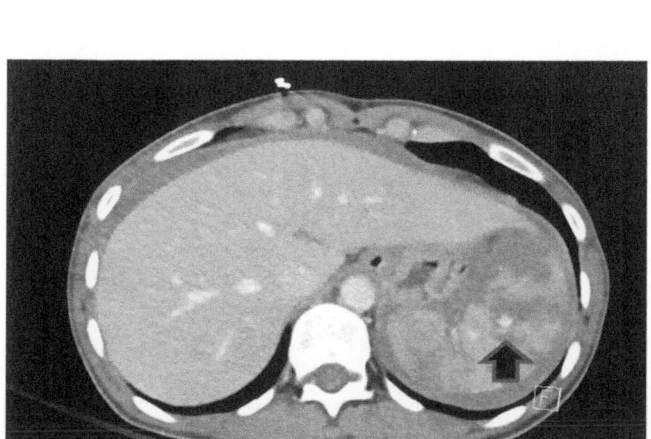

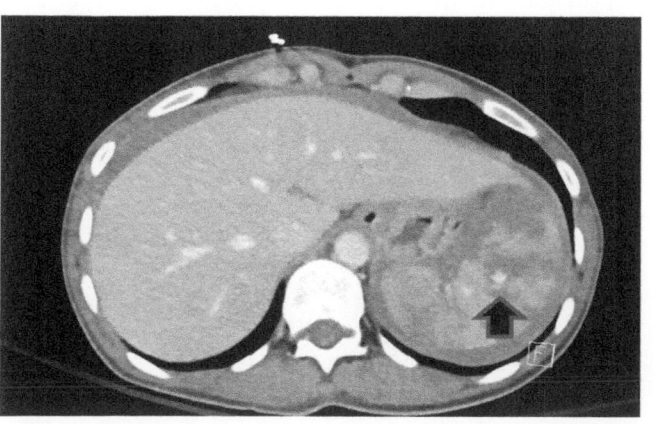

Answer: A

Zarzaur BL, Kozar R, Myers JG, et al. The splenic injury outcomes trial: an American association for the surgery of trauma multi-institutional study. *J Trauma & ACS* 2017; 79: 335–342.

Coccolini F, Montori G, Catena F, et al. Splenic trauma: WSES classification and guidelines for adult and pediatric patients. *W J Emerg Surg* 2017; 12: 40.

Cotton BA, Dossett LA, Haut ER, et al. Multi-center validation of a simplified score to predict massive transfusion in trauma. *J Trauma* 2010; 69: s33–s39.

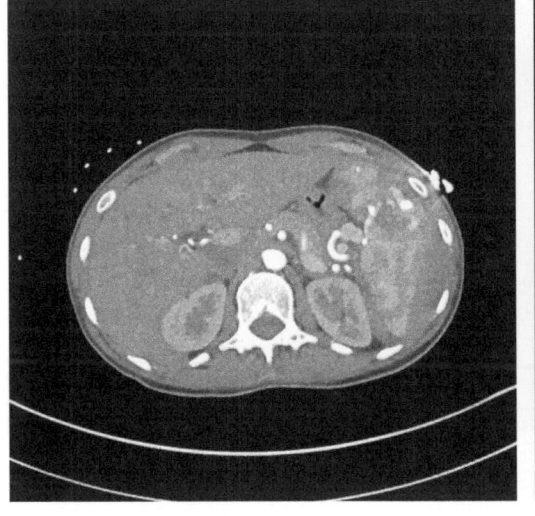 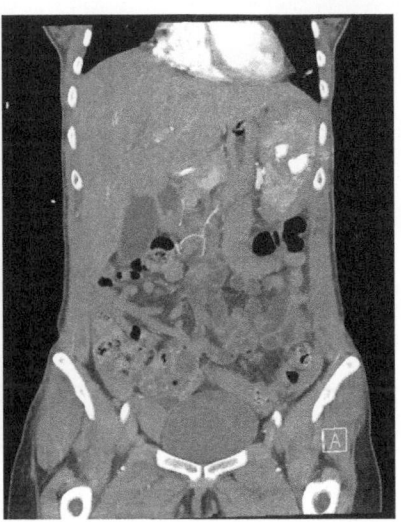

13 *On admission, the above patient in Question 12 underwent a successful coil IR embolization of the pseudoaneurysm and was admitted to the hospital. One week later while she remained in the hospital, she underwent a follow-up repeated CTA of the abdomen/pelvis. The CT findings are shown below. Which of the following statement is INCORRECT?*

A *The CT scan demonstrates multiple pseudoaneurysms.*

B *The incidence of a delayed splenic vascular injury (DSVI) is real and can be as high as 23% especially after a high-grade splenic injury.*

C *A routine follow-up repeating a CT angiography will help identify DSVI.*

D *The failure rate incidence after the initial IR embolization is underreported.*

E *This patient should undergo another repeated angiography and embolization.*

Timing for follow-up and repeating CT scan after the initial CT after a nonoperative management (NOM) of splenic injury remains debatable. However, literature support that the incidence of delayed splenic vascular injury (DSVI) after blunt splenic injury is real and can be as high as 23% in certain series. This patient's finding is interesting in that her initial admission CT scan did demonstrate a pseudoaneurysm and she underwent a successful IR embolization. Despite the success of the initial IR embolization, a follow-up and repeated CT scan did demonstrate still multiple pseudoaneurysm in various arterial branches (arrow). A repeated IR embolization (choice E) after failed attempt would probably be unwise, especially with a multiple pseudoaneurysms, and hence this patient should undergo splenectomy. The incidence and failure rate after the initial IR embolization are rare and probably underreported (choice D).

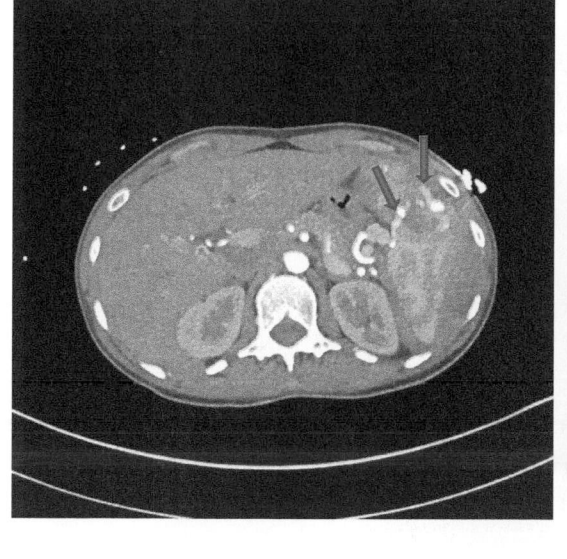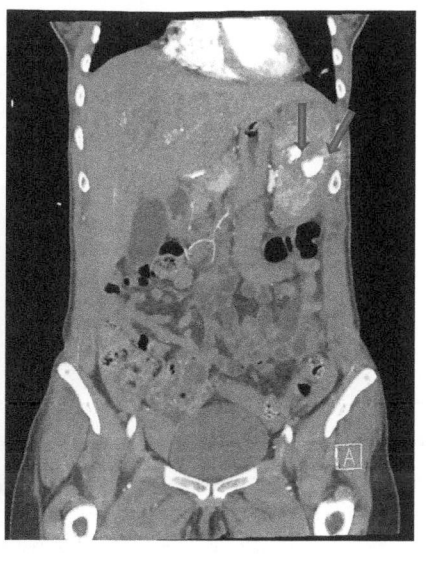

Answer: E

Furlan A, Tublin ME, Rees MA, et al. Delayed splenic vascular injury after nonoperative management of blunt splenic trauma. *AJS* 2017; 211: 87–94.

Coccolini F, Montori G, Catena F, et al. Splenic trauma: WSES classification and guidelines for adult and pediatric patients. *W J Emerg Surg* 2017; 12: 40.

Leeper WR, Leeper TJ, Ouellette D, et al. Delayed hemorrhagic complications in the operative management of blunt splenic trauma: early screening leads to a decrease failure rate. *J Trauma & ACS* 2014; 76: 1349–1353.

14 *Which of the following statement is the most correct regarding red blood cell (RBC)-related hemolytic anemia?*

  A *Thalassemia is an autosomal dominant genetic disorder. A heterozygous which is common in North America patient (Thalassemia minor) often has a mild form. Splenectomy is often not required unless patient has hypersplenism.*

  B *Glucose-6-Phosphate deficiency is an* <u>X-linked</u> *genetic disorder. Hemolytic anemia is triggered by an oxidative stress; therefore, splenectomy is usually required.*

  C *Elliptocytosis is an inherited heterogeneous red blood cell (RBC) disorder, characterized by elongated, oval, or elliptical-shaped red blood cells that are trapped and removed by the spleen resulting in hemolytic anemia.*

  D *Spherocytosis is the most uncommon congenital anemia but splenectomy can be curative.*

  E *Autoimmune hemolytic anemia (AHA) is an inherited disorder in women and splenectomy does not treat this disorder.*

Splenectomy is mainly performed for hematologic disorders along with traumatic injuries. Hemolytic anemia develops when there are not now red blood cells because the body destroys them sooner than it should. Splenectomy is often performed for hematological diseases which may be red blood cell (RBC), platelets, or lymphoproliferative and myeloproliferative disorders related. Of the RBC-related, autoimmune hemolytic anemia (AHA) is probably the less frequent disorder that requires splenectomy. AHA in children is often viral-induced and self-limited. They respond effectively to steroid treatment. Splenectomy is reserved for adult who is resistant to steroid treatment. Spherocytosis is the most common congenital anemia that results from decreased deformability of the RBC which leads to destruction within the spleen; hence, splenectomy is often curative. Elliptocytosis has similar pathophysiology to spherocytosis, it is autosomal dominant and common among Mediterranean and African descents. Hereditary elliptocytosis (HE), also known as hereditary ovalocytosis, is an inherited heterogeneous red blood cell (RBC) disorder, characterized by elongated, oval, or elliptical-shaped red blood cells on the peripheral blood smear. These elliptocytes are trapped and removed by the spleen resulting in hemolytic anemia.

Most of the cases of hereditary elliptocytosis are asymptomatic and require no treatment. However, symptomatic patients should be managed with blood transfusion and splenectomy. Similar to spherocytosis, splenectomy is often curative. Thalassaemia is a genetic disease of the hemoglobin protein in red blood cells. It is classified into thalassaemia minor, intermedia, and major, depending on the severity of the disease and the genetic defect. Thalassemia is an autosomal recessive. In the United States, most carry one gene which makes them less symptomatic (Thalassemia minor). Splenectomy is often not required unless they have a severe form (Thalassemia major) and hypersplenism. Glucose-6-Phosphate deficiency is an x-linked genetic disorder. Anemia is often triggered by oxidative stress (acute infection, oxidant medication, and fava beans). Splenectomy is often not required. Management focuses on the avoidance of trigger food and medications.

Answer: C

Cameron JL, Cameron AL. (2017) Current Surgical Therapy, 13th Edition. In John L. Cameron and Andrew M Cameron *Splenectomy for Hematologic Disorders.* Philadelphia, PA: Elsevier, p. 605–607.

Easow Mathew M, Sharma A, Aravindakshan R. Splenectomy for people with thalassaemia major or intermedia. *Cochrane Database Syst Rev.* 2016; 6: CD010517. doi: 10.1002/14651858.CD010517.pub2. Update in: Cochrane Database Syst Rev. 2019 Sep 17;9:CD010517. PMID: 27296775.

Barcellini W, Zaninoni A, Giannotta JA, Fattizzo B. New insights in autoimmune hemolytic anemia: from pathogenesis to therapy stage 1. *J Clin Med.* 2020; 9(12): 3859. doi: 10.3390/jcm9123859. PMID: 33261023; PMCID: PMC7759854.

15 *During a splenectomy, which ligament most always contains vessels?*
  A *Splenocolic ligament*
  B *Splenorenal ligament*
  C *Splenogastric ligament*
  D *Splenoomental ligament*
  E *Splenophrenic ligament*

The spleen has three constant ligament attachments (splenogastric, splenorenal, and splenocolic) that must be divided in order to mobilize the spleen. Occasionally, there may be additional ligament attachments to the surrounding structures including splenophrenic and splenoomental. Most ligament attachments are avascular except the splenogastric which contains the short gastric vessels that must be ligated when performing a splenectomy. Once spleen is mobilized, the last step is to ligate the hilar splenic vessels that should be done as close to the spleen as possible to avoid injury to the tail of the pancreas.

Answer: C

Sabiston Chapter 56: The Spleen. In CM Townsend, RD Beauchamp, BM Evers and KL Mattox *Textbook of Surgery: The Biologic Basis of Modern Surgical Practice,* April 2016,Elsevier, 20th edition.

16 *A 35-year-old man known intravenous drug user with a known HIV infection is admitted for endocarditis and bacteremia. He continues to have fever. Further workup including abdominal computed tomography (CT) scan demonstrated multiple fluid collection within the spleen, the largest of which is 3 cm. What is the next best step in management?*

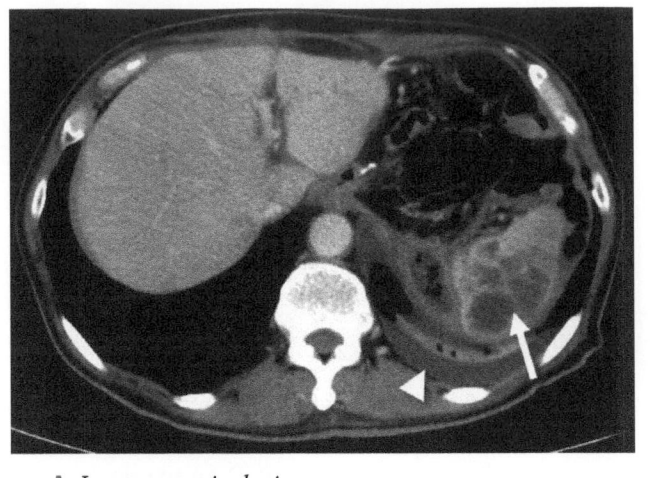

  A *Laparoscopic drainage*
  B *Cyst wall fenestration*
  C *IR-guided drainage*
  D *Splenectomy*
  E *Continued observation and repeat CT scan in 1 week*

Differential diagnosis in this patient includes splenic cyst and abscess, but in this setting of IVDA with endocarditis and bacteremia, splenic abscess is the most likely diagnosis. Definitive management of splenic abscess with a percutaneous drainage has had a good success in most recent studies; however, for patient with multiple abscesses such as this person, splenectomy is indicated. Splenic abscesses in general are uncommon. The known risk factors include immunocompromised states such as human immunodeficiency virus (HIV) or neoplasms, metastatic infection, diabetes, splenic infarction, and previous interventional radiologist embolization for trauma. Splenic abscesses have also been associated with parasitic infections of the spleen.

Answer: D

Sabiston Chapter 56: The Spleen, Splenectomy, Miscellaneous Benign Conditions, Splenic Abscess. In: CM Townsend, RD Beauchamp, BM Evers and KL Mattox *Textbook of Surgery: The Biological Basis of Modern Surgical Practice,* April 2016, Elsevier, 20th edition.

Cameron JL, Cameron AL. (2017) Current Surgical Therapy, 13th Edition. In: John L. Cameron and Andrew M Cameron *Splenectomy for Hematologic Disorders.* Philadelphia, PA: Elsevier, p. 605–607.

Coco D, Leanza S. Indications for surgery in non-traumatic spleen disease. *Open Access Maced J Med Sci.* 2019; 7(17): 2958–2960. doi: 10.3889/oamjms.2019.568. PMID: 31844464; PMCID: PMC6901870.

17 *An African-American man is concerned about the risk for hemolytic anemia from anesthesia and drug-induced during his planned elective inguinal hernia repair. His father has glucose-6-phosphate dehydrogenase (G6PD) deficiency. His mother had genetic testing in the past that confirmed she is not a carrier of G6PD deficiency. The patient has never been tested. Knowing the manner of G6PD deficiency inheritance, what is the risk of him having perioperative complications?*

   A *0%*
   B *25%*
   C *50%*
   D *75%*
   E *100%*

Glucose-6-phosphate dehydrogenase (G6PD) deficiency is the most common enzymatic disorder of red blood cells in humans. It is estimated that about 400 million people are affected by this deficiency. G6PD deficiency is an X-linked genetic disorder of the glutathione pathway, which leads to damage of RBCs by toxin oxygen products. It causes acute hemolytic accidents during oxidative stress such as acute infections, oxidant medication, and fava beans. Transfusion and splenectomy are often not required unless patient has severe hypersplenism. In this patient, since his mother is not a carrier and cannot pass the x-gene to her son, the patient has zero chance of having this genetic disorder.

Answer: A

Elyassi AR, Rowshan HH. Perioperative management of the glucose-6-phosphate dehydrogenase deficient patient: a review of literature. *Anesth Prog.* 2009; 56(3): 86–91. doi: 10.2344/0003-3006-56.3.86. PMID: 19769422; PMCID: PMC2749581.

Frank JE. Diagnosis and management of G6PD deficiency. *Am Fam Physician.* 2005; 72(7): 1277–82. PMID: 16225031.

18 *A trauma patient underwent successful traumatic splenectomy after motorcycle-related crash. Postoperatively, he received pneumococcal PPV23 vaccine and was told to receive more vaccines in 2 weeks. What are other appropriate vaccines required at that time?*

   A *Varicella*
   B *H. influenza type B and Meningococcus*
   C *Hepatitis A & B*
   D *Measles, mumps, rubella*
   E *Tetanus*

Overwhelming post-splenectomy infection (OPSI) is often cited complication post-splenectomy, particularly in the Western world. It is extremely rare, however, following a splenectomy for trauma in adults compared to a splenectomy for hematologic diseases in young children, but it is still a potential concern and clinician must beware. It is our traditional practice that patient receives a vaccination against encapsulated organisms such as Pneumococcus, Meningococcus, and Haemophilus. The timing of receiving vaccination postoperatively varies and is controversial, but from an immunological response, it suggests that 2 weeks post-splenectomy gives the best immunological response to the vaccination. However, for a practical reason in dealing with trauma patient who is often noncompliant with follow-up, most splenectomy trauma patients will receive their vaccination just prior to discharge from the hospital. Since this patient has already received a pneumococcus vaccine, he should still receive a vaccination for the other encapsulated organisms such as *H. influenza* and Meningococcus at his 2-week clinic follow-up.

Answer: B

Bianchi FP, Stefanizzi P, Spinelli G, Mascipinto S, Tafuri S. Immunization coverage among asplenic patients and strategies to increase vaccination compliance: a systematic review and meta-analysis. *Expert Rev Vaccines.* 2021; 14: 1–12. doi: 10.1080/14760584.2021.1886085. Epub ahead of print. PMID: 33538617.

Hammerquist RJ, Messerschmidt KA, Pottebaum AA, Hellwig TR. Vaccinations in asplenic adults. *Am J Health Syst Pharm.* 2016; 73(9):e220–e228. doi: 10.2146/ajhp150270. PMID: 27099328.

Schimmer JA, van der Steeg AF, Zuidema WP. Splenic function after angioembolization for splenic trauma in children and adults: a systematic review. *Injury.* 2016; 47(3): 525–30. doi: 10.1016/j.injury.2015.10.047. Epub 2015 Nov 19. PMID: 26772452.

19 *A 24-year-old man otherwise healthy presents with recurrent nosebleeds, petechiae of his lower extremities, and new-onset bleeding gums. He denies taking any medication. Exam shows hepatomegaly. Laboratory demonstrates platelets of 42 000/uL. Urine analysis is negative for hematuria and viral panel is unremarkable. What is the best initial treatment?*

   A *Platelet transfusion*
   B *Prednisone 1 mg/kg/day*
   C *Intravenous immunoglobulin*
   D *Rituximab*
   E *Splenectomy*

This patient has immune thrombocytopenic purpura (ITP). Management of ITP depends on the history of treatment and severity of thrombocytopenia. Asymptomatic patients with platelet counts > 50 000/uL may be simply observed. Symptomatic patients usually have platelets lower than 50 000/uL usually responds to high-dose steroid (e.g., prednisone 1 mg/kg/day) 7–10 days and then tapered. Studies have shown a 66% improvement in platelets in 1–3 weeks, and 25% of patients experience a complete response. Platelets transfusion is indicated only in patients with severe hemorrhage. Intravenous immunoglobulin is also useful in acute bleeding or for patients being prepped for splenectomy. Rituximab is reserved for patients who are refractory to steroids. Splenectomy is reserved for patients who fail medical management.

Answer: B

Sukumar S, Lämmle B, Cataland SR. Thrombotic thrombocytopenic purpura: pathophysiology, diagnosis, and management. *J Clin Med.* 2021; 10(3): 536. doi: 10.3390/jcm10030536. PMID: 33540569; PMCID: PMC7867179.

Dubois L, Gray DK. Case series: splenectomy: does it still play a role in the management of thrombotic thrombocytopenic purpura? *Can J Surg.* 2010; 53(5): 349–355. PMID: 20858382; PMCID: PMC2947115.

20 *Which of the following medical conditions is splenectomy is not recommended?*
   A *Spherocytosis*
   B *Elliptocytosis*
   C *Immune (idiopathic) thrombocytopenia purpura (ITP)*

D *Thrombotic thrombocytopenic purpura (TTP)*
E *Felty's syndrome*

Several hematological diseases often require surgical splenectomy for treatment. Spherocytosis and elliptocytosis are two congenital red blood cell morphology abnormality that led to an increase in RBC elimination in the spleen. Splenectomy therefore is curative. Immune (idiopathic) thrombocytopenia purpura (ITP) is a diagnosis of exsclusion for thrombocytopenia. Patient's initial treatment often responds to steroid; however, if medical treatment fails, splenectomy is indicated. Thrombotic thrombocytopenic purpura (TTP) classically presents with thrombocytopenia, fever, hemolytic anemia, renal disease, and central nervous system dysfunction, and is quite similar to hemolytic uremic syndrome. Plasmapharesis is, however, the treatment of choice. Felty's syndrome is the clinical triad of thrombocytopenia, cutaneous leg ulcers, and rheumatoid arthritis. The syndrome is not well understood, but sometimes patients will benefit from splenectomy if medical therapy fails.

Answer: D

Dubois L, Gray DK. Case series: splenectomy: does it still play a role in the management of thrombotic thrombocytopenic purpura? *Can J Surg.* 2010; 53(5): 349–355. PMID: 20858382; PMCID: PMC2947115.

Kappers-Klunne MC, Wijermans P, Fijnheer R, Croockewit AJ, van der Holt B, de Wolf JT, Löwenberg B, Brand A. Splenectomy for the treatment of thrombotic thrombocytopenic purpura. *Br J Haematol.* 2005; 130(5): 768–776. doi: 10.1111/j.1365-2141.2005.05681.x. PMID: 16115135., PA.

40

Incarcerated Hernias and Abdominal Wall Reconstruction

Michael C. Smith, MD[1] and Richard S. Miller, MD[2]

[1] *Division of Trauma and Surgical Critical Care, Vanderbilt University Medical Center, Nashville, TN, USA*
[2] *Department of Surgery, TCU & UNTHSC School of Medicine, John Peter Smith Health, Fort Worth, TX, USA*

1 *A 52-year-old man presents with abdominal pain and fever. He is found to have diverticulitis with feculent peritonitis, for which he undergoes sigmoidectomy. Which suture material is associated with the lowest rate of dehiscence for fascial closure of a midline laparotomy in a contaminated field?*
   A *Looped polydioxanone (PDS)*
   B *Triclosan-coated looped PDS*
   C *Polypropylene*
   D *Braided polyester*
   E *Barbed triclosan-coated PDS*

In a recent multicenter, randomized controlled trial, a barbed, triclosan-coated PDS suture outperformed both triclosan-coated loop PDS and uncoated PDS. Previous studies have demonstrated improved outcomes with long-term absorbable suture as compared to permanent suture. Both the monofilament nature of this suture as well as its antimicrobial coating are thought to decrease microbial colonization and thus fascial dehiscence.

van't Riet M, Steyerberg EW, Nellensteyn J, Bonjer HJ, Jeekel J. Meta-analysis of techniques for closure of midline abdominal incisions. *Br J Surg.* 2002;89(11):1350–1356. doi: 10.1046/j.1365-2168. 2002.02258.x. PMID: 12390373.

Ruiz-Tovar J, Llavero C, Jimenez-Fuertes M, Duran M, Perez-Lopez M, Garcia-Marin A. Incisional surgical site infection after abdominal fascial closure with triclosan-coated barbed suture vs triclosan-coated polydioxanone loop suture vs polydioxanone loop suture in emergent abdominal surgery: a randomized clinical trial. *J Am Coll Surg.* 2020;230(5):766–774. doi: 10.1016/j. jamcollsurg.2020.02.031. Epub 2020 Feb 27. PMID: 32113031.

2 *Which fascial closure technique is associated with a decreased rate of incisional hernia?*
   A *Simple interrupted*
   B *Continuous suture with ≥ 4:1 suture: wound length ratio*
   C *Interrupted figure of eight with retention suture*
   D *Continuous, locked closure*
   E *Continuous suture with internal retention suture*

B. Incisional hernia is a complication of laparotomy, with rates in excess of 20% at long-term follow-up. Of the listed techniques, a continuous suture, with a long-term absorbable suture is preferable to the other options. This was highlighted by the STITCH Trial, which showed using a long-term absorbable suture with 5 mm bites and 5 mm advancement resulted in a greater than 4:1 suture-to-wound length ratio and a significantly decreased rate of incisional hernia.

Deerenberg EB, Harlaar JJ, Steyerberg EW, Lont HE, van Doorn HC, Heisterkamp J, Wijnhoven BP, Schouten WR, Cense HA, Stockmann HB, Berends FJ, Dijkhuizen FPH, Dwarkasing RS, Jairam AP, van Ramshorst GH, Kleinrensink GJ, Jeekel J, Lange JF. Small bites versus large bites for closure of abdominal midline incisions (STITCH): a double-blind, multicentre, randomised controlled trial. *Lancet.* 2015;386(10000):1254–1260. doi: 10.1016/S0140-6736(15)60459-7. Epub 2015 Jul 15. PMID: 26188742.

3 *When performing an incisional hernia repair with mesh, which mesh position is associated with the lowest risk of recurrence?*
   A *Onlay*
   B *Inlay*
   C *Sublay*

Surgical Critical Care and Emergency Surgery: Clinical Questions and Answers, Third Edition.
Edited by Forrest "Dell" Moore, Peter M. Rhee, and Carlos J. Rodriguez.
© 2022 John Wiley & Sons Ltd. Published 2022 by John Wiley & Sons Ltd.
Companion website: www.wiley.com/go/surgicalcriticalcare3e

D *Preperitoneal*

E *Underlay*

C. When performing a mesh repair, one may utilize the onlay (anterior to the anterior rectus sheath), inlay (sewn as a "bridge" between fascial edges), sublay or retrorectus (between the rectus abdominis muscle and posterior rectus sheath), preperitoneal (between the peritoneum and posterior rectus sheath), or underlay (intraperitoneal) techniques. In a meta-analysis, the sublay or retrorectus mesh position was associated with the lowest rate of hernia recurrence. Though technically challenging, the preperitoneal repair may be useful in patients who have undergone multiple prior repairs.

Sosin M, Nahabedian MY, Bhanot P. The perfect plane: a systematic review of mesh location and outcomes, update 2018. *Plast Reconstr Surg.* 2018;142(3 Suppl):107S–116S. doi: 10.1097/PRS.0000000000004864. PMID: 30138278.

Novitsky YW, Porter JR, Rucho ZC, Getz SB, Pratt BL, Kercher KW, Heniford BT. Open preperitoneal retrofascial mesh repair for multiply recurrent ventral incisional hernias. *J Am Coll Surg.* 2006;203(3):283–9. doi: 10.1016/j.jamcollsurg.2006.05.297. Epub 2006 Jul 13. PMID: 16931299.

4 *A 54-year-old woman with a history of multiple incisional hernia repairs, both laparoscopic and open, presents for consideration of repair. Her defect at maximum width measures 15 cm. Which of the below may be injected into the abdominal wall musculature to facilitate a tension-free approximation of the linea alba?*

A *Botulinum Toxin A*

B *Rocuronium*

C *Nitroglycerin*

D *Lidocaine*

E *Verapamil*

A. Botulinum Toxin A injection under ultrasound or EMG guidance can temporarily paralyze the abdominal wall musculature in the perioperative period. This may allow an increase in abdominal domain and thus less tension on the linea alba approximation when repairing a ventral hernia. Other techniques, such as pneumoperitoneum and tissue expanders, have also been utilized for this purpose.

Motz BM, Schlosser KA, Heniford BT. Chemical components separation: concepts, evidence, and outcomes. *Plast Reconstr Surg.* 2018;142(3 Suppl):58S–63S. doi: 10.1097/PRS.0000000000004856. PMID: 30138269.

5 *Which of the following is the most appropriate indication for the consideration of biologic mesh in place of synthetic mesh?*

A *Body mass index $\geq 35\,kg/m^2$*

B *Hemoglobin A1C ≥ 8*

C *Contaminated operative field*

D *Recurrent hernia*

E *Colonization with methicillin-resistant* Staphylococcus aureus

C. While all of the above choices raise the risk of surgical site occurrences and/or hernia recurrence, only the contaminated field merits the consideration for a repair with a biologic mesh over a synthetic mesh. Efforts to identify these risk factors and modify them preoperatively can reduce this risk.

Rosen MJ, Bauer JJ, Harmaty M, Carbonell AM, Cobb WS, Matthews B, Goldblatt MI, Selzer DJ, Poulose BK, Hansson BM, Rosman C, Chao JJ, Jacobsen GR. Multicenter, prospective, longitudinal study of the recurrence, surgical site infection, and quality of life after contaminated ventral hernia repair using biosynthetic absorbable mesh: the COBRA study. *Ann Surg.* 2017;265(1):205–211. doi: 10.1097/SLA.0000000000001601. PMID: 28009747; PMCID: PMC5181129.

Liang MK, Goodenough CJ, Martindale RG, Roth JS, Kao LS. External validation of the ventral hernia risk score for prediction of surgical site infections. *Surg Infect (Larchmt).* 2015;16(1):36–40. doi: 10.1089/sur.2014.115. PMID: 25761078; PMCID: PMC4363797.

6 *A 42-year-old woman presents with a recurrent incisional hernia. It measures 18 cm wide at maximum width. When performing a transversus abdominis release (TAR), where is the transversus abdominis incised?*

A *At the linea alba*

B *At the linea semilunaris*

C *Just medial to the neurovascular bundles*

D *Just lateral to the neurovascular bundles*

E *At the arcuate line*

C. To perform a transversus abdominis release (TAR), one first must incise the posterior rectus sheath just lateral to the linea alba and develop the retrorectus space. Upon reaching the neurovascular bundles, one must incise the transversus abdominis muscle to expose the underlying transversalis fascia. This dissection can then be continued laterally and posteriorly in order to achieve approximation of the linea alba and facilitate large mesh placement. This maneuver is not possible from the linea alba. If attempting this maneuver at the linea semilunaris or lateral to the neurovascular bundles, it would result in oblique muscle weakness.

Novitsky YW, Elliott HL, Orenstein SB, Rosen MJ. Transversus abdominis muscle release: a novel approach to posterior component separation during complex abdominal wall reconstruction. *Am J Surg*. 2012;204(5):709–716. doi: 10.1016/j.amjsurg.2012.02.008. Epub 2012 May 16. PMID: 22607741.

7   *A 32-year-old man undergoes a laparotomy for a gunshot wound to the liver. This is treated with packing and a temporary abdominal closure device is placed. Which of the following is an indication for abdominal wall closure?*
    A *pH of 7.41*
    B *Ongoing blood product requirements*
    C *Peak inspiratory pressure of 42 cm H_2O upon fascial approximation*
    D *Core temperature 34 °C*
    E *Escalating pressor dosage*

A. Damage control laparotomy is utilized in patients whose physiology is deranged to the point that an abbreviated laparotomy is deemed more appropriate. In this patient, packing in an attempt to control bleeding, with the potential for angioembolization, is an indication for a temporary abdominal closure. Once the underlying "lethal triad" of acidosis, coagulopathy, and hypothermia is corrected, closure is permissible. However, if the patient's peak inspiratory pressure is elevated upon fascial approximation, then closure will cause the abdominal compartment syndrome.

Coccolini F, Roberts D, Ansaloni L, Ivatury R, Gamberini E, Kluger Y, Moore EE, Coimbra R, Kirkpatrick AW, Pereira BM, Montori G, Ceresoli M, Abu-Zidan FM, Sartelli M, Velmahos G, Fraga GP, Leppaniemi A, Tolonen M, Galante J, Razek T, Maier R, Bala M, Sakakushev B, Khokha V, Malbrain M, Agnoletti V, Peitzman A, Demetrashvili Z, Sugrue M, Di Saverio S, Martzi I, Soreide K, Biffl W, Ferrada P, Parry N, Montravers P, Melotti RM, Salvetti F, Valetti TM, Scalea T, Chiara O, Cimbanassi S, Kashuk JL, Larrea M, Hernandez JAM, Lin HF, Chirica M, Arvieux C, Bing C, Horer T, De Simone B, Masiakos P, Reva V, DeAngelis N, Kike K, Balogh ZJ, Fugazzola P, Tomasoni M, Latifi R, Naidoo N, Weber D, Handolin L, Inaba K, Hecker A, Kuo-Ching Y, Ordoñez CA, Rizoli S, Gomes CA, De Moya M, Wani I, Mefire AC, Boffard K, Napolitano L, Catena F. The open abdomen in trauma and non-trauma patients: WSES guidelines. *World J Emerg Surg*.

2018;13:7. doi: 10.1186/s13017-018-0167-4. PMID: 29434652; PMCID: PMC5797335.

8   *A 65-year-old man presents with a ruptured abdominal aortic aneurysm. This is repaired successfully with an open, midline laparotomy approach. Given his high hernia risk, a prophylactic onlay mesh is placed using permanent material. What is the most common complication of the mesh implantation?*
    A *Infection*
    B *Recurrence*
    C *Chronic pain*
    D *Seroma*
    E *Skin necrosis*

D. While all of the above are possible complications of mesh placement in an onlay position, whether for a hernia repair or for prophylaxis, the most common complication is seroma. This is usually a self-limiting issue. There have been a multitude of studies examining prophylactic mesh for midline laparotomies, which show a reduction in incisional hernia rates.

Rhemtulla IA, Messa CA 4th, Enriquez FA, Hope WW, Fischer JP. Role of prophylactic mesh placement for laparotomy and stoma creation. *Surg Clin North Am*. 2018;98(3):471–481. doi: 10.1016/j.suc.2018.01.003. PMID: 29754617.

9   *In patients at high risk for superficial surgical site infection (SSI) of a midline laparotomy, which of the below is associated with decreased risk of SSI?*
    A *Extended (72 hour) antibiotic prophylaxis*
    B *Incisional negative pressure wound therapy*
    C *Topical antimicrobial ointment*
    D *Polypropylene fascial suture*
    E *Subcuticular sutured closure*

B. Incisional negative pressure wound therapy is associated with a decreased rate of SSI in a high-risk population. Extended prophylaxis, topical ointment, permanent suture, and subcuticular closure are not associated with improvement in midline laparotomy, though subcuticular closure has been shown to be effective in sternotomy and Pfannenstiel closures.

Hall C, Regner J, Abernathy S, Isbell C, Isbell T, Kurek S, Smith R, Frazee R. Surgical site infection after primary closure of high-risk surgical wounds in emergency general surgery laparotomy and closed negative-pressure wound therapy. *J Am Coll Surg*. 2019 228(4):393–397. doi: 10.1016/j.jamcollsurg.2018.12.006. Epub 2018 Dec 23. PMID: 30586643.

10 *Perioperative outcomes following minimally invasive retro-muscular abdominal wall reconstruction comparing patients with a BMI < 35 to BMI > 35 have:*
   A *Shorter hospital length of stay*
   B *Less hospital charges*
   C *Lower postoperative complications*
   D *Shorter operative times*
   E *No difference in outcomes*

E. Advances in minimally invasive surgery (MIS) using laparoscopy or robotics have proven to benefit more patients with abdominal wall hernias, including those with morbid obesity. MIS using laparoscopy and/or robotics has shown significant benefits for the obese patient population. Extraperitoneal approaches for dissection, component separation, and mesh placement have substantially reduced complications. A recent study demonstrated statistically equivalent outcomes comparing patients above and below a BMI of 35. The technical choice of hernia repair is based most importantly on the contamination of the surgical field, then the size of the hernia and finally on the experience of the surgeon with both open and MIS techniques.

Addo A, Lu R, Broda A, George P, Huerta N, Park A, Zahiri HR, Belyansky I. Impact of Body Mass Index (BMI) on perioperative outcomes following minimally invasive retromuscular abdominal wall reconstruction: a comparative analysis. *Surg Endosc.* 2020. doi: 10.1007/s00464-020-08069-3. Epub ahead of print. Erratum in: Surg Endosc. 2020 Nov 2;: PMID: 33051760.

Soliani G, De Troia A, Portinari M, Targa S, Carcoforo P, Vasquez G, Fisichella PM, Feo CV. Laparoscopic versus open incisional hernia repair: a retrospective cohort study with costs analysis on 269 patients. *Hernia* 2017;21(4):609–618. doi: 10.1007/s10029-017-1601-3. Epub 2017 Apr 10. PMID: 28396956.

11 *According to the Centers of Disease Control and Prevention, a Class III wound is defined as:*
   A *An old traumatic wound and retained devitalized tissue or those that involve existing clinical infection or perforated viscera.*
   B *Open, fresh, accidental wound or operations with gross spillage from the GI Tract or incisions in which acute, non-purulent inflammation is encountered.*
   C *Open fracture with gross contamination of dirt and debris.*
   D *An uninfected wound in which no inflammation is encountered in the respiratory, alimentary, genital, or uninfected urinary tract is not entered.*
   E *An operative wound in which the respiratory, alimentary, genital, or urinary tract is entered under controlled conditions and without unusual contamination.*

B. The Center of Disease Control and Prevention wound classifications stratifies wounds as follows:

   Class I = Clean- choice d
   Class II = Clean, contaminated- choice e
   Class III = Contaminated- choice b
   Class IV = Dirty or infected- choice a
   Choice c is part of the Gustillo classification of open fractures

De Simone B, Birindelli A, Ansaloni L, Sartelli M, Coccolini F, Di Saverio S, Annessi V, Amico F, Catena F. Emergency repair of complicated abdominal wall hernias: WSES guidelines. *Hernia* 2020;24(2):359–368. doi: 10.1007/s10029-019-02021-8. Epub 2019 Aug 12. PMID: 31407109.

12 *A 77-year-old man presents to the emergency department with a one-day history of severe right groin pain after lifting a heavy object. Physical exam reveals an erythematous, severely tender mass in the right inguinal area. He is febrile, pulse is 110, WBC of 18 K. Arterial lactate is 6. CT scan reveals a right inguinal hernia with reduced small bowel wall enhancement and no free fluid. The next step in management should include:*
   A *Pain control, fluid resuscitation, antibiotics, delayed repair.*
   B *Attempt to reduce the incarcerated hernia under conscious sedation followed by delayed repair.*
   C *Immediate operative intervention via an open groin incision and/or laparoscopic approach to assess for bowel viability and to repair hernia.*
   D *Immediate operative intervention via an open lower midline incision.*
   E *Immediate operative exploration with laparoscopy via preperitoneal approach (TEP).*

C. Patients should undergo emergent operative intervention when intestinal strangulation is suspected. The physical exam, lab values, and CT findings in this case combined are highly suspicious for strangulation. Diagnostic laparoscopy is a useful tool to assess bowel viability after operative reduction. An acceptable surgical approach to minimize an open midline laparotomy is hernioscopy, a mixed open groin incision with laparoscopy to verify the viability of the incarcerated bowel. For patients with strangulation that require bowel resection without gross contamination, surgical repair with synthetic mesh can be performed. Biologic mesh use is reserved for contaminated-dirty wounds (peritonitis with bowel spillage) and/or when the hernia repair by direct suture repair is not possible and the biologic mesh is used as a bridge. Unless the peritoneum is violated, it is not possible to visualize bowel sufficiently utilizing the preperitoneal approach (TEP) and should be avoided when strangulation is suspected.

De Simone B, Birindelli A, Ansaloni L, Sartelli M, Coccolini F, Di Saverio S, Annessi V, Amico F, Catena F. Emergency repair of complicated abdominal wall hernias: WSES guidelines. *Hernia*. 2020;24(2):359–368. doi: 10.1007/s10029-019-02021-8. Epub 2019 Aug 12. PMID: 31407109.

Sajid MS, Ladwa N, Colucci G, Miles WF, Baig MK, Sains P. Diagnostic laparoscopy through deep inguinal ring: a literature-based review on the forgotten approach to visualize the abdominal cavity during emergency and elective groin hernia repair. *Surg Laparosc Endosc Percutan Tech*. 2013 Jun;23(3):251–254. doi: 10.1097/SLE.0b013e31828dacc5. PMID: 23751987.

Bessa SS, Abdel-fattah MR, Al-Sayes IA, Korayem IT. Results of prosthetic mesh repair in the emergency management of the acutely incarcerated and/or strangulated groin hernias: a 10-year study. *Hernia* 2015;19(6):909–914. doi: 10.1007/s10029-015-1360-y. Epub 2015 Mar 3. PMID: 25731947.

De Simone B, Catena F, Biondi A, Baiocchi G, Campanile F, Coccolini F, Testini M, Di Saverio S, Sartelli M, Heyer A, Ansaloni L. Incisional Hernia Repair in Contaminated Surgical fields (I.H.R.C.S.) study using biological prostheses in emergency surgery setting with contaminated hernias: a multicenter prospective observational study. *J Peritoneum (and other serosal surfaces)*. 2016. https://doi.org/10.4081/joper.2016.26.

13 *Which one of the following is NOT an acceptable management plan for a symptomatic end-colostomy parastomal hernia?*

  A *Suture repair*

  B *Laparoscopic mesh repair*

  C *Open repair with a keyhole technique*

  D *Re-siting of the stoma reinforced with synthetic mesh*

  E *Retrorectus biologic mesh repair*

Parastomal hernias are common and cause a substantial amount of distress for a patient with a permanent stoma. Open or laparoscopic repairs with permanent synthetic mesh have comparative results. However, mesh repair without a hole is preferred to a keyhole mesh repair when laparoscopic repairs are performed. Re-siting of the stoma is an acceptable approach especially when dealing with multiple recurrences and very large parastomal hernias. The use of prophylactic synthetic mesh upon construction of a permanent end-colostomy is strongly recommended. There is no data comparing the use of permanent synthetic mesh with biologic mesh to reinforce the repair of a parastomal hernia. However, the cost of biologic mesh is substantially higher without any evidence of infection reduction. Suture repair, while the most technically simple solution, is associated with a high recurrence and wound complication rate.

Antoniou SA, Agresta F, Garcia Alamino JM, Berger D, Berrevoet F, Brandsma HT, Bury K, Conze J, Cuccurullo D, Dietz UA, Fortelny RH, Frei-Lanter C, Hansson B, Helgstrand F, Hotouras A, Jänes A, Kroese LF, Lambrecht JR, Kyle-Leinhase I, López-Cano M, Maggiori L, Mandalà V, Miserez M, Montgomery A, Morales-Conde S, Prudhomme M, Rautio T, Smart N, Śmietański M, Szczepkowski M, Stabilini C, Muysoms FE. European hernia society guidelines on prevention and treatment of parastomal hernias. *Hernia*. 2018;22(1):183–198. doi: 10.1007/s10029-017-1697-5. Epub 2017 Nov 13. PMID: 29134456.

14 *A 57-year-old woman presents to the emergency department with nausea and vomiting for 2 days. Past surgical history includes a sigmoid colon resection for diverticulitis via a midline incision. On physical exam, there is a tender mass in the supra-umbilical area. CT scan confirms a fascial defect of 6 cm with incarcerated small bowel causing a complete obstruction. BMI is 33. What is the BEST operative repair of the hernia if the ischemic, incarcerated small bowel requires resection?*

  A *Primary fascial repair without mesh.*

  B *Primary fascial repair with the use of an onlay synthetic mesh.*

  C *Wide underlay biologic mesh bridge repair.*

  D *Primary fascial repair reinforced with the use of lightweight mesh placed in the retrorectus space.*

  E *Temporary abdominal closure using a vacuum-assisted closure with mesh-mediated traction.*

D. For patients that require a concomitant bowel resection without gross contamination, surgical repair with a synthetic mesh can be performed without any increased morbidity and has a significantly lower rate of recurrence than primary repair, regardless of the size of the defect. Retrorectus placement of a lightweight mesh is the superior repair in this case, keeping the mesh outside of the peritoneal cavity or subcutaneous space, both of which would have higher infection and recurrence rates. While primary repair is an option, it is associated with a significant recurrence rate. A temporary abdominal closure with the use of a VAC system would be reserved for a hemodynamically unstable patient with diffuse peritonitis and vasopressor support and/or where the bowel is left in discontinuity, the abdominal cavity is washed out and the patient brought to the ICU for ongoing resuscitation.

De Simone B, Birindelli A, Ansaloni L, Sartelli M, Coccolini F, Di Saverio S, Annessi V, Amico F, Catena F. Emergency repair of complicated abdominal wall hernias: WSES guidelines. *Hernia*. 2020;24(2):359–368. doi: 10.1007/s10029-019-02021-8. Epub 2019 Aug 12. PMID: 31407109.

15 *The best management of an umbilical hernia in patients with compensated cirrhosis and ascites is:*
   A *Immediate repair when identified*
   B *Conservative management until symptomatic*
   C *Repair at the time of a liver transplant*
   D *Elective umbilical hernia repair after reduction*
   E *Preoperative TIPS procedure*

A. Cirrhosis complicated with ascites is associated with a 20% risk of developing an umbilical hernia. These hernias tend to enlarge over time. Major complications of untreated umbilical hernias in this patient population include incarceration, strangulation, rupture of the hernia sac and bacterial peritonitis, all of which cause extremely high mortality rates. Multiple recent studies have shown that early repair of umbilical hernias in compensated cirrhosis with ascites offers an acceptable morbidity and substantial reduction in mortality. Therefore, it is recommended that repair should be performed when identified rather than waiting until the hernia is symptomatic or at the time of liver transplant. In patients with ascites, reduction of the hernia is not helpful as it will recur almost immediately in most cases. Preoperative TIPS procedure is reserved for patients with uncompensated cirrhosis.

Hill CE, Olson KA, Roward S, Yan D, Cardenas T, Teixeira P, Coopwood BT, Trust M, Aydelotte J, Ali S, Brown C. Fix it while you can . . . Mortality after umbilical hernia repair in cirrhotic patients. *Am J Surg*. 2020;220(6):1402–1404. doi: 10.1016/j.amjsurg.2020.08.022. Epub 2020 Sep 1. PMID: 32988606.

Pinheiro RS, Andraus W, Waisberg DR, Nacif LS, Ducatti L, Rocha-Santos V, Diniz MA, Arantes RM, Lerut J, D'Albuquerque LAC. Abdominal hernias in cirrhotic patients: surgery or conservative treatment? Results of a prospective cohort study in a high volume center: cohort study. *Ann Med Surg (Lond)*. 2019;49:9–13. doi: 10.1016/j.amsu.2019.11.009. PMID: 31853365; PMCID: PMC6911966.

Hew S, Yu W, Robson S, Starkey G, Testro A, Fink M, Angus P, Gow P. Safety and effectiveness of umbilical hernia repair in patients with cirrhosis. *Hernia*. 2018;22(5):759–765. doi: 10.1007/s10029-018-1761-9. Epub 2018 Mar 27. PMID: 29589135.

16 *The inguinal ligament, pectineal ligament, and the lacunar ligament comprise the borders of which potential hernia site?*
   A *Direct inguinal hernia*
   B *Indirect inguinal hernia*
   C *Obturator hernia*
   D *Femoral hernia*
   E *Richter's hernia*

D. Femoral hernias occur through an opening in the inferior triangle beneath the inguinal ligament. This differentiates this hernia from direct and indirect inguinal hernias. The borders of the femoral canal are the inguinal ligament anteriorly, the pectineal ligament posteriorly, and the lacunar ligament medially. The femoral vein marks the lateral border.

An obturator hernia is a rare hernia of the pelvic floor in which the pelvic or abdominal contents protrude through the obturator foramen which lies inferiorly to the acetabulum and is an opening between the ischium and the pubic bones. A Richter's hernia occurs when the anti-mesenteric wall of the intestines protrudes through a defect in the abdominal wall.

Hogan S, Skanes M, Hartery A. Groin hernias: a pictorial essay outlining basic anatomy with illustration of interesting cases on computed tomography. *SN Compr Clin Med*. 2020;2:2738–2748. https://doi.org/10.1007/s42399-020-00615-3.

17 *An 83-year-old frail woman presents to the emergency department with a history of sudden epigastric pain and intractable retching without vomiting. The ED team attempts to place a nasogastric tube unsuccessfully and orders a CT scan (below). The next step in management should be:*

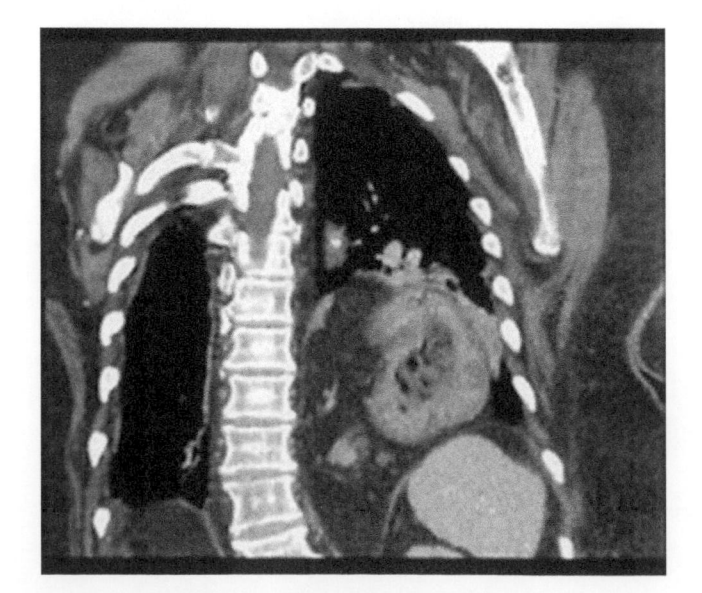

A *Medical management with IV hydration, antiemetics, and continued attempts to place an NG for decompression.*

B *Open, laparoscopic, or robotic fundoplication*

C *Primary repair of the paraesophageal hernia*

D *Emergent intervention, detorsion, and gastropexy*

E *Collis gastroplasty*

F *D. Gastric volvulus most often occurs in the elderly population. Risk factors include other diaphragmatic abnormalities (hiatal and paraesophageal hernias), phrenic nerve weakness, and bariatric surgery. Symptoms are variable depending on the degree of rotation of the volvulus. In the acute setting, patients often present with severe vomiting, chest and upper abdominal pain. The clinician is often unable to pass a nasogastric tube.*

The triad of acute pain, vomiting, and inability to pass an NGT is known as Borchardt's triad and is present in up to 70% of the acute cases reported. Major complications include strangulation, ischemia, and gastric perforation. Mortality can be as high 50% without prompt intervention.

Detorsion and gastropexy are essential components of treatment. Endoscopy is a necessary first step to determine the optimal treatment strategy, and endoscopic reduction is often effective. Open or laparoscopic technique for gastropexy with or without repair of the diaphragmatic defect prevents recurrence. Decisions on operative technique are dependent on the clinical skills of the surgeon and the comorbidities of the patient.

A Collis gastroplasty is a surgical procedure performed to lengthen the esophagus when the surgeon desires to create a Nissen fundoplication, but the portion of esophagus inferior to the diaphragm is too short.

Zuiki T, Hosoya Y, Lefor AK, Tanaka H, Komatsubara T, Miyahara Y, Sanada Y, Ohki J, Sekiguchi C, Sata N. The management of gastric volvulus in elderly patients. *Int J Surg Case Rep*. 2016;29:88–93. doi: 10.1016/j.ijscr.2016.10.058. Epub 2016 Oct 27. PMID: 27835806; PMCID: PMC5107685.

Verde F, Hawasli H, Johnson PT, Fishman EK. Gastric volvulus: unraveling the diagnosis with MPRs. *Emerg Radiol*. 2019;26(2):221–225. doi: 10.1007/s10140-019-01669-0. Epub 2019 Jan 14. PMID: 30644001.

Wu MH, Chang YC, Wu CH, Kang SC, Kuan JT. Acute gastric volvulus: a rare but real surgical emergency. *Am J Emerg Med*. 2010;28(1):118.e5–118.e7. doi: 10.1016/j.ajem.2009.04.031. PMID: 20006232.

18 *A healthy, muscular 30-year-old man presents to your office with chronic pain on the right side of his abdomen. You can palpate a vague mass that is tender. He has had no previous surgery. All labs are normal. A representative slice of the CT scan is illustrated. The BEST treatment option for this patient is?*

A *Laparoscopic appendectomy*

B *Non-steroidal anti-inflammatories and avoid weight-lifting for 6 weeks*

C *Laparoscopic or robotic hernia repair reinforced with mesh*

D *Primary suture repair*

E *Mindfulness meditation*

C. The CT scan illustrates an example of a Spigelian hernia. The defect is located in the transversalis fascia at the level of the arcuate line where the aponeuroses are at their weakest. This defect is covered by the external oblique aponeurosis, thus often making the diagnosis difficult. Patients often present with abdominal pain with or without a painful vague abdominal mass or lump. Diagnosis can be made with CT, ultrasound, or diagnostic laparoscopy.

Treatment traditionally has been by an open technique over the area of tenderness, reducing the hernia and primarily repairing the defect with or without mesh. More recently, with the advantages of minimal access, laparoscopic or robotic approaches are favored. Advantages include less pain, quicker recovery, and visualization of the contralateral side. Multiple laparoscopic techniques have been described with the majority utilizing synthetic mesh for repair.

Barnes TG, McWhinnie DL. Laparoscopic spigelian hernia repair: a systematic review. *Surg Laparosc Endosc Percutan Tech*. 2016;26(4):265–270. doi: 10.1097/SLE.0000000000000286. PMID: 27438174.

Ferris M, Diegidio P, Loflin C, Nottingham J. Laparoscopic management of the spigelian hernia. *Am Surg*. 2014;80(12):E329–E330. PMID: 25513898.

Polistina FA, Garbo G, Trevisan P, Frego M. Twelve years of experience treating Spigelian hernia. *Surgery*. 2015;157(3):547–550. doi: 10.1016/j.surg.2014.09.027. Epub 2015 Feb 3. PMID: 25656692.

41

Necrotizing Soft Tissue Infections and Other Soft Tissue Infections

MAJ Jacob Swann, MD[1] and Joseph DuBose, MD[2]

[1] *Regions Hospital, Saint Paul, MN, USA*
[2] *Department of Surgery, Dell School of Medicine, University of Texas Austin, Austin, TX, USA*

1   *An 18-year-old patient presents to the emergency room after being involved in a motor vehicle collision. He suffers a mild traumatic brain injury (TBI) and a 4% total body surface area (TBSA) abrasion of his right arm. The patient remains as an inpatient for 5 days for topical wound care and TBI evaluations. On the day of discharge, the patient reports worsening erythema at the proximal aspect of the right arm abrasion. The patient has approximately 4 cm of erythematous skin that has mild tenderness to palpation. The patient has normal vitals and normal labs. No bullae, fluctuance, or crepitus is present, and there is no pain-out-of-proportion to exam. Some mild induration is appreciated around the wound bed, and a bedside ultrasound fails to reveal an organized fluid collection. What is the appropriate next step in management of this patient?*

   A   *Discharge home with typical outpatient follow up in 2 weeks*
   B   *Bedside incision and drainage*
   C   *Cephalexin*
   D   *Vancomycin IV, piperacillin/tazobactam IV, and clindamycin IV*
   E   *Emergent surgical exploration and debridement*

This patient is presenting with uncomplicated cellulitis. The patient has an open wound that became subsequently infected likely secondary to skin flora. This patient warrants a course of antibiotics to treat the cellulitis. First-line therapy for cellulitis is an assessment to ensure no evidence of a drainable fluid collection is present. Once significant occult pathology is ruled out, initiation of antibiotics is appropriate. If there are no systemic signs of inflammation (i.e. fever, tachycardia, or leukocytosis), a 5-day course of oral antibiotics is recommended by the Infectious Disease Society of America

(IDSA); appropriate therapy includes cephalexin, or clindamycin if the patient has a severe penicillin allergy. This course can be extended based on the patient's response to therapy. If the patient has a history of methicillin-resistant *Staphylococcus aureus* (MRSA) positivity or is high risk for MRSA infection (i.e. positive screening nasal swab, prior MRSA wound cultures, or a personal history of IV drug abuse), then using a medication with MRSA coverage is first-line therapy.

In this scenario, with no fluctuance on exam and an ultrasound showing no fluid collection, there is no need for an incision and debridement at the site. Similarly, the patient does not appear to have a necrotizing soft tissue infection (no bullae, crepitus, or pain out of proportion to exam); as such, emergent exploration, debridement, or broad-spectrum antibiotics are not indicated. Discharge home without intervention is inappropriate as the patient has active cellulitis. Thus, the correct answer is to start cephalexin.

Answer: C

Stevens, DL, Bisno AL, Chambers HF, et al. "Practice guidelines for the diagnosis and management of skin and soft tissue infections: 2014 updated by the infectious diseases society of America." *Clinical Infectious Diseases.* 2014; 59 (2): e10–e52.

2   *A 20-year-old college athlete presents to the emergency room with a 1 cm abscess on his right medial thigh 10 cm inferior to the inguinal ligament. There is no associated cellulitis. The patient has normal vital signs, an unremarkable physical exam other than appropriate tenderness around the abscess, and unremarkable labs. He has a history of MRSA infections. What is the next step in management?*

Surgical Critical Care and Emergency Surgery: Clinical Questions and Answers, Third Edition.
Edited by Forrest "Dell" Moore, Peter M. Rhee, and Carlos J. Rodriguez.
© 2022 John Wiley & Sons Ltd. Published 2022 by John Wiley & Sons Ltd.
Companion website: www.wiley.com/go/surgicalcriticalcare3e

A *Incision and drainage*

B *Incision and drainage with a course of oral cephalexin*

C *Incision and drainage with a course of oral trimethoprim-sulfamethoxazole (TMP-SMX)*

D *Computed tomography (CT) scan with IV contrast of the right lower extremity*

E *Wide local excision and operative exploration*

This patient has a simple abscess without evidence of systemic inflammation. Traditional teaching would recommend incision and drainage alone is likely adequate therapy for this patient with no evidence of systemic inflammation or superimposed cellulitis. However, emerging literature supports a short course of therapy with oral TMP-SMX or clindamycin for simple abscesses. Several recent studies have shown a decreased rate of treatment failure (i.e. recurrent abscess) or recurrence. However, with the use of antibiotics, there is an increased risk of side effects, namely, an increase in GI symptoms and diarrhea. In these studies, cephalosporins did not reduce treatment failure risk.

While the IDSA has not published new guidelines on this subject, it appears likely that a recommendation will change in the coming guidelines for skin/soft tissue infections. Referencing the latest IDSA guidelines, collecting abscess fluid cultures are ideal for any drainable fluid collection, however the IDSA does not support culturing wounds in the setting of simple abscesses as it will not guide antibiotic therapy.

In this question stem, further imaging for a simple abscess is not indicated given the well-circumscribed nature of the abscess. There is no role for wide local excision of a simple abscess as this is not an NSTI. Cephalexin is suboptimal when compared to TMP-SMX or clindamycin. Simple incision and drainage is associated with a higher treatment failure rate.

Answer: C

Duam, RS, Miller LG, Immergluck L, et al. "A placebo-controlled trial of antibiotics for smaller skin abscesses." *The New England Journal of Medicine.* 2017; 376 (26): 2545–2555.

Vermandere, M., Aertgeerts B, Agoritsas T, et al. "Antibiotics after incision and drainage for uncomplicated skin abscesses: a clinical practice guideline." *The British Medical Journal.* 2018; 360: k243.

Wang, W., Chen W., Liu Y., et al. "Antibiotics for uncomplicated skin abscesses: systemic review and network meta-analysis." *BMJ Open.* 2018; 8: e020991.

3 *A 38-year-old patient presents to the emergency room with a chief complaint of right arm pain. The patient reports that he is an IV drug abuser and uses dirty needles. The injection site has become more and more painful. There is significant erythema and induration along the majority of the right arm around the wound site for several centimeters circumferentially. The patient reports that these changes have happened rapidly over the previous 6 hours. The patient has pain-out-of-proportion to exam with light touch eliciting a vigorous pain response. The patient does not have bullae or palpable crepitus on exam. The patient is febrile, tachycardic, and normotensive. What is the next best step in management?*

A *Bedside incision and drainage*

B *Perform a laboratory assessment and a CT scan with IV contrast of the right arm*

C *Admit the patient to the floor and start cefazolin IV*

D *Admit the patient to the ICU and start vancomycin, clindamycin, and piperacillin/tazobactam IV*

E *Emergency incision, drainage, and wide local excision of all devitalized tissues*

The patient is presenting with many signs and symptoms concerning for a necrotizing soft tissue infection (NSTI). The patient has signs of systemic inflammation as evidenced by the vital sign abnormalities. On exam, the patient has pain-out-of-proportion to exam with a rapidly spreading cellulitis. The patient also has a high-risk exposure history with use of dirty needles for his IV drug abuse. With this constellation of symptoms, the patient has a presumptive diagnosis of an NSTI and needs to proceed to the operating room emergently for exploration and wide debridement. Early debridement and sufficient debridement are the two best predictors of survival in this disease process.

Bedside incision and drainage of the wound site is unlikely to obtain adequate source control of the rapidly spreading bacterial infection. Insufficient debridement is associated with a higher mortality. Further workup with laboratory and imaging workups will not add any additional data that would make the patient a nonoperative candidate. This would only delay his time to the operating room (OR). Initiation of appropriate antibiotics (vancomycin, clindamycin, and piperacillin/tazobactam) is important for this patient; however, doing so should not delay going to the operating room. Moreover, admitting the patient to the ICU or a lower level of care in lieu of the operating room will add mortality to this patient as the patient needs to be emergently operated on to obtain surgical source control.

Answer: E

Nawijn F, Smeeing DPJ, Houwert RM, et al. "Time is of the essence when treating necrotizing soft tissue infections: a systemic review and meta-analysis." *World Journal of Emergency Surgery.* 2020; 15: 4.

4 *A 64-year-old patient presents to the emergency department with increasing pain at a left leg venous stasis ulcer site. The patient has dealt with venous stasis disease for years and has developed a venous stasis ulcer on the medial aspect of his medial malleolus. This wound has been present for weeks. Three days ago the patient reported onset of pain, redness, and induration at the site, and over the last 12 hours, the pain is worsening and the redness has progressed. The patient has pain with passive flexion/extension of the ankle. Laboratory testing is performed in the emergency department and reveals the following data:*

White blood cell count (WBC): 23.8 cell/mm^3
Hemoglobin: 10.6 g/dL
Hematocrit: 29.4 g/dL
Platelets: 445
Sodium: 132 mmol/L
Potassium: 4.2
Chloride: 102
Bicarbonate: 20
Blood urea nitrogen (BUN): 58
Creatinine: 2.3 mg/dL
Glucose: 224 mg/dL
C-reactive protein (CRP): 228 mg/L

Which of the above laboratory values is most predictive of a diagnosis of NSTI?
　A *WBC*
　B *Hemoglobin*
　C *Sodium*
　D *Creatinine*
　E *CRP*

The Laboratory Risk Indicator for Necrotizing Fasciitis (LRINEC) score can be used to assist in medical decision-making when the diagnosis is not clear. This score uses weighted scores for six laboratory results as follows:

C-reactive protein, mg/L
　<150　　　0
　≥150　　　4
Total white cell count, cells/mm^3
　<15　　　　0
　15–25　　　1
　>25　　　　2
Hemoglobin, g/dL
　>13.5　　　0
　11–13.5　　1
　<11　　　　2
Sodium, mmol/L
　≥135　　　0
　<135　　　2
Creatinine mg/dL
　≤1.6　　　0
　>1.6　　　2

Glucose, mg/dL
　≤180　　　0
　>180　　　1

The maximum score is 13; a score of ≥6 should raise suspicion of necrotizing fasciitis, and a score of ≥8 is strongly predictive of this disease.

CRP is the most heavily weighted component of the LRINEC score, and—as such—it is the most predictive of NSTI. The results of the LRINEC are not generalizable for all patients with a skin/soft tissue infection. For patients with a clinical exam not concerning for NSTI, LRINEC can be elevated due to underlying comorbidities. If the patient has simple cellulitis without concerning signs or symptoms of NSTI (i.e. no rapid spread, no pain-out-of-proportion to exam, no bullae) but has an elevated LRINEC, there is a high likelihood of having a negative exploration. The opposite is also true; if a patient has an exam highly concerning for NSTI, the patient warrants operative exploration even if the LRINEC score is not elevated. The LRINEC is best applied in patients who have significant cellulitis but who do not have worrisome signs of an NSTI to aid in the determination of whether operative exploration is warranted or not.

Answers A, B, C, and D do not have as high of a weighted score as CRP and are not as predictive of NSTI as CRP.

Answer: E

Wong CH, Khin LW, Heng KS, et al. "The LRINEC (Laboratory Risk Indicator for Necrotizing Fasciitis) score: a tool for distinguishing necrotizing fasciitis from other soft tissue infections." *Critical Care Medicine.* 2004; 32 (7): 1535–1541.
Abdullah M, McWilliams B, Khan SU. "Reliability of the Laboratory Risk Indicator in Necrotising Fasciitis (LRINEC) score." *The Surgeon: Journal of the Royal Colleges of Surgeons of Edinburgh and Royal College of Surgeons in Ireland.* 2019; 17 (5): 309–318.

5 *A 2-year-old patient presents with signs and symptoms consistent with a diagnosis of NSTI. Which of the following is the best way of diagnosing an NSTI?*
　A *CT scan*
　B *Laboratory risk stratification*
　C *Operative exploration*
　D *Bedside physical exam*
　E *History consistent with NSTI*

NSTI is a diagnosis that is often suspected based on a number of clinical criteria. A patient presenting with a history of rapid onset of pain-out-of-proportion to exam, rapidly spreading cellulitis, or a chronic wound that changes in severity and rapidity of progression are generally concerning for NSTI, but these do not establish the diagnosis definitively. Similarly, physical exam with significant erythema, induration, and bullae are also concerning for NSTI, but other diagnoses exist, which can have similar symptoms. LRINEC is a risk stratification model, which assists in medical decision-making for questionable cases of severe cellulitis to guide therapy (operative exploration versus antibiotics). However, patients can have NSTI with a negative LRINEC or have a positive LRINEC but no NSTI. CT scan—which can reveal edema, organized fluid collections, and air in the subcutaneous space—does not definitively diagnose all cases of NSTI. Operative exploration carried down to the fascia and muscle remains the gold standard of determining if the fascia and muscle are viable, as well as to determine if the overlying soft tissue is normal and healthy as evidenced by bleeding from the surrounding tissues.

Answer: C

Kiat HJ, Natalie YH, Fatimah L. "Necrotizing fasciitis: how reliable are the cutaneous signs?" *Journal of Emergencies, Trauma, and Shock*. 2017; 10 (4): 205–210.

6   *A 52-year-old man presents with pain, erythema, and edema of the groin and perineum. The patient has boggy tissue that has exquisite tenderness to palpation on exam. The patient has copious amounts of foul-smelling discharge coming from an unroofed abscess along the proximal-medial aspect of the right thigh near the perineum. A plan is made for operative exploration due to concern for Fournier's gangrene. What is the ideal first-line choice of antibiotic regimen for this patient?*
   A   *Cefazolin*
   B   *Gentamicin + linezolid*
   C   *Imipenem + piperacillin/tazobactam + clindamycin*
   D   *Vancomycin + piperacillin/tazobactam + clindamycin*
   E   *Linezolid + penicillin G*

Empiric antibiotic choice is important in NSTI as the causative organisms can be quite broad. MRSA coverage is necessary as the most common single organism isolated in NSTI is MRSA. This necessitates vancomycin, linezolid, or ceftaroline depending on allergy history for MRSA coverage. Polymicrobial infections are very common with NSTI and necessitate anaerobic coverage and gram-negative coverage for causative organisms. These two groups of bacteria can be covered with piperacillin/tazobactam or a carbapenem adequately. Lastly, group A *Streptococcus* (GAS) is also a common cause of NSTI and is treated with high-dose

penicillin; Group A *Streptococcus* is adequately covered with the above empiric antibiotics, but narrowing to high-dose penicillin is an option pending final speciation/sensitivities of wound cultures. Clindamycin has the added theoretical benefit of blocking the 50s subunit of the bacterial ribosomes, thus decreasing the production and downstream secretion of exotoxin helping to aid in the direct tissue damage associated with NSTI infections.

Of the examples above, the only antibiotic regimen that adequately covers for an NSTI empirically is vancomycin + piperacillin/tazobactam + clindamycin. Option A has inadequate coverage for MRSA, polymicrobial infections, and GAS. Option B lacks adequate GAS coverage. Option B also is using gentamicin for anaerobic and gram-negative coverage. While adequate coverage for gram-positive cocci and gram-negative rods, gentamicin would be less favored than piperacillin/tazobactam as gentamicin carries the added risk of systemic toxicities (e.g. nephrotoxicity and ototoxicity) with marginal benefit to first-line therapy as the likelihood of encountering a piperacillin/tazobactam resistant, gentamicin-sensitive organism is unlikely. While use of an aminoglycoside may be necessary based on clinical deterioration or final culture results, empiric first-line use is not recommended. Moreover, gentamicin is effective at treating anaerobes due to an oxygen-dependent active transport into the bacteria demonstrating that option B has inadequate anaerobic coverage. Option C lacks adequate MRSA coverage. Option E lacks adequate gram-negative and anaerobic coverage.

Answer: D

Giuliano A, Lews F, Hadley K, et al. "Bacteriology of necrotizing fasciitis." *American Journal of Surgery*. 1977; 134 (1): 52–57.

Zimbelman J, Palmer A, Todd J. "Improved outcome of clindamycin compared with beta-lactam antibiotic treatment for invasive Streptococcus pyogenes infection." *The Pediatric Infectious Disease Journal*. 1999; 18 (12): 1097–100.

Jaggi P, Beall B, Rippe J, et al. "Macrolide resistance and emm type distribution of invasive pediatric group A streptococcal isolates: three-year prospective surveillance from a children's hospital." *The Pediatric Infectious Disease Journal*. 2007; 26 (3): 253–255.

7   *A 72-year-old diabetic patient presents with a medical history of a chronic left foot ulcer. The patient has been performing wound care at home intermittently for the past several weeks. The patient presents*

to the emergency department today with rapid progression of pain, erythema, and edema spreading proximally over the previous 12 hours. A full workup is performed, and the patient is diagnosed with an NSTI. Plans are made to take the patient to the operating room. The patient has had anaphylactic reactions to penicillin and vancomycin in the past. What is the ideal antibiotic regimen to start this patient on in preparation for the operating room?

A *Cefazolin + penicillin G*

B *Imipenem + linezolid + clindamycin*

C *Metronidazole + clindamycin*

D *Piperacillin/tazobactam + linezolid + clindamycin*

E *Ceftaroline + metronidazole + clindamycin*

Drug allergies provide significant issues with antibiotic regimens, and second-line therapies due to allergies are high yield for the surgical critical care boards. The four main categories of antibiotic coverage required are (1) MRSA coverage, (2) gram-negative coverage, (3) anaerobic coverage, and (4) group A *Streptococcus* coverage. For MRSA coverage, vancomycin is often used first line. In the setting of a vancomycin allergy, linezolid or ceftaroline can be used. For gram-negative coverage, piperacillin/tazobactam is often used as it also has effective coverage against anaerobes. Using cefepime or a carbapenem in the setting of a penicillin allergy is appropriate. If using cefepime, keep in mind that metronidazole is needed to provide adequate anaerobic coverage. Lastly, GAS coverage is best provided by clindamycin in the setting of a penicillin allergy.

Answer A provides inadequate anaerobic and MRSA coverage. Answer C provides inadequate gram negative and MRSA coverage. Answer D cannot be used due to the patient's anaphylactic penicillin allergy as piperacillin/tazobactam are contraindicated. Answer E does not provide adequate gram-negative coverage.

Answer: B

Stevens, DL, Bisno AL, Chambers HF, et al. "Practice guidelines for the diagnosis and management of skin and soft tissue infections: 2014 updated by the infectious diseases society of America." *Clinical Infectious Diseases.* 2014; 59 (2): e10–e52.

8 *In a patient with NSTI who is decompensating despite aggressive debridement, antibiotics, and resuscitation, which of the following causative organisms may benefit from IVIG therapy?*

A *Staphylococcus aureus*

B *Streptococcus pyogenes*

C *Clostridium perfringens*

D *Vibrio cholera*

E *Pseudomonas aeruginosa*

IVIG can act to help bind exotoxin secreted by group A *Streptococcus*. By binding the exotoxin via IVIG, clearance of the toxin and limiting the local tissue damage and systemic inflammatory response can be assisted. Data on using IVIG to treat NSTI has shown no benefit for use in any of the other causative organisms and is not recommended except in group A *Streptococcus* infections. Data on IVIG is largely based on generalizing data from toxic shock syndrome patients and patients in septic shock from disseminated group A *Streptococcus* infections. As such, consideration of using IVIG for patients with group A *Streptococcus* NSTIs is warranted.

Answer: B

Cocanour CS, Chang P, Huston JM, et al. "Management and novel adjuncts of necrotizing soft tissue infections." *Surgical Infections.* 2017; 18 (3): 250–272.

Madsen MB, Hjortrup PB, Hansen MB, et al. "Immunoglobulin G for patients with necrotizing soft tissue infection (INSTINCT): a randomized, blinded, placebo-controlled trial." *Intensive Care Medicine.* 2017; 43 (11): 1585–1593.

9 *A 59-year-old patient presents to the surgical critical care unit with a diagnosis of NSTI. Appropriate empiric antibiotics are started. Resuscitation with IV fluids are given, and vasopressors are required in order to maintain a mean arterial pressure > 65 mm Hg. The patient is taken urgently to the operating room for wide local debridement. Postoperatively, the patient continues to require vasopressor support. A member of the care team asks if the patient is a candidate for hyperbaric oxygen therapy (HBOT). Which of the following is true regarding HBOT in patients with NSTI?*

A *HBOT affords increased oxygen delivery to end-organs thus limiting the SIRS response.*

B *HBOT increases bacterial clearance by leukocytes.*

C *HBOT is beneficial in anaerobic bacterial infections.*

D *HBOT decreases time to surgical debridement.*

E *There has been no high-quality trials to support HBOT universal use in NSTI patients.*

HBOT has been an area of controversy. Initially, HBOT was thought to assist with management of NSTI via multiple hypothetic mechanisms. One animal model study demonstrated a suppression in *Clostridium perfringens* growth when exposed to HBOT; however, other *Clostridium* species showed no growth suppression. While a few small, retrospective, observational case series have been published, none have shown a discrete patient population where HBOT has clearly been of benefit. HBOT requires equipping a dive chamber to provide ICU-level support for prolonged periods of time as the patient will need an extensive period of time to reach the appropriate atmospheric pressure, be sustained at that pressure, and then brought back to a normal, external air pressure. These will keep the patient in the dive chamber for several minutes if not hours.

A clear mechanism of action of HBOT in NSTI has not been demonstrated, thus answers A and B are incorrect. *Clostridium perfringens* is the only organism thought to be suppressed by HBOT; thus, answer C is incorrect. Diving a patient in a HBOT chamber increases time to surgical debridement making answer D incorrect.

Answer: E

Levett DZ, Bennett MH, Millar I. "Using oxygen at high pressure (in a compression chamber) for the treatment of individuals with severe soft tissue infection (necrotizing fasciitis)." *Cochrane Database of Systematic Reviews.* 2015; 1.

Thrane JF, Oversen T. "Scare evidence of efficacy of hyperbaric oxygen therapy in necrotizing soft tissue infection: a systematic review." *Infectious Diseases.* 2019; 57 (7): 485–492.

10 *A 58-year-old patient presents to the emergency department with right lower extremity pain. The patient has diabetes mellitus complicated by microvascular disease, peripheral neuropathy, and end-stage renal disease. The patient has a past surgical history of a left lower extremity below-the-knee amputation for multiple non-healing diabetic wounds. The patient presents with altered mental status, hypotension, tachycardia, and is febrile. On exam, the patient has a large wound on the plantar surface of the right foot with associated erythema, bullae, and induration extending up to the knee. The patient is diagnosed with a necrotizing soft tissue infection and is taken to the operating room. The patient undergoes a wide local excision and is admitted to the SICU postoperatively for further management. Which of the following is a risk factor for increased mortality in this patient?*

A *BMI > 29.9*
B *History of type II diabetes mellitus*
C *History of end-stage renal disease requiring dialysis*
D *Age > 50*
E *Normal vital signs on presentation*

Risk factors for mortality in the setting of an NSTI are varied and include septic shock on presentation, age > 74, malnutrition (BMI < 18.5), need for dialysis, pre-existing cancer diagnoses, MRSA antibiotic use, severe peripheral arterial disease, and hospital-acquired infections.

Presumed risk factors that have not correlated with an NSTI include: gender, pre-existing type II diabetes, IVIG use, or antithrombin III use.

Answer: C

Suzuki H, Muramatsu K, Kubo T, et al. "Factors associated with mortality among patients with necrotizing soft tissue infections: an analysis of 4597 cases using the diagnosis procedure combination database." *International Journal of Infectious Diseases.* 2020. 102: 73–78.

Hua C, Sbidian E, Hemery F, et al. "Prognostic factors in necrotizing soft-tissue infections (NSTI): a cohort study." *Journal of the American Academy of Dermatology.* 2015; 73 (6): 1006–1012.

11 *A 63-year-old patient presents to the hospital in profound septic shock. On arrival to the emergency department, the patient is noted to be hypotensive, tachycardic, febrile, and has altered mental status. The patient is intubated, IV access is obtained, cultures are obtained, empiric antibiotics are initiated, and resuscitation is started. On evaluation of NGT placement, the portable abdominal films show markedly dilated small bowel and subcutaneous emphysema of the right flank abdominal wall. Exam is significant for abdominal distension, profound cellulitis of the right flank, and palpable crepitus. The patient is taken to the operating room where a large debridement is needed to treat presumptive necrotizing fasciitis. Final culture results from the abdominal wound reveal the causative organism. The final etiology of the patient's small bowel obstruction is discovered to be a near obstructing right-sided colon cancer. Which of the following organisms is associated with NSTI with an underlying malignancy*

A *Clostridium novyi*
B *Clostridium perfringes*
C *Vibrio vulnificus*
D *Psuedomonas aeruginosa*
E *Clostridum septicum*

Traditionally, the three most common causes of NSTI infection are divided into three types: type 1 is polymicrobial, type 2 is group A *Streptococcal*, and type 3 is gas gangrene due to clostridial myonecrosis. That said, several unique bacteria species are associated with particular clinical scenarios that the astute clinician should be aware of.

Clostridium novyi is associated with IV drug abuse with resultant local or hematologic spread of an NSTI. *Clostridium perfringes* is seen in injuries suffered due to disasters or wartime. *Vibrio vulnificus* is associated with injuries suffered in or near bodies of water (both salt and freshwater) with subsequent infection. *Pseudomonas aeruginosa* is a rare cause of NSTI without classic associations with underlying disease processes. *Clostridium septicum* is associated with underlying malignancies. Several case studies have shown occult malignancy of multiple organ systems in association with infection by *C. septicum*. A recent review showed that in patients with *C. septicum* NSTIs, 71% had known or occult malignancy in association with their infection.

Answer: E

Srivastava I, Aldape MJ, Bryant AE, Stevens DL. Spontaneous C. septicum gas gangrene: a literature review. *Anaerobe*. 2017; 48: 165–171. doi: 10.1016/j.anaerobe.2017.07.008. Epub 2017 Aug 2. PMID: 28780428.

Sidhu JS, Mandal A, Virk J, Gayam V. Early detection of colon cancer following incidental finding of clostridium septicum bacteremia. *Journal of Investigative Medicine High Impact Case Reports*. 2019; 7: 2324709619832050. doi: 10.1177/2324709619832050. PMID: 30857430; PMCID: PMC6415464.

Gray KM, Padilla PL, Sparks B, Dziewulski P. Distant myonecrosis by atraumatic *Clostridium septicum* infection in a patient with metastatic breast cancer. *IDCases*. 2020; 20: e00784. doi: 10.1016/j.idcr.2020.e00784. PMID: 32420030; PMCID: PMC7218154.

Saunders RN, Hayakawa E, Gibson CJ, Chapman AJ. Clostridium septicum myonecrosis secondary to an occult small bowel adenocarcinoma. *Journal of Gastrointestinal Cancer*. 2019; 50 (4): 1001–1004. doi: 10.1007/s12029-018-0168-2. PMID: 30198050.

Cullinane C, Earley H, Tormey S. Deadly combination: *Clostridium septicum* and colorectal malignancy. *BMJ Case Reports*. 2017; 2017: bcr2017222759. doi: 10.1136/bcr-2017-222759. PMID: 29197851; PMCID: PMC5720338.

42

Obesity and Bariatric Surgery

Thomas A. O'Hara, DO[1] and Gregory S. Peirce, MD[2]

[1] Dwight D. Eisenhower Army Medical Center, Fort Gordon, GA, USA
[2] Womack Army Medical Center, Fort Bragg, NC, USA

1 *Which of the following statements regarding obesity and COVID-19 is true?*
   A *Obese patients who contract COVID-19 have a decreased rate of severe infection compared to non-obese patients who contract COVID-19.*
   B *The mortality rate of COVID-19 is comparable between obese and nonobese patient populations.*
   C *Obesity is only a risk factor for severe COVID-19 infection in patients older than 60 years of age.*
   D *Obese patients are twice as likely to develop a severe COVID-19 infection as nonobese patients.*
   E *All overweight patients have similar COVID-19 outcomes regardless of BMI.*

Answer: D

Multiple studies have shown that obesity significantly increases the risk of severe COVID-19 infection, with odds ratios ranging from 1.84 to 3.6. The mortality rate also significantly increased in obese patients, with an odds ratio up to 8.43. Also, obesity is an independent risk factor for hospital and ICU admission in COVID-19 patients less than 60 years of age. Furthermore, the severity of the COVID infection appears to worsen within the overweight population with increasing BMI. As seen in Table 42.1 below, there exists a significant difference in rates of ICU admission between patients with BMI 30–34 and BMI > 35.

Cai Q, Chen F, Wang T, Luo F, Liu X, Wu Q, He Q, Wang Z, Liu Y, Liu L, Chen J, Xu L. Obesity and COVID-19 severity in a designated hospital in shenzhen. *China Diabetes Care.* 2020;43(7):1392–1398. doi: 10.2337/dc20-0576. Epub 2020 May 14. PMID: 32409502.

Lighter J, Phillips M, Hochman S, Sterling S, Johnson D, Francois F, Stachel A. Obesity in patients younger than 60 years is a risk factor for COVID-19 hospital admission. *Clin Infect Dis.* 2020;71(15):896–897. doi: 10.1093/cid/ciaa415. PMID: 32271368; PMCID: PMC7184372.

Peng Y, Meng K, He M, Zhu R, Guan H, Ke Z, Leng L, Wang X, Liu B, Hu C, Ji Q, Keerman M, Cheng L, Wu T, Huang K, Zeng Q. Clinical characteristics and prognosis of 244 cardiovascular patients suffering from coronavirus disease in Wuhan. *China J Am Heart Assoc.* 2020;9(19):e016796. doi: 10.1161/JAHA.120.016796. Epub 2020 Aug 14. PMID: 32794415.

2 *A 55-year-old man status-post gastric bypass 8 weeks ago presents to the emergency department with confusion and numbness in the hands and feet. She has had prolonged vomiting and poor oral hydration for 3 weeks. Which of the following will best treat her symptoms?*
   A *Normal saline bolus*
   B *Broad-spectrum antibiotics*
   C *"Banana bag" of fluids*
   D *Bolus of D5 half normal saline*
   E *Endoscopic dilation*

Answer: C

Peripheral neuropathy and confusion are consistent with thiamine or vitamin B_1 deficiency. Thiamine has a half-life of 18 days and is an essential vitamin. Its deficiency can result in Wernicke's encephalopathy (WE) and beriberi. This patient needs thiamine—the standard content of a "banana bag," which typically contains 100 mg thiamine, 1 mg folate, 3 g magnesium, and other

Table 42.1 Adult patients who tested positive for COVID-19 during 3 March–4 April 2020 (*N* = 3615).

BMI, kg/m^2	No. (%)	Admission to acute (vs discharge From ED), OR (95% CI)	*P* value	No. (%)	ICU admission (vs discharge from ED), OR (95% CI)	*P* value
Age ≥ 60 years						
BMI 30–34	141 (19)	0.9 (0.6–1.2)	0.39	57 (22)	1.1 (0.8–1.7)	0.57
BMI ≥ 35	99 (14)	0.9 (0.6–1.3)	0.59	50 (19)	1.5 (0.9–2.3)	0.10
Age < 60 years						
BMI 30–34	173 (29)	2.0 (1.6–2.6)	<0.0001	39 (23)	1.8 (1.2–2.7)	0.006
BMI ≥ 35	134 (22)	2.2 (1.7–2.9)	<0.0001	56 (33)	3.6 (2.5–5.3)	<0.0001

Abbreviations: BMI, body mass index; CI, confidence interval; COVID-19, coronavirus disease 2019; ED, emergency department; ICU, intensive care unit; OR, odds ratio.

daily vitamins. Afterward, the patient may need additional thiamine. For WE, patients should receive 500 mg IV thiamine three times a day until symptoms abate. In most cases, symptoms improve within 24 hours of administration.

Patients who undergo malabsorptive procedures are particularly at risk of thiamine deficiency, as it is mostly absorbed in the duodenum and proximal jejunum. All bariatric patients should take a daily multivitamin (which contains thiamine) and have regular thiamine level checks. Most importantly, any bariatric patient with prolonged vomiting and poor intake should be treated empirically with thiamine supplementation to prevent irreversible neurologic complications.

The patient is dehydrated and would benefit from normal saline, but this will not reverse her neurologic symptoms. As with alcoholics, thiamine should be given prior to any glucose-containing fluids. Broad-spectrum antibiotics would be important if an infection, leak, or perforated marginal ulcer was suspected. The patient may soon need endoscopic dilation, as she could have a stricture at the gastro-jejunal anastomosis, but her encephalopathy must be addressed first.

Oudman E, Wijnia JW, van Dam M, Biter LU, Postma A. Preventing wernicke encephalopathy after bariatric surgery. *Obes Surg.* 2018;28(7):2060–2068.

Raziel A Thiamine deficiency after bariatric surgery may lead to Wernicke encephalopathy. *Isr Med Assoc J.* 2012;14:692–694.

3 *A 50-year-old woman presents to the emergency department with severe abdominal pain and PO intolerance. She had a laparoscopic Roux-en-Y gastric bypass (RYGB) 2 years ago and now weighs 100 pounds less than her preoperative weight. Contrast-enhanced CT abdomen reveals portions of the small bowel to be dilated with vascular rotation at the mesenteric root. Which of the following is true regarding her condition?*

A *This is more likely to occur with an antecolic Roux limb.*

B *An appropriate management option is nasogastric decompression and observation.*

C *Definitive diagnosis of this condition can only be achieved through surgical exploration.*

D *Due to the high sensitivity of CT scans, a lack of dilated small bowel and mesenteric rotation almost always rules this condition out.*

E *Closure of the mesenteric defects at her index surgery does not decrease the possibility of this condition.*

Answer: C

This patient has an internal hernia. Internal hernias may occur following any procedure in which the mesentery is divided—such as a RYGB or duodenal switch with biliopancreatic diversion. The small bowel may herniate through mesenteric defects created by the procedure. For an antecolic-oriented RYGB, the two possible sites of herniation are at the jejunojejunostomy or between the Roux limb mesentery and the transverse mesocolon (Peterson's defect). For a retrocolic RYGB, an additional site of herniation is at the mesocolic defect. Patients with internal hernias typically present with intermittent nonspecific abdominal pain and PO intolerance, but symptoms may worsen if the hernia incarcerates. CT imaging will often show a circular rotation of the vasculature (i.e. a "swirl sign"), as well as dilated small bowel. However, these findings are neither sensitive or specific and their absence does not rule out internal hernia.

Internal hernias more commonly occur with a retrocolic Roux limb. The lowest incidence of internal hernia occurs with an antecolic approach with closure of the mesenteric defects. Observation and decompression is not a viable option in bariatric patients with an internal hernia. If concerned for an internal hernia, exploration must be performed to diagnose the condition, assess the viability of the intestines, reduce the hernia, and close the defect.

Geubbels N, Lijftogt N, Fiocco M, van Leersum NJ, Wouters MW, de Brauw LM. Meta-analysis of internal herniation after gastric bypass surgery. *Br J Surg.*

2015;102(5):451–460. doi: 10.1002/bjs.9738. Epub 2015 Feb 24. PMID: 25708572.

Santos EPRD, Santa Cruz F, Hinrichsen EA, Ferraz ÁAB, Campos JM. Internal hernia following laparoscopic Roux-en-Y gastric by-pass: indicative factors for early repair. *Arq Gastroenterol.* 2019;56(2):160–164. doi: 10.1590/S0004-2803.201900000-32. PMID: 31460580.

Lockhart ME, Tessler FN, Canon CL, Smith JK, Larrison MC, Fineberg NS, Roy BP, Clements RH. Internal hernia after gastric bypass: sensitivity and specificity of seven CT signs with surgical correlation and controls. *AJR Am J Roentgenol.* 2007;188(3):745–750. doi: 10.2214/ AJR.06.0541. PMID: 17312063.

Altinoz A, Maasher A, Jouhar F, Babikir A, Ibrahim M, Al Shaban T, Nimeri A. Diagnostic laparoscopy is more accurate than computerized tomography for internal hernia after Roux-en-Y gastric bypass. *Am J Surg.* 2020;220(1):214–216. doi: 10.1016/j.amjsurg.2019. 10.034. Epub 2019 Oct 19. PMID: 31668708.

Blockhuys M, Gypen B, Heyman S, Valk J, van Sprundel F, Hendrickx L. Internal hernia after laparoscopic gastric bypass: effect of closure of the petersen defect - single-center study. *Obes Surg.* 2019;29(1):70–75. doi: 10.1007/ s11695-018-3472-9. PMID: 30167987.

4   *For the above patient, you perform a laparoscopic exploration. You reduce the hernia by running the small bowel from the ileocolic valve toward the jejuno-jejunostomy. You find 40 cm of the common channel to be of questionable viability. This starts about 20 distal to the jejunojejunostomy. During the case, the patient was started on norepinephrine for hypotension and a blood gas showed her pH to be 7.15. Which of the following is most appropriate in the management of this patient?*

   A *Convert to a laparotomy, resect the questionable portion, and perform a small bowel anastomosis to place the common channel back in continuity*

   B *Resect the concerning portion, perform a small bowel anastomosis to place the common channel in continuity, and reverse the gastric bypass to prevent short gut syndrome*

   C *Plan for a "second look" procedure to assess bowel viability*

   D *Leave bowel intact, terminate the procedure, administer antibiotics, and follow the patient clinically to assess the need for future intervention.*

   E *Perform a transoral intraoperative endoscopy to assess bowel viability and visualize the mucosa*

Answer: C

An internal hernia can result in small bowel ischemia and/or necrosis. The treatment principles for this are similar to managing bowel of questionable viability with damage control surgery. This patient became

hypotensive and acidotic after the hernia reduction – a poor time to perform any anastomosis. A planned reoperation, or "second look" after resuscitation is the best of the choices. This could be done either laparoscopically or through a temporary abdominal closure if the procedure had been converted to open. Reversing the gastric bypass would involve the creation of an anastomosis between the gastric pouch to gastric remnant. This may be needed if the patient had necrosis of a much longer portion of her small intestine. However, the common channel averages near 400 cm and losing 40 cm will not result in short gut syndrome. During reoperation for a previous malabsorptive procedure, one should measure the separate small intestinal limbs (i.e. Roux limb, bilio-pancreatic limb, and the common channel) and document the lengths. Leaving the bowel intact and following clinically is wrong without a planned reassessment of the bowel. Performing an intraoperative endoscopy to assess the small bowel distal to the jejunojejunostomy has no utility in this context.

Bradley JF 3rd, Ross SW, Christmas AB, Fischer PE, Sachdev G, Heniford BT, Sing RF. Complications of bariatric surgery: the acute care surgeon's experience. *Am J Surg.* 2015;210(3):456–461. doi: 10.1016/j. amjsurg.2015.03.004. Epub 2015 May 8. PMID: 26070377.

5   *A 45-year-old woman presents to the emergent department complaining of severe abdominal pain and nausea. The patient had a Roux-en-Y gastric bypass 5 days prior. Her heart rate remains in the 120s, and her systolic blood pressure is in the 80s. What is the most appropriate next step in management for this patient?*

   A *Operative washout and drainage*

   B *Barium swallow*

   C *CT scan with oral contrast*

   D *Broad spectrum antibiotics only*

   E *Nasogastric tube decompression*

Answer: A

This patient is presenting with an anastomotic leak. A leak occurs in 1–3% of patients following a Roux-en-Y gastric bypass. Leaks can occur at any of the staple lines (gastric pouch, remnant stomach, gastrojejunostomy and jejunojejunostomy) but most commonly occur at the gastrojejunostomy. Leaks typically present within 5 days of surgery, as postoperative edema subsides. Patients most commonly present with tachycardia, fevers, and abdominal pain. Patients may also present with nausea, emesis, purulent drainage from incision sites, hypotension, oliguria, or tachypnea.

Because this patient is presenting with signs of sepsis, the most appropriate for this patient is operative intervention.

The tenets of operative management of anastomotic leaks include washout and wide drainage. The leak site may also be primarily oversewn or an omental patch may be placed. Placement of enteral feeding access with jejunostomy tube or gastric tube in the remnant stomach should also be considered for postoperative nutrition. Barium swallow and CT scan with oral contrast are appropriate diagnostic studies to diagnose anastomotic leak in hemodynamically stable patients but are inappropriate in an unstable patient. Broad-spectrum antibiotics and nasogastric decompression are also appropriate, but source control must be obtained for definitive management.

Wernick B, Jansen M, Noria S, Stawicki SP, El Chaar M. Essential bariatric emergencies for the acute care surgeon. *Eur J Trauma Emerg Surg*. 2016;42(5):571–584. doi: 10.1007/s00068-015-0621-x. Epub 2015 Dec 15. PMID: 26669688.

Contival N, Menahem B, Gautier T, Le Roux Y, Alves A. Guiding the non-bariatric surgeon through complications of bariatric surgery. *J Visc Surg*. 2018;155(1):27–40. doi: 10.1016/j.jviscsurg.2017.10.012. Epub 2017 Dec 23. PMID: 29277390.

6 *A 65-year-old man presents to the emergency room complaining of worsening abdominal pain. The patient had a sleeve gastrectomy 6 days ago. The patient has a sustained heart rate in the low 100s and is normotensive. The patient's abdomen is tender in the left upper quadrant, without guarding or rebound. CT scan with oral contrast shows a fluid collection posterior to the stomach, with a small amount of contrast extravasation from the proximal staple line. Which of the following is true regarding this patient's condition?*

A *This patient's condition is likely due to a technical error.*

B *CT scan has a sensitivity of > 95% for diagnosing this condition.*

C *The most appropriate management for this patient is emergent surgical exploration.*

D *Endoluminal stenting eliminates the need for drainage of the fluid collection.*

E *Endoscopy with fluoroscopy and contrast injection is the most accurate diagnostic method.*

Answer: E

This patient has a leak at the staple line after a gastric sleeve. Leaks after a sleeve occur in approximately 1–2% of sleeve gastrectomy patients. Leaks that occur within the first 2 postoperative days are due to technical failures, while leaks due to ischemia occur around postoperative days 5 and 6. Leaks typically occur at the staple line in the proximal

stomach due to ischemia, though they may be exacerbated by high pressures created by distal sleeve stenosis. Upper GI series and CT are often used for diagnosis, though these tests are unreliable, with sensitivities of approximately 30 and 56%, respectively. Endoscopy with fluoroscopy is a more reliable diagnostic method, with the benefit of allowing for interventions during the same procedure.

The management of sleeve leaks is a combination of drainage, broad-spectrum antibiotics, and supplemental nutrition. Stable patients can be managed with percutaneous drainage and bowel rest; however, patients with peritonitis or evidence of hemodynamic instability should be taken to the operating room for surgical exploration. Endoluminal stenting, in conjunction with percutaneous drainage and antibiotics, is another possible management option. Stenting allows the patient to resume a liquid diet, though stent migration is a common complication.

Wernick B, Jansen M, Noria S, Stawicki SP, El Chaar M. Essential bariatric emergencies for the acute care surgeon. *Eur J Trauma Emerg Surg*. 2016;42(5):571–584. doi: 10.1007/s00068-015-0621-x. Epub 2015 Dec 15. PMID: 26669688.

Shehab H. Enteral stents in the management of post-bariatric surgery leaks. *Surg Obes Relat Dis*. 2018;14(3):393–403. doi: 10.1016/j.soard.2017.12.014. Epub 2017 Dec 16. PMID: 29428690.

Tsai YN, Wang HP, Huang CK, Chang PC, Lin IC, Tai CM. Endoluminal stenting for the management of leak following sleeve gastrectomy and loop duodenojejunal bypass with sleeve gastrectomy. *Kaohsiung J Med Sci*. 2018;34(1):43–48. doi: 10.1016/j.kjms.2017.08.004. Epub 2017 Sep 1. PMID: 29310815.

7 *Which of the following is true concerning the baseline respiratory physiology of obese individuals when compared to those of normal weight?*

A *Obese patients have no change in baseline oxygen saturation.*

B *Obese patients have a decreased respiratory rate.*

C *Obese patients have increased pulmonary compliance.*

D *Obese patients have no change in functional residual capacity.*

E *Obese patients have an increased oxygen consumption.*

Answer: E

Obesity increases the risk of respiratory complications and failure. Obese patients can be slightly hypoxemic. They have increased metabolic demands and, as such, have an increased oxygen consumption and carbon dioxide production—both of which lead to an increased respiratory rate. Obese individuals have a decreased pulmonary compliance secondary due to adipose tissue deposits on the chest wall and in the abdomen. Increased abdominal adiposity reduces the pulmonary volumes—specifically the expiratory reserve volume (ERV) and functional residual capacity (FRC). In sitting patients, the ERV and FRC in patients with a BMI of $30\,kg/m^2$ are reduced 47 and 75%, respectively, when compared to patients with a BMI of $20\,kg/m^2$.

Jubber AS. Respiratory complications of obesity. *Int J Clin Pract*. 2004;58:573–580.

Kuchta KF Pathophysiologic changes of obesity. *Anesthesiol Clin North Am*. 2005;23:421–429.

Levi D, Goodman ER, Patel M, Savransky Y Critical care of the obese and bariatric surgical patient. *Crit Care Clin*. 2003;19:11–32.

Jones RL, Nzekwu MM. The effects of body mass index on lung volumes. *Chest*. 2006;130(3):827–833.

8 *You are covering the surgical and trauma intensive care unit. An obese patient just became hypoxic and lost consciousness. You mask ventilate him with 100% oxygen in preparation for intubation. Which of the following is true with respect to intubating obese patients?*

   A *Obesity itself is an independent risk factor for difficult intubation.*

   B *Placing the head of the bed at 25° does not assist with intubation.*

   C *Obstructive sleep apnea is not a risk factor for difficult mask ventilation.*

   D *Obesity is a risk factor for difficult mask ventilation.*

   E *Obese patients with a large neck circumference, excessive pre-tracheal adipose tissue, and high Mallampati classification do not have an increased risk for a difficult intubation.*

Answer: D

Obesity itself is not an independent risk factor for a difficult intubation. However, many features associated with obesity do increase the likelihood of a difficult intubation—such as a large neck circumference, excessive pre-tracheal adipose tissue, and a high Mallampati classification. Additionally, obesity and obstructive sleep apnea increase the probability of having difficulty with mask ventilation. Elevating the torso of obese patients 25–30° can increase the functional residual volume by offsetting the abdominal mass. Additionally, the use of videolaryngoscopy can significantly improve the visualization of the larynx in obese patients and should be rapidly available when intubating obese patients.

Brodsky JB, Lemmens H, Brock-Utne JG, Vierra M, Saidman LJ. Morbid obesity and tracheal intubation. *Anesth Analg*. 2002;94(3):732–736.

Marrel J, Blanc C, Frascarolo P., Magnusson L.; Videolaryngoscopy improves intubation condition in morbidly obese patients. *Euro J Anaesth*. 2007;24(12):1045–1049.

9 *Which of the following is true regarding the placement and care of a tracheostomy in obese patients?*

   A *There is no difference in procedural time between obese and nonobese patients.*

   B *Obese patients have a higher rate of surgical site infection.*

   C *Obese patients have a higher risk of perioperative mortality associated with decannulation.*

   D *Performing a percutaneous tracheostomy is a relative contraindication in obese patients.*

   E *The complication rate of placing a tracheostomy does not correlate with the degree of obesity.*

Answer: C

Obese patients typically have a longer tracheostomy tract due to increased neck circumference. In addition, obese patients tend to have a significantly increased amount of anterior cervical adipose tissue, which can lead to stoma collapse. These factors can increase the difficulty of replacing the tracheostomy tube in the event of decannulation, leading to an increased risk of mortality.

Tracheostomy procedural times are significantly longer in obese patients for both open surgical tracheostomy and percutaneous tracheostomy. The rates of surgical site infection are equivalent for the obese and nonobese patient populations. Complication rates for percutaneous tracheostomy are increased in obese patients; however, complications rates are similarly increased for obese patients in open tracheostomy, and both procedures can be safely performed. Obese patients have increased complication rates following tracheostomy compared to normal weight and overweight patients, but this difference is even more significant for patients with a BMI > 40.

Cordes SR, Best AR, Hiatt KK. The impact of obesity on adult tracheostomy complication rate. *Laryngoscope*. 2015;125(1):105–110. doi: 10.1002/lary.24793. Epub 2014 Jun 17. PMID: 24939326.

Clark M, Greene S, Reed MJ. Tracheostomy in critical ill morbidly obese. *Crit Care Clin*. 2010;26(4):669–670. doi: 10.1016/j.ccc.2010.09.003. PMID: 20970055.

10 *A 55-year-old woman presents to the emergency department complaining of right upper quadrant*

pain. The patient had a Roux-en-Y gastric bypass 1 year ago. Laboratory evaluation shows an elevated conjugated bilirubin and alkaline phosphatase. Right upper quadrant ultrasound demonstrates a dilated common bile duct. Which of the following will not treat the cause of her abdominal pain?

A *Balloon-assisted ERCP*

B *Laparoscopic-assisted ERCP*

C *EUS-directed trans-gastric ERCP*

D *Percutaneous transhepatic drainage*

E *Laparoscopic cholecystectomy*

Answer: E

Choledocholithiasis is a difficult problem to manage in patients with altered gut anatomy. The primary goal of initial management is biliary compression and, ideally, simultaneous stone removal. A standard ERCP cannot be performed in Roux-en-Y patients due to the creation of the gastric pouch and exclusion of the biliopancreatic limb. An ERCP may be performed in a bypass patient in multiple ways. A balloon-assisted ERCP allows the endoscope to gain access to the common bile duct via the gastric pouch, the Roux limb, and then retrograde through the biliopancreatic limb. However, this approach is technically very difficult. A laparoscopic-assisted ERCP requires a gastrotomy to be made in the remnant stomach to allow the endoscope to pass into the duodenum. An EUS-directed trans-gastric ERCP is performed by passing a needle from the gastric pouch to the gastric remnant to facilitate biliary stent placement, though there is a significant risk of a persistent gastrogastric fistula following this procedure. If all ERCP techniques are unavailable, percutaneous biliary drainage is an appropriate initial management to provide decompression. Laparoscopic cholecystectomy may be performed, but simultaneous common bile duct exploration should also be performed to provide biliary decompression.

Narula VK, Fung EC, Overby DW, Richardson W, Stefanidis D; SAGES Guidelines Committee. Clinical spotlight review for the management of choledocholithiasis. *Surg Endosc.* 2020;34(4):1482–1491. doi: 10.1007/s00464-020-07462-2. Epub 2020 Feb 24. PMID: 32095952.

Williams E, Beckingham I, El Sayed G, Gurusamy K, Sturgess R, Webster G, Young T. Updated guideline on the management of common bile duct stones (CBDS). *Gut* 2017;**66:**765–782.

García M, Esquivel C, Palermo M. Common bile duct stones after Roux-en-Y gastric bypass: *same issue, different ways to deal with. J Laparoendosc Adv Surg Tech A.* 2020;30(8):900–906. doi: 10.1089/lap.2020.0269. Epub 2020 May 18. PMID: 32423282.

11 *A 45-year-old man with a BMI of 50 kg/m^2 is undergoing an elective laparoscopic ventral hernia repair. She has no additional hypercoagulable risk factors. What is the most appropriate initial postoperative dosing to prevent venous thromboembolism?*

A *Subcutaneous heparin 5000 units every 8 hours*

B *Subcutaneous enoxaparin 40 mg once daily*

C *Subcutaneous enoxaparin 40 mg twice daily*

D *Warfarin 5 mg twice daily*

E *Placement of an inferior vena cava filter*

Answer: C

Obesity is an independent risk factor for venous thromboembolism (VTE). The higher risk of VTE in obese patients is explained by enhanced platelet activity, a procoagulant state due to increased thrombotic factors (including tissue factor, fibrinogen, factor VII, factor VIII, and thrombin), and impaired fibrinolysis. Additional risk factors for VTE in this patient population include a BMI > 40, older age, male sex, obstructive sleep apnea, obesity of hypoventilation syndrome, and a history of VTE. High-dose enoxaparin has been shown to decrease VTE in patients with BMI > 40 undergoing non-bariatric surgery (compared to unfractionated heparin or standard dose enoxaparin), without an increased risk of bleeding complications. Neither warfarin nor an inferior vena cava filter is indicated in this context. Additionally, these patients should receive a preoperative dose of chemoprophylaxis.

Venclauskas L, Maleckas A, Arcelus, JI; for the ESA VTE Guidelines Task Force. European guidelines on perioperative venous thromboembolism prophylaxis. *Eur J Anaesthesiol.* 2018;35(2):147–153. doi: 10.1097/EJA.0000000000000703.

Gould MK, Garcia DA, Wren SM, Karanicolas PJ, Arcelus JI, Heit JA, Samama CM. Prevention of VTE in nonorthopedic surgical patients: antithrombotic therapy and prevention of thrombosis, American college of chest physicians evidence-based clinical practice guidelines. *Chest.* 2012;141(2 Suppl):e227S–e277S. doi: 10.1378/chest.11-2297. Erratum in: Chest. 2012 May;141(5):1369. PMID: 22315263; PMCID: PMC3278061.

12 *A 35-year-old woman presents to the emergency department with severe abdominal pain. The patient had a Roux-en-Y gastric bypass 10 months prior. She reports smoking one pack of cigarettes daily. On exam, she has peritonitis. Chest x-ray reveals air under the diaphragm. What is the most likely diagnosis?*

A *Intussusception at the jejuno-jejunostomy*

B *Perforated marginal ulcer*

C *Incarcerated internal hernia*

D *Obstruction of the gastro-jejunal anastomosis*

E *Candy cane syndrome*

Answer: B

This patient has a perforated marginal ulcer. Marginal ulcers are ulcerations on the jejunal aspect of the gastro-jejunal anastomosis following a Roux-en-Y gastric bypass. Marginal ulcers occur in up to 25% of Roux-en-Y patients. Though ulceration may occur at any time postoperatively, it most commonly occurs within 1 year. Patients are often treated with empiric proton pump inhibitors for 6–12 months to prevent ulceration. Smoking and NSAID use are known risk factors for development of marginal ulcers. Typical presenting symptoms of a nonperforated marginal ulcer include abdominal pain, nausea, anemia, hematemesis, and dysphagia. Standard medical therapy includes 8 weeks of high-dose PPI therapy, with a possible cytoprotective barrier medication such as sucralfate. Patients with ulcers refractory to medical management may require revisional surgery to achieve full mucosal healing.

Perforated marginal ulcers occur in approximately 1–2% of all Roux-en-Y patients. Patients present with acute onset abdominal pain, peritonitis, tachycardia, tachypnea, and fevers. With a high clinical suspicion, free air under the diaphragm on upright chest x-ray is sufficient to confirm diagnosis. The treatment of a perforated marginal ulcer is resuscitation, broad-spectrum antibiotics, and surgical intervention.

Intussusception at the jejuno-jejunostomy and an internal hernia can cause obstruction, ischemia, and free air – but are much less likely than a perforated marginal ulcer. Obstruction of the gastro-jejunostomy can occur from stricture – which stricture is often caused by an associated marginal ulcer. However, the stricture will not cause free air unless a perforation occurs. The so-called Candy cane syndrome occurs when food falls into an excessively long blind jejunal limb at the gastro-jejunostomy causing postprandial pain, bloating, and nausea.

Choi J, Polistena C. (2018) Management of Marginal Ulceration. In: Camacho D., Zundel N. (eds) *Complications in Bariatric Surgery*. Springer, Cham. https://doi.org/10.1007/978-3-319-75841-1_4.

Moon RC, Teixiera AF, Goldbach M, Jawad MA. Management and treatment outcomes of marginal ulcers after Roux-en-Y gastric bypass at a single high volume bariatric center. *Surg Obes Relat Dis*. 2014;10:229–234.

13 *The above patient is given broad-spectrum antibiotics and taken to the operating room. A diagnostic laparoscopy is performed, and a large perforated marginal ulcer with a significant amount of friable tissue at the gastro-jejunal anastomosis is found. The patient is becoming increasingly hypotensive with an increasing pressor requirement. What is the most appropriate surgical management?*

A *Irrigation and wide drainage*

B *Revision of the gastro-jejunal anastomosis*

C *Placement of an omental patch*

D *Creation of an esophago-jejunal anastomosis*

E *Primary repair of the defect*

Answer: A

Operative treatment for a perforated marginal ulcer can be done from a laparoscopic or open approach. The tenets of surgical repair include irrigation and wide drainage, with either primary repair, omental patch repair, or both, depending on the size of the defect. Additionally, placement of a feeding tube in the remnant stomach should be strongly considered. This patient is hemodynamically unstable, and obtaining source control with a definitive repair at a later date is the most appropriate management.

Revision of the gastro-jejunal anastomosis is not advised in the context of a perforation, as it is associated with increased blood loss and operative times. Creation of an esophago-jejunal anastomosis is usually not the best option for the management of a marginal ulcer.

Choi J, Polistena C. (2018) Management of Marginal Ulceration. In: Camacho D., Zundel N. (eds) *Complications in Bariatric Surgery*. Springer, Cham. https://doi.org/10.1007/978-3-319-75841-1_4.

Carr WR, Mahawar KK, Balupuri S, Small PK. An evidence-based algorithm for the management of marginal ulcers following Roux-en-Y gastric bypass. *Obes Surg*. 2014;24(9):1520–1527. doi: 10.1007/s11695-014-1293-z. PMID: 24851857.

14 *A 65-year-old man patient with a BMI 45 has been intubated for several days after aspirating. His chest x-ray shows bilateral pulmonary infiltrates. Arterial blood gas collected while on 70% inhaled oxygen demonstrates a partial pressure of oxygen of 65. Which of the following management options improves this patient's mortality risk?*

A *Positive end-expiratory pressure of 20 cm H_2O*

B *Tidal volume of 6 mL/kg body weight*

C *Trendelenberg position*

D *Discontinue paralyzing agents*

E *Supine positioning*

Answer: A

This patient has severe ARDS, with a P/F ratio < 100. Obese ventilated patients have a higher incidence of

ARDS compared to nonobese patients; however, they have similar mortality risk. The increased thoracic wall weight and increased intra-abdominal pressure due to abdominal fat mass lead to decreased pulmonary compliance and a diminished functional residual capacity. As a result, inadequate PEEP in obese ventilated patients can cause additional atelectrauma, worsening hypoxemia. To optimize end-expiratory lung volume, a PEEP of 18–20 cm H_2O is often required. Titration of PEEP is associated with improved gas exchange and improve 30-day mortality.

Optimal tidal volumes are based on ideal body weight, as opposed to actual body weight. Obese ARDS patients benefit from prone positioning, which allows for more homogenous lung inflation, which can improve V/Q mismatch. Reverse Trendelenberg position has been shown decreased time to vent liberate in this patient population. Neuromuscular blocking agents can improve patient-ventilator synchrony, have been shown to improve oxygenation with lower PEEPs, and to improve mortality. However, prolonged using of these agents is associated with increased risk of diaphragmatic dysfunction.

De Jong A, Verzilli D, Jaber S. ARDS in obese patients: specificities and management. *Crit Care.* 2019;23(1):74. doi: 10.1186/s13054-019-2374-0. PMID: 30850002; PMCID: PMC6408839.

Hibbert K, Rice M, Malhotra A. Obesity and ARDS. *Chest.* 2012;142(3):785–790. doi: 10.1378/chest.12-0117. PMID: 22948584; PMCID: PMC3435141.

Chiumello D, Brioni M. Severe hypoxemia: which strategy to choose. *Crit Care.* 2016;20(1):132. doi: 10.1186/s13054-016-1304-7. PMID: 27255913; PMCID: PMC4891828.

15 *A 35-year-old woman presents to the emergency department complaining of lethargy and dizziness. She had a Roux-en-Y gastric bypass 5 years ago. She denies any abdominal pain. She also denies any melena or hematochezia. Labs reveal a hemoglobin of 8.0 mg/dL. Which associated lab abnormality does this patient likely have?*

A *Increased mean corpuscular volume*
B *Decreased folate levels*
C *Decreased thiamine levels*
D *B12 deficiency*
E *Decreased ferritin levels*

Answer: E

The most likely cause of this patient's anemia is iron deficiency. Up to 58% of Roux-en-Y gastric bypass patients develop postoperative anemia, with up to 90% of these

due to iron deficiency anemia. Reasons for iron deficiency include lack of dietary iron, hypochlorhydria associated with their altered gastric anatomy, which decreases the bioavailability of dietary iron, and bypass of the duodenum and jejunum where a majority of iron absorption occurs. Preoperative risk factors for iron deficiency anemia include preoperative anemia and premenopausal women. Notably, iron deficiency anemia in Roux-en-Y patients is characterized by decreased ferritin levels with normal serum iron levels.

Although Roux-en-Y patients can become deficient in folate, thiamine and B12, these deficiencies are significantly less common than iron deficiency. Deficiency in these nutrients would result in a macrocytic anemia, as opposed to the microcytic anemia found in iron deficiency anemia. Marginal ulcers must also be considered as a cause of anemia in bariatric patients.

Weng TC, Chang CH, Dong YH, Chang YC, Chuang LM. Anaemia and related nutrient deficiencies after Roux-en-Y gastric bypass surgery: a systematic review and meta-analysis. *BMJ Open.* 2015;5(7):e006964. doi: 10.1136/bmjopen-2014-006964. PMID: 26185175; PMCID: PMC4513480.

Engebretsen KV, Blom-Høgestøl IK, Hewitt S, Risstad H, Moum B, Kristinsson JA, Mala T. Anemia following Roux-en-Y gastric bypass for morbid obesity; a 5-year follow-up study. *Scand J Gastroenterol.* 2018;53(8):917–922. doi: 10.1080/00365521.2018.1489892. PMID: 30231804.

Kotkiewicz A, Donaldson K, Dye C, Rogers AM, Mauger D, Kong L, Eyster ME. Anemia and the need for intravenous iron infusion after Roux-en-Y gastric bypass. *Clin Med Insights Blood Disord.* 2015;8:9–17. doi: 10.4137/CMBD.S21825. PMID: 26078589; PMCID: PMC4462165.

McCracken E, Wood GC, Prichard W, Bistrian B, Still C, Gerhard G, Rolston D, Benotti P. Severe anemia after Roux-en-Y gastric bypass: a cause for concern. *Surg Obes Relat Dis.* 2018;14(7):902–909. doi: 10.1016/j.soard.2018.03.026. Epub 2018 Mar 28. PMID: 29735346.

16 *A 45-year-old man presents to the emergency department complaining of severe abdominal pain. He had a duodenal switch performed 3 years ago. On exam, he has a non-reducible incisional hernia with overlying skin changes. Which of the following will be found in the operating room?*

A *A remnant stomach*
B *100 cm common channel*
C *Gastro-ileal anastomosis*
D *50 cm alimentary limb*
E *50 cm biliopancreatic limb*

Answer: B

An understanding of the revisional structure of bariatric surgery is essential for any surgeon who undertakes an abdominal procedure on these patients. Many variations of even the most common bariatric procedures exist. If possible, reviewing the initial bariatric operative report can yield valuable information to a surgeon—such as the lengths of the limbs, the types of anastomoses, and closure of potential spaces.

The traditional biliopancreatic diversion with a duodenal switch combines a sleeve gastrectomy, duodeno-jejunostomy and distal ileo-ileostomy. The ileo-ileostomy is usually performed 100–150 cm proximal to the ileocecal valve, with an alimentary limb of approximately 150 cm – creating a common channel of 100–150 cm in length. A common channel shorter than 100 cm will result in nutritional deficiencies and diarrhea often seen in patients with short gut syndrome. The remnant stomach is removed in the duodenal switch procedure. The biliopancreatic limb is typically not measured when performing the duodenal switch, but would be several hundred centimeter long as the majority of the intestine is bypassed prior to the ileo-ileal anastomosis.

Biertho L, Lebel S, Marceau S, Hould FS, Julien F, Biron S. Biliopancreatic diversion with duodenal switch: surgical technique and perioperative care. *Surg Clin North Am.* 2016;96(4):815–826. doi: 10.1016/j.suc.2016.03.012. PMID: 27473803.

Conner J, Nottingham JM. (2020) Biliopancreatic Diversion With Duodenal Switch. In: *StatPearls [Internet].* StatPearls Publishing, Treasure Island (FL); 2020 Jan–. PMID: 33085340.

Anderson B, Gill RS, de Gara CJ, Karmali S, Gagner M. Biliopancreatic diversion: the effectiveness of duodenal switch and its limitations. *Gastroenterol Res Pract.* 2013;2013:974762. doi: 10.1155/2013/974762. Epub 2013 Nov 21. PMID: 24639868; PMCID: PMC3929999.

Dorman RB, Rasmus NF, Al-Haddad BJ, Serrot FJ, Slusarek BM, Sampson BK, Buchwald H, Leslie DB, Ikramuddin S. Benefits and complications of the duodenal switch/biliopancreatic diversion compared to the Roux-en-Y gastric bypass. *Surgery.* 2012;152(4):758–765; discussion 765-7. doi: 10.1016/j.surg.2012.07.023. Epub 2012 Sep 6. PMID: 22959653.

17 *A 43-year-old woman is one postoperative day from a laparoscopic Roux-en-Y gastric bypass. The nurse calls you to the patient's bedside because she is tachycardic to 120 and hypotensive with a blood pressure of 80/40. On exam, the patient's abdomen is moderately tender. The most recent labs show a decrease in the patient's hemoglobin by 4 g/dL compared to her pre-operative value. VTE prophylaxis is discontinued. She receives 2 units of packed red blood cells without improvement in her blood pressure. What is the most appropriate next step in management?*

A *Evaluation by interventional radiology*
B *Upper endoscopy*
C *Diagnostic laparoscopy*
D *Initiation of vasopressors*
E *Administer 2 additional units of packed red blood cells*

Answer: C

This patient is presenting with postoperative hemorrhage, which typically presents within the first 48 hours postoperatively. After Roux-en-Y gastric bypass, patients may present with intraluminal or extraluminal hemorrhage. Intraluminal hemorrhage typically occurs along a staple line (gastric pouch, gastric remnant, gastrojejunostomy, or jejunojejunostomy) and presenting symptoms include hematemesis, hemoptysis, and melena. Extraluminal bleeding may occur from staple lines, retro-gastric vessels, the short gastric vessels, the omentum, splenic or liver injuries, or trocar sites. Signs and symptoms of postoperative hemorrhage include tachycardia, hypotension, decreased urine output, increased sanguineous drain output, sanguineous drainage from incisional sites, and increased abdominal pain.

Initial management of postoperative hemorrhage in stable patients includes administration of blood products and cessation of chemical DVT prophylaxis agents. An EGD can be considered in stable patients if an intraluminal source is suspected. Any hemodynamic instability mandates prompt surgical exploration to control further hemorrhage.

Vasopressors will not definitively treat a bleeding patient. Interventional radiology will not be able to stop any bleeding at the staple lines and may delay ultimate control of hemorrhage. Giving additional blood will help resuscitate the patient but will not stop the source of bleeding.

Chand B, Prathanvanich P. Critical care management of bariatric surgery complications. *J Intensive Care Med.* 2016;31(8):511–528. doi: 10.1177/0885066615593067. Epub 2015 Jun 25. PMID: 26115959.

Ferreira LE, Song LM, Baron TH. Management of acute postoperative hemorrhage in the bariatric patient. *Gastrointest Endosc Clin N Am.* 2011;21(2):287–294. doi: 10.1016/j.giec.2011.02.002. PMID: 21569980.

18 *A 55-year-old man presents to the emergency department complaining of several days of worsening abdominal pain and erythema. He had a laparoscopic gastric band placed 7 years ago, and had an injection at the*

port site 1 week ago. On exam, there is significant erythema overlying his port site with palpable fluctuance. What is the most appropriate initial management?

A Upper endoscopy
B Incision & drainage of port site abscess with band removal
C Deflation of band
D IV antibiotics
E Conversion to Roux-en-Y gastric bypass

Answer: B

This patient has erosion of his gastric band causing an acute port infection. Late band erosion may be due to high band pressure, band over-inflation, or dietary noncompliance. Symptoms include chronic melena, anemia, and possible weight regain. Exsanguinating hemorrhage may also occur secondary to erosion. Port-site infection is a sequelae of band erosion with bacteria traveling from the gastric lumen to the subcutaneous port. Acute port infection often presents as local inflammation, an abscess or cutaneous fistula. Port-site infection requires urgent surgical drainage.

Upper endoscopy is the best test to evaluate if an erosion is present. Deflation of the band can decrease the band pressure, but does not address the existing erosion. IV antibiotics are appropriate, but antibiotics alone will not clear the port-site infection, which must be done with band removal. Typically, removal of the gastric band and port is performed laparoscopically, with an omental patch placed on the gastric erosion. Conversion to a Roux-en-Y gastric bypass can be considered several months later, if the patient recovers appropriately.

Chand B, Prathanvanich P. Critical care management of bariatric surgery complications. *J Intensive Care Med.* 2016;31(8):511–528. doi: 10.1177/0885066615593067. Epub 2015 Jun 25. PMID: 26115959.
Quadri P, Gonzalez-Heredia R, Masrur M, Sanchez-Johnsen L, Elli EF. Management of laparoscopic adjustable gastric band erosion. *Surg Endosc.* 2017;31(4):1505–1512. doi: 10.1007/s00464-016-5183-4. Epub 2016 Aug 23. PMID: 27553794.

19 A 57-year-old man with a BMI of 60 undergoes laparoscopic Roux-en-Y gastric bypass. The case took 6 hours due to prolonged lysis of adhesions from multiple previous abdominal surgeries. In the PACU, the patient complains of low back and gluteal pain. He has tea-colored urine draining from his Foley catheter. Which of the following tests will confirm the suspected diagnosis?

A EKG
B Urinalysis
C Basic metabolic panel
D Serum creatinine phosphokinase
E Arterial blood gas

Answer: D

This patient developed rhabdomyolysis. Bariatric patients are at risk of developing rhabdomyolysis intraoperatively, particularly in super-obese male patients during procedures that last more than 5 hours. The incidence of rhabdomyolysis is as high as 6% after bariatric surgery, with acute renal failure developing in up to one third of those patients. Patients may complain of lumbar or gluteal discomfort. Diagnosis may be delayed due to postoperative analgesia, late extubation, or pre-existing musculoskeletal symptoms.

A serum creatinine phosphokinase (CPK) elevated five times the normal value is considered a biochemical diagnosis of rhabdomyolysis. Elevation of CPK is the most sensitive diagnostic evidence of muscle injury and is present in 100% of cases of rhabdomyolysis. A basic metabolic panel would show elevations of potassium, creatinine, and BUN; however, these elevations are not specific to rhabdomyolysis. An EKG may show peaked T waves associated with hyperkalemia but does not confirm the diagnosis. A urinalysis will show an elevated urine myoglobin, protein, brown casts, and uric acid crystals. An arterial blood gas may demonstrate hypoxemia (due to myoglobinemia) or metabolic acidosis, but does not confirm the diagnosis of rhabdomyolysis.

Chand B, Prathanvanich P. Critical care management of bariatric surgery complications. *J Intensive Care Med.* 2016;31(8):511–528. doi: 10.1177/0885066615593067. Epub 2015 Jun 25. PMID: 26115959.
Matłok M, Major P, Małczak P, Wysocki M, Hynnekleiv L, Nowak M, Karcz K, Pędziwiatr M, Budzyński A. Reduction of the risk of rhabdomyolysis after bariatric surgery with lower fluid administration in the perioperative period: a cohort study. *Pol Arch Med Wewn.* 2016;126(4):237–242. doi: 10.20452/pamw.3368. Epub 2016 Apr 13. PMID: 27074693.

20 Which of the following is true regarding these essential nutrients?

A Vitamin B_{12} can be stored in the liver for 3–5 years. Additionally, low levels can result in microcytic anemia and neurologic symptoms.
B Folate is mostly absorbed in the ileum, has low body stores, and a deficiency will result in macrocytic anemia.
C The half-life of thiamine is 90 days and acute deficiency can cause life-threatening cardiovascular and neurologic complications.

D *The ferrous form of iron (Fe^{2+}) is primarily absorbed, while the ferric form (Fe^{3+}) is the primary form found in foods. Fe^{3+} must be reduced to Fe^{2+} by acid for absorption.*

E *Calcium absorption is enhanced by calcitriol and it is primarily absorbed in the terminal ileum.*

Answer: D

Bariatric patients are prone to several nutritional deficiencies secondary to the rearrangement of normal intestinal anatomy. Understanding the physiology of these deficiencies will aide in caring for any critical care patient.

Vitamin B_{12} is stored in the liver for 3–5 years. Low levels can result in macrocytic anemia and neurologic symptoms. Bariatric patients are prone to a deficiency secondary to lack of intrinsic factor, hydrochloric acid, and decreased dietary intake of foods rich in vitamin B_{12}. Vitamin B_{12} is absorbed in the terminal ileum.

Folate is primarily absorbed in the duodenum and jejunum. Like vitamin B_{12}, low levels of folate will result in macrocytic anemia. Unlike vitamin B_{12}, very low levels of folate are stored in the body and constant intake is needed to maintain sufficient levels.

Thiamine has a short half-life (around 10–20 days) and is primarily absorbed in the duodenum and proximal jejunum. As with alcoholics, any bariatric patient presenting to the hospital with poor oral intake should be given thiamine, as an acute deficiency case result in life-threatening complications.

Iron deficiency in bariatric patients can result from a decreased intake of iron-rich foods, decreased gastric acid (which converts Fe^{3+} to the absorbable Fe^{2+}), and a bypass of the proximal intestines where iron is primarily absorbed.

Active absorption of calcium occurs primarily in the duodenum and proximal jejunum. Its absorption is enhanced by calcitriol – an active form of vitamin D (1,2 5-dihydroxycholecalciferol).

Bronner F, Pansu D. Nutritional aspects of calcium absorption. *J Nutr.* 1999;**129**(1):9–12

Aills L, Blankenship J, Buffington C, Furtado M, Parrott J. ASMBS allied health nutritional guidelines for the surgical weight loss patient. *Surg Obes Relat Dis.* 2008;**4**(5 Suppl):S73–S108.

43

Burns, Inhalational Injury, and Lightning Injury

MAJ Jacob Swann, MD and William Mohr, III, MD

Regions Hospital, Saint Paul, MN, USA

1 *A 26-year-old petroleum engineer presents after suffering burns from an explosion at his worksite. The patient has a mixture of burns over his body as follows: superficial burns to the anterior half of his face, superficial partial thickness burns of the anterior chest, deep partial thickness burns of the anterior bilateral lower extremities, and full thickness burns of the right upper extremity circumferentially. What percentage of the patient's total body surface area is burned?*

   A *9%*
   B *18%*
   C *27%*
   D *45%*
   E *54%*

Calculating total body surface area (TBSA) for burns is critical to adequate resuscitation following injury. TBSA involvement dictates whether a patient needs intravenous (IV) fluid resuscitation, protocolized resuscitation via a burn formula (e.g. the Parkland formula, USAISR calculator, or Burn Navigator system), and acts as a guide for severity of injury. Calculation of TBSA is performed by using the "rule of nines."

Chest: 18%
Back: 18%
Right upper extremity (RUE): 9%
Left upper extremity (LUE): 9%
Right lower extremity (RLE): 18%
Left lower extremity (LLE): 18%
Head: 9%
Perineum: 1%

Only superficial partial thickness, deep partial thickness, and full thickness burns are counted in the "rule of 9s." Red skin that is not blistered (i.e. superficial burns) are not counted. For burns that don't encompass the whole 9% allotted, a provider measures the palmer surface of the patient's hand and uses this size as an estimate of 1% TBSA.

In our stem, the patient has superficial burns of the anterior half of the face (0% TBSA), superficial partial thickness burns of the anterior chest (18% TBSA), deep partial thickness burns of the anterior BLE (9% on the RLE and 9% on the LLE), and circumferential full thickness burns of the RUE (9% TBSA). Therefore, the patient has 0 + 18 + 9 + 9 + 9 = 45% TBSA.

Answer: D

Pham TN, et al. *Advanced Burn Life Support Course: Provider Manual 2018 Update.* Chicago, IL. American Burn Association. 2018.

2 *A 64-year-old woman presents after suffering a scald injury. The patient was boiling water to cook pasta with and she slipped, fell, and spilled the boiling water on herself. Her trauma survey is negative for any associated traumatic injury. On evaluation, she has mixed superficial partial thickness, deep partial thickness, and scattered areas of full thickness burns to her chest, back, and BLE for a total involved TBSA of 40%. Her body weight is 100 kg. What should her initial IV fluid rate be?*

   A *500 mL/h of LR*
   B *1000 mL/h of NS*
   C *1500 mL/h of LR*
   D *2000 mL/h of NS*
   E *2000 mL/h of LR*

Patients with large TBSA burns (>20%) require IV fluid resuscitation and choosing an initial fluid type and rate is critical. The systemic inflammatory response leads to systemic capillary leakage and loss of vascular oncotic pressure. Interstitial edema causes changes in the structural proteins leading to less resistance to further edema. Both under- and over-resuscitation of burns can promote conversion of partial thickness burns to full thickness burns, burn shock, and end-organ damage. Anasarca can result in extremity and abdominal compartment syndrome with mortality rates as high as 80% in burn patients.

Major burn resuscitation will require large volumes of crystalloid fluid. The important difference between LR and NS is the chloride content; LR has 109 mEq/L, while NS has 154 mEq/L. Even 3–5 L of NS can produce hyperchloremic metabolic acidosis, as bicarbonate shifts intracellularly to maintain electric neutrality throughout the body. Due to the large volumes needed in burn resuscitation, NS is contraindicated due to the high risk of developing a hyperchloremic metabolic acidosis compromising the patient's likely strained metabolic status. LR is the preferred resuscitation formula for this patient. Thus, answers B and D are incorrect.

The calculation of the initial fluid rates for burned patients is a topic of debate. But recently the American Burn Association (ABA) has endorsed a consensus formula utilizing the most beneficial aspects of the Parkland and modified Brooke formulae. This formula is now taught in both the Advanced Burn Life Support and Advanced Trauma Life Support programs. The ABA formula uses the patient's body weight and TBSA to estimate their 24-hour fluid requirement with the starting rate half of the traditional Parkland formula: Initial rate = 2 mL/hr * body weight in kg * TBSA divided by 16. This is because the physiologic fluid requirements are not linear with time; they create a Bell-shaped curve that is shifted toward the early resuscitation period making more volume needed up front than at the end of the initial 24-hour resuscitation period. Burn patients need roughly half of their resuscitation volume over an 8-hour period between hours 4 and 12 postburn.

In our example, the patient's body weight is 100 kg and TBSA is 40%. The initial fluid rate is:

$$2 * 100 \text{ kg} * 40 = 8000 \text{ mL as the estimated}$$
$$\text{24-hour fluid requirement.}$$

8 L/16 (this is half of the volume divided by 8 per the initial Parkland calculation) is 500 mL/h as the starting rate. Although older teaching tried to make up or reduce fluid rates based upon volumes given prior to admission, the capillary fluid loss does not allow for fluid already given or not given to be made up or carried forward. For instance, you cannot give our patient 8 L over 4 hours and expect them to not need further fluids for the next 4 hours. In our patient, the volume of resuscitation was 500 mL/h and would not change your calculations.

Answer: A

Greenhalgh DG. Burn resuscitation: the results of the ISBI/ABA survey. *Burns*. 2010; 36 (2): 176–182.

Pham TN, et al. *Advanced Burn Life Support Course: Provider Manual 2018 Update*. Chicago, IL. American Burn Association. 2018.

3 *You are the on-call surgical intensivist at a geographically remote level 2 trauma center. The nearest ABA accredited burn center is several hours away. A 42-year-old farmer presents to your emergency room after suffering a 62% TBSA flame burn to his chest, back, BUE, and BLE from a fire on his farm. You initiate IVF resuscitation. You call the regional burn center who accepts the patient for transfer; however, the weather prohibits aeromedical evacuation for the next several hours. While waiting for transport, what is the best marker for adequacy of fluid resuscitation in this patient?*
   A *Urine output*
   B *Base deficit*
   C *Serum lactate*
   D *Blood pressure*
   E *Tachycardia*

End-markers of resuscitation can be misleading during burn resuscitation in that traditional markers can be normal or improved from presentation while total body volume status is relatively low. When inadequate resuscitation occurs, partial thickness burns can convert to deep burns. Moreover, burn shock can occur due to progressive third-space fluid sequestration later in the course of the initial burn resuscitation. Conversely, over-resuscitation also leads to downstream consequences with development of abdominal compartment syndrome, conversion of partial thickness burns to deep burns, and anasarca. Given this, it is important to achieve appropriate resuscitation without over- or under-resuscitating.

Tachycardia can be elevated persistently due to pain from burns and—if used to guide resuscitation—could lead to over-resuscitation as fluid rates are increased in the face of a heart rate that is not responding to expanded intravascular volumes. Similarly, blood pressure can often be maintained early in a resuscitation even if inadequate resuscitation is initiated. It is not until burn shock develops 24–48 hours after presentation that blood pressure issues will likely arise. Serum lactate can be elevated for many reasons in a burn patient (i.e. carbon monoxide poisoning, cyanide toxicity, burn shock); therefore, normalization of the lactate should not be used to determine if a patient is adequately resuscitated. Moreover, trending lactates on an hourly basis to guide IV fluid resuscitation rates is not supported by the American Burn Association or Advanced Burn Life Support. For similar reasons, normalization of the base deficit is not appropriate to guide adequacy of resuscitation as this may be falsely elevated from pathologies that have nothing to do with the patient's fluid status. Similarly, a normal base deficit should not prompt decreasing IV fluid rates. As such, these traditional end-point markers used in other ICUs to guide resuscitation are inadequate or inappropriate to use for hourly titration of fluid resuscitation. Urine output (UOP) of 0.5 mL/kg/hr is the most sensitive and appropriate end point to guide resuscitation. UOP should be followed hourly, and IVF titrated based on UOP.

Answer: A

Guilabert P, Usua G, Matin N, et al. Fluid resuscitation management in patients with burns: update. British Journal of Anaesthesia. 2016; 117 (3): 284–296.

Pham TN, Cancio LC, and Gibran NS. "American burn association practice guidelines burn shock resuscitation. *Journal of Burn Care and Research.* 2008; 29 (1): 257–266.

4   *A 36-year-old man presents to the emergency department after EMS removed them from a house fire. The patient suffered a 38% TBSA thermal burn to his posterior trunk and posterior aspects of all extremities. On initial evaluation in the emergency room, the patient has altered mental status with a GCS of 11, a cough productive of carbonaceous sputum, a hoarse voice, and diffuse bilateral wheezing appreciated on auscultation. Which of the following is an appropriate step in management in the first 24 hours of resuscitation after burn injury?*

   A   *Open tracheostomy*
   B   *Increasing IV fluid resuscitation beyond what is calculated by the Parkland formula*
   C   *Using high-flow nasal cannula in lieu of intubation*
   D   *Intubation with low tidal volume ventilation to assist with secretion evacuation*
   E   *Initiation of systemic corticosteroids*

The patient presents following a house fire with prolonged extraction from the building and has suffered an inhalational injury. Edema of the upper airways and vocal cords causes the hoarse voice. Carbonaceous sputum is due to inhalation of particulate matter from incompletely burned materials. This matter builds in the lower airways causing copious amounts of secretions. Wheezing is consistent with mucus narrowing the bronchioles of the lower airways. Lastly, incomplete combustion of carbon and nitrogen-based materials produce carbon monoxide, hydrogen cyanide, and other toxic gases. With exposure to these gases, patients develop altered mental status due to poor oxygen delivery and utilization within the cells of the central nervous system demonstrated by altered mental status.

With a clinical diagnosis of inhalational injury producing symptoms of respiratory distress, proceeding with intubation is most appropriate for this patient. Performing a tracheostomy within 24 hours is not appropriate at this time. In a recent survey of burn centers, the average time to tracheostomy was approximately 2 weeks. Some patients with severe head and neck burns will progress more quickly to a surgical airway, but this patient has none of these indications. There is no role for systemic corticosteroids in the treatment of inhalational injury. While data on the optimal ventilator management of burned and inhalation injury patients is limited, consensus across burn centers is to use ARDSNet-style ventilation with low tidal volumes (LTV) to limit ventilator-associated lung injury. It is important to note that, due to fibrin casts, extensive chest wall thermal injuries, or high volumes of fluid resuscitation, LTV strategies can be ineffective in the burn population. After suffering an inhalational injury, patients will require a large volume of resuscitation in their initial hospital course. While some patients with smoke inhalation require increased fluid volumes, targeting 0.3–0.5 mL/kg/hr of urine output remains the goal in these patients. The surgical intensivist should be aware that the amount of IV fluids may exceed that predicted by standard formula in these patients.

Answer: D

Dries DJ and Endorf FW. Inhalation injury: epidemiology, pathology, and treatment strategies. *Scandanavian Journal of Trauma, Resuscitation, and Emergency Medicine.* 2013; 21: 31–46.

Chung KK, et al. A survey of mechanical ventilator practices across burn centers in North America. *Journal of Burn Care and Research.* 2016; 37: e131–e139.

Walker PF, et al. Diagnosis and management of inhalation injury: an updated review. *Critical Care.* 2015; 19: 351–363.

5   *A 72-year-old woman is brought into the emergency room after being involved in a house fire. The patient suffered a 38% TBSA burn while smoking in bed. The patient was unable to self-extricate from the house, but firefighters were able to remove her from the house. She was intubated in the field due to altered mental status with a Glasgow Coma Scale of 6. On arrival, she is intubated, has copious soot-colored secretions, has flushed red skin diffusely including skin that is not burned, is hypotensive, and bradycardic. Appropriate support lines, IVF, labs, and a chest x-ray are obtained. The x-ray shows appropriately placed support lines. The laboratory workup is significant as follows:*

pH: 6.9
PaO_2: 280
$PaCO_2$: 30

HCO₃⁻: 12

HCO_3^-: 12
Lactate: 16

What is the most appropriate treatment for her acidosis?
A *Increase LR resuscitation rate*
B *Change IVF from LR to bicarbonate infusion*
C *Increase respiratory rate*
D *Emergent hemodialysis*
E *Hydroxycobalamin*

Cyanide toxicity is an uncommon presenting issue outside of industrial accidents, wartime casualties, and house fires. Cyanide is liberated from nitrogen-containing polymers when ignited; both natural (wool, silk, paper) and synthetic (nylon, polyvinyl chloride) sources can release cyanide. Cyanide causes cellular asphyxia by blocking the electron transport chain in the mitochondria of the cells, preventing oxidative phosphorylation with resultant anaerobic metabolism throughout the body. This causes a markedly elevated lactate and glucose resulting in profound metabolic acidosis. Urgent reversal of this is required to restart ATP generation. High-dose hydroxycobalamin is the preferred agent to correct this. The dosing is 5 mg of hydroxycobalamin IV, and it may be repeated once. Less preferred agents are sodium thiosulfate or sodium nitrite.

Increasing the LR infusion rate, changing LR to bicarbonate, increasing the respiratory rate, or starting hemodialysis will not affect the root cause of the patient's metabolic acidosis.

Answer: E

MacLennan L and Moiemen N. Management of cyanide toxicity in patients with burns. *Burns.* 2015; 41 (1): 18–24.

Walker PF, et al. Diagnosis and management of inhalation injury: an updated review. *Critical Care.* 2015; 19: 351–363.

Anseeuw K, Delvau N, Burillo-Putze G, et al. Cyanide poisoning by fire smoke inhalation: a European expert consensus. *European Journal of Emergency Medicine.* 2013; **20** (1): 2–9.

Mintegi S, Clerigue, N, Tipo, V, et al. Pediatric sign poisoning by fire smoke in elation: a European expert consensus. *Pediatric Emergency Care.* 2013; **29** (11): 1234–1240.

6 *A 22-year-old woman presents to the emergency room after being involved in a house fire. At the scene, the patient crawled out of the house and suffered no thermal injuries. However, the patient reports having a significant headache. On exam, the patient's vital signs are normal. Pulse oximetry is 100% on RA. Physical exam shows faint wheezing in the lower*

airways, a slight cough, and diffuse hyperemia of the skin with a flushed appearance of all visualized dermatomes. What is the next most appropriate step in management of this patient?
A *Discharge from the emergency room*
B *Application of 100% FiO₂ via nonrebreather mask*
C *Chest x-ray*
D *Treatment with an albuterol inhaler*
E *IV fluid resuscitation*

Carbon monoxide poisoning is common after being involved in a fire in a confined space, and it is a by-product of incomplete combustion of organic products. This odorless, colorless gas binds to the heme subunit of the hemoglobin molecule at a much higher affinity than oxygen (200x stronger) forming carboxyhemoglobin (COHb) leading to poor oxygen delivery to end-organs. Moreover, when carbon monoxide binds to the heme molecule, it causes a conformational change to the heme molecule making it appear bright red when exposed to light. Thus, a pulse oximeter may read 100% saturated but will falsely estimate oxygen content carried in these patients. This patient presents with classic findings of carbon monoxide poisoning: namely, the patient has a red appearance, is complaining of CNS symptoms (headache), and has some findings concerning for exposure to this gas (cough, wheezing, and involvement in a house fire).

Treatment for carbon monoxide poisoning requires application of 100% oxygen to competitively displace carbon monoxide off of the hemoglobin molecules. Mild intoxication (COHb levels of 10–30%) present with symptoms such as headache, nausea, vomiting, and visual complaints. More severe intoxication (>30%) can present with syncope, coma, and cardiovascular collapse. Some research on hyperbaric oxygen therapy (HBO) has been performed to assess if there is a role in HBO use for carbon monoxide poisoning. HBO can more rapidly eliminate CO with the added atmospheres of pressure delivered to the patient, but HBO use requires specialized centers. Delays in secondary transport from a burn center to a dive chamber typically negates the elimination advantage. Meta-analysis has not shown a benefit for HBO with smoke inhalation patients.

For this question, discharge is clearly inappropriate as the patient warrants treatment of their COHb given their CNS symptoms. A chest x-ray would not be necessary to aid in making the diagnosis, and it is not the next most appropriate step as increasing the pO₂ for the patient. While bronchodilators may assist with their airway symptoms, this will not improve COHb clearance. The patient does not have any burned tissue; starting IV fluids is likely unnecessary and not the next best step in management of this patient.

Answer: B

Ekhbaatar P, Sousse LE, Cox R, Herndon DN et al. "Chapter 16: The Pathophysiology of Inhalation Injury." In David Herndon *Total Burn Care*, 5th Edition. Elsevier, 2018.

7   *A 53-year-old man suffers a 22% TBSA scald burn to the back and BLE after slipping and falling while carrying a pot of boiling water. He presents to an emergency room where he is treated with local wound debridement and application of a topical antibiotic. He then is transferred to his local burn center for definitive care. The topical antibiotic agent is continued. On hospital day 6, he is noted to have developed a significant metabolic acidosis. Which of the following topical antibiotics is the most likely causative agent for the metabolic acidosis?*
   A *Silver sulfadiazine*
   B *Silver nitrate*
   C *Mafenide acetate*
   D *Hypochlorous acid*
   E *Bacitracin + neomycin + polymyxin B*

Topical antibiotics are a mainstay of burn treatment. Key to preparing wounds for skin grafting is keeping the bacterial count low so that the bacteria do not damage subsequent grafts. Using topical agents is done routinely in burn care. While side effects from topical agents are rare, they are classic questions that are often asked about on in-service and certifying examinations.

For this clinical presentation, the most likely agent is mafenide acetate. This antibiotic has excellent coverage of gram-negative and gram-positive bacteria, as well as good eschar penetration. However, it can cause discomfort with application. Moreover, mafenide acts as a carbonic anhydrase inhibitor putting the patient at risk for development of a metabolic acidosis in a dose-dependent manner (amount and time of exposure).

Answer: C

Church D, Elsayed S, Reid O, et al. Burn wound infections. *Clinical Microbiology Reviews*. 2006; 19 (2): 403–434.

Liebman PR, Kennelly MM, and Hirsch EF. Hypercarbia and acidosis associated with carbonic anhydrase inhibition: a hazard of topical mafenide acetate use in renal failure. *Burns Including Thermal Injury*. 1982; 8 (6): 395–398.

White MG, Asch MJ. Acid-base effects of topical mafenide acetate in the burned patient. *New England Journal of Medicine*. 1971; 284 (23): 1281–1286.

Cambiaso-Daniel J, Gallagher JJ, Norbury WB, et al. "Chapter 11: Treatment of Infection in Burn Patients."

Total Burn Care, 5th Edition. Edited by Herndon D. Elsevier, 2018, pp. 93–113.

8   *A 48-year-old homeless man presents to the emergency room with 12% TBSA of the BLE. The patient was acutely intoxicated, and he fell asleep by a fire. Subsequently, his pant legs caught fire. The patient woke up later, and they came to the emergency room for evaluation. On exam, the patient's burns are mostly deep partial thickness and full thickness burns. The patient is admitted, resuscitated, and placed on a topical antibiotic. On a routine daily CBC, the patient is noted to have a WBC of $500/mm^3$. On review of previous lab tests, the patient is noted to have had a gentle decrease in his WBC over the previous several days. Which of the following antibiotics is most likely the cause of the patient's leukopenia?*
   A *Silver sulfadiazine*
   B *Silver nitrate*
   C *Mafenide acetate*
   D *Hypochlorous acid*
   E *Bacitracin + neomycin + polymyxin B*

Leukopenia is associated with silver sulfadiazine. While the incidence of leukopenia is quite low, the degree of leukopenia can be startling as in this clinical scenario. Risk of leukopenia occurring appears to be a dose-dependent response with longer periods of use, as well as larger amounts of silver sulfadiazine being used. When leukopenia occurs (defined by WBC less than normal for the institution's laboratory reference range), it does not put the patient at an increased risk of infection. Moreover, a change in antibiotic therapy is often not required.

Answer: A

Greenhalgh DG. Topical antimicrobial agents for burn wounds. *Clinics in Plastic Surgery*. 2009; 36 (4): 597–606.

Choban PS and Marshall WJ. Leukopenia secondary to silver sulfadiazine: frequency, characteristics and clinical consequences. *The American Surgeon*. 1987; 53 (9): 515–517.

Cambiaso-Daniel J, Gallagher JJ, Norbury WB, et al. "Chapter 11: Treatment of Infection in Burn Patients." *Total Burn Care*, 5th Edition. Edited by Herndon D. Elsevier, 2018, pp. 93–113.

9   *A 25-year-old man is admitted for a necrotizing soft tissue infection of his left lower extremity. Serial operative debridements are needed to obtain definitive surgical source control. The total TBSA of the involved wound is approximately 14%. The patient undergoes*

skin grafting with a 3:1 meshed split thickness skin graft for reconstruction. Approximately 1 week after skin grafting, hyper-granulation tissue is noted to be forming in the interstices of the skin graft. Also, there are some areas of skin graft loss noted near the areas of hyper-granulation with associated biofilm concerning for a bacterial infection. The patient is put in a topical antibiotic solution to treat for the presumptive wound infection, as well as to aid in the treatment of the hyper-granulation tissue. On a routine lab check 3 days later, the patient is noted to have hyponatremia and hypochloremia ($Na^+ = 129$ and $Cl^- = 88$). Which of the following topical antibiotics is associated with the laboratory abnormalities noted above?

A Silver sulfadiazine

B Silver nitrate

C Mafenide acetate

D Hypochlorous acid

E Bacitracin + neomycin + polymyxin B

Multiple topical antibiotic solutions can cause electrolyte disturbances. In this case, the patient has been treated with silver nitrate solution. Silver nitrate acts as a topical antibiotic and aids in microscopic source control of the wound bed. Moreover, silver nitrate assists in decreasing hyper-granulation tissue height due to desiccation of the edematous tissues allowing for the tissue to flatten and smooth out. This allows for improved filling of the wound interstices and a flatter, more functional, and more cosmetic wound bed. However, a known side effect of silver nitrate is direct chelation of sodium and chloride from the tissues. When using this antibiotic, it is important to obtain serial laboratory tests to monitor these levels while the solution is in use.

Answer: B

Greenhalgh DG. Topical antimicrobial agents for burn wounds. *Clinics in Plastic Surgery*. 2009; 36 (4): 597–606.

Cambiaso-Daniel J, Gallagher JJ, Norbury WB, et al. "Chapter 11: Treatment of Infection in Burn Patients." *Total Burn Care*, 5th Edition. Edited by Herndon D. Elsevier, 2018, pp. 93–113.

10 Five burn patients present to a rural emergency department during the same shift. A verified ABA regional burn center is available to transfer the patients that meet ABA burn center referral. Of these patients, which one can be treated locally?

A 22-year-old patient with a 8% TBSA flame burn of the BLE that spares the joints

B 6-year-old patient with a 4% TBSA scald burn to the bilateral feet

C 82-year-old patient with ESRD, DM2, and COPD with a 2% TBSA flame burn to the RUE

D 44-year-old patient with a 3% TBSA acid chemical burn to the chest

E 32-year-old patient with a 6% TBSA electrical burn to the RUE and LLE

ABA burn referral criteria is critical for appropriate triage of patients. Patients who meet burn center referral criteria are best suited to receive definitive care at burn centers. At a burn center, patients can have a large, specialized, multidisciplinary care team provide their care in a more efficient manner than can often be delivered in non-burn centers. The specialized wound care, initial resuscitation, burn nursing, psychologic support, and intensive physical therapy (PT) and occupational therapy (OT) requirements all create an environment where complex burns require care at a burn center. However, for patients with minor burns that can be treated locally should be treated locally as over-utilization of referrals to burn centers because added strain on the burn center for resources and personnel, added healthcare costs to the patient and safety net programs, and added discomfort and imposition on the patient and their families.

That said, a good guiding principle is that complex or uncommon burns are best served at a burn center. Thus, complex burns that are large (>10% TBSA), involve sensitive areas (face, joints, genitals, hands, feet), occur at the extremes of age (elderly and children), or that are medically complex (multiple comorbidities, significant underlying psychiatric disease) all warrant referral to a burn center. Similarly, uncommon mechanisms of burn injury often require specialized burn care; chemical burns (acid and base), electrical burns, burns associated with an inhalational injury, or burns that will cause extensive rehabilitation requirements also all require transfer to an ABA burn center.

Of the patients above, only the first patient should be treated locally. Their burn is small, they have no medical comorbidities, and their burns spare the joints. The second patient – while having a small burn – cannot be treated locally as no inpatient pediatric support is available. The third patient has multiple comorbidities and – even though their burns are small – referral to the local burn center is appropriate. The fourth patient warrants referral as does the fifth patient as their mechanisms of injury (chemical/electrical burns) require additional specialty care that is best done in a high-volume center.

Answer: A

American Burn Association. (2006). "Burn Center Referral Criteria." https://ameriburn.org/public-resources/burn-center-referral-criteria/. Accessed 7 FEB 2021.

11 *Which of the following statements is true about early excision and grafting?*

   A *Results in increased blood loss but decreased mortality*

   B *Results in decreased scar formation but increased metabolic rate*

   C *Results in decreased risk of systemic sepsis but increased overall risk of infection*

   D *Results in increased mortality but decreased hospital length of stay*

   E *Complete excision is beneficial but should be avoided within 24 hours postburn*

A meta-analysis of randomized controlled trials evaluating early excision of burn injuries found a significant reduction in mortality and decreased hospital length of stay. Individual studies have shown that early excision results in improved rates of early wound coverage, decreased metabolic demands, and reduction in the rate of sepsis. Reduced risk of burn-wound infection was seen in children but not in adults. There is no evidence that the early excision and coverage technique results in improved cosmetic outcomes. Complete excision within 24 hours has been demonstrated to be safe and effective in adults and children.

Answer: A

Sheridan RL and Chang P. Acute burn procedures. *Surgical Clinics of North America*. 2014; 94 (4): 755–764.

Ong YS, Samuel M, Song C. Meta-analysis of early decision of burns. *Burns*. 2005; 32 (2): 145–150.

Moussa A, Lo CH, and Cleland H. Burn wound excision within 24 h: a 9-year review. *Burns*. 2020; S0305-4179 (20): 30642.

12 *Burn patients with blood stream infections due to Pseudomonas aeruginosa are most commonly associated with?*

   A *Central venous catheters*

   B *Patient age > 65 years*

   C *Concurrent pneumonia with P. aeruginosa*

   D *Burn wound infection*

   E *Diabetes mellitus*

Bloodstream infections occur in 3–12% of burn patients, is associated with inhalation injury, and has a 13–36% reported mortality. Early infections (<7 days) were mostly due to methicillin-resistant *Staphylococcus aureus*. While *P. aeruginosa* bacteremia tends to develop later in the hospital course, it is frequently drug-resistant (86% after 30 days), and it has the highest mortality rate for any organism. Overall, catheter-associated (36%), bloodstream (25%), and urinary tract (24%) act as the predominate sources for bacteremia in burn patients. Although the respiratory tract is a much less frequent (3%) source, most *P. aeruginosa* bacteremia events occur with a concurrent *P. aeruginosa* pneumonia.

Answer: C

Sousa D, Ceniceros A, Galeiras R, et al. Microbiology in *burn patients with bloodstream infections colon trends over time and during the course of hospitalization. Infectious Diseases*. 2018; **50** (4): 289–296.

Patel BM, Paratz JD, Mallet A, et al. Characteristics of bloodstream infections in burn patients: an 11-year retrospective study. *Burns*. 2012; **38** (5): 685–690.

13 *Which of these statements about 24-hour volume of resuscitation in burn patients are true?*

   A *The use of IV narcotic and sedation infusions result in decreased fluid volume.*

   B *Over-estimation of burn size does not alter the total fluid volume.*

   C *Delay in transport of patients to burn centers does not alter the total fluid volume.*

   D *The use of crystalloid boluses for low urine output increases total fluid volume.*

   E *The use of goal-directed fluid therapy using $ScVO_2$ decreases fluid volume.*

As narcotic and sedative medications tend to cause vasodilation, a significant association has been shown between opioid dosages and escalating fluid requirements. Over-estimation of the burn size is common and results in increased fluid administration, especially in children, where it occurs in almost 60% of patients. Patients who have a delay in resuscitation typically require more fluid and have increased rates of complications. The use of goal-directed therapies have been shown to increase the volume of resuscitation. Bolus administration is advocated for treatment for hypotension or to correct a known volume deficit (i.e. blood loss) but not to correct low urine output as it will contribute more to tissue edema due to the profound capillary leak from the patient's burns without improving the patient's resuscitation.

Answer: D

Cancio LC, Bohanon FJ, and Kramer GC. "Burn Resuscitation." *Total Burn Care*, 5th edition. Edited by Herndon D. Elsevier, Chicago, 2018, pp. 77–86.

Goverman J, Bittner EA, and Friedstat JS, et al. Discrepancy in initial pediatric burn estimates and its impact on fluid resuscitation. *Journal of Burn Care and Research*. 2015; 36 (5): 574–579.

Malbrain ML, Langer T, Annane D, et al. Intravenous fluid therapy in the preoperative and critical care setting:

executive summary of the International Fluid Academy (IFA). *Annals Intensive Care.* 2020; 10 (64): 1–19.

14 *Which is the correct statement about smoke inhalation injury?*

    A *Direct heat injury to the alveoli is the most common pathology.*

    B *A normal CXR and gas exchange on admission effectively rules out an inhalation injury.*

    C *A PaO_2:FiO_2 ratio of < 350 correlates with increased fluid requirements.*

    D *SpO_2 decreases as the CO levels increase.*

    E *Fibrin deposition in the alveolar space is rare.*

With rare exceptions such as inhalation of steam, the injury to the airway is usually from chemicals in the smoke and not heat, as the bronchial circulation is very efficient in regulating the temperature of inhaled gases. A normal chest x-ray and gas exchange on admission do not rule out a significant inhalation injury. A P:F ratio of less than 350 has been shown to be a reliable predictor of increased fluid requirements with smoke inhalation. The inability to differentiate oxyhemoglobin from carboxyhemoglobin limits the use of the standard pulse oximeter (SpO_2), although a co-oximetry monitoring device can give a COHb level. Protein-rich exudate is the response to the airway inflammatory response resulting in fibrin casts, necrotic debris, and loss of surfactant.

Answer: C

Enkhbaatar P, Sousse LE, Cox R, Herndon DN. "The Pathophysiology of Inhalation Injury." In David Herndon *Total Burn Care*, 5th Edition. Edited by Herndon D. Elsevier, Chicago. 2018, pp. 174–83.

Endorf FW and Gamelli RL Inhalation injury, pulmonary perturbations, and fluid resuscitation. *Journal of Burn Care Research.* 2007; **28** (1): 80–83.

15 *Which statement regarding red blood cell transfusions in burn patients is true?*

    A *Transfusion triggers are higher in burn patients due to the 60% decrease in microcirculation in the skin.*

    B *Patients are more likely to have a myocardial event with a hemoglobin of 8 versus a level of 10.*

    C *Increased red cell transfusions decrease the rate of acute respiratory distress syndrome.*

    D *Patients transfused at a hemoglobin of 7 versus a level of 10 have longer healing times and length of stay.*

    E *Compared to a 4:1 ratio of RBC to FFP, a 1:1 ratio results in decreased red cell transfusions.*

The red cell flow in the microcirculation after burn is reduced by 60% compared to unburned skin but is unrelated to transfusion indications. A multicenter randomized trial of large burns (≥20% TBSA) reported that a restrictive transfusion protocol (hemoglobin ≤ 7 gm/dL) compared to a liberal protocol (hemoglobin ≤ 10 gm/dL) demonstrated no difference in mortality, cardiac complications, bloodstream infections, ventilator days, or time to wound healing. There is a well-defined relationship between increasing blood transfusions and the development of acute respiratory distress syndrome in burn patients. A prospective randomized trial of 4:1 versus 1:1 ratio of packed red blood cells to fresh frozen plasma performed in burn patients undergoing early excision and skin grafting showed a 1:1 ratio resulted in lower red cell transfusion volumes and was as safe as a 4:1 ratio.

Answer: E

Wolf SE, Sterling JP, Hunt JL, et al. The year in burns 2010. *Burns.* 2011; 37 (8): 1–13.

Palmieri TL, Holmes JH, Arnoldo B, et al. Transfusion requirement in burn care evaluation (TRIBE): a multicenter randomized prospective trial of blood transfusion in major burn injury. *Annals of Surgery.* 2017; 266 (4): 595–602.

Dries DJ. Key questions in ventilator management of the burn-injured patient (first of two parts). *Journal of Burn Care and Resuscitation.* 2009; 30 (1): 128–138.

Palmieri TL, Greenhalgh DG, and Sen S. Prospective comparison of packed red blood cell-to-fresh frozen plasma transfusion ratio of 4:1 versus 1:1 during acute massive burn excision. *Journal of Trauma and Acute Care Surgery.* 2013; 74 (1): 76–83.

16 *Which statement regarding electrical injury and the heart is true?*

    A *The most common cause of death is hyperkalemia-induced cardiac arrest.*

    B *Non-specific ST changes are uncommon abnormalities noted on initial ECG.*

    C *Atrial fibrillation is the most common dysrhythmia*

    D *Ventricular fibrillation is the most common late (>24 hours after injury) fatal arrhythmia.*

    E *Asystole is the most common fatal arrhythmia in high-voltage injuries.*

The most frequent reason for death after electrical injury is cardiac pathology. Nonspecific ST changes are the most common ECG abnormality, and atrial fibrillation is the most common dysrhythmia. However, ventricular fibrillation is the most common cause of death at the scene of injury. Asystole is seen with high-voltage injuries and lightning strikes.

Answer: E

Bernal E and Arnoldo BD. "Electrical Injuries." *Total Burn Care*, 5th Edition. Edited by Herndon D. Elsevier, Chicago, 2018. pp. 396–402.

17 *Which statement about inhaled treatments for smoke inhalation injury is true?*
   A *Heparin, N-acetylcysteine, and albuterol have been shown to decrease lung injury but not mortality.*
   B *Heparin, N-acetylcysteine, and albuterol have been shown to decrease mortality but have an increased risk of bleeding.*
   C *N-acetylcysteine should only be used if secretions are thick.*
   D *Heparin helps control airway inflammation and prevents free radical-induced cell injury in the airways.*
   E *Heparin should be combined with N-acetylcysteine for administration.*

Nebulized heparin and N-acetylcysteine have been advocated for use to treat inhalational injuries. A recent meta-analysis of nine published trials showed nebulized heparin can reduce lung injury and improve lung function in burn patients with inhalation injury without abnormal coagulation or bleeding. Mortality was lower, duration of mechanical ventilation was shorter, and length of hospital stay was significantly shorter than that of the traditional treatment group. In addition to the mucolytic effects, N-acetylcysteine plays an important role in production of the antioxidant glutathione and decreases inflammation in the lung tissue. Heparin is combined with normal saline for inhalation, while N-acetylcysteine is given along with albuterol due to compatibility issues. The two inhalation treatments are each given every 4 hours with alternating treatments every 2 hours.

Answer: D

Desai MH, Mlcak R, et al. Reduction in mortality in pediatric patients with inhalation injury with aerosolized heparin/N-acetylcystine therapy. *The Journal of Burn Care and Research*. 1998. 19 (3): 210–212.
Lan X, Huang Z, Richardson J et al. Nebulized heparin for inhalation injury in burn patients: a systematic review and meta-analysis. *Burns & Trauma*. 2020; 8: 1–10.

18 *Which of the following statements about hydrofluoric acid is true?*
   A *Irrigation is not effective due to the rapid penetration of the fluoride ion.*
   B *Hypokalemia, hypercalcemia, and hypomagnesemia lead to QT prolongation and ventricular fibrillation.*
   C *Dialysis does not remove the fluoride ions.*
   D *High concentrations of HF can cause death with as low as 5% TBSA involvement.*
   E *5% HF concentrations cause immediate pain.*

Hydrofluoric acid (HF) is a corrosive used in industrial applications, but it is also common in materials such as dyes, cleaning agents, and rust removers. HF concentrations greater than 50% cause immediate tissue destruction and pain. For 20–50% concentrations, damage occurs within several hours; less than 20% concentrations may take up to 24 hours to become apparent. Hydrofluoric acid can be lethal as the fluoride ions penetrate until completely chelated by positively charged ions such as calcium and magnesium. This chelation results in severe hypocalcemia and hypomagnesemia. Manganese may be affected as a bivalent cation but is not a factor in the cause of the Q–T interval prolongation, which is the typical ECG change seen from the chelation of these cations. Treatment for hydrofluoric acid exposure is copious irrigation for at least 30 minutes. Topical, subcutaneous, or intra-arterial mixtures of calcium gluconate are often required. The fluoride ions can be removed by hemodialysis or cation exchange resins.

Answer: D

Williams FN and Lee JO. "Chemical Burns." *Total Burn Care*, 5th Edition. Edited by Herndon D. Elsevier, Chicago, 2018, pp. 408–413.

19 *What is the most common infectious complication after thermal injury?*
   A *Wound-site infection*
   B *Surgical-site infection*
   C *Bacteremia*
   D *Catheter-associated urinary tract infection*
   E *Respiratory tract infections*

The data analysis from a five-year review of infections showed the most common healthcare-associated infections were respiratory tract (44%), urinary tract (22%), other site infections (21%), bloodstream (12%), and surgical-site infections (1%).

Answer: E

Weber DJ, van Duin D., DiBiase LM Healthcare-associated infections among patients in a large burn intensive care unit: incidence and pathogens, 2008-2012. *Infection Control and Hospital Epidemiology*. 2014; 35 (10): 1304–1306.

20 *Which statement about pharmacologic interventions for the burn hypermetabolic response is true?*

A *Oxandrolone has no effect on net protein balance and improves insulin resistance.*

B *Propranolol improves net protein balance and insulin resistance.*

C *Insulin has no effect on net protein balance and improves insulin resistance.*

D *Metformin improves net protein balance and improves insulin resistance.*

E *Recombinant growth hormone has no effect on net protein balance and improves insulin resistance.*

Severe burns result in a 50-fold increase in catecholamine levels, increased resting energy expenditure, and contributes to profound catabolism. Cortisol levels are elevated, and testosterone is decreased. This leads to a loss of lean body mass of up to 25% of body weight for a 20% TBSA burn. Treatment of the hypermetabolic state decreases that loss to only 10%. Catecholamines, glucagon, and glucocorticoid surge resulting in increased gluconeogenesis. The resulting hyperglycemia results in protein catabolism, reduced graft take, and increased risk for infection, morbidity, and mortality.

Oxandrolone is a testosterone analog that has been shown to improve that muscle protein synthesis and metabolism while also improving insulin resistance. Propranolol is a non-selective beta-1 and beta-2 receptor antagonist that reduces the hyperdynamic circulation, blocks peripheral lipolysis, helps to reverse hepatic dysfunction, increases lean body mass, and decreases skeletal muscle wasting. It also downregulates the genes involved with gluconeogenesis and insulin resistance. Insulin improves protein balance by increasing glucose uptake in tissues, increasing amino acid use, and initiating protein translation. Metformin suppresses gluconeogenesis and improves glucose uptake by the peripheral muscles without causing hypoglycemia. Metformin does not improve net protein balance; despite some improvement in protein synthesis, it does not decrease muscle protein breakdown. Recombinant growth hormone (rhGH) administration increases nitrogen retention, cellular uptake of amino acids, and protein synthesis. Hyperglycemia is the most notable side effect of rhGH.

Answer: B

Williams FN and Herndon DN Metabolic and endocrine considerations after burn injury. *Clinics in Plastic Surgery*. 2017; 44 (3): 541–553.

21 *Which statement about nutritional support after a 40% TBSA thermal injury is true?*

A *Tube feeding should wait until the initial resuscitation is complete due to gastroparesis.*

B *Post-pyloric feeding tubes have the advantage of continued use in the operating room.*

C *Targets for large TBSA burns: 2.0 × BEE and 1.5 g/ kg protein.*

D *Targets for large TBSA burns: 2.0 × BEE and 2.0 g/ kg protein.*

E *Targets for large TBSA burns: 1 × BEE and 1.5 g/kg protein and 0.5 × BEE parenteral nutrition.*

Patients with very large burns have metabolic rates of 1.5 × BEE at 40% TBSA and 1.8 × BEE for the most severely injured. This increased metabolic demand does not return to normal even at 1 year postburn. Enteral nutrition is routinely started within hours of being burned, and goal feedings are reached within the typical 12–48 hours of the initial resuscitation. Intraoperative feeding using post-pyloric placed feeding tubes has been shown to be safe and avoids large periods of time without goal nutrition. The non-protein calorie target would be 1.5 × BEE and the protein goal would be 1.5–1.7 g/kg. Parenteral nutrition has no demonstrated benefit in burn patients who can tolerate enteral feedings.

Answer: B

Greenhalgh DG Management of burns. *New England Journal of Medicine*. 2019; 380 (24): 2349–2359.

Williams FN and Herndon DN. Metabolic and endocrine considerations after burn injury. *Clinics in Plastic Surgery*. 2017; 44 (3): 541–553.

44

Gynecologic Surgery

Joshua Klein, DO

Department of Surgery, Trauma & Acute Care Surgeon, Westchester Medical Center, Division of Trauma & Acute Care Surgery, New York Medical College, Valhalla, NY, USA

1 *A 38-year-old woman is undergoing an abdominal hysterectomy for a uterine leiomyoma. When preparing to ligate the uterine artery, there is an iatrogenic transection injury to the distal ureter. What is the next appropriate step in management?*
   A *Nephrostomy tube placement*
   B *Ureteral resection with end-end anastomosis*
   C *Ureteroneocystostomy*
   D *Antibiotics and drainage*
   E *Ureteral ligation*

Iatrogenic ureteral injury is a potential complication of surgery, and management depends on the location of the injury. Gynecologic, colorectal, and vascular pelvic surgery have been shown to have higher rates of iatrogenic injury compared to other surgical procedures. The distal ureter is the most common site of injury, and the treatment depends on which part of the ureter is injured. Distal ureteral injury is best managed by debridement of the ureter and re-implantation (correct choice C). An anterior or posterior location on the dome of the bladder is the preferred site of the ureteroneocystostomy as lateral re-implantation is prone to kinking of the ureter leading to a partial or complete outflow obstruction. A vesico-psoas hitch can be performed in conjunction with the ureteroneocystostomy if there is a large defect in the distal ureter that would result in tension on the anastomosis. Nephrostomy tube placement may be used in conjunction with repair but it by itself would not be sufficient (choice A). Upper and mid-ureteral injuries can be managed with ureteral debridement and primary ureteroureterostomy (choice B). Ureteral repairs should be performed in conjunction with stenting and indwelling urinary catheter drainage. Antibiotics and drainage alone would also not be a viable alternative (choice D). Ureteral ligation may be a last ditch damage control

option, but a nephrostomy tube would be required. Also in a damage control scenario, externalization of the ureter with an internal drain is also an option.

Answer: C

Burks F, Santucci R. Management of iatrogenic ureteral injury. *Therapeutic Advances in Urology.* 2014; 6(3):115–24.

Sharp HT, Adelman MR. Prevention, recognition, and management of Urologic Injuries during gynecologic surgery. *Obstetrics & Gynecology.* 2016; 127(6):1085–96

2 *A 32-year-old, G2P2 woman undergoes laparoscopy for chronic pelvic pain despite medical management. A 5-cm cyst containing dark brown fluid is removed from the right ovary. Pathologic examination reveals ovarian parenchyma, as well as endometrial glands and stroma. B-HCG screen was negative. Which of the following is the most likely diagnosis?*
   A *Ectopic pregnancy*
   B *Endometriosis*
   C *Hemorrhagic cyst*
   D *Ovarian torsion*
   E *Adenomyosis*

Endometriosis is characterized by the presence of endometrial tissue outside of the uterine cavity. Endometriosis affects 10–15% of all women of reproductive age and 70% of women with chronic pelvic pain. Ultrasound and magnetic resonance imaging have low sensitivity and specificity for deep infiltrating endometriosis, and there are no serum markers to aid in diagnosis. Laparoscopy is the gold standard for the diagnosis, and surgical biopsies allow for histological confirmation. Management involves surgical debulking and hormonal treatment to suppress recurrence and progression. Ectopic pregnancy should be suspected in patients with B-HCG greater than 1500 mIU/mL and a transvaginal ultrasound not showing an intrauterine gestational sac (choice A). Ovarian torsion is characterized by acute pelvic pain and caused when the ovary and its vascular pedicle twists on its suspensory ligament (choice D). Ultrasound will show an enlarged ovary with absence of Doppler flow. Adenomyosis is a benign gynecologic condition in which there is the presence of ectopic endometrial glands and stroma within the myometrium of the uterus (choice E). Hemorrhagic cysts are formed after ovulation with spontaneous bleeding into a corpus luteum cyst. There would not be endometrial glands present in hemorrhagic cysts (Choice C).

Answer: B

Parasar P, Ozcan P, Terry K. Endometriosis: Epidemiology, diagnosis, and clinical management. *Current Obstetrics and Gynecology Reports.* 2017; 6(1):34–41

Protopapas A, Grimbizis G. Adenomyosis: disease, uterine aging process leading to symptoms, or both. *Facts, Views and Vision in OBGYN.* 2020; 12(2):91–104.

3   *A 28-year-old woman with placenta accreta is scheduled for a cesarean section (C-section). After delivery of the fetus, there is significant bleeding that is uncontrollable despite bimanual pressure, uterotonic agents, and suture ligation. The patient becomes hemodynamically unstable with hypotension and a massive transfusion protocol is activated. Which of the following is true regarding the use of resuscitative endovascular balloon occlusion of the aorta (REBOA) in this patient?*

   A *Vascular access should be obtained via the right femoral vein.*

   B *The optimal location for balloon deployment is in Zone II.*

   C *Planned C-section with the use of REBOA results in lower intraoperative blood loss in women with placenta accreta compared to those who had C-section alone.*

   D *The REBOA balloon can safely remain inflated for up to 5 hours.*

   E *All patients who undergo REBOA require prophylactic lower extremity fasciotomies to prevent reperfusion injury and lower extremity compartment syndrome.*

REBOA is a minimally invasive procedure in which a balloon occlusion catheter is introduced into the aorta through a percutaneous groin puncture in the femoral artery (choice A). REBOA can be a temporary measure that serves as a bridge to definitive control of hemorrhage. In order to facilitate proper balloon placement, the aorta is divided into three functional zones; Zone I, which extends from the left subclavian artery to the celiac trunk; Zone II, which lies between the celiac truck and renal artery; Zone III, which is comprised of the infra-renal aorta. Zone II is not a recommended balloon inflation zone due to risk of dissection and/or perforation of visceral and renal vessels (choice B). Total aortic occlusion is not without potential risks to other organ

systems. Animal studies have shown that occlusion time greater than 40 minutes can result in irreversible organ injury and death; therefore, balloon deflation should occur as soon as life-threatening bleeding has been controlled (choice D). Prolonged ischemia followed by reperfusion can result in multisystem organ failure, limb ischemia, and myonecrosis. While prophylactic lower extremity fasciotomies are not recommended, comprehensive neurovascular exams along with the patient's overall physiologic status should guide post-REBOA procedures (choice E). Studies have shown that prophylactic use of REBOA deployed to Zone III under fluoroscopy or x-ray during elective c-sections for patients with morbidly adherent placenta, resulted in lower overall blood loss and fewer blood transfusions as compared to c-sections performed without REBOA. In patients with morbidly adherent placenta, REBOA may serve as an adjunct to minimize blood loss intraoperatively. Placenta previa is classified by the degree of encroachment upon the internal cervical os. In total placenta previa, the cervical os is completely covered by the placenta. In partial placenta previa, the cervical os is partly covered by the placenta. Invasive placentas are classified according to the degree of myometrial invasion. In placenta accreta, the abnormally adherent placental villi are attached directly into the myometrium, but do not invade it. In a placenta increta, the villi invade the myometrium. When the placental villi penetrate through the myometrium, reaching the serosal surface of the uterus, then a placenta percreta is present.

Answer: C

Source: From Robert, J.N., et. al, Resuscitative endovascular balloon occlusion of the aorta with a low profile, wire free device: A game changer?, *Trauma Case Reports*, Vol. 7, 2017, 11–14, with permission.

Manzano-Nunez R, Vidarte M. Resuscitative endovascular balloon occlusion of the aorta deployed by acute care surgeons in patients with morbidly adherent placenta: a feasible solution for two lives in peril. *World Journal of Emergency Surgery.* 2018; 13:44.

Ribeiro M, Feng C, Nguyen A. The complications associated with Resuscitative Endovascular Balloon Occlusion of the Aorta (REBOA). *World Journal of Emergency Surgery.* 2018; 13:20.

4 *A 25-year-old woman presents to the emergency department with complaints of right lower quadrant abdominal pain and fevers over the past 48 hours. She reports anorexia and is nauseous. She has two sexual partners and uses an intrauterine device for contraception. Vital signs are BP 86/50 mmHg, HR 112 beats/ min, and a temperature of 39.8 °C. On pelvic exam, there is purulent cervical discharge, cervical motion tenderness, and a right adnexal mass that is tender to palpation. Which of the following is the most appropriate initial management.*

A *Obtain ultrasound and CT abdomen*

B *Removal of intrauterine contraceptive device*

C *Inpatient treatment with intravenous cefotetan and doxycycline*

D *Outpatient treatment with intramuscular ceftriaxone and doxycycline*

E *Exploratory laparotomy with drainage of tubo-ovarian abscess*

Pelvic inflammatory disease (PID) is caused by an ascending infection from the cervix that is frequently related to an untreated sexually transmitted infection. The primary pathogens include *Neisseria gonorrhoeae* and *Chlamydia trachomatis*, although other cervical microbes including *Mycoplasma genitalium*, and *Peptostreptococcus* species have been implicated as well. Risk factors for development of PID include multiple sexual partners, previous history of PID, intrauterine device implantation, and tubal ligation. Patients typically present with lower abdominal or pelvic pain, vaginal discharge, dyspareunia, cervical motion tenderness, and vaginal bleeding. Ultrasound and computed tomography have a low sensitivity for PID diagnosis; therefore, early treatment should be started based on clinical suspicion (choice A). Initial treatment will depend upon the patient's physiologic status, with indications for hospitalization including pregnancy, failed outpatient treatment, and severe clinical illness or signs of sepsis. Removal of an intrauterine device is only recommended in cases of PID, which show no clinical improvement in the first 48–72 hours when treated with antibiotics (choice B). A patient with suspected PID should be treated with either intravenous cefotetan or cefoxitin

plus doxycycline. In patients with cephalosporin or tetracycline allergies, clindamycin plus gentamicin is an appropriate substitution. Outpatient treatment with intramuscular ceftriaxone and oral doxycycline should be reserved for those patients with mild disease (choice D) but this patient has hypotension and septic shock. Tubo-ovarian abscess is a complication of PID in which an abscess forms involving the tubes and ovaries (choice E). Initial management consists of antibiotics; however, uncontrolled infection may require percutaneous drainage or surgical intervention.

Answer: C

Centers for Disease Control and Prevention. Pelvic Inflammatory Disease. 2015 Sexually Transmitted Diseases Treatment Guidelines. Cdc.gov/std/tg2015/pid.htm.

5 *A 28-year-old woman is undergoing a diagnostic laparoscopy due to chronic lower abdominal and pelvic pain. Which finding on laparoscopy would indicate a prior history of pelvic inflammatory disease?*

A *Diverticulosis*

B *Ovarian cyst*

C *Endometriosis*

D *Peri-hepatic adhesions*

E *Free intraperitoneal fluid in pelvis*

Fitz-Hugh-Curtis syndrome is a chronic manifestation of pelvic inflammatory disease (PID). Spread of PID is hypothesized to occur in three ways: (1) ascending infection from the cervix or vagina travel to the endometrium, through the fallopian tubes, and into the peritoneal cavity; (2) lymphatic spread; (3) hematogenous spread. Diagnosis can be made via laparoscopy or laparotomy by direct visualization. The classic "Violin string" adhesions can be visualized on the hepatic capsule. Treatment consists of antibiotics covering *Chlamydia trachomatis, Neisseria gonorrhea*, and gram-negative organisms. Abscesses visualized during laparoscopy can be surgically drained. Endometriosis is the presence of endometrial tissue outside of the uterine cavity and laparoscopy will identify bluish or red spots on the peritoneal surface (choice C). Diverticula can either be "false" diverticula in which the mucosa and submucosa herniate through a defect in the muscularis layer, or "true" diverticula, which involves outpouching of all layers of the intestinal wall (choice A). Causes of intraperitoneal fluid are multifactorial and not specifically related to PID (choice E). Ovarian cysts can range from physiologically normal to an ovarian malignancy. Risk factors for development of ovarian cysts include infertility treatment, pregnancy, hypothyroidism, and tobacco use. PID is not a risk factor for ovarian cyst development (choice B).

Answers: D

Das B, Ronda J, Trent M. Pelvic inflammatory disease: improving awareness, prevention, and treatment. *Infection and Drug Resistance*. 2016; 9:191–97.

Khine H, Wren SB, Rotenberg O. Fitz-hugh-curtis syndrome in adolescent females: a diagnostic dilemma. *Pediatric Emergency Care*. 2019; 35(7):121–23.

6   A 32-year-old woman presents to the emergency department with right-sided abdominal pain. Ultrasound shows no Doppler flow to the right ovary, and she is taken to the operating room for adnexal torsion. During laparoscopy, the right ovary is noted to be torsed and has a dusky appearance. What is the first best step in management?
   A   Removal of the right ovary
   B   Detorsion of the right ovary and observation
   C   Removal of the right ovary and fallopian tube
   D   Detorsion of the right ovary and bilateral oophorectomy
   E   Hysterectomy and bilateral salpingo-oophorectomy

Adnexal torsion may involve twisting of the ovary alone, ovary and fallopian tube together, or the fallopian tube alone. Ovarian torsion occurs when the ovary folds over the adnexal ligaments compromising the blood flow from the ovarian and uterine arteries. Any ovarian mass will predispose an individual to torsion. In adults, a cyst is typically the precipitant mass that may lead to the torsion. Other conditions and masses leading to torsion include ovarian cysts and tumors, corpus luteum cysts, tubal pregnancies, and hemo/hydrosalpinx. Torsion is more likely to occur on the right than the left as the right-sided ureteral ovarian ligament is longer. Some authors speculate that the presence of the sigmoid colon reduces space of the left pelvis and decreases the likelihood of left-sided torsion. Presentation is variable, ranging from lower abdominal pain in early stages to overt sepsis once the ovary undergoes necrosis. Patients present with sudden onset of intense unilateral pelvic pain, which may radiate to the lumbar area. The pain episodes may be intermittent if the adnexal structures spontaneously torsed and detorsed. Ultrasound is typically used for diagnosis; however, it is specific but not sensitive for adnexal torsion. Ultrasound findings, which may be suggestive of adnexal torsion, includes the absence of flow to the affected side and asymmetry of the ovaries. Treatment consists of surgical detorsion and observation of the ovary for viability as the first step (choice B). If the ovary appears necrotic, management should include salpingo-oophorectomy (choice C). If after detorsion, the cause of torsion is secondary to an ovarian cyst, cystectomy can

be performed if benign appearing; if there are concerns for malignancy or if the woman is postmenopausal, salpingo-oophorectomy should be performed. Bilateral oophorectomy would not be recommended as there is no indication to remove the contralateral ovary as torsion on one side does not predict torsion on the other (choice D). Hysterectomy would obviously not be indicated in this case (choice E).

Answer: B

Ashwal E, Hiersch L, Krissi H. Characteristics and management of ovarian torsion in premenarchal compared with postmenarchal patients. *Obstetrics and Gynecology*. 2015; 126(3):514–20.

Oelsner G, Cohen SB, Soriano D. Minimal surgery for the twisted ischaemic adnexa can preserve ovarian function. *Human Reproduction*. 2003; 18(12):2599–602.

7   A 20-year-old woman is brought into the emergency department after being assaulted. On physical exam, she is noted to have facial fractures, rib fractures, and a copious amount of blood at the vaginal introitus. She is taken up to the operating room where she is found to have a perineal laceration extending through the perineal fascia, internal and external anal sphincters, and the anal mucosa. Which of the following perineal lacerations does this patient have?
   A   First-degree laceration
   B   Second-degree laceration
   C   Third-degree laceration subclass 3a
   D   Third-degree laceration subclass 3b
   E   Fourth-degree laceration

Perineal lacerations are classified based on the tissues and musculature that are disrupted. First-degree lacerations involve injury to the skin and subcutaneous tissue of the perineum. Second-degree lacerations extend into the fascia and perineal body musculature. Third-degree lacerations are subclassified into 3a, in which less than 50% of the external anal sphincter is torn, 3b where greater than 50% of the external anal sphincter is torn, and 3c where there is involvement of both external and internal anal sphincters. Fourth-degree lacerations extend through the anal sphincters and into the rectal mucosa. Repair of perineal lacerations are performed with polyglactin suture. The muscles of the perineal body should be reapproximated. Studies have demonstrated that 20–50% of patients have anal incontinence or rectal urgency after repair of third-degree lacerations. Colostomy is often not required during the index operation; however, in patients requiring muscular flaps for anal incontinence or treatment of complications including colovesical and colovaginal fistulas, it may be considered.

Answer: E

Goh R, Goh D, Ellepola H. Perineal tears- A review. *Australian Journal of General Practice*. 2018; 47(1–2):35–8.

Monteiro M. Pereira G, Aguiar R. Risk factors for severe obstetric perineal lacerations. *International Urogynecology Journal*. 2016; 27(1):61–7.

8 *A 40-year-old woman is undergoing a Cesarean-section for malpresentation. After delivery of the fetus, the patient becomes acutely hypoxic requiring emergent intubation, and hypotensive necessitating vasopressor initiation. She is transferred to the intensive care unit where labs reveal a hypercarbic respiratory failure and coagulopathy. Which of the following should be administered?*
   A *Broad spectrum antibiotics*
   B *Hydrocortisone*
   C *Methotrexate*
   D *Intravenous immunoglobulin*
   E *Mifepristone*

Amniotic fluid embolism syndrome (AFES) occurs when amniotic fluid and fetal cells enter the maternal pulmonary circulation. While the pathophysiology of AFES is incompletely understood, the entry of amniotic fluid into the maternal circulation activates inflammatory mediators leading to a humoral immune response. AFES is a clinical diagnosis that is based upon the constellation of clinical findings. To make the diagnosis, four criteria are needed to be present: acute hypoxia, hypotension, coagulopathy or hemorrhage, and signs/symptoms occurring during labor, cesarean section, or dilation and evacuation. The mainstay of treatment is cardiopulmonary supportive care. Steroids to mediate the immune response are recommended. There is no role for antibiotics as this is not an infectious process. Methotrexate and mifepristone are used in clinical practice for medical abortions (choices A and E). Intravenous immunoglobulin has not shown to be beneficial in treating AFES (choice D). This syndrome can be extremely severe, and there have been case reports of use of nitric oxide, right ventricular assist device with right heart failure, as well as the use of extracorporeal membrane oxygenation and intra-aortic balloon pump for severe left ventricular failure and hypoxemia.

Answer: B

Society for Maternal-Fetal Medicine (SMFM) with the assistance of Pacheco LD, Saade G, et al. Amniotic fluid embolism: diagnosis and management. *American Journal of Obstetrics and Gynecology* 2016; 215:B16–24.

9 *A 25-year-old woman presents to the emergency department and workup is concerning for an ectopic pregnancy. In discussing her management, which of the following is an absolute contraindication to medical management of an ectopic pregnancy?*
   A *Ruptured ectopic pregnancy*
   B *3 cm ectopic pregnancy visualized on transvaginal ultrasonography*
   C *B-hCG 4500 mIU/mL*
   D *Refusal to accept blood and blood product transfusion*
   E *History of prior cesarean section*

Ectopic pregnancy is a complication of pregnancy that carries a high rate of morbidity and mortality when not identified and treated early. Patients with ectopic pregnancy typically present with history of abdominal pain and amenorrhea. Irregular vaginal bleeding may also raise suspicion, and some patients may present with peritonitis. Irritation of the diaphragm by hemoperitoneum may also result in complaint of neck or shoulder pain. The rate of ectopic pregnancy in the general population is under 2%, however increases to 5% in patients who undergo assisted reproductive technology. A positive pregnancy test and transvaginal ultrasound can confirm the diagnosis of ectopic pregnancy by identifying a fetal heartbeat outside the uterine cavity. Absence of an intrauterine pregnancy along with findings of a complex adnexal mass and echogenic-free fluid supports the diagnosis of ruptured ectopic pregnancy. Management can be either medical or surgical, with intramuscular methotrexate utilized in patients with no contraindications. Methotrexate is a folic acid antagonist and is contraindicated in pregnancy because it is an abortive and has teratogenic effects. It is a way to treat pregnancy that is implanted outside the uterus and administered in a single-dose injection. Intrauterine pregnancy, ruptured ectopic pregnancy, hemodynamic instability, hepatic or pulmonary disease, allergy to methotrexate, and immunodeficiency are all absolute contraindications to methotrexate administration, and treatment with salpingectomy or salpingostomy should be performed. Relative contraindications to medical treatment of ectopic pregnancy includes a high initial B-hCG (>5000 mIU/mL), ectopic pregnancy > 4 cm in size, and refusal to accept blood transfusion (choices B, C, and D).

Answer: A

Barash J, Buchanan E, Hillson C. Diagnosis and management of ectopic pregnancy. *American Family Physician*. 2014; 90(1):34–40.

10 *A 23-year-old, G1P0 woman who is 32 weeks pregnant is scheduled to undergo a laparoscopic cholecystectomy. She is undergoing a preoperative evaluation by the anesthesiologist. Which is true regarding the physiologic changes of pregnancy?*

  A *Cardiac output decreases in order to compensate for an increase in systemic vascular resistance.*

  B *There is a 25% increase in expiratory reserve volume.*

  C *Permeability of the blood–brain barrier decreases.*

  D *There is an increase in both plasma volume and red cell mass.*

  E *Pregnancy decreases the risk of thrombotic events.*

Pregnancy causes multiple physiologic changes within the body, which are summarized in the table below:

Neurologic	Epidural vein engorgement ↑ Maternal blood–brain barrier permeability ↑ Sensitivity to opioids and sedatives
Cardiovascular	↓ Peripheral vascular resistance ↑ Heart rate ↑ Cardiac output
Respiratory	↓ Residual volume ↓ Expiratory reserve volume ↑ Minute ventilation
Gastrointestinal	Delayed gastric emptying ↑ Gastric pH
Renal	↑ Glomerular filtration rate ↑ Renal plasma flow
Hematologic	↑ Plasma volume ↑ Red cell volume ↓ Fibrinolytic activity ↑ Factors VII, VIII, IX, X, XII, vWF

Answer: D

Hill C, Pickinpaugh J. Physiologic changes in pregnancy. *Surgical Clinics of North America.* 2008 88(2):391–401.

Nejdlova M, Johnson T. Anaesthesia for non-obstetric procedures during pregnancy. *Continuing Education in Anaesthesia Critical Care & Pain.* 2012; 12(4):203–06.

11 *A 23-year-old, 36-week pregnant woman is brought into the emergency department in extremis following a motor vehicle crash. During the primary survey, the patient goes into cardiac arrest. Which of the following is true regarding her management?*

  A *Emergent cesarean section should be considered if life support interventions fail to restore maternal circulation within 4 minutes.*

  B *Manual right lateral uterine displacement improves advanced cardiac life support maneuvers.*

  C *Perimortem delivery does not improve maternal mortality.*

  D *Defibrillation is contraindicated in pregnant patients.*

  E *Chest compressions should be performed at a rate of 60 per minute to optimize blood flow to the fetus.*

Advanced cardiac life support (ACLS) during pregnancy has distinct differences compared to those in their nongravid counterparts. The normal supine positioning of a patient undergoing CPR can lead to significant aortocaval compression in the pregnant patient. Left lateral uterine displacement can offload the vena cava, thus optimizing venous return to the heart. There are no changes to the ACLS recommendations for defibrillation in the setting of ventricular fibrillation or pulseless ventricular tachycardia in the pregnant vs nonpregnant patient, and defibrillation should be performed if clinically warranted. However, cardiac arrest after blunt trauma is typically due to exsanguination and defibrillation is futile. Chest compressions should be performed as per ACLS protocol of 100 compressions/min. If interventions are unable to restore maternal circulation within 4 minutes of cardiac arrest, emergent cesarean section should be considered in patients who have a uterus ≥20 weeks in size. Even if the fetus is nonviable, delivery can decrease the aortocaval compression and improve the effectiveness of CPR, thus decreasing maternal mortality. The primary goal is the resuscitation of the mother.

Answer: A

Rose C, Faksh A, Traynor K. Challenging the 4- to 5-minute rule: from perimortem cesarean to resuscitative hysterotomy. *American Journal of Obstetrics and Gynecology.* 2015; 213(5):653.

Zelop C, Einav S, Mhyre J. Cardiac arrest during pregnancy: ongoing clinical conundrum. *American Journal of Obstetrics and Gynecology.* 2018;219(1): 52–61.

12 *A 23-year-old woman presents to the emergency department after sustaining a straddle injury while trying to skateboard down a handrail. She is complaining of severe vulvar pain. Physical exam reveals a 2-cm hematoma. On re-examination 1 hour later, the hematoma is now 5 cm. What is the next best step in management?*

  A *Analgesia and ice pack*

  B *Manual compression*

  C *Uterine artery embolization*

  D *Surgical exploration*

  E *Needle aspiration*

Genital hematomas occur secondary to a vascular injury to the lower genital tract. Risk factors for hematoma formation include primiparity, instrumental delivery, pudendal nerve block, macrosomia, and coagulopathic disorders. Conservative management with analgesia and compression may be appropriate for small, non-expanding hematomas (choices A and B), whereas expanding hematomas necessitate operative exploration in order to identify any source and obtain hemorrhage control (choice D). Large vulvar hematomas that are left undrained may continue to expand leading to ischemia to the skin and subcutaneous tissue and subsequent necrosis. Vulvar hematomas typically are secondary to bleeding from a branch of the internal pudendal artery; therefore, uterine artery embolization would not be effective (choice C). Needle aspiration will decrease the size of the hematoma, however, will not address the underlying cause of bleeding (choice E).

Answer: D

Rani S, Verma M, Pandher DK. Risk factors and incidence of puerperal genital haematomas. *Journal of clinical and diagnostic research: JCDR.* 2017; 11(5):QC01–03.

Benrubi G, Neuman C, Nuss RC. Vulvar and vaginal hematomas: a retrospective study of conservative versus operative management. *Southern Medical Journal.* 1987;80(8): 991–4.

13 *A 40-year-old woman presents to the hospital with diffuse abdominal pain 8 days following a laparoscopic hysterectomy. She complains of bleeding and a sensation of vaginal pressure. You are called to see this patient in the ED because the physical exam revealed the presence of small bowel within her vagina. Which is true of her condition?*

A *Couples may safely resume coitus 2 weeks following a laparoscopic hysterectomy.*

B *Preoperative treatment of bacterial vaginosis decreases the risk of vaginal cuff dehiscence.*

C *Rates of vaginal cuff dehiscence are higher with transvaginal cuff closure following laparoscopic hysterectomy.*

D *Perioperative estrogen therapy increases wound complications.*

E *Higher BMI increases the risk of vaginal cuff dehiscence following hysterectomy.*

Vaginal cuff dehiscence is a serious postoperative complication following a hysterectomy that causes significant patient morbidity. Vaginal atrophy, prior or current radiation therapy, early resumption of coitus, and perioperative gynecologic infections can predispose an individual to cuff dehiscence. Following a hysterectomy, it is recommended to abstain from coitus or deep vaginal penetration for 6–8 weeks following the surgery (choice A). Patients who are found to have bacterial vaginosis or trichomonas vaginitis should be treated prior to surgery to minimize the risk of dehiscence (choice B). Total laparoscopic hysterectomy is associated with higher rates of cuff dehiscence compared to patients who undergo abdominal hysterectomy or vaginal hysterectomy; however, in patients who do undergo laparoscopic hysterectomy, transvaginal suturing reduces the risk of vaginal dehiscence (choice C). Perioperative estrogen therapy can assist with wound healing, and studies examining pelvic floor reconstruction found that patients who were prescribed estrogen cream had higher levels of mature collagen and vaginal wall thickness after treatment for 6 weeks (choice D). Patients with higher BMI were found to have lower rates of cuff dehiscence than their counterparts with lower BMI (choice E).

Answer: B

Uccella S, Ceccaroni M, Cromi A. Vaginal cuff dehiscence in a series of 12,398 hysterectomies: effect of different types of colpotomy and vaginal closure. *Obstetrics and Gynecology.* 2012; 120(3):516–23.

Weizman N, Einarsson J, Wang K. Vaginal cuff dehiscence: risk factors and associated morbidities. *Journal of the Society of Laparoscopic & Robotic Surgeons.* 2015; 19(2):e20013.00351.

14 *A 19-year-old woman presents to the emergency department with a 3-day history of lower abdominal pain, fevers, and purulent vaginal discharge. One week ago she found out she was pregnant after she missed her period. She was afraid to tell her parents about her pregnancy at which time she travelled to Mexico where she found a practitioner who performed a vacuum-assisted aspiration abortion. In the emergency department, the patient is hypotensive, tachycardic, and febrile. Her physical exam reveals a tender uterus with sanguinopurulent discharge from the cervix. Which of the following is the next best step in management?*

A *Methotrexate*

B *CT guided drainage of uterine contents*

C *Broad-spectrum antibiotics*

D *Dilation and curettage with broad-spectrum antibiotics*

E *Mifepristone-misoprostol*

A septic abortion is a uterine infection caused by improper, non-sterile, or inadequate removal of products of conception during an induced or spontaneous abortion. Septic abortions are frequently associated with induced abortions performed by untrained practitioners or those using non-sterile technique. A detailed history and physical exam can often lead to a clinical diagnosis; however, ultrasound should be utilized to examine for retained products of conception. Treatment consists of broad-spectrum antibiotics and uterine evacuation. Thus, antibiotics alone will not suffice (choice C). Typical causative agents include Staphylococci, Proteus, Enterobacter, and anaerobic organisms. CT-guided drainage will be unable to fully evacuate retained products of conception and will not eliminate the source of infection (choice B). The patient has already had a vacuum-assisted aspiration; therefore, there is no role for medications utilized for medical abortion as this will not clear the uterus of retained products of conception (choices A and E).

Answer: D

Eschenback D. Treating spontaneous and induced septic abortions. *Obstetrics and Gynecology.* 2015; 125:1042–8.

Sedgh G, Singh S, Shah IH. Induced abortion: incidence and trends worldwide from 1995 to 2008. *Lancet.* 2006; 369(9550):1887–92.

15 *A 24-year-old woman presents to the emergency department with fevers, RLQ, and pelvic pain. She also has vaginal discharge for 3 days. An ultrasound reveals a complex right cystic adnexal structure with multiple septations. She is started on broad-spectrum antibiotics; however, after 48 hours she is showing no clinical improvement. Which of the following is true regarding the management of this patient?*

 A *The most commonly isolated organism is Chlamydia trachomatis.*

 B *Fluoroquinolones are effective empiric antibiotics.*

 C *CT-guided aspiration should only be considered in postmenopausal women.*

 D *Patients treated with ultrasound-guided drainage have a lower hospital length of stay than those treated with IV antibiotics alone.*

 E *Surgery is required for all tubo-ovarian abscess > 8 cm*

Tubo-ovarian abscess (TOA) is an adnexal infection secondary to pelvic inflammatory disease. The most common cause is secondary to pathogens, which ascend from the vagina and/or cervix through the endometrium and fallopian tubes into the peritoneal cavity. Risk factors for TOA are similar to those of pelvic inflammatory disease. While there is an association with sexually transmitted infections, the most commonly cultured organisms from TOA include *Escherichia coli, Bacteroides*

fragilis, and *Peptostreptococcus* (choice A). Initial management consists of a second-generation cephalosporin and doxycycline. Patients with cephalosporin allergies can be managed with clindamycin and gentamicin. Patients who fail to show any clinical improvement over 24 hours should be considered candidates for image-guided drainage. Patients who are treated with image-guided drainage and antibiotics have a faster resolution of symptoms and decreased hospital length of stay. Image-guided drainage can be performed transabdominal, transrectal, transvaginal, and transgluteal. Menopausal status does not preclude drainage of TOA (choice C). Surgery should be reserved for hemodynamically unstable patients, as well as those patients with TOA that do not respond to initial treatment measures (choice E). In one study, the average abscess size for those treated successfully with conservative management was 6.3 cm versus those requiring drainage and/or surgery (7.7 cm). Abscesses greater than 8 cm were associated with an increased risk of complications.

Answer: D

Lareau SM, Beigi RH. Pelvic inflammatory disease and tubo-ovarian abscess. *Infectious Disease Clinics of North America.* 2008; 22(4):693–708.

Fouks Y, Cohen A, Shapira U, Solomon N, Almog B, Levin I. Surgical intervention in patients with tubo-ovarian abscess: clinical predictors and a simple risk score. *Journal of Minimally Invasive Gynecology.* 2019; 26(3):535–543.

16 *A 32-year-old, G1P0 woman presents with right lower quadrant pain. Ultrasound reveals a noncompressible tubular structure with periappendiceal fluid, and a diagnosis is made of acute appendicitis. In regards to laparoscopy during pregnancy, which of the following is true?*

 A *Optical trocar entry is contraindicated during pregnancy.*

 B *Gravid patients in their third trimester should be placed in a partial right lateral decubitus position.*

 C *Veress needle entry provides safe abdominal access when adjusted for fundal height.*

 D *There is increased rate of fetal mortality with bipolar energy during laparoscopy during pregnancy.*

 E *Routine tocolytics are recommended for all pregnant patients undergoing laparoscopic surgery.*

Abdominal access during pregnancy can be accomplished via both open and closed techniques. Optical trocar and Veress entry techniques can be performed safely if the initial port location is adjusted according to fundal height (choice A). A subcostal approach at

Palmer's point with abdominal wall elevation can provide abdominal access without causing an increase in maternal or fetal complications. Gravid patients past the first trimester should be positioned in a partial left lateral decubitus position to decrease compression of the vena cava and optimize cardiac venous return (choice B). Ultrasound, bipolar, and monopolar energy sources are safe to use during laparoscopic procedures and cause no increase in fetal mortality (choice D). Tocolytics should not routinely be used prophylactically and instead should only be considered in patients who have signs of preterm labor (choice E).

Answer: C

Pearl J, Price R. Guidelines for the use of laparoscopy during pregnancy- *A SAGES Publication*. 2017.

Ball E, Waters N, Cooper N. Evidence-based guideline on laparoscopy in pregnancy. *Facts, Views Vis OBGYN*. 2019; 11(1):5–25.

17 *A 29 year old woman presents to the ED with a 2 day history of right lower quadrant pain. She is diagnosed with acute appendicitis and consented for surgery. At the time of laparoscopy, she is found to have appendicitis, as well as a 5-cm cystic mass on her right ovary that is concerning for malignancy. In addition to an appendectomy, what is the most appropriate management for this patient?*

A *No further intervention unless patient becomes symptomatic*

B *Postoperative transvaginal ultrasound to evaluate the right ovary*

C *Biopsy of mass, cytology of pelvic washings, evaluation of pelvic lymph nodes, and examination of upper abdomen and omentum for metastases*

D *Right oophorectomy*

E *Total abdominal hysterectomy with bilateral salpingo-oophorectomy*

During abdominal surgery, incidental gynecologic processes may be encountered for which a patient may be unaware of or asymptomatic from. Management of ovarian masses found during laparoscopy must take into account not only the morphological features of the mass but additionally the patient's age and menopausal status. In premenopausal patients with a suspicious ovarian mass, a staging procedure consisting of a biopsy, peritoneal washing cytology, evaluation of intra-abdominal organs, and examination of pelvic lymph nodes should be performed, and the patient should have a postoperative referral to a gynecologist (choice C). In postmenopausal patients with a suspicious ovarian mass found incidentally, an oophorectomy is preferred rather than a biopsy. A total abdominal hysterectomy with bilateral salpingo-oophorectomy can be performed if intraoperative frozen section is consistent with malignancy (answers D and E). Suspicious features of an ovarian mass, which should prompt these considerations, include size greater than 4 cm, solid components, septations, and involvement of the ipsilateral fallopian tube. Delaying management will only result in the need for additional tests and procedures for the patient (Choice A&B).

Answer: C

Boyd C, Riall T. Unexpected gynecological findings during abdominal surgery. *Current Problems in Surgery*. 2012; 49(4):195–251.

18 *A 68 year-old woman with ovarian cancer with metastases to the liver presents to the emergency department with a 3-day history of abdominal distension, nausea, and emesis. A CT scan of her abdomen and pelvis reveals dilated, fluid-filled loops of small and large bowel with a transition point in the sigmoid colon. Concerning malignant bowel obstructions (MBO) in advanced ovarian cancer, which of the following is true?*

A *There is a higher incidence of large bowel obstruction compared to small bowel obstruction.*

B *Venting gastrostomy insertion for inoperable but symptomatic patients reduces visceral symptoms and decreases the number of hospital re-admissions.*

C *Self-expandable metallic colonic stents are contraindicated in MBO from a gynecologic source.*

D *Platinum-based chemotherapy should be offered to all patients presenting with MBO secondary to ovarian cancer.*

E *Somatostatin analogues improve progression-free survival in patients with MBO.*

Malignant bowel obstruction is a complication of and often the end-stage of advanced gynecologic malignancy. Management of MBO must take into account the patients symptoms in relation to the disease histology, tumor burden, presence of recurrent or progression of disease, and the patients physiologic status. Small bowel obstruction is more common than large bowel obstruction, with external compression from peritoneal carcinomatosis or functional occlusion from tumor infiltration being the most common etiologies (answer A). Discussions regarding goals of care and limitations of surgery must be discussed with patients in order to set realistic expectations as there is significant risk of hospital readmission, re-obstruction, and operative mortality in patients managed surgically. Surgical intervention can be successful in re-establishing bowel function patients with good base-line functional status and available oncologic treatment options. Large bowel obstruction secondary to ovarian cancer has significant risk of subsequent perforation; therefore, a diverting proximal ostomy should be considered. Additionally, self-expandable metallic stents can be utilized in select patients with large bowel obstruction and act as either a palliative procedure or a bridge for surgery (answer C). Chemotherapy can be considered in certain patients with advanced gynecologic cancers causing MBO; however, since MBO is often an end-stage consequence of the malignancy, the majority of patients will have already received multiple lines of chemotherapy and are unlikely to mount a significant clinical response (answer D). Studies investigating use of somatostatin analogues to reduce symptoms related to secretions and endoluminal pressure have found no observed benefits (answer E). For inoperable patients that are symptomatic, venting gastrostomy for digestive decompression has been shown to reduce visceral symptoms. Patients who underwent gastrostomy placement were able to avoid repeated hospital admissions, as well as consume a diet for comfort and should be considered in patients with protracted nausea and emesis as their main symptom.

Answer: B

Yeh Chen L, Jivraj N, O'Brien C. Malignant bowel obstruction in advanced gynecologic cancers: an updated review from a multidisciplinary perspective. *Obstetrics and Gynecology International.* 2018 May; 2018:17.

DeEulis T, Yennurajalingam S. Venting gastrostomy at home for symptomatic management of bowel obstruction in advanced/recurrent ovarian malignancy: a case series. *Journal of Palliative Medicine.* 2015; 18(8):722–8.

19 *A 25-year-old, G0P0 woman presents with a 5-month history of left lower pelvic pain and heavy menses. The pain is most pronounced 2 days prior to the start of her menses and associated with increased discomfort during defecation and sexual intercourse. She is diagnosed with endometriosis and ordered for confirmatory testing. Regarding the evaluation and management of endometriosis, which of the following is true?*

   A *Late menarche increases the risk of developing endometriosis.*
   B *Discontinuation of oral contraceptives can improve symptoms associated with endometriosis.*
   C *Endometriomas are most commonly located within the uterosacral ligaments.*

   D *MRI has a higher sensitivity than ultrasonography in diagnosing deep infiltrating endometriosis.*
   E *Risk of ovarian cancer is lower in patients with endometriosis.*

Endometriosis is an estrogen-dependent gynecologic disease in which endometrial tissue is present outside of the uterus. Risk factors for development of endometriosis include: nulliparity, early menarche (before 11–13 years old), late menopause, consumption of high amounts of trans-unsaturated fats, and in utero exposure to diethylstilbestrol (answer A). Patients will frequently present with pelvic pain, painful menses, dyschezia, dysuria, and dyspareunia. Endometriomas can typically be visualized on imaging, with laboratory evaluations providing limited clinical benefit. Ultrasound, computed tomography, and magnetic resonance imaging can all be utilized to identify endometriomas. MRI has been shown to have a higher sensitivity for detecting deep infiltrating endometriosis; however, due to cost, ultrasound is more commonly used. Laparoscopy remains the gold standard for the diagnosis of endometriosis as there is direct visualization of the endometrial implant, and the lesion can be biopsied at the time of surgery. The most common site of endometriosis are the ovaries; however, fallopian tubes, uterosacral ligaments, gastrointestinal tract, and soft tissue may also have endometrial implants (Answer C). While the overall risk of cancer related to endometriosis is low, studies have demonstrated that women with endometriosis have a higher incidence of clear cell and endometrioid ovarian cancer (Answer E)

Answer: D

Vercellini P, Viganò P, Somigliana E, Fedele L. Endometriosis: pathogenesis and treatment. *Nature Reviews Endocrinology.* 2014; 10(5):261–75.

Johnson NP, Hummelshoj L. World Endometriosis Society Montpellier Consortium: consensus on current management of endometriosis. *Human Reproduction.* 2013; 28(6):1552–68.

20 *A 49-year-old woman with a history of pelvic pain and heavy menses is diagnosed with uterine leiomyomas. Transvaginal ultrasound reveals two intramural fibroids, both 5 cm in size. Regarding laparoscopic myomectomy and hysterectomy for uterine leiomyoma, which of the following is true?*

   A *Power morcellation should be contained within a bag to prevent potential dissemination of occult malignancy during laparoscopic hysterectomy.*
   B *Uterine artery embolization for uterine leiomyoma is associated with a lower rate of re-intervention compared to myomectomy.*

C *Administration of oxytocin reduces intraoperative blood loss during laparoscopic myomectomy.*

D *Laparoscopic myomectomy has similar reproductive outcomes compared to hysterectomy.*

E *Laparoscopic hysterectomy is associated with higher mortality rates than myomectomy.*

Uterine leiomyomata (fibroids) are the most common benign tumor affecting women. Fibroids originate from the uterine smooth muscle and are dependent on levels of circulating estrogen. Patients present with menorrhagia, metrorrhagia, pelvic pain, and in severe cases symptoms associated with anemia. Treatment options can include medical management with nonsteroidal anti-inflammatory drugs, hormonal contraceptives, or GnRH agonists. Surgical therapy offers the patient definitive management in those patients who undergo a hysterectomy; however, other options including endometrial ablation, uterine artery embolization, and myomectomy can be used in appropriately selected patients. Uterine artery embolization acts to decrease the total blood supply to the uterus thereby decreasing bleeding symptoms associated with fibroids. Myomectomy is a surgical procedure, which can be performed either open or laparoscopically to remove uterine fibroids while preserving the uterus. Both myomectomy and uterine artery embolization preserve a patient's fertility (choice D); however, myomectomy has a lower rate of re-intervention for recurrent symptoms comparatively (choice B). Myomectomy and hysterectomy have similar rates of mortality (choice E). Studies looking at minimizing intra-operative blood loss have shown no benefit after administration of oxytocin and benefits of preventing hemorrhage are limited (choice C). Power morcellators are a tool to break up the tissue specimen into smaller pieces facilitating removal through small incisions. The Food and Drug Administration recommends morcellation take place within a tissue containment system or specimen bag in order to reduce the risk of dissemination of undiagnosed uterine sarcoma throughout the abdomen when performing a laparoscopic hysterectomy (choice A).

Answer: A

Zimmermann A, Bernuit D, Gerlinger C, Schaefers M, Geppert K. Prevalence, symptoms and management of uterine fibroids: an international internet-based survey of 21,746 women. *BMC Womens Health*. 2012; 12(6). https://doi.org/10.1186/1472-6874-12-6.

Wallace K, Zhang S, Thomas L. Compartive effectiveness of hysterectomy versus myomectomy on one-year-health-related quality of life in women with uterine fibroids. *Fertil and Sterility*. 2020; 113(3):618–26.

Winner B, Biest S. Uterine morcellation: fact and fiction surrounding the recent controversy. *Missouri Medicine*. 2017; 114(3):176–80.

45

Cardiovascular and Thoracic Surgery

Kristine Tolentino Parra, MD[1], Theodore Pratt[1], and Matthew J. Martin, MD[2]

[1] *Naval Medical Center, San Diego, CA, USA*
[2] *Trauma and Acute Care Surgery Service, Scripps Mercy Hospital, San Diego, CA, USA*

A 63-year-old woman is transferred to the intensive care unit (ICU) for shortness of breath and a new oxygen requirement. She is postoperative day 2 (POD2) from hip arthroplasty. She requires intubation for acute hypoxia. EKG shows sinus tachycardia and chest x-ray is pending. Arterial blood gas (ABG) shows PaO$_2$ of 55 mm Hg on FiO$_2$ of 100%. She requires norepinephrine (20ug/kg/min) to maintain adequate blood pressure. A bedside echocardiogram shows a hyperkinetic left ventricle, right ventricular free wall akinesis, and normal motion of the RV apex. Pulmonary artery pressures are mildly elevated.

1   *What is the most likely explanation of the patient's hemodynamic instability?*
    A *Acute myocardial infarction*
    B *Fat embolism*
    C *Pulmonary embolism*
    D *Tension pneumothorax*
    E *Sepsis secondary to prosthetic implant*

2   *EKG is performed. The most common finding on EKG with this condition is:*
    A *ST-segment elevation indicating right ventricular infarction*
    B *Q-wave and inverted T-wave in lead III*
    C *Prominent S-wave in lead I*
    D *Sinus tachycardia*
    E *Normal EKG*

3   *Which of the following interventions should be considered next?*
    A *Surgical or transvenous pulmonary embolectomy*
    B *Cardiac catheterization*
    C *Systemic intravenous thrombolytics*
    D *IV antibiotics*
    E *Tube thoracostomy*

4   *One hour after successful intervention, her heart rate is 90 beats/min, blood pressure is 90/50 mm Hg, and central venous pressure (CVP) is 20 mm Hg. Vasopressin has been added. She is anuric. CXR shows good endotracheal tube position and no pneumothorax. Bedside echocardiogram demonstrates worsening function and increased dilation of the right ventricle. What is the next step in management?*
    A *Milrinone drip*
    B *Veno-venous extracorporeal membrane oxygenation (ECMO)*
    C *Placement of a ventricular assist device*
    D *Furosemide drip*
    E *Addition of epinephrine*

Orthopedic surgery carries a significant risk for pulmonary emboli (PE). The patient is demonstrating signs of an acute pulmonary embolism with shortness of breath, hypoxia, and hypotension. Pulmonary embolism leads to increased pulmonary resistance and increased right ventricular (RV) afterload and wall stress. The distribution of wall stress in the RV is not uniform, which can lead to localized free wall ischemia and dysfunction. The associated decreased RV cardiac output produces decreased left ventricular (LV) preload. Decreased LV output results in hypotension. The combination of regional RV dysfunction (RV free wall akinesis or bulging), normal RV apex, and hyperkinetic left ventricle is referred to as McConnell's sign.

Although the patient is at risk of a postoperative myocardial infarction, which can cause cardiogenic shock, this is unlikely given the patient's preserved left ventricular function. Fat embolism would present in the operating room or shortly after surgery and typically features a syndrome including kidney injury, neurologic changes, and petechial rash. Tension pneumothorax can cause hypotension and hypoxia, but unlikely to have spontaneously developed in this patient 2 days after surgery. Sepsis is a very unlikely cause in this case.

The purpose of performing an EKG is to exclude myocardial infarction, not necessarily aid in the diagnosis of pulmonary embolism. The most common EKG finding in pulmonary embolism is sinus tachycardia. McGinn-White Sign (S1Q3T3), demonstrating cor pulmonale, is a classic finding that is not common.

The mainstay of treatment for stable patients with acute pulmonary embolism is systemic anticoagulation with intravenous heparin drip or subcutaneous low-molecular-weight-heparin.

The patient described has a massive PE causing hemodynamic instability and hypotension.

In addition to anticoagulation, this patient should be immediately considered for a surgical or transvenous pulmonary embolectomy.

Patients with massive PE can also be treated with intravenous thrombolytic therapy; however, this patient has an increased risk of bleeding from her orthopedic surgery 2 days ago. The patient is unlikely to have an acute MI given her preserved LV function, therefore heart catheterization would be inappropriate. The patient is not in septic shock and therefore does not require IV antibiotics. Tube thoracostomy would be the treatment for a pneumothorax/hemothorax, which the patient does not have.

Milrinone, a phosphodiesterase inhibitor, is an inotrope that improves right ventricular contractility and is a potent pulmonary artery dilator, which would decrease pulmonary pressures. This would be the best next therapeutic to administer among the choices, as it would act to reduce afterload on the right heart and improve right-sided cardiac output. Caution should be taken when using milrinone in hypotensive patients, as it can also produce a significant decrease in systemic vascular resistance and worsen a patient's hypotension.

Veno-venous ECMO would be inappropriate as this would only unload the right heart and improve oxygenation but would not address the patient's hypotension. A patient with significant cardiac dysfunction and hypotension would require veno-arterial ECMO, which can be used effectively to stabilize patients with massive pulmonary embolism as a bridge to surgical or percutaneous treatment or to aide in RV recovery after treatment. In the event that maximal medical management and milrinone was not effective, veno-arterial ECMO would be a salvage option. Ventricular assist devices (such as the Impella) are now available but would not be a first-line option in this patient. The patient's elevated CVP and low UOP is due to her right heart failure, not fluid overload making diuresis inappropriate.

Answers: 1) C 2) D 3) A 4) A

Kearon C, Akl EA, Ornelas J, et al. Antithrombotic therapy for VTE disease: CHEST guideline and expert panel report. *Chest.* 2016;149(2):315–352. doi:https://doi.org/10.1016/j.chest.2015.11.026.

Lualdi JC, Goldhaber SZ. Right ventricular dysfunction after acute pulmonary embolism: pathophysiologic factors, detection, and therapeutic implications. *Am Heart J.* 1995;130(6):1276–1282. doi:https://doi.org/10.1016/0002-8703(95)90155-8.

Bryce YC, Perez-Johnston R, Bryce EB, Homayoon B, Santos-Martin EG. Pathophysiology of right ventricular failure in acute pulmonary embolism and chronic thromboembolic pulmonary hypertension: a pictorial essay for the interventional radiologist. *Insights Imaging.* 2019;10(1). doi:https://doi.org/10.1186/s13244-019-0695-9.

A 64-year-old man with type 2 diabetes and hypertension presented to the emergency department with chest pain, shortness of breath, and hypotension. His electrocardiogram (EKG) shows an ST-elevation myocardial infarction (STEMI), and his cardiac catheterization demonstrates an acute thrombotic occlusion of the mid-left anterior descending (LAD) artery.

5 *What is the best option for acute treatment of this patient?*
  A *Consult for emergency coronary artery bypass graft (CABG) surgery*
  B *Systemic fibrinolytic therapy*
  C *Percutaneous coronary intervention and stent placement*
  D *Dual antiplatelet therapy*
  E *Warfarin only*

After treatment with placement of an intra-aortic balloon pump and inotropic medications, the patient is transferred to the ICU in guarded condition. A Swan-Ganz catheter is placed for monitoring. He has elevated troponins, and a bedside echocardiogram demonstrates a left ventricular ejection fraction (LVEF) of 25% with a dyskinetic anterolateral wall. On hospital day 5, the patient has an acute drop in blood pressure with decreased cardiac output and elevated ventricular filling pressures. A repeat bedside echocardiogram demonstrates a new moderate-sized effusion.

6 *Which of the following is the likely cause of the patient's acute change in condition?*
  A *Papillary muscle rupture with acute mitral regurgitation*
  B *Ventricular free wall rupture*
  C *Acute stent thrombosis*
  D *Atrial septal rupture*
  E *Ventricular septal rupture*

The patient presented with a STEMI. Cardiac catheterization demonstrated occlusion of the left anterior descending artery and should be treated with percutaneous stent placement. Options for revascularization include percutaneous coronary intervention (PCI) or coronary artery bypass grafting (CABG). Surgical revascularization in the acute setting carries a significant mortality risk and would not be indicated in this case with single vessel disease.

Systemic fibrinolytic therapy can be considered for reperfusion in patients with STEMIs where PCI is not available if the patient does not have contraindications. Patients requiring systemic fibrinolytic therapy due to limitations of the facility should be transferred to a center with specialty capabilities expeditiously. The patient will likely require dual antiplatelet therapy with aspirin and clopidogrel; however, he requires an intervention to revascularize the LAD. Systemic anticoagulation with warfarin for acute treatment in this case is not indicated.

Mechanical complications of an acute myocardial infarction (AMI) include ventricular septal rupture, free wall rupture, and ischemic mitral regurgitation. The incidence of these is quite low, but significantly contribute to the total mortality of AMI. Classically these complications occur 3–7 days after an acute MI. With the advent of thrombolytics and PCI, they can present as soon as 24 hours after presentation. There should be a high level of suspicion for mechanical complications in a patient after an MI who becomes acutely hypotensive. Emergent surgical repair usually will be required. Free wall rupture is the most common major mechanical complication of an acute MI and carries a high fatality rate, oftentimes resulting in immediate death. The patient above has a ventricular free wall rupture with tamponade based on the presence of a new effusion and will require emergency surgery.

Papillary muscle rupture will result in severe mitral regurgitation, which will be visualized on echo. Typically, these patients present with fulminant heart failure and pulmonary edema and would not have an acute effusion. Ventricular septal rupture will cause an acute left-to-right shunt seen on echo and will cause pulmonary vascular congestion. Atrial septal rupture does not occur in this setting. Acute stent thrombosis would present with an EKG consistent with large MI in the distribution of the coronary artery with the stent.

Answers: 5) C 6) B

Manhart JD. Acute myocardial infarction. *McGill Med J.* 1954;23(3):161–168. doi:https://doi.org/10.1056/NEJMra1606915.

Farina P, Gaudino MFL, Taggart DP. The eternal debate with a consistent answer: CABG vs PCI. *Semin Thorac Cardiovasc Surg.* 2020;32(1):14–20.

A 64-year-old man underwent left pneumonectomy for non-small-cell lung carcinoma. Five weeks after surgery, he presented to the Emergency Department with tachycardia and tachypnea. CT scan of the chest demonstrates irregular pleural thickening, and air-filled pockets throughout the left hemithorax (Figure 45.1).

7   *Which of the following interventions is appropriate definitive management?*
   A *Placement of a large-bore right tube thoracostomy to 20cm H₂O suction*
   B *Thoracotomy and Eloesser flap*
   C *Video-assisted thoracoscopic (VATS) debridement*
   D *IV antibiotics alone*
   E *Placement of a large bore right tube thoracostomy to water seal*

The patient has a post-pneumonectomy empyema (Figure 45.1) likely caused by a bronchopulmonary fistula, and the space will require drainage in the short term, but will not be definitive treatment. Because of the late presentation and the complexity of the empyema, definitive management can be achieved with a thoracotomy and Eloesser flap. An Eloesser flap is a single-staged operation with placement of a U-shaped incision and the resection of several adjacent posterolateral ribs, creating a permanent communication. This can be done after initial drainage and stabilization of the mediastinum. Although VATS can be considered, it is unlikely to be successful given the expected postoperative changes and diffuse nature of the disease process as described.

IV antibiotics will be included in this patient's care but will not be enough to resolve the patient's empyema alone. Minimally invasive approaches for infected post-pneumonectomy spaces have a high incidence of failure.

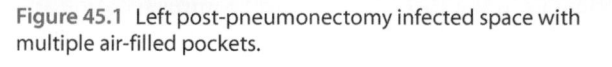

Figure 45.1 Left post-pneumonectomy infected space with multiple air-filled pockets.

Answer: 7) B

Groth SS, Burt BM, Sugarbaker DJ. Management of complications after pneumonectomy. *Thorac Surg Clin.* 2015;25(3):335–348. doi:https://doi.org/10.1016/j.thorsurg.2015.04.006.

Clark JM, Cooke DT, Brown LM. Management of complications after lung resection: prolonged air leak and bronchopleural fistula. *Thorac Surg Clin.* 2020;30(3):347–358. doi:https://doi.org/10.1016/j.thorsurg.2020.04.008.

A 44-year-old man with longstanding hypertension presents to the emergency department with acute, severe, ripping chest pain. The patient has a heart rate of 96 beats/min with a systolic blood pressure of 110/60 mm Hg. CXR reveals a widened mediastinum. Bedsides echo shows preserved ventricular function with no wall motion abnormalities, moderate aortic valve insufficiency, and a large pericardial effusion.

8   *The best diagnostic test to confirm the cause of the patient's hypotension is:*
   A *CT angiogram chest*
   B *CT pulmonary embolism protocol*
   C *Transthoracic echocardiogram*
   D *Transesophageal echocardiogram*
   E *Diagnostic catheterization*

9   *Which of the following would constitute appropriate definitive management?*
   A *Blood pressure control with intravenous sodium nitroprusside infusion alone*
   B *Blood pressure control with intravenous esmolol infusion alone*
   C *Immediate operative repair*
   D *Heart rate control with intravenous infusion of amiodarone*
   E *Blood pressure control with nitroglycerin*

Accurate and timely diagnosis of acute aortic dissection is necessary. The current patient's presentation is suspicious for a dissection complicated by a pericardial effusion and tamponade. The best imaging modality for diagnosis, if patient stability allows, would be CT angiogram of the chest. The accuracy of CT in diagnosing an aortic dissection is 98–100%. In addition, CT provides vital information for operative planning.

Although transthoracic echocardiography can be a quick and adequate assessment of the aorta, it has limitations even with skilled technicians visualizing the proximal aorta. Transesophageal echocardiogram can provide clear anatomical imaging due to the proximity of the esophagus to the aorta, but the test requires sedation and expertise. In a patient with presentation suggestive of dissection, instability, and CXR showing widened mediastinum, a TEE can be performed under general anesthetic in the operating room just prior to cardiac surgery. CT PE protocol would be the diagnostic test of choice for pulmonary embolism. Diagnostic catheterization in this setting is not indicated.

Initial management of the aortic dissection should be directed at immediate blood pressure control with beta blockade to decrease heart rate (and the stress on the aortic wall defined as the change in pressure over time (Dp/Dt). This patient has a proximal or type A aortic dissection as evidenced by the aortic valve pathology and pericardial effusion. Patients with type A dissection require emergent surgical consultation and operative repair for definitive management. Proximal propagation of the dissection can occur, causing rupture and cardiac tamponade, coronary compression, or aortic valve insufficiency. This is in contrast to patients with a type B dissection and stable hemodynamics, who can largely be managed nonoperatively.

Answers: 8) A 9) C

Hiratzka LF, Bakris GL, Beckman JA, et al. ACCF/AHA/AATS/ACR/ASA/SCA/SCAI/SIR/STS/SVM guidelines for the diagnosis and management of patients with thoracic aortic disease: executive summary: a report of the american college of cardiology foundation/american heart association task force on practice guidelines, american association for thoracic surgery, american college of radiology, american stroke association. *Circulation.* 2010;121(13):266–369. doi:https://doi.org/10.1161/CIR.0b013e3181d4739e.

Stevens LM, Madsen JC, Isselbacher EM, et al. Surgical management and long-term outcomes for acute ascending aortic dissection. *J Thorac Cardiovasc Surg.* 2009;138(6):1349–1357.e1. doi:https://doi.org/10.1016/j.jtcvs.2009.01.030.

Thrumurthy SG, Karthikesalingam A, Patterson BO, Holt PJE, Thompson MM. The diagnosis and management of aortic dissection. *BMJ.* 2012;344(7839). doi:https://doi.org/10.1136/bmj.d8290.

A 48-year-old woman has an aortic valve replacement with a mechanical valve. Three hours after surgery she develops decreasing cardiac index despite inotropes and low urine output. She has 700 mL total of serosanguinous output from the chest tube, which has decreased to 50 mL over the last hour. Swan-Ganz catheter demonstrates low cardiac index, increased pulmonary capillary wedge pressure, and a central venous pressure of 20 mm Hg. Labs demonstrate a hemoglobin 7 gm/dL, platelets 241 × 109/L, partial thromboplastin time 68 seconds, and INR 2.7. On telemetry, she has a paced rhythm at 86 bpm.

10 What is the best next step in management of the patient?

    A Transfuse 2U packed red blood cells (PRBCs)

    B Administer fresh frozen plasma (FFP)

    C Stat bedside echocardiogram

    D Bolus albumin

    E Stat CXR

11 Which of the following measures would constitute appropriate treatment?

    A Urgent bedside pericardial window

    B Image-guided catheter drainage of the pericardium

    C Administer FFP

    D Urgent reoperation

    E Place chest tube to wall suction

The patient above recently underwent cardiac surgery and now demonstrates a decreased cardiac output with elevation and equalization of filling pressures. Prompt bedside echocardiogram should be performed to confirm the diagnosis of tamponade. Although the patient's coagulopathy is contributing to the problem and should be addressed, it is not definitive management of the tamponade. Chest x-ray has low sensitivity for diagnosing cardiac tamponade. The patient's low cardiac output is primarily caused by cardiac tamponade and not hypovolemia secondary to hemorrhage; therefore, the patient is not in current need of blood transfusion or volume resuscitation.

Cardiac tamponade after open-heart surgery is considered "early," typically within the first 24 hours and no later than 5–7 days after surgery. Early cardiac tamponade is an indication for immediate reoperation. Bedside drainage via a pericardial window or image-guided drainage could lead to immediate hemodynamic instability and the inability to directly visualize and address the patient's source of bleeding. Placement of the chest tube to suction may dislodge the clot contributing to the tamponade and cause acute worsening of the patient's hemodynamic status by draining the pericardium and not addressing the source of bleeding. Administration of FFP will correct the patient's coagulopathy but will not address the source of bleeding.

Answers: 10) C 11) D

Khan NK, Loisa EL, Sutinen JA, Laurikka JO, Khan JA. Incidence , presentation and risk factors of late postoperative pericardial effusions requiring invasive treatment after cardiac surgery. 2017;24(February): 835–840. doi:https://doi.org/10.1093/icvts/ivx011.

Kuvin JT, Harati NA, Pandian NG, Bojar RM, Khabbaz KR. Postoperative cardiac tamponade in the modern surgical era. *Ann Thorac Surg.* 2002;74(4):1148–1153. doi:https://doi.org/10.1016/S0003-4975(02)03837-7.

A 44-year-old man with 60-pack-year smoking history presents to the ED with new onset hemoptysis. In the emergency department, he has expectorated 200 mL of bright red blood. His vitals are HR 95 beats/min, BP of 110/80 mm Hg, RR 20 breaths/min, SpO2 93% on 2 L/min nasal cannula. While a CT scan is being performed, he acutely worsens with a heart rate of 115 beats/min, BP 89/65 mm Hg, and SpO2 of 90% on 8L nasal cannula and expectorates another 400 mL of bright red blood.

12 What is the next step in management of this patient?

    A Transfuse blood

    B Complete the CT scan

    C Angiography and embolization

    D Intubation

    E Emergent thoracotomy

13 Which of the following would constitute appropriate therapeutic considerations?

    A Emergent rigid and flexible bronchoscopy in the operating room

    B Emergent bronchial artery embolization (BAE)

    C Immediate tracheostomy

    D Placement of emergent chest tube

    E Thoracotomy for lung resection

Airway control is very important and should be the initial step when managing a patient with massive hemoptysis. Hemoptysis of 200–1000 mL within a 24-hour period can meet the criterion of massive hemoptysis, but more importantly any volume which causes significant hypotension or respiratory failure from obstruction is considered life-threatening. The patient should be intubated with an endotracheal tube of at least 8.5 mm inner diameter to allow for therapeutic flexible bronchoscopy. Rigid bronchoscopy, if available, can be useful for airway management, diagnosis, and possibly be therapeutic. In addition to controlling the patient's airway, if the laterality is known, then the patient should be placed with the bleeding side in the dependent position as these patients often die from asphyxiation and not exsanguination. Although lateralizing the source of bleeding will be necessary for treatment, imaging should not precede airway protection. The patient will require eventual treatment with rigid bronchoscopy or bronchial artery embolization, but the patient should be intubated first for airway control. Laterality of the source of bleeding has not yet been determined, so emergent thoracotomy would be premature and should not precede airway protection.

Bronchial arterial embolization is an effective therapy for hemoptysis if the bronchial artery has been determined as the source of bleeding and if the patient is stable enough to undergo angiography. Thoracotomy for lung resection is no longer considered first-line treatment of massive hemoptysis with advances in bronchoscopy and interventional radiology. Surgical treatment should be considered salvage therapy if other bronchoscopy or IR methods fail. Tracheostomy is not indicated as intubation with a large diameter endotracheal tube should be sufficient for airway protection and to allow for passage of both rigid and flexible bronchoscopes for diagnostic and therapeutic purposes. Chest tube placement will not treat massive hemoptysis

Answers: 12) D 13) A

Davidson K, Shojaee S. Managing massive hemoptysis. *Chest.* 2020;157(1):77–88. doi:https://doi.org/10.1016/j.chest.2019.07.012.

Jougon J, Ballester M, Delcambre F, et al. Massive hemoptysis: what place for medical and surgical treatment. *Eur J Cardio-thoracic Surg.* 2002;22(3):345–351. doi:https://doi.org/10.1016/S1010-7940(02)00337-8.

Sakr L, Dutau H. Massive hemoptysis: an update on the role of bronchoscopy in diagnosis and management. *Respiration.* 2010;80(1):38–58. doi:https://doi.org/10.1159/000274492.

A 35-year-old woman with metastatic renal cell cancer presents with worsening dyspnea over the last week. Her chest x-ray shows a very large left pleural effusion. She is transferred to the intensive care unit where a left tube thoracostomy is placed with immediate drainage of two liters of straw-colored fluid. Fifteen minutes after chest tube placement, her respiratory status worsens with a RR 24 breaths/min and SpO$_2$ 90% on 8L NC. She is intubated for hypoxia. A chest x-ray is obtained that demonstrates a complete white-out of the left chest. Inspection of the chest tube reveals it is in good position and not obstructed.

14 *What is the likely cause of the patient's condition?*
   A *Tension pneumothorax*
   B *Re-accumulation of the effusion*
   C *Mucous plugging*
   D *Pneumonia*
   E *Re-expansion pulmonary edema*

15 *Which of the following constitute the appropriate maneuvers at this time?*
   A *Respiratory support by increasing positive end expiratory pressure (PEEP)*
   B *Immediately clamp the patient's chest tube*
   C *Replacement of the patient's pleural drainage chamber and continued suction evacuation*
   D *Intravenous fluid challenge*
   E *Placement of a second left chest tube*

The patient above has re-expansion pulmonary edema (RPE). It is a rare complication that occurs with expansion of the lung after drainage of large chronic pleural effusion (Figure 45.2). It can also occur with re-expansion of a pneumothorax with chronically collapsed lung. Risk factors to developing RPE include degree of lung collapse, rapid re-expansion, and use of negative pressure causing increased speed of lung re-expansion. Symptomatic chronic pleural effusions should be drained in small increments over several hours.

Although tension pneumothorax can cause hypoxemic respiratory failure, a chest x-ray would not show white out of the left lung, but rather absence of lung markings in the left chest. Re-accumulation of the effusion can cause a white out of the chest x-ray, but this is unlikely due to the rapid time course and considering that the chest tube continues to function. Pneumonia can be seen as dense consolidations on chest x-ray but would not result from drainage of the pleural fluid.

Treatment of re-expansion pulmonary edema is supportive. This patient requires ongoing respiratory support and improvement of oxygenation with positive airway pressure by increasing PEEP. Other possible treatment options include diuresis, steroids, and inotropic agents.

Placing another chest tube will not improve the patient's symptoms as the white out of the left chest is caused by pulmonary edema and not increased pleural fluid around the lung. Placement of the chest tube's drainage chamber to suction could worsen the patient's condition by increasing the rate of expansion of the lung. Fluid challenge could also potentially worsen the patient's pulmonary edema, rather diuresis would be an option to treat the patient's condition. Although decreasing the rate of drainage of the pleural fluid could potentially

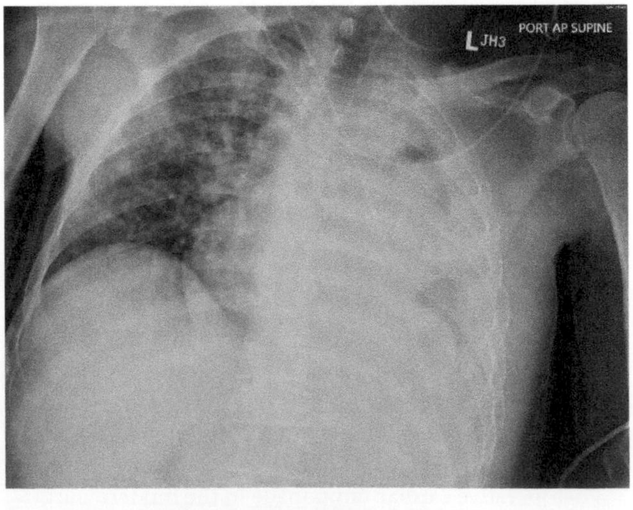

Figure 45.2 Left pleural effusion causing white-out on chest x-ray.

improve the patient's symptoms, clamping the chest tube is not recommended as this could result in tension pneumothorax/hemothorax physiology. A decreased rate of drainage is obtained by placing the chest tube immediately to water seal and avoiding using additional suction (which increased the rate of evacuation).

Answers: 14) E 15) A

Feller-Kopman D, Berkowitz D, Boiselle P, et al. Large-volume thoracentesis and the risk of reexpansion pulmonary edema. *Ann Thorac Surg.* 2007;(84):1656–1662. doi:https://doi.org/10.1016/j.athoracsur.2007.06.038.

A 22-year-old man with multi-organ injury and paraplegia due to a high-speed motor vehicle collision underwent tracheostomy 10 days ago. You are called to the bedside because of a report of bright red blood from the tracheostomy site. You immediately note pulsatile bleeding at the tracheostomy site. After applying increased cuff inflation, the bleeding does not stop and becomes more significant.

16   *What is the next appropriate maneuver to manage this patient?*
  A *Rigid bronchoscopy after tracheostomy removal in the operating room*
  B *Emergent angiography*
  C *Orotracheal intubation, tracheostomy removal, and digital compression*
  D *CT scan of the neck and chest*
  E *Flexible bronchoscopy at the bedside*

17   *What is the definitive management of the patient?*
  A *Emergent angiography*
  B *Median sternotomy and repair of the innominate artery*
  C *Median sternotomy and repair of the innominate artery with interposition graft*
  D *Rigid bronchoscopy and bronchial stent placement*
  E *Relocate tracheostomy in more superior location*

Significant bleeding from a tracheostomy site must be assumed to be a trachea-innominate fistula (TIF) until proven otherwise. Erosion into the innominate artery is the most common fatal complication of tracheostomy. Airway protection is the priority when hemorrhage occurs from a TIF. Patients are subject to both massive hemorrhage and asphyxiation from aspiration of blood. Hyperinflating the tracheostomy cuff is usually an effective initial maneuver to temporarily decrease the bleeding. After initial maneuvers fail, then the patient should be orotracheally intubated to re-establish an airway. The tracheostomy should be removed and digital compression

of the innominate artery against the sternum can be performed, while preparations for emergency surgery are made.

In the setting of massive hemorrhage, measures to stop the bleeding and airway control should be attempted prior to transfer to the operating room for rigid bronchoscopy. Emergent angiography is not appropriate treatment for TIF. There is no role for imaging in setting of hemorrhage from a TIF. Flexible bronchoscopy for diagnosis of tracheostomy bleeding should not take priority over bleeding and airway control.

Definitive repair of TIF is approached via an upper hemi-sternotomy or complete median sternotomy. Proximal and distal control of the innominate artery is the initial step prior to removal necrotic tissue. There are various methods to manage the innominate artery. In the setting of emergent bleeding and potential infected space, ligation of the innominate artery is recommended as first choice of treatment, with prior studies demonstrating no significant neurologic or vascular deficits due to collateral flow through the external carotid artery, thyrocervical trunk, and vertebral vessels.

Median sternotomy and patch repair have been performed, but the use of grafts in a potentially infected space is not recommended. Emergent angiography and embolization are not recommended in this scenario as the patient has active bleeding requiring immediate surgical hemorrhage control. Angiography could be considered in a scenario where bedside interventions are able to achieve temporary hemostasis, and there is no ongoing large volume bleeding. Rigid bronchoscopy and bronchial stent will not control the bleeding of the innominate fistula. Relocating the tracheostomy is not necessary at this time because the patient's definitive airway is achieved by replacing an endotracheal tube and priority should be placed on stopping the hemorrhage from the innominate artery.

Answers 16) C 17) B

Shamji FM, Deslauriers J, Nelems B. Recognition and management of life-threatening tracheovascular fistulae and how to prevent them. *Thorac Surg Clin.* 2018;28(3):403–413. doi:https://doi.org/10.1016/j.thorsurg.2018.05.005.
Wang X, Xu Z, Tang P, Yu Y. Tracheo-innominate artery fistula: diagnosis and surgical management. *Head Neck.* 2014;36(10):1391. doi:https://doi.org/10.1002/HED.

A 30-year-old woman suffered a severe traumatic brain injury after being struck by motor vehicle. On hospital day 9, she underwent a tracheostomy placement. The night of the procedure you are called to the bedside because after repositioning the patient, she is now unable to be ventilated. On arrival, the patient is unable to be manually ventilated using an Ambu bag by the respiratory therapist. Suctioning through the tracheostomy is attempted, which is unsuccessful.

18 What is the next step in the management of this patient?
   A Flexible bronchoscopy to reposition tracheostomy
   B Remove tracheostomy and replace with smaller tracheostomy tube utilizing bronchoscopy
   C Emergent orotracheal intubation and return to the operating room
   D Remove tracheostomy to locate the cause of the obstruction
   E Chest x-ray to rule out pneumothorax

Inadvertent decannulation of a freshly placed tracheostomy can result in loss of an airway. Airway protection should be the first priority when the first attempt to replace the tracheostomy is unsuccessful in ventilating the patient. Complete healing of the stoma typically takes about 7 days. Tracheostomies that are accidentally dislodged, usually when moving the patient, especially in the immediate postoperative period before the tract has matured, can result in tissue planes covering the entry into the trachea. When the cannula is pushed back in, a false passage is created. If a false tract has been created, bronchoscopy through the stoma will not be successful and may cause bleeding. Replacing the previous tracheostomy with a smaller tracheostomy or an endotracheal tube blindly may worsen the creation of a false passage. The patient should be immediately intubated with a standard orotracheal tube and returned to the operating room for exploration of the wound and replacement or revision of the tracheostomy.

Answers: 18) C

Morris LL, Afifi MS. The dreaded false passage: management of tracheostomy tube dislodgement. *Emerg Med News*. 2011;33:1. doi:https://doi.org/10.1097/01. eem.0000399883.10405.3d.

Morris LL, Whitmer A, Mcintosh E. Tracheostomy care and complications in the intensive care unit. *Crit Care Nurse*. 2013;33(5):18–30. doi:https://doi.org/10.4037/ccn2013518.

A 69-year-old woman presents with facial swelling, fatigue, and weight loss. She has distension of the superficial vessels of her neck. She is admitted for further workup. CT scan reveals a large mediastinal mass located in the right apical hemithorax. She is transferred to the intensive care unit for worsening facial and upper extremity edema, and mild dyspnea.

19 What is the likely cause of the patient's condition?
   A Cardiac tamponade
   B Heart failure
   C Upper extremity deep vein thrombosis (DVT)
   D Tumor causing superior vena cava syndrome
   E Pulmonary embolism

20 Which of the following modalities are appropriate for initial management?
   A Stent placement
   B Urgent surgical bypass between the innominate vein and right atrium
   C Inferior vena cava filter placement
   D Immediate institution of radiation treatment
   E Sternotomy and mediastinal mass removal

Superior vena cava syndrome (SVCS) is an obstruction of the superior vena cava due to external compression or internal thrombus. Malignancy is the most common cause of SVCS, but it can have benign causes as well. The patient has superior vena cava (SVC) syndrome likely from a lung malignancy causing external compression and obstruction of her SVC.

Cardiac tamponade could present with distended neck veins but is typically accompanied with hypotension and muffled heart sounds. An effusion would also be seen on cross-sectional imaging of the chest. Heart failure can cause edema, but it would not be limited to the face and upper extremities. An upper extremity (DVT) will cause unilateral extremity swelling of the affected side. Acute symptoms of pulmonary embolism do not present with facial or upper extremity swelling.

SVCS typically presents with facial and upper extremity swelling that can be distressful for the patient. Most patients have developed multiple venous collaterals at the time of presentation. Immediate institution of radiation or appropriate cancer chemotherapy is the best treatment option to relieve the patient's symptoms.

SVCS is a true emergency when the patient presents with hypotension, laryngeal or cerebral edema. Endovascular stenting should be considered for these patients as it is shown to provide faster symptomatic improvement. Surgical bypass or surgical mass resection should not be considered first line treatment. Surgical bypass is considered for patients not amenable to medical or percutaneous treatment. IVC filter placement would be treatment for lower extremity DVTs in patients with contraindication to coagulation, and inappropriate for treatment of SVCS.

Answers: 19) D 20) D

Friedman T, Quencer KB, Madoff DC, Winokur RS. Malignant venous obstruction: superior vena cava syndrome and beyond. 2017;1(212):398–408.

Straka C, Ying J, Kong FM, Willey CD, Kaminski J, Kim DWN. Review of evolving etiologies , implications and treatment strategies for the superior vena cava syndrome. *Springerplus*. Published online 2016. doi:https://doi.org/10.1186/s40064-016-1900-7.

A 65-year-old man with diabetes, congestive heart failure (CHF), and previous history of an anterior myocardial infarction presents to emergency department for fevers and ulceration of his left heel. He is febrile to 101 °C, heart rate of 115 bpm, and blood pressure of 88/65 mm Hg. His EKG demonstrates LBBB and slightly prolonged QRS complex. He is given 2L bolus of crystalloid and started on IV antibiotics. He is admitted to the ICU where a pulmonary artery catheter is placed for his hemodynamic instability. During its placement, the patient becomes bradycardic with a rate of 40 beats/min and hypotensive at 88/60 mm Hg.

21 *What is the likely cause of the patient's change in status?*

   A *Tension pneumothorax*
   B *Air embolus*
   C *Cardiac tamponade*
   D *Pulmonary artery rupture*
   E *Complete heart block*

22 *What should have been done prior to placement of the PA catheter?*

   A *Prophylactic placement of pacing pads*
   B *Have equipment prepared for chest tube placement*
   C *Have equipment ready for pericardiocentesis*
   D *Intubate the patient*
   E *Initiate dopamine drip*

The placement of the Swan Ganz catheter or pulmonary artery catheter caused a complete heart block. The patient had a left bundle branch block (LBBB) prior to placement of the PA catheter. A relative contraindication to placement of a PA catheter is LBBB as there is a risk of creating complete heart block as the balloon is floated to the proper position. Indications for PA catheter include diagnosis of shock, pulmonary edema, left ventricular function/cardiac output, tamponade, ventricular septal defect (VSD), mitral regurgitation, and pulmonary hypertension. Absolute contraindications for placement of PA catheter are the presence of thrombus, right-sided endocarditis, and right heart mechanical valves. In addition to LBBB, other relative contraindications are recent permanent pacemaker/implantable cardioverter defibrillator placement, bioprosthetic right-sided valve, and user inexperience.

Risk of central catheter placement include pneumothorax/hemothorax, air embolus, and arterial stick. There is no other evidence of respiratory change to suggest pneumothorax. Air emboli are a rare complication, and symptoms can be nonspecific like chest pain, difficulty breathing, and altered mental status.

Risks of advanced catheter placement include those of central catheters, as well as additional risk of arrythmias, complete heart block in pre-existing LBBB, cardiac perforation/tamponade, and pulmonary artery rupture. There is no indication that this patient is having cardiac tamponade with decreased heart sounds or distended neck veins. Symptoms of PA rupture vary from slight cough to massive hemorrhage, which the patient is not experiencing.

This patient has a relative contraindication for a PA catheter placement due to his left bundle branch block and the potential risk of causing a complete heart block. If placement of the PA catheter is absolutely necessary, it is recommended that pacing pads be placed on the patient in anticipation of potential arrythmias.

Answers: 21) E 22) A

Chatterjee K. The Swan-Ganz catheters: past, present, and future: a viewpoint. *Circulation*. 2009;119(1):147–152. doi:https://doi.org/10.1161/CIRCULATIONAHA.108.811141.

Gidwani UK, Mohanty B, Chatterjee K. The pulmonary artery catheter. A critical reappraisal. *Cardiol Clin*. 2013;31(4):545–565. doi:https://doi.org/10.1016/j.ccl.2013.07.008.

A 58-year-old man was admitted with left-sided hemiparesis. CT of the head demonstrates a right middle cerebral artery stroke. During his hospital stay, he undergoes a transesophageal echocardiogram (TEE) as part of his embolic stroke workup. Several hours after the procedure, the patient develops fever, tachycardia, and crepitus in the neck. Esophagram demonstrates extravasation of contrast at the mid-esophagus into the left chest. An endoscopic stent is placed over the perforation, but the patient's condition worsens.

23 *The best next step for this patient:*
   A *IV antibiotics and left tube thoracostomy*
   B *Repeat esophagram*
   C *Operative repair via left thoracotomy*
   D *Operative repair via right thoracotomy*
   E *Operative repair via laparotomy*

Esophageal perforation is a life-threatening condition that requires early recognition, diagnosis, and treatment to minimize patient morbidity and mortality. Esophageal perforations are most commonly iatrogenic as a complication of a TEE or esophagogastroduodenoscopy (EGD). Treatment of esophageal perforation is dependent on various factors such as hemodynamic stability, time to recognition of injury, location of perforation, size of injury and degree of contamination. The next step in the management would be to provide drainage of contaminated material from the left chest. This should be followed by radiographic or endoscopic evaluation of the stent to ensure no further contamination or leakage is occurring. This patient is at a very high risk of morbidity and mortality with major surgical interventions, and treatment with an esophageal stent and tube thoracostomy is highly successful.

Endoscopic treatment options for esophageal perforations are currently evolving. Patients who have contained leaks, hemodynamic stability, and a white blood cell count below $12\,000/mm^3$ may be considered for nonoperative management. Injuries to the upper two thirds of the esophagus are best approached via a right posterolateral thoracotomy. Perforations of the distal third esophagus are best approached via a left thoracotomy. Perforations of the abdominal esophagus will require a laparotomy for surgical repair.

Answers: 23) A

Soukiasian HJ, Luketich JD. *Management of Esophageal Perforation*. Thirteenth Edition. Elsevier; 2010. doi:https://doi.org/10.1016/B978-1-4160-3993-8.00058-1.

Lampridis S, Mitsos S, Hayward M, Lawrence D, Panagiotopoulos N. The insidious presentation and challenging management of esophageal perforation following diagnostic and therapeutic interventions. *J Thorac Dis*. 2020. doi:https://doi.org/10.21037/jtd-19-4096.

Raff LA, Schinnerer EA, Maine RG, et al. Contemporary management of traumatic cervical and thoracic esophageal perforation: the results of an Eastern Association for the Surgery of Trauma multi-institutional study. *J Trauma Acute Care Surg*. 2020. doi:https://doi.org/10.1097/TA.0000000000002841.

Chen S, Shapira-Galitz Y, Garber D, Amin MR. Management of Iatrogenic cervical esophageal perforations: a narrative review. *JAMA Otolaryngol - Head Neck Surg*. 2020. doi:https://doi.org/10.1001/jamaoto.2020.0088.

A 59-year-old man underwent a transhiatal esophagectomy 1 day ago for esophageal adenocarcinoma. While on rounds, the patient is complaining of mild chest pain. He has a heart rate of 102 bpm and is normotensive. His chest tube output is dark and bilious. He is taken back to the operating room for repair of a presumed anastomotic

leak. Immediately after induction, there was a large volume of bilious emesis and aspiration.

24 *Which of the following is the best maneuver to prevent this?*
A *Rapid sequence intubation (RSI) and cricoid pressure*
B *RSI and nasogastric (NG) tube decompression*
C *RSI in the head up position after NG tube decompression*
D *Nasotracheal intubation*
E *Minimize bag mask ventilation*

Patients who have undergone an esophagectomy have a high risk of aspiration. Anatomic changes from the surgery require resection of the lower esophageal sphincter, creation of an anastomosis in either the neck (transhiatal esophagectomy) or within the chest (Ivor Lewis esophagectomy), and pyloroplasty. The proximally relocated stomach relies on gravity for drainage. If a postoperative esophagectomy patient requires intubation, then maneuvers should be done to lower their aspiration risk. RSI in the head up position is the best option for the patient after fully decompressing the conduit with NGT.

Other maneuvers that can be employed to protect the patient from aspiration include RSI with cricoid pressure, pre-induction NG decompression, and awake intubation. Cricoid pressure is presumed to occlude the esophageal lumen by compression between the cricoid and cervical vertebrae. However, multiple studies have found cricoid pressure to be largely ineffective at reducing aspiration events. In addition, this patient recently underwent a transhiatal esophagectomy, and cricoid pressure may be less effective due to displacement of the cervical esophagus to the left for the anastomosis. Nasotracheal intubation and minimizing bag mask ventilation will not reduce aspiration risk.

Answers: 24) C

Blank RS, Huffmyer JL, Jaeger JM. Principles and practice of anesthesia for thoracic surgery. *Princ Pract Anesth Thorac Surg*. Published online 2011. doi:https://doi.org/10.1007/978-1-4419-0184-2.

A 60-year-old man is in the ICU on veno-arterial extracorporeal membrane oxygenation (VA ECMO) via femoral artery and vein cannulation for cardiopulmonary failure. While rounding you note pink frothy secretions within the endotracheal tube. You obtain a portable chest x-ray, which demonstrates diffuse pulmonary infiltrates. The pulmonary artery catheter monitor demonstrates elevated central venous and pulmonary artery pressures.

25 *What is the best choice in management of the patient?*
  A *Increase the ECMO flow rates*
  B *Diuresis with furosemide infusion*
  C *Replace arterial cannulation to more proximal location*
  D *Percutaneous trans-aortic ventricular assist device*
  E *Replace venous cannulation to more proximal location*

This patient is showing signs of left ventricular overload while on veno-arterial extracorporeal membrane oxygenation. VA ECMO is a temporary mechanical circulatory support device. The basic circuit consists of venous cannulation for drainage, a pump, an oxygenator, and arterial cannulation for inflow. Cannulation can be done centrally in the operating room, as well as peripherally. Peripheral configurations include arterial access via femoral artery with venous drainage into the femoral vein or internal jugular vein and/or arterial cannulation via the axillary artery or subclavian. A consequence of arterial cannulation is left ventricular distension as the flow into the aorta is retrograde. With inflow into the aorta, there is effectively an increase in left ventricular afterload. When there is suspicion of left ventricular distension then considerations to vent the LV should be made. Options for LV venting include percutaneous trans-aortic ventricular assist device (Impella), intra-aortic balloon pump, percutaneous left ventricular vent, percutaneous left atrial vent, and surgical LV vent.

The patient is showing signs of LV dilation with evidence of pulmonary edema. Increasing the flow within the closed system will still require some method to vent the circuit. Weaning the patient now with signs of LV dilation will worsen the patient's condition. Diuresis may initially improve the patient's pulmonary edema on chest x-ray, but patient will eventually need interventions to decrease the LV distension. Relocating the cannulas will not address the LV distension.

Answers: 25) D

Abrams D, Brodie D. Extracorporeal membrane oxygenation for adult respiratory failure: 2017 update. *Chest.* 2017;152(3):639–649. doi:https://doi.org/10.1016/j.chest.2017.06.016.
Rao P, Khalpey Z, Smith R, Burkhoff D, Kociol RD. Venoarterial extracorporeal membrane oxygenation for cardiogenic shock and cardiac arrest. *Circ Heart Fail.* 2018;11(9):e004905. doi:https://doi.org/10.1161/CIRCHEARTFAILURE.118.004905.
Xie A, Forrest P, Loforte A. Left ventricular decompression in veno-arterial extracorporeal membrane oxygenation.

Ann Cardiothorac Surg. 2019;8(1):9–18. doi:https://doi.org/10.21037/acs.2018.11.07.

A 69-year-old woman with small-cell-lung cancer is completing her staging workup with a cervical mediastinoscopy after a PET-CT demonstrated an FDG-avid R4 lymph node. As the scope was advanced to the right paratracheal region, a pinch forceps biopsy was performed followed by immediate active bleeding with obscuration of the visual field through the endoscope.

26 *What is the initial step to management of the problem?*
  A *Abort the procedure and perform a right thoracotomy*
  B *Abort the procedure and perform a left thoracotomy*
  C *Abort the procedure and perform a median sternotomy*
  D *Irrigate the scope and proceed with lymph node biopsy*
  E *Pack the wound cavity tightly and remove the scope*

Cervical mediastinoscopy is a procedure that is proven to be safe and effective for staging of bronchogenic carcinomas. As dissection occurs in the mediastinum in proximity to the great vessels, hemorrhage is one of the most feared complications during the procedure. When significant hemorrhage is encountered during the procedure, the surgeon should immediately pack the wound and apply pressure if possible. Anesthesia should assist in ensuring placement of large bore IV access for resuscitation. In addition, preparations should be made for either sternotomy or thoracotomy. Irrigating the scope and proceeding with the lymph node biopsy is inappropriate until the hemorrhage has been controlled. Most bleeding during mediastinoscopy can be controlled conservatively with packing and local pressure; however, if bleeding does not stop or the patient shows signs of hemodynamic instability, then surgical exploration is required.

Explanation: 26) E

Park BJ, Flores R, Downey RJ, Bains MS, Rusch VW. Management of major hemorrhage during mediastinoscopy. *J Thorac Cardiovasc Surg.* 2003;126(3):726–731. doi:https://doi.org/10.1016/S0022-5223(03)00748-7.
Hung JJ, Wu YC, Hsu HS, Wang KM, Hsu WH. Major hemorrhage and subsequent cardiac tamponade during mediastinoscopy. *J Thorac Cardiovasc Surg.* 2007. doi:https://doi.org/10.1016/j.jtcvs.2006.08.064.
Córdova H., Cubas G, Boada M, et al. Adverse events of NOTES mediastinoscopy compared to conventional

video-assisted mediastinoscopy: a randomized survival study in a porcine model. *Endosc Int Open*. 2015. doi:https://doi.org/10.1055/s-0034-1392599.

A 55-year-old patient with history of hypertension and congestive heart failure has a left ventricular assist device (LVAD) placed 7 days ago. He has increasing complaints of shortness of breath especially when supine and developed a cough with white foamy sputum. His urine output has become darker in color and slowly decreased to 15 mL/hr. Labs demonstrate a drop in hemoglobin, rising creatinine, and a sharp increase in LDH. After investigating the device, you note there is drag on the rotor requiring increased power.

27 *Which of these is the likely cause of the patient's condition?*
A *Cannula migration*
B *Outflow obstruction*
C *Aortic regurgitation*
D *Pump thrombosis*
E *Tamponade*

Left-sided heart failure can be a complication of a left ventricular assist device with many causes. The patient above has evidence of hemolysis with down-trending hemoglobin, dark urine, and increased LDH. The combination of left heart failure, increased power of the LVAD, and evidence of hemolysis, there should be a high level of suspicion for pump thrombosis. Pump thrombosis with mild left-sided heart failure can be treated with intensifying anticoagulation or antiplatelet therapy. With increased pump power, the device may need exchanging.

Outflow obstruction or kink of the device would show a decrease in power of the LVAD; diagnosis can be confirmed with CT imaging. Aortic regurgitation can show increased left ventricle dilation and heart failure with increased power of the pump; however, there would not be evidence of hemolysis. Cannula migration could cause heart failure, but the pump would likely have decreased power with increased turbulent flow. Cardiac tamponade would demonstrate pump parameters with decreased power and flow.

Answer: 27) D

Fryer ML, Balsam LB. Mechanical circulatory support for cardiogenic shock in the critically Ill. *Chest*. 2019;156(5):1008–1021. doi:https://doi.org/10.1016/j.chest.2019.07.009.

46

Pediatric Surgery

Brandt Sisson, MD[1], Matthew J. Martin, MD,[2] and Romeo Ignacio, MD,[3]

[1] Naval Medical Center, San Diego, CA, USA
[2] Trauma and Acute Care Surgery Service, Scripps Mercy Hospital, San Diego, CA, USA
[3] Division of Pediatric Surgery, Rady Children's Hospital, San Diego, CA, USA

1 *A 5-year-old child is struck by a car while crossing the street, and he sustains multiple abrasions and lacerations to his face. On arrival to the trauma bay his GCS is 6, and his oxygen saturation is 88% on room air. Multiple attempts at placing an endotracheal tube have been unsuccessful and he remains at 88% saturation with bag-valve-mask ventilation. What is the next best step for this patient?*

A *Reattempt endotracheal intubation*
B *Needle cricothyroidotomy with jet insufflation*
C *Surgical cricothyroidotomy*
D *Tracheostomy*
E *Place the patient on ECMO (extracorporeal membrane oxygen)*

Management of the pediatric airway in trauma patients represents unique challenges. Lack of oxygenation and ventilation due to the inability to establish an airway can lead to increased morbidity and potentially cardiac arrest in these patients. Anatomical differences between pediatric and adult patients include a larger head-to-total body surface area, as well as a shorter neck. The soft tissues of the oropharynx are also relatively larger than the oral cavity making the larynx and vocal cords difficult to visualize. The trachea is relatively more anterior, shorter, and narrower than those of adults and predisposes to possible airway challenges. Some of the airway problems that can occur in pediatric patients include right mainstem intubation, inadvertent extubation with small degrees of tube movement, and airway occlusion from mucous or blood. Many of the same principles in airway management are similar in children, including supplemental oxygenation, suctioning, and use of airway adjuncts.

Bag-mask ventilation is a helpful adjunct in ventilating patients; however, in a scenario where a patient is decompensating, a definitive airway needs to be obtained. Emergent surgical airways in children carry a higher risk of complications compared with adults. These include injury to the airway or esophagus, tube misplacement or dislodgment, and longer-term risks of subglottic stenosis. In particular, a surgical cricothyroidotomy should be avoided in children <12 years old due to the higher risk of iatrogenic complications, as this is the narrowest part of the airway and is also immediately adjacent to the vocal cords. In this scenario, needle cricothyroidotomy with jet insufflation is the next best step to oxygenate the patient until a definitive airway can be established. If an endotracheal tube or needle cricothyroidotomy is unsuccessful, then a surgical tracheostomy should be performed to secure the airway in an emergent setting. ECMO is not indicated for this patient and would not be available as an immediate intervention.

Answer: B

Pediatric Trauma in American College of Surgeons *Advanced Trauma Life Support Student Course Manual, 10th Ed.* 2018, Chicago, IL, American College of Surgeons.

Chameides L, Samson RA, Schexnayder SM, Hazinski MF (Eds) *Pediatric Advanced Life Support Provider Manual.* 2012, American Heart Association, Dallas.

Apfelbaum JL, Hagberg CA, Caplan RA, et al. Practice guidelines for management of the difficult airway: an updated report by the American Society of Anesthesiologists Task Force on Management of the Difficult Airway. *Anesthesiology.* 2013;118(2):251–70.

TEACHING POINT: Definitive airway for children is an endotracheal tube. However, if placing and endotracheal tube is unsuccessful, other approaches such as needle cricothyroidotomy with jet insufflation, surgical cricothyroidotomy, and tracheostomy should be considered.

Surgical Critical Care and Emergency Surgery: Clinical Questions and Answers, Third Edition.
Edited by Forrest "Dell" Moore, Peter M. Rhee, and Carlos J. Rodriguez.
© 2022 John Wiley & Sons Ltd. Published 2022 by John Wiley & Sons Ltd.
Companion website: www.wiley.com/go/surgicalcriticalcare3e

Surgical cricothyroidotomy and tracheostomy are rarely indicated for children, especially <12 years of age.

2 *A 2-year-old girl requires emergent intubation for severe traumatic brain injury. Which of the following is the best method to confirm correct placement of a definitive airway?*
   A *Auscultation of bilateral breath sounds*
   B *Chest x-ray appearance*
   C *End-tidal CO_2*
   D *Symmetrical chest rise*
   E *Oxygen saturation >90%*

Orotracheal intubation is considered the most effective way of establishing a definitive airway in a child. A definitive airway is defined as a CUFFED endotracheal tube below the vocal cords. Cuffed endotracheal tubes provide the benefit of improving oxygenation and ventilation in these patients. Previous recommendations were for uncuffed tubes in pediatric patients due to cuffed endotracheal tubes causing tracheal necrosis or stenosis; however, this is no longer an issue due to improvements in cuff design with low-pressure balloons. The gold standard for confirming correct tube placement is visualization of the tube passing through the vocal cords and confirmation with capnography demonstrating end-tidal CO_2. Although auscultation of breath sounds, symmetrical chest rise, and chest x-ray are all important primary confirmation techniques, only end-tidal CO_2 using waveform capnography or colorimetric detector is considered the gold standard for confirmation of correct placement. Well-oxygenated patients can maintain high oxygen saturations for several minutes even with esophageal intubation.

Answer: C

Pediatric Trauma in American College of Surgeons *Advanced Trauma Life Support Student Course Manual, 10th Ed.* 2018, Chicago, IL.
Bano S, Akhtar S, Zia N, Khan UR, Haq AU. Pediatric endotracheal intubations for airway management in the emergency department. *Pediatr Emerg Care.* 2012;28(11):1129–31.
Sagarin MJ, Chiang V, Sakles JC, et al. Rapid sequence intubation for pediatric emergency airway management. *Pediatr Emerg Care.* 2002;18(6):417–23.

TEACHING POINT: Definitive airway must be confirmed in good placement by end-tidal CO_2 using waveform capnography or colorimetric detector.

3 *Which of the following statements is TRUE regarding spinal cord injury without radiographic abnormality (SCIWORA)?*
   A *It is defined as a traumatic myelopathy with evidence of ligamentous instability but no fracture on plain radiography or CT scans.*
   B *SCIWORA injuries are more common in the thoracic and lumbar spine than the cervical spine.*
   C *SCIWORA injuries typically show no abnormalities on magnetic resonance imaging (MRI) and MRI provides no benefit in predicting the prognosis of the injury.*
   D *A SCIWORA injury does not require further immobilization since there is no fracture or ligamentous damage.*
   E *Younger children (<9 years) with SCIWORA are more likely to have severe or complete spinal cord injuries due to increased spinal elasticity.*

SCIWORA is a clinical diagnosis that is defined as a traumatic myelopathy or spinal cord injury with NO evidence of fracture or ligamentous instability on plain radiography or CT scans. It is an injury that occurs primarily in children, especially those <9 years old. This is due to several anatomical differences in the pediatric spine causing increased elasticity with significant, self-reducing injuries of the spinal column. Younger children also have a disproportionately larger head with weaker cervical musculature that permits greater flexion and extension of the cervical spine, leading to more injuries in this region. MRI is useful in diagnosis of ligamentous and/or spinal cord injury in these patients and helps to predict outcomes. Patients with SCIWORA who have a normal MRI, minor hemorrhage, or edema only have an improved prognosis compared to that predicted by the initial neurological examination. The mechanism of injury occurs through hyperextension, flexion, distraction, and spinal-cord ischemia. This allows the spinal cord to stretch beyond its ability to withstand injury and to create a significant injury without associated bony fracture of the vertebral column. Pooled data from multiple studies estimates that 63% of children with spinal cord injury (SCI) age 0–9 have SCIWORA, whereas 20% of children with SCI age 10–17 have SCIWORA. Younger children also have a higher incidence of upper level cervical spine injuries (C1–C4 level). Furthermore, cervical spine immobilization plays a key role in limiting repeated mobility of an already injured spinal cord and helps to limit further injuries.

Answer: E

Grabb PA, Pang D. Magnetic resonance imaging in the evaluation of spinal cord injury without radiographic abnormality in children. *Neurosurgery.* 1994;35(3):406–14; discussion 414.
Carroll T, Smith CD, Liu X, et al. Spinal cord injuries without radiologic abnormality in children: a systematic review. *Spinal Cord.* 2015;53(12):842–8.
Pang D, Pollack IF. Spinal cord injury without radiographic abnormality in children--the SCIWORA syndrome. *J Trauma.* 1989;29(5):654–64.
Pang D. Spinal cord injury without radiographic abnormality in children, 2 decades later. *Neurosurgery.* 2004;55:1325–43.
Liao CC, Lui TN, Chen LR, et al. Spinal cord injury without radiological abnormality in preschool-aged children: correlation of magnetic resonance imaging

findings with neurological outcomes. *J Neurosurg (Pediatr 1).* 2005;103:17–23.

TEACHING POINT: Due to the increase elasticity of the spinal cord in children, SCIWORA is a unique finding in pediatric trauma patients, especially in those <9 years of age.

4   *An 11-year-old girl is the restrained backseat passenger in a high-speed motor vehicle collision. On arrival to the trauma bay, she is noted to have a seatbelt sign over her neck with no hematoma. Her GCS is 15 with no neurologic deficits. What is the next best step for this patient in evaluating for a possible blunt cerebrovascular injury?*
    A   *Ultrasound of the neck*
    B   *Magnetic resonance angiography (MRA)*
    C   *Computed tomography angiography (CTA)*
    D   *Cerebral angiography*
    E   *Observation*

Pediatric patients with blunt cerebral vascular injury are generally asymptomatic at presentation. Early detection and management in these patients can prevent further neurological disabilities such as stroke or seizure. Several hard signs of vascular injury include an expanding hematoma, bruit, or focal neurological deficits, which all require further imaging and/or treatment. Furthermore, there are two well-recognized screening guidelines for blunt cerebral vascular injury to include the Denver and Memphis guidelines. There are two modifications for evaluating

BCVI in pediatric patients: the Utah and McGovern criteria (see below). These guidelines take into account certain injuries sustained, as well as injury mechanism for selection of patients for further imaging. Because of the lack of any of these variables, no imaging is warranted in this patient even with the presence of a seat belt sign. Even with the patient's mechanism of injury, her score is <3.

There are also several imaging modalities used to screen patients for BCVI. These include duplex ultrasonography, standard catheter-based cerebral angiography, MRA, and CT angiography (CTA). In adult patients, CTA has become the current standard for evaluation and has largely replaced catheter-based angiography. In pediatric patients, there is no clear data on the utility or benefit of aggressive screening with CTA, and there are heightened concerns with the risks associated with exposure to ionizing radiation from CT scans. Both duplex ultrasound and MRA have a lower sensitivity and specificity for detecting BCVI in adult and pediatric populations. Furthermore, operative intervention plays a limited role in these patients due to the nature and location of the injuries, except for patients with select high-grade injuries or bleeding injuries in zone II of the neck. Endovascular treatment is the preferred approach for zone I and zone III injuries that are not readily accessible via an operative approach. Antithrombotic therapy with either an antiplatelet agent or anticoagulation plays a key role in management of these patients. The goal of therapy is to prevent propagation of thrombosis and avoid secondary injuries such as stroke or seizure.

Denver criteria	Modified Memphis criteria	EAST criteria
Focal neurological deficit	Petrous temporal bone fracture	Cervical hyperextension associated w/displaced midface or complex mandibular fracture or closed head injury consistent with diffuse axonal injury
Arterial hemorrhage	Carotid canal fracture	Anoxic brain injury due to hypoxia as a result of squeezed arteries
Cervical bruit in patients <50 years	Le Fort fracture II or III	Seatbelt abrasion or other soft-tissue injury resulting in swelling or altered mental status
Expanding neck hematoma	Cervical spine fracture	Cervical vertebral body fracture or carotid canal fracture in proximity to the internal carotid or vertebral arteries
Neurological exam findings inconsistent w/ head CT scan	Horner's syndrome	
Cerebrovascular accident on follow-up head CT scan not seen on initial head CT scan	Neck soft-tissue injury (seatbelt sign, hypoxia as a result of squeezed arteries, or hematoma)	
Presence of Le Fort II or III fractures	Focal neurologic deficit not explained by imaging	
Cervical spine fracture w/ subluxation		
C1–C3 cervical spine fracture		
Cervical spine fracture extending into the transverse foramen		
Basilar skull fracture w/ carotid involvement		
Diffuse axonal injury w/ GCS score <6		
Hypoxic ischemia due to squeezed arteries		

For each of these 3 screening tools, if any of the screening criteria are met, the recommendation is to perform further workup with angiographic imaging.

Variable	No. of points
Utah score	
GCS score ≤8	1
Focal neurological deficit	2
Carotid canal fracture	2
Petrous temporal bone fracture	3
Cerebral infarction on CT	3
McGovern score	
GCS score ≤8	1
Focal neurological deficit	2
Carotid canal fracture	2
MOI	2
Petrous temporal bone fracture	3
Cerebral infarction on CT	3

A score ≥ 3 points on both scales signifies high risk for BCVI and indicates that the patient should undergo angiography.*Source*: Tables above cited from: Herbert JP, Venkataraman SS, Turkmani AH, et al. Pediatric blunt cerebrovascular injury: The McGovern screening score. *J Neurosurg Pediatr*. 2018;21(6):639–49.

Answer: E

Bromberg WJ, Collier BC, Diebel LN, et al. Blunt cerebrovascular injury practice management guidelines: The Eastern Association for the Surgery of Trauma. *J Trauma*. 2010;68(2):471–7.

Burlew CC, Biffl WL, Moore EE, et al. Blunt cerebrovascular injuries: redefining screening criteria in the era of noninvasive diagnosis. *J Trauma Acute Care Surg*. 2012;72(2):330–5.

Grigorian A, Dolich M, Lekawa M, et al. Analysis of blunt cerebrovascular injury in pediatric trauma. *J Trauma Acute Care Surg*. 2019;87(6):1354–9.

Rossidis AC, Tharakan SJ, Bose SK, Shekdar KV, Nance ML, Blinman TA. Predictors of pediatric blunt cerebrovascular injury. *J Pediatr Surg*. 2017;S0022-3468(17)30659-0.

Savoie KB, Shi J, Wheeler K, Xiang H, Kenney BD. Pediatric blunt cerebrovascular injuries: A national trauma database study. *J Pediatr Surg*. 2020;55(5):917–20.

TEACHING POINT: A cervical seatbelt sign is not an indication for imaging to evaluate for BCVI. The Utah and McGovern criteria can be utilized for suspected BCVI to consider if CTA is warranted.

5 *A 15-year-old girl sustains a gunshot wound (GSW) to her right chest.*

On arrival to the trauma bay, she is noted to be tachycardic and hypotensive. Intravenous access is obtained, and she receives two 20 mL/kg boluses of lactated ringer's (LR), as well as 1 unit of packed red blood cells (PRBC). A right chest tube is placed with immediate output of 750 mL of bright red blood. She remains tachycardic and hypotensive despite this initial resuscitation. Which of the following is the optimal approach to continued fluid resuscitation in this patient?

A *Give another 20 mL/kg bolus of crystalloid fluid.*
B *Initiate massive transfusion with 1:1:1 ratio resuscitation.*
C *Administer tranexamic acid (TXA).*
D *Administer 10 units of cryoprecipitate.*
E *Administer 2 additional units of PRBC.*

This patient has clear evidence of ongoing hemorrhage and physiologic shock as defined by persistent hypotension and tachycardia despite resuscitation. Trauma remains a major source of blood loss in pediatric, as well as adult patients. In comparison to adult patients, pediatric patients can better maintain a normal blood pressure by compensating with higher heart rates. Pediatric patients who are hypotensive may have lost already 30–45% of their blood volume. Initial management consists of fluid resuscitation with initial fluid boluses of crystalloid at 20 mL/kg. Most guidelines recommend two crystalloid boluses at 20 mL/kg, followed by a transfusion of one unit of packed red blood cells. After the initial blood transfusion, the next step is for balanced resuscitation with a 1:1:1 ratio of red blood cells, plasma, and platelets. The current blood replacement guidelines consist of 10 mL/kg of pRBCs, 1 unit of platelets per 10 kg, and 10 mL/kg of plasma. Furthermore, balanced resuscitation has led to improved survival of pediatric trauma patients that require large volume transfusions. The current definition of a massive transfusion in a pediatric trauma patient is debated but is often defined as administration of 40 mL/kg (approximately half of the pediatric circulating volume) of blood products in a 24-hour period. The most important point in the initiation of a massive transfusion protocol (MTP) is for each hospital to have an established protocol and to expeditiously implement the MTP when required. Balanced resuscitation also has proven benefits in preventing coagulopathy. Cryoprecipitate has been added to some massive transfusion protocols to provide higher concentrations of fibrinogen. TXA showed a reduction in all-cause mortality in the CRASH-2 trial; however, no large studies have been conducted on pediatric trauma patients. Recent studies have now evaluated the benefits of whole blood as an initial resuscitation in trauma patients, and this would be an appropriate alternative to a 1:1:1 approach if available.

Answer: B

Pediatric Trauma in American College of Surgeons *Advanced Trauma Life Support Student Course Manual, 10th Ed.* 2018, Chicago, IL.

Dehmer JJ, Adamson WT. Massive transfusion and blood product use in the pediatric trauma patient. *Semin Pediatr Surg.* 2010;19(4):286–91.

Parker RI. Transfusion in critically ill children: indications, risks, and challenges. *Crit Care Med.* 2014;42(3):675–90.

Neff LP, Cannon JW, Morrison JJ, et al. Clearly defining pediatric massive transfusion: cutting through the fog and friction with combat data. *J Trauma Acute Care Surg.* 2015;78(1):22–8; discussion 28-9.

CRASH-2 trial collaborators, Shakur H, Roberts I, et al. Effects of tranexamic acid on death, vascular occlusive events, and blood transfusion in trauma patients with significant haemorrhage (CRASH-2): a randomised, placebo-controlled trial. *Lancet.* 2010;376(9734):23–32.

TEACHING POINT: Trauma patients that require a massive transfusion protocol should be considered for a balanced resuscitation of 1:1:1 blood, FFP, and platelets.

6 *Which of the following mechanisms of injury is responsible for the most pediatric deaths?*
   A *Motor vehicle crash*
   B *Drowning*
   C *Non-accidental trauma (NAT)/child abuse*
   D *Falls*
   E *Gunshot wounds*

Trauma-related injury remains the most common cause of death and disability in childhood. Morbidity and mortality related to injury surpasses all major diseases in children and young adults, making trauma the most serious and preventable disease in this population. Motor vehicle crashes (MVC) continue to be the leading cause of pediatric deaths worldwide. This is related to blunt trauma causing multi-organ system injury and the unique characteristics of pediatric trauma patients. More importantly, the majority of injured pediatric trauma patients have no hemodynamic abnormalities, and those with multisystem injuries can rapidly deteriorate, prompting immediate recognition and intervention. After MVC, pediatric mortality is due to drowning, house fires, homicides, and falls. In children <1 year of age, the majority of homicides are due to child abuse/NAT, whereas in children >1 year of age, the majority of homicides are related to firearm injuries. Firearm-related deaths are the second leading cause of death overall among US children aged 1–17 years and the second leading cause of injury-related death. Firearm-related fatality is 49 TIMES higher for 15–24 year olds in the United States than any other high-income country. Lastly, falls are the most common pediatric injury, but rarely result in mortality or severe injury.

Answer: A

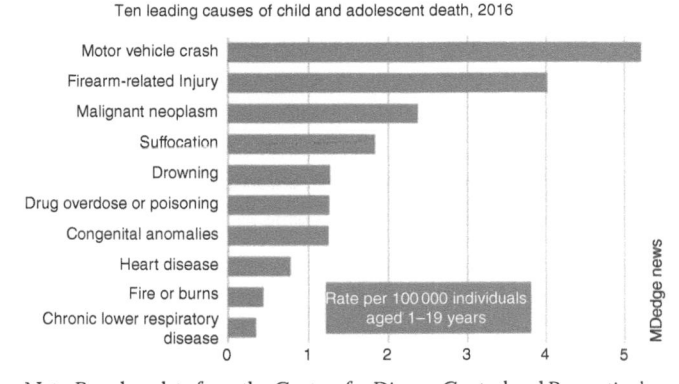

Ten leading causes of child and adolescent death, 2016

Note: Based on data from the Centers for Disease Control and Prevention's Wide-ranging Online Data for Epidemiologic Research system.
Source: Cunningham, RM, Walton, MA, Carter, PM. The major causes of death in children and adolescents in the United States. *N Engl J Med.* 2018;379(25): 2468–75.

Pediatric Trauma in American College of Surgeons *Advanced Trauma Life Support Student Course Manual, 10th Ed.* 2018, Chicago, IL.

Centers for Disease Control and Prevention (CDC). Vital signs: Unintentional injury deaths among persons aged 0-19 years - United States, 2000-2009. *MMWR Morb Mortal Wkly Rep.* 2012;61:270–6.

Cotton, BA, Nance ML. Penetrating trauma in children. *Semin Pediatr Surg.* 2004;13(2):87–97.

TEACHING POINT: Motor vehicle collisions and firearm-related injuries are the leading causes of death in children.

7 *Which child below would be considered both hypotensive and tachycardic based on the admission vital signs?*
   A *10-year-old girl with HR 110 beats/min and SBP 85 mm Hg*
   B *8-month-old boy with HR 155 beats/min and SBP 65 mm Hg*
   C *5-year-old boy with HR 142 beats/min and SBP 70 mm Hg*
   D *14-year-old girl with HR 98 beats/min and SBP 100 mm Hg*
   E *2-year-old girl with HR 148 beats/min and SBP 75 mm Hg*

When caring for pediatric trauma patients, the normal range for vital signs can vary between certain age groups, as well as the characteristic hemodynamic response of children to injury and hemorrhage. Children have an increased physiologic reserve that allows for maintenance of their systolic blood pressure even in the presence of shock. The response to ongoing hemorrhage will typically result in worsening tachycardia with preserved systolic blood pressure. Some children can lose approximately 40–50% of their blood volume before they manifest signs of hypotension; therefore, early identification of the subtle changes is paramount with initiation of fluid resuscitation.

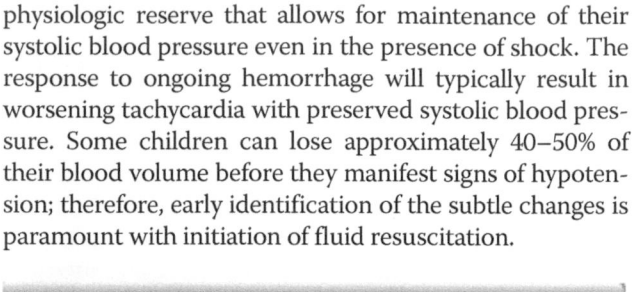
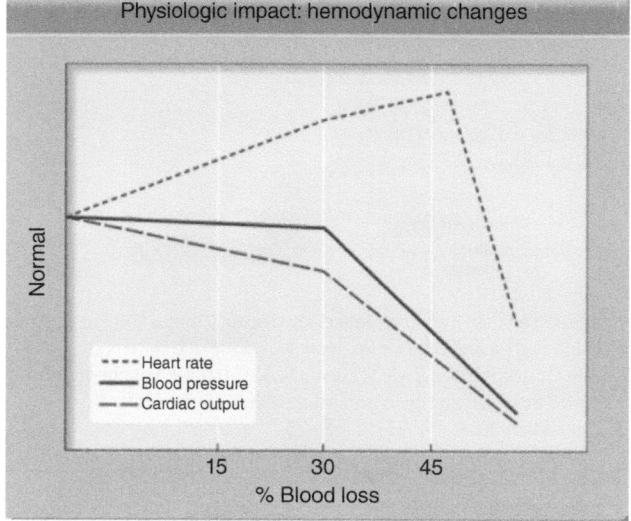

Source: Pediatric Trauma in American College of Surgeons *Advanced Trauma Life Support Student Course Manual, 10th Ed.* 2018, Chicago, IL. Page 195.

A quick method of determining a child's weight, normal vital signs, medication doses, and fluid volume is by using a length-based resuscitation tape, commonly known as the Breslow tape. A more recent method in determining early signs of shock in a pediatric patient is the Shock Index Pediatric Adjusted (SIPA) is calculated as heart rate/systolic blood pressure. SIPA has recently been published as a method to determine if a pediatric patient with blunt abdominal injury requires transfusion. A paper by Acker et al. noted that SIPA of 1.22 (age 4–6), >1.0 (7–12), and >0.9 (13–16) predictive of patients that require transfusion and also have a high risk of mortality.

Answer: C

Pediatric Trauma in American College of Surgeons *Advanced Trauma Life Support Student Course Manual, 10th Ed.* 2018, Chicago, IL.

Gaines BA, Scheidler MG, Lynch JM, Ford HR (2008) Pediatric trauma. In Peitzman AB, Rhodes M, Schwab CW, et al. (eds) *The Trauma Manual: Trauma and Acute Care Surgery, 3rd Ed*, Lippencott, Williams & Wilkins, Philadelphia, PA, pp. 499–514.

Nordin A, Coleman A, Shi J, Wheeler K, Xiang H, Acker S, et al. Validation of the age-adjusted shock index using pediatric trauma quality improvement program data. *J Pediatr Surg.* 2017:S0022-3468(17)30645-0.

Acker SN, Bredbeck B, Partrick DA, Kulungowski AM, Barnett CC, Bensard DD. Shock index, pediatric age-adjusted (SIPA) is more accurate than age-adjusted hypotension for trauma team activation. *Surgery.* 2017;161(3):803–7.

TEACHING POINT: The normal ranges for vital signs vary on the age of a pediatric patient. In comparison to adults, pediatric patients can compensate for early signs of shock and can lose significant blood volumes before becoming hypotensive.

8 *A 7-year-old boy arrives to the emergency department after falling out of a second story window. He was immobilized on a spine board with a cervical collar in place. His initial vital signs are within normal limits and his GCS is 15. He denies any neck pain or tenderness, has no pain with neck rotation or flexion/extension, and his neurological exam shows no sensory or motor deficits. Cervical spine x-rays reveal mild anterior displacement of C2 on C3. What is the next best step in management of this patient?*

A *Cervical spine immobilization with repeat x-rays in 4–6 weeks*

B *MRI to evaluate for spinal cord injury*

C *Flexion and extension cervical spine films*

D *Cervical spine clearance and collar removal*

Pediatric vital sign normal ranges

Age group	Respiratory rate	Heart rate	Systolic blood pressure	Weight in kilos	Weight in pounds
Newborn	30–50	120–160	50–70	2–3	4.5–7
Infant (1–12 months)	20–30	80–140	70–100	4–10	9–22
Toddler (1–3 years)	20–30	80–130	80–110	10–14	22–31
Preschooler (3–5 years)	20–30	80–120	80–110	14–18	31–40
School age (6–12 years)	20–30	70–110	80–120	20–42	41–92
Adolescent (13+ years)	12–20	55–105	110–120	>50	>110

E *CT scan to evaluate for C-spine fracture or ligamentous injury*

It is important to understand the anatomical differences in children with potential spinal injuries. Pediatric patients have relatively larger heads and weaker musculature, which accounts for higher cervical spine injuries. The interspinous ligaments are also more flexible and their growth plates are not closed leading to more elasticity in the spinal column. Normal variants such as pseudo-subluxation of the pediatric cervical spine are common radiographic findings. Pseudo-subluxation often occurs at the C2-C3 junction and is seen in approximately 20–40% of pediatric patients <7 years of age. It is less common at the C3-C4 junction. When subluxation is seen, clinicians must determine whether it is a true subluxation or pseudo-subluxation. A true dislocation of C2 on C3 can be differentiated from pseudo-subluxation by drawing Swischuk's line. Swischuk's line is drawn along the anterior aspect of the spinous processes of C1 and C3. A true dislocation is present if the line is more than 2 mm anterior to the anterior process of C2. Because the patient has no neurological symptoms or neck pain, further x-rays or immobilization are not necessary. Routine CT in pediatric patients following trauma is not recommended unless x-ray studies are inadequate, show suspicious findings, or are abnormal. MRI would be recommended if neurological symptoms were present, x-rays were abnormal, or the c-collar could not be cleared due to neck pain or instability. In this patient with a normal exam and no distracting injuries or complicating factors, the cervical spine can be cleared, and the collar removed if the x-ray review is consistent with pseudo-subluxation. Repeating the evaluation in the next 24 hours can be done to assess his cervical spine if there are any additional concerns or equivocal findings on examination.

Answer: D

Lustrin ES, Karakas SP, Ortiz AO, et al. Pediatric cervical spine: normal anatomy, variants, and trauma. *Radiographics*. 2003;23(3): 539–60.

Pediatric Trauma in American College of Surgeons *Advanced Trauma Life Support Student Course Manual, 10th Ed.* 2018, Chicago, IL.

Shaw M, Burnett H, Wilson A, Chan O. Pseudo-subluxation of C2 on C3 in polytraumatized children prevalence and significance. *Clin Radiol*. 1999;54(6):377–80.

Nigrovic LE, Rogers AJ, Adelgais KM, et al. Utility of plain radiographs in detecting traumatic injuries of the cervical spine in children. *Pediatr Emerg Care*. 2012;28(5):426–32.

TEACHING POINT: Pseudo-subluxation of the cervical spine is a normal variant found in pediatric patients but must be correlated with the patient's clinical symptoms and physical exam.

9 *An 11-year-old girl was the restrained backseat passenger in a motor vehicle collision. On initial presentation, she was noted to be tachycardic and hypotensive with an abdominal seat belt sign present. Her abdomen was noted to be distended, and the FAST scan was positive for intraperitoneal fluid. She was taken to the operating room where she was noted to have a grade 5 splenic laceration, and a splenectomy was performed. Which of the following statements is true regarding her postoperative care?*
A *She should be revaccinated within 10 years.*
B *She should be treated with daily antibiotic prophylaxis until age 16.*
C *Vaccines should be administered 21 days postoperatively.*
D *Vaccines should be administered prior to hospital discharge.*
E *She requires no vaccinations.*

There are numerous studies discussing the use of vaccines and antibiotic prophylaxis for pediatric patients undergoing a splenectomy. Failure to give vaccinations could result in overwhelming postsplenectomy infection (OPSI) leading to increased morbidity and mortality in these patients. All patients >2 years of age should be vaccinated against pneumococcus, meningocooccus, and *Haemophilus influenza* type B. A single revaccination with pneuomococcal vaccine should be given 5 years after the first dose. Ideally, patients should be vaccinated 14 days postsplenectomy; however, a majority of patients are discharged prior to this time period. Therefore, it is important to vaccinate patients prior to discharge. Regarding antibiotic prophylaxis after splenectomy, the current recommendations state that children <5 years of age should receive daily prophylaxis with oral penicillin V. Once these children reach age 5, they may stop daily prophylaxis if they have not experienced a pneumococcal infection.

Answer: D

Howdieshell TR, Heffernan D, Dipiro JT, et al. Surgical infection society guidelines for vaccination after traumatic injury. *Surg Infect (Larchmt)*. 2006;7(3):275–303.

Robinson CL, Bernstein H, Romero JR, Szilagyi P. Advisory committee on immunization practices recommended immunization schedule for children and adolescents aged 18 years or younger - United States, 2019. *MMWR Morb Mortal Wkly Rep*. 2019;68:112.

Chong J, Jones P, Spelman D, et al. Overwhelming post-splenectomy sepsis in patients with asplenia and hyposplenia: a retrospective cohort study. *Epidemiol Infect* 2017;145:397.

Luoto TT, Pakarinen MP, Koivusalo A. Long-term outcomes after pediatric splenectomy. *Surgery.* 2016;159:1583.

TEACHING POINT: Pediatric patients who undergo a splenectomy secondary to trauma require vaccinations after splenectomy. Children <5 years of age should receive daily antibiotic prophylaxis with oral penicillin.

10 *A 3-year-old boy is brought into the emergency room by his mother for a scalp laceration after he reportedly fell off the top bunk in his bedroom. This is his third ED visit in the past month for similar complaints related to blunt trauma. The mother reports she was not present when he fell, and you are concerned for child physical abuse (CPA). Which of the following physical examination findings is most suggestive of CPA?*
    A *Small bruising on anterior lower leg*
    B *Radius fracture*
    C *Facial abrasions*
    D *Well healed scar over left knee*
    E *Frenulum tear*

Clinicians caring for pediatric trauma patients should always remain vigilant for potential signs of child abuse/maltreatment. Oftentimes, the signs can be subtle, and it is important to note that children who suffer from CPA can significantly have a higher injury severity that potentially leads to increased mortality in these patients. Potential signs of child abuse include inconsistencies in the history, implausible mechanism of injury based on child's age, history of repeated trauma with multiple ED visits, bruising or fractures in various stages of healing, and significant delay between injury and initial presentation. More subtle exam findings include perioral injuries (such as frenulum tears), bruising behind the ear, subdural hematomas, and retinal hemorrhages. These injuries may often not be apparent, and it is important for physicians to maintain a high level of suspicion in cases of child abuse. **TEN-4 FACES P** is a helpful mnemonic for abnormal bruising patterns suggestive of child abuse. It includes any bruising on the **T**runk, **E**ars, **N**eck, any bruising on a child **<4** months-old, **F**renulum, **A**uricular area, **C**heek, **E**yes, **S**clera, and **P**atterned bruising. Management of these patients warrants admission and notification to child protective services. Further workup includes a CT scan of the head, skeletal survey

for patients under 2 years, optical exam for those under 3 years, and any additional studies tailored to specific clinical concern.

Answer: E

Wildeman C, Emanuel N, Leventhal JM, et al. The prevalence of confirmed maltreatment among US children, 2004 to 2011. *JAMA Pediatr.* 2014;168(8):706–13.

Pediatric Trauma in American College of Surgeons *Advanced Trauma Life Support Student Course Manual, 10th Ed.* 2018, Chicago, IL.

Ten-4 bruising rule. Face It website. https://faceitabuse.org/ten4rule/ (accessed 2 December 2020).

Pierce MC, Kaczor K, Aldridge S, et al. Bruising characteristics discriminating physical child abuse from accidental trauma. *Pediatrics.* 2009;125(1):67–74.

Sheets LK, Leach ME, Koszewski IJ, et al. Sentinel injuries in infants evaluated for child physical abuse. *Pediatrics.* 2013;131(4):701–7.

TEACHING POINT: **TEN-4 FACES P** is a helpful mnemonic for abnormal bruising patterns suggestive of child abuse: **T**runk, **E**ars, **N**eck, any bruising on a child **<4** months-old, **F**renulum, **A**uricular area, **C**heek, **E**yes, **S**clera, and **P**atterned bruising.

11 *A 6-year-old restrained male back seat passenger was involved in a high-speed motor vehicle collision and complains of significant chest and upper abdominal pain. The primary survey is remarkable for significant contusions, a thoracoabdominal seat belt sign and left-sided tenderness. Which of the following chest x-ray findings warrants a CT scan of the chest?*
    A *Multiple rib fractures*
    B *Hemothorax/pneumothorax*
    C *Pulmonary contusion*
    D *Widened mediastinum*
    E *All of the above*

Thoracic injuries are relatively uncommon in children and account for roughly 8% of all traumatic injuries to the chest. The majority of these injuries are due to blunt force trauma and commonly involve multiple organ system injuries. This is due to anatomical differences in the child's chest wall that cause increased pliability from increased cartilage and incomplete ossification. This allows for significant energy to be transmitted to the underlying lung parenchyma and soft tissues without an associated bony injury. As a result, pulmonary contusions are more common in the pediatric population, and if there are associated fractures, it signifies a greater force involved in the mechanism of injury. Furthermore, as part of the primary survey, a chest x-ray is very useful in diagnosis and management. A chest x-ray may show pneumothorax, hemothorax, rib fractures or lung contusion. Management of most of these conditions can be treated with supportive care or placement of a chest tube. These patients rarely require a thoracostomy and do not require CT imaging; however, a widened mediastinum or questionable diaphragmatic rupture are concerning for a possible aortic injury or peritoneal contents in the left chest, respectively. This requires a CT scan of the chest for confirmation and guiding the need for any further evaluation or interventions.

Answer: D

Holscher CM, Faulk LW, Moore EE, et al. Chest computed tomography imaging for blunt pediatric trauma: not worth the radiation risk. *J Surg Res.* 2013;184(1):352–7.

Yanchar NL, Woo K, Brennan M, et al. Chest x-ray as a screening tool for blunt thoracic trauma in children. *J Trauma Acute Care Surg.* 2013;75(4):613–9.

Pediatric Trauma in American College of Surgeons *Advanced Trauma Life Support Student Course Manual, 10th Ed.* 2018, Chicago, IL.

Sartorelli KH, Vane DW. The diagnosis and management of children with blunt injury of the chest. *Semin Pediatr Surg.* 2004;13(2):98–105.

TEACHING POINT: Chest radiography should be the initial screening tool for suspected intrathoracic trauma in children. Selective use of CT scan of the chest should be reserved for suspected major vascular injuries (i.e. widened mediastinum) or a questionable diaphragmatic injury in a stable pediatric patient.

12 *Which of the following statements is TRUE regarding nutrition in pediatric trauma patients?*

  A *Infants have less nutritional reserve than older children and require initiation of supplemental nutrition earlier.*

  B *Pediatric patients have a similar overall energy expenditure compared to adults.*

  C *Albumin is the best lab value to monitor acute changes in protein status.*

  D *The majority of calories in daily nutrition should come from lipids.*

  E *Enteral nutrition increases gut mucosal atrophy leading to bacterial translocation.*

There are multiple important differences between nutritional requirements of critically ill adult and pediatric trauma patients. Optimizing nutritional status is an important component for treatment of pediatric trauma patients. During the post-trauma phase, the metabolic response is broken down into two phases. The first phase is characterized by a decreased metabolism and decreased oxygen requirements. This is followed by hyper-metabolic phase that varies based on the mechanism and severity of injury. There is increased turnover of protein, carbohydrates, and lipids often as much as 2–3 times the normal resting state. Compared to adult trauma patients, children have a higher protein requirement per kilogram and higher baseline expenditure. Children also have decreased protein reserves and during the catabolic phase, this can lead to increased complications such as infection, respiratory failure, and poor wound healing. Supplemental nutrition such as enteral or parenteral nutrition also plays a key role in management of these patients. Most guidelines recommend initiating nutrition if greater than 3 days without a diet is anticipated; however, infants require initiation of nutrition earlier due to low energy reserves. Enteral nutrition is the preferred route to avoid the complications of parenteral nutrition such as central venous catheter complications, infection, and bacterial translocation from gut mucosal atrophy. Furthermore, when calculating the caloric distribution of nutrition, 50% carbohydrates, 40% fats, and 10% protein is recommended. Although albumin may be a useful nutritional marker in the outpatient or elective setting, it has little value during acute severe illness or injury; however, prealbumin, transferrin, and retinol binding protein have shorter half-lives and are more indicative of acute changes and may be useful for monitoring nutritional status and response to therapy.

Answer: A

Martindale RG, Warren M. Should enteral nutrition be started in the first week of critical illness? *Curr Opin Clin Nutr Metab Care.* 2015;18(2):202–6.

Cook RC, Blinman TA. Nutritional support of the pediatric trauma patient. *Sem Pediatr Surg.* 2010;19:242–51.

Jaksic T. Effective and efficient nutritional support for the injured child. *Surg Clin North Am.* 2002;82:379–91.

Goday PS, Mehta NM. *Pediatric Critical Care Nutrition.* 2014, McGraw-Hill Education.

TEACHING POINT: There are unique nutritional needs in children compared to adults.

13 *A 6-year-old boy is admitted to the PICU with sepsis and respiratory failure secondary to pneumonia. He is intubated and sedated on the ventilator and broad-spectrum antibiotics are initiated. Which of the following parameters should be closely monitored regarding early goal-directed therapy in this patient?*

  A *Capillary refill < 5 seconds*

  B *Cardiac index > 2.5 L/min/m^2*

C *Central venous O_2 saturation (ScvO$_2$) >/= 50%*
D *Hemoglobin levels > 10 g/dL*
E *Urine output >1 mL/kg/hr*

Sepsis is a leading cause of morbidity and mortality worldwide, and prompt recognition and treatment are vital in these patients. The Surviving Sepsis Campaign was formed in 2001 to develop evidenced-based guidelines and recommendations for the resuscitation and management of patients with sepsis. Pediatric sepsis resuscitation generally follows similar guidelines to adults, with several considerations that take into account the unique pediatric physiology and response to infection. These include initiation of broad-spectrum antibiotics (preferably after cultures have been obtained), fluid resuscitation, and source control. Initial endpoints of resuscitation for septic shock include:

1) Capillary refill </= 2 seconds
2) Normal blood pressure for age
3) Normal pulse exam with no differential between peripheral and central pulses and warm extremities
4) Urine output >/= 1 mL/kg/hr, normal mental status
5) ScvO$_2$ >/= 70% and cardiac index between 3.3 and 6.0 L/min/m^2

Furthermore, alternative endpoints of resuscitation such as lactate or dynamic ultrasound assessment may be substituted. Similar hemoglobin targets to adults are recommended in pediatric patients, and a hemoglobin target of >7 g/dL is appropriate after initial resuscitation and stabilization. The key points to remember are early recognition of the shock state, early fluid resuscitation and initiation of antibiotics, monitoring endpoints of resuscitation, and finally treating the source of the infection.

Answer: E

Weiss SL, Peters MJ, Alhazzani W, et al. Surviving sepsis campaign international guidelines for the management of septic shock and sepsis-associated organ dysfunction in children. Pediatr Crit Care Med. 2020;21(2):e52–106.
Rivers EP, Katranji M, Jaehne KA, et al. Early interventions in severe sepsis and septic shock: a review of the evidence one decade later. *Minerva Anestesiol.* 2012;78(6):712–24.

TEACHING POINT: Pediatric sepsis requires broad-spectrum antibiotics, fluid resuscitation, and source control. Assessment of resuscitation can be performed using targeted endpoints such a capillary refill, blood pressure, urine output, and cardiac index.

14 *A 2-month-old boy presents to the ED with persistent bilious emesis. On physical exam, he appears dehydrated, and his abdomen is non-distended and non-tender. An abdominal x-ray is performed and shows a paucity of gas but no evidence of free air. What is the best next step in management of this patient?*
A *Abdominal ultrasound*
B *Contrast enema*
C *CT abdomen/pelvis*
D *Proceed to the operating room*
E *Upper GI contrast series*

Bilious emesis in a child should immediately raise suspicion for intestinal malrotation. Malrotation is defined as a failure of normal intestinal rotation during embryogenesis and can be associated with other congenital anomalies such as gastroschisis, omphalocele, duodenal or jejunal atresia, anorectal malformations, and Hirschsprung's disease. Due to this failure of rotation, adhesions can form, commonly called Ladd's band, and can create fixed points of rotation around the narrowed pedicle of the superior mesenteric vessels. The majority of cases occur within the first year of life but can occur at an older age. The typical clinical findings of a child with malrotation include bilious emesis, dehydration, and abdominal distention. This can lead to intestinal obstruction or volvulus with vascular compromise and eventual bowel necrosis leading to perforation; therefore, prompt diagnosis and intervention are warranted.

The initial work up begins with a plain radiograph of the abdomen. If no signs of perforation are present, the next step is an upper GI series with oral contrast. Findings suggestive of malrotation include a misplaced duodenum with the ligament of Treitz on the right side of the abdomen and small bowel predominantly in the right abdomen (see image below). Volvulus can appear as the duodenum with a "corkscrew" appearance or duodenal obstruction. Other imaging modalities such as ultrasound, CT, and contrast enema can be useful to aid in diagnosis of intestinal rotational anomalies and other associated disorders but are not considered the best initial screening tool. Signs of peritonitis, hypotension, or free air on radiographs warrant emergent exploration. The surgical procedure, called a Ladd procedure, involves (1) detorsion of the volvulus (2) division of Ladd's bands, (3) orientation of the small bowel on the right abdomen and the colon on left side, and (4) an appendectomy. This can be done either laparoscopically or open depending on surgeon preference and patient status.

Answer: E

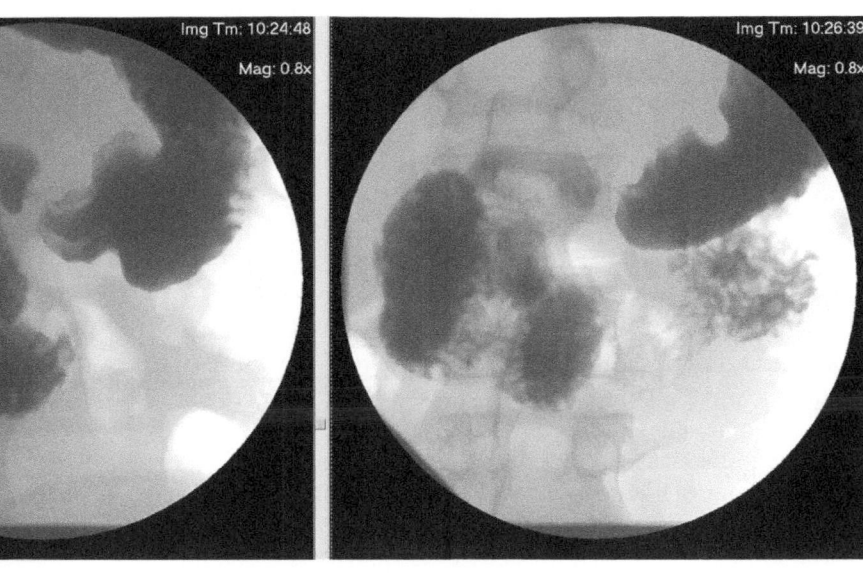

Upper GI study demonstrating small bowel on the right side of the abdomen.

Mehall JR, Chandler JC, Mehall RL, et al. Management of typical and atypical intestinal malrotation. *J Pediatr Surg.* 2002;37(8):1169–72.

Graziano K, Islam S, Dasgupta R, et al. Asymptomatic malrotation: Diagnosis and surgical management: An American Pediatric Surgical Association outcomes and evidence based practice committee systematic review. *J Pediatr Surg.* 2015;50:1783.

Hsiao M, Langer JC. Surgery for suspected rotation abnormality: selection of open vs laparoscopic surgery using a rational approach. *J Pediatr Surg* 2012;47(5):904–10.

Lodwick DL, Minneci PC, Deans KJ. Current surgical management of intestinal rotational abnormalities. *Curr Opin Pediatr.* 2015;27(3):383–8.

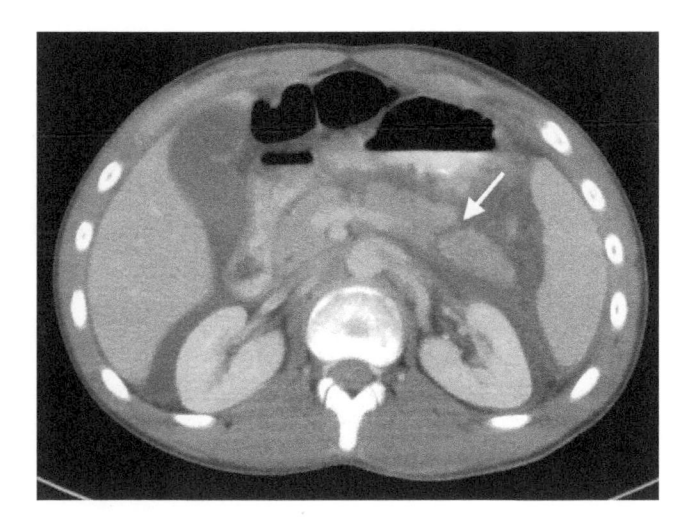

TEACHING POINT: Bilious emesis in an infant should raise suspicion for intestinal malrotation. Workup includes an abdominal x-ray to rule out any free air or perforation followed by an upper GI contrast series. Treatment is a Ladd's procedure.

15 *An 11-year-old male is riding his bicycle and sustains a handlebar injury to the upper abdomen. He presents to the ED the next day complaining of persistent epigastric pain, nausea, and early satiety. On exam, he is noted to have bruising and tenderness around his umbilicus. Labs show an elevated serum lipase and leukocytosis. A CT scan is shown below and demonstrates a near-complete pancreatic transection in the distal body.*

Which of the following statements is TRUE regarding management of this blunt pancreatic injury?

A *Grade V injuries can be safely managed with ERCP and pancreatic duct stenting.*

B *Injuries to the distal pancreas always mandate surgical exploration.*

C *Low-grade injuries that damage the main pancreatic duct can be managed with drain placement only.*

D *Nonoperative intervention has a higher risk of pseudocyst formation.*

E *Delayed operative intervention results in superior outcomes compared to early operative intervention.*

Blunt abdominal injuries occur in approximately 10–15% of pediatric trauma patients, and pancreatic injuries account for 3–4% of those injuries. Blunt force trauma to the epigastrium such as a sharp blow or a sudden acceleration/deceleration injury are common mechanisms of injury to the pancreas and duodenum, with bicycle crashes being a common mechanism. There are also physical exam findings such as Cullen's sign (peri-umbilical bruising) or Grey Turner's sign (flank bruising) that indicate retroperitoneal hemorrhage from pancreatic injury although these are not commonly seen. This patient has a classic presentation for a pancreatic injury, and a CT scan is performed to help with grading of the injury and potential management pathways. The two most important factors in determining prognosis and optimal management are (1) the location of the injury and (2) the integrity of the main pancreatic duct. This is outlined in the AAST Organ Injury Scale for pancreatic injuries (see Table below).

Grade I and II injuries without duct disruption can be safely treated with nonoperative management. Grade III injuries (with duct disruption) can be treated with ERCP and stent placement or distal pancreatectomy with splenic preservation if possible. Grade IV and V injuries are located in the head of the pancreas and are associated with high-energy mechanisms. These generally require operative management to address the main pancreatic duct and frequent presence of associated injuries. Recent literature has also shown fewer complications such as pseudocyst formation, length of stay, infection, and days on parenteral nutrition with operative intervention versus nonoperative management. The most important thing to remember is that injuries that have a better prognosis and are most amenable to nonoperative management are injuries to the body/tail that do not involve the main pancreatic duct. Managing a pancreatic injury with drains only would be most appropriate for a grade 1 or 2 injury that involves parenchyma and not injuries involving the main pancreatic duct or injuries to the pancreatic head.

Answer: D

Mahajan A, Kadavigere R, Sripathi S, et al. Utility of serum pancreatic enzyme levels in diagnosing blunt trauma to the pancreas: A prospective study with systematic review. *Injury*. 2014;45(9):1384–93.

Mora MC, Wong KE, Friderici J, et al. Operative vs nonoperative management of pediatric blunt pancreatic trauma: evaluation of the National Trauma Data Bank. *J Am Coll Surg*. 2015;222(6):977–82.

Iqbal CW, St Peter SD, Tsao K, et al. Operative vs nonoperative management for blunt pancreatic transection in children: Multi-institutional outcomes. *J Am Coll Surg*. 2014;218(2):157–62.

Beres AL, Wales PW, Christison-Lagay ER, McClure ME, Fallat ME, Brindle ME. Non-operative management of high-grade pancreatic trauma: Is it worth the wait? *J Pediatr Surg*. 2013;48(5):1060–4.

TEACHING POINT: Management of blunt pancreatic injuries is based on grade, which is determined by location of injury and integrity of the main pancreatic duct. High-grade injuries are managed operatively and carry a lower risk of pseudocyst formation when compared with nonoperative management.

16 *A 6-year-old girl is the restrained backseat passenger in a low-speed motor vehicle accident. She presents to the ED with complaints of abdominal pain, nausea, and two episodes of non-bilious, non-bloody emesis. On physical exam, she alert, and awake with a GCS of 15. She is hemodynamically stable, and her abdomen is non-tender and non-distended. CBC, LFTs, lipase, and urinalysis are all within normal limits. What is the most appropriate next step in management of this patient?*

   A *Admit for observation with serial abdominal exams*
   B *Abdominal ultrasound exam (FAST)*
   C *CT abdomen/pelvis*

Pancreas injury scale

Grade[*]	Type of injury	Description of injury
1	Hematoma	Minor contusion without duct injury
	Laceration	Superficial laceration without duct injury
II	Hematoma	Major contusion without duct injury or tissue loss
	Laceration	Major laceration without duct injury or tissue loss
III	Laceration	Distal transection or parenchymal injury with duct injury
IV	Laceration	Proximal[?] transection or parenchymal injury involving ampulla
V	Laceration	Massive disruption of pancreatic head

[*]Advance one grade for multiple injuries up to grade III.
Source: Moore, EE, Cogbill TH, Malangoni MA, et al. Table showing the American Association for the Surgery of Trauma Organ Injury Scale (AAST-OIS) for pancreatic injuries. Reproduced with permission from Moore et al., *J Trauma*. 1990;30:1427–9.

D *Proceed to the operating room for urgent laparotomy*

E *Trial oral diet in the ED and discharge to home*

Most pediatric abdominal injuries that result from blunt trauma are primarily due to motor vehicle collisions and falls. There is a current debate regarding the management of blunt abdominal trauma such as when to order a CT scan or when operative intervention is necessary. The PECARN (Pediatric Emergency Care Applied Research Network) has developed a clinical predictive tool for children with an abdominal injury. The low-risk rule is based on the following findings:

- Glasgow coma scale ≥14
- No evidence of abdominal wall trauma or seat belt sign
- No abdominal tenderness
- No complaints of abdominal pain
- No vomiting
- No thoracic wall trauma
- No decreased breath sounds

If patients have none of these findings, then a CT scan could be avoided due to the very low risk of an intra-abdominal injury. Routine laboratory screening for these trauma patients varies but should include a CBC, LFTs, lipase/amylase, coagulation studies, and UA. The FAST exam is not as useful in pediatric patients due to the inability to detect intra-parenchymal injuries, and clinically significant injuries can be present in the absence of any free fluid. Observation with serial abdominal exams in a hemodynamically stable patient without laboratory findings of intra-abdominal injury is the next best step for this patient and is effective at detecting low likelihood abdominal injuries without added morbidity. In addition, it avoids unnecessary exposure to radiation. She is not safe for discharge home due to her emesis and complaints of abdominal pain. If her abdominal exam changes or she becomes hemodynamically unstable, then further imaging or proceeding to the operating room is warranted.

Answer: A

Mahajan P, Kuppermann N, Tunik M, et al. Comparison of clinician suspicion versus a clinical prediction rule in identifying children at risk for intra-abdominal injuries after blunt torso trauma. *Acad Emerg Med.* 2015;22(9):1034–41.

Streck CJ, Jewett BM, Wahlquist AH, et al. Evaluation for intra-abdominal injury in children after blunt torso trauma: Can we reduce unnecessary abdominal computed tomography by utilizing a clinical prediction model? *J Trauma Acute Care Surg.* 2012;73(2):371–6; discussion 376.

Holmes JF, Lillis K, Monroe D, et al. Identifying children at very low risk of clinically important blunt abdominal injuries. *Ann Emerg Med.* 2013;62(2): 107–16.

Holmes JF, Sokolove PE, Brant WE, et al. Identification of children with intra-abdominal injuries after blunt trauma. *Ann Emerg Med.* 2002;39(5):500–9.

TEACHING POINT: A selective use of CT scan in pediatric trauma patients is recommended to avoid unnecessary tests and exposure to radiation.

17 *A 2-year-old, 12-kg boy is brought to the ED after falling into a fire pit. On exam, he is noted to have burns to face, entire right upper extremity, and anterior torso. The burns on his face are mildly erythematous and painful, but no blistering is present. The burns on his right upper extremity and anterior torso are pink, blistered, and blanch to the touch. According to the Parkland formula, which of the following is the most appropriate fluid resuscitation regimen for this patient in the first 8 hours?*

A *D5 0.25% saline at 81 mL/hr*

B *D5 lactated ringers at 81 mL/hr*

C *Lactated ringers at 81 mL/hr plus D5 lactated ringers at 44 mL/hr*

D *Lactated ringers at 101 mL/hr*

E *Normal saline at 101 mL/hr plus D5 normal saline at 12 mL/hr*

The initial management of burn patients follows the resuscitation of any trauma patient, starting with the airway first. After addressing the patient's airway and treating any life-threatening injuries, immediate management begins with appropriate fluid resuscitation. The principles of burn management in pediatric patients generally follow those of adult patients with a few key differences. The "rule of nines" is a practical guide in determining total body surface area (TBSA) burned and is the preferred tool for calculating the extent of a burn injury. Furthermore, body surface area (BSA) differs in children due to a disproportionately larger head; therefore, the most accurate measurement of BSA is with the modified "rule of nines" (see graph below).

The American Burn Association recently updated their initial fluid rate used for burn resuscitation due to concerns of over-resuscitation using the traditional Parkland formula. Resuscitation of pediatric burn patients should begin at 3 mL/kg/%TBSA of LR, with 50% of the total volume administered over 8 hours and the other 50% administered over the next 16-hour period. The goal is to balance a higher resuscitation volume requirement due to larger surface area of body mass with smaller intravascular volume. Children <30 kg should also receive dextrose containing isotonic fluids such as D5LR at a maintenance rate because of the limited glycogen stores and the avoidance of hyponatremia. Also, when calculating the TBSA, only second- and third-degree burns should be counted. Fluid rates should be adjusted to a target urine output of 1 mL/kg/hr. The goal is to avoid under-resuscitation resulting in hypoperfusion and end-organ injury, as well as over-resuscitation that results in increased edema leading to potential respiratory distress syndrome or compartment syndrome. It is also important to note that the 24-hour timeframe is from the time of injury, not presentation. In patients who present several hours after injury, higher initial rates of resuscitation are indicated to make up for the time lapsed since injury.

For this patient, only the burns on the right upper extremity and torso are calculated for a total of 36%, with 18% for the anterior torso, 9% for the anterior arm, and 9% for the posterior arm. The facial burns are not included because they are first-degree burns. Using the Parkland formula for this patient: 3 mL LR × 12 kg × 36% TBSA = 1296 mL. This is the total for a 24-hour period with half (648 mL) being administered in the first 8 hours to give an hourly rate of 81 mL/hr LR. This is in addition to the maintenance rate of intravenous fluid, which can be calculated using the 4:2:1 rule where for the first 10 kg, one receives 4 mL × kg/hr, the second 10 kg, one adds 2cc × kg/hr ,and after 20 kg, the patient will receive 1 mL × kg/hr. For our patient with a weight of 12 kg ((4 mL × 10 kg for first 10 kg) + (2 mL × 2 kg for next 2 kg) = 44 mL/hr of D5LR).

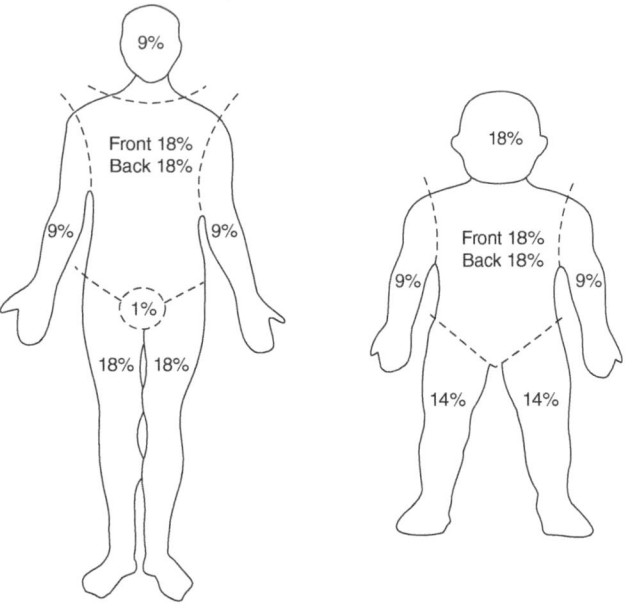

Source: Graph taken from Sojka J, Krakowski AC, Stawicki SP. "Burn Shock and Resuscitation: Many Priorities, One Goal." *IntechOpen*, IntechOpen, 30 May 2019, www.intechopen.com/books/clinical-management-of-shock-the-science-and-art-of-physiological-restoration/burn-shock-and-resuscitation-many-priorities-one-goal.

Answer: C

Gonzalez R, Shanti CM. Overview of current pediatric burn care. *Semin Pediatr Surg.* 2015;24(1):47–9.
Barrow RE, Jeschke MG, Herndon DN. Early fluid resuscitation improves outcomes in severely burned children. *Resuscitation.* 2000;45(2):91–6.

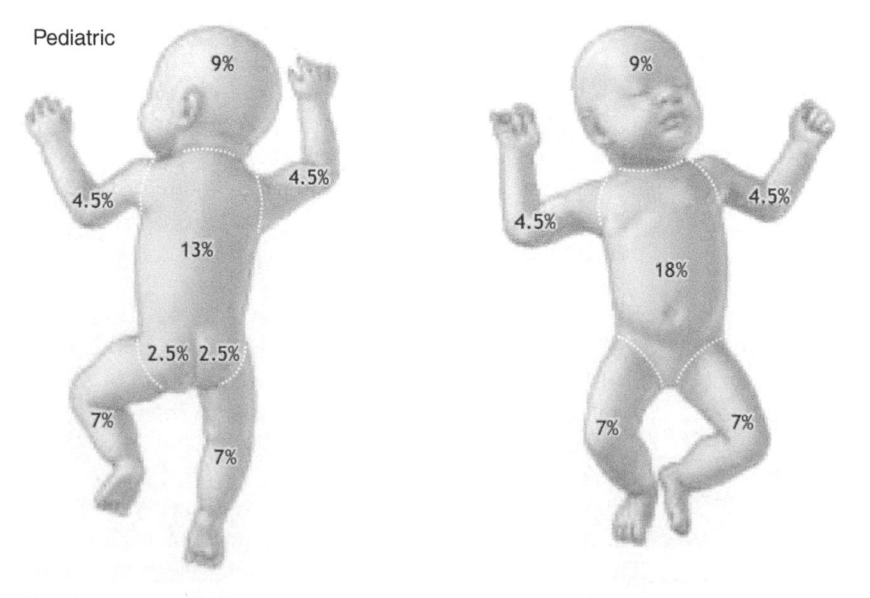

Source: Graph taken from Pediatric Trauma in American College of Surgeons *Advanced Trauma Life Support Student Course Manual, 10th Ed.* 2018, Chicago, IL. Page 175.

Pediatric Trauma in American College of Surgeons
*Advanced Trauma Life Support Student Course Manual,
10th Ed.* 2018, Chicago, IL.
Herndon DN, Spies M. Modern burn care. *Semin Pediatr
Surg.* 2001;10(1):28–31.

TEACHING POINT: Fluid resuscitation in pediatric
burns is 3 mL/kg/%TBSA of LR in addition to maintenance fluids. TBSA is based on second- and third-degree
burns.

18 *A 36-week gestation male infant is born with the following defect below (see picture). The infant was intubated immediately and an orogastric tube was
inserted. Intravenous antibiotics and fluids are
administered. On exam, the bowel appears viable
with no signs of ischemia or necrosis. What is the next
best step in management of this patient?*

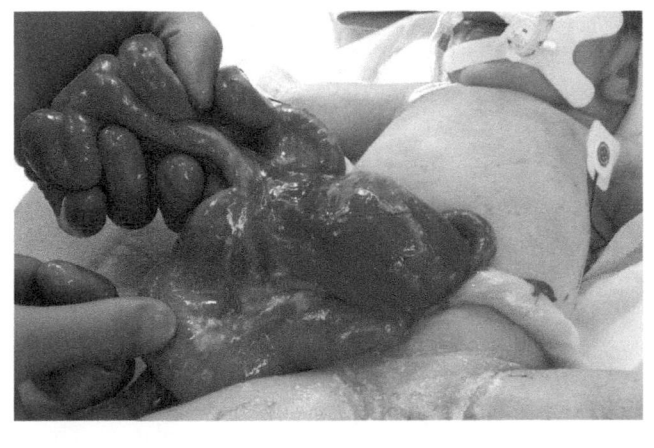

A *Initiate enteral feeds via the OG tube*
B *Wrap the bowel with a sterile dressing or cover*
C *Placement of a silastic silo*
D *Skin closure only at the bedside*
E *Proceed immediately to the operating room for pri-
mary closure*

This patient has a classic presentation for gastroschisis
with an abdominal wall defect and evisceration of bowel
to the right of the umbilical cord with no covering membrane. Another common abdominal wall defect is an
omphalocele, which occurs at the umbilicus and is covered by a membrane and frequently associated with
other congenital abnormalities. Gastroschisis commonly
occurs in premature infants and in younger mothers
while omphalocele infants are full-term infants.
Omphalocele patients may have associated cardiac,
chromosomal, genitourinary, renal, facial, and skeletal
abnormalities.
    The most important first step in management of these
patients is securing an airway, if needed, and initiating

adequate fluid resuscitation. Patients that have a larger
abdominal wall defect with no peritoneal covering are
more prone to heat and fluid losses from the bowel, often
2.5 times more than a healthy newborn. The next best
step for this patient is to wrap the bowel in a sterile dressing to preserve body heat, minimize fluid losses, and
protect the bowel. Patients should also have an orogastric tube placed to decompress the stomach. Fluid resuscitation should begin at 2–3 times the normal
maintenance rate. The size of the defect, the abdominal
domain, and clinical status of the patient will determine
the best approach in closing the defect. If feasible, primary closure is preferred in the first few hours of life and
is successful in approximately 70% of patients. If primary
closure is not feasible, then placement of a silastic silo is
the next step in management. This allows for serial
reductions to increase abdominal domain and a staged
closure at a later time. A newer approach in closing the
defect is the sutureless closure. This approach involves
reducing the abdominal contents (with or without a silo)
and then placing the umbilical cord over the defect without fascial suturing. Current data is promising with high
rates of spontaneous closure, less requirement for general anesthesia, and decreased wound complications and
infections. The overall important aspects of management include minimizing fluid loss while protecting the
bowel and early closure of the defect when possible.
Enteral feedings should not start until the defect has
been repaired or adequately covered.

Answer: B

Skarsgard ED. Management of gastroschisis. *Curr Opin
Pediatr.* 2016;28:363.
Kunz SN, Tieder JS, Whitlock K, et al. Primary fascial
closure versus staged closure with silo in patients with
gastroschisis: a meta-analysis. *J Pediatr Surg.*
2013;48:845.
Fraser JD, Deans KJ, Fallat ME, et al. Sutureless vs sutured
abdominal wall closure for gastroschisis: Operative
characteristics and early outcomes from the Midwest
Pediatric Surgery Consortium. *J Pediatr Surg*
2020;55:2284.

TEACHING POINT: Gastroschisis and omphalocele are
two common congenital abdominal wall defects. The initial approach is airway control, aggressive fluid resuscitation, intravenous antibiotics, gastric decompression, and
abdominal wall closure.

19 *A 7-year-old skateboarder falls onto the concrete and
strikes his head. He had a brief loss of consciousness at
the scene and one episode of emesis. On arrival to the
ED, he is hemodynamically stable with a GCS of*

15 with no neurological deficits. He has some small abrasions to the right side of his face, a forehead hematoma, and no gross facial deformities. Which of the following is the next best step in management of this patient?

A *Admission for observation*
B *Skull radiographs*
C *Neurosurgery consultation*
D *CT scan of the head*
E *Hypertonic saline infusion*

Head injuries are one of the most common injuries in the pediatric trauma population, and they are the leading cause of morbidity and mortality. These injuries commonly result from motor vehicle accidents, falls, bicycle crashes, and child abuse. Most of these injuries are minor and do not require any intervention; however, children with moderate and severe head injuries require immediate CT scan imaging to evaluate whether medical or surgical intervention is indicated. The main goal in treating patients with severe head trauma is to minimize secondary brain injury due to hypoxemia and hypoperfusion.

For children that have minor head injuries, PECARN (Pediatric Emergency Care Applied Research Network) has developed a set of clinical guidelines that outline parameters for imaging versus observation. According to the guidelines in patients >2 years of age, CT imaging is recommended if the GCS </= 14, signs of altered mental status, or palpable skull fracture. For patients with a history of loss of consciousness, vomiting, severe headache, or severe mechanism (such as this patient), then observation is recommended. Based on the guidelines, this patient has an approximate 0.9% risk of clinically important TBI. If the patient has any neurological decline (such as a change in GCS or persistent vomiting or headache), then a CT is indicated. Furthermore, it is not safe to discharge this patient home due to his loss of consciousness and emesis. Neurosurgical consultation and hypertonic saline infusion is not indicated in this patient. Skull radiographs are indicated only if there is suspected child abuse and otherwise have little utility in modern trauma evaluations.

Answer: A

Bell MJ, Kochanek PM. Pediatric traumatic brain injury in 2012: The year with new guidelines and common data elements. *Crit Care Clin*. 2013;29(2):223–38.

Kuppermann N, Holmes JF, Dayan PS, et al. Identification of children at very low risk of clinically important brain injuries after head trauma: A prospective cohort study. *Lancet*. 2009;374(9696):1160–70.

Babl FE, Borland ML, Phillips N, et al. Accuracy of PECARN, CATCH, and CHALICE head injury decision rules in children: A prospective cohort study. *Lancet*. 2017;389(10087):2393-2402.

Singh S, Hearps SJC, Borland ML, et al. The effect of patient observation on cranial computed tomography rates in children with minor head trauma. *Acad Emerg Med*. 2020;27(9):832-843.

TEACHING POINT: CT imaging of the head is recommended in pediatric trauma if the GCS </= 14, signs of altered mental status, a palpable skull fracture or a deterioration in neurologic status.

20 *A 5-year-old girl is involved in a multiple car crash on the highway. She sustains multiple injuries and requires CT scans of the head, chest, abdomen, and pelvis to aid in diagnosis and management. Which of the following statements is TRUE in reducing overall radiation dose and risks in this patient?*

A *Decreasing the pitch during CT scan will decrease radiation exposure.*
B *Increasing the beam current will decrease radiation exposure.*
C *There is no association with increased cancer risk related to CT scans.*
D *Utilizing thinner slice thicknesses will decrease radiation exposure.*
E *Using weight-based protocols will decrease radiation exposure.*

CT scans are used for the diagnosis and management of majority of trauma patients. They allow for the quick and accurate identification of injuries; however, they are not without risk especially in the pediatric population. There is small increase in the lifetime risk of cancers, and some studies have shown decreased long-term cognitive function. In order to mitigate this risk, CT scans should be avoided unless absolutely necessary. If imaging is indicated, then radiation must be kept As Low As Reasonably Achievable (ALARA). This concept is based on:

- Using weight-based protocols and shielding as needed
- Alternative imaging modalities such as MRI that have no radiation risk
- Using focused or limited review studies as appropriate
- Avoiding repeat CT scans unless absolutely necessary

Furthermore, radiation exposure can be reduced by altering the tube current and pitch of the machine. This is achieved by decreasing the tube current and increasing the pitch. Increasing the pitch allows the table to move through the scanner faster without decreasing the quality of the images. Using thicker cuts is also preferred to thin cuts as this also decreases radiation exposure, although this will result in lower resolution images. Clinicians should follow ALARA to achieve the lowest radiation doses possible and perform CT scans only when medically necessary and when it will change management.

Answer: E

Donnelly LF. Reducing radiation dose associated with pediatric CT by decreasing unnecessary examinations. *AJR Am J Roentgenol*. 2005;184:655.

Shah NB, Platt SL. ALARA: is there a cause for alarm? Reducing radiation risks from computed tomography scanning in children. *Curr Opin Pediatr*. 2008;20:243.

Boone JM, Geraghty EM, Seibert JA, Wootton-Gorges SL. Dose reduction in pediatric CT: A rational approach. *Radiology*. 2003;228:352.

Goske MJ, Applegate KE, Boylan J, et al. The image gently campaign: Working together to change practice. *AJR Am J Roentgenol*. 2008;190:273.

TEACHING POINT: If imaging is indicated, then radiation must be kept As Low As Reasonably Achievable (ALARA).

47

Geriatrics
Douglas James, MD[1] and Kartik Prabhakaran, MD[2]

[1] Section of Trauma and Acute Care Surgery, Westchester Medical Center, Valhalla, NY, USA
[2] New York Medical College, Westchester Medical Center, Valhalla, NY, USA

The following vignette applies to questions 1–5. An 88-year-old man is admitted to the intensive care unit after sustaining a fall down a flight of stairs. On presentation, he has a GCS of 13, a heart rate of 78 beats/min, blood pressure of 152/76, and oxygen saturation of 94% on 4 L of oxygen by nasal cannula. His medical history is significant for atrial fibrillation for which he takes metoprolol and warfarin. His international normalized ratio (INR) is 2.5. Imaging studies reveal a 4-mm right-sided subdural hematoma, and fracture of right ribs 3–10.

1   *Which of the following is the most effective treatment for reversing the patient's hypocoagulopathy?*
    A *Fresh frozen plasma*
    B *Vitamin K*
    C *Platelets*
    D *Prothrombin Complex Concentrate*
    E *Cryoprecipitate*

Elderly patients are at particular risk of poor outcomes after traumatic brain injury given the frequency of prescribed anticoagulant medications superimposed upon underlying frailty and other comorbidities. Therapeutic anticoagulation with warfarin poses an increased risk of mortality in these patients. Fresh frozen plasma (FFP) (*answer A*) and Vitamin K (*answer B*) have long been standard therapy for reversing the anticoagulant effects of warfarin. However, more recent literature and guidelines demonstrate increased rapidity and greater efficacy of prothrombin complex concentrate (PCC) in reversing warfarin, as well as a reduction in mortality associated with bleeding (***answer D***). Therefore, use of prothrombin complex concentrate has become the recommended guideline for reversing the coagulopathy caused by warfarin in bleeding patients. Although platelets (*answer C*) and cryoprecipitate (*answer E*) are useful as part of overall hemostatic resuscitation in the bleeding patients, they do not specifically reverse the effects of warfarin. Fresh frozen plasma, while effective at reversing the effects of warfarin, takes significantly longer to achieve its effect and may be beneficial in settings where volume resuscitation of the bleeding patient is also required due to its colloid properties. Vitamin K is also useful in counteracting the effects of warfarin, but its effects are not only delayed when compared to PCC but also long-lasting, which can complicate the need to resume therapeutic anticoagulation with warfarin.

Answer: D

Frontera JA, Gordon E, Zach V et al. (2014) Reversal of coagulopathy using prothrombin complex concentrates is associated with improved outcome compared to fresh frozen plasma in warfarin-associated intracranial hemorrhage. *Neurocritical Care.* 2014 Dec;21(3):397–406.

Chai-Adisaksopha C, Hills C, Siegal DM et al (2016) Prothrombin complex concentrates versus fresh frozen plasma for warfarin reversal. A systematic review and meta-analysis. *Thrombosis and Haemostasis.* 2016 Oct 28;116(5):879–890.

Edavettal M, Rogers A, Rogers F et al (2014) Prothrombin complex concentrate accelerates international normalized ratio reversal and diminishes the extension of intracranial hemorrhage in geriatric trauma patients. *American Surgeon.* 2014 Apr;80(4):372–376.

2   *Which of the following represents the optimal analgesic regimen for treatment of the patient's rib fractures?*
    A *Patient Controlled Analgesia (PCA) with intravenous morphine*

B *Regional (thoracic epidural, intramuscular, or paravertebral) anesthesia*

C *Oral opioid analgesia supplemented by intravenous acetaminophen*

D *Nonsteroidal anti-inflammatory drugs (NSAID)*

E *Oral opioid analgesia supplemented by transdermal lidocaine*

Although opioids form the cornerstone of analgesia in the treatment of pain arising from trauma-associated injuries, the elderly are particularly vulnerable to the deleterious effects of opioids including respiratory depression and delirium. A PCA with morphine (*answer A*) can be used, but with significant risks of long-acting opioid side effects due to the long half-life of morphine. Oral opioid analgesia (*answer C*) may be effective in the subacute phase of injury associated pain but cannot be easily titrated to effect, and intravenous acetaminophen is ineffective as a primary agent. NSAIDS (*answer D*) are not recommended as primary agents of analgesia due to the potential for exacerbating coagulopathy and causing acute kidney injury. Transdermal lidocaine (*answer E*) is not effective for the treatment of rib fractures as it does not produce enough of a systemic effect. Although often prescribed, the only approved indication for transdermal lidocaine is for herpetic lesions. Transdermal lidocaine does not penetrate tissues to the bony level to produce local anesthesia. Regional techniques in the form of thoracic epidural, paravertebral, and intercostal analgesic delivery have become evidence-based, favored approaches to providing optimal pain control, while reducing the delirium associated with systemic opioid analgesics (***answer B***).

Answer: B

O'Connell KM, Quistberg DA, Tessler R et al. (2018) Decreased risk of delirium with use of regional analgesia in geriatric trauma patients with multiple rib fractures. *Annals of Surgery* 2018 Sep;268(3):534–540.

Jensen CD, Stark JT, Jacobson LL et al. (2017) Improved outcomes associated with the liberal use of thoracic epidural analgesia in patients with rib fractures. *Pain Medicine*. 2017 Sep 1;18(9):1787–1794.

Peek J, Smeeing DPJ, Hietbrink F et al. (2019) Comparison of analgesic interventions for traumatic rib fractures: a systematic review and meta-analysis. *European Journal of Trauma and Emergency Surgery*. 2019 Aug;45(4):597–622.

3 *Twenty-four hours after admission to the ICU, the patient becomes agitated and confused, with an increase in heart rate to 110 beats/min. Repeat CT scan of the head demonstrates no worsening of the subdural hematoma. Which of the following medications should be avoided in managing this agitated, delirious elderly patient?*

A *Risperidone*

B *Quetiapine*

C *Lorazepam*

D *Haloperidol*

E *Dexmedetomidine*

Delirium among elderly patients, particularly those admitted to an ICU setting, is often underdiagnosed and multifactorial in etiology. Sun-downing and delirium in the elderly patient is often unavoidable, but the hallmark of treatment is understanding of the etiology and symptomatic management. Investigating the underlying cause (e.g. inadequate analgesic effect) and prevention strategies remain the cornerstones of treatment approaches. Assessment and screening for delirium is recommended at regular intervals using measures such as the Confusion Assessment Method for the ICU (CAM-ICU). When prevention strategies such as reorientation, optimizing analgesia and nutrition, reducing physical restraints, and promoting good sleep hygiene are not sufficient, pharmacologic therapy may be required for managing acute episodes of delirium. Atypical antipsychotic medications such as haloperidol (*answer D*) (recommended for short term treatment of acute delirium by the Society of Critical Care Medicine), risperidone (*answer A*), and quetiapine (*answer B*) may provide short-term benefit in the acute setting, albeit requiring caution with respect to polypharmacy and cardiac side effects. In ICU patients with delirium unrelated to alcohol and benzodiazepine withdrawal, continuous infusions of dexmedetomidine (*answer E*) may be used for sedation to reduce the duration of delirium. Benzodiazepines such as lorazepam, however, are associated with significant risk in the elderly given its amnestic properties, effects on respiratory drive, its long half-life and active metabolites and should be avoided (***answer C***).

Answer: C

Devlin JW, Skrobik Y, Gelinas C et al. (2018) Executive summary: clinical practice guidelines for the prevention and management of pain, agitation/sedation, delirium, immobility, and sleep disruption in adult patients in the ICU. *Critical Care Medicine*: September 2018;46(9):1532–1548.

Girard TD, Pandharipande PP, Ely EW. (2008). Delirium in the intensive care unit. *Critical Care*;12(suppl. 3):S3.

Ouimet S, Kavanagh BP, Gottfried SB et al. (2007) Incidence, risk factors and consequences of ICU delirium. *Intensive Care Medicine*;33:66–73.

4 *Despite optimizing analgesia, pulmonary hygiene measures, and management of delirium, the patient's respiratory function and his ability to protect his airway deteriorate to the point of requiring endotracheal intubation and the initiation of mechanical ventilation.*

Twelve hours after the initiation of mechanical ventilation, arterial blood gas demonstrates a p/f ratio of 190. When managing the patient's mechanical ventilator, which of the following is true?

A *Chest wall compliance will be increased due to weakening of connective tissue and loss of muscle strength.*

B *Higher tidal volumes should be utilized in order to overcome the loss of alveolar elasticity.*

C *Positive end-expiratory pressure (PEEP) is important to overcome the greater tendency of alveolar collapse at higher volumes.*

D *Airway pressure release ventilation (APRV) is unlikely to increase alveolar recruitment for the treatment of ARDS in the elderly.*

E *Positioning of the patient (prone or semi-prone) to ameliorate V/Q mismatch is contraindicated in the elderly.*

Aging is associated with changes in pulmonary physiology, which includes blunting of the mucociliary reflex, decline in vital capacity, and reduction in chest wall compliance (*answer A*). Positive end-expiratory pressure (PEEP) is helpful, particularly in the elderly, as the loss of airway and alveolar elasticity results in closure of alveoli at higher volumes (**answer C**). Alveolar recruitment in the form of airway pressure release ventilation (APRV) (*answer D*) has not been shown to improve mortality particularly when begun late after the diagnosis of acute respiratory distress syndrome (ARDS), but can be of benefit in improving oxygenation when used within the first 24 hours after diagnosis, and there is no limitation of APRV based upon age or the physiology of aging lungs. Positioning of the patient (particularly upright positioning with early mobilization) has been demonstrated to decrease oxygen consumption, and prone positioning (*answer E*) has been shown to be of benefit in improving oxygenation particularly in patients with ARDS, and there is no contraindication to prone positioning based on age. However, the use of high tidal volumes (*answer B*), particularly over a prolonged period of time, has been shown to result in over aeration of healthy lung tissue and barotrauma, which results in progressive lung injury and impaired pulmonary function.

Answer: C

Zhou Y, Jin X, Lv Y et al. (2017) Early application of airway pressure release ventilation may reduce the duration of mechanical ventilation in acute respiratory distress syndrome. *Intensive Care Medicine* 017 Nov;43(11): 1648–1659. doi: 10.1007/s00134-017-4912-z.

Villar J, Kacmarek RM, Perez-Mendez L et al. (2006). A high positive end-expiratory pressure, low tidal volume ventilatory strategy improves outcome in persistent acute respiratory distress syndrome: a randomized, controlled trial. *Critical Care Medicine* 2006 May; 34(5):1311–8.

Gee MH, Gottlieb JE, Albertine KT, et al. (1990). Physiology of aging related to outcome in the adult respiratory distress syndrome. *Journal of Applied Physiology*;69:822–829.

5 *Ten days after the initiation of mechanical ventilation, the patient's delirium has significantly improved. His pulmonary function has improved to the point of tolerating a spontaneous breathing trial, and he is extubated after meeting established parameters and criteria. However, 6 hours after extubation, the patient is noted to have poor respiratory effort and is unable to effective expectorate resulting in tachypnea and desaturation. He is re-intubated successfully, is maintained on light sedation, and his family is informed. Which of the following should guide the decision-making process of whether the patient should be considered for tracheostomy?*

A *The patient is intubated and therefore unable to participate in decision-making. Therefore, the providers should act in the patient's best interest.*

B *The patient is likely to fail repeated attempts at extubation, and therefore, a tracheostomy is the preferred approach irrespective of the patient's previously expressed wishes.*

C *The patient's health care proxy should make decisions on behalf of the patient in conjunction with the patient's family, irrespective of the patient's wishes.*

D *A shared decision model should be employed that is based on choice, option, and decision talk with both the patient and his health care proxy/family.*

E *A tracheostomy is unlikely to improve the patient's overall quality of life and should not be offered.*

Decision-making in the elderly can often be challenging, particularly in critical care settings where patients may require end-of-life decision-making with limited capacity to fully engage in the process. Whereas patient autonomy is the overriding principle in medicine at large, end-of-life decision-making for critically ill elderly patients with limitations in communication and sensorium can make the process difficult for patients, their families, and providers. Although providers are always tasked with acting in the best interest of the patient, a patient's own wishes must be investigated using all means available including temporary cessation of stimuli and medications that can alter sensorium (*answer A*). The judgment of the treating health care provider team, while important in helping to guide and counsel patients and their families, cannot constitute the overriding rationale for decision-making without focusing on the patient's wishes (*answers B and E*).

Discussions with health care proxies and surrogates, as well as the patient's families, are of the utmost importance both ethically and legally. However, such discussions should be patient-centered and actively involve the patient to the greatest extent that is possible (*answer C*). The shared decision-making model that is based on choice, option, and decision talk rests on a process of deliberation and understanding that decisions should be influenced based on exploring and respecting the patient's preferences, whether previously expressed or evolving (*answer D*).

Answer: D

Elwyn G, Frosch D, Thomson R et al (2012). Shared decision making: A model for clinical practice. *Journal of General Internal Medicine*, Oct;27(10):1361–1367.

Ma J, Chi S, Buettner B et al (2019). Early palliative care consultation in the medical ICU: A cluster randomized crossover trial. *Critical Care Medicine*. Dec;47(12):1707–1715.

White DB, Angus DC, Shields AM et al. (2018). A randomized trial of a family-support intervention in intensive care units. *New England Journal of Medicine*. Jun 21;378(25):2365–2375.

The following vignette applies to questions 6–8. A 79-year-old woman presents to the emergency department with progressive left lower quadrant abdominal pain for a period of 5 days that has worsened over the last 24 hours. On presentation, she has a heart rate of 88, a blood pressure of 84/45, and oxygen saturation of 92% on 3 L of oxygen by nasal cannula. Her medical history is significant for hypertension, diabetes, peripheral vascular disease, and hyperlipidemia for which she takes atenolol, metformin, clopidogrel, and a statin. She is afebrile and her white blood cell count is 17 k/mm3. A CT scan was obtained prior to surgical consultation and reveals pneumoperitoneum and intra-abdominal free fluid. On exam, the patient has diffuse abdominal tenderness with guarding in the left lower quadrant.

6 Which of the following is true regarding the patient's cardiac physiology?
   A For patients with chronic hypertension, a normal mean arterial blood pressure improves organ perfusion.
   B Tachycardia in response to shock can be blunted by β-adrenergic blocking medications.
   C Chronic atherosclerotic disease reduces systemic vascular resistance.
   D Intravenous fluid hydration should be limited in this patient due to risks of cardiac dysfunction associated with aging.
   E Cardiac afterload is decreased due to decreased elastin in large arteries.

The natural aging process is accompanied by several important structural and physiologic changes in the cardiovascular system. Progressive arteriosclerosis and decreased elastin in the aorta and major vessels lead to increased systemic vascular resistance (*answer C*) and chronic hypertension. For patients with chronic hypertension, a typically "normal" mean arterial blood pressure may be inadequate to support organ perfusion (*answer A*). These same processes also lead to increased afterload (*answer E*), which in turn make the heart dependent on preload and even minor changes in volume status. In a state of sepsis, patients have cytokine-mediated reduction in systemic vascular resistance owing to impaired capillary integrity. Irrespective of age, patients in states of sepsis and distributive shock require resuscitation of their intravascular volume (*answer D*), which is even more important in the elderly patient that is preload dependent. The typical response to sepsis and other inflammatory states is accompanied by tachycardia. However, patients being treated chronically with β-adrenergic blocking medications may have heart rates that appear more "normal." This blunted response to sepsis must be treated with caution as a "normal" heart rate in these instances is not indicative of the disease process at hand and cannot be used as an end-point of resuscitation (*answer B*).

Answer: B

Nagappan R, Parkin G. (2003). Geriatric critical care. *Critical Care Clinics*;**19**:253–270.

Menaker J., Scalea, TM. (2010). Geriatric care in the surgical intensive care unit. *Critical Care Medicine*;38(9):S452–S459.

7 *The patient is taken to the operating room where she is found to have perforated diverticulitis with feculent peritonitis. She undergoes abdominal washout and sigmoid colon resection. Postoperatively, the patient is admitted to the ICU and is hypotensive despite 4 L of crystalloid bolus requiring the initiation of vasopressors. Her serum lactate is 4.*
   Which of the following statements is correct?
   A *The addition of albumin to volume resuscitation in sepsis improves outcomes.*
   B *There is benefit to hydrocortisone and fludrocortisone in the setting of septic shock with respect to improving mortality.*
   C *Early use of a pulmonary artery catheter in the setting of severe sepsis reduces mortality.*
   D *Antimicrobial therapy should be terminated after source control.*
   E *Systemic vascular resistance is increased in the elderly with septic shock.*

The initial phase of shock resulting from sepsis is distributive in nature, irrespective of age or underlying cardiac pathophysiology. The hallmarks of treatment center around timely and effective source control with concomitant resuscitation guided by the Surviving Sepsis campaign. Albumin resuscitation (*answer A*) in addition to crystalloid resuscitation has not been shown to confer a benefit when compared to crystalloids alone. Similarly, the use of pulmonary artery catheters (*answer C*), although potentially helpful in guiding resuscitation, has not been demonstrated to be associated with a reduction in mortality. Although systemic vascular resistance is generally higher in the elderly (when compared to younger cohorts) due to athcrosclerosis, sepsis causes an overall decrease in systemic vascular resistance due to cytokine-induced increases in vascular permeability (*answer E*). Antimicrobial therapy, in settings of severe intra-abdominal sepsis, should be continued for between 3 and 5 days (*answer D*) after source control in patients without severe organ dysfunction. More recent literature does indicate that a combination of hydrocortisone and fludrocortisone can lower mortality in septic shock, when compared to placebo (***answer B***).

Answer: B

Rhodes A, Evans LE, Dellinger RP. (2017) Surviving sepsis campaign: international guidelines for management of sepsis and septic shock: 2016. *Intensive Care Medicine*;43:304–377(2017).

Ciaroni P, Tognoni G, Masson S et al. (2014) Albumin replacement in patients with severe sepsis or septic shock. *New England Journal of Medicine* 2014;370:1412–1421.

Annane D, Renault A, Brun-Buisson C et al. (2018) Hydrocortisone plus fludrocortisone for adults with septic shock. *New England Journal of Medicine* 2018; 378:809–818.

8   Which of the following is most correct regarding nutrition in this critically ill, elderly patient with septic shock?

A   Early parenteral nutrition should be initiated in this patient.

B   Early trophic enteral nutrition is contraindicated in this patient due to the use of vasopressors.

C   Changes in total energy expenditure are related to increases in ATPase and triiodothyronine.

D   Early enteral nutrition initiation is associated with a reduction in the duration of mechanical ventilation.

E   Nutrition should be deferred until the resolution of septic shock.

Nutrition in the care of the critically ill elderly patient is of the utmost importance, particularly when taking into account the effects of aging upon underlying changes in nutrient balance and deficits. After age 60, mean body weight and BMI tend to decrease, as does the resting metabolic rate. In catabolic states such as sepsis, the early initiation of nutrition is essential in enhancing recovery and reducing mortality (*answer E*). Decrease in resting metabolic rate in geriatric patients is multifactorial and is related to a decline in Na^+K^+ adenosine triphosphatase (ATPase) activity, a decline in triiodothyronine, and a decrease in food intake (*answer C*). Early initiation of trophic enteral nutrition is both safe in the face of low-dose vasopressors (*answer B*) and of benefit in reducing the duration of mechanical ventilation (***answer D***) in patients suffering from septic shock. In contrast, late initiation of parenteral nutrition (*answer A*) has been associated with faster recovery and fewer complications when compared to early initiation.

Answer: D

Casaer MP, Mesotten D, Hermans G et al. (2011) Early versus late parenteral nutrition in critically ill adults. *New England Journal of Medicine* 2011; 365:506–517.

Mancl EE, Muzevich KM. (2013) Tolerability and safety of enteral nutrition in critically ill patients receiving intravenous vasopressor therapy. *Journal of Parenteral and Enteral Nutrition* 2013 Sep;37(5):641–651.

Patel JJ, Kozeniecki M, Biesboer A et al. (2016) Early trophic enteral nutrition is associated with improved outcomes in mechanically ventilated patients with septic shock: A retrospective review. *Journal of Intensive Care Medicine*. 2016 Aug;31(7):471–477.

9   *A 78-year-old female presents to the emergency department after a ground level fall. On presentation she has a heart rate of 80 beats/min, a blood pressure of 140/70 mm Hg, and an oxygen saturation of 98% on room air. She has a medical history of hypertension. She has pain over her left hip without noticeable deformity. Radiograph demonstrates a left femoral neck fracture. She is functionally independent, walks without assistance, and manages her own activities of daily living. Which of the following is true regarding hip fractures in the elderly?*

A   *Geriatric consultation improves survival.*

B   *Geriatric consultation improves functional outcomes at 1 year.*

C   *All in-hospital complications are similar regardless of geriatric consultation.*

D   *Select patients with decompensation of comorbid conditions require preoperative cardiac workup.*

E   *Most patients return to previous functional status following operative fixation.*

Ground-level falls are the most common mechanism of traumatic injury in the elderly. Isolated hip fractures account for 340 000 hospitalizations annually in the United States. One-year mortality from hip fractures ranges from 12 to 37%. Coordinated care from a multidisciplinary team has been shown to improve outcomes in these patients. Specifically, the role of a formal pathway with consultation of or management by a geriatric medical service has been proposed. Though some retrospective case series have shown a mortality benefit with geriatric consultation, randomized control trials have not shown a mortality benefit (*answer A*). Geriatric consultation has shown improvement in functional outcomes such as mobility, cognitive status, and functional status post injury up to 6 months (*answer B*). Geriatric consultation has been shown to result in a lower rate of pressure ulcers and delirium in this population (*answer C*), though many in-hospital complications appear to be unaffected. Patients do not necessarily require additional cardiac workup unless they have an acute decompensation of chronic medical problems (**answer D**), and their preoperative evaluation should follow those recommended by the ACC/AHA Guideline on Perioperative Cardiac Evaluation and Management of Patients Undergoing Noncardiac Surgery. Following a hip fracture, many patients develop functional and self-care limitations despite operative fixation (*answer E*).

Answer: D

Mukherjee K, Brooks SE, Barraco RD, et al. (2020) Elderly adults with isolated hip fractures- orthogeriatric care versus standard care: A practice management guideline from the Eastern Association for the Surgery of Trauma. *Journal of Trauma and Acute Care Surgery*. 2020 Feb;88(2):266–278.

Swart E, Kates S, McGee S, Ayers DC. (2018) The case for comanagement and care pathways for osteoporotic patients with a hip fracture. *Journal of Bone and Joint Surgery American* 2018 Aug 1;100(15):1343–1350.

10 *An 86-year-old male presents from a nursing home after a ground level fall. He has a heart rate of 96 beats/min, a blood pressure of 142/74 mmHg, an oxygen saturation of 94% on 2 L nasal cannula, and a GCS of 7. He has a medical history of hypertension, stroke, and atrial fibrillation. He takes warfarin, aspirin, metoprolol, and simvastatin. His INR is 2.6. He is intubated in the trauma bay. Head CT reveals diffuse subarachnoid hemorrhage and subdural hemorrhage without significant midline shift. He receives prothrombin complex concentrate for reversal. The paperwork from the nursing home identifies his code status as full code and his daughter as the health-care proxy. How should further medical decisions be made for this patient?*

A *Patient should receive aggressive medical care regardless of health-care proxy's wishes as he currently lacks decision-making capacity.*

B *Patient should remain full code as this was his previous code status.*

C *An explanation of best-case, worst-case, and most likely case scenarios for the patient will promote shared decision-making for patient's surrogate.*

D *Shared decision-making promotes aggressive medical therapy.*

E *There is no benefit to early palliative care consultation.*

Patients 65 years of age and older make up 20% of trauma-related admissions in the United States. It is estimated that 10–20% of those admitted to the intensive care unit in this age group die from their injuries. With high morbidity and mortality in this age group, it is important to ensure therapeutic interventions are in alignment with the patient's wishes as early as possible. This patient lacks decision-making capacity due to his traumatic brain injury and should initially receive aggressive medical care. However, his health-care proxy should be involved in decision-making as soon as possible (*answer A*). Though the patient's code status was full code in the nursing home, his traumatic injury has significantly changed his prognosis and may be changed by his health-care proxy (*answer B*). A thorough discussion of projected outcomes utilizing a best-case/worst-case framework improves shared decision-making for patients and families presented with difficult treatment decisions (***answer C***). Shared decision-making engages patients and/or their surrogate decision makers to better understand the likely outcomes and options for medical care in order to integrate the patient's preferences into a recommendation that is most consistent with their long-term goals (*answer D*). Evidence suggests that early involvement of palliative care can decrease length of stay and hospital costs without affecting mortality (*answer E*).

Answer: C

Taylor LJ, Nabozny MJ, Steffens NM et al. (2017). A framework to improve surgeon communication in high-stakes surgical decisions: Best case/worst case. JAMA Surgery. 2017 Jun 1;152(6):531–538. doi: 10.1001/jamasurg.2016.5674. PMID: 28146230; PMCID: PMC5479749.

Aziz HA, Lunde J, Barraco R, et al. (2019). Evidence-based review of trauma center care and routine palliative care processes for geriatric trauma patients; A collaboration from the American Association for the Surgery of Trauma Patient Assessment Committee, the American Association for the Surgery of Trauma Geriatric Trauma Committee, and the Eastern Association for the Surgery of Trauma Guidelines Committee. *Journal of Trauma and Acute Care Surgery*. 2019 Apr;86(4):737–743.

11 *An 82-year-old male suffers a fall while getting out of bed. He was discovered on the floor by his son and was last seen well over 12 hours ago. His heart rate is 83 beats/min, blood pressure is 82/41 mmHg, respiratory rate is 14 breaths/min, and oxygen saturation is 94% on room air. He has a medical history of hypertension. He is confused with GCS 14, has right wrist pain, and right chest pain. His hemoglobin is 16 g/dL, base deficit is -6 mEq/L, and creatinine is 1.8 mg/dL. Imaging reveals a right distal radius/ulna fracture and multiple right-sided rib fractures without pneumothorax or hemothorax. Which statement best describes changes in cardiovascular physiology in the elderly?*

A *Increased number of myocytes*
B *Increased vascular compliance*
C *Decrease in collagen deposition*
D *Increased coronary artery blood flow*
E *Decreased response to β-adrenergic stimulation*

Older adults have lower physiologic reserve of major organ systems. The number of cardiac myocytes decreases with age (*answer A*). Changes in cardiac structure and function occur with advanced age. Structural changes include decreased number of myocytes, increased arterial wall thickness, increase in collagen deposition and reduced vascular compliance (*answer B*). Throughout life, there is an increase in collagen deposition (*answer C*). Due to increased prevalence of coronary artery disease and widening of pulse pressure in this population, blood flow to the coronary arteries is diminished (*answer D*). Elderly patients are also at higher risk of developing arrhythmias, most commonly atrial fibrillation. It is important to recognize that the elderly have a diminished response to β-adrenergic stimulation (***answer E***). The maximal heart rate possible is 220 minus the age. A patient in hypovolemic shock may not develop significant tachycardia and cardiac output is largely dependent on increased preload and stroke volume. The base deficit is a useful indicator of "occult shock" and can help identify those elderly patients in need of further resuscitation and intensive monitoring. When resuscitating the hypovolemic elderly patient, care must be taken to avoid hypervolemia, which can precipitate pulmonary edema.

Answer: E

Darden DB, Moore FA, Brakenridge SC, et al. (2021). The effect of aging physiology on critical care. Crit Care Clinics. 2021 Jan;37(1):135–150.
Jacobs DG, Plaisier BR, Barie PS, et al. (2003). EAST Practice Management Guidelines Work Group. Practice management guidelines for geriatric trauma: the EAST Practice Management Guidelines Work Group. *Journal of Trauma.* 2003 Feb;54(2):391–416.

12 *A 76-year-old male presents from a nursing home with 5 days of periumbilical abdominal pain that has migrated to the right lower quadrant. He has lost his appetite and reports some emesis. He has a medical history of stroke, hypertension, and hyperlipidemia. On exam, he has right lower quadrant tenderness. Which of the following is true regarding acute appendicitis in the elderly?*

A *The Alvarado score is not helpful in elderly patients.*
B *Ultrasound is the diagnostic test of choice in the elderly.*
C *Open appendectomy is associated with lower morbidity than laparoscopic appendectomy.*
D *Colonoscopy should be performed following treatment for acute appendicitis in the elderly.*
E *Nonoperative management is contraindicated in the elderly.*

The incidence of acute appendicitis peaks in the second or third decade of life. Though acute appendicitis is less common in the elderly, approximately 15% of patients older than 50 years of age presenting to the emergency department with abdominal pain will have acute appendicitis. Patients 65 years of age and older with acute appendicitis have a mortality rate of 8%, considerably larger than the 0–1% mortality associated with younger populations. The elderly are also more likely to present with complicated acute appendicitis.

Clinical scoring systems such as the Alvarado score can be useful in stratifying the risk of acute appendicitis in elderly patients (*answer A*). The Alvarado score is a 10-point score, which includes symptoms (nausea/vomiting, anorexia, migration of pain to right lower quadrant), signs (pain in right lower quadrant, rebound tenderness, body temperature $\geq 37.3\,°C$), and laboratory signs (leukocytosis shift, white blood cell count $> 10 \times 10^9/L$) of acute appendicitis. An Alvarado score less than 5 is helpful in excluding acute appendicitis but is not sufficiently specific to confirm the diagnosis. CT scan is the preferred diagnostic study due to its high sensitivity and specificity; however, ultrasound can be helpful in workup in patient at risk for contrast-induced nephropathy (*answer B*). Laparoscopic appendectomy is the operation of choice in the elderly due to reduced hospital length of stay, morbidity, and costs (*answer C*). The incidence of cecal/appendiceal cancer in patients older than 55 presenting with acute appendicitis range from 1.6 to 24%; therefore, elective colonic screening should be performed after treatment (***answer D***). Nonoperative management may be offered to select elderly patients who wish to avoid surgery, are willing to take on risk of recurrence, and do not have evidence of complicated appendicitis with diffuse peritonitis or suspected free-perforation (*answer E*).

Answer: D

Fugazzola P, Ceresoli M, Agnoletti V, et al. (2020). The SIFIPAC/WSES/SICG/SIMEU guidelines for diagnosis and treatment of acute appendicitis in the elderly (2019 edition). *World Journal of Emergency Surgery*. 2020 Mar 10;15(1):19.

Bhangu A, Søreide K, Di Saverio S, et al. (2015). Acute appendicitis: modern understanding of pathogenesis, diagnosis, and management. Lancet. 2015 Sep 26;386(10000):1278–1287.

Segev L, Keidar A, Schrier I, et al. (2015). Acute appendicitis in the elderly in the twenty-first century. *Journal of Gastrointestinal Surgery*. 2015 Apr;19(4):730–735.

13 *A 75-year-old female presented with perforated diverticulitis. She has a medical history of hypertension and diabetes. She takes amlodipine and metformin at home. She initially presented in septic shock. After preoperative resuscitation and antibiotics, she is taken to the operating room for exploratory laparotomy. There was feculent peritonitis. She undergoes a sigmoidectomy. Postoperatively she is taken to the surgical intensive care unit. Despite aggressive fluid resuscitation, she requires norepinephrine drip for hypotension. Her urine output drops to 0–10 mL/hr. Her creatinine increases to 3.2 mg/dL, blood urea nitrogen is 100 mg/dL, and potassium is 5.6 mmol/L. Which of the following best describes age-related changes in renal function and acute kidney injury?*

  A *The mean glomerular filtration rate (GFR) is < 60 mL/min/1.73 m2 in individuals over the age of 70.*

  B *Kidney volume increases with advanced age.*

  C *Creatinine is a reliable marker of renal function in the elderly.*

  D *Age is not an independent risk factor for acute kidney injury (AKI)*

  E *Renal replacement therapy should be avoided in the elderly as there is little chance of return to baseline renal function.*

Physiologic changes occur as a natural process of aging. The term senescence delineated the predictable progressive anatomic and physiologic changes associated with aging as opposed to those induced by diseases. A normal part of aging is a gradual decline in renal function. In individuals over the age of 70, the mean GFR is less than 60 mL/min/1.73 m^2 (***answer A***). Structural changes that

Table 47.1 KDIGO staging of AKI.

Stage	Serum creatinine	Urine output
Stage 1	1.5–1.9 times baseline OR ≥0.3 mg/dL increase	<0.5 mL/kg/h for 6–12 hours
Stage 2	2.0–2.9 times baseline	<0.5 mL/kg/h for ≥ 12 hours
Stage 3	3.0+ times baseline OR Increase in serum creatinine to ≥ 4.0 mg/dL OR Initiation of renal replacement therapy OR In patients <18 years, decrease in eGFR to <35 mL/min/1.73 m^2	<0.3 mL/kg/h for ≥ 24 hours OR Anuria for ≥12 hours

occur with the aging kidney include nephrosclerosis, nephron hypertrophy, decrease in number of functional nephrons, decrease in kidney volume, and increase in kidney cysts/masses (*answer B*). Functional changes that occur with the aging kidney include decreased GFR, impaired ability to regulate urine concentration, impaired clearance of renally excreted drugs, and impaired response to hypovolemia. Creatinine is a less reliable biomarker for AKI in the elderly as they have lower lean muscle mass, and creatinine is formed almost exclusively in the muscle (*answer C*).

Age greater than 65 is an independent risk factor for AKI (*answer D*). AKI can be caused by ischemia, hypovolemia, urinary obstruction, drug-induced nephrotoxicity, or contrast-induced nephrotoxicity. The preferred criteria for acute kidney injury is based on serum creatinine levels and urine output as defined by the 2012 Kidney Disease: Improving Global Outcomes (KDIGO) guidelines as defined in Table 47.1. In a randomized control trial comparing early versus delayed renal-replacement therapy in intensive care unit patients with stage 3 AKI found no mortality benefit in the early intervention group. The mean age of the study population was 65 years old, and many of the patients in this study had a return of renal function (*answer E*). Therefore, renal-replacement therapy should be administered with the same indications utilized in younger patients.

Answer: A

Denic A, Glassock RJ, Rule AD. Structural and functional changes with the aging kidney. *Advances in Chronic Kidney Disease* 2016;23(1):19–28. doi: 10.1053/j.ackd. 2015.08.004.

Gaudry S, Hajage D, Schortgen F, et al. (2016). Initiation strategies for renal-replacement therapy in the intensive care unit. *New England Journal of Medicine*. 2016 Jul 14;375(2):122–133.

14 *An 81-year-old male cattle rancher presents with acute onset upper abdominal pain. He has a medical history of peptic ulcer disease for which he occasionally takes famotidine. He works daily on his family ranch and requires no assistance for daily activities. His heart rate is 100 beats/min, blood pressure is 114/64 mm Hg, and oxygen saturation is 98% on room air. Upright chest radiograph demonstrates pneumoperitoneum. How does age affect outcomes following emergency surgery?*

 A *Frailty is stronger predictor of mortality following surgery compared to age or American Society of Anesthesiologists (ASA) physical status classification.*

 B *Frailty is purely a "phenotype" manifested by decline in lean body mass, strength, endurance, balance, and activity.*

 C *The use of frailty measurement is not useful in emergency surgery as scores are difficult to calculate.*

 D *All patients over the age of 75 years are frail.*

 E *Elderly patients who are considered frail are at similar risk for postoperative complications compared to their non-frail counterparts.*

In the United States, over one third of all operations are performed on adults over the age of 65 years. Age alone does not seem to predict surgical outcomes in the elderly population. Frailty is a biologic syndrome characterized by a decreased homeostatic reserve and diminished resistance to stressors due to a decline in multiple physiologic organ systems. Frailty has been shown to be a stronger predictor of postoperative morbidity and mortality as compared to chronologic age or ASA classification (**answer A**). Currently there is no standardized method to measure frailty with various instruments described and validated in the literature. There are two main models, the "phenotype" model and the cumulative deficit model (*answer B*). The "phenotype model" measures frailty utilizing physical indicators such as decline in lean body mass, strength, endurance, balance, and activity level. The cumulative deficit model, or Frailty Index (FI), utilizes components of physiologic, cognitive, social and psychological deficits in measuring frailty. Frailty instruments have been shown to be useful in predicting outcomes in emergency general surgery as frail patients are at higher risk for postoperative complications compared to their non-frail counterparts (*answer E*). Some instruments can be incorporated into electronic medical record systems allowing scores to be rapidly calculated prior to emergency surgery (*answer C*). Not all patients over the age of 75 years are considered frail and utilizing a frailty assessment preoperatively can help guide discussion of postoperative expectations and outcomes with patients (*answer D*).

Answer: A

Nidadavolu LS, Ehrlich AL, Sieber FE, Oh ES (2020). Preoperative evaluation of the frail patient. *Anesthesia & Analgesia* 2020 Jun;130(6):1493–1503.

Joseph B, Zangbar B, Pandit V, et al. (2016). Emergency general surgery in the elderly: Too old or too frail? *Journal of American College of Surgeons*. 2016 May;222(5):805–13.

Lin HS, Watts JN, Peel NM, Hubbard RE (2016). Frailty and post-operative outcomes in older surgical patients: a systematic review. BMC Geriatrics. 2016 Aug 31;16(1):157.

15 *A 91-year-old nursing home patient presents with severe abdominal pain and vomiting for 4 hours. She has a medical history of atrial fibrillation, hypertension, and stroke. Her heart rate is 95 beats/min, blood pressure is 98/62 mm Hg, and respiratory rate is 20 breaths/min. Her abdominal pain is out of proportion to physical exam findings of mildly distended abdomen without rigidity. Her white blood cell count is 12 000, and lactate is elevated at 2.4 mmol/L. A CT angiogram of the abdomen demonstrates occlusion of the proximal superior mesenteric artery with thickening of the small bowel. Which of the following statements is true regarding acute mesenteric ischemia?*

 A *The incidence of acute mesenteric ischemia decreases with age.*

 B *Mesenteric venous thrombosis is the most common etiology of mesenteric ischemia.*

 C *Duplex ultrasonography is the preferred diagnostic study for acute mesenteric ischemia.*

 D *Initial management of non-occlusive mesenteric ischemia is non-operative in absence of peritonitis.*

 E *On exploratory laparotomy, if the majority of the small bowel is necrotic, it must be resected.*

Acute mesenteric ischemia (AMI) is an uncommon cause of abdominal pain accounting for less than 1 of every 1000 hospital admission. However, it is associated with a 60–80% mortality; therefore, it is necessary to maintain a high index of suspicion of this disease process. The incidence of AMI increases with advanced age (*answer A*). There are various causes of AMI, which are important to differentiate as the management is different. Mesenteric arterial embolism is the most common etiology accounting for 50% of cases and is associated with cardiac arrhythmias and dysfunction (*answer B*). Mesenteric arterial thrombosis accounts for approximately 25% of cases and patients may have a previous history of chronic mesenteric ischemia. Mesenteric venous thrombosis accounts for approximately 20% of cases. Nonocclusive mesenteric ischemia accounts for approximately 5–15% of cases and is often associated with cardiac insufficiency or low-flow states occurring in relation to cardiac surgery, hypovolemia, or heart failure.

A patient presenting with excruciating abdominal pain with an unrevealing abdominal exam should be presumed AMI until ruled out. Laboratory biomarkers are not specific, and though leukocytosis, metabolic acidosis, hyperkalemia and elevated lactate can be present with bowel ischemia, their absence does not rule-out AMI. CT angiography with arterial and venous phase are the diagnostic modalities of choice (*answer C*). AMI due to arterial embolism/thrombosis should be treated operatively with the following goals addressed:

1) Re-establishment of blood supply to ischemic bowel
2) Resection of all non-viable regions of bowel
3) Preservation of all viable bowel

A combination of open and endovascular can be considered depending on capabilities at the treating institution. A "second-look" operation should be considered to reassess bowel viability. Mesenteric venous thrombosis can often be managed with anticoagulation alone with approximately 5% requiring additional intervention. The management of nonocclusive mesenteric ischemia focuses on management of the underlying cause without immediate surgery, but may require operative intervention if peritonitis or perforation develops (**answer D**). It is important to counsel patients and their families regarding the possibility that nearly all the small intestine may not be viable and that depending on patients comorbidities and functional status, comfort care rather than bowel resection with parenteral nutrition would be a more humane treatment plan (*answer E*).

Answer: D

Clair DG, Beach JM. (2016). Mesenteric ischemia. *New England Journal of Medicine.* 2016 Mar 10;374(10): 959–968.

Bala M, Kashuk J, Moore EE, et al. (2017). Acute mesenteric ischemia: guidelines of the World Society of Emergency Surgery. World Journal of Emergency Surgery. 2017 Aug 7;12:38. doi: 10.1186/s13017-017-0150-5. PMID: 28794797; PMCID: PMC5545843.

16 *The following vignette applies to questions 16 and 17. A 78-year-old woman presents after a fall from standing. She felt palpitations and briefly lost consciousness before the fall. She has a medical history of hypertension and hyperlipidemia, but no history of arrhythmias. Her heart rate is 152 beats/min, blood pressure is 75/35 mmHg, and oxygen saturation is 94% on 2 L via nasal cannula. On secondary survey, she has some bruising and swelling over the right side of her face. Her Glasgow Coma Score is 13. Electrocardiogram demonstrates an irregularly irregular rhythm consistent with atrial fibrillation with rapid ventricular rate. She has negative chest x-ray and pelvic x-ray, and her FAST is negative. She has no external signs of trauma. What is the appropriate next step in management?*

A *Electrical cardioversion*
B *Diltiazem intravenous drip*
C *Metoprolol intravenous push*
D *Amiodarone bolus followed by amiodarone intravenous drip*
E *Fluid resuscitation and heparin drip*

Atrial fibrillation (AF) is a supraventricular arrhythmia with uncoordinated atrial conduction leading to irregular ventricular response, which is often rapid. Key electrocardiographic findings are a loss of P waves, erratic activation of ventricles, and an irregular rapid heart rate. It is the most common arrhythmia in the elderly as aging myocytes lose their normal biochemical conductive properties. Given a patient presenting with hemodynamically unstable AF, the treatment should be with electric cardioversion regardless of duration of arrhythmia (***answer A***). Non-emergent cardioversion can be performed if duration is less than 48 hours. If duration > 48 hours or unknown, the patient must be anticoagulated for 4 weeks before electrical/pharmacologic cardioversion. Chemical cardioversion with amiodarone is advised in the normotensive patient but is not the treatment of choice in the acutely hypotensive patient (*answer D*). Beta-blockers and non-dihydropyridine calcium channel blockers are first-line agents for rate control in the hemodynamically stable patient but do not aid in the conversion to sinus rhythm and caution is advised as both agents can cause or exacerbate hypotension (*answers B and C*). Hypovolemia (including hemorrhagic shock) may be an inciting factor for the development of rapid atrial fibrillation but unlikely in this patient after a ground level fall. Volume resuscitation is important in the hypotensive patient, and anticoagulation may be indicated for long-term prevention of stroke particularly if the arrhythmia is sustained. However, neither intravenous fluids nor heparinization will aid in the immediate resolution of the unstable arrhythmia (*answer E*). Though exacerbating causes of atrial fibrillation may include hypovolemia, trauma and sepsis; however, this patient is hypotensive and requires immediate cardioversion.

Answer: A

Gutierrez C, Blanchard DG. (2016). Diagnosis and treatment of atrial fibrillation. American Family Physician2016 Sep 15;94(6):442–452. PMID: 27637120.

Riley AB, Manning WJ. (2011). Atrial fibrillation: an epidemic in the elderly. *Expert Review of Cardiovascular Therapy*. 2011 Aug;9(8):1081–1090.

17 *The above patient has successful cardioversion but thereafter has recurrences of atrial fibrillation, which are managed by her cardiologist with beta-blockers for rate control. In addition, she is placed on apixaban (Eliquis®) for therapeutic anticoagulation to decrease her risk of stroke. Six months later, she presents to the hospital again after a mechanical fall. She has a GCS of 14 and is found on CT scan to have a subdural hemorrhage. Which of the following is true regarding apixaban?*

A *Apixaban functions as a direct thrombin inhibitor.*

B *Traumatic brain injuries have worse outcomes in the setting of therapeutic anticoagulation with apixaban, when compared to heparin and Coumadin.*

C *Apixaban can be reversed effectively with pro-thrombin complex concentrate or andexanet alfa.*

D *Direct oral anticoagulants such as apixaban can safely be resumed 1 week after traumatic brain injuries.*

E *Patients receiving apixaban will have elevated partial thromboplastin time (PTT).*

Direct oral anticoagulants (DOAC's) have become more popular and widespread in use, when compared to traditional oral vitamin K antagonists, for the treatment of chronic conditions (such as atrial fibrillation and venous thromboembolism) requiring therapeutic anticoagulation. The direct oral anticoagulants fall into different categories based on mechanism of action. The two major classes are direct thrombin inhibitors (dabigatran) and factor Xa inhibitors such as apixaban and rivaroxaban (*answer A*). As specific antidotes and reversal agents have become available, DOACs have been deemed to be equally safe when compared to more traditional anticoagulants such as warfarin. Studies examining the outcomes of patients with traumatic brain injury have shown contradictory results but have overall failed to show consistently worse outcomes with DOACs compared to warfarin (answer B). For reversal of Factor Xa inhibitors, andaxanet alfa (Andexxa) is an FDA-approved antidote that carries a relatively high rate of thromboembolic events when compared to four-factor prothrombin complex concentrate, which also effective in reversing the effects of these medications (*answer C*). There is no consensus on resuming full anticoagulation following TBI, high-risk patients can generally be restarted within 10–14 days and low to moderate risk patients can be restarted within 4–8 weeks (answer D). One of the challenges in using the direct oral anticoagulants is the difficulty in titrating the medication based on laboratory testing or measured effect. Unlike unfractionated heparin or warfarin, traditional laboratory coagulation profiles such as prothrombin time and partial thromboplastin time are not affected in a dose-dependent fashion by direct oral anticoagulants (*answer E*). It remains to be seen if other parameters such as viscoelastic testing can be used to measure these effects.

Answer: C

Wiegele M, Schöchl H, Haushofer A, et al (2019). Diagnostic and therapeutic approach in adult patients with traumatic brain injury receiving oral anticoagulant therapy: an Austrian interdisciplinary consensus statement. *Critical Care* 2019;23(1):62. Published 2019 Feb 22. doi: 10.1186/s13054-019-2352-6.

Shin SS, Marsh EB, Ali H et al (2020). Comparison of traumatic intracranial hemorrhage expansion and outcomes among patients on direct oral anticoagulants versus vitamin K antagonists. Neurocritical Care 2020 Apr;32(2):407–418.

Kobayashi LM, Brito A, Barmparas G et al. Laboratory measures of coagulation among trauma patients on NOAs: results of the AAST-MIT. Trauma Surgery and Acute Care Open 2018 Oct 15;3(1):e000231.

18 *A 73-year-old man is brought to the hospital after sustaining a 35% deep partial thickness and full thickness burn to his extremities following a house fire. He has no evidence of inhalation injury. He is admitted to the ICU, undergoes IV fluid resuscitation, and wound care. Which statement is most true regarding burn care in the elderly population?*

A *The elderly and children have similar mortality from burn injuries.*

B *The elderly tend to have less full thickness burn injuries.*

C *The LD50 burn size in the elderly is around 35% total body surface area (TBSA).*

D *Resuscitative fluids should be reduced in half in elderly burn patients to avoid fluid overload.*

E *Increased mortality in elderly burn patients is only seen with inhalation injury.*

Despite advances in burn care over the past few decades having improved outcomes in children and adults, there has not been as much improvement in outcomes in the elderly. The elderly are at increased risk for burn injury due to physiologic changes including decreased physical strength, impaired protective mechanisms, decreased reaction times, and poor vision. Mortality from burns seems to increase in a linear fashion with advanced age (*answer A*). In patients over the age of 65 years, the LD50 has remained around 35% for the past few decades (***answer C***). The elderly tend to have a higher percentage of full thickness burns due to atrophic skin with thinning of the dermis and a decrease in epidermal appendages (*answer B*). Despite increased risk of volume overload in this population, patients will still require aggressive intravenous fluid resuscitation with careful monitoring of resuscitative end-points (*answer D*). Though there is increased mortality associated with inhalation injury, age related increases in mortality are seen in the absence of inhalation injury (*answer E).*

Answer: C

Goei H, van Baar ME, Dokter J, et al. (2020) Dutch burn Repository group. Burns in the elderly: a nationwide study on management and clinical outcomes. Burns & Trauma. 2020 Oct 22;8:tkaa027.

Gregg D, Patil S, Singh K, et al. (2018). Clinical outcomes after burns in elderly patients over 70 years: A 17-year retrospective analysis. *Burns.* 2018 Feb;44(1):65–69.

Jeschke MG, Pinto R, Costford SR, Amini-Nik S. (2016). Threshold age and burn size associated with poor outcomes in the elderly after burn injury. *Burns.* 2016 Mar;42(2):276–281.

19 *The following vignette applies to questions 19 and 20. An 80-year-old female with a history of hypertension, chronic obstructive pulmonary disease, and non-insulin-dependent diabetes undergoes open cholecystectomy for management of acute, gangrenous cholecystitis. Postoperatively, the patient is continued on intravenous antibiotics, but on postoperative day 4, she develops a fever to 102.5 °F with a heart rate of 110. A presumptive diagnosis of intraperitoneal abscess is made, and a CT of the abdomen/pelvis with intravenous contrast is ordered. The patient has a baseline creatinine of 0.9 mg/dL. Which of the following is accurate regarding the prevention of contrast-induced nephropathy?*

A *Intravenous fluids should be minimized prior to CT scan in order to prevent volume overload.*

B *The elderly are not at elevated risk for contrast-induced nephropathy when compared to younger patients if the baseline creatinine is normal.*

C *Intravenous contrast is contraindicated in the elderly when performing CT scans.*

D *Intravenous fluid hydration and statin administration can be protective against contrast-induced nephropathy.*

E *Sodium bicarbonate should be administered before and after intravenous contrast administration.*

Though the risk of contrast-induced nephropathy is overall relatively low in the general population, the geriatric population is particularly vulnerable given the relative decrease in functional nephrons with advancing age (*answer B*). Intravenous contrast is helpful in CT scans obtained with the intent of diagnosing abscesses and bleeding, and there is no need to eliminate the diagnostic accuracy in the elderly population particularly with the imaging studies may lead to a higher chance for source control (*answer C*). Therefore, in the elderly, normal baseline creatinine is not indicative of normal glomerular filtration rate and renal function. Avoiding prerenal azotemia in the elderly by optimizing intravascular volume status is of particular importance as this can predispose patients to contrast-induced nephropathy (*answer A*). While the role of sodium bicarbonate and N-acetylcysteine remain unclear (answer E), a recent large meta-analysis demonstrated a protective effect of statins with intravenous fluids, when compared to intravenous fluids alone in reducing the risk of contrast-induced nephropathy (***answer D***).

Answer: D

20 *A CT scan was obtained with intravenous contrast, demonstrating an abscess that has been treated with percutaneous drainage and intravenous antibiotics. The patient has developed leukocytosis and continues to be febrile, while developing oliguria and elevation of creatinine to 2.1 mg/dL. In this elderly patient with sepsis and acute kidney injury:*

A *A trial of furosemide should be administered in addition to intravenous fluids to increase urine output.*

B *The choice of antibiotics should be based on treating sepsis, irrespective of the risks of exacerbating acute kidney injury.*

C *The initiation of renal replacement therapy in the elderly leads to irreversible loss of nephrons and dialysis dependence.*

D *Determination of the patient's intravascular volume status is critical in optimizing the plan for volume administration.*

E *Protein administration should be limited to prevent further kidney injury.*

After the onset of acute kidney injury, determination of the patient's intravascular volume status is essential for treatment. Although furosemide is often administered in an effort to increase urine output and convert oliguric renal failure to non-oliguric renal failure, doing so in the setting of potential hypovolemia and prerenal azotemia can have deleterious consequences and do not translate to improved clinical outcomes or reduced mortality (*answer A*). Careful monitoring of a patient's urine output and intravascular volume status, in addition to calculating the fractional excretion of sodium, are helpful in determining whether a patient requires further intravenous fluid resuscitation (***answer D***). The prevention of iatrogenic exacerbation of acute kidney injury is of the utmost importance, and all medications should be dosed based on creatinine clearance. Antibiotics are common offending agents in such iatrogenic exacerbation and should be chosen carefully while balancing appropriate coverage of organisms and nephrotoxicity (*answer B*). The decision to initiate renal replacement therapy in the geriatric patient is fraught with complexity, but the indications remain the same as in younger patients. Moreover, many patients (both elderly and young) have complete return of baseline renal function after resolution of the inciting physiologic insult (*answer C*). Particularly in the setting of acute kidney injury superimposed upon sepsis, adequate nutrition including the requisite amount of protein is essential to patient recovery and should not be withheld (*answer E*).

Answer: D

Pannu N, Weibe N, Tonelli M, et al (2006). Prophylaxis strategies for contrast –induced nephropathy. *Journal of the American Medical Association* Surgery;295(23):2765–2779.

Subramaniam RM, Wilson RF, Turban S, et al (2016). *Contrast-Induced Nephropathy: Comparative Effectiveness of Preventive Measures. Comparative Effectiveness Review No. 156. (Prepared by the Johns Hopkins University Evidence-based Practice Center under Contract No. 290-2012-00007-I.). AHRQ Publication No. 15(16)-EHC023-EF*. Agency for Healthcare Research and Quality, Rockville, MD.

Cheung CM, Ponnusamy A, Anderton JG. (2008). Management of acute renal failure in the elderly patient. *Drugs and Aging*;25(6):455–476.

48

Statistics

Alan Cook, MD, MS

University of Texas at Tyler, Tyler, TX, USA

1 *A federal healthcare payer is considering incentive payments to trauma centers based on patient survival. The leadership wants to make sure the comparison is fair, so they are developing a risk adjustment model. They plan to incorporate injury severity into the model. They are choosing between the Injury Severity Score (ISS) (Baker, et al., 1974) and the Trauma Mortality Prediction Model (TMPM) (Osler, et al., 2008). One method of comparing the ISS and TMPM is to estimate the area under the receiver operating characteristic curve (AUROC) for each model with death as the outcome. The results are shown in Figure 48.1.*
Which of the following statements is the most correct?
   A *The payer should chose TMPM because the AUROC is higher than the ISS.*
   B *The payer should chose ISS because the AUROC is lower than the TMPM.*
   C *The horizontal line represents the "perfect" AUROC score.*
   D *The Y-axis can also be considered the False Negative Rate.*
   E *The ISS can discriminate survivors from fatalities 16.9% of the time (1 − AUROC).*

The area under the receiver operating characteristic curve originated as a measure of radio signal detection or discrimination of signal from noise. It also gained a great deal of traction in psychology then radiology and medical decision-making. The AUROC can be interpreted as a measure of a model's ability to discriminate patients with an outcome from those without. Here, the outcome was death from traumatic injury. The construct of the graph is the sensitivity (y-axis) over 1-the specificity (x-axis) for each point computed by the model or at predetermined cut points. This can also be described as the true-positive rate (y-axis) over the false-positive rate

(x-axis). The AUROC for the ISS indicates the ISS can discriminate survivors from fatalities 83.1% of the time. Whereas the TMPM can make such discrimination 87.5% of the time. As such, the TMPM compares favorably over the ISS. In this analysis, the closer the curve is to the point [0, 1] (left upper corner) the greater the area under the curve indicating better discrimination capability. Thus, the diagonal line represents an AUROC of 0.5 where the model predicts no better than a coin toss.

Answer: A

Hanley J, McNeil B. The meaning and use of the area under a receiver operating characteristic (ROC) curve. *Radiology.* 1982;143:29–36.

2 *An academic trauma surgeon is studying the effect of cigarette smoking on the actual versus predicted inspiratory volume in elders with rib fractures. Trauma centers are required to record the chronic medical conditions of the patients, including smoking. Other pertinent clinical data will be included in the final, published article.*
Select the best answer from the following:
   A *The term for the proportion of patients who smoke is "incidence."*
   B *The proper study design is a randomized trial in this study and all others.*
   C *This would be considered a cohort study as elderly patients with rib fractures are selected for the study, and the exposure is whether or not they are an active smoker.*
   D *This study would not require participant consent since no intervention is involved.*
   E *The study is considered a longitudinal study because the patients are elderly and if they smoke have likely done so for a long time.*

Surgical Critical Care and Emergency Surgery: Clinical Questions and Answers, Third Edition.
Edited by Forrest "Dell" Moore, Peter M. Rhee, and Carlos J. Rodriguez.
© 2022 John Wiley & Sons Ltd. Published 2022 by John Wiley & Sons Ltd.
Companion website: www.wiley.com/go/surgicalcriticalcare3e

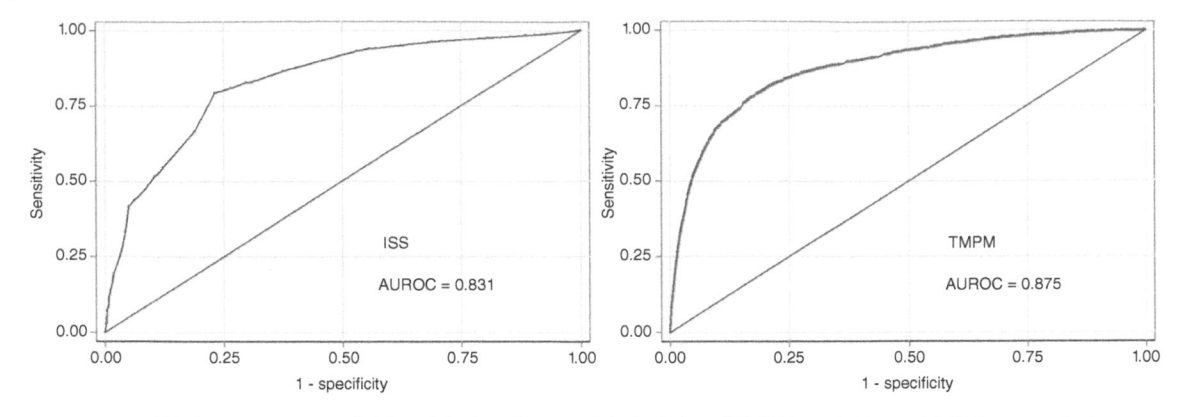

Figure 48.1 AUROC comparison of ISS and TMPM. The AUROCs for ISS and TMPM are 0.831 and 0.875, respectively.

This study should be considered cohort study as the patients are selected for the study, and the outcome is compared according to smoking status (the exposure). If the study sought to describe the proportion of smokers among elderly trauma patients, it could be considered a prevalence study or a cross-sectional study. Prevalence is a measure of the number of subjects in a population who have a condition at the time of the study and can be thought of as a "snapshot-in-time," much like a survey or poll. While a randomized study is considered the epitome of study designs, it is not feasible in all studies. Here, we cannot ethically randomize elderly patients to smoke or not, and the physiological phenomenon of interest is deterioration of pulmonary function, which takes a significant amount of time to accumulate before an effect would be manifest clinically (choice C). The long follow-up time would be prohibitively resource intensive. Although no intervention is being studied, the study would require consent from the participant as the protocol will entail medical testing and include the analysis of other clinical data. Since no new intervention is involved, the study may qualify for expedited review by the Institutional Review Board (choice D). If the study began with a group of teenagers and followed their pulmonary function over their lifetime at 5-year intervals, the study would be a longitudinal study (choice E). The quintessential cohort study is the Framingham Heart Study.

Answer: C

Dawber TR, Meadors GF, Moore Jr FE. Epidemiological approaches to heart disease: the Framingham study. *American Journal of Public Health and the Nations Health*. 1951;41(3):279–86.

3 *Confounding is a term frequently bandied about in research. Select the item below, which accurately describes confounding.*
  A *A confounder is a variable (G) directly affected by two other variables, namely, the exposure (X) and the outcome (Y).*

  B *The effects of a confounder cannot be mitigated in an observational study.*
  C *Including the confounder in the analysis exaggerates the effect sizes of the variables of interest, i.e. the odds ratio for the outcome due to the exposure is larger than the "true" effect.*
  D *A confounder is equally distributed between groups of subjects in a study.*
  E *Confounding describes the circumstance when the measure of effect of the exposure on the outcome is primarily due to a third variable related to both the exposure and the outcome.*

Confounding results when a third variable is responsible for the effect of the exposure (X) on the outcome (Y). The third variable, the confounder, is related to the exposure and the outcome. A classic example is the effect of alcohol consumption on lung cancer. The effect may be accounted for by the confounder of smoking. Oftentimes, people smoke while drinking or drink in places where smoking is present, like bars. Here, smoking is not equally distributed among the alcohol drinkers. Confounding is shown schematically in the following diagram:

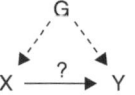

The effects of confounding can be mitigated or adjusted for by including the confounding variable in a multivariable model, for example. The result of including smoking status in the analysis would likely mitigate or completely negate any observed association between alcohol consumption and lung cancer.

Answer: E

Williamson EJ, Aitken Z, Lawrie J, Dharmage SC, Burgess JA, Forbes AB. Introduction to causal diagrams for confounder selection. *Respirology*. 2014;19(3):303–11.

4 *Randomized, controlled trial is regarded as the epitome of study designs. However, not all studies are suitable for this particular design. Please select the most correct answer from the following, regarding randomization.*

A *Randomized trials are relatively inexpensive compared to other study designs.*

B *Randomized trials, like other study designs, cannot infer causality between the exposure or intervention and the outcome.*

C *Randomization essentially guarantees significant p-values for the effect of the intervention on the outcome.*

D *Randomization removes the potential for selection bias in terms of allocating patients to the intervention or control group.*

E *Randomization is the most ethical approach to clinical research.*

Randomization is the process in a randomized control trial where the participants are allocated to intervention or control groups through a formal randomization process. A trial that includes a randomization step as part of the protocol is, by definition, a prospective study that requires an intervention, follow-up time, and staff to collect data. These characteristics of randomized trials tend to make them expensive compared to other study designs. A key strength of randomization is the removal of selection bias in the allocation of subjects to intervention and control groups. The removal of selection bias and the prospective nature of the study provide strong justification to infer causality between the intervention and outcome of a study. The randomization process tends to produce relatively balanced groups of participants in terms of characteristics important to the study. However, since p-values are influenced by the effect size of the intervention and the number of observations in the analysis, the mere act of randomization does not assure statistical significance. Finally, not all studies lend themselves to a random allocation of subjects to the treatment or control groups. This is the case when treatments have become established as the standard of care despite the lack of prospective randomized trials.

Answer: D

Greenland S. Randomization, statistics, and causal inference. *Epidemiology.* 1990;1(6):421-9.

5 *An investigator wishes to study the association of chlorhexidine oral rinse compared to saline rinse on the incidence of ventilator-associated pneumonia (VAP, yes/no) at any point in the patient's ICU stay. The other risk factors for VAP include patient age, gender, injury severity, GCS on ED arrival, days of mechanical ventilation, traumatic brain injury (yes/no), face frac-*tures *(yes/no), etc. Since the incidence of VAP can be confounded by the presence or absence of other factors, several variables must be controlled for simultaneously to estimate the effect of chlorhexidine oral rinse.*

The proper test for this analysis is:

A *Paired Student's t-test*

B *Multivariable logistic regression*

C *Multivariable linear regression*

D *Cox proportional hazard ratio*

E *The Mann-Whitney U test*

In a previous question, we discussed the phenomenon of confounding. One method of adjusting for one or more confounders in the analysis phase of a study is to control for them in a multivariable model. Here, the outcome of interest is binary, VAP (yes/no). Therefore, the paired Student's *t*-test, which compares the means of a variable for a group of individuals measured before and after an intervention, like subjects' weight before and after a diet change is not appropriate (choice A). The Mann-Whitney U test is another name for the Wilcoxon Rank Sum test where one can compare the means of a variable between two independent groups of subjects when the distribution of the variable is not normally distributed. Additionally, the Mann-Whitney U test is a bivariate test and cannot accommodate the nine variables necessary to the study (choice E). The Cox proportional hazard ratio is a multivariable model that incorporates a time-to-event component, e.g. the number of ICU days until discharge or death. The study in question is simply interested in whether or not VAP develops, not how long it takes to develop (choice D). The multivariable linear regression would be an appropriate multivariable model if the outcome of interest is continuous and linear, like hospital length of stay. The multivariable logistic regression is the model of choice for the analysis at hand (choice C). The logistic regression model is used to describe the relationship between a binary outcome variable, VAP, and a set of independent predictor variables whether they are continuous, categorical, or binary. The results are reported as odds ratios with 95% CIs and p-values for the predictors.

Answer: B

Peng C-YJ, So T-SH. Logistic regression analysis and reporting: a primer. *Understanding Statistics: Statistical Issues in Psychology, Education, and theSocial Sciences.* 2002;1(1):31–70.

6 *A group of investigators conducted a multicenter survey study of 27 trauma centers across three states. They hypothesized that the number of trauma and acute care surgery (TACS) consults and activations was associated with the number of cases done by TACS residents per month. The data are as follows:*

	Mean (SD)	Minimum, maximum	Median (IQR)
Activations	199.7 (110.5)	60, 408	160 (200)
Resident cases	22.1 (6.8)	12, 32	23.2 (11.6)

Describe the variable activations in terms of data type.
A *Binary*
B *Nominal*
C *Ordinal*
D *Continuous*
E *Ratio*

Numerical data can take several forms. The type of numerical data in a variable can determine the appropriate tests of significance and regression model to choose. The simplest type is binary or dichotomous. Binary data contain two mutually exclusive values like 1 or 0 for alive or dead (choice A). Nominal data represents categories of a phenomenon like blood type, for example 1 = A+, 2 = A–, . . ., 6 = O–. There is no quantitative difference between the categories. A+ ≠ 2 × A–. Moreover, the blood types aren't ordered. The numeric values are contiguous as a matter of convenience (choice B). Ordinal data can be placed in meaningful order, e.g. the order of finishers in a race (1st place, 2nd place, and so on). However, there is no information about how far apart the runners finished (0.01 seconds between 1st and 2nd place, 0.07 seconds between 2nd and 3rd place) (choice C). If the variable was named "Total Time" and contained each racer's course time in milliseconds, the variable would be considered continuous just as the variable "Activations." Note that continuous data are presented as discrete values rounded to a convenient decimal place (choice D). Most biometric data belong on the ratio scale. The ratio scale is like the continuous numeric scale with the limitation that it includes zero but does not include negative numbers (choice E).

Answer: C

Barkan H. Statistics in clinical research: important considerations. *Annals of Cardiac Anaesthesia.* 2015;18(1):74.

7 *One fundamental analytic technique is to compare dichotomous variables and outcomes using a 2 × 2 contingency table. Only one of the following can be computed from this construct.*
A *Spearman's correlation coefficient*
B *Odds ratio*
C *Cox Hazard Ratio*
D *Pearson's rho*
E *β coefficient*

The 2 × 2 contingency table is a fundamental construct in biostatistics. It can represent a test result (positive or negative) and the disease state (present or absent), a risk factor and the disease, etc.

	Disease	No disease
Exposure	*a*	*B*
No exposure	*c*	*D*

All of the following can be calculated from the 2 × 2 table as follows:

Risk ratio $= \dfrac{a/(a+b)}{c/(c+d)}$ or the ratio of risk of an outcome in the exposed to that in the unexposed. Odds ratio (OR) is the ratio of <u>odds</u> of an outcome in the exposed to the odds in the unexposed. $OR = \dfrac{ad}{bc}$ Sensitivity and specificity are common terms in scientific literature. Sensitivity is the proportion of true positive cases (*a*) among all who develop the disease (*a* + *c*). While specificity is the proportion of true negative cases (*d*) among all who do not have the disease (*d* + *b*).

$$\text{Sensitivity} = \frac{a}{a+c} \quad \text{Specificity} = \frac{d}{b+d}$$

Positive and negative predictive values (PPV and NPV, respectively) represent the degree to which a disease is present or absent given positive or negative test results.

$$\text{PPV} = \frac{a}{a+b} \quad \text{NPV} = \frac{d}{c+d}$$

The β coefficient is the measure of effect size and direction from a regression model, e.g. least squares linear regression. Spearman's correlation coefficient and Pearson's rho are measures of how the value of one continuous variable changes in response to the amount of change in another continuous variable, or the *covariance (choices A and D)*. Correlation coefficients range between –1 and +1, where –1 represents a perfectly negative relationship and +1 indicates a perfectly positive relationship. A value of 0 represents the absence of a linear relationship between the two variables. The Cox hazard ratio is a statistic used in survival analysis (choice C).

Answer: B

Mosteller F. Association and estimation in contingency tables. *Journal of the American Statistical Association.* 1968;63(321):1–28.

8 *Speaking of contingency tables. Which of the following is the appropriate test of significance for the following table?*

	Women, *n* (%)	Men, *n* (%)
Commercial insurance	*41(57.8)*	*61 (31.4)*
Medicare/medicaid	*30 (42.2)*	*133 (68.6)*

  A *Wilcoxon's Rank Sum test*
  B *Mann-Whitney U test*
  C *ANOVA*
  D *Kruskal-Wallis test*
  E *Chi-squared (X2) test*

A contingency table is an essential part of biostatistical analyses. In its most general form, it is a row x column (*r x c*) table where the rows are the values of a categorical variable and the columns are the values of another categorical variable. The variables can consist of 2 or more categories. As such, the current table is obviously a 2 × 2 table though if we had two more categories of insurance coverage, for example it would be a 4 × 2 table. The chi-square test is used to test the null hypothesis that proportions are equal between groups. Here, the null hypothesis is that the proportions of insurance categories are equivalent between women and men. The chi-squared test is the appropriate test to reject the null hypothesis if the p-value is less than the predetermined alpha (0.05) (choice C). The Wilcoxon's Rank Sum test is a means of testing two independent samples with ordinal or continuous data, if the data follow a nonparametric distribution. An example would be hospital length of stay (see question 15) compared between men and women. The Mann-Whitney U test is another name for the Wilcoxon's Rank Sum test (choices A and B). The ANOVA is a test to determine if a difference exists between two or more groups with regard to a normally distributed continuous variable (choice C). An example would be comparing resting heart rate between Olympic marathon runners, cross country skiers, and swimmers. The Kruskal-Wallis test is the nonparametric equivalent to the ANOVA (choice D).

Answer: E

Winters R, Winters A, Amedee RG. Statistics: a brief overview. *Ochsner Journal.* 2010;10(3):213–6. Also see Barkan, 2015.

9 *Recall the TACS activation/consult study from question 6.*

The data are as follows:
The analysis included a linear regression model.

	β **Coefficient**	**95% CI**	**P-value**
Total activations & consults	0.06	0.04–0.07	<0.001
Constant	11.05	8.49–13.62	<0.001
R-squared: 0.80			

Select the best answer regarding the regression model.
  A *The β coefficient indicates that for each additional TACS activation/consult, the residents are doing 11 more operative cases per month.*
  B *For every 1000 activations/consults per month, the residents operate on 6 cases.*
  C *The average resident should expect to do 11 cases per month of the TACS service.*
  D *For every increase of 100 activations/consults per month the residents operate on about 6 more cases.*
  E *The 95% confidence interval (95% CI) indicates 95% of all of the data values in the population fall within the interval.*

Linear regression modeling fits a line through the data points via several methods, the simplest is the least squares linear regression. The line takes the form of $y = c + \beta x$, where y is the number of resident OR cases, x is the number of activations and consults, β is the regression coefficient, and c is the intercept of the line on the y-axis. Here, the minimum value for activations and consults is 60, so the number of resident cases is predicted to be 11 based on the model of the entire data set. The β coefficient represents the slope of the line. In this model, the value of 0.06 indicates each increase of 100 activations, and consults is associated with an increase of 6 resident operative cases, on average. See Figure 48.2. The 95% CI is a means to quantify the uncertainty of the measurement and variability of the phenomena in the population. The equation for the 95% CI includes terms for the sample mean μ, the standard deviation σ, which measures the variability, and the cohort size n. the equation for the upper and lower bounds of the confidence interval is given below.

$$95\%\text{CI} = \mu \pm 1.96 \times \frac{\sigma}{\sqrt{n}}$$

Answer: D

Marill KA. Advanced statistics: linear regression, part I: simple linear regression. *Academic Emergency Medicine.* 2004;11(1):87–93.

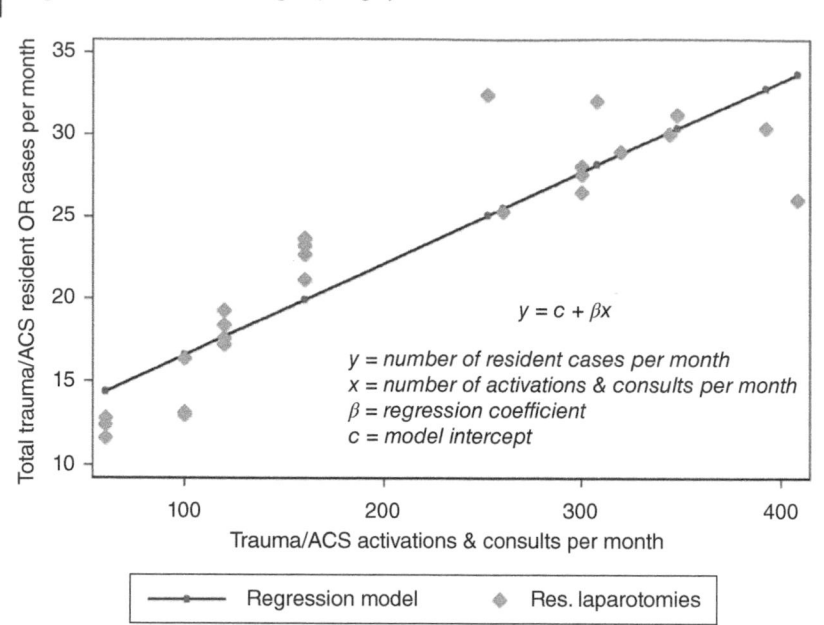

Figure 48.2 Diamonds represent data values gathered from the responding trauma centers. The diagonal line is the line computed by the model that intercepts the y-axis at *c* and has the slope *β* for each increment of *x*.

10 *A different group of academic clinician/investigators is interested in the advances in acute surgical care of patients with feculent peritonitis treated in 2018 (most recent data in this fictional registry) to a group treated in 1990 (earliest data in the registry). They used registry data from a professional organization, The American Fecal Peritonitis Society. The group has hospital administrative data from the 38 surgical intensive care units across the United States. They hypothesize the difference in patient care for over the last 28 years has improved survival from sepsis. One aspect of their study is a comparison of each group's time to death from sepsis. Their results are illustrated in the graph below. Which of the following is the correct interpretation of the graph?*

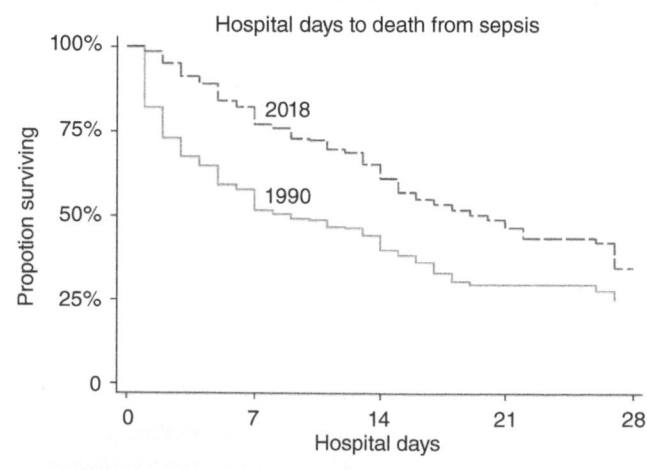

A *The death rate of abdominal sepsis has not improved over 28 years.*

B *The mortality rate from abdominal sepsis is constant over time.*

C *The line drops down when someone dies from abdominal sepsis.*

D *We are seeing fewer cases of feculent abdominal peritonitis in 2018 compared to 1990.*

E *None of the above.*

The graph depicts a Kaplan-Meier survival curve (Kaplan and Meier, 1958), which can be thought of as a time-to-event analysis. Here, the event is the death from abdominal sepsis but the event could be resolution of shock, liberation from the ventilator, or some other discrete event. Note that the events are binary, yes or no. The analysis describes the proportion of subjects who have not experienced the event of interest. The distribution of survival times is characterized by the survival function. The survival function is the probability a patient will remain event-free beyond a point in time. When an event occurs, the line drops down at which point the survival function recalibrates. In this fashion, the Kaplan-Meier estimator accommodates the variation of incidence rates over time. This model allows subjects to leave the group at risk, or in this example die from abdominal sepsis. This is known as censoring. The inclusion of censored data distinguishes survival analysis from other types of analysis. Here, we see a greater mortality rate from abdominal sepsis in 1990 compared to 2018 because a lower proportion of patients are event-free beginning on hospital day 1. Also, a greater proportion of patients died earlier in the process in 1990, while the patients in 2018 demonstrated a more consistent death rate over time. The investigators cannot infer if the number of patients with feculent abdominal peritonitis is different between the two time periods. The model only concerns the proportion of each group having the event.

Answer: C

Clark TG, Bradburn MJ, Love SB, Altman DG. Survival analysis part I: basic concepts and first analyses. *British Journal of Cancer.* 2003;89(2):232–8.

11 *A university and a large pharmaceutical company have partnered in the development of a very promising new drug to treat hemorrhoid disease, hemorrhoidumab. In accordance with the Food and Drug Administration's (FDA) protocols for new drug development, the sponsors are required to conduct a series of clinical trials, Phases I through IV. Which phase is conducted to evaluate whether the drug has any biological activity/effect?*
  A *Phase I*
  B *Phase II*
  C *Phase III*
  D *Phase IV*
  E *Plasma phase*

There are four phases of drug trials that must be conducted before and after a drug goes to market in the United States. Phase I trials are aimed at estimating the safety and tolerability of the drug pharmacokinetics (what the body does to the drug) and pharmacodynamics (what the drug does to the body). Phase II studies evaluate if the drug has any biological activity. Phase II trials are not powered to define the effect on the important clinical end points. Phase III trials are aimed to assess the effectiveness of new interventions or new indications for existing treatments. These are the large, randomized, double-blinded trials we read about in the big journals. These are the career-makers. Not for the scientists so much, but for the CEOs and stockholders of big pharma. Long-term surveillance of a medication or intervention is often needed after regulatory approval. These long-term studies are referred to as Phase IV studies. The plasma phase is not a type of study design; it is a state of matter which is frequently mistaken as a subset of gases. Like gas, plasmas have no fixed shape or volume and are less dense than liquids or solid matter. However, plasmas are made up of atoms though most or all of their electrons have been stripped away and the nuclei are positively charged.

Answer: B

Mahan VL. Clinical trial phases. *International Journal of Clinical Medicine.* 2014;5(21):1374.

12 *An academic surgeon is planning to conduct a retrospective study using the surgery chairman's personal registry of 10 000 open cholecystectomy operations over 47 years. The researcher is hoping to find a significant difference in the rates of incisional dehiscence based on the type of suture used to close the fascia. Which of the following choices are true regarding sample size?*
  A *As the sample size decreases, the power to detect an actual difference increases.*
  B *Studies with dichotomous predictors require fewer subjects to reject the null hypothesis.*
  C *The power of a sample ($1 - \beta$) is the ability to detect a true significant difference between groups.*
  D *Statements of sample size calculation only need to be reported in studies that report significant differences between groups (positive studies).*
  E *With such a large group of patients, only clinically important differences between groups will be significant.*

The size of a study sample is known as power and is expressed mathematically as $1 - \beta$, where β is the probability of a Type II error. The estimation of sample size is of paramount importance when planning any study, especially studies testing an intervention. In prospective trials, the cost of the study is proportional to the number of subjects in the study, as is the ability to detect a true (significant) difference between groups. Thus, the accurate estimation of the number of study subjects is a matter of scientific and economic necessity. Dichotomizing continuous predictors, or dividing a continuous predictor variable into two mutually exclusive categories, results in a substantial loss of power to detect real relationships. As such, more subjects are needed to compensate for the loss of power. Sample size calculation should be stated in research manuscripts, especially in studies that report no difference between groups, the so-called negative study. The reader needs to know if the null result is simply a matter of an insufficient sample size, a Type II error. Large data sets are becoming common. While the ability to study rare disease processes is an attractive feature of such abundant data, researchers must be careful to differentiate statistically significant results from clinically important ones since p-values are influenced by sample size.

Answer: C

Guyatt G, Jaeschke R, Heddle N, Cook D, Shannon H, Walter S. Basic statistics for clinicians: 1. Hypothesis testing. *CMAJ: Canadian Medical Association Journal.* 1995;152(1):27.

13 *In a comparison of time from ED arrival to incision in hypotensive penetrating trauma patients who arrive by helicopter versus those who arrive by ground* *ambulance, the investigator observes a difference in the mean time to incision. The alpha was set at p < 0.05. The manuscript reports the helicopter transport group was associated with a mean of 12 minutes (95% confidence interval (95%CI) 10.2–14.6 minutes). The mean of the ground transport group was 18 minutes (95% CI 12.5–20.0). The p-value was 0.07. The result is reported as a real (significant) difference. What type of error was committed in this manuscript?*

A *Type II error*

B *Type I error*

C *Beta error*

D *No error has occurred. The authors correctly rejected the null hypothesis.*

E *Gamma error*

The authors set the alpha, or level of significance at $p < 0.05$. The study results were associated with a p-value of 0.07. When the p-value of the result is greater than the alpha value, the null hypothesis is correct in that no real difference is present. When the null hypothesis is incorrectly rejected, a type I error has occurred. Type I error is also referred to as alpha error because it occurs at the frequency of alpha. When the null hypothesis is incorrectly retained, a type II error has occurred. Type II error is also referred to as beta error because it occurs at the frequency of beta (usually 0.8). Type II errors are frequently due to very small effect size for the predictor variable, as well as small sample sizes. Also note that the 95% CIs overlap as substantially. This is also an indication that the two groups differ insufficiently for a statistical significance.

Answer: B

Guyatt G, Jaeschke R, Heddle N, Cook D, Shannon H, Walter S. Basic statistics for clinicians: 1. Hypothesis testing. *CMAJ: Canadian Medical Association Journal.* 1995;152(1):27.

14 *Cross-sectional studies analyze data from a group of subjects collected at a single point in time.*

A *They are the design of choice to study the prevalence of a disease.*

B *Cross-sectional studies have two groups while group 1 gets the study intervention, group 2 serves as the control. Then, the groups switch to group 1 is now the control and group 2 gets the intervention, i.e. they cross over.*

C *Investigators can infer causality from this kind of study data.*

D *Cross-sectional studies are very expensive to conduct.*

E *The inherent difficulty with cross-sectional studies is the selection of the control group.*

Cross-sectional studies analyze data gathered at a single point in time, e.g. a survey or poll. Due to the "snapshot in time" nature of this study design, we can only make inferences regarding the exposure (present or absent) and disease state (present or absent) at the same point in time. We cannot say which came first. When erroneous inferences about the proper temporal sequence of cause and effect are made, this is known as temporal bias. This study design cannot produce disease incidence rate data. We can only study disease prevalence in a cross-sectional study. When two groups are compared with one group receiving a treatment and the other serving as the control, then the roles are reversed is called a cross-over study design. Since cross-sectional studies are a kind of observational study, they are relatively inexpensive to conduct.

Answer: A

Mann C. Observational research methods. Research design II: cohort, cross sectional, and case-control studies. *Emergency Medicine Journal* 2003;20(1):54–60.

15 *One of the first steps in data analysis is describing characteristics of the study cohort in terms of basic differences between exposed and unexposed groups. Select the correct choice from the following.*

A *A multivariable logistic regression model is a typical approach in this task.*

B *This is the step where confounders are controlled.*

C *The distributions of the variables are not taken into consideration at this point in the analysis.*

D *Tests for descriptive analyses include chi-square, t-test, and Wilcoxon's Rank Sum test.*

E *None of the above choices are true.*

Describing the characteristics of the study cohort is an important first step in the analysis of research data. Usually this is found in Table 1 and formatted to compare basic differences in the exposed and unexposed groups. Multivariable analyses are not considered descriptive tests, per se. Multivariable analyses allow us to appraise the effect size of a predictor in the context of other predictors and confounders in the data. The tests like those listed in answer D serve to identify differences between groups. The distribution of the variables is central to selecting the proper test of significance.

Answer: D

Ambrosius WT. *Topics in bio-statics.* Switzerland: Springer; 2007.

16 *There are myriad statistical tests being used to analyze data. One-way biostatisticians earn their* *paycheck by understanding the underlying statistical assumptions in order to choose and correctly interpret the appropriate test for the data. Select the correct answer from the following.*

A *The distribution of the data refers to the minimum and maximum values of a variable.*

B *The distribution of the data does not play a role in selecting the proper statistical test.*

C *Hospital length of stay among trauma patients and shoe size among all the women in the United States exhibit the same distribution.*

D *Distribution refers to the values of a variable along with the frequency of their occurrence.*

E *The distribution of a variable is the product of a number by an addition is equal to the sum of products of that number by each of the addends.*

One key assumption of choosing the appropriate statistical test is understanding the assumption regarding the distribution of the variables under consideration. The distribution of a variable refers to the values of a variable along with the frequency of their occurrence. Consider the example of the shoe sizes of all adult women in the United States. We would find that the physical makeup of adult women in the United States is about the same with variation around the average (mean) shoe size. The shoe sizes at the extremes occur with decreasing frequency as the sizes becomes more extreme. (Women's shoes were selected for the example but the same idea applies to men's shoes as well.) The terms mean, median, and mode refer to the "average" of all sizes, the middle value of the range of sizes, and the shoe size that occurs most frequently, respectively. When the mean, median, and mode occur at the same value and the extreme values occur with decreasing frequency, and the rates of

decrease are symmetric, we say the distribution is normal or parametric (also called Gaussian). As such, the minimum and maximum values do not describe the distribution. Many phenomena do not exhibit normal distributions of their measurements. For example, hospital length of stay is skewed to the right in that the majority of patients leave the hospital after a day or two and as the hospital days add up, fewer patients remain. Here, the mode would be to the far left, then the median to the right and the mean will be farther to the right. Answer E is the definition of the distributive property of multiplication, which is frequently applied in mathematics (Figure 48.3).

Answer: D

Winters R, Winters A, Amedee RG. Statistics: a brief overview. *Ochsner Journal.* 2010;10(3):213–6. Also see Barkan, 2015.

17 *The p-value gives us information about the results of a test. Which of the following is true regarding p-values?*

A *The importance of a finding is determined solely on the basis of a p-value less than 0.05.*

B *P-values less than 0.05 indicate there is a less than 5% chance that a difference as big or bigger that the one observed will be the product of random chance.*

C *Under ideal circumstances, all p-values in a study would be significant (p < 0.05).*

D *The p-value is based on the prespecified beta term.*

E *The p-value is calculated before the test.*

The p-value in statistical analyses is a measure of the probability of obtaining a result as large of larger than that observed if the null hypothesis is true. That is, the

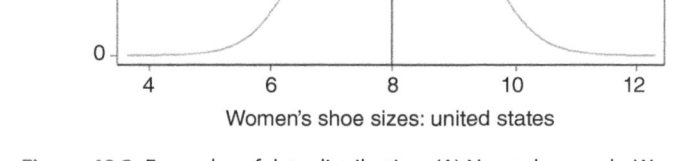

(a)

Normal (parametric) distribution

(b)

Nonparametric, right skewed data

Figure 48.3 Examples of data distribution: (A) Normal example, Women's shoe sizes. Note mean, median, and mode are size 8. (B) Nonparametric, right skewed: Hospital length of stay. Mode 2 days (solid line), median 3 days (dashed line), mean 5 days (dotted line).

probability of incorrectly rejecting a true null hypothesis by random chance alone. When a study involves a sufficiently large cohort of subjects, even extremely small differences, including clinically or practically insignificant ones will have p-values less than 0.05. There are times when results with p-values greater than 0.05 are preferred. One example is testing the results of randomizations when groups are intended to be identical. It is calculated after the statistical test. The p-value is based on the alpha, which is traditionally set at 0.05, or the probability of incorrectly rejecting the null hypothesis when it is actually true.

Answer: B

Guyatt G, Jaeschke R, Heddle N, Cook D, Shannon H, Walter S. Basic statistics for clinicians: 1. Hypothesis testing. *CMAJ: Canadian Medical Association Journal.* 1995;152(1):27.

18 *Question 17 addresses p-values. Another measure we often see in research publications is the 95% confidence interval (95% CI). Which of the following statements is true of p-values and 95% CIs?*
   A *P-values and 95% CIs are redundant measures of significance because the two add to 100.*
   B *A p-value of 0.05 means that 5% of the time the result will be wrong.*
   C *P-values less than 0.05 indicate there is a less than 5% chance that a difference as big or bigger than the one observed will be the product of random chance.*
   D *The 95% CI indicates 95% of all of the data values in the population fall within the interval.*
   E *The 95% CI indicates that if the population were randomly sampled repeatedly and 95% CIs were calculated for each sample, 95% of those CIs would contain the true population mean.*
   F *C and E.*
   G *None of the above.*

The p-value and 95% CI are often the subjects of misinterpretation. To be valid and meaningful, the results of statistical tests must take into account the uncertainty of the measure and the variability within the population of the measure in question, for example the time required to place a chest tube for a new approach compared to the clinical standard. The most common measures of such requirements are the p-value and 95% CI. The p-value is discussed above. The 95% CI is a method of accounting for the variability of the phenomenon of interest (time of chest tube placement) in the target population (blunt trauma patients). The equation for the 95% CI includes terms for the sample mean μ, the standard deviation σ, which measures the variability of chest tube placement in the cohort, and the cohort size n. For the sake of completeness, the equation for the upper and lower bounds of the confidence interval is given below.

$$95\%CI = \mu \pm 1.96 \times \frac{\sigma}{\sqrt{n}}$$

Answer: F

Winters R, Winters A, Amedee RG. Statistics: a brief overview. *Ochsner Journal.* 2010;10(3):213–6. Also see Barkan, 2015.

19 *Clinical research is fraught with pitfalls and threats to relevance at every turn. It also is the only path to improving clinical practice and patient outcomes. The internal and external validity of a study are foundational to the relevance of the study. Select the true statement from the following choices.*
   A *Internal validity reflects the conduct of the study but represents no threat beyond the reputations of the scientists involved.*
   B *Internal and external validity are important tradeoffs that must be reconciled in the design phase of the study.*
   C *Bias is an important area of concern and potential pitfall separate from validity.*
   D *Confounding is also unrelated to validity as it is strictly a statistical computation issue.*
   E *Internal validity and external validity represent mutually exclusive concepts, both of which must be optimized for the study to be relevant.*

Internal and external validity each represent threats to the credibility of a study. Oftentimes, they pose important tradeoffs that must be reconciled at the outset of a study. Internal validity represents an essential criterion of clinical research. It refers the ability of the study to measure what it aims to measure. The consequences when a study lacks internal validity can render the results irrelevant or potentially dangerous. For example, an observational study shows a benefit to strenuous exercise following myocardial infarction because the participants who did such exercise lived longer than those who did not follow this routine. A critical error was a lack of attention to confounding variable reflecting exercise tolerance prior to the heart attack. Indeed unmeasured confounding poses an important threat to internal validity. Bias, in all its forms, is another threat to internal validity. Consider the bias introduced by flawed case selection such that the exposure of interest is systematically distributed unevenly between the cases and controls of a case-control study. External validity reflects the degree to which the findings and inferences of a study can be extrapolated to groups beyond the study cohort. Say you are creating a statistical model for predicting death due to sepsis among patients with a hepatic abscess from perforated diverticulitis. In this group, the model is associated with an area under the receiver operating characteristic curve of 0.92. Will that model also predict death from sepsis in patients with a hepatic abscess and neutropenia from cancer chemotherapy? The excellent model performance in the perforated diverticulitis group is unlikely to function as well in the neutropenic patients. Hence, there is a similar tradeoff made in most if not all clinical studies.

Answer: B

Grimes DA, Schulz KF. Bias and causal associations in observational research. *The Lancet.* 2002;359(9302):248–52.

20 *Bias presents a serious threat to the internal validity of clinical research studies. In the research context, the definition of bias differs from its use in public discourse, i.e. prejudice. Select the true statement from the following choices.*

   A *Ideally, in a cohort study, cases and controls are similar in all relevant aspects except for the exposure of interest, i.e. free of selection bias.*

   B *Confounding and bias are synonymous terms.*

   C *Bias can result from random chance.*

   D *Information bias includes publication bias or the decreased likelihood that a paper with equivocal findings, a "negative study," will be published.*

   E *Selection bias, like confounding, can be remedied in the statistical analysis.*

Bias significantly compromises the internal validity of studies. Bias is defined as a systematic error in the sampling or measurement of study participants and their data. Two major classes of bias are known as selection bias and information bias. Selection bias results when membership in the treatment or control arm is unevenly distributed with respect to a characteristic important to the phenomenon under study. That is a systematic flaw that causes a dissimilarity in one or more important participant aspect between groups. Information bias occurs when information is gathered in systematically different ways between groups. In a case-control study, participants who have the disease under investigation, the "cases," may have clearer memories of the exposure than those who have not manifested the disease. This is referred to as recall bias, and is an example of information bias. The word "systematic" is key in the distinction of bias from random chance. Differential effects of exposures may be the result of random chance, which does not constitute bias. Selection bias cannot be remedied in the analytic phase of a study. The damage has already been done. Confounding can be addressed in the analyses of the data. Publication bias is not a form of information bias and does not impact the internal validity of a study.

Answer: B

Grimes DA, Schulz KF. Bias and causal associations in observational research. *The Lancet.* 2002;359(9302):248–52.

49

Ethics, End-of-Life, and Organ Retrieval

Lewis J. Kaplan, MD[1,2]

[1] *Division of Trauma, Surgical Critical Care and Emergency Surgery, Department of Surgery, Perelman School of Medicine, University of Pennsylvania, Philadelphia, PA, USA*
[2] *Corporal Michael J. Crescenz VA Medical Center, Philadelphia, PA, USA*

1 *An elderly woman is brought to the emergency depart-ment from her nursing home with obvious septic shock. She is intubated, sedated, fluid resuscitated, and placed on a norepinephrine infusion. The patient's sole surviving relative is her daughter. When the daughter arrives, she indicates that her mother would not want the care she is currently receiving and would instead wish to pursue comfort care. Which of the fol-lowing principles is the care team using in pursuing the daughter's statement of her mother's wishes for comfort care?*
   A *Substituted judgment*
   B *Distributive justice*
   C *Ethical parity*
   D *Non-malfeasance*
   E *Respect*

Since the patient is intubated, sedated, and cannot state her desires, one must obtain outside input. Using a fam-ily member who can articulate the patient's desires is appropriate. Accepting that family member's input is termed substituted judgment. Distributive justice is the principle that applies the concept of justice across sev-eral individuals or groups of individuals instead of a sin-gle person. Ethical parity implies the equally appropriate application of ethical principles across different cultures and circumstances. Non-malfeasance indicates a lack of wrongdoing by a public official, often in a financial undertaking. Respect is linked with the concept of autonomy but does not address accepting another's rep-resentation of what individuals' wishes would be if they were only able to share them.

Answer: A

Thompson IE (1987) Fundamental ethical principles in healthcare. *British Medical Journal* **295**, 1461–5.

2 *A 67-year-old man has a potentially resectable colon cancer and has a tumor type that is thought to be favorably responsive to chemotherapy administration. After a lengthy discussion with you, his surgeon, he declines operative therapy, as well as chemotherapy. What principle is being utilized in his decision to decline indicated and potentially life-saving therapy?*
   A *Nonrational thinking*
   B *Deontology*
   C *Autonomy*
   D *Munificence*
   E *Principlism*

This question addresses the role of patient autonomy in medical decision-making. Autonomy is a key principle in Western medical ethics, which preserves a patient's ability to engage in self-determination with regard to goals of therapy, as well as diagnostic or therapeutic undertakings. If the physician believes that the patient has appropriate decisional capacity and understands the implications of the decisions being made, then respecting their informed and autonomous decision to decline medically indicated therapy is appropriate. Nonrational thinking is decision-making based on obedience, imitation, feeling, desire, intuition, or habit. Deontology is rules-based decision-making. Munificence is generosity in giving and does not apply here. Principlism, generally a Western approach, embraces beneficence, non-maleficence, and autonomy, as well as justice, and as such is too broad an answer.

Answer: C

Surgical Critical Care and Emergency Surgery: Clinical Questions and Answers, Third Edition.
Edited by Forrest "Dell" Moore, Peter M. Rhee, and Carlos J. Rodriguez.
© 2022 John Wiley & Sons Ltd. Published 2022 by John Wiley & Sons Ltd.
Companion website: www.wiley.com/go/surgicalcriticalcare3e

Limentani AE (1999) The role of ethical principles in health care and the implications for ethical codes. *Journal of Medical Ethics* **25**, 394–8.

Kilbride MK, Joffe S (2018) The new age of patient autonomy: implications for the patient-physician relationship. *JAMA*;**320** (19), 1973–4.

3 *A 24-year-old motorcyclist arrives with a severe traumatic brain injury (TBI) and within 48 hours has an examination and supportive investigations consistent with brain death. Which of the following strategies is associated with the greatest likelihood that his family's legally authorized representative will consent to organ donation on his behalf?*

A *A structured interview with an organ donation recipient and family*

B *Approach and consent obtained by the physician and nurse care team*

C *Approach and consent by the organ procurement surgeon*

D *Combined approach by the care team and organ procurement network team*

E *Combined approach by nursing, social service, and chaplaincy representatives*

One of the challenges in organ procurement has been obtaining consent from the legally authorized representative of a potential donor patient. Components cited as contributing to failure in obtaining consent include lack of consistent messaging between clinicians; lack of readily understood language; lack of understanding of organ donation in general; concerns regarding costs of organ donation; concerns regarding mutilation; and faith-based concerns or objections. Perhaps the most readily addressable set of concerns are those that impact clear and consistent communication. A prefamily "huddle" consisting of physicians, nurses, and representatives of the organ procurement organization to discuss the best approach for a given family has been demonstrated to significantly improve consent rates. Other members of the care team may also participate in the "huddle" as appropriate. Engaging a donor recipient and family is ideal for recipients and their families but not necessarily the donor family. The organ procurement surgeon is ethically constrained from participating in the consent process due to a conflict of interest. Similarly, the care team members are constrained from participating in organ procurement for the same reason.

Answer: D

Rady MY, Verheijde JL, McGregor JL (2010) Scientific, legal and ethical challenges of end-of-life organ procurement in emergency medicine. *Resuscitation* **81** (9), 1061–2.

Witjes M, Kruijff PE, Haase-Kromwijk BJ, van der Hoeven JG, Jansen NE, Abdo WF (2019) Physician experiences with communicating organ donation with the relatives: a Dutch nationwide evaluation on factors that influence consent rates. *Neurocritical Care* **31** (2), 357–64.

4 *The ethical and humane treatment of prisoners of war (POW) by physicians is specifically addressed by which of the following:*

A *Hastings Center report*

B *Nuremberg proceedings*

C *North Atlantic Treaty Organization*

D *World Health Organization*

E *Geneva Conventions*

The ethical treatment of POWs is explored in detail within the Geneva Conventions. The tenets are embraced and further articulated within a variety of military field manuals as well. Physicians are specifically constrained from being active combatants but are expected to be able to defend themselves and the patients for whom they actively provide care. The Geneva Convention also prohibits the deliberate attack of medical care providers and the torture of prisoners. Provision of nourishment, medical and surgical care, and humane holding conditions are also explicitly required within the document. The Hastings Center mission is to address fundamental ethical issues in the areas of health, medicine, and the environment as they impact individuals, communities, and societies. This center focuses ethical issues addressing end-of-life, public health, and new and emerging technology. Periodic reports are generated on these topics, but not treatment of POWs. The Nuremberg Proceedings addressed war crimes. NATO is a collection of allied countries with similar aims and who have signed mutual aid and intent treaties. The WHO is an organization that addresses world health issues. NATO and the WHO both endorse the Geneva Conventions.

Answer: E

Carter BS (1994) Ethical concerns for physicians deployed to operation desert storm. *Military Medicine* **159** (1), 55–9.

Barilan YM, Asman O (2017) Research ethics, military medical ethics, and the challenges of international law. *The American Journal of Bioethics* **17** (10), 53–5.

5 *If one argues that principles and moral rules are not absolutely binding, but are instead prima facie, this means that the principles and moral rules are:*

A *Self-evident and are context independent when rendering moral judgment*

B *Duties that are binding unless in conflict with an equal or stronger duty*

C *Unable to be equally applied across the same circumstance in different cultures*

D *Only able to be understood within the context of virtue ethics and behavior*

E *Rooted in Western culture and interwoven within the rules for social behavior*

Prima facie means that principles and moral rules are duties that are binding unless in conflict with an equal or stronger duty. In this way, *prima facie* recognizes that principles may come into conflict with one another and that there is a context-sensitive nature to principles that may not translate from one culture to another. Therefore, *prima facie* allows one to allow contextual influences to help shape a moral judgment, instead of strictly adhering to a single set of rules. Thus, a need for overall balance is embedded in the concept of *prima facie*. Virtue ethics asserts that decision-maker characteristics are reflected in their behavior, and ethics may be interpolated from a behavior set. This type of ethics implies that virtuous behavior is a type of moral excellence.

Answer: B

Limentani AE (1999) The role of ethical principles in health care and the implications for ethical codes. *Journal of Medical Ethics* **25**, 394–8.

Jones A. (2020) Principlism in medicine–a philosopher's view. *Medicine.***48** (10), 637–9.

6 *Which of the following ethical principles may be used as a justification for performing scientific and medical research?*
   A *Non-maleficence*
   B *Distributed justice*
   C *Beneficence*
   D *Autonomy*
   E *Pluralism*

Beneficence is acting for the greater good and implies a sense of moral and ethical correctness in the assignation of good to a particular behavior or activity. Research may be justified using this concept in that the discovery of new knowledge may be applied to others with similar conditions to enable recovery, survival, or mitigate the consequences of that particular, as well as other related, illnesses. Non-maleficence is different in that it constrains one from willfully doing harm. Distributed justice implies equality in a particular element in either equal share, or in proportion to need, effort, contribution, or merit. Autonomy relates to an individual's right to self-determination. Pluralism is the philosophy that it is desirable and beneficial to have several distinct ethnic, religious, or cultural groups thrive within a single society. Pluralism also holds that no single explanatory or belief system may reliably and definitively account for all the phenomena of life. In this way, pluralism supports many different ethical viewpoints and contextually specific moral judgments.

Answer: C

Limentani AE (1999) The role of ethical principles in health care and the implications for ethical codes. *Journal of Medical Ethics* **25**, 394–8.

Beauchamp TL, Childress JF (eds) (2009) *Principles of Biomedical Ethics,* 6th edn, Oxford University Press, New York.

7 *A patient with metastatic colorectal cancer, with symptomatic bony and brain metastases, is critically ill in the ICU with sepsis and impending acute respiratory failure. As the intensivist, you have a discussion with the patient regarding his goals of care. He states that although he is aware that he has only a limited time to live based on his malignancy, he wishes to receive intubation, mechanical ventilation, and CPR if he has a pulmonary or cardiac arrest. His wife is on her way to the ICU but has not yet arrived. As the intensivist, you do not believe that those therapies are reasonable to pursue for this patient. The next most appropriate course of action is to:*
   A *Accept the patient's decisions to respect his autonomy*
   B *Enter a DNR/DNI order to respect your autonomy*
   C *Contact the hospital legal/risk management department*
   D *Discuss with the wife and accept her substituted judgment*
   E *Convene an ethics committee consultative visit*

This patient is critically ill and has brain metastasis. Therefore, his judgment may be compromised, and he may not be able to appropriately interpret the consequences of his decisions. Moreover, as it is an emergency situation, asking a patient to articulate goals of therapy may be viewed as coercive. Furthermore, since you do not believe that intubation will help the patient achieve a reasonable goal, it is appropriate to discuss goals of therapy with an individual who is not physiologically compromised and with impending respiratory failure. The next most appropriate individual is his wife. Were she not alive, then an adult child would be the next most appropriate individual. Others may have a legally authorized representative empowered by a durable healthcare power of attorney designation. Still others have a court appointed conservator when there are no kin to help make healthcare decisions—or when those who are present are unwilling or incapable of making such decisions. Accepting the goals as articulated by the most appropriate individual as those of the patient is known as substituted judgment. Substituted judgment relies on the perspective that the goals being related are those that the patient would most likely share with the care team if they were able to do so. The clinician must be careful to ensure that the goals do not instead reflect what the individual stating the goals wants for the patient, but rather what the patient would want for his or herself. Respecting autonomy also implies that the patient is competent to render a decision. Entering a DNR/DI order to respect your autonomy is inappropriate and violates the patient's right to self-determination—either autonomously or via substituted judgment. Hospital agencies including Clinical Ethics Committees generally act slowly to render a rapid decision regarding care, but are very helpful when there is the luxury of time to have an outside agency (not the primary healthcare team), review the case, and share input regarding difficult ethical decisions.

Answer: D

Mazur DJ (2006) How successful are we at protecting preferences? Consent, informed consent, advance directives and substituted judgment. *Medical Decision Making* **26** (2), 106–9.

Seckler AB, Meier DE, Mulvihill M, Paris BE (1991) Substituted judgment: how accurate are proxy predictors? *Annals of Internal Medicine* **115** (2), 92–8.

Kayser J, Kaplan LJ (2020) Conflict management in the intensive care unit: a concise definitive review. *Critical Care Medicine* **48** (9), 1349–57.

8 *While on call at night in the ICU, one of the surgeons brings up a patient from the OR after performing an adhesiolysis and small bowel resection for a small-bowel obstruction. The operation reportedly went smoothly. As the surgeon is discussing the patient with you in the ICU, it is clear to you that the surgeon's breath smells of alcohol and the surgeon appears to be intoxicated. Your most appropriate course of action is to:*

A *Have a private conversation with the surgeon once the surgeon is sober*

B *Do nothing as you do not have laboratory evidence of intoxication*

C *Immediately contact the surgeon's Chairman with your concerns*

D *Disenfranchise the surgeon from the patient's care due to incompetence*

E *Discuss your observations with the patient's family to provide full disclosure*

Using the principle of non-maleficence (do no harm), one is compelled to act in order to support patient safety. Operating while under the influence of alcohol is clearly unsafe, unethical, and morally unsupportable. The most appropriate action is to engage the hierarchical power structure that can directly intervene to protect the patient from harm. From the standpoint of beneficence (doing good), one must also act in the surgeon's best interest as if the surgeon is operating while intoxicated, it may be a powerful marker of a personal health issue. While "blowing the whistle" may be superficially construed as damaging, it is the most appropriate action to undertake from any perspective. A private conversation will not support patient safety, nor will inaction. One cannot unilaterally disenfranchise a surgeon from their patient's care. Providing disclosure without evidence that supports your suspicion of intoxication is also not appropriate at this time, especially if there is no direct evidence of harm.

Answer: C

Beauchamp TL, Childress JF (eds) (2009) *Principles of Biomedical Ethics*, 6th edn, Oxford University Press, New York.

Gay D, Steratore A, Hoffman A, Neidhardt J, Cundiff C, Shaver E, Kiefer A, Kiefer C (2020) What do you do if your relief comes to work intoxicated: an impaired provider scenario. *Journal of Education and Teaching in Emergency Medicine* **5** (4).

9 *A 36-year-old woman was involved in a motorcycle crash 2 days ago. She has severe TBI, and the neurosurgeon believes it to be a nonsurvivable injury. She has a physical examination that describes the absence of brain stem reflexes by two physicians and has a transcranial Doppler assessment through an ocular insonation window that demonstrates no optic flow. Her temperature is 32.8C, HR 102 beats/min, BP 96/42 mm Hg (MAP = 60 mm Hg), SaO2 98% on AC/VCV, and FIO2 0.40 on fentanyl at 0.5 µg/kg/hour, and propofol at 0.25 mg/kg/hour. She breathes only with the ventilator. The next most appropriate action is to:*

A *Start a norepinephrine infusion to raise her MAP*

B *Perform an apnea test to assess CO_2 responsivity*

C *Disconnect her from the ventilator as she is brain dead*

D *Obtain a radionuclide cerebral blood flow scan*

E *Change to fentanyl and dexmedetomidine to minimize sedation*

This patient may have a nonsurvivable brain injury in the neurosurgeon's opinion, but she does not meet criteria for the declaration of brain death. The absence of brainstem reflexes is supportive, but she is still on sedating agents that need to be discontinued to render the examination valid; changing to a different sedative will not enable the determination of brain death. Transcranial Doppler examination is similarly insufficient to determine cerebral blood flow as a universally agreed upon standard. Universal standards include four-vessel cerebral angiography and cerebral radionuclide scanning. There remains controversy regarding cerebral computed tomogram angiography for the declaration of brain death. One does need to be euthermic as well to be declared brain dead. Given the low temperature and the analgesic and sedative agents, a radionuclide scan is the most appropriate method of supporting the determination of brain death of the choices offered as it is temperature and sedative independent, unlike an apnea test – which may be significantly influenced by sedative agents. Raising the MAP will also not help address whether or not she is brain dead, and MAP manipulation is best done in conjunction with determining cerebral perfusion pressure (MAP − ICP), and there is no ICP monitor in this patient. EEG testing may be useful to exclude sub-clinical status epilepticus as well.

Answer: D

Greer DM, Straczyk D, Schwamm LH (2009) False positive CT angiography in brain death. *Neurocritical Care* **11** (2), 272–5.

Tibbalis J (2010) A critique of the apneic oxygenation test for the diagnosis of "brain death". *Pediatric Critical Care Medicine* **11** (4), 475–8.

Zuckier LS, Kolano J (2008) Radionuclide studies in the determination of brain death: criteria, concepts and controversies. *Seminars in Nuclear Medicine* **38** (4), 262–73.

Greer DM, Shemie SD, Lewis A, Torrance S, Varelas P, Goldenberg FD, Bernat JL, Souter M, Topcuoglu MA, Alexandrov AW, Baldisseri M (2020) Determination of brain death/death by neurologic criteria: the World Brain Death Project. *JAMA* **324** (11), 1078–97.

10 *A patient is declared brain dead, and you have shared the news with the family. It is Wednesday evening and they request that you do not remove their father from the ventilator until Saturday as they want family to arrive from across the country. However, Friday is their father's wedding anniversary and their mother died only 8 months ago. Which of the following paradigms best described the basis for the family members' thought process in requesting the 3-day delay?*
  A *Consequentialism*
  B *Principlism*
  C *Nonrationalism*
  D *Virtue ethics*
  E *Deontologism*

This patient's family is making an unsupportable request. It is superficially logically to the family but is inconsistent with appropriate medical care and legal rulings. Once one is declared brain dead, then one is legally dead and may be disconnected from life support devices. The family has articulated a desire to delay disconnection, which is a nonrational request as they apparently understand that he is medically and legally dead. Nonrationalism identifies that decision and requests stem from feelings, desires, intuition, habit, obedience, or imitation. Consequentialism renders decisions based on the downstream effects of each individual decision. Principlism frames decisions within autonomy, beneficence, nonmaleficence, justice, and respect. Virtue ethics derives ethical values from the behavior of an individual who is believed to be virtuous as a kind of moral excellence. Deontologism renders ethical decisions based on adherence to predefined and accepted rules.

Answer: C

Limentani AE (1999) The role of ethical principles in health care and the implications for ethical codes. *Journal of Medical Ethics* **25**, 394–8.

Thompson IE (1987) Fundamental ethical principles in healthcare. *British Medical Journal* **295**, 1461–5.

Vordermark II JS The Elements of Medical Decision-Making. In: Vordermark JS, *An Introduction to Medical Decision-Making* 2019 (pp. 51–61). Springer, Cham.

11 *A 72-year-old man underwent a left inguinal hernia repair. Post-operatively, he is admitted to the surgical service due to unanticipated hypoxia requiring supplemental oxygen. He has underlying COPD, CAD, DM-II, and CKD (baseline creatinine = 2.4); he is DNR but not DNI. You are called at 02:00 as part of your hospital's rapid response team for severe hypoxemia. When you arrive, the patient has a HR of 126 beats/min, RR of 36 breaths/min, BP of 98/52 mm Hg (baseline 142/82 mm Hg), and a SpO2 of 90% on 100% O2 by nonrebreather while sitting bolt upright. Before proceeding with intubation, the anesthesiologist wants to obtain consent from the patient. Which of the following is the most appropriate course of action?*
  A *Engage in a discussion of intubation to obtain an informed consent*
  B *Obtain a CXR to evaluate for treatable causes of hypoxemia*
  C *Administer furosemide 80 mg IVP as well as nebulized albuterol*
  D *Establish phone contact with a family member to obtain consent*
  E *Proceed with intubation as consent in this situation is coercive*

The concept of informed consent embraces a plethora of issues including the clarity and scope of the discussion, the patient's ability to comprehend the discussion, the ability of the clinician to explain the intervention, and the ability of the patient to understand the consequences of agreeing or disagreeing to the intended intervention.

Truly informed consent must embrace adequate time for questions, answers, discussion, and perhaps reflection as well. Emergency situations such as the one described preclude that process for the patient as well as with family members. It also underscores the importance of having discussions that impact goals of care prior to elective hospitalization and early within the course of unplanned admission. Diagnostic or therapeutic undertakings that do not immediately address impending respiratory arrest are inappropriate compared with rapid airway and work of breathing control. While furosemide may treat pulmonary edema, it is not clear that the etiology of hypoxemia stems from fluid overload based on the available data.

Answer: E

Brendel RW, Wei MH, Schouten R, Edersheim JG (2010) An approach to selected legal issues: confidentiality, mandatory reporting, abuse and neglect, informed consent, capacity decisions, boundary issues, and malpractice claims. *Medical Clinics of North America* **94** (6), 1229–40.

Suah A, Angelos P (2018) How should trauma patients' informed consent or refusal be regarded in a trauma bay or other emergency settings?. *AMA Journal of Ethics* **20** (5), 425–30.

12 *You are caring for an injured patient who is being nonoperatively managed for a grade II liver injury and a grade III splenic injury but who also has a right femur fracture. The orthopedic surgeon on call, and who is ready to operate on the patient, is one whom you believe is less technically and cognitively competent than any of the other surgeons who take orthopedic trauma panel call. The patient's family asks you for your opinion of the orthopedic surgeon who is intending to operate on their mother. Your most appropriate course of action is to:*

A *Suggest that the family search for social media reviews of the surgeon*

B *State that since you are not an orthopedist, you cannot comment*

C *Suggest that the family might want to obtain a second opinion*

D *Find a reason to delay the OR until a more skilled surgeon is available*

E *Offer that it is their comfort with the surgeon that is important*

This question addresses both patient autonomy (the right to choose therapy and who will deliver it) and surgeon autonomy (the right to practice in an unrestricted fashion) in the setting of medical professionalism (professional conduct in patient care). Reassuring the family that "all is well" if one does not believe it to be so is patently lying and not to be condoned as appropriate behavior. Suggesting that the family peruse social media for information directs them to use an unreviewed source to make an informed decision – an approach that is internally inconsistent and medically unprofessional. Declining to comment about the surgeon since you have expertise in different aspects of the field is similarly untruthful and deceitful. Suggesting a second opinion may also infringe upon the orthopedist's practice autonomy. Delaying an indicated operation on the basis of personal bias is medically inappropriate and morally incorrect. Therefore, the only appropriate answer is to identify that it is not your opinion that matters, but rather the family's comfort and confidence in the surgeon that is paramount. If you truly believe that the orthopedist is practicing below an acceptable standard of care, then there are performance improvement data-driven mechanisms that one may engage to evaluate performance. Engaging your hospital's peer-review process is the professional and appropriate means to address your concerns regarding the orthopedist's skill set and professional judgment.

Answer: E

Lantos J, Matlock AM, Wendler D (2011) Clinical integrity and limits to patient autonomy. *Journal of the American Medical Association* **305** (5), 495–9.

Egener BE, Mason DJ, McDonald WJ, Okun S, Gaines ME, Fleming DA, Rosof BM, Gullen D, Andresen ML (2017) The charter on professionalism for health care organizations. *Academic Medicine* **92** (8), 1091.

Bennett KG, Berlin NL, MacEachern MP, Buchman SR, Preminger BA, Vercler CJ (2018) The ethical and professional use of social media in surgery—a systematic review of the literature. *Plastic and Reconstructive Surgery* **142** (3), 388e.

13 *A 14-year-old boy is struck by a vehicle at high speed and brought to the Emergency Department. On evaluation, the child has a GCS of 4, no pupillary responses and a palpable open, depressed skull fracture. While the trauma team does not feel that there is a reasonable hope of survival, the patient is intubated and resuscitated in the hopes that he could be an organ donor. Which of the following actions is the most appropriate?*

A *Providing futile care to an adolescent with an unsurvivable injury is unethical, and all efforts should be halted.*

B *Resuscitative efforts should be provided to give the family a chance to come to terms with the prognosis and decide on organ donation.*

C *The local organ procurement organization (OPO) should be immediately called for consultation.*

D *Resuscitation should proceed with set limits to give the appearance to the family that every effort was made.*

E *The patient should be transitioned to V-A ECMO to provide the best opportunity for organ perfusion.*

The appropriateness of continuation of care is predicated on the determination of futility in further care of this patient and the intent of the actions behind those actions. Given the lack of certainty in the patient's prognosis in the acute setting, discontinuation of care would be premature at this stage. Contacting the OPO at this stage is reasonable and appropriate as the injury is assessed as essentially non-survivable, and there is loss of some brainstem reflexes. When prognosis is definitively established, nonbeneficial procedures such as CPR may be considered in limited circumstances as a compassionate act for the benefit of the family, providing comfort and reassurance that everything possible was done for their child. For patients in whom organ transplantation is considered, the United States Uniform Anatomic Gift Act was revised in 2006 to permit the use of life support systems at or near death in order to maximize the potential for organ procurement. The utility of ECMO for organ support is inappropriate for this patient as he has no clinical need for that therapy.

Answer: C

Sachdeva R, Jefferson L, Coss-Bu J, Brody BA (1996) Resource consumption and extent of futile care among patients in a pediatric intensive care unit setting. *Journal of Pediatrics* **128** (6), 742–7.

Truog RD (2010) Is it always wrong to perform futile CPR? *New England Journal of Medicine* **362**, 477–9.

Verheijde JL, Rady MY, McGregor JL (2007) The United States Revised Uniform Anatomical Gift Act (2006): new challenges to balancing patient rights and physician responsibilities. *Philosophy, Ethics, and Humanities in Medicine* **2**, 19.

Kotloff RM, Blosser S, Fulda GJ, Malinoski D, Ahya VN, Angel L, Byrnes MC, DeVita MA, Grissom TE, Halpern SD, Nakagawa TA (2015) Management of the potential organ donor in the ICU: society of critical care medicine/American college of chest physicians/ association of organ procurement organizations consensus statement. *Critical Care Medicine* **43** (6), 1291–325.

14 *During a routine preoperative chest x-ray in a 68-year-old woman, a suspicious nodule is identified that is concerning for malignancy. The reviewing physician feels that a CT scan is warranted, and she refers the patient to a radiology center that the reviewing physician's husband owns and manages. Which of the following is the most accurate description of this event?*

A *The patient can be referred so long as the physician's financial ties are disclosed to the patient.*

B *There is no violation of conflict of interest since the reviewing physician has no direct financial ties to the center.*

C *The patient can be referred since the center is an external facility, and regulations against self-referral only apply to internal facilities.*

D *Referring to this center is a violation of Stark laws unless there are no other nearby appropriate facilities.*

E *The physician cannot make the referral herself, but can have her physician's assistant fill out the referral form.*

Physician self-referral occurs when physicians refer patients to medical facilities in which they have a financial interest. Such arrangements are ethically questionable due to the potential for over-utilization of medical resources and subsequently, increased healthcare costs. The Stark laws, enacted in 1992, state that a physician cannot refer a Medicare or Medicaid patient to a facility in which he or she (or an immediate family member) has a financial relationship. An exception to this rule exists for rural settings in which no other facility is reasonably available. A Physician's Assistant operates under the supervision of the physician within the practice and therefore is not exempt from the tenets for the Stark laws. Advanced practice nurses (APRN's) are similarly incorporated when they are working within the confines of the physician's practice. Importantly, Stark Law imperatives have also been explored within the realm of Telemedicine and referrals for specific care resulting from remote evaluations.

Answer: D

Department of Health and Human Services, Centers for Medicare & Medicaid Services (2007) 42 CFR Parts 409, 410, *et al.* Medicare Program; Proposed Revisions to Payment Policies Under the Physician Fee Schedule, and Other Part B Payment Policies for CY 2008; July 12.

Manchikanti L, McMahon EB (2007) Physician refer thyself: is Stark II, phase III the final voyage? *Pain Physician* **10** (6), 725–41.

Feldt KS (2010) Ethical Issues in Advanced Practice Nursing. In: Blair KA, Jansen MP. *Advanced Practice Nursing: Core Concepts for Professional Role. Development*, Springer.

Nittari G, Khuman R, Baldoni S, Pallotta G, Battineni G, Sirignano A, Amenta F, Ricci G (2020) Telemedicine practice: review of the current ethical and legal challenges. *Telemedicine and e-Health* **26** (12), 1427–37.

15 *A 45-year-old man suffers a massive intracranial hemorrhage from a previously undiagnosed aneurysm. Despite aggressive medical and surgical management, his condition is deemed unsalvageable. The surgical critical care fellow has been taking care of this patient and is very involved in the discussions with the family. The family shares that the patient would want to pursue comfort care and would desire to pursue organ donation. At the time of organ procurement, the transplant surgeon invites the fellow to join the team in the operating room since this is a good "teaching opportunity." The fellow should do which of the following?*

A *Accepting the invitation could be seen as a conflict of interest, and the fellow should therefore decline*

B *Accept this because as a trainee, there is no conflict of interest, and it would be an educational opportunity*

C *Accept this but as an observer only since he is a critical care fellow and not a transplant fellow*

D *Accept the invitation but go to the operating room only after obtaining the written consent of the family*

E *Accept and participate in the procedure since it is educational, but without informing the family*

Perceived conflict of interest can occur when there is overlap or confusion regarding patient care responsibility between the treating team and the transplantation team, including the organ procurement organization. Indeed, consent rates have been shown to be up to three times greater when an optimal request pattern was pursued, including clear separation between the treatment team and the donation affiliated team. The surgical critical care fellow is a member of the treating team, and although he may be involved in the discussion of potential outcomes – including organ donation – he must be clearly separated from and obtaining consent for organ procurement, as well as the OR procedure to do so due to a conflict of interest. Indeed, the fellows "contract" is with the patient and the patient's family, not the OPO, the organ procurement team nor the recipient or the recipient's family.

Answer: A

Siminoff LA, Arnold RM, Hewlett J (2001) The process of organ donation and its effect on consent. *Clinical Transplantation* **15**, 39–47.

Prabhu A, Parker LS, DeVita MA (2017) Caring for patients or organs: new therapies raise new dilemmas in the emergency department. *The American Journal of Bioethics* **17** (5), 6–16.

16 *A trainee places an enteral access catheter to provide nutritional support for an elderly, debilitated patient in the ICU. On confirmatory chest X-ray, the catheter is noted to traverse the right mainstem bronchus and is located curled in the right pleural space with an accompanying large pneumothorax. The family is informed, the catheter is removed, and a chest tube is placed. The patient remains stable throughout, and the chest tube is removed 5 days later without complications. The family is irate and threatens to sue. Which is the most appropriate course of action?*

A *Conduct further discussions only in the presence of a representative from the Legal department*

B *Request the input of the Palliative Care Medicine team to determine the best course of action and to counsel the family*

C *Say as little as possible since the trainee was unsupervised at the time*

D *Ignore the family's threat, since there is no medical liability due to the fact that no harm was done*

E *Schedule a family meeting to ensure that the family is fully informed and to discuss their concerns*

Mistakes are common in medicine. Full disclosure of medical errors can be difficult due to embarrassment and concerns over legal liability and erosion of the patient–physician relationship. However, studies have shown that when a policy of full disclosure is followed, no clear increases in lawsuits or healthcare costs occur. Moreover, the provider–patient relationship is strengthened with a policy of openness and honesty. Models for medical error compensation have been proposed and may lead to decreases in overall healthcare costs.

Answer: E

Hebert PC (2001) Disclosure of adverse events and errors in healthcare: An ethical perspective. *Drug Safety* **24** (15), 1095–104.

Kachalia A, Kaufman SR, Boothman R, Anderson S, Welch K, Saint S, Rogers MA (2010) Liability claims and costs before and after implementation of a medical error disclosure program. *Annals of Internal Medicine* **153** (4), 213–21.

O'Connor E, Coates HM, Yardley IE, Wu AW (2010) Disclosure of patient safety incidents: a comprehensive review. *International Journal for Quality in Health Care* **22** (5), 371–9.

Hannawa AF (2019) When facing our fallibility constitutes "safe practice": further evidence for the Medical Error Disclosure Competence (MEDC) guidelines. *Patient Education and Counseling* 102 (10), 1840–6.

Lane AS, Roberts C (2020) Developing open disclosure strategies to medical error using simulation in final-year medical students: linking mindset and experiential learning to lifelong reflective practice. *BMJ Simulation and Technology Enhanced Learning* 7, 345–351.:bmjstel-2020.

17 *A 12-year-old girl falls onto a glass table with a deep laceration to her thigh and loses a significant volume of blood before being found. She is brought into the Emergency Department tachycardic, hypotensive, and profoundly anemic. Her parents, who are Jehovah's Witnesses, refuse to consent to blood transfusion based on their religious beliefs. What is the most appropriate course of action?*

A *Try to obtain the patient's consent for transfusion*
B *Respect the wishes of the parents since the patient is a minor*
C *Transfuse the patient, since her condition is life-threatening*
D *Obtain a court order to override the wishes of the parents*
E *Contact the congregation elder to negotiate with the family*

The Jehovah's Witness Society is notable for their religious stance against transfusion of blood, even in the face of life-threatening anemia. In the competent adult patient, adherence to the patient's wishes is in accordance with *respect for persons* and the patient's right to self-determination. However, in the case of the child, the patient is incapable of formulating a rational, informed choice and expressing those views, therefore transfusion is justified by our societal obligation to the child's best interests, based on the principle of *beneficence.*

Answer: C

Gillon R (1994) Medical ethics: four principles plus attention to scope. *British Medical Journal* **309**, 184–8.
Gillon R (2003) Four scenarios. *Journal of Medical Ethics* **29** (5), 267–8.
Woolley S (2005) Children of Jehovah's witnesses and adolescent Jehovah's witnesses: what are their rights? *Archives of Disease in Childhood* **90** (7), 715–19.
Woolley S (2005) Jehovah's witnesses in the emergency department: what are their rights? *Emergency Medicine Journal* **22** (12), 869–71.
Bester JC, Smith M, Griggins C (2017) A Jehovah's witness adolescent in the labor and delivery unit: should patient and parental refusals of blood transfusions for adolescents be honored?. *Narrative Inquiry in Bioethics* **7** (1), 97–106.
Conti A, Capasso E, Casella C, Fedeli P, Salzano FA, Policino F, Terracciano L, Delbon P (2018). Blood transfusion in children: the refusal of Jehovah's Witness parents'. *Open Medicine* **13** (1), 101–4.

18 *On review of his monthly billings, a physician notices that he billed for the incorrect procedure on a patient. The claim had already been accepted and paid by the insurance company. What is the appropriate course of action?*

A *Nothing, since the RVUs between the two procedures are similar*
B *If the claim amount is less than $10,000, no correction is necessary*
C *Report the error, refund the monies, and resubmit with justification*
D *Report the error to the insurance company and refund the claim*
E *Nothing can be done since the claim is already paid to the physician*

Policies differ between insurance carriers and Medicare/Medicaid in terms of correction of incorrect claims. Review and understanding of these agreements is important in minimizing the exposure to liability and prosecution. In general, failure to report errors in billing is subject to repayment of claims and imposed fines. Reporting, refunding, and resubmitting an honest error with justification will cover all of the requirements for full disclosure and accuracy in correcting incorrect billing claims. This strategy may not ensure that there is not an associated fine but is consistent with the concept of distributed justice across the healthcare system and is internally consistent with the concept of virtuous behavior. The worst course of action is to do nothing and hope that the incorrect billing is not noticed.

Answer: C

Vogel RL (2010) The False Claims Act and its impact on medical practices. *Journal of Medical Practice Management* **26** (1), 21–4.
Stowell NF, Schmidt M, Wadlinger N (2018) Healthcare fraud under the microscope: improving its prevention. *Journal of Financial Crime* 25 (4), 1039–61.
Grioux W, Maul J, Delaplane A, Hane F, Josephy D, Pfeiffer N, Safirstein P (2018) Health care fraud. *American Criminal Law Review* **55**, 1333.

19 A 72 year-old woman suffers an out of hospital cardiac arrest and achieves return of spontaneous circulation with bystander CPR. She receives targeted temperature management at the hospital but fails to recover neurologic function. She then suffers a major territory ischemic stroke and is declared brain dead by neurologic criteria. She is an affirmed organ donor (as per her state driver's license), and the OPO is engaged for organ procurement. Her husband is against organ donation and does not want to proceed. Which of the following is most accurate regarding this situation?

A *Donation should be abandoned since the husband is her surviving next of kin and the team should respect his wishes.*

B *Donation should proceed since organ donation is governed by gift law and the patient has opted-in for gift giving.*

C *Donation should be placed on hold until a Conflict Management arbitrator can help both sides reach an acceptable solution.*

D *Donation should be placed on hold until the facilities Clinical Ethics Committee may be assembled and identify the ethical next step.*

E *Representatives from the OPO should be engaged to have a discussion with the husband to help him agree to donation.*

Indeed, the US Uniform Anatomical Gift Act reflects gift law and as such, declaration of organ donor status on a driver's license is an effective way of opting-in to the process. Once an individual has opted-in, the family does not have the right to override the decision. The other way to opt-in is for a surrogate to authorize donation for a previously unregistered individual. There is no need to pursue any kind of arbitration or ethics discussion since the decision for donation has been made in accordance with federal law. The role of the OPO is to provide information for surrogates who are considering decision-making, as well as to provide information for family members whose loved one has already declared their intent to donate. The OPO has no need to help the husband agree to donation as the wife has already agreed.

Answer: B

Glazier A, Mone T (2019) Success of opt-in organ donation policy in the United States. *JAMA* **322** (8), 719–20.

20 You are consulted to care for a patient with a reducible but symptomatic ventral hernia in the Emergency Department. You and the patient agreed to admission and repair as it interferes with his work and lifestyle. As part of your institution's approach to SARS-CoV-2 surveillance and screening, you order a rapid test to be obtained before inpatient admission. The patient, a 34-year-old male, refuses to be tested. Which of the following actions is most appropriate?

A Admit the patient regardless to respect autonomy since he has decisional-capacity

B Decline to admit the patient to the facility unless he agrees to testing

C Transfer him to another facility if another surgeon will accept the patient

D Provide moderate sedation in the ED to obtain the COVID-19 sample

E Proceed directly to the OR and obtain the COVID-19 sample under anesthesia

While autonomy is a key pillar of Western Ethics, during a pandemic, the safety of others must also be taken into consideration. Therefore, for those with emergency conditions, care should be undertaken while treating the patient as if they are SARS-CoV-2 positive. For those without emergency needs, refusal to participate in safe practices may be addressed by declining to provide nonemergent care without testing. This patient is not obstructed nor strangulated and his care may be deferred to a later date. It is always wrong to obtain sampling that the patient has refused by using sedatives or taking advantage of the patient's inability to refuse during general anesthesia. While some may consider transferring to another facility, in the midst of a pandemic, that approach may also place other vulnerable patients at risk and is therefore also inappropriate.

Answer: B

Kopar PK, Kramer JB, Brown DE, Bochicchio GV (2021) Critical ethics: how to balance patient autonomy with fairness when patients refuse coronavirus disease 2019 testing. *Critical Care Explorations* **3** (1), e0326 doi: 10.1097/CCE.0000000000000326.

Index

Note: Page numbers in *italic* indicate Figures and those in **bold** indicate Tables.

Surgical Critical Care and Emergency Surgery: Clinical Questions and Answers, Third Edition.
Edited by Forrest "Dell" Moore, Peter M. Rhee, and Carlos J. Rodriguez.
© 2022 John Wiley & Sons Ltd. Published 2022 by John Wiley & Sons Ltd.
Companion website: www.wiley.com/go/surgicalcriticalcare3e